O9-ABH-697

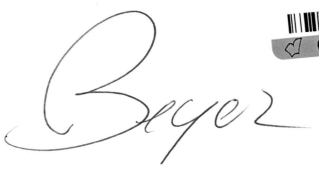

Yochum and Rowe's

ESSENTIALS
OF
SKELETAL
RADIOLOGY

Third Edition

Volume Two

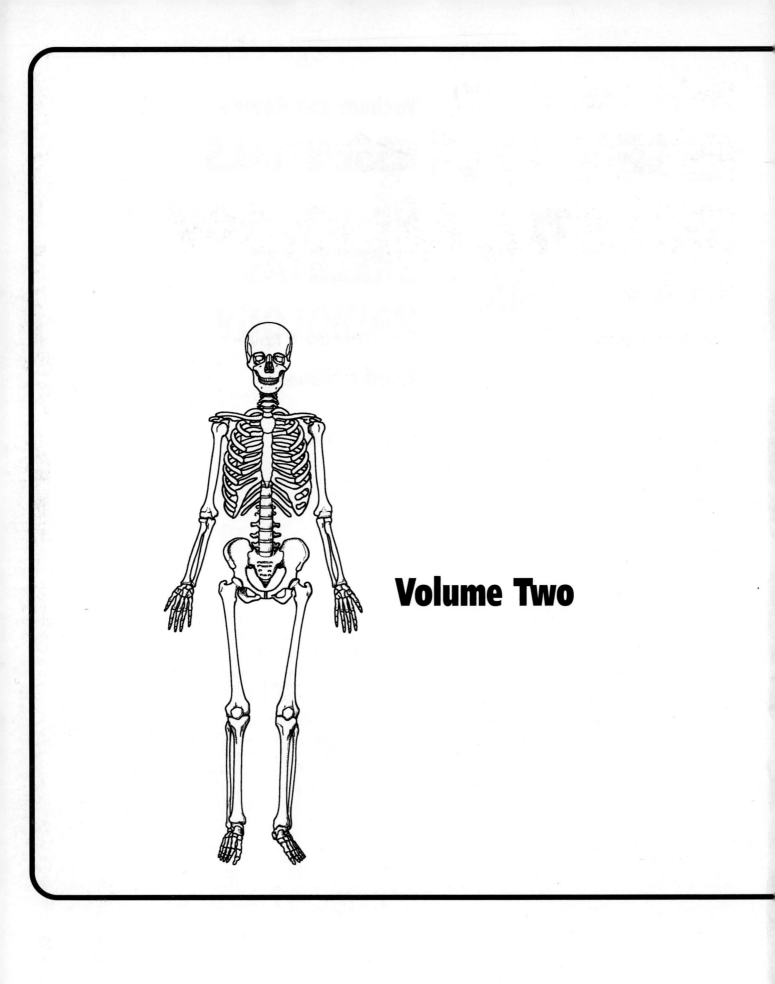

Volume Two

Yochum and Rowe's
ESSENTIALS OF SKELETAL RADIOLOGY

Third Edition

Terry R. Yochum
B.S., D.C., D.A.C.B.R., F.C.C.R. (C), F.I.C.C., Fellow, A.C.C.R

Director
Rocky Mountain Chiropractic Radiological Center
Denver, Colorado

Adjunct Professor of Radiology
Southern California University of Health Sciences
Los Angeles, California

Instructor of Skeletal Radiology
Department of Radiology
University of Colorado School of Medicine
Denver, Colorado

Formerly:
Professor of Radiology
Colorado College of Chiropractic
Marycrest International University
Denver, Colorado

Senior Lecturer
Department of Diagnostic Sciences

Division Head
Department of Radiology
Phillip Institute of Technology—School of Chiropractic
Melbourne, Australia

Professor and Chairman
Department of Radiology
Logan College of Chiropractic
St. Louis, Missouri

Assistant Professor of Radiology
National College of Chiropractic
Lombard, Illinois

Lindsay J. Rowe
M.App.Sc (Chiropractic), M.D., D.A.C.B.R., F.C.C.R. (C), F.A.C.C.R., F.I.C.C., F.R.A.N.Z.C.R.

Associate Professor, Diagnostic Radiology
Faculty of Medicine
University of Newcastle
Newcastle, Australia

Senior Staff Specialist Radiologist
Department of Medical Imaging
John Hunter Hospital
Newcastle, Australia

Consultant Radiologist
Pittwater Imaging
Gosford, Australia

Formerly:
Research Fellow in Musculoskeletal Radiology
Veterans Administration Hospital
University of California
San Diego, California

Associate Professor and Chairman
Department of Radiology
Northwestern College of Chiropractic
Minneapolis, Minnesota

Associate Professor and Chairman
Department of Radiology
Canadian Memorial Chiropractic College
Toronto, Canada

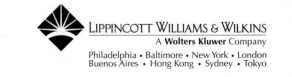

LIPPINCOTT WILLIAMS & WILKINS
A **Wolters Kluwer** Company

Philadelphia • Baltimore • New York • London
Buenos Aires • Hong Kong • Sydney • Tokyo

Executive Editor: Pete Darcy
Managing Editor: Karen Gulliver
Senior Project Editor: Karen Ruppert
Marketing Manager: Christen DeMarco
Designer: Doug Smock
Compositor: Circle Graphics
Printer: Edwards Brothers

351 West Camden Street
Baltimore, MD 21201

530 Walnut St.
Philadelphia, PA 19106

Printed in the United States of America

First Edition, 1987

Second Edition, 1996

Library of Congress Cataloging-in-Publication Data

CIP data available from the Library of Congress

To purchase additional copies of this book, call our customer service department at
(800) 638-3030 or fax orders to **(301) 824-7390.** International customers should call
(301) 714-2324.

Visit Lippincott Williams & Wilkins on the Internet: http://www.LWW.com.
Lippincott Williams & Wilkins customer service representatives are available from
8:30 am to 6:00 pm, EST.

04 05 06 07 08

1 2 3 4 5 6 7 8 9 10

In a profession now 100 years old, a few giants rise above the crowd. While each giant stands with unique distinction, a common underlying principle unites them. Longfellow captured the essence:

> *The heights of great men reached and kept*
> *Were not attained by sudden flight,*
> *But they, while their companions slept,*
> *Were toiling upward through the night.*
>   *Henry Wadsworth Longfellow,*
>   *"The Ladder of St. Augustine"*

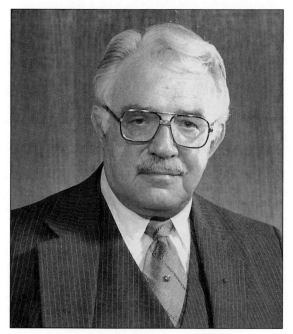

Joseph (Jozias) Janse, D.C.
(1909–1985)

Through the hectic hallowed halls of college, first as a student, then as a resident, and finally as a faculty member, Dr. Joseph Janse was before us as the example of dedication and commitment to a cause. He was more than a college president (National College of Chiropractic 1945–1983). He was more than a person of international renown in politics, education, research, and chiropractic. Foremost, he was a teacher! Always concerned, "Did you get that?" he would ask, arms raised, elbows bent, and a stiffened right forefinger pointing toward heaven. You would think he was asking a higher power if it understood what he was explaining until he brought his eyes back to focus on his students. He studied their faces waiting for the lights to go on inside. The English language never received such an exercise as when he spoke. Uncommon words pierced reality and definitions always followed with clear examples that even his grandchildren could understand. An artisan of the highest order, no one could experience his tutelage without being edified while being educated.

From his humble beginnings in Holland, Joe Janse experienced poverty and hard times. Supported by the toils of a dedicated father and mother, two older sisters, and an older brother hampered with a severe kyphoscoliosis of the spine, "Jozias" never complained because they were no worse off than anyone else. The family migrated to Huntsville, Utah, after converting to Mormonism in Holland. Father Pieter left in advance of the family by nearly a year to work and earn their passage to the New World. Their newfound religion instilled lasting values of self-worth and compassion without prejudice and added an eternal perspective to life. Coupled with forced frugality associated with near frontier farm life, hard work, and a keen desire for excellence, Joe excelled in school. He returned to Europe for 3 years as a self-supported missionary for the Mormon church. Upon his return, he sought direction for his secular life.

Janse's mother had experienced severe migraine headaches and relief came only from the hands of a chiropractor. Intrigued, young Joe investigated. Soon convinced that chiropractic had a place, he enrolled at the National School of Chiropractic (Chicago). The Utah townsfolk, including prominent church leaders whom he respected, discouraged the decision. Undaunted, J.J. (as so many affectionately called him) excelled as a student and was invited to join the faculty after his graduation and marriage in 1938. For the next 7 years he would excite and guide his students in the field of chiropractic. He served as Dean of Students, and stories abound regarding his willingness to help individuals with their studies, their dissections, and their manipulative techniques.

By 1945, the business manager of the school (the president had passed away) asked Janse to assume the role of president and was charged to lead the college out of proprietorship into a nonprofit status, a bold move at the time. In the 1950s, Dr. Janse was brought up short by a talented lawyer challenging the validity of chiropractic education because of the absence of an educational standard developed and maintained by a nationally recognized accrediting body. As a result, Janse pioneered the creation of the Council on Chiropractic Education (CCE) and led the charge to gain accreditation from the North Central Accrediting Association in 1974. He also pioneered, with his close friend Dr. Fred W. Ilii, from Geneva, Switzerland, the early research on the movement of the sacroiliac joints. This work served as a foundation for additional study to document true movement of these joints and describe their relationship to gait and posture. He generated the motivation for the development of specialty councils and specialty certification boards on a national level and was one of the first three board-certified chiropractic radiologists. He placed the school in deep debt to finance a new campus in Lombard,

Illinois, in the 1960s and then proceeded to become the most prolific fund-raiser in the history of the National College to meet the financial challenge. A beautiful campus, debt free, now stands as a monument to his dedicated stewardship, leadership, and untiring efforts.

Some memorable quotes come to mind when we think back to the times of his motivational lectures on life's principles and chiropractic philosophy. When asked, "What is it that you do?" Janse would respond, "I am a chiropractor, nothing more, but incidentally, my friend, nothing less." Perhaps his most memorable quote came from Rudyard Kipling, which speaks of the great spirit of understanding and fellowship that Joseph Janse held for his chiropractic colleagues.

> Here's to the men and women of my own breed,
> Good or bitter bad, as though they may be,
> At least they hear the things I hear,
> And see the things I see.

The accolades could continue, but the legacy is clear. His inspiring example allowed no room for mediocrity or compromise. His commitment to excellence remains unparalleled. How well he is represented by one of his favorite poems:

> Oh for the silent doer of the deed,
> One who is happy with the deed's own reward,
> One who in people's plight of night
> has solitary certitude of that which is right.

Similarly, the creators of this book and its revisions have been driven to bring to pass a text worthy of his emulation. We dedicate the product of our labors to the life of Dr. Joseph Janse in the hope that its readers may come to understand the value of "toiling upward through the night."

TERRY R. YOCHUM
LINDSAY J. ROWE

Few children have the privilege of entering the same profession as their father. I consider it a real honor to be a second-generation chiropractor following in my father's footsteps. Kenneth Emil Yochum, D.C., my father and best friend, provided the impetus to enter this great profession of chiropractic.

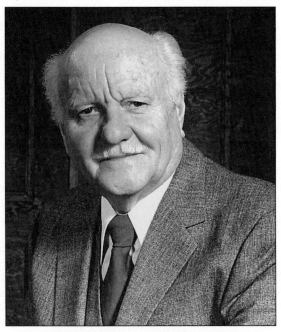

Kenneth E. Yochum, D.C.
(1914–1989)

Kenneth E. Yochum was a resident of South St. Louis, Missouri. He graduated from Cleveland High School in 1933 and the Missouri Chiropractic College in 1936. He was married to Cecelia G. Yochum for 48 years, father of Kay and Terry, and grandfather to five children. He practiced in South St. Louis at the Wilmington Chiropractic Clinic for 45 years. Dr. Yochum presented many lectures at the National College of Chiropractic and Logan College of Chiropractic in the area of clinical practice, nutrition, and the Nimmo technique. He had a keen interest in orthopedics and nutrition, with a special love for radiology. In 1980, Dr. Yochum was honored to be invited to present a lecture for the International College of Chiropractic in Melbourne and Sydney, Australia. He was one of the first five certified instructors in the receptor tonus (RT) technique (Nimmo technique), a topic on which he frequently lectured.

Dr. Yochum's untimely death in 1989 deprived his family of his love and guidance and many students of his great clinical expertise. Kenneth E. Yochum was a man of great character and integrity who always put the best interest of his patients before any personal need or gain. What a privilege it was to have been raised in a chiropractic family with such a great role model as a father and leader in the chiropractic profession. He lived his life by a number of spirited commitments. I can remember him saying many times, "Son, right is right and wrong is nobody." He spent his life attempting to always do the right thing for his patients and family. A leader in his community in every way, he stood as the pillar of his practice and family. So many times he told me that "chiropractic was worth making a difference for—extend yourself to make it better." His most memorable quotation involves living one's life as a reflective leader. He said that I, as his son, should "make dust—not eat dust." How thankful I am to have had a father who cared so much about the chiropractic profession and his family to have extended himself so sincerely, seemingly at every turn within his personal life.

A motivated student of radiology and an excellent radiographic technician, he produced radiographs of the finest quality in his clinical practice in St. Louis. In fact, his name follows many films in all three editions of this book, cases that came directly from his practice.

Kenneth E. Yochum was a very proud man and this was reflected in all aspects of his professional and personal life. His commitment to excellence was untiring and that driving spirit was given to me by this great man. His influence upon my life still continues. He is greatly missed by the entire Yochum family and it is befitting that the third edition of the Yochum and Rowe textbook be dedicated to his memory.

TERRY R. YOCHUM

Within a lifetime, a few select individuals will significantly affect the life of another. For both of us, Bryan Hartley, M.D., was one of those individuals. He was a person who seemed to achieve whatever he wanted in life: an extraordinary professional career, diversified personal interests, and close ties with family and friends. Bryan was born in Aldershot, England, in 1926 and studied medicine at Guy's Hospital Medical School in London. He was appointed house surgeon at the Royal Infirmary, Edinburgh, in 1950, following which he emigrated to Australia. He became a flight lieutenant in the R.A.A.F. medical branch and was a Fulbright traveling scholar. He was appointed medical officer in the Northern Territory Medical Services in Western Australia and was a resident medical officer at General Hospital in Tasmania.

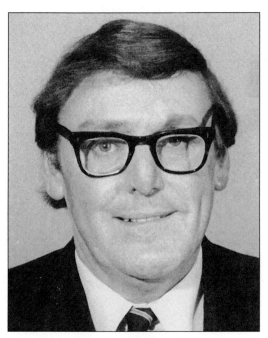

Bryan Hartley, M.D.
(1926–1984)

Bryan Hartley's early postgraduate training appointments alternated between the fields of surgery and radiology. He held appointments in surgery at the Union Memorial Hospital in Baltimore, Maryland; Launceston General Hospital in Tasmania; the Royal Children's Hospital in Melbourne, Victoria; and as Surgeon Superintendent at the Lyell District Hospital, Tasmania. His appointments in radiology were at the Launceston General Hospital, St. Vincent's Hospital, Melbourne, and the Royal Hobart Hospital in Tasmania. After a short appointment in Rome as a radiologist for the Department of Immigration, Bryan returned to Melbourne to become the director of the Department of Radiology at the Repatriation General Hospital and held this position until 1981. At that time, he accepted a position as staff radiologist in the Department of Radiology at the Austin Hospital also in Melbourne, the post he occupied until his death.

In his chosen career of medicine, Bryan Hartley excelled in both surgery and radiology, holding specialist qualifications in both fields. This interest in surgery was of considerable advantage to him in radiology, as it enabled him to see a diagnostic problem in its proper clinical perspective. A unique combination of clinical understanding, experience, and aptitude for clear expression made Bryan an outstanding teacher for his many students, residents, and colleagues. His boundless enthusiasm and wry humor provided for stimulating and informative discussions on almost any topic. His opinions were highly valued, particularly in patient evaluation and treatment.

For both of us, it was Bryan who, by example, provided the stimulus for developing our knowledge and abilities and advancing the standards of our profession. His influence on our careers is reflected not only in the use of his personal case material in this text but, more important, in the knowledge, expertise, and teaching methods he so freely shared with us. His untimely death in 1984 now deprives us and others of the opportunity of sharing his special gifts. He is survived by his wife, Beverley, and their children, Lynne and John.

In gratitude we have dedicated the first edition of this book to Bryan Hartley, M.D.

TERRY R. YOCHUM
LINDSAY J. ROWE

It is my privilege to once again provide a foreword for this remarkable new edition of the text *Essentials of Skeletal Radiology,* by Terry R. Yochum and Lindsay J. Rowe. As with the previous editions, this work is characterized by impeccable organization, a text that is extremely user friendly, supplemented by vivid illustrations and tabular material that provides summaries of the important points discussed in the adjacent paragraphs. What sets this book apart from others is the completeness of the coverage of the various disease processes that affect the musculoskeletal system. Tumors, infections, metabolic and articular disorders, traumatic conditions, and developmental abnormalities among other things—it is all here in the pages of this work. The manifestations of these processes are illustrated through the use of all imaging methods, ranging from conventional radiography to MRI. The legends that accompany this illustrative material are clear and to the point.

The quality of this text comes as no surprise to me. Both of the authors are experienced and knowledgeable in the ways of musculoskeletal diseases, both are gifted writers, and both share a bond of enthusiasm and energy that is required to complete the task. I have known both Terry and Lindsay for many, many years, and they are formidable clinicians and educators. They have a message and a desire to have others hear that message and, through careful and thoughtful planning, they present that message throughout the pages of this text. I know full well what is required to maintain one's focus during the months and years of the publication process, to stay focused and on time, and I am aware that both of these authors had the drive to see the process through. The result is a text that will bring ample reward to the reader, providing him or her with information that will ensure a more complete understanding of the disease process and the ability to provide correct diagnoses in a more timely fashion. The result will be improved patient care, something we all desire.

Terry and Lindsay, congratulations again on a job well done. To the potential readers, here is critical information, now at your fingertips, presented in a painless fashion. Enjoy!

DONALD RESNICK, M.D.
Professor of Radiology
University of California, San Diego
Chief of Osteoradiology Section
Veterans Affairs Medical Center
San Diego, California

FOREWORD to the Third Edition

We are all so busy in our lives that I often ponder how we accomplish the everyday things we must do, let alone also find time for new or additional endeavors. Well, Terry R. Yochum and Lindsay J. Rowe have an extraordinarily busy daily schedule and, again, they have found the time and energy to produce a third edition to their highly successful *Essentials of Skeletal Radiology.*

This new edition represents the pinnacle of Terry's and Lindsay's knowledge and compilation of work in this field. Today, they have added four more contributing authors for a total of 11. Incredibly, they have added 500 new illustrations and more than 1000 new references.

The reader will greatly appreciate the use of a new bolder color and shadings to highlight and enhance those important points that are seen in the headings, tables, diagrams, and figure captions. The quality of the reproductions is excellent, and there is no question of what the authors wish to demonstrate with well-placed arrows at the areas of interest. Of course, this text follows the wonderful fluid writing style previously seen in their earlier editions. I particularly enjoy the capsule summaries, which are a welcome highlight of the text.

I believe you will like their new chapter, "Masqueraders of Musculoskeletal Disease." Here, they have utilized plain films, CT, and MRI in areas of the head, neck, chest, and abdomen to provide an insight to other abnormalities that could mimic musculoskeletal complaints.

I am very impressed with this new and wonderful text, just as I was when I reviewed the earlier editions. *Essentials of Skeletal Radiology* is for every student in the field. I believe the blending of the new material and additions into the solid foundation of the second edition has produced a masterful harmony of needed core skeletal information with the newer imaging of the twenty-first century.

Thank you, Terry and Lindsay, for a wonderful work and a job well done.

M. BRUCE FARKAS, D.O., J.D.
Professor of Radiology (Retired)
Midwest University College of
    Osteopathic Medicine
Chief, Radiology, Military Entrance
    and Processing Station (Retired)
Chicago, Illinois

FOREWORD to the Third Edition

As the saying goes, "The third time is the charm." In skeletal radiology, the third edition of *Yochum and Rowe's Essentials of Skeletal Radiology* will become the gold standard.

It is no easy task to improve upon a work that has received acclaim worldwide but this third edition does more than improve upon the second edition. With its expanded material and featured new chapter, "Masqueraders of Musculoskeletal Disease," this third edition brings together inside a single cover all one needs to know to be an effective skeletal radiologist and clinician. If by some circumstance all skeletal radiology texts were burned to ashes, this edition would be a stand-alone, worthy of the risk and sacrifice required to preserve it from the fires of ignorance.

Chiropractic representatives invited to write a foreword are proud that such a well-used text has arisen from within our own ranks. The authors have distinguished themselves as radiologists in both the chiropractic profession and the medical profession. They have worked with, walked with, and talked on the same programs with the world's greatest. We hope the chiropractic profession recognizes the great contribution they have made, not only to the practice of skeletal radiology but to enhance the image of chiropractic.

We have been close enough to the action to know that creating this third edition has been a monumental task. The same commitment of sweat and tears that went into the first and second editions are evident between the lines and around every picture on every page. If any errors are present, it can only be blamed on computers.

The golden thread that weaves this third edition together, strengthening the authors' skill in conveyance of subject matter, is their love of teaching. They are master teachers, and their skill in holding an audience on the front of the seat in a darkened conference room has been incorporated into this lively text. Whether or not skeletal radiology is your love, *Essentials* will become your nightly reading companion.

We salute the work of these great teachers with Lee Iacocca's sentiment:

> In a completely rational society, the best of us would aspire to be teachers and the rest of us would have to settle for something less, because passing civilization along from one generation to the next ought to be the highest honor and the highest responsibility anyone could have.

REED B. PHILLIPS, D.C., D.A.C.B.R., PH.D.
President
Southern California University of Health Sciences
Whittier, California

JOSEPH W. HOWE, D.C., D.A.C.B.R., F.I.C.C., FELLOW, A.C.C.R.
Emeritus Professor of Radiology
Southern California University of Health Sciences
Whittier, California
Faculty
Department of Radiology
Logan College of Chiropractic
St. Louis, Missouri

PREFACE to the Third Edition

The overwhelming success of the first and second editions of *Essentials of Skeletal Radiology* has now given us the opportunity to publish the third edition. We believed in our work and were convinced of its merits from the beginning. What we did not fully perceive was the magnitude of the need for this text. We have been startled by the widespread acceptance of this publication. Although initially targeted to fill a need in the chiropractic educational system, it has also been adopted into the curricula of various medical and osteopathic teaching institutions worldwide. We have often seen the worn and torn covers on our books as a testimony to its use. The number of citations of the book in many scientific publications has been quite rewarding to see, and although morally and financially distressing, a form of compliment was offered by the numerous illegal and counterfeit copies that have surfaced here and abroad.

The most common question asked of any author in preparing a new edition is, "Are there any differences from the previous edition?" This text has undergone significant structural and content changes. Each chapter has been revised, some more extensively than others, and a new chapter (Chapter 18, **"Masqueraders of Musculoskeletal Disease"**) has been added to this edition. We feel these modifications and additions will provide the reader with a more "clinical" based text with respect to understanding the approach to radiology as it relates to practice. In addition, a sample CD of cervical spine anatomy, range of motion testing, and demonstration of orthopedic and neurological tests has been included with this text. This CD was created in association with Primal Pictures, Ltd., of London, England.

Our approach to a more clinical text will be evident early, as the reader notices the modifications made to Chapter 1. In this chapter, carefully selected radiographs displaying commonly found pathologies have been added for comparison with the normal radiographs. These images have been labeled **"clinicoradiologic correlations,"** and we feel they will emphasize the importance of being able to identify normal in order to better identify abnormal. These insertions will allow the reader to understand that many radiologic findings may be subtle and that careful attention to detail must be applied when reviewing radiographs. This comparison approach has been made easy by images displayed in close approximation. Also, a new **"common pitfalls"** section has been added to provide helpful information in hopes of preventing the clinician from making the most frequently seen exposure, positioning, and technological errors.

Chapter 3 has grown significantly with the addition of many new figures, references, and considerable expansion of the text. The addition of a **"synonym section"** should be very helpful. The normal variant segment has had many new images added to both the spine and extremities section.

A quick glance at Chapter 6 again demonstrates our efforts in not only compiling an informative text but also providing a clinical reference book. Remarkable new technologies continue to emerge, sometimes complementing and occasionally supplanting the existing modalities. The sheer volume of knowledge and the rate at which the knowledge base expands are both increasing rapidly. This has resulted in numerous areas of imaging specialties and subspecialties based on anatomy, imaging technology, or both. However, the edges of these specialty areas are not always black and white. While the focus of an individual practitioner may be specialized, it cannot be so narrow as to eliminate the need for an "overview" perspective capable of recognizing findings that may indicate an abnormality in a different anatomical system, or necessitate the application of a different imaging technology. In this chapter we have incorporated sections on the technological advances made in the areas of magnetic resonance angiography, DEXA osteoporosis scanning, musculoskeletal diagnostic ultrasound, and upright (stand-up) MRI of the spine.

Further progression through the text will make evident the changes to Chapter 15, which will enable the clinician to create a competent report and to better understand the importance of report writing. A **report commentary** section has been added to each case study in this chapter to critique the reports provided. This approach emphasizes the common errors people make while creating a report and reiterates the proper format of report writing.

The new chapter, **"Masqueraders of Musculoskeletal Disease,"** has been added to present an overview of the clinical findings and imaging applications for areas other than the musculoskeletal system. This new chapter emphasizes plain films as well as CT and MRI of the more common disorders involving the head, soft tissues of the neck, chest, and abdomen that can mimic musculoskeletal complaints. It follows the usual format of our textbook with the clinical and radiological features emphasized.

Despite the numerous additions and modifications, there has been a vigilant effort to maintain the hallmark features and core material of the first and second editions, so familiarity in this third edition may be evident. As we outlined in the preface of the first and second editions, the emphasis has been placed on constructing a clear and concise presentation. Significant effort has been directed at containing the size of this text to maintain its usefulness in the classroom, while attempting to provide a comprehensive review that incorporates the phenomenal technological advances in diagnostic imaging that have occurred in the interim.

Subsequent editions are like retouching original works of art. Though there is always the risk of spoiling it, the challenge of constructing a revision that is better than our previous works provided inspiration for this third edition.

The existing format has been enhanced by numerous design and color changes. We believe these changes will improve readability and accentuate important points. Most of the diagrams have been highlighted to emphasize key radiologic features. Headings and figure captions have been selectively colored. Some aspects of the book have remained the same owing to an overwhelming positive response to their appearance in the previous edition. For example, the structure of Chapters 5, 8, 10, 11, 12, 13, and 14 using progressive headings of **"general considerations," "clinical features," "pathologic features," "radiologic features,"** and **"treatment and prognosis"** has been maintained. The **"capsule summary"** remains an integral component to assist the reader in quick review for examination or to expedite differential considerations. A key addition to the second edition that has been repeated in this third edition is the **"medicolegal implications"** section that follows many of the conditions discussed. This reflects the increasing emphasis that diagnostic imaging has assumed in clinical practice and is designed to complement the case management decision-making process in a way that will reduce liability. The use of imaging and treatment **algorithms** in Chapter 5 will significantly impact the treatment of many patients with spondylolisthesis. In addition, the special section on **mnemonics** continues to appear as an appendix at the end of each volume.

Numerous favorable comments have been relayed to us regarding how the references in the first and second editions have been used as the basis for various research and other scientific articles and case reports. Although a vast amount of relevant literature was again systematically reviewed for this third edition, we have attempted to limit additional citations to those of significant merit. All owners of this third edition, whether student, teacher, researcher, or practitioner, should find these additions useful to their clinical and scientific endeavors.

The photographic reproductions and diagrams have always been listed as one of the most attractive and valuable characteristics of the book. New diagrams have been added and improvements on existing ones have been made, such as the skeletal distribution diagrams that incorporate new localizing symbols to identify most common and less common sites of involvement. We have selectively removed some images and replaced them with new ones when better examples could be found. We have also continued with the teaching principle of placing arrows on images that correlate with the descriptive caption and direct the readers to important facets of the case. When possible, the case material has been augmented with bone scans, CT, and MRI to reflect the technological revolution in musculoskeletal diagnosis.

As with the first and second editions, this text is meant to be used for at least three purposes: as a ***teaching text*** aimed at all those who seek knowledge and expertise in musculoskeletal disorders, as a ***reference text*** when information is sought, and as a ***clinical aid*** to assist you with those patients who seek your care. In this regard, we encourage you to read this text carefully and use it for its intended purposes.

We also hope the book will help the reader avoid the many pitfalls of clinical decision making—one of the most obvious being addressed in a quote from an unknown author, *"You see what you look for and recognize what you know."*

TERRY R. YOCHUM
LINDSAY J. ROWE

The release of *Essentials of Skeletal Radiology* in 1987 was a dream fulfilled for both of us. We had hardly blinked an eye before the publishers were requesting us to consider a second edition, and now we have completed the third. This edition has been a monumental task, which has taken approximately 3 years to research, write, and publish. A task of this magnitude is never accomplished without significant support from numerous people assisting in many different ways.

Our contributing authors have provided a distinct and unique contribution to this third edition and we wish to recognize their efforts:

Michael S. Barry, D.C., D.A.C.B.R., Denver, Colorado
Gary M. Guebert, B.S., D.C., D.A.C.B.R., St. Louis, Missouri
Bryan Hartley, M.D., Melbourne, Australia
Claude Pierre-Jerome, M.D., PhD., Oslo, Norway
Norman W. Kettner, D.C., D.A.C.B.R., F.I.C.C.,
  St. Louis, Missouri
Robert J. Longenecker, D.C., D.A.C.B.R., Dallas, Texas
Chad J. Maola, B.S., D.C., Denver, Colorado
Melanie D. Osterhouse, D.C., D.A.C.B.R., St. Louis, Missouri
Margaret A. Seron, D.C., D.A.B.C.O., D.A.C.B.R.,
  Denver, Colorado
David P. Thomas, M.D., Melbourne, Australia
Jeffrey R. Thompson, D.C., D.A.C.B.R., Houston, Texas

Their assistance in numerous chapters in this edition is greatly appreciated.

We would also like to thank Leon L. Wiltse, M.D., Long Beach Memorial Hospital, Long Beach, California, and Lyle J. Micheli, M.D., Children's Hospital, Harvard Medical School, Department of Orthopedics, Boston, Massachusetts, for their expert review and editing of Chapter 5 ("The Natural History of Spondylolysis and Spondylolisthesis.")

There have been several new topics added to Chapter 6 ("Diagnostic Imaging of the Musculoskeletal System"), the nucleus of which has been provided by Norman W. Kettner, D.C., D.A.C.B.R., Robert J. Longenecker, D.C., D.A.C.B.R., and Melanie D. Osterhouse, D.C., D.A.C.B.R. We wish to thank them for their outstanding contribution. Thanks also to Steven Gould, D.C., D.A.C.B.R., who provided us a number of musculoskeletal diagnostic ultrasound images used in this chapter.

Dr. Thomas H. Berquist, of the Mayo Clinic, provided excellent review and editorial comments for the new "Masqueraders" chapter and we thank him. Gratitude is expressed to two radiology residents, Dr. Gregory Bathurst and Dr. Thanh Vu, from the University of Colorado Health Sciences Center for their extraordinary efforts in proofreading this new chapter.

A special thank you to those physicians who have graciously provided the forewords for the third edition:

Joseph W. Howe, D.C., D.A.C.B.R, Fellow, A.C.C.R.
M. Bruce Farkas, D.O., J.D.
Reed B. Phillips, D.C., D.A.C.B.R., Ph.D.
Donald Resnick, M.D.

Several people were involved at varying levels in the editorial process of the production of the third edition of this textbook. Special thanks are offered to Drs. Michael S. Barry, Gary M. Guebert, John K. Hyland, Norman W. Kettner, Chad J. Maola, Melanie D. Osterhouse, Jeffrey R. Thompson, and William M. Ursprung. They were of great assistance to this project, conducting endless literature searches, proofreading, and offering editorial comments. The extensive updating of the references was facilitated by Mr. Bob Snyder, Public Services/Reference Librarian of the Logan College of Chiropractic. We thank him for his endless efforts on our behalf. A special thank you is due to Ms. Erica L. Collier, able assistant and secretary to Dr. Kettner at the Logan College of Chiropractic. Erica received endless phone calls and helped in locating the Logan radiology staff, always on short notice. Her pleasant attitude and quick response to our needs with faxing and e-mailing numerous documents has been most appreciated.

Special thanks to Michael L. Manco-Johnson, M.D., F.A.C.R., Professor of Radiology and Medicine, Chairman of the Department of Radiology, University of Colorado Health Science Center, Denver, Colorado, and Ray F. Kilcoyne, M.D., Professor of Radiology, Department of Radiology, University of Colorado Health Science Center, Denver, Colorado, for allowing their valuable case material from various departments at the university to be photographed and utilized in this third edition. Thanks also to the many radiology residents at this university who have secured unique skeletal radiology cases for our teaching file and, in particular, this third edition. Many of those residents' names appear scattered throughout various chapters following their case material.

Chapter 8 ("Skeletal Dysplasias") of this book provided a particular challenge in upgrading the case material. The staff of Children's Hospital, Department of Radiology, Denver, Colorado, was most cooperative in allowing us to photograph their skeletal teaching file. These cases are dispersed throughout the textbook, particularly in the area of dysplasias. Our gratitude goes specifically to John D. Strain, M.D., Chairman of the Department of Radiology, Children's Hospital, Denver, Colorado, for his assistance in obtaining this case material.

The majority of the new photographs for this third edition were skillfully processed and perfected by the able staff at the Pro Lab, Inc., Denver, Colorado. The quality of their work is evident by the end product.

Thanks to those who assisted us at Lippincott Williams & Wilkins in the production of this book, including all who worked behind the scenes and whom we never met or interacted with.

Special thanks to Karen K. Gulliver, freelance managing editor, for her diligent, thorough review and processing of this huge manuscript. She did a great job in the second edition and equally outstanding work in the third edition.

Finally, our gratitude is expressed to Joseph Janse, D.C., and Kenneth E. Yochum, D.C., in our dedications.

TERRY R. YOCHUM
LINDSAY J. ROWE

With a deep sense of gratitude, I wish to thank my devoted wife, companion, and best friend, Inge. Her understanding, support, and unconditional love fashioned the vehicle that carried me as I traveled the difficult road of this third edition. Special thanks to my children, Kimberley Ann, Philip Andrew, and Alicia Marie. They have readily forgiven their father's frequent absences during this project. I want to especially acknowledge my most devoted follower, Cecelia G. Yochum, my mother, who gave me life and nurtured and encouraged me throughout my entire career. She knew of this third edition and inspired me to work hard to finish it. Unfortunately, she passed away on August 22, 2001. I hope she would have been proud of my efforts and the finished product.

I wish to acknowledge and thank the following special individuals who have shaped my professional career and touched my personal life:

- Dr. M. Bruce Farkas, an exceptional osteopathic radiologist, who helped me greatly in the beginning of my career.
- Dr. Joseph W. Howe, my professor, after whom a progeny of radiology diplomates emerged.
- Dr. Joseph Janse, modern-day father of chiropractic.
- Dr. William E. Litterer, who spared no detail and forgot no face.
- Dr. Reed B. Phillips, a critical thinker, man of great integrity and leadership, and one of my very best friends.
- Dr. Donald B. Tomkins, who is remembered for knowledge tempered by wisdom, and one of my teachers at National College who inspired me early in my career to enter into radiology.
- Dr. James F. Winterstein, one of my original teachers and an outstanding radiologist who provided inspiration for me to enter the radiology residency program at National College.

For the development and production of this book I express sincere gratitude to:

- my associate, Chad J. Maola, B.S., D.C., who has co-authored five chapters in this edition. There are no adequate words to express my sincere thanks for his exceptional devotion to this entire project. When this revision was at risk of not being finished, he stepped in and assisted me day and night to bring this project to fruition. Chad is an outstanding individual who has gone above and beyond the call of duty for me.
- my adopted resident and loyal friend, Norman W. Kettner, D.C., D.A.C.B.R., F.I.C.C., who has co-authored three chapters in this edition. His untiring efforts for this project and support of me personally will forever by appreciated.

- my resident and good friend, Jeffrey R. Thompson, D.C., D.A.C.B.R., who has co-authored one chapter in this edition and who once again responded graciously to my request for help. His literary expertise and superior effort on behalf of this entire project has been most appreciated.
- my associate, Michael S. Barry, D.C., D.A.C.B.R., who has co-authored three chapters in this edition. His support was exceptional. He proofread and edited many of these chapters and our friendship is forever strengthened as a result.
- my staff, Connie L. Jones, R.T.(R), Lanna L. Gosage, R.T.(R), and Wanda I. Hidy. My gratitude is extended to these three wonderful women who have worked closely with me for many years. They supported me through the arduous task of the daily workloads of my radiology practice and the revision of this textbook. I could not have gotten through this without their unflagging support.
- my able typist, Debbie K. Schlosser, for the time she freely gave when her energy was needed to type and repeatedly review chapters and manuscript submissions. Debbie typed the second edition and had a significant impact on the third edition. Her efforts are most appreciated.
- a family friend, Joshua Rohleder, who provided assistance in the organization of many new photos throughout this text.

I express particular thanks to five very distinguished individuals:

- Mr. Kent S. Greenawalt, President, Foot Levelers, Inc, Roanoke, Virginia
- Mr. Rodney Moulder, President, HCMI, Springfield, Missouri
- Dr. Reed B. Phillips, President, Southern California University of Health Sciences, Whittier, California
- Dr. Mark Sanna, President, Breakthrough Coaching, Miami, Florida
- Mr. George Stamathis, experienced medical publisher and publishing consultant, Bel Air, Maryland

These dear friends were never too busy to receive a late-night phone call or to be a sounding board for my concerns and woes. They carried me over hard, rocky places as I proceeded down the long road of this project.

The inspiration to undertake the third edition of this text came from the many doctors and students who have attended my lectures from coast to coast, and I wish to thank them for providing this motivation.

And finally, thanks to my co-author, Dr. Lindsay J. Rowe, for his efforts on behalf of this third edition, particularly his work on our new chapter, "Masqueraders of Musculoskeletal Disease."

TERRY R. YOCHUM

With a few words much needs to be acknowledged. This book was born in the early 1980s out of an idea to do things better, to consolidate, to explain, to bring logic to just one area of human disease. Along the way many contributed—patients, students, colleagues, publishers, and all of our ancillary staff. Many went to extraordinary lengths to make these volumes better, for which we all benefit. All manner of obstacles have been overcome. With this third edition all of these ideals continue with but a few exceptions.

My thanks go to Stephen Heaney of the Medical Communication Unit at John Hunter Hospital, Newcastle, for their fine photographic reproductions. To the radiographic technologists at our Newcastle Hospitals for their fine work in obtaining examinations of the highest quality and bringing cases of interest to my attention is greatly appreciated. Similarly, the many radiology, medical, and surgical residents who ensured all manner of cases come to me for review I am indebted.

For the students of Medicine in Newcastle and Chiropractic throughout the world who I teach, they provide the perpetual fertile environs and impetus to write, research, and understand this subject area. Similarly, at the medical and chiropractic meetings that I address domestically and throughout the world, I glean a great deal that is directly reapplied back to teaching. A large proportion of the case material contained in this third edition has been derived from these interactions.

Thanks to Professor Joe Ghabriel, M.D., orthopedist and spine surgeon; Eric Ho, M.D., pediatric orthopedist; and Martin Epstein, M.D., endocrinologist and bone mineral specialist, for securing additional case material and allowing me to review their patients' studies on a regular basis and for providing me with great stimulus to increase my expertise and knowledge.

To James Brandt, M.S., D.C., F.A.C.O., in Minneapolis, Minnesota, for his perceptive insight, encouragement, guidance, and friendship over many years I am very grateful to have him and his family as part of my life. Special recognition goes to Brian Nook, D.C., C.C.S.P., of Perth, Australia, Associate Professor, School of Chiropractic Murdoch University. As we shared an office in 1985–86 during the genesis of this text he provided a sense of direction, purpose, and vision, which has been rekindled for this third edition. My long-term friends and colleagues from different parts of the globe Michael Buna, B.S., D.C., from Victoria, Canada; Shane Carter, B.S., D.C., of Inverarie, Scotland; and Wayne Minter, B.S., D.C., in Sydney, Australia, have given that much needed sense of perspective, balance, and humor continuing through all previous and present editions.

Finally, to my extraordinary wife, Anne Baxter, B.S., M.D., and my son, Ryan, the time given to this project is time lost for us but much gained for others. You are indelibly entwined throughout these pages more than anyone could know. You are my life.

I hope in some way these books will assist all of those who use them and will make a difference to those patients that seek their care. I dedicate my last contribution to this book to these patients.

LINDSAY J. ROWE

Michael S. Barry, D.C., D.A.C.B.R.
Private Radiology Practice
Private Chiropractic Practice
Denver, Colorado

Postgraduate Faculty Member
Logan College of Chiropractic
Chesterfield, Missouri

Gary M. Guebert, B.S., D.C., D.A.C.B.R.
Private Radiology Practice
St. Louis, Missouri

Assistant Professor of Radiology
Logan College of Chiropractic
Chesterfield, Missouri

Formerly:
Assistant Professor and Chairman, Radiology Department
Texas Chiropractic College
Pasadena, Texas

Bryan Hartley, M.D. (deceased)
Staff Radiologist
Austin Hospital
Melbourne, Australia

Head, Department of Radiology
Heidelberg Repatriation Hospital
Melbourne, Australia

Claude Pierre-Jerome, M.D., Ph.D.
Associate Professor of Radiology—MRI section
Ulleval University Hospital
Oslo, Norway

Norman W. Kettner, D.C., D.A.C.B.R., F.I.C.C.
Chairman, Department of Radiology
Logan College of Chiropractic
Chesterfield, Missouri

Professor, Clinical Science Division
Logan College of Chiropractic
Chesterfield, Missouri

Robert J. Longenecker, D.C., D.A.C.B.R.
Private Radiology Practice
Dallas, Texas

Post Graduate Faculty Member
Parker College of Chiropractic
Dallas, Texas

Chad J. Maola, B.S., D.C.
Orthopedic and Radiology Consultant
Denver, Colorado

Formerly:
Instructor in Orthopedics and Radiology
Colorado College of Chiropractic
Marycrest International University
Denver, Colorado

Melanie D. Osterhouse, D.C., D.A.C.B.R.
Instructor, Clinical Science Division
Logan College of Chiropractic
Chesterfield, Missouri

Margaret A. Seron, D.C., D.A.B.C.O., D.A.C.B.R.
Private Radiology Practice
Denver, Colorado

Postgraduate Faculty Member
Southern California University of Health Sciences
Whittier, California

Formerly:
Assistant Professor of Radiology
Los Angeles College of Chiropractic
Whittier, California

David P. Thomas, M.D. (retired)
Formerly:
Head, Department of Radiology
Austin Hospital
Melbourne, Australia

Jeffrey R. Thompson, D.C., D.A.C.B.R.
Private Radiology Practice
Houston, Texas

Associate Professor, Diagnostic Imaging
Texas Chiropractic College
Pasadena, Texas

CONTENTS

B. App. Sc. (Chiro)
Bachelor of Applied Science (Chiropractic)
This is the chiropractic qualification issued by the Royal
Melbourne Institute of Technology, School of Chiropractic,
Melbourne, Australia

B.S.
Bachelor of Science

C.C.S.P.
Certified Chiropractic Sports Physician

D.A.B.C.O.
Diplomate of the American Board of Chiropractic Orthopedists

D.A.C.B.N.
Diplomate of the American Chiropractic Board of Nutrition

D.A.C.B.S.P.
Diplomate of the American Chiropractic Board of
Sports Physicians

*D.A.C.B.R.
Diplomate of the American Chiropractic Board of Radiology

D.A.C.B.R. (Hon.)
Honorary Diplomate of the American Chiropractic Board
of Radiology

D.C.
Doctor of Chiropractic

D.O.
Doctor of Osteopathy

D.P.M.
Doctor of Podiatric Medicine

Ed.D.
Doctor of Education

F.A.C.C.R. (Aus)
Fellow of the Australian Chiropractic College of Radiology
(Australia)

F.A.C.O.
Fellow of the Academy of Chiropractic Orthopedists

*F.C.C.R. (C)
Fellow Chiropractic College of Radiologists (Canada)

*Fellow, A.C.C.R.
Fellow American Chiropractic College of Radiology

F.I.C.C.
Fellow of the International College of Chiropractors

J.D.
Juris Doctor

*M.D.
Doctor of Medicine

M.I.R.
Member of the Institute of Radiography

M.Sc. or M.S.
Master of Science

Ph.D.
Doctor of Philosophy

R.T. (R.)
Radiological Technologist (Radiology)

---

*Physicians referred to in this text holding these degrees are radiologists.

Skeletal Radiology: An Historical Perspective

Lindsay J. Rowe and Terry R. Yochum

All disciplines within the health sciences have undergone enormous change and technological development throughout the last century, with radiology being at the forefront of innovation and discovery. The subspecialty of musculoskeletal imaging has been an integral part of these advances, experiencing a long and intricate history, with great changes witnessed over the last 20 years. (1) For those involved in musculoskeletal imaging, it is a demanding challenge to keep abreast of the ever-changing technology and knowledge base and to develop the new skills necessary to serve the demands of those who seek their services. Clinicians of musculoskeletal medicine face similar demands of selecting appropriate imaging modalities for the clinical situation, interpreting the clinically important findings, and integrating them into the delivery of patient care. Given this crescendo of increasing demands on musculoskeletal radiologists and clinicians, the need to interact, consult, and discuss patients on a regular basis is paramount to optimizing patient care. The purpose of this prelude is to reflect on key achievements of the past and provide a descriptive overview of where we are in the new millennium.

In 1995, the 100-year anniversary of the discovery of x-rays was celebrated. As the first x-ray was that of a hand, so too was it the centenary of the subspecialty of musculoskeletal radiology. Such anniversaries present the opportunity to reflect on the past: beginnings, leaders, martyrs, innovators, and advancements in technology. So rapid and spectacular has been the acceleration of knowledge and technology within radiology, it is arguably one of the most dynamic and challenging specialties within the health disciplines. Testament to this are the evolving terms describing the specialty, from the early beginnings as *roentgenology,* honoring the original discoverer Roentgen; to *radiology,* encompassing both the diagnostic and therapeutic applications; and to the more recent *imaging,* including the non-x-ray producing modalities of ultrasound and magnetic resonance. (1–4)

THE EVOLUTION OF IMAGING

The history of the development of radiology is long and intricate. As with so many other significant advancements in science, x-rays were discovered accidentally. In 1895, Wilhelm Conrad Roentgen, a professor at the University of Würzburg in Germany, was working on experiments in his laboratory. (Fig. A) He was investigating the properties of an early cathode-ray tube, called a Crookes' tube, which accelerated electrons in a manner similar to

today's x-ray apparatus. While conducting a stream of electrons from the cathode through the evacuated tube, he noticed that a plate covered with barium platinocyanoide located at some distance away began to fluoresce. Not knowing what to call these invisible rays from the Crookes' tube that induced fluorescence, he named them "x-rays," *x* standing for the unknown quantity. Roentgen then feverishly began experimenting and defining their characteristics, and in little more than a month he had described all the major properties of the x-ray as they are recognized today.

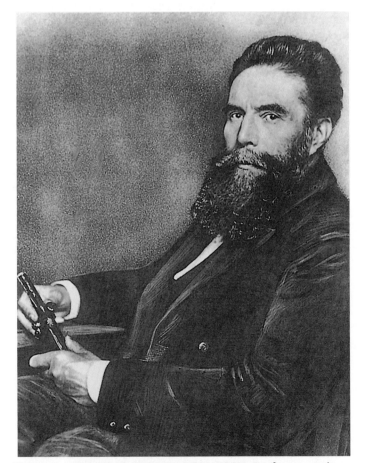

Figure A **WILHELM CONRAD ROENTGEN.** Professor at the University of Würzburg in Germany, winner of the first Nobel Prize for Physics in 1901 for his discovery of the x-ray.

Professor Roentgen produced the first clinical radiograph, an image of his wife's hand, on November 8, 1895, and first reported his findings on December 8, 1895, to the Würzburg Physico-Medical Society. (2–4) (Fig. B) In recognition of his discovery, he received the first Nobel Prize for Physics in 1901. Others soon recognized the potential role of the x-ray in industry and the healthcare professions. Examples of the earliest diagnostic x-rays are those made in 1896 by Pupin of a hand imbedded with multiple shotgun pellets, those made by Frost of a fractured wrist, and a case of osteosarcoma imaged by Manell. (2)

Thereafter, a global technological revolution began. Pupin developed the first intensifying screen, and Edison, the first fluoroscope, to mention only two developments. In 1921, Potter and Bucky introduced a moving grid mechanism. Sausser, a chiropractor, in 1934 was the first to produce a single-exposure, anteroposterior, full-spine radiograph. The cumulative result of all of these refinements was the production of diagnostic images of improved quality, which depicted abnormalities directing more effective treatment. (2) (Figs. C–E)

These early advancements were tempered with the recognition of the harmful nature of radiation. Many severe and often fatal injuries occurred to those who pioneered the research in radiology. As a result, the use of the x-ray came under close bureaucratic scrutiny and control. Despite these complications, and in the face of increasingly poor publicity, the usefulness of this new diagnostic tool could not be ignored, and innovations in imaging technology continued, aimed at dose reduction, personnel and patient protection, and improving image quality. Previously, the use of rare earth screens, compensating filtration, and high-frequency generators were some of the significant advancements.

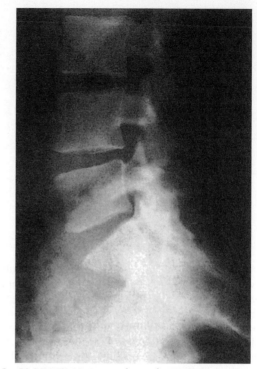

Figure C **PLAIN FILM. Lateral Lumbar.** Observe the excellent bony detail along with the depth of the lumbar lordosis and lumbosacral disc angle. The intervertebral disc spaces are outlined; however, no details concerning the internal substance of the disc or adjacent neural structures can be assessed.

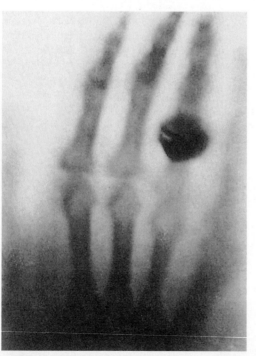

Figure B **ROENTGEN'S FIRST RADIOGRAPH.** Professor Roentgen's historic first radiograph of his wife's hand taken November 8, 1895, in Würzburg, Germany. (Courtesy of Deutsches Roentgen-Museum, Remscheid-Lennep, West Germany.)

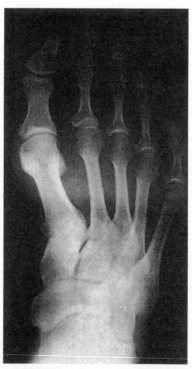

Figure D **PLAIN FILM. Dorsoplantar Foot.** Bony alignment, as well as joint spaces, are adequately assessed through the foot and tarsal bones. Observe the filtration of the forefoot and toes used to obtain a uniform exposure. This is done with a compensating filter of copper and aluminum.

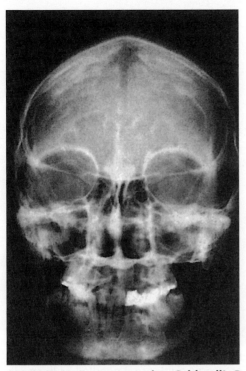

Figure E PLAIN FILM. Posteroanterior, Caldwell's Projection, Skull. The complexity of the anatomy requires careful attention to detail and anatomic landmarks. Supplemental imaging, such as CT or MRI, not only clarifies these structures but also provides depiction of clinically important intracranial structures.

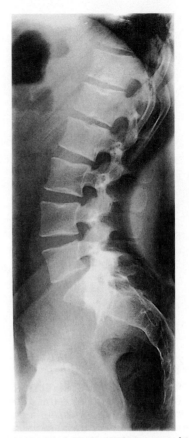

Figure F COMPENSATING FILTRATION. Lateral Lumbar. A single-exposure standing lateral radiograph from the lower sacrum to the T11 level has been achieved by the placement of a number of aluminum filters in the primary beam at the collimator. These have included 2 mm to the level of the iliac crest, a curved tapered filter into the lumbar lordosis to enhance detail of the spinous processes and neural arch, and a curved filter conforming to the diaphragmatic contour to eliminate overexposure of the lower thoracic segments. (Courtesy of Lloyd Wingate, DC, Dapto, New South Wales, Australia.)

(Fig. F) Today, updated technology leading to digital imaging has virtually eliminated the need for darkroom procedures and x-ray cassettes in hospital and smaller private practice environments.

The dynamics of joint motion have been extensively investigated with various imaging methods. Spinal mechanics have been depicted with single views performed at the extremes of motion (dynamic or stress radiography) and with compression–distraction forces. Obtaining simultaneous views at 90° to each other (biplanar radiography) has been employed for complex computer analysis of motion patterns. Continuous spinal and peripheral joint motion can be observed with fluoroscopy and videotaped for retrospective analysis (videofluoroscopy). (3,4)

The use of radiopaque contrast media within hollow organs and body spaces improved the diagnostic evaluations. Introduction of radiopaque substances into the subarachnoid space of the spine (myelography) provided information not previously available, especially in regard to intraspinal and intervertebral disc lesions. (Figs. G and H) Injection of the nucleus pulposus of the intervertebral disc, which can be performed in conjunction with CT (discography, CT discography), has provided both a morphological evaluation of disc integrity and become a clinical provocational tool for isolating a discogenic cause for spinal pain syndromes. In the skeletal system, an opaque medium placed into the joint space of a peripheral or spinal facet articulation (arthrography) has allowed demonstration of cartilage, synovium, and ligamentous structures. (Fig. I) Introduction of contrast into a peripheral lymphatic vessel will opacify both lymphatic channels and lymph nodes (lymphangiogram). Injection of contrast can also be made into sinus infection or pilonidal tracts to trace their

course (sinogram). (Fig. J) In some bone lesions, such as simple bone cysts, details of internal structure can be identified.

The inherent lack of sensitivity of conventional radiography was countered by the administration of selective radioisotopes (nuclear medicine) that seek out specific tissues and areas of cellular activity. In skeletal disorders the administration of isotopes such as technetium-99m and gallium provided information on bone activity (bone scan) not recognizable with conventional procedures. These are usually performed as a triphasic study consisting of an initial "flow" study, a "blood pool," and a "delayed" study. (Fig. K) This has been particularly important in the early detection of many skeletal disorders. The combination of computed tomograms with nuclear medicine has added a third dimension to musculoskeletal imaging (single-photon emission computed tomography; SPECT).

In the early 1970s, computed tomograms (CT scans, CAT scans) were first produced, combining the technology of the computer with the advances in x-ray technology. With refinements in machine and computer technology, exquisite sectional images are now produced in almost every anatomic plane. CT studies have had a particular impact on the evaluation of spinal and neurological diseases (Figs. L–O) Three-dimensional images depict anatomy

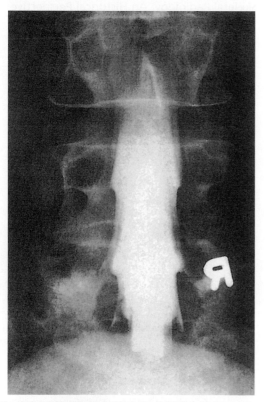

Figure G **METRIZAMIDE LUMBAR MYELOGRAM.** Placement of water-soluble contrast media into the subarachnoid space allows demonstration of the normal cauda equina, dural sleeves, and caudal sac. This contrast media is eliminated through the filtration of the kidneys and excreted in the urine.

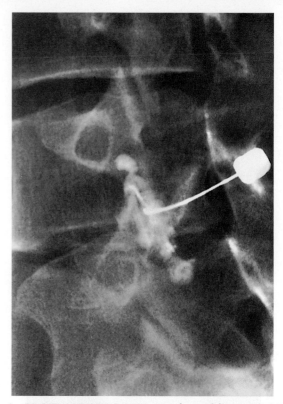

Figure I **FACET ARTHROGRAM. Lumbar Oblique L4–L5.** Under fluoroscopic guidance a needle has been placed into the facet joint space, which has been injected with a contrast agent. This reveals the integrity of the joint capsule and identifies correct needle placement before injection of a local anesthetic, irritant, or anti-inflammatory agent for diagnostic or therapeutic purposes.

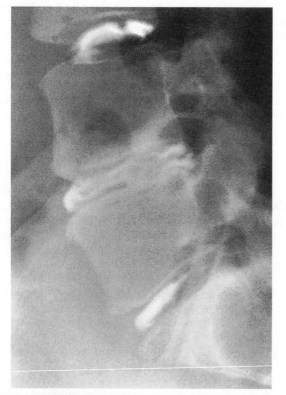

Figure H **DISCOGRAM. L3–L5.** Contrast media has been injected into the nucleus pulposus at three levels. Only the L3 disc is normal in morphology, with both L4 and L5 demonstrating migration of contrast posteriorly and anteriorly through discal tears. (Courtesy of Inger F. Villadsen, DC, Newcastle, New South Wales, Australia.)

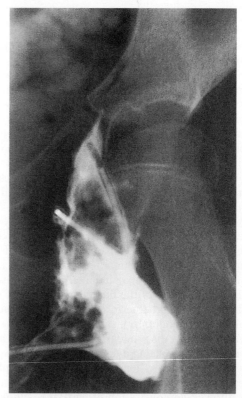

Figure J **HIP SINOGRAM: PSOAS ABSCESS.** A draining inguinal sinus was cannulated and opaque contrast media was introduced. Observe the tracking of the contrast cephalad outlining the course of the sinus, which proved later to be continuous with a tuberculous infective focus in the spine at the L2–L3 level.

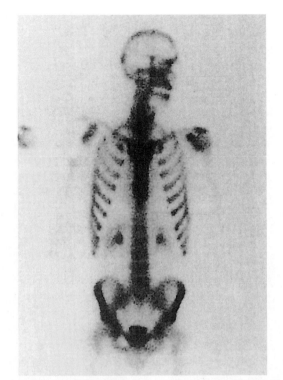

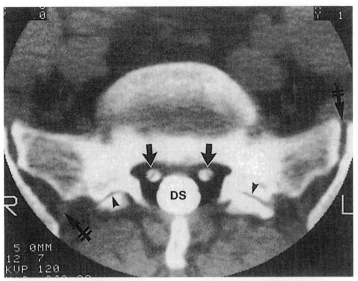

Figure M   **CONTRAST-ENHANCED (MYELOGRAM) CT STUDY. S1 Level.** The dural sac (*DS*) and the S1 spinal nerve roots (*arrows*) are accurately depicted. In addition, the lumbo-sacral (*arrowheads*) and sacroiliac (*crossed arrows*) articulations are demonstrated.

Figure K   **FULL-BODY DELAYED NUCLEAR BONE SCAN.** This study is designated as "delayed" because the image is obtained some hours after intravenous injection of the isotope. This is usually preceded by an immediate postinjection study and within minutes another set of images obtained to evaluate capillary "pooling." The delayed study demonstrates the normal uptake of radioactive isotope in metabolically active areas of the skeleton, demonstrated as dark regions (*hot spots*) that require only a 3–5% change in activity to be detectable. (Courtesy of Nuclear Medicine Department, M.D. Anderson Hospital, Houston, Texas.)

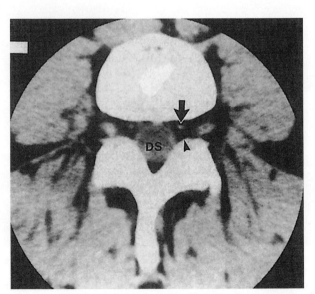

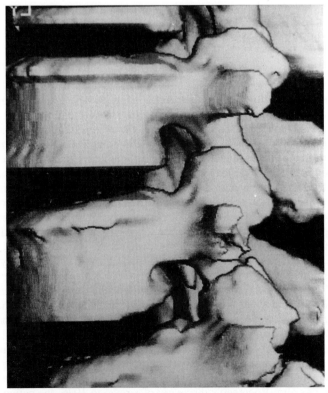

Figure L   **CT STUDY. Axial L4 Level.** Observe the exquisite details of the dural sac (*DS*), nerve roots (*arrow*), perineural fat (*arrowhead*), paravertebral musculature, and bony confines.

Figure N   **THREE-DIMENSIONAL CT: A 1985 STUDY. Sagittal Lumbar Spine.** Observe the lumbar anatomy on this surface-rendered CT image. The more recent CT scans with helical imaging render images of greater detail. This is a normal study.

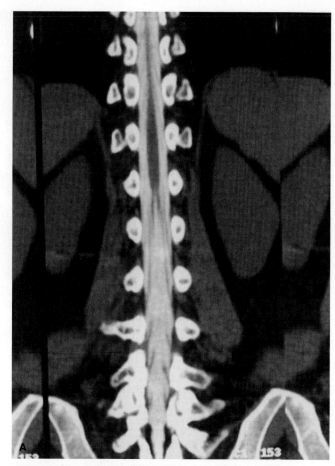

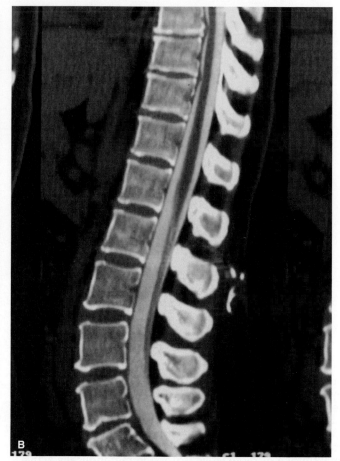

Figure O **CT MYELOGRAM. A. Coronal Lumbar Spine. B. Sagittal Lumbar Spine.** This patient had a dorsal column stimulator that prevented him from having an MRI scan.

Observe the exquisite detail of the spinal cord and vertebral segments on these multislice CT myelograms.

and abnormalities in exquisite detail. (Fig. P) The use of strong magnetic fields (MRI) has revolutionized body-imaging capabilities and the identification of abnormalities previously unrecognizable. (Figs. Q–V) The use of gadolinium-enhanced MRI delivers information on vascularity and the inflammatory nature of a lesion. Ultrasound has expanded its applications in musculoskeletal disorders. Evaluation of soft tissue lesions provides some limited information on its characteristics that can assist in management. Ultrasound screening for pediatric hip dysplasia has been a particularly notable contribution to a common problem that has considerable delayed morbidity if undetected.

Further progression of CT and MRI has allowed detailed analysis of the entire human body, including the vascular system. (Figs. W and X) However, in spite of all these technological advances, many fundamental principles of imaging remain unchanged. The plain film radiograph still forms the foundation for a large portion of the diagnostic investigations in clinical practice, especially in the evaluation of skeletal disorders. This is demonstrated with an example from the past. The radiograph shown in Figure Y was taken in 1897 at the John Sealy Hospital in Galveston, Texas, just 2 years after Roentgen's discovery of x-rays. In 1976, the patient, Mrs. Minne Powell Bowers, consulted a chiropractor in Conroe, Texas, for evaluation of a low back complaint. When questioned about prior x-rays, she stated that she had fallen at the age of 14 and her father, a medical doctor, had decided to transport her from

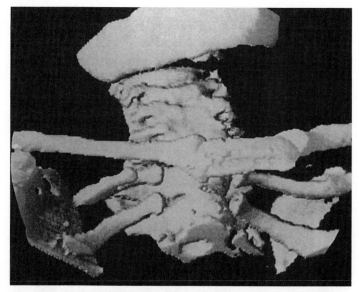

Figure P **THREE-DIMENSIONAL CT STUDY. Thoracic Outlet.** The image was reconstructed from thin axial images and then tilted to allow greater visualization of the bony thorax. Soft tissues could similarly be detected by selecting a different "window" setting. (Courtesy of Kenneth B. Heithoff, MD, Minneapolis, Minnesota.)

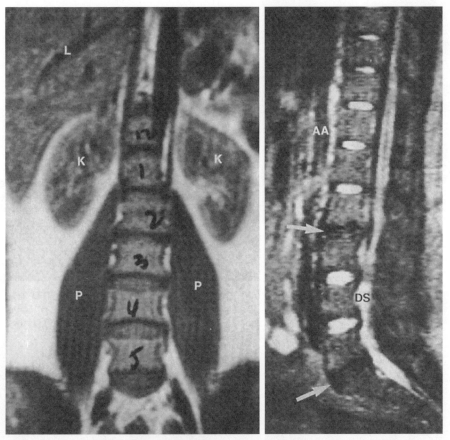

Figure Q   **OLDER-GENERATION MRI. Coronal and Sagittal Lumbar Spine.**
Details of the posterior abdomen can be defined, including the liver (*L*), kidneys (*K*), and psoas muscles (*P*). The dural sac (*DS*) and the abdominal aorta (*AA*) are also visible. Note the bright signal intensity of the nucleus of the discs indicating adequate hydration and lack of degeneration. However, the L2 and L5 discs are low in signal (*arrows*), representing underlying degenerative disc desiccation (dehydration).

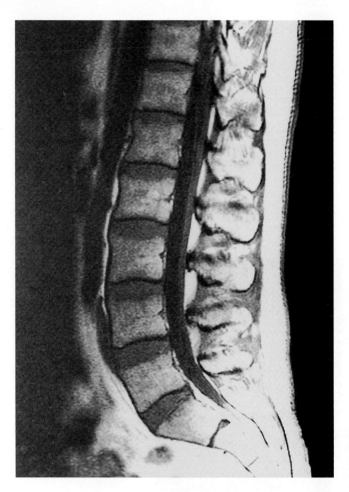

Figure R   **NEWER-GENERATION MRI. T1-Weighted MRI, Sagittal Lumbar.** Exquisite anatomic detail is depicted, including the cauda equina, vertebral bodies, and intervertebral discs. (Courtesy of Kenneth B. Heithoff, MD, Minneapolis, Minnesota.)

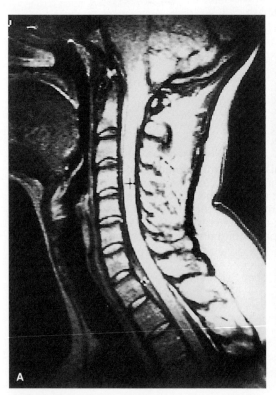

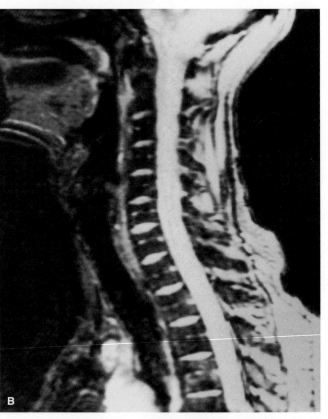

Figure S   **MRI STUDIES. A. T1-Weighted MRI, Sagittal Cervical. B. T2-Weighted MRI, Sagittal Cervical.** These images represent a normal cervical spine. Observe the difference in appearance of the vertebral bodies and spinal cord on the T1- and T2-weighted imaging sequences.

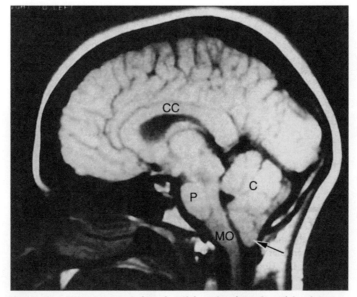

Figure T **MRI. T1-Weighted, Midsagittal Brain.** This view clearly shows the normal pons (*P*), medulla oblongata (*MO*), cerebellum (*C*), and corpus callosum (*CC*). Observe the cerebellar tonsils below the foramen magnum (*arrow*)—Arnold-Chiari malformation type II.

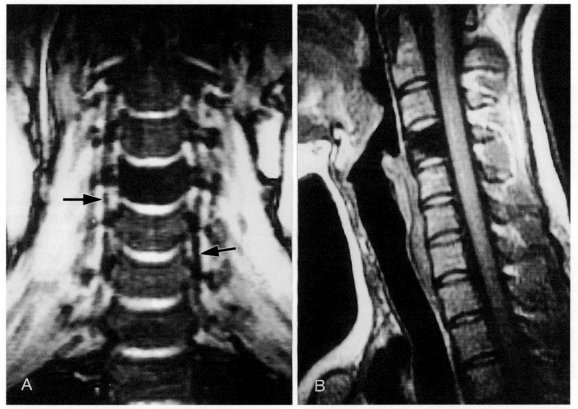

Figure U **MRI. A. T2-Weighted MRI, Coronal Cervical. B. T1-Weighted MRI, Sagittal Cervical.** Observe the low signal intensity of the C4 vertebral body. This has occurred as a result of significant marrow replacement—cause unknown. The most likely diagnosis with this appearance on MRI is metastatic bone disease. Observe the vertebral arteries (*arrows*). (Courtesy of Todd M. Aordkian, DC, Astoria, New York.)

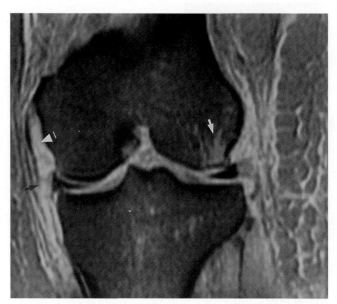

Figure V **T2-WEIGHTED MRI, CORONAL KNEE.** Observe the disruption of the medial collateral ligament (*black arrow*) as a result of a recent severe knee injury. There is significant joint effusion (*white arrowhead*) associated with a medial collateral ligament tear. In the subarticular surface of the lateral femoral condyle, there is bright signal intensity indicating bone marrow edema (*white arrow*). The small black triangular densities seen on the medial and lateral joint spaces represent the respective menisci.

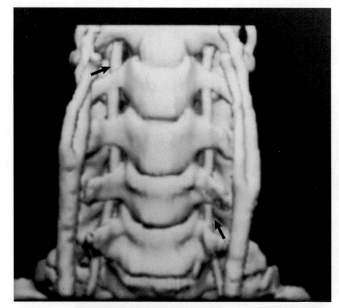

Figure W **SURFACE-RENDERED CT ANGIOGRAM: POST-INTRAVENOUS CONTRAST. Coronal Neck.** This intravenous contrast scan beautifully demonstrates the blood vessels of the neck, particularly the vertebral arteries (*arrows*) and the bony anatomy. This is a normal study.

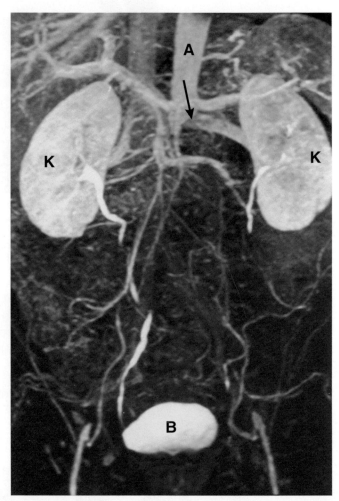

Figure X **MAGNETIC RESONANCE ANGIOGRAPHY. Coronal Abdomen.** There has been an acute and complete occlusion of the aorta, which extends from the aortic bifurcation to almost the renal arteries (*arrow*). This atherosclerotic occlusion of the aorta at its bifurcation has been referred to as *Leriche's syndrome.* This image was obtained with gadolinium injection. Observe the aorta (*A*), kidneys (*K*), and bladder (*B*), along with other vessels within the abdomen. Magnetic resonance angiography provides a non-invasive imaging modality as an alternative to traditional angiography, with its use of catheters and inherent risks.

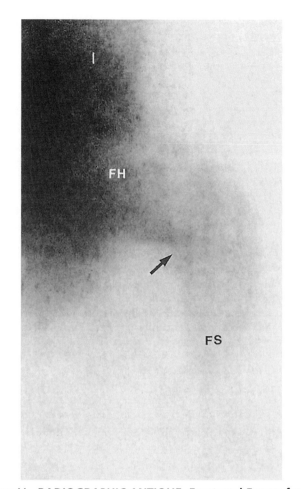

Figure Y **RADIOGRAPHIC ANTIQUE. Fractured Femur from 1897.** Despite the crude radiographic image, observe the ilium (*I*), femoral head (*FH*), and femoral shaft (*FS*). Careful observation reveals an acute angular deformity of the femoral neck caused by a fracture (*arrow*). (Courtesy of Michael L. Davis, DC, Conroe, Texas.)

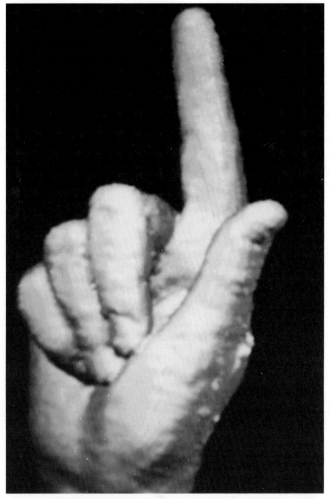

Figure Z **THREE-DIMENSIONAL SURFACE-RENDERED MRI. Hand.** What does the future hold in terms of further applications of MRI when an actual three-dimensional image of the hand can be produced as demonstrated here?

Willis, Texas, to Galveston in a horse-drawn wagon to have her hip pain evaluated with this new x-ray procedure. Mrs. Bowers brought on her next visit to the chiropractor the radiograph shown in Figure Y. Although the radiograph has aged and lacks technical clarity, careful observation of the image reveals an acute angular deformity of the femoral neck owing to a displaced fracture. Even today, some 100 years later, the initial diagnostic examination of choice for a similar case is still the same: *the plain film radiograph.*

For examinations of the skeleton, there is no modality to match the time and cost-effectiveness of the plain film radiograph. It is from this "plain film" perspective that *Essentials of Skeletal Radiology* has been written and integrated with examples of more complex sophisticated imaging technologies.

THE FUTURE OF IMAGING

The immense advances made in musculoskeletal imaging technology have placed greater demands on professions that use these procedures. The future applications of many of these imaging modalities are yet to be defined, particularly MRI. (Fig. Z) For the clinician and radiologist alike, there must be a commensurate understanding of anatomy, physics, morbidity, economics, advantages, and disadvantages of each modality to correctly choose those procedures that best suit the particular clinical problem being investigated. It is the role of the musculoskeletal radiologist to complement these demands and assist colleagues and patients in making such decisions. (1,2)

■ *References*

1. **Feldman F:** *Musculoskeletal radiology: Then and now.* Radiology 216:309, 2000.
2. **Yochum TR:** *1895–1995: Diagnostic imaging in its first century.* J Manipulative Physiol Ther 18(9):618, 1995.
3. **Grigg ERN:** *The trail of the invisible light.* Springfield, IL, Charles C Thomas, 1965.
4. **Eisenberg RL:** *Radiology: An illustrated history.* St. Louis, Mosby-Yearbook, 1992.

Arthritic Disorders 10

Lindsay J. Rowe and Terry R. Yochum

INTRODUCTION TO RADIOLOGIC INTERPRETATION IN JOINT DISEASE

Arthritis has the distinction of being the foremost crippler in the United States. Arthritis costs the American economy > $14 billion yearly and affects one in every seven people. (1) The most prevalent types are osteoarthritis (degenerative joint disease), rheumatoid arthritis, lupus erythematosus, ankylosing spondylitis, gout, juvenile rheumatoid arthritis, and scleroderma. The role of radiology in the diagnosis of these joint diseases is undisputed. A number of diagnostic imaging modalities, including arthrograms, arthroscopy, isotopic scans, CT, and even MRI, can be used in the evaluation of these joint abnormalities; however, it is the conventional radiograph that is usually the first and most extensively used method. (2) Proper inspection and interpretation of the visualized articulations frequently render important diagnostic information that otherwise would remain unrecognized and lead to incorrect diagnosis and treatment regimes.

PERSPECTIVES IN INTERPRETATION OF JOINT DISEASE

Over 100 rheumatic conditions have been identified and classified. Roentgen recognition of these individual entities is often difficult and confusing; however, by understanding joint anatomy,

pertinent clinical features, pathophysiology, and important roentgen signs, a single diagnosis or short list of differential diagnoses can usually be made. (1,2)

Incidence of Individual Arthritides

The overall population frequency of individual disorders makes the probability of encountering them variable. (Table 10-1) For example, degenerative joint disease (osteoarthritis) is so prevalent that in a normal practice it will be confronted on almost a daily basis. Conversely, a rarity such as ochronosis will almost never be seen. As a result a relative diagnostic priority should be placed on the arthritic conditions that present in clinical practice.

Clinical Information

Obtaining clinical information is the most important aspect of a patient's evaluation. Pertinent background data consists of age, sex, family history, and previous diseases, diagnoses, and therapies. (3) (Tables 10-2 and 10-3) Patients should be questioned in detail regarding symptoms, especially the type of onset, locations involved, description of pain, as well as any local and systemic effects. One should search for signs that will give important clues to the most likely diagnostic considerations. Careful laboratory investigations for inflammatory or metabolic disturbance should also be considered. (2)

Table 10-1	General Guide to Relative Frequency of Arthritis Diagnosed in Practice[a]	
Weekly	**Monthly**	**Yearly**
Degenerative joint disease (osteoarthritis)	Ankylosing spondylitis	Gout
	CPPD crystal deposition (pseudo-gout)	Infection
	DISH	Lupus erythematosus
	Osteitis condensans ilii	Reiter's syndrome
	Psoriatic arthritis	Scleroderma
	Rheumatoid arthritis	
	Synoviochondrometaplasia	

[a] The arthritises not listed should be considered rare and should be diagnosed with caution.
CPPD, calcium pyrophosphate dihydrate; *DISH,* diffuse idiopathic skeletal hyperostosis.

Table 10-2	General Age of Onset of Arthritis	
0–20 Years	**20–40 Years**	**≥ 40 Years**
Juvenile rheumatoid arthritis	Ankylosing spondylitis	Degenerative joint disease
	Osteitis condensans ilii	DISH
	Lupus erythematosus	Gout
	Psoriatic arthritis	Hypertrophic osteoarthropathy
	Reiter's syndrome	Pseudo-gout (CPPD)
	Rheumatoid arthritis	
	Scleroderma	
	Synoviochondrometaplasia	

Adapted with permission from **Wood, PHN:** *Age and the rheumatic diseases. Population studies of the rheumatic diseases.* Congress ser 148:26, 1968.
CPPD, calcium pyrophosphate dihydrate; *DISH,* diffuse idiopathic skeletal hyperostosis.

Table 10-3	Arthropathies Associated with Distinct Sex Predilection	
Male	**Female**
Ankylosing spondylitis	Juvenile rheumatoid arthritis
Gout	Lupus erythematosus
Hypertrophic osteoarthropathy	Osteitis condensans ilii
Reiter's syndrome	Primary osteoarthritis
Secondary osteoarthritis	Rheumatoid arthritis
	Scleroderma

Table 10-4	Anatomic Classification of Joints	
Type[a]	**Example**
Fibrous	Cranial sutures; syndesmoses (tibia–fibula, radius–ulna)
Cartilaginous	Symphysis pubis; intervertebral discs; manubriosternal junction
Synovial	Fingers, toes, knees, hips; apophyseal joints; sacroiliac joints

[a] Based on intervening tissue type.

ANATOMIC CONSIDERATIONS

A fundamental understanding of joint anatomy and histology is paramount in the understanding of the roentgen manifestations of normal and abnormal joints. Essentially, three broad categories of articulations exist in the body and are classified according to the tissue type at the junctional region: fibrous, cartilaginous, and synovial. (Table 10-4)

Fibrous Joints

The major interposed tissue is fibrous in nature such as in sutures, between the radius and the ulna, or between the tibia and the fibula. Radiographically, the opposing surfaces remain essentially parallel and have distinct cortices but often may be irregular in contour, which should not be interpreted as evidence of abnormality. (Fig. 10-1)

Cartilage Joints

The predominant tissue is cartilage, which histologically is usually of the fibrocartilage variety. Hyaline cartilage, however, may also be present, especially at the bone–cartilage interface. Examples of cartilage joints are the symphysis pubis, sternoclavicular joint, and intervertebral disc.

Intervertebral Disc. The unique anatomy of the intervertebral disc warrants special attention. (Fig. 10-2) The opposing surfaces of each vertebral body are composed of a 1-mm thickness of cortical bone that is readily identifiable radiographically. On its discal surface is a similar thickness of hyaline cartilage. Located centrally but slightly posterior is the initially gelatinous, but later fibrocartilaginous, nucleus pulposus. Peripherally, the annulus fibrosus encircles the disc; the inner fibers are made up of fibrocartilage, the outer fibers of collagen. Attachment of the annulus to the vertebral body margin, and internally, is by way of penetrating fibers and Sharpey's fibers. Radiographically, the normal annulus, nucleus, and cartilage endplates are not visible.

Synovial Joints

Synovial joints are characterized by the presence of a number of individual structures, including joint capsule, articular cartilage, synovial membrane, synovial fluid, joint space, and opposing smooth bony surfaces. (Fig. 10-3)

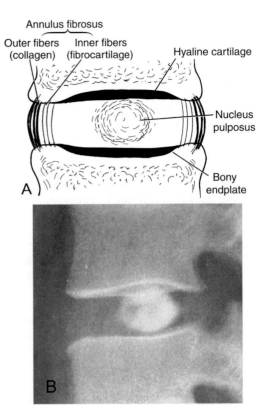

Figure 10-2 **ANATOMY OF THE INTERVERTEBRAL DISC. A. Diagram.** Note the outer annular fibers consist primarily of collagen and insert by way of Sharpey's fibers into the vertebral body margin. The inner fibers are fibrocartilaginous. Note the hyaline cartilage endplate that covers the bony surface centrally. **B. Discogram.** Note that the nucleus pulposus has been injected with a radiopaque contrast medium. Notice its position and shape and the intervening lucent space beneath the endplate, representing the cartilaginous endplate.

Figure 10-1 **EXAMPLES OF FIBROUS JOINTS. A. Radius–Ulna. B. Tibia–Fibula.**

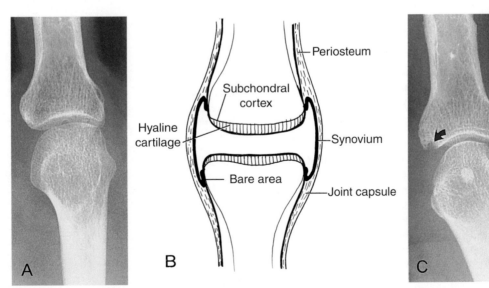

Figure 10-3 **SYNOVIAL JOINT. A. Normal Appearance.** Note the thin articular cortex and uniform joint space. **B. Joint Components. C. Marginal Erosion.** Note that at the bare area, where synovium directly opposes the articular cortex, synovial erosion from pannus produces a characteristic excavation at the articular margin (*arrow*). *COMMENT:* This is an important early sign of synovial disease, especially rheumatoid arthritis.

Joint Capsule. The predominant tissue type is fibrous in nature, essentially serving the function of a ligament, and is not normally visible radiographically. Notably, the fibers penetrate and are continuous with the adjacent periosteum. Variable degrees of intra-capsular bone will be present, depending on the joint. In some joints, including the knee, the wrist, the temporomandibular, acromioclavicular, sternoclavicular, and costovertebral joints, a fibrocartilaginous disc (meniscus) extends into the joint from the capsule.

Synovial Membrane. The synovium, which adheres to the overlying fibrous capsule and non-articular bone, consists of a loose, vascular connective tissue and secretes the synovial fluid. Regions where the synovium lies in direct contact with intra-articular bone that is not covered with articular cartilage are called *bare areas* and constitute anatomically predisposed regions of bone erosion from synovial disease. (Fig. 10-3*C*)

Synovial Fluid. Synovial fluid is a direct dialysate of blood plasma to which is added a mucoid substance secreted by the synovium. Its function is to provide lubrication and nutrition for the joint.

Articular Cartilage. Hyaline cartilage is the most common type of intra-articular cartilage. It is composed of chondrocytes embedded in a matrix of collagen fibrils and a ground substance. The latter is made up of mucopolysaccharides, particularly chondroitin sulfate, highly concentrated in water. The thickness of the cartilage varies between 1 and 7 mm, depending on the joint. Generally, the most stressed region of a joint will exhibit the thickest layer of cartilage. A number of layers are histologically evident within the cartilage.

The chondro-osseous junction demonstrates interdigitations, allowing for adequate mechanical adherence between the two tissues. Notably, at non-articulating intra-articular bone surfaces, the cartilage becomes thin and may be almost absent at the joint margin, constituting the intra-articular bare area. The cartilage depends for most of its nutrition on the synovial fluid owing to its relatively avascular nature.

Subchondral Bone Plate. Bony tissue beneath the articular cartilage is composed of a thin cortex and underlying cancellous trabeculae. Metabolically, the tissue is quite active with an abundant blood supply. Generally, there is no periosteum found around intracapsular cortices, which explains the lack of periosteal reaction of this bony structure.

RADIOLOGIC CONSIDERATIONS

Technologic Aspects

The most important structures scrutinized in the evaluation of joint disease are the individual joint components and bone insertions of tendons and ligaments (entheses). Radiographic examination of a joint requires a minimum of two views perpendicular to each other, with at least one view clearly demonstrating the opposing articular surfaces. Normally, a joint will not be fully visible unless the penetrating x-ray beam passes parallel to these joint surfaces, and the angle of the beam may vary according to the anatomic location. (Table 10-5)

Film quality must be optimum to observe fine details of articular anatomy. In the extremities, this is enhanced by the use of single-screen, single-emulsion films, as well as other techniques. Wherever possible, closely collimated projections of the area of abnormality should supplement the general radiologic examination. In the instances of multiple joint involvement, single views may be obtained to minimize radiation dose to the patient, but each must be the optimum view.

Anatomic–Radiologic Correlation

A sequential method in the evaluation of joint disease is critical to the recognition and subsequent interpretation of abnormalities. A simple, effective method is to examine, serially, alignment (A), bone (B), cartilage (C), and soft tissue (S). The *ABCs approach* allows a systematic routine examination to be followed. (1)

Alignment. Evaluation of joint relationships is an important diagnostic procedure because subtle and often characteristic misalignments and deformities may be overlooked. Wherever possible, orthopedic lines and measurements should be applied to aid the visual inspection.

Bones. The key osseous structure analyzed in joint disease is the subchondral bone plate, consisting of the articular cortex and underlying cancellous bone. The articular cortex is distinctively thinner than cortices in other locations. It is also smooth and invariably parallel with the opposing articular surface. The subarticular cancellous bone consists of supporting trabeculae distributed according to stresses traversing the joint. Within a single

Table 10-5	Anatomic–Technologic Correlation in Joint Evaluation
Joint	**Optimum Views**
Spine	
Intervertebral disc	
Cervical, thoracic, and lumbar	Lateral,* AP
Apophyseal	
Cervical	Lateral,* oblique, pillar
Thoracic	Oblique (70°)
Lumbar	Oblique,* lateral
Costovertebral	AP
Sacroiliac	AP cephalad angulation* (25–30°)
	PA caudad angulation (20–25°)
	Obliques
Symphysis pubis	AP
Hip	AP, frog leg
Knee	
Femorotibial	AP*
Patellofemoral	Lateral, skyline*
Ankle	
Tibiotalar	AP, oblique*
Subtalar	Oblique, special views
Foot	Dorsiplantar,* obliques
Shoulder	
Acromioclavicular	AP cephalad angulation 10°*
Glenohumeral	AP internal, external rotation*
Sternoclavicular	PA (computed tomography)*
Elbow	AP,* oblique, lateral
Wrist	PA,* PA ulnar flexion, oblique, lateral
Fingers	
Metacarpophalangeal	PA,* oblique, Norgaard
Interphalangeal	PA,* oblique, lateral

*Denotes most optimum single view.

bone the subarticular region of the epiphysis often appears the most radiolucent. The remaining bone of the metaphysis and diaphysis should also be evaluated for density, periosteal response, and changes at bone–ligament or bone–tendon junctions.

Cartilage. Cartilage is normally not visible on radiographic examination; however, the width of the joint cavity between the two opposing articular surfaces is a direct manifestation of the cartilage thickness. Because joint diseases act to destroy this intra-articular cartilage in different ways, recognition of joint space alterations is a key diagnostic sign of articular disease.

Soft Tissue. Articular and periarticular soft tissues are important structures to be observed. The joint capsule and synovium are normally not visible; however, a layer of pericapsular fat often renders the margin of the capsule visible, especially when intra-articular effusion is present. Fat between muscle planes and tendons can also be identified and may be distended and obliterated with edema, particularly following trauma, infection, and inflammatory changes. In addition, the overall thickness and density of the soft tissue, especially adjacent to a joint, should be assessed.

Basic Terminology in Joint Disease

The jargon employed in the description of abnormal articulations is varied and often quite specific for individual disorders; however, a number of terms should be recognized and defined to aid in the understanding of basic roentgen signs.

Glossary

enthesis—Anatomic term for the transition zone between bone and ligament or tendon.

enthesopathy—Inflammatory cellular infiltrate at the bone–ligament or bone–tendon junction. Seen in inflammatory arthritides, especially ankylosing spondylitis, as cortical erosion and periostitis.

erosion—Loss of bone owing to pressure atrophy or active breakdown of bone tissue.

hyperostosis—Exuberant ossification of a ligament or tendon, characteristically seen in diffuse idiopathic skeletal hyperostosis.

monoarticular—A single joint is involved in the disease process.

non-uniform loss of joint space—Localized decrease in the joint cavity, owing to isolated loss of cartilage, usually at the most stressed site. This is a sign of degenerative arthritis.

osteophyte—Degenerative bony outgrowth continuous with underlying cortex, covered with a cartilaginous cap, occurring at the insertion of a ligament near a joint.

pauciarticular—Two to four joints are involved in the disease process.

periostitis—Elevation of the periosteum results in localized periosteal new bone and is seen in inflammatory arthritides.

polyarticular—More than four joints are involved in the disease process.

rheumatoid variants—Inflammatory arthropathies that may simulate rheumatoid arthritis clinically but lack rheumatoid factor and show different pathologic and radiographic features.

seronegative arthritis—Inflammatory arthritis that lacks the presence of rheumatoid factor, including ankylosing spondylitis, psoriatic arthritis, Reiter's syndrome, and enteropathic arthritis.

seronegative spondyloarthropathy—Inflammatory arthritis of the spine that lacks the presence of rheumatoid factor, including ankylosing spondylitis, psoriatic arthritis, Reiter's syndrome, and enteropathic arthritis.

spondyloarthropathy—Inflammatory arthritis involving the spine.

spondylophyte—Degenerative spinal osteophyte.

symmetric pattern of joint involvement—When comparing one side of the body with the other, or one joint to another, the changes appear similar.

syndesmophyte—Inflammatory ossification within a spinal ligament, especially ankylosing spondylitis (marginal type) and, less commonly, psoriasis or Reiter's syndrome (nonmarginal type).

uniform loss of joint space—The entire joint cavity is decreased owing to complete loss of the cartilage independent of stressed areas: This is a sign of inflammatory arthritis.

DIFFERENTIAL DIAGNOSIS OF ARTHRITIS

A successful differential diagnosis among arthritic disorders is based on the correlation of clinical, pathologic, and radiographic findings. From an overall perspective, a useful categorization based on these findings has delineated three basic types: inflammatory, degenerative, and metabolic. (1,2) (Table 10-6) When combined with the patterns and characteristics of these disorders, a differential approach to a presenting joint abnormality can be formulated. (Fig. 10-4)

Inflammatory

The general radiographic features of inflammatory joint disease consist of soft tissue swelling and edema, uniform loss of joint space, bone erosions, juxta-articular osteoporosis, and occasionally periostitis of the adjacent metaphysis. (Fig. 10-5) These findings may be monoarticular or polyarticular. When polyarticular, a symmetric pattern of involvement is more frequent. (Fig. 10-6) There is a greater predisposition to bony ankylosis with inflammatory arthritis than in any other type of arthropathy. Inflammatory arthropathies include rheumatoid arthritis, psoriasis, ankylosing spondylitis, and Reiter's syndrome.

Degenerative

In contrast to the inflammatory diseases, a degenerating joint exhibits a non-uniform loss of joint space, osteophytes, subchondral sclerosis, subchondral cysts, and a predilection for being distinctly asymmetric. (Fig. 10-5)

Metabolic

The radiologic findings of metabolic arthritis are the notable presence of soft tissue masses within the periarticular soft tissues, well-marginated bone lesions, and a relative preservation of the joint space. (Fig. 10-7) However, overlapping degenerative changes may occur if the nutrition to the articular cartilage is disturbed as in gout and pseudo-gout (calcium pyrophosphate dihydrate crystal disposition). In addition, some features of inflammatory changes will be apparent if a reactive synovitis is induced. The most characteristic disease associated with metabolic arthritis is gout and, far less commonly, amyloidosis.

Table 10-6	General Radiologic Differential Features of Joint Disease		
Feature	**Inflammatory**	**Degenerative**	**Metabolic**
Symmetry	Symmetric	Asymmetric	Asymmetric
Joints involved	Polyarticular	Monoarticular	Monoarticular or pauciarticular
Alignment	Abnormal	Abnormal	Normal
Bone density	Decreased	Normal or increased	Normal
Erosions	Poorly defined	Absent	Sharply defined
Osteophytes	Absent	Present	Absent
Periostitis	Present	Absent	Absent
Example	Rheumatoid arthritis	Degenerative joint disease	Gout

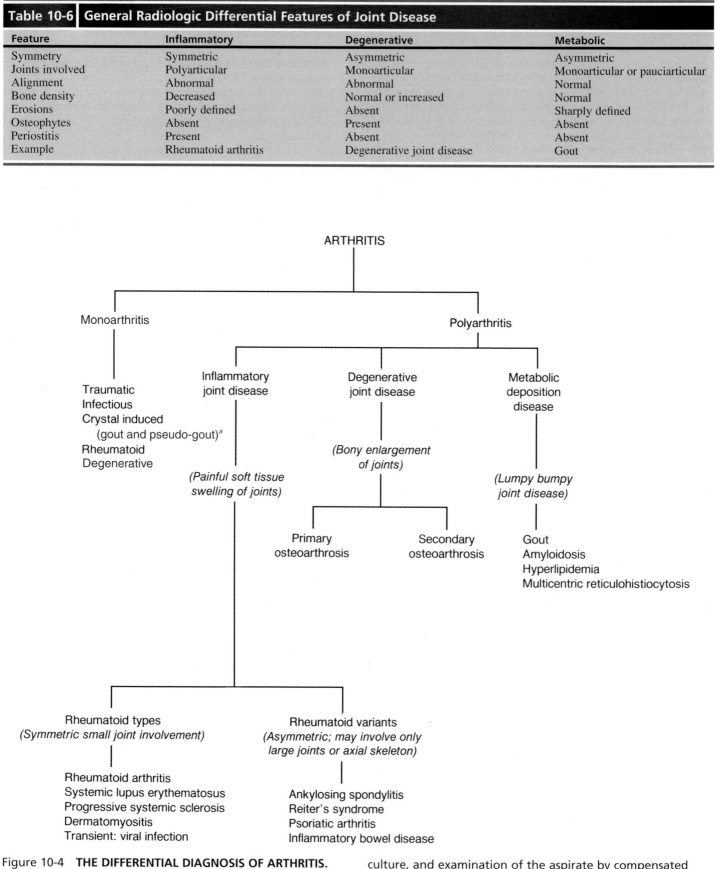

Figure 10-4 **THE DIFFERENTIAL DIAGNOSIS OF ARTHRITIS.**
[a]Occasionally, more than one joint may be involved by an infectious process or acute crystal-induced synovitis. These are differentiated by joint aspiration, followed by Gram staining, culture, and examination of the aspirate by compensated polarizing microscopy for crystals. (Reprinted with permission from **Forrester DM, Brown JC, Nesson JW:** *The Radiology of Joint Disease,* ed 2. Philadelphia, WB Saunders, 1978.)

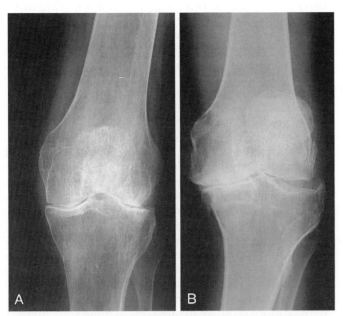

Figure 10-5 **INFLAMMATORY VERSUS DEGENERATIVE ARTHRITIS. A. Inflammatory Arthritis (Rheumatoid Arthritis).** The most prominent feature is the uniform bicompartmental loss of joint space. **B. Degenerative Arthritis (Degenerative Joint Disease).** In contrast, selective loss of a single compartment joint space in a non-uniform manner is apparent. *COMMENT:* This is an important differential feature between inflammatory and degenerative joint changes.

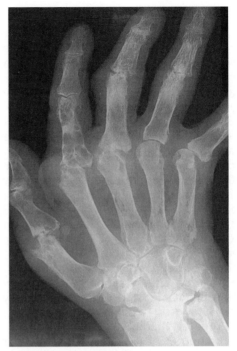

Figure 10-6 **POLYARTICULAR DISEASE, INFLAMMATORY (RHEUMATOID) ARTHRITIS. PA Hand.** Note that distinctive multiple joint disease is evident in the radiocarpal, intercarpal, metacarpophalangeal, and proximal interphalangeal articulations. Observe the extensive intraosseous rheumatoid cysts within the proximal phalanx of the second digit.

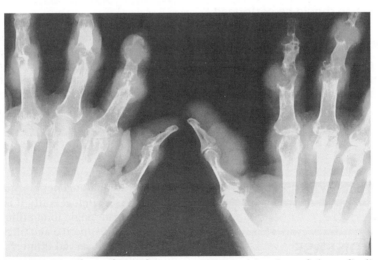

Figure 10-7 **METABOLIC JOINT DISEASE. Bilateral Hands.** Note the large, prominent periarticular soft tissue densities in association with joint disease (*lumpy bumpy joint disease*). The combination of these findings strongly suggests a metabolic joint disorder—in this case, gout.

Medicolegal Implications

ARTHRITIS

Degenerative Joint Disease

- Any condition that predisposes to degenerative joint disease should be recognized to improve the long-term prognosis. This may include slipped femoral capital epiphysis and Perthes disease. Good-quality film studies with adequate views of appropriate areas are crucial to making the correct diagnosis and implementing a management strategy.
- Degenerative diseases of the spine have complex medicolegal ramifications owing to the high prevalence of asymptomatic degenerative findings. In the lumbar spine up to 50% of asymptomatic individuals will have disc abnormalities as demonstrated on MRI, and 35–50% with degenerative disease are found on CT scan. (3,4) In the cervical spine, similar figures have been formulated in asymptomatic patients, with 25–60% showing degenerative features on MRI. (5)
- Recognition of degenerative conditions that may precipitate a cauda equina syndrome (large central disc herniation, synovial cyst) and compression myelopathy (spinal stenosis, ossified posterior longitudinal ligament) have the greatest medicolegal risk.
- Vascular complications such as vertebral artery disease should be screened for clinically, especially before manual therapy. Co-existence of aortic aneurysms should be noted in a degenerative spine.
- In diffuse idiopathic skeletal hyperostosis, clinical correlation for unsuspected diabetes mellitus should be considered.
- In the peripheral joints, differentiation from other arthropathies should be made. The correct diagnosis is critical. The presence of loose bodies may accelerate the degenerative process if not recognized and removed. If joint prostheses are in situ, evaluation for loosening, fracture, dislocation, or infection should be performed.

Inflammatory Joint Diseases

- A multitude of problem scenarios exist relating to imaging. Six key issues with inflammatory joint disease are apparent: the need for quality films of appropriate body areas, the need to clinically correlate and use sensitive tests (bone scan, blood, etc.), atlantoaxial instability, cortico-steroid osteoarthropathy, propensity to fracture, and other direct known complications of the disease.
- Early in the natural history of the disease, diagnosis is often delayed owing to non-specific symptoms. Good-quality radiographs often suggest the diagnosis. Back pain in a young adult male with loss of bilateral sacroiliac joint definition suggests ankylosing spondylitis. Multiple arthralgias of the upper and lower joints may be the first manifestation of a thoracic or abdominal neoplasm, suspected by the presence of long-bone periostitis (hypertrophic osteoarthropathy).
- A key radiologic issue is assessment for atlantoaxial instability with a flexion view. Rheumatoid arthritis, juvenile rheumatoid arthritis, psoriasis, Reiter's disease, and ankylosing spondylitis all are associated with atlantoaxial instability even early in the disease. (6) Measurement of the atlantodental interspace (ADI) and posterior cervical lines are critical to this assessment.
- Corticosteroid changes need to be ascertained. Osteopenia and fractures, especially of the spine, often co-exist and should be investigated. In addition, avascular necrosis should be considered as a cause of hip, knee, or shoulder pain, which should be examined with plain films or more sensitive means such as bone scan. Steroid-induced diabetes may occur.
- Osteopenia in an ankylosed spine places the person at considerable risk for pathologic fracture (carrot-stick fracture),which can be catastrophic. In ankylosing spondylitis with a neurological complaint one should consider a carrot-stick fracture, compression fracture, atlantoaxial instability, or arachnoid diverticula as a potential cause. The connection with inflammatory bowel disease should also be considered.

Metabolic Joint Disease

- Crystal-associated arthropathies in their acute phases often have to be differentiated from septic arthritis. If clinical doubt exists and plain films are not helpful, aspiration of the joint is the key differential test. The radiographic latent period for peripheral septic arthritis is a minimum of 10 days. The finding of chondrocalcinosis is a differential sign, and its cause should be sought. (Table 10-7)

DEGENERATIVE DISORDERS

DEGENERATIVE JOINT DISEASE

Degenerative joint disease (DJD) is a progressive, non-inflammatory disease characterized by degenerative pathologic changes in articular cartilage and its related components. Typically, the small joints of the hands and larger weight-bearing joints are involved. The exact cause of DJD is essentially unknown, although the pathogenetic sequence of changes is well documented. As a clinical entity it is by far the most commonly encountered pathologic joint affliction. Although the radiographic features are distinctive and often pronounced, a great disparity exists in the observed clinical and radiologic findings in any given patient.

Few orthopedic and radiographic abnormalities have enjoyed such a wide variation in nomenclature as degenerative joint disease. Tarnopolsky (1) collected 54 terms applied to this disease. The most common terms include osteoarthritis, osteoarthrosis, degenerative arthritis, degenerative arthrosis, and degenerative joint disease. (Table 10-7)

Table 10-7	Descriptive Terminology in Degenerative Joint Disease	
Common		**Uncommon**
Degenerative arthritis		Arthritis deformans
Degenerative arthrosis		Kellgren's arthritis
Degenerative joint disease		Hypertrophic arthritis
Osteoarthritis		
Osteoarthrosis		

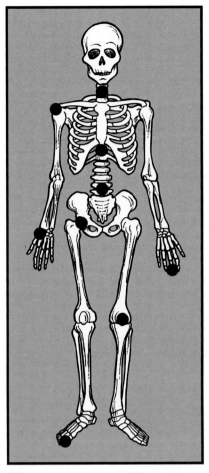

● More common ● Less common

Figure 10-8 **SKELETAL DISTRIBUTION OF DEGENERATIVE JOINT DISEASE.**

Osteoarthritis has been the term traditionally identified with DJD; however, it is no longer considered accurately descriptive. In reality it is a misnomer because the suffix *-itis* implies an inflammatory condition, which is not substantiated by the observed pathologic alterations. Consequently, the term *degenerative joint disease* has gained the most universal acceptance in the literature.

A classification system based on origin is commonly encountered. Primary (idiopathic) DJD is used when no proven factor or groups of factors are directly attributable to the arthropathy, although numerous factors have been hypothesized. Secondary DJD, conversely, is applied when a known factor or event has caused the resultant degenerative changes.

Degenerative joint disease is not without its eponyms derived from original and historical published works. In the early literature, von Bechterew's reports were so ambiguous that at one time his name had been associated with degenerative-related spinal ankylosis, senile kyphosis, and ankylosing spondylitis. (2) Kellgren et al. (3–5), in the 1950s and 1960s, investigated epidemiologic and anatomic distributions of articular involvement. Subsequently, Kellgren's name has become associated with polyarticular DJD seen mainly in middle-aged and elderly women involving the interphalangeal joints of the hand, first carpometacarpal and first metatarsophalangeal joints, knees, and spinal apophyseal articulations, with sparing of the wrists and hips. Kashin-Beck disease, an endemic metabolic variant of degenerative joint disease associated with an ingested fungus found only in eastern Siberia, China, and Korea, derives its name from two of its pioneering investigators. (6)

Clinical Features

A poor correlation exists among the extent of radiologic changes and clinical signs and symptoms. (7) Patients with radiologic signs of advanced DJD are often remarkably asymptomatic. Generally, this arthropathy is more common in males until the age of 45, with a reversal of this sex predilection in later decades of life.

The most common sites of involvement in degenerative joint disease are the weight-bearing articulations of the spine, hips, and knees, and the acromioclavicular, first metatarsophalangeal, first metacarpal–trapezium, and distal interphalangeal (DIP) joints of the hands; however, any joint may develop this arthropathy. (Fig. 10-8)

Invariably, the onset is insidious with intermittent exacerbations of mild to moderate aching pain, stiffness, and swelling of the affected joint. Stiffness typically occurs on rest, particularly in the morning, but gradually disappears with activity. Environmental changes such as cold and lowered barometric pressures may aggravate joint symptoms. A work history may reveal an oc-

cupation of repetitive movements or recurrent chronic injury. The non-inflamed joint reveals crepitus, reduced motion, and palpable excrescences, and there may be evidence of adjacent muscle atrophy. An inflammatory episode is characterized by articular swelling and increased pain. There is always a lack of signs to suggest systemic involvement, with normal blood chemistries and body temperature. Research currently supports the use of the nutriceutical glucosamine as both a pain-relieving agent and source of protection for cartilaginous surfaces. (8)

Signs of spinal stenosis and lateral nerve entrapment syndromes may also be evident. Vertebral artery stenosis from compressive osteophytes in the lower cervical spine may give rise to signs and symptoms of positional vertebrobasilar ischemia. (9)

Pathologic Features

Degenerative joint disease is pathologically characterized by a discrete sequence of individual histologic events that eventually lead to cartilage destruction and secondary alterations in the related tissues. (10) (Fig. 10-9) Initially, degeneration begins as a focal process, gradually spreading to involve a greater proportion of the joint surface. Once the process is initiated, degenerative changes appear to be irreversible, although the rate of change may be modified.

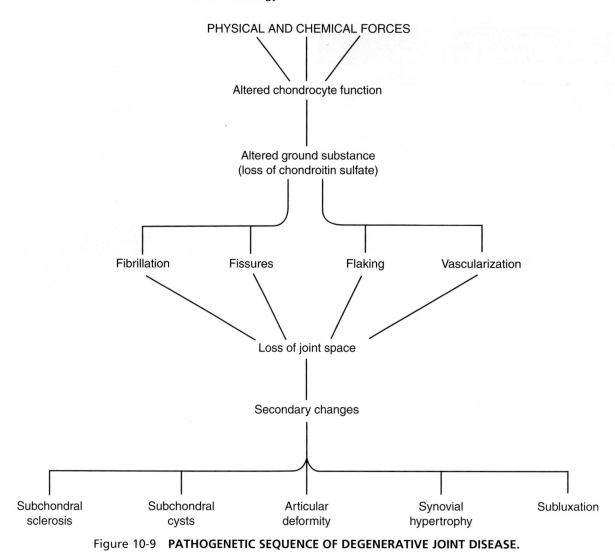

Figure 10-9 **PATHOGENETIC SEQUENCE OF DEGENERATIVE JOINT DISEASE.**

Normal cartilage essentially consists of collagen fibers embedded within a mucopolysaccharide (proteoglycan) ground substance, predominantly chondroitin sulfate. The main physiologic functions of the ground substance are to supply support for collagen fibers and to provide the articular cartilage with resilience to mechanical forces. The hypothesized trigger mechanism in DJD is thought to be abnormal articular physical forces that promote loss of this chondroitin sulfate by interfering with normal chondrocyte function. Once the ground substance is altered, the exposed collagen fibers undergo destruction with subsequent fissure and crevice formation. This initially involves the cartilage surface and later extends deeper toward the subchondral bone. With progression of the degenerative process, vascular infiltration, ulcer formation, cartilage shedding, and fibrillation occur, exposing the underlying subchondral bone. This process of cartilage degradation is the radiographic correlation of loss of joint space.

Until recently, the pathologic sequelae to this cartilage degradation process was believed to be only a secondary phenomena related to altered joint function; however, more recent research has identified a genetic predisposition of the chondrocytes to this alteration. (11) The synovium hypertrophies and thickens as cartilaginous debris causes irritation. Osteophytes develop from a combination of cartilage metaplasia at the joint margin and increased capsular insertion stress.

An osteophyte invariably is characterized by a distinct bony cortex and normal internal trabecular architecture continuous with its site of origin. The distal, unattached surface is invariably capped with a layer of cartilage of variable thickness and is analogous to a long-bone growth plate (physis), contributing to the progressive growth of the osteophyte.

In the subarticular bone, there is augmentation of the structural capacity with an increase in the number and thickness of supporting trabeculae. Weakness of the overlying joint cartilage and cortical microfractures allow synovial fluid intrusion into the subarticular bone, which eventually becomes replaced with fibrous or myxoid tissue, resulting in subchondral cysts. These lesions have also been called *geodes,* a geologic term used to describe gas-filled spaces in rocks. Articular surface deformities result from altered stress trajectories and remodeling as surface incongruity and joint instability ensue.

The end stage of this degenerative process may be complete or incomplete osseous fusion across the joint and variable degrees of loss of function, depending on the site.

The pathologic sequence in degenerative disc disease has been the subject of intensive investigation in recent times and is complex. The implicated initiating factors are numerous, although three major mechanisms appear crucial: mechanical, immunologic, and vascular. The mechanical factors revolve around axial torsion, as well as other forces acting on the annulus, resulting in initially circumferential tears that become confluent with connecting radial tears (internal disc disruption). This disturbs the mechanics of the disc, leading to degradation of the nucleus pulposus. (12) The immunologic mechanism focuses on the embryologic basis that the nucleus pulposus has not been exposed to blood and therefore is not recognized by the immune system as "self." A breach in the discovertebral junction allows immunocompetent cells to come into contact with nuclear material, which initiates a cascade of autoimmune events, leading to progressive degradation of the disc. (13) The vascular theory encompasses the concept of a decreased vascular perfusion to the endplate, either owing to aortic atherosclerosis or microvascular changes secondary to discovertebral changes. (14,15)

Radiologic Features

There are eight essential roentgen signs of degenerative joint disease: asymmetric distribution, non-uniform loss of joint space, osteophytes, subchondral sclerosis, subchondral cysts, intra-articular loose bodies, intra-articular deformity, and joint subluxation. (Figs. 10-10 and 10-11)

These roentgen signs may suggest the degree of underlying pathologic sequences involving the joint components; however, recent correlations have suggested that radiographic findings should not be used as an indicator or representation of the degree of cartilaginous destruction. (16) (Table 10-8) All signs will not necessarily be present in every case of DJD.

Asymmetric Distribution. Characteristically, when comparing an involved articulation with its contralateral counterpart, a recognizable disparity exists in the extensiveness and general characteristics of the disease. This is often seen in the hip, where one articulation is extensively involved yet the other remains relatively normal. Asymmetric involvement serves as a useful differential feature from inflammatory arthropathies, such

as rheumatoid arthritis, which tend to exhibit a symmetric type of distribution.

Non-Uniform Loss in Joint Space. Diminution in joint space tends to be at the regions of greatest intra-articular stress. This results in a phenomenon of joint space preservation in those intra-articular areas that are not exposed to these stresses and is

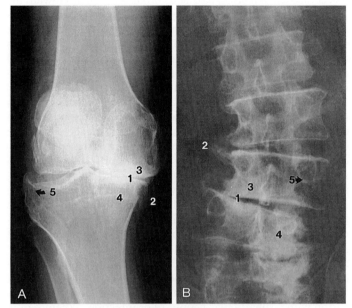

Figure 10-11   **GENERAL RADIOLOGIC FEATURES OF DEGENERATIVE JOINT DISEASE. A. AP Knee. B. AP Lumbar Spine.** Observe the following: non-uniform loss of joint space (*1*), osteophytes (*2*), subchondral sclerosis (*3*), deformity (*4*), and subluxation (*5*).

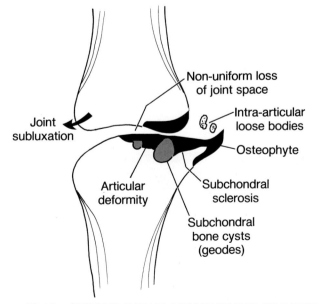

Figure 10-10   **GENERAL RADIOLOGIC FEATURES OF DEGENERATIVE JOINT DISEASE.** The cardinal features of a degenerative joint are shown.

Table 10-8	Radiologic-Pathologic Correlation in Degenerative Joint Disease
Radiologic Features	**Pathologic Features**
Asymmetric distribution	Site predilection modified by local and systemic factors
Non-uniform loss of joint space (selective compartmental loss of joint space)	Fibrillation and destruction of joint cartilage
Osteophytes (spurs) (bony outgrowths at joint margins)	Metaplasia of joint cartilage or ligamentous traction
Subchondral sclerosis (eburnation) (increased subarticular density)	Increased thickness and number of trabeculae
Subchondral cysts (geodes) (geographic radiolucencies in bone)	Intraosseous synovial fluid intrusion through fissured cartilage
Intra-articular loose bodies (joint mice)	Fragmentation of cartilage, bone, and synovium
Articular deformity (articular structures altered in shape)	Altered joint mechanics with redistribution of forces and bone deformation
Joint subluxation (instability)	Altered planes of joint surfaces and ligamentous laxity

especially true of the weight-bearing articulations such as the spine, hip, and knee. This pattern of joint space loss is a fundamental roentgen sign of DJD in these locations.

Osteophytes. Of all roentgen signs of DJD, osteophytes are the most easily recognized alteration. Their exact pathogenesis has remained a point of conjecture for many decades. (17) Radiographically, an osteophyte is seen as a bony outgrowth from the adjacent bone in the locality of the capsular insertion. Usually it is composed of a broad base at its origin and extends toward the joint space, tapering at its distal extent. If these bony excrescences are large enough, trabeculae can be seen in the internal matrix with an outline of distinct cortical bone. Infrequently, osteophytes may completely bridge a joint space, creating bony ankylosis. All osteophytes are covered with a cartilaginous cap of variable thickness that is not visible radiographically.

Subchondral Sclerosis (Eburnation). Subchondral sclerosis is usually most prominent in those areas of subchondral bone where the joint space shows the greatest cartilage loss. The pathologic changes of bony sclerosis are secondary to the increased mechanical forces being transmitted to the joint surfaces without the stress-absorbing effect of the normal resilient cartilage. Consequently, existing trabeculae thicken and new ones appear to counteract these increased stresses. This localized compensatory increase in bone mass is seen radiographically as increased radiopacity in the subchondral bone. Usually, no subchondral sclerosis is present without radiographic evidence of diminution in joint space.

Subchondral Cysts (Geodes). Depending on location, geodes, or focal regions of loss in bone density within subarticular bone, may be absent, small, or at times large enough to cause confusion with a subarticular neoplasm or infection. When seen in combination with consistent signs of joint degeneration, the diagnosis is usually apparent. (Fig. 10-12) Essentially, these cysts parallel the location of the previously described subchondral sclerosis because their origin is related to increased mechanical stress on the joint surface. The radiographic features consist of an ovoid or rounded geographic loss of bone density of 2–20 mm in diameter, often with a sclerotic margin. They are invariably close to a joint surface that has lost its normal articular space. The formation of these cysts may be owing to intraosseous synovial fluid intrusion through the exposed articular plate or may occur secondary to trabecular fractures that subsequently necrose and are replaced with fibrous or myxoid tissue. (18) Large and numerous cysts may predispose to fractures and deformation of the involved articular surfaces, particularly in weight-bearing articulations such as the hip, but are rare in the spine.

Intra-Articular Loose Bodies. Inherent with cartilage degeneration is a flaking or fragmentation phenomenon that results in intra-articular accumulations of cartilage and occasionally pieces of subchondral bone. (Fig. 10-13) This phenomenon is most commonly encountered in the knee. In addition, the synovium may undergo metaplasia to produce cartilaginous and osseous debris (synoviochondrometaplasia). These osteochondral lesions are usually round or ovoid and smoothly marginated and may appear laminated. Cartilaginous loose bodies are not seen on plain film radiographic examinations and require a contrast arthrogram or arthroscopic inspection.

Articular Deformity. The denuded subarticular bone, with time and continual repetitive stress, will deform secondary to trabecular remodeling, fracture, and collapse. Progressive deformation of the articular surfaces may result in secondary vascular disturbances, precipitating further necrosis, collapse, and joint degeneration.

Joint Subluxation. Progressive loss of joint space, capsular and ligamentous laxity, and joint surface deformation render the joint unstable and prone to non-physiologic displacement, thus increasing the abnormal stresses on the joint and accelerating the degenerative process. Weight-bearing and functional stress films are often useful to demonstrate early or latent instability, particularly in the spine.

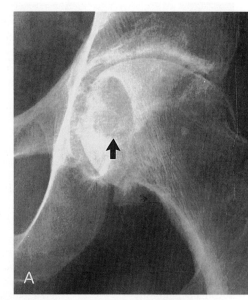

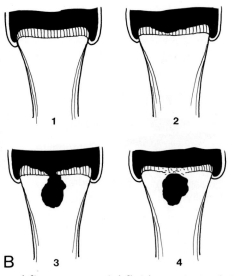

Figure 10-12 **SUBCHONDRAL BONE CYST (GEODE).**
A. AP Hip: Femoral Head. Note the circumscribed geographic lucency (*arrow*). This simulates a neoplasm such as chondroblastoma or even a Brodie's abscess. **B. Pathogenesis: Synovial Fluid Intrusion Theory.** As the joint cartilage cracks and fissures, synovial fluid penetrates into the subchondral bone. The point of communication is subsequently obstructed with fibrous tissue, producing the cyst. (Panel A courtesy of Mahinder Lall, BSc (Hon), MSc, DC, Melbourne, Australia.)

Cervical Spine

The most common locations for degenerative changes to occur are in the lower cervical spine, particularly at the C5 and C6 interspaces. (19) (Fig. 10-14) Single or multiple levels may be involved simultaneously, with different degrees of severity. The incidence of DJD in the cervical spine in asymptomatic adults with no past symptoms, injury, or organic disease is almost 45%. (20)

Below the atlantoaxial joint, each segment has three joint complexes that potentially can undergo degeneration either separately or simultaneously: apophyseal, uncovertebral, and intervertebral disc. (Table 10-9)

Atlantoaxial Joint Arthrosis. Osteoarthritis of the lateral mass joints is uncommon and rarely produces symptomatic spinal stenosis, but it can be the source of occipitocervical pain, especially in elderly patients. (21–23) (Fig. 10-15) Degenerative changes in the median atlanto-odontoid joint are best shown on CT as osteophytes from the superior and inferior aspects of the atlas anterior arch, facet, and odontoid apex and as cysts, ossicles, and calcification of the transverse ligament. (24)

Apophyseal Joints (Facet Arthrosis). Degeneration of the apophyseal joints usually is confined to the lower cervical spine, al-

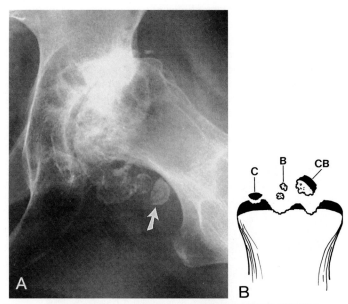

Figure 10-13   INTRA-ARTICULAR LOOSE BODIES (JOINT MICE). A. Frog-Leg Hip. Note the degenerative joint changes and multiple loose bodies (*arrow*). **B. Pathogenesis.** Loose bodies may be produced from cartilage (*C*), bone (*B*), or both (*CB*). On occasion synovial metaplasia may also propagate loose body formation.

Table 10-9	Radiologic Features of Degenerative Joint Disease in the Spine
Cervical spine	
C5–C6	
Apophyseal joints	
Osteophytes, sclerosis, subluxation	
von Luschka's joints	
Osteophytes, foraminal encroachment	
Intervertebral disc	
Decreased height, vacuum phenomenon, osteophytes, canal stenosis	
Thoracic spine	
T6–T12	
Costovertebral joints	
Osteophytes	
Intervertebral disc	
Decreased height, osteophytes (unilateral, right), kyphosis	
Lumbar spine	
L4–L5	
Apophyseal joints	
Decreased space, sclerosis, osteophytes, subluxation (instability)	
Intervertebral disc	
Decreased height, vacuum phenomenon, osteophytes, canal stenosis, body sclerosis	

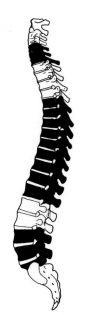

Figure 10-14   SPINAL DISTRIBUTION OF DEGENERATIVE JOINT DISEASE. The preferred sites are shown.

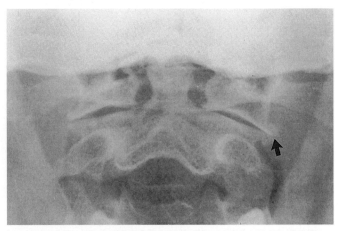

Figure 10-15   ARTHROSIS OF THE ATLANTOAXIAL JOINT. AP Open Mouth. Note the loss of joint space in conjunction with lateral osteophytes (*arrow*). *COMMENT:* This is an unusual location for arthrosis to occur.

though not exclusively, and is frequently overlooked. Facet arthrosis is characterized by loss of joint space, subchondral sclerosis, osteophytes, and on occasion anterolisthesis (degenerative spondylolisthesis). The most diagnostic radiographs are frontal (anteroposterior; AP) and oblique projections. (Fig. 10-16) On the AP projection the normally smooth lateral contour of the articular pillars shows sharp osteophytic projections and sclerosis. The oblique projection may demonstrate posterior foraminal encroachment from protruding osteophytes.

Uncovertebral (Neurocentral) Joints (von Luschka's Joint Arthrosis). The neurocentral joints also show predilection for degenerative changes in the lower segments of C5 and C6. Anatomically, they occupy the posterolateral portions of the vertebral bodies, contributing to the anterior border of the intervening intervertebral foramen and lateral recess. Degenerative changes consist predominantly of osteophytic formation, particularly of the uncinate process. This is optimally observed on the AP and oblique projections. (Fig. 10-17)

Uncovertebral arthrosis can precipitate an apparent fracture line (pseudo-fracture, split vertebral body) across the inferior margin of a lower cervical vertebral body on the lateral projection. (25,26) This most commonly occurs at C5–C6 and C6–C7 and is invariably associated with a loss in disc height. (25)

The AP projection will show an initial sharpening of the tip of the uncinate process, with a progressive bulbous enlargement, especially in a lateral direction. The superior fossa of the joint at a later stage may also show this lateral osteophytic formation. Oblique views will frequently demonstrate uncovertebral arthrosis with osseous foraminal encroachment when AP and lateral views appear normal. Osteophytes of uncovertebral origin invariably project directly posterior into the anterior aspect of the intervertebral foramen, creating stenosis of the adjacent lateral recess and, at times, may interfere with vertebral artery blood flow. (9,27) (Figs. 10-18 and 10-19) The combination of anterior uncovertebral and apophyseal joint arthrosis may result in a foraminal configuration analogous to an hourglass. (Fig. 10-16C)

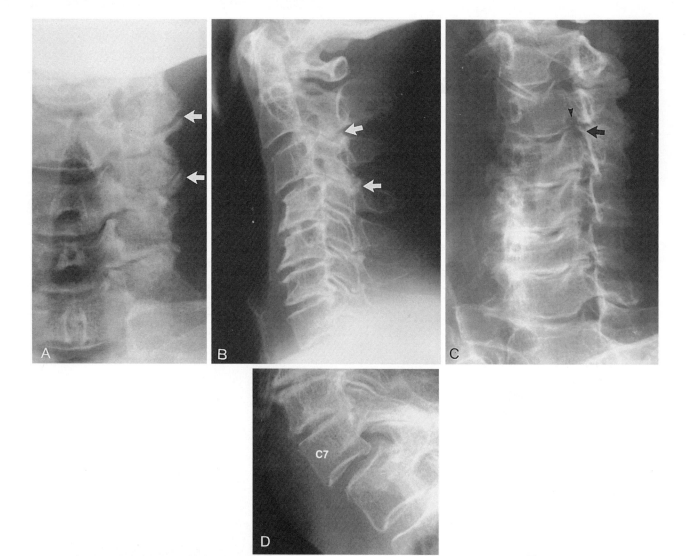

Figure 10-16 **FACET ARTHROSIS: CERVICAL SPINE. A. AP Lower Cervical.** Observe the projecting osteophytes (*arrows*). **B. Lateral Cervical.** Note the loss of joint space, sclerosis, and osteophytes (*arrows*). **C. Oblique Cervical.** Note the osteophytes projecting posteriorly and anteriorly into the neural foramina (*arrow*). Note the hourglass shape of the third foramen (*arrowhead*) owing to facet and von Luschka's joint osteophytes. **D. Degenerative Anterolisthesis, Lateral Cervical.** Observe the loss of joint space and progressive facet remodeling, which have precipitated an anterolisthesis of the C7 vertebra.

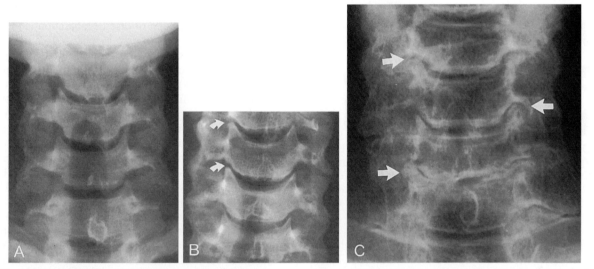

Figure 10-17 **VON LUSCHKA'S JOINT DEGENERATION, AP LOWER CERVICAL. A. Normal Appearance. B. Early Changes.** Note the flattened, bulbous appearance to the uncinate processes (*arrows*). **C. Advanced Changes.** Note that the un-cinate processes and adjacent fossae show sclerosis and large osteophyte formation (*arrows*). At this stage there will always be loss of disc height.

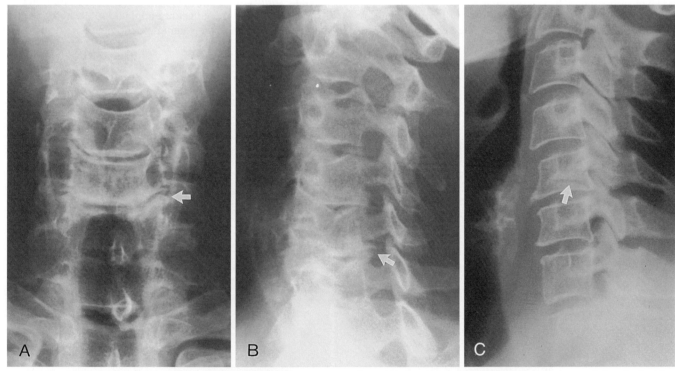

Figure 10-18 **VON LUSCHKA'S JOINT DEGENERATION: CHARACTERISTIC FINDINGS. A. AP Lower Cervical.** Note the degeneration (*arrow*). **B. Oblique Cervical.** Note the anterior foraminal encroachment (*arrow*). **C. Lateral Cervical.** Observe the radiolucent pseudo-fracture (*arrow*) owing to sclerosis of the uncinate process and opposing fossa.

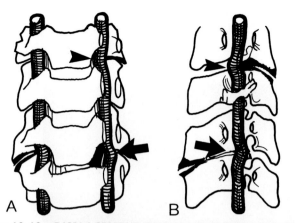

Figure 10-19   DISPLACEMENT OF THE VERTEBRAL ARTERY FROM CERVICAL OSTEOPHYTES. A. AP Cervical: Diagram. B. Oblique Cervical: Diagram. The most frequent sites of origin are the von Luschka's (*arrows*) and facet joints (*arrowheads*). These may produce symptoms of vertebrobasilar ischemia.

The degree of anatomic reduction in foraminal dimensions cannot be accurately assessed owing to a 1- to 3-mm radiolucent cartilage cap. This accounts for the frequent discrepancy between radiographically visible degenerative changes and directly related clinical abnormalities. (28) CT bone window remains the optimum method for accurate assessment, though MRI with thin sections may also be used. (29)

Intervertebral Disc (Spondylosis). Of the three joints in the cervical spine, the intervertebral disc is the most readily visible site of DJD. The most common levels of involvement are C5 and C6. Signs of intervertebral disc degeneration are, pre-dominantly, loss of disc height, osteophytes, and endplate sclerosis. (Fig. 10-20) An occasional accessory sign is the *vacuum phenomenon,* which is more frequently observed in the lumbar spine. The appearance of a lucent vacuum cleft adjacent to an endplate on an extension film following trauma may indicate annular tearing. (30)

The most reliable sign of disc degeneration is the presence of varying degrees of loss in disc height. Above the degenerating disc, the lordosis is frequently diminished as the uncovertebral joint surfaces approximate and act as a fulcrum to produce segmental flexion. (28) Flexion–extension stress films may demonstrate initial instability with increased anterior and posterior movement. Later, intersegmental fixation manifests radiographically as a loss of segmental movement. Osteophytes initially may be nonmarginal in origin and large in the absence of visible disc disease. Usually, however, the combination of loss in disc height and osteophyte formation is seen isolated to the involved level. Anteriorly projecting osteophytes rarely result in dysphagia. (31) Posterior osteophytes projecting into the spinal canal are usually smaller, owing to their type of posterior longitudinal ligament attachment, but they can produce central canal stenosis with resultant myelopathy. (32) The most common levels for degenerative spinal stenosis in the cervical spine are C5 and C6, when the sagittal canal measurement is < 12 mm. (Fig. 10-21)

Another prominent sign often observed is varying degrees of endplate sclerosis, occasionally extending into the midportion of the vertebral body. (Fig. 10-22A) This may simulate an osteoblastic neoplasm or infection. Sclerosis beneath an osteophyte may simulate the inflammatory sclerosis of ankylosing spondylitis (*pseudo-shiny corner sign*). (Fig. 10-22B) The differential key in DJD is to observe the adjacent endplate, associated loss of disc space, and, if present, the vacuum phenomenon. (Fig. 10-23) The

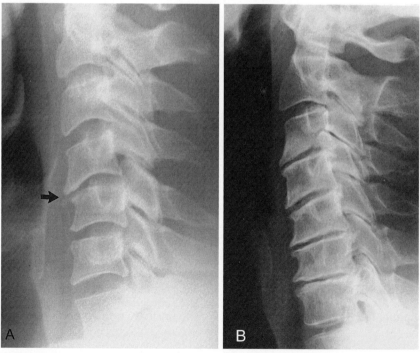

Figure 10-20   CERVICAL SPONDYLOSIS. A. Lateral Cervical Unisegmental Involvement. Observe the loss of disc height and osteophytes at the C4 disc (*arrow*). **B. Lateral Cervical Multisegmental Involvement.** Note that all intervertebral discs are narrowed and exhibit osteophytes, vacuum phenomena, and loss of lordosis.

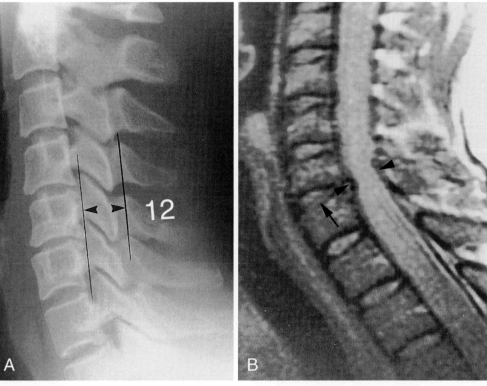

Figure 10-21   **CERVICAL SPONDYLOSIS: CENTRAL CANAL STENOSIS. A. Lateral Cervical.** Note the sagittal canal dimension is at the lower limits of normal (12 mm) (*arrowheads*) owing to posterior osteophyte formation. **B. T2-Weighted MRI, Sagittal Cervical.** Observe the decreased signal of the C6 disc consistent with dehydration (*arrow*). Observe the front–back narrowing owing to disc and ligamentum flavum bulging (*arrowheads*). (Courtesy of Geoffrey G. Rymer, DC, Sydney, Australia.)

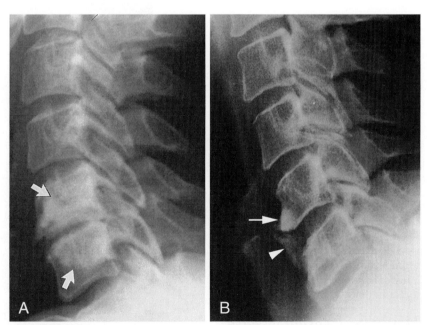

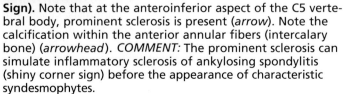

Figure 10-22   **PROMINENT DEGENERATIVE SCLEROSIS. A. Lateral Cervical Vertebral Body.** Note the increased density adjacent to the level of disc narrowing within the vertebral bodies (*arrows*). COMMENT: This appearance, called hemispheric spondylosclerosis, is more common in the lumbar spine, and may be confused with an osteoblastic neoplasm. **B. Lateral Cervical Osteophyte (Pseudo-Shiny Corner Sign).** Note that at the anteroinferior aspect of the C5 vertebral body, prominent sclerosis is present (*arrow*). Note the calcification within the anterior annular fibers (intercalary bone) (*arrowhead*). COMMENT: The prominent sclerosis can simulate inflammatory sclerosis of ankylosing spondylitis (shiny corner sign) before the appearance of characteristic syndesmophytes.

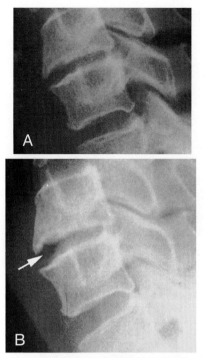

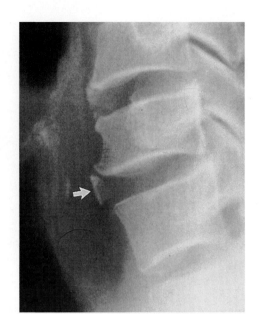

Figure 10-24 INTERCALARY BONE, LATERAL CERVICAL. Note that a frequent accompanying sign of degenerative disc disease is calcification within the annular fibers (*arrow*).

Figure 10-23 VACUUM PHENOMENON. A. Neutral Lateral. Note that no evidence for the vacuum sign is seen, though loss of disc height and anterior osteophytes are apparent. **B. Extension Lateral.** Observe the intradiscal radiolucency representing nitrogen accumulation in a cracked and fissured disc (*arrow*). *COMMENT:* Extension is the best view to form a vacuum. The presence of a vacuum phenomenon can be interpreted in three ways: It is a reliable plain film sign for excluding infection; it indicates that the disc is degenerative; and it indicates that intersegmental motion is occurring.

presence of a vacuum phenomenon and a normal endplate strongly suggests a degenerative rather than infective cause. Calcification of the anterior annulus (intercalary bone) is a common finding of degenerative disc disease. (Fig. 10-24)

Thoracic Spine

Diseases of degenerative origin in the thoracic spine are localized to three joint complexes: apophyseal articulations, costal articulations, and intervertebral disc.

Apophyseal Articulations (Facet Arthrosis). Facet arthrosis is infrequently observed in the thoracic spine, except in the lower thoracic segments. The changes are best observed on the AP film and consist of joint space loss and sclerosis. (Table 10-9) Pain may be referred one segment inferior and lateral to the involved joint, although the lower thoracic joints can refer to the lower lumbar spine (thoracolumbar syndrome, Maigne's syndrome). (33,34)

Costal Articulations (Costovertebral, Costotransverse Arthrosis). As with cervical apophyseal arthrosis, changes in the costal articulations are often overlooked. They are most commonly involved in the lower thoracic segments and have been implicated in pain production, simulating upper gastrointestinal disease (Robert's syndrome). (35–37) (Fig. 10-25) Infrequently, an exuberant degenerative costal articulation may simulate a *coin*

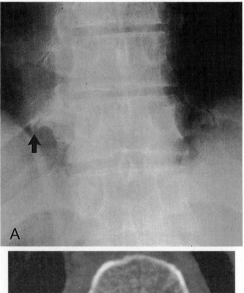

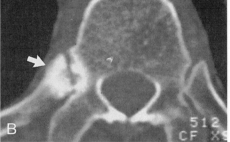

Figure 10-25 COSTAL JOINT ARTHROSIS. A. AP Thoracic Costotransverse Joints. Note the sclerosis and osteophytes (*arrow*). **B. Axial CT: Costovertebral Joint.** Note the prominent sclerosis (*arrow*). *COMMENT:* Costotransverse arthropathies can be implicated in the simulation of pseudo-visceral abdominal pain (Robert's syndrome). (Panel A courtesy of Mark McEwan, BAppSc (Chiro), Sydney, Australia.)

lesion of the lung in the AP projection and can usually be confirmed only with computed tomography.

Intervertebral Disc (Spondylosis, Senile Kyphosis). Degenerative disc changes are less pronounced in the thoracic spine than in any other spinal region. Developmentally, the height of normal thoracic disc spaces gradually decreases in a cephalad direction, with the thinnest disc interspaces present between the T2 and the T4 regions. The most common sites for disc-related degenerative changes to occur are the middle and lower thoracic levels. The major radiographic features in the thoracic spine are osteophytes, minimal sclerosis, and mild disc narrowing. There is a notable absence of osteophyte formation on the left side of the thoracic spine, thought to be related to a pulsation–inhibition effect of the closely approximated descending aorta. (38,39) (Fig. 10-26) This phenomenon may be reversed in situs inversus. (40)

Infrequently, usually in patients > 70 years of age, anterior disc degeneration in multiple segments in the midthoracic spine may lead to ankylosis across the anterior disc space, with an associated localized kyphosis (senile kyphosis). (41)

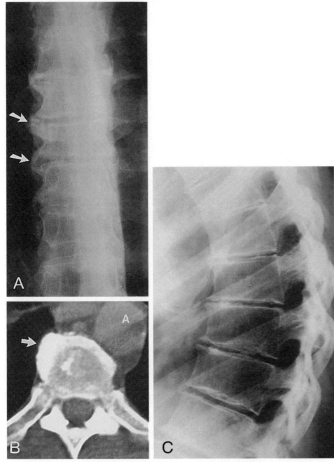

Figure 10-26 **THORACIC SPINE SPONDYLOSIS. A. AP Thoracic.** Note that the right-sided osteophytes are striking (*arrows*). **B. Axial CT: Thoracic Spine.** Note the proximity of the aorta (*A*) to the left side of the vertebral body and the projecting osteophyte (*arrow*) on the right. **C. Lateral Thoracic.** Note that the generalized loss of disc height, small anterior osteophytes, and increased kyphosis are distinctive. *COMMENT:* The transmitted pulsations of the thoracic aorta are thought to inhibit the production of left-sided osteophytes in the thoracic spine.

Lumbar Spine

Only two joint complexes in the lumbar spine undergo degenerative changes: the apophyseal articulations and intervertebral discs. (Table 10-9)

Apophyseal Articulations (Facet Arthrosis). The most common locations for facet arthrosis are the L4 and the L5 articulations. A correlation of the orientation of the facet joints with the development of arthrosis has been identified. Sagittally oriented facet joints are significantly more prone to degenerative changes. (42) Arthrosis in these locations is characterized by loss of joint space, sclerosis, osteophytes, and subluxation, particularly anterolisthesis. (Fig. 10-27) The most diagnostic projections are the AP and oblique films, although degenerative spondylolisthesis and intersegmental instability may require lateral films in flexion and extension.

The AP film will show loss of joint space, although this is an unreliable sign in this projection owing to common anatomic variations in facet planes and projectional distortions. Sclerosis may be evident in the subchondral bone. (Fig. 10-27A) Osteophytes usually arise at the superior aspect of the joint, but they too are difficult to identify. By far the most diagnostic film is the oblique, which allows accurate visualization of most of the lumbar apophyseal joints. (Figs. 10-27C and 10-28) Less than 25% of degenerative facets will be shown on the obliques when compared with CT. (43) With an oblique projection, all of those signs seen on the AP will be readily seen, in addition to facet subluxation, as shown by a disturbance in Hadley's S curve. (See Chapter 2.) Often, this degenerative facet subluxation is evidenced as subchondral sclerosis in the adjacent pars region, which is being mechanically impacted, particularly at L4 and L5.

The lateral radiograph may reveal an increase in density in the region of the apophyseal joints, but this is often relative owing to decreased beam penetration through the overlying pelvis. (Fig. 10-27B) Caution should also be used if a single foramen appears decreased in size owing to the anatomic projection of the normal lower lumbar foramina. An additional common radiographic projectional artifact seen at the L4 and L5 levels is the superimposition of the superior articulating process into the foramen, simulating osseous encroachment. Facet arthrosis may produce anterolisthesis (degenerative spondylolisthesis) and, less frequently, retrolisthesis of an individual segment. (Fig. 10-29)

Intervertebral Disc (Spondylosis). Radiographically visible changes of the intervertebral disc and vertebral body represent a chronic and irreversible state of DJD. The CT and MRI features of degenerative syndromes are dealt with in Chapter 6.

The most common locations for disc degeneration are at the L4 and L5 levels. As in the cervical spine, the major radiographic signs consist of decrease in disc height, osteophyte formation, endplate sclerosis, vacuum phenomenon, and subluxation. Each of these features may be present or absent in varying degrees. The most diagnostic radiograph for the detection of degenerative disc disease is the lateral projection, supplemented with AP and oblique studies.

Early signs of a degenerating disc are retrolisthesis, mild loss in disc height, small anterior traction spurs, and vacuum phenomenon. Endplate sclerosis is difficult to interpret in early spondylosis. Additionally, beneath an osteophyte the sclerosis may simulate the *shiny corner sign* of ankylosing spondylitis. Retrolisthesis often occurs early, with loss of disc height owing to the posterior orientation of the apophyseal joints, drawing the segment posteriorly as the segment displaces inferiorly. However, not all retrolistheses

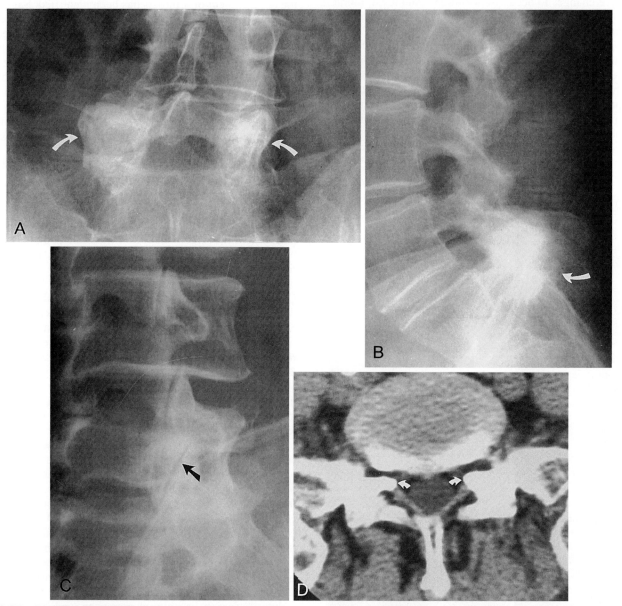

Figure 10-27 FACET ARTHROSIS: LUMBOSACRAL JUNCTION. A. AP Lumbar. Note the considerable increase in density of the articular processes (*arrows*). **B. Lateral Lumbar.** Note that similar findings are exhibited on this view (*arrow*). **C. Oblique Lumbar.** Note the decreased joint space and adjacent sclerosis (*arrow*). **D. Axial CT: L5/S1.** Observe that protruding osteophytes from the facet joints (*arrows*) have created lateral canal stenosis bilaterally.

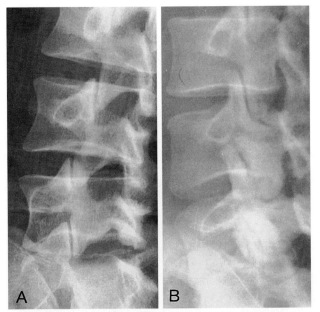

Figure 10-28 **FACET ARTHROSIS: OBLIQUE LUMBAR.**
A. Normal Facets. Note that the joint spaces are smooth and uniform; the articular processes are of a triangular shape.
B. Facet Arthrosis. Observe that the joint spaces are narrowed and the articular processes sclerotic and altered in shape owing to osteophytes.

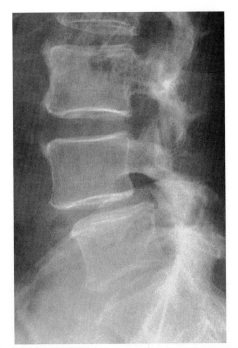

Figure 10-29 **DEGENERATIVE SPONDYLOLISTHESIS LATERAL LUMBAR.** Observe the anterolisthesis of the L4 body secondary to facet remodeling and arthrosis. (Courtesy of Daryl D. Wills, DC, Gering, Nebraska.)

are caused by disc degeneration, particularly if the disc space is normal. A wide apophyseal joint space or an offset in the articular surfaces, as seen in the oblique projection, has been implicated as an early sign of degenerative disc disease. (44)

The osteophytes seen are of two types: (45) (Fig. 10-30)

- *Traction osteophytes.* These occur in the early phase of disc degeneration, typically originate about 2 mm from the anterior vertebral body margin, and are horizontal and tapered at their distal extent. (46) (Fig. 10-30, A–C) Discography shows a marked correlation between loss in disc height and disc disruption with these osteophytes. They have not correlated with the level of symptomatic disc pathology. (47) Posterior body osteophyte formation is infrequent in the lumbar spine owing to a less adherent posterior longitudinal ligament and annulus fibrosus. (Fig. 10-30C)
- *Claw osteophytes.* These have a broader base, climb vertically in a curvilinear fashion, and are tapered. (Fig. 10-30, D and E) They appear to be derived from traction spurs after the shear forces have reduced to more compressive loads. (45)

The vacuum sign (of Knuttsen) is an important early radiographic finding. (48) Essentially, this represents collections of nitrogen gas in nuclear and annular fissures and presents as an area of linear radiolucency in the disc space. (49) (Fig. 10-31) Studies have shown this to be a common sign of disc aging and degeneration, with an incidence of 2–3% in the general population. (50) The collection of nitrogen in the discal fissures is thought to originate from adjacent extracellular fluid. In movements of the spine that produce a lowered pressure in the disc, such as in extension, nitro-

gen is released from the adjacent extracellular fluid and, owing to the pressure gradient, accumulates in the discal fissures. On MRI the disc shows diminished signal intensity owing to dehydration and a signal void at the vacuum site. (Fig. 10-32) This collection of gas can be made to disappear with spinal flexion and reappear with spinal extension. (48,51,52) (Fig. 10-33) Disc infections do not demonstrate this sign owing to fluid collections in the fissures. (52,53) Central vacuum phenomena correspond to fissuring of the nucleus pulposus, whereas peripheral lesions represent rim lesions in which the anulus fibrosus has been disrupted from its attachment to the vertebral body margin. (52)

In the peripheral joints, especially the hip, shoulder, and knee, a vacuum sign does not denote degenerative joint changes. (54) (Fig. 10-34; Table 10-10) The vacuum sign is produced as an accompanying physiological phenomenon, usually induced by the position of the patient in a position of traction when the exposure was made. Gas in the symphysis pubis is a normal finding during pregnancy and up to 3 weeks postpartum and may be seen as a vertical, thin radiolucency. (55)

As the disease process progresses in the disc, the degenerative signs become more severe. Subluxations are more readily recognizable, and lateral, anterior, and posterior vertebral body displacements of a measurable degree occur. (Fig. 10-33) Flexion–extension films usually reveal decreased motion in these displaced segments. Disc height is markedly diminished, with > 25% loss of its vertical dimension. Loss of disc height can also be the result of infection, which should be excluded by careful scrutiny for the loss of the vertebral body endplates. (56)

Large osteophytes may completely bridge the intervertebral disc space or may be in close apposition to the adjacent segment. These osteophytes exhibit a broad base that extends from the vertebral body margin to a few millimeters away. The distal extension of

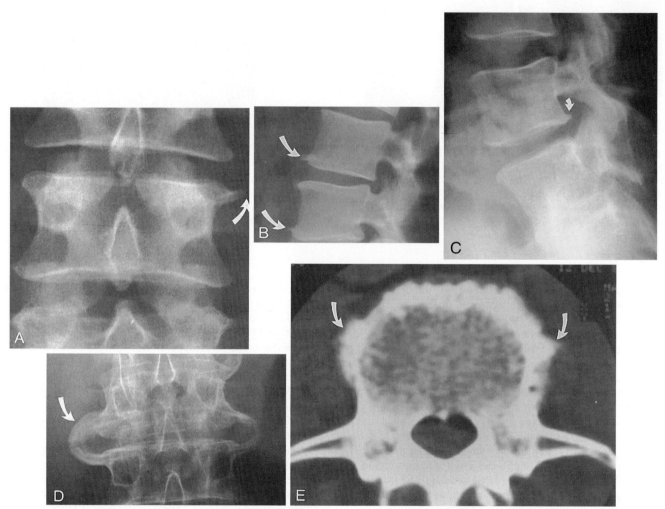

Figure 10-30 **OSTEOPHYTES: LUMBAR SPINE. A–C. Traction Osteophytes.** Note that the origin of the osteophytes is non-marginal, and they tend to be horizontal (*arrows*). **D. Claw Osteophyte.** Note that these osteophytes also tend to be non-marginal and project horizontally but are larger, curve superiorly or inferiorly, and taper distally (*arrow*). **E. Axial CT: Thoracic Spine, Claw Osteophyte.** Note that the bony outgrowths are circumferential but rarely involve the posterior body (*arrows*).

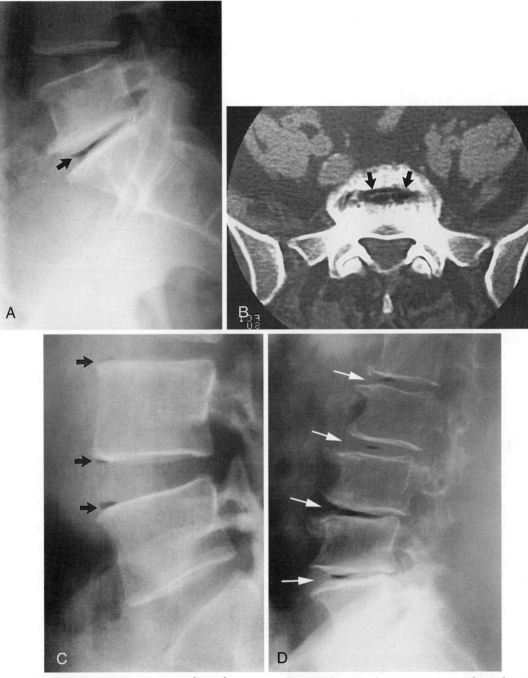

Figure 10-31   **VACUUM PHENOMENON. A. Lateral Lumbar Nuclear Degeneration.** Note the thin, wafer-like radiolucency (*arrow*). **B. Axial CT: L5/S1 Nuclear Degeneration.** Note the central location of the radiolucency (*arrows*). **C. Lateral Lumbar Annular Degeneration.** Observe the localized lucencies (*arrows*), which are thought to be the result of rupture of the annular attachments. **D. Lateral Lumbar Multilevel Central Vacuum Phenomenon.** Note that in concert with varying degrees of disc degeneration multiple levels of intradiscal gas can be observed (*arrows*). (Panel C courtesy of John K. Hyland, DC, DACBR, DABCO, Denver, Colorado. Panel D courtesy of Richard L. Green, DC, Winthrop, Massachusetts.)

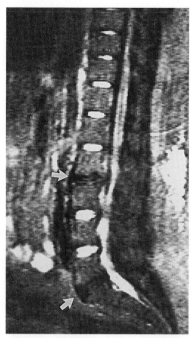

Figure 10-32 DISC DEGENERATION. T2-Weighted MRI: Sagittal Lumbar. Note that the normal disc spaces appear white (high signal intensity) owing to their high water content. Degenerating discs at the L2 and L5 levels, which have reduced water levels, fail to be highlighted (low signal intensity) (*arrows*). (Courtesy of Steven P. Brownstein, MD, Springfield, New Jersey.)

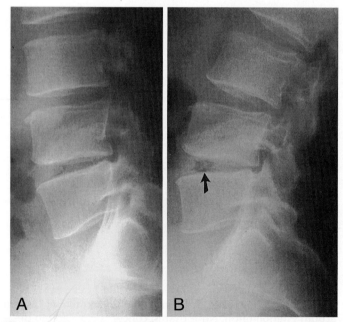

Figure 10-33 VACUUM PHENOMENON: FLEXION–EXTENSION. A. Flexion. Note that the vacuum is almost obliterated at the L4 disc. **B. Extension.** Observe that the vacuum is now more apparent (*arrow*). Note the accompanying L4 retrolisthesis, indicating intersegmental instability. *COMMENT:* Extension is the best view to form a vacuum. The presence of a vacuum phenomenon can be interpreted in three ways: it is a reliable plain film sign for excluding infection, it indicates that the disc is degenerative, and it indicates that intersegmental motion is occurring.

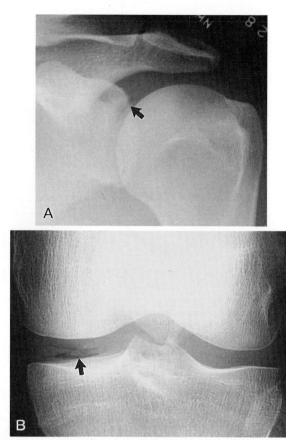

Figure 10-34 PHYSIOLOGIC VACUUM PHENOMENA. A. External Rotation, Shoulder. Note the vacuum phenomenon (*arrow*). **B. Stress Study, Knee.** Note the vacuum phenomenon (*arrow*). *COMMENT:* The presence of a vacuum phenomenon in these locations is not indicative of degenerative joint disease.

Table 10-10	Vacuum Phenomenon: Anatomic/ Radiologic Correlation	
Joint	**Patient Position**	**Appearance**
Shoulder	External rotation, abduction, or traction	Lucent crescent parallels humeral head surface 1–2 mm from articular bone
Hip	Frog leg or longitudinal traction	Lucent crescent parallels femoral head surface 1–2 mm from articular bone
Knee	Abduction stress	Medial joint space parallel to femoral condyle surface 1–2 mm from articular bone
Spine		
Disc	Extension or neutral	Central or peripheral linear lucency paralleling endplate
Facet	Oblique with torsion	Linear lucency in facet joint space
Sacroiliac	AP, recumbent or upright	Linear lucency in sacroiliac joint space
Symphysis pubis	AP, frog leg	Vertical, linear central

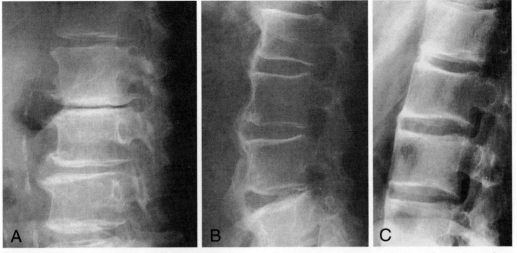

Figure 10-35 **DIFFERENTIATION OF SPINAL OUTGROWTHS: LUMBAR SPINE. A. Osteophytes.** Observe their thick base, horizontal orientation, and associated loss of disc height, distinctive of degenerative joint disease. **B. Hyperostosis.** Note that thick new bone formation within the anterior longitudinal ligament gives the spine a bumpy contour characteristic of diffuse idiopathic skeletal hyperostosis. **C. Syndesmophytes.** Observe the thin vertical ossifications within the outer annulus fibers, typical of ankylosing spondylitis.

the osteophyte exhibits a gentle curve laterally and superiorly or inferiorly, gradually tapering to a slightly rounded, pointed apex, simulating the claw of an animal (claw osteophyte); it is best seen on the anterior and lateral body margins. (46) (Fig. 10-30) These degenerative bony excrescences should not be confused with the thin, bridging, vertical syndesmophytes of ankylosing spondylitis. (Fig. 10-35)

Associated Degenerative Syndromes

Degenerative Spondylolisthesis. Degenerative changes of the apophyseal joints allow for up to 10–30% anterolisthesis of the involved vertebral segment. Such changes are most common at the L4 level and are more common in females > 40 years of age. In the cervical spine it is most frequent at the C7 level. (57)

- *Lumbar spine.* This entity is discussed in more depth in Chapters 5 and 6. Anterolisthesis occurs as a combination of loss of joint space, loss of disc height, remodeling of the facet surfaces to a more sagittal orientation, and broadening of the pedicle facet angle. It frequently is associated with lateral and central canal stenosis.
- *Cervical spine.* Co-existence of anterolisthesis with facet arthrosis is a frequent occurrence (degenerative spondylolisthesis). The most common levels are C7–T1, C6–C7, and C5–C6, in order of frequency, although any level can be involved. The key features include loss of facet joint and disc space, sclerosis, a more horizontal plane of the articulation, and even diminished height of the articular pillar. It may be associated with significant lateral and central stenosis as well as considerable instability, requiring decompression and fusion. The presence of a cervical anterolisthesis should initiate the search for a posterior arch defect, either congenital (cleft pillar, pedicle agenesis), fracture (pillar, pedicle), or dislocation (unilateral or bilateral facet), before considering a degenerative entity. (58,59)

Instability. The term *instability* has been loosely applied to the demonstration of increased movement or loss of stiffness between two vertebral segments. (60) It is, however, poorly understood and imprecisely defined. Radiographically, the diagnosis has focused on comparing intersegmental movements at extremes of physiologic motion: sagittal (flexion–extension), coronal (lateral bending), and axial (compression–distraction). (61,62) Stereoradiographic methods have also been applied. (63)

In the cervical spine, sagittal intersegmental motion > 3.5 mm or more than 11° is considered unstable. (64) In the lumbar spine, flexion–extension radiographs may demonstrate early intersegmental instability, with or without visible changes of facet or disc degeneration. Signs of instability in these projections are largely anterior or posterior displacement of one vertebral body in relation to another and a single foramen that appears markedly smaller than the adjacent foramina, particularly in extension. (65) A wide facet joint space at one level on an oblique extension film may correlate with an abnormal disc at the same level (unstable apophyseal joint sign). (44) Lateral bending is assessed for interbody shear and offset spinous processes. (62)

The clinical importance of the above-described degenerative changes involving the posterior joints and instability is their close relationship to the development of lateral nerve entrapment syndromes, which are best demonstrated by CT scanning. (Fig. 10-27D) This type of syndrome often shows an excellent response to chiropractic spinal manipulative therapy. (66,67)

Spinal Stenosis. Narrowing of the spinal canal and intervertebral foramina is a common finding associated with spinal degenerative changes. Narrowing of the central canal can be the result of hypertrophy of the ligamentum flavum, facet and vertebral body osteophytes, and disc bulging. Stenosis of the lateral canal is most commonly owing to osteophytes from the superior articular process. These entities are discussed in detail in Chapter 6.

Synovial (Ganglion, Juxta-Articular) Cysts. Synovial cysts characteristically occur in conjunction with degenerative facet arthropathy, most commonly at L4–L5. (68) They are rare in the cervical spine. (69) The cause remains obscure but may be either a herniation of synovium from the facet joint or mucinous degen-

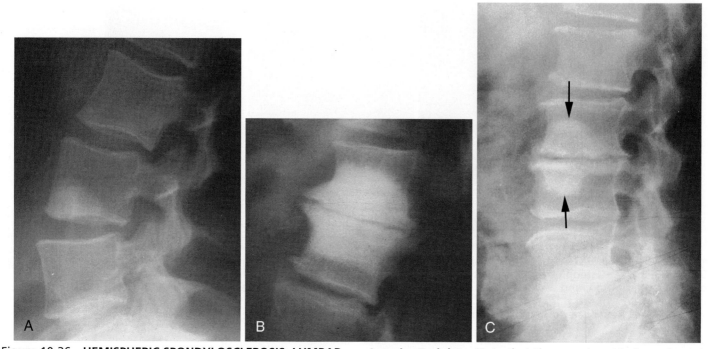

Figure 10-36 HEMISPHERIC SPONDYLOSCLEROSIS: LUMBAR SPINE. A. Unisegmental. Note the localized sclerotic focus adjacent to the endplate. The peripheral convex border is characteristic. **B. Multisegmental, Entire Endplate.** Note that a similar sclerotic reaction of both opposing surfaces is evident at a severely degenerated disc. **C. Multisegmental,** **Anterior Endplate.** Note that the prominent helmet-shaped sclerosis extends into the L3 and L4 vertebral bodies (*arrows*). Note within the disc a small vacuum phenomenon exists, assisting in distinguishing this discovertebral abnormality from infection. (Panel A courtesy of David E. Friedman, DC, Denver, Colorado.)

eration of connective tissue adjacent to the joint. These cysts are rarely visible on plain film examination. On myelography an extradural mass is found near the facet joint. On CT, a soft tissue mass within the canal near the facet joint can be seen, sometimes with a low-attenuation central zone or even containing gas. (70) Erosion of the lamina and facet surface can be observed. (68) MRI shows a mass that on T2-weighting has a hyperintense central area surrounded by a peripheral thin rim of low intensity. (68) If the central zone is hyperintense relative to the cerebrospinal fluid (CSF), then hemorrhage into the cyst is likely; if this zone is isointense with the CSF, then a high protein content fluid is more likely. (71)

Hemispheric Spondylosclerosis (HSS). Prominent subchondral sclerosis may be seen in the bone adjacent to the endplate. The most common locations are at the L4 and L5 vertebral bodies. Occasionally, this may be so dense and large as to simulate a blastic neoplasm or infection. (Fig. 10-36) Key radiologic signs of degenerative subchondral sclerosis include a hemispheric contour of density usually adjacent to the inferior endplate, osteophytes, Schmorl's nodes, and loss of contiguous disc height. (72,73) (See Chapter 6.)

Baastrup's Syndrome (Kissing Spine Syndrome). Impingement between adjacent spinous processes owing to excessive lordosis resulting in interspinous osteoarthrosis was first described by Baastrup in the 1930s. (74,75) Additional factors may include enlarged spinous processes, degenerative disc disease, facet arthrosis, neuromuscular disorders, thoracic kyphosis, thoracolumbar gibbus, obesity, and congenital hip dysplasia. (76) Its clinical significance is controversial, as similar changes are noted in asymptomatic individuals. (76) On frontal radiographs the spinous processes are closely opposed and at their points of contact exhibit a distinct articular cortex, which may be planar,

oblique, or curved. At the lateral margins of these neoarthroses, osteophytes can often be seen, and occasionally degenerative cysts create 1- to 5-mm rounded lucencies in the spinous processes.

Sacroiliac Joint

Age-related degenerative changes of the sacroiliac joint are common. (77) Generally, until the 4th decade these changes remain as a histologic phenomena only with no radiographic manifestations. (55) Premature degenerative abnormalities are often seen in altered weight-bearing situations such as scoliosis, leg deficiencies, and disruption of the pelvic ring from trauma. (Fig. 10-37) Radiographic abnormalities accompanying sacroiliac joint degeneration are limited to the lower two thirds of the joint, corresponding to the synovial compartment. The major characteristic signs are loss of joint space, subchondral sclerosis, and osteophytes. (Fig. 10-38)

The normal articular interspace ranges between 2 and 5 mm. Diminution is the radiographic manifestation of loss of articular cartilage, which may be generalized or focal. A generalized loss of articular space < 2 mm is confined to the lower two thirds of the joint. (78) Focal areas of diminution are also confined to this lower region and more frequently are located at the superior and inferior extents of the synovial portion of the joint.

Sclerosis of 1–2 mm in thickness invariably is most obvious on the iliac margin, owing to the anatomically thinner iliac surface cartilage. This may be generalized or localized to the superior and inferior extents of the synovial portion of the joint.

Osteophytes occur at the anterior aspect of the synovial portion of the joint, either at its superior or inferior extent. Anteroinferior

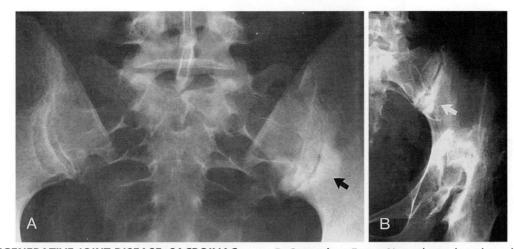

Figure 10-37   DEGENERATIVE JOINT DISEASE: SACROILIAC JOINT. A. Primary Form. Note the loss of joint space and subchondral sclerosis in the lower (synovial) two thirds of the joint (*arrow*). Compare with the normal contralateral side.

B. Secondary Form. Note that sclerosis and loss of joint space (*arrow*) have occurred in the sacroiliac joint from abnormal stress created by a congenital hip dislocation.

spurs are most often visible as a triangular density that may completely or incompletely bridge the articular cavity. (Fig. 10-39A) Anterosuperior spurs usually have to be large before they manifest radiographically. When present, the typical osteophytic configuration is not usually visible; the only sign is an increase in density overlying the superior portion of the joint space, which may simulate an active neoplastic or infectious process. (Fig. 10-38) Rarely, osteophytic formation may impinge on the sciatic nerve, producing neurological symptoms. (79)

Infrequently, joint surface erosions and ligamentous calcification, especially of the iliolumbar and interosseous ligaments, may be apparent. Ankylosis with advancing age may be bilateral and indistinguishable radiographically from ankylosing spondylitis (senile ankylosis). (Fig. 10-39B) Occasionally, a vacuum phenomenon may be seen as a linear radiolucency in the center of the articular cavity, paralleling but separated from the subchondral

bone; however, the appearance of the vacuum sign is not diagnostic of degenerative changes in this articulation. (Fig. 10-39)

Hip

Distinctive radiographic signs consist of non-uniform loss in joint space, osteophytes, prominent subchondral bone cysts, sclerosis, cortical buttressing, and joint deformity. (Fig. 10-40; Table 10-11) Advanced DJD in this location has also been called such terms as *coxarthrosis* and *malum coxae senilis*. Hip degeneration is an indicator of reduced risk for osteoporosis. (80)

Non-Uniform Loss of Joint Space. Depending on location, decreased cartilage thickness allows for varying directions of femoral head migration. These patterns of migration have been classified into three types: superior, medial, and axial. (81,82) (Fig. 10-41) There is no evidence that upright (weight-bearing)

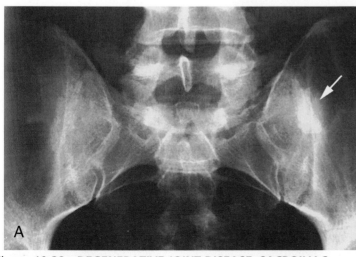

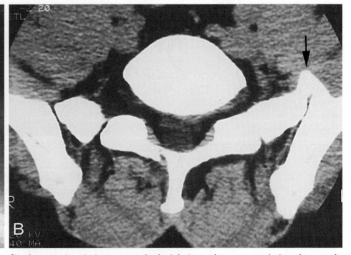

Figure 10-38   DEGENERATIVE JOINT DISEASE: SACROILIAC JOINT. A. AP Sacrum. Observe the focal blastic lesion toward the upper part of the synovial portion of the joint (*arrow*). **B. Axial CT: S1.** Note the opacity, which is owing to a calci-

fied anterior joint capsule bridging the upper joint (*arrow*). (Courtesy of Donald E. Freuden, DC, DABCO, Denver, Colorado.)

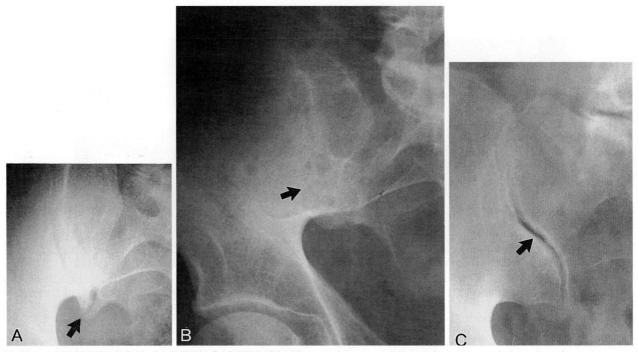

Figure 10-39 **ACCESSORY SIGNS: SACROILIAC JOINT DISEASE.**
A. Anteroinferior Osteophyte. Note the osteophyte (*arrow*).
B. Senile Ankylosis. Note that the joint has been completely
obliterated (*arrow*). **C. Normal Vacuum Phenomenon.** Note
that this vacuum phenomenon (*arrow*) should not be mistaken as an accessory sign of sacroiliac degenerative change.

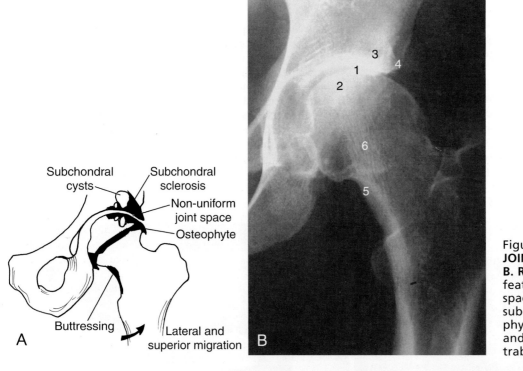

Figure 10-40 **DEGENERATIVE
JOINT DISEASE: HIP. A. Diagram.
B. Radiograph.** Note the following
features: non-uniform loss of joint
space (*1*), subchondral sclerosis (*2*),
subchondral bone cysts (*3*), osteophytes (*4*), cortical buttressing (*5*),
and thickened weight-bearing
trabeculae (*6*).

Table 10-11	Radiologic Signs of Degenerative Joint Disease of the Hip (Malum Coxae Senilis)
	Cortical buttressing
	Lateral femoral shift
	Non-uniform decrease in joint space
	Osteophytes
	Prominent subchondral cysts
	Remodeling of joint
	Sclerosis

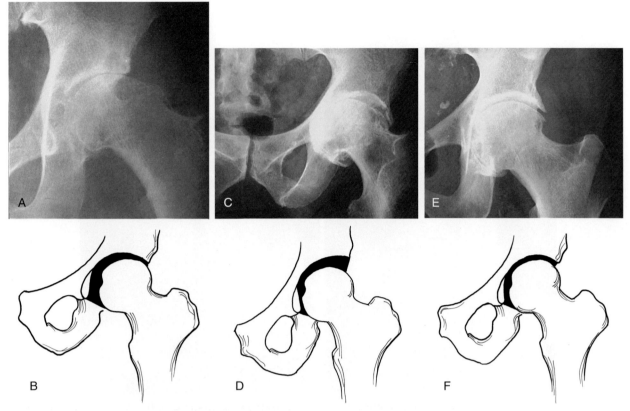

Figure 10-41 **PATTERNS OF HIP MIGRATION: DEGENERATIVE JOINT DISEASE. A and B. Superior.** Note that this is the most common pattern. **C and D. Medial. E and F. Axial.** Note that this is the least common pattern and is usually seen in inflammatory hip disease.

views of the hip have any benefit in the identification of joint space loss when compared with supine views. (83) In view of this information, it is recommended that supine views be used in the assessment of hip arthritis to improve image quality. (83)

- *Superior migration.* Loss of cartilage in the superior joint compartment allows the femur to move superiorly and laterally, with the medial joint space being comparatively widened (*Waldenstrom sign*). This is by far the most common pattern seen. It usually occurs in combination with anterior migration as determined on CT. (82)
- *Medial migration.* Cartilage loss in the medial compartment of the joint results in displacement of the femoral head medially. Occasionally, a mild degree of protrusio acetabuli may be seen. The superior joint space is distinctively normal. On CT there usually is an associated posterior migration. (82)
- *Axial migration.* This pattern of displacement is characterized by a diminution in joint space involving the whole articular cavity with no compartmental preference. Consequently, the femoral head displaces superomedially in the same plane as the femoral neck. This is a rarely encountered variant of DJD and is more typical of rheumatoid arthritis or infection.

Osteophytes. Characteristically, osteophytes are observed in the outer supra-acetabular margin and the lateral and inferomedial surfaces of the femoral head.

Subchondral Bone Cysts. Subchondral bone cysts are often large and typically found adjacent to the reduced joint space. (Fig. 10-42) Most commonly, these are present in the ilium at the supra-acetabular margin and the superior portion of the femoral head. When large, these may simulate a destructive neoplasm. In the femoral head these cysts make differentiation from avascular necrosis at times impossible. (Fig. 10-43)

Subchondral Sclerosis. Subchondral sclerosis parallels those locations where the greatest articular surface stress occurs. (Fig. 10-44) Most commonly, the areas of greatest condensation are found in the acetabular margin of the ilium when compared with the adjacent superior femoral head. (84) Localized areas of radiolucency in this sclerosis invariably represent subchondral bone cysts.

Buttressing. Frequently, buttressing is visible on the medial side of the femoral neck as thickening of the cortex. (Fig. 10-44) This is purely a stress-related thickening owing to the altered joint mechanics from the degenerative process.

Joint Deformity. Flattening of the femoral head at its superior portion is usually associated with a similar alteration in the acetabular roof. (Fig. 10-44) In long-standing DJD, remodeling of the femoral head results in the *tilt deformity.* (85) This abnormality is a combination of flattening of the superior head surface and prominent osteophyte formation of the inferomedial surface. This remodeling process gives the femoral head the appearance of "slipping" inferiorly.

Knee

The knee is a common site of DJD. This is most likely associated with its weight-bearing function and susceptibility to injury. Sev-

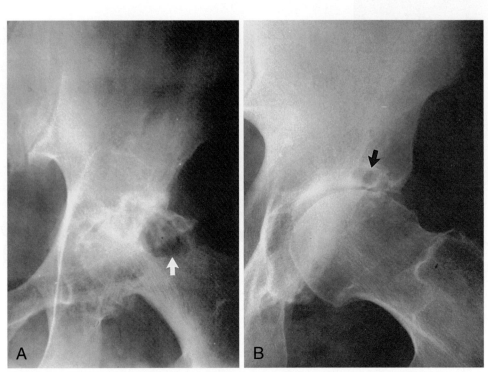

Figure 10-42 **SUBCHONDRAL CYSTS. A. AP Hip, Femoral Head.** Note that the large geographic lucency simulates a destructive neoplasm (*arrow*). **B. Frog-Leg Hip, Acetabulum.** Note the cyst (*arrow*).

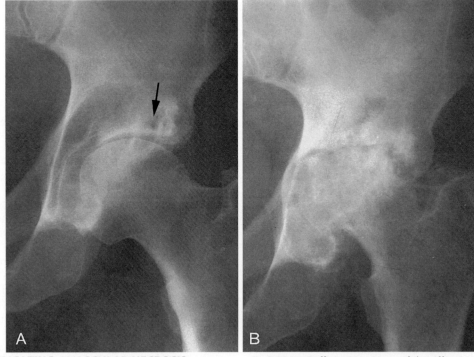

Figure 10-43 **COMPLICATING AVASCULAR NECROSIS: DEGENERATIVE JOINT DISEASE. A. Initial Film.** Note the loss of joint space and subchondral cyst formation (*arrow*).

B. 3-Year Follow-Up. Note the collapse of the femoral head with an irregular contour. This signifies the presence of osteonecrosis. A mild protrusio acetabuli has also developed.

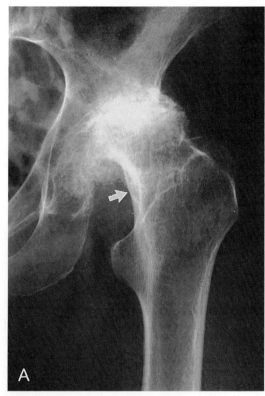

Figure 10-44 ADVANCED DEGENERATIVE JOINT DISEASE: HIP (MALUM COXAE SENILIS). A. AP Hip. Note the prominent sclerosis, cortical buttressing (*arrow*), and deformity. A tilt deformity is also seen. **B. Diagram: Tilt Deformity.** Resorption at the lateral femur (*arrow*) and deposition medially from osteophytes (*arrowhead*) produce an appearance that simulates a slipped epiphysis.

eral factors have been implicated in the predisposition of the knee to arthritis, including altered knee extension mechanisms (86) and the use of wide-heeled shoes. (87) In the early phases of degeneration, radiographic examination is often unrewarding. When degenerative changes are radiographically visible, they are characterized by selective involvement of the knee compartments, with non-uniform loss of joint space, sclerosis, small osteophytes, loose bodies, and deformity. (Table 10-12) MRI shows degeneration well before it becomes apparent on plain film and is especially useful in the depiction of meniscal abnormalities. (88)

Three compartments of the knee are radiographically visible: medial, lateral, and patellofemoral. Degenerative joint disease is characterized by its relative selectivity of one or, less commonly, two of these compartments. The most common compartment involved is the medial femorotibial joint. It is distinctly unusual to see uniform bicompartmental or tricompartmental joint disease.

Femorotibial Joint. Non-uniform loss of femorotibial joint space is typified by the decreased medial joint space. (Fig. 10-45) Erect weight-bearing AP films are essential to accurately evaluating diminution in joint space in this location. (Fig. 10-46) Sclerosis is usually not prominent and is limited to the subchondral bone adjacent to the loss of joint space. This is usually more evident in the tibia than in the femur. Osteophytes are usually quite small and also not a prominent feature. When present, they arise from the tibial and femoral margins on the side of decreased articular space. Sharpening of the tibial eminences is a manifestation of femorotibial joint degeneration.

Loose bodies frequently are encountered in this articulation. (Fig. 10-47) They may be singular but more often are multiple.

Table 10-12	Radiologic Findings in Degenerative Joint Disease of the Knee	
Femorotibial	**Patellofemoral**	**Chondromalacia Patellae**
Medial compartment	Loss of joint space—	Normal study
Loss of joint space	lateral facet	Medial facet
Small osteophytes	Small patellar	osteoporosis
Small bone cysts	osteophytes	Patella alta
Sclerosis:	Sclerosis	
tibia > femur	Anterior femoral	
Genu varus	erosion	
	Anterior patellar	
	surface roughening	

Their distinctive radiographic morphology allows easy differentiation from the fabella, a sesamoid bone in the lateral head of the gastrocnemius tendon. These loose bodies commonly calcify and ossify in concentric laminations, reminiscent of radio-positive gallstones. In addition, their borders are smooth and sometimes faceted at points of contact with adjacent loose bodies. If these loose bodies do not contain calcium, they are not visible on routine radiographic examinations, requiring contrast arthrograms or arthroscopy for diagnosis.

Subchondral cysts occur in < 10% of degenerative femorotibial joints, with the majority located beneath the tibial plateau, especially near the tibial eminences. (89,90) These may be > 1 cm and mimic a proximal tibial neoplasm. On CT the depiction of gas within the lesion is diagnostic of a degenerative cyst. (90)

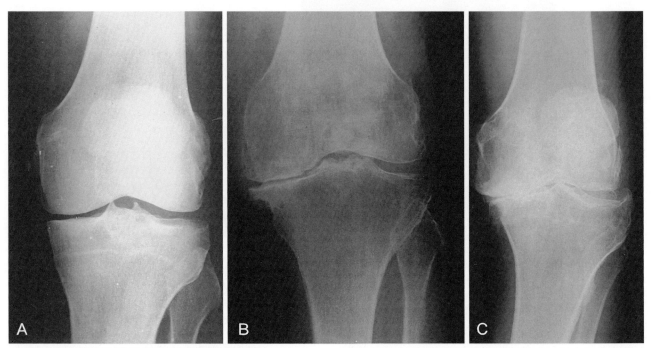

Figure 10-45 DEGENERATIVE JOINT DISEASE: KNEE (FEMOROTIBIAL JOINT). A. Early Changes. Note the decreased medial joint space and sharpened tibial eminences. **B. Moderate Changes.** Observe the more severe loss of medial joint space, sclerosis, and osteophytes. **C. Advanced Changes.** Note the complete loss of medial joint space, sclerosis, osteophytes, and lateral tibial shift (genu varus).

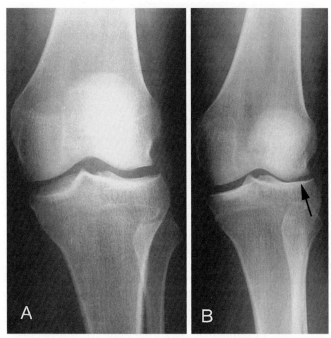

Figure 10-46 DEGENERATIVE JOINT DISEASE: KNEE. A. Recumbent. B. Erect. Observe the loss of lateral joint space not seen on the recumbent film (*arrow*).

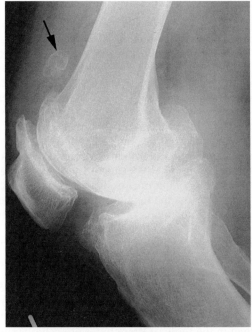

Figure 10-47 DEGENERATIVE JOINT DISEASE: LOOSE BODY. Lateral Knee. Note the solitary lesion in the suprapatellar pouch (*arrow*).

Deformity typically is a late manifestation and is usually a varus type with a relative medial shifting of the femur in relation to the tibia. Cyst formation is usually absent, although small cysts are occasionally seen beneath the tibial spines and posterior tibia. Chondrocalcinosis of the ipsilateral cartilage is also infrequently seen.

Patellofemoral Joint. Patellofemoral changes are usually found in combination with varying degrees of femorotibial DJD. Isolated patellofemoral joint degeneration is uncommon and should arouse suspicion of underlying calcium pyrophosphate dihydrate (CPPD) crystal deposition disease or significant previous trauma.

The most prominent signs are loss of joint space, osteophytes, sclerosis, and anterior femoral erosion. (Fig. 10-48) Loss of joint space in the early stages is usually more pronounced in the lateral aspect of the joint. Later, there may be close apposition of the patellar and femoral surfaces. Sclerosis usually accompanies the sites of closest apposition, especially on the patellar surface. Typically, osteophytes are seen arising near the articular surfaces at the inferior, superior, medial, and lateral poles of the patella.

A smooth, well-circumscribed, extrinsic erosive defect is occasionally observed in advanced patellofemoral degeneration 2–3 cm above the superior pole of the patella. This is secondary to a mechanical pressure effect on the anterior femoral surface after loss of the patellofemoral joint space. The anterior surface of the patella often appears irregular owing to bony excrescences (*tooth sign*). (91) (Fig. 10-49)

Chondromalacia Patellae. *Chondromalacia patellae* is the term applied to the syndrome of pain and crepitus arising from the patellofemoral articulation. As a distinct entity, it was first described by Budinger in 1906. (92) Plain film radiography is for the most part unrewarding and usually acts to exclude other underlying pathologic alterations.

Clinical Features. Considerable confusion exists as to the actual nature and cause of this condition. The term *chondromalacia patellae* is often haphazardly used to encompass a wide variety of patellofemoral syndromes, and this has contributed greatly to the confusion. Typically, chondromalacia patellae is a disease of the adolescent and young adult. Causal factors include trauma, patellar dislocation, malalignment syndrome, primary cartilage vulnerability, and occupation. (93) Many consider it a normal part of patellofemoral joint aging. It is often confused clinically with symptoms arising from a meniscal injury.

The most often used clinical criteria for applying the diagnosis of chondromalacia patellae are anteromedial knee pain associated with crepitus, buckling, locking, stiffness, swelling, and tenderness. Pain is usually aggravated by sitting in a confined space with the knee flexed (*movie sign*) and by walking up stairs. (94) A distinctive physical sign is retropatellar pain elicited by direct patellofemoral compression with the knee slightly flexed.

Measurement of the Q angle has received attention as a method to detect patellar malalignment, which may predispose the patient

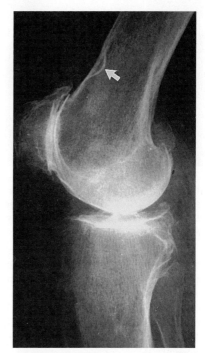

Figure 10-48 DEGENERATIVE JOINT DISEASE: PATELLO-FEMORAL JOINT. Lateral Knee: Note the loss of the retropatellar joint space, osteophytes, and sclerosis. Note the smooth, concave anterior femoral erosion (*arrow*), caused by mechanical extrinsic pressure of the superior patellar osteophyte.

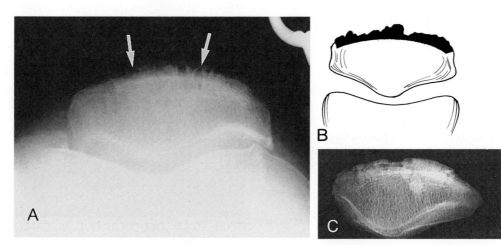

Figure 10-49 PATELLAR DEGENERATIVE ENTHESOPATHY (PATELLA TOOTH SIGN). A. Skyline Projection. B. Diagram. C. Specimen Radiograph. Observe the irregular bony spicules (*arrows*). COMMENT: The serrated surface and vertical linear lucencies can be readily misinterpreted as evidence of stress or acute fractures.

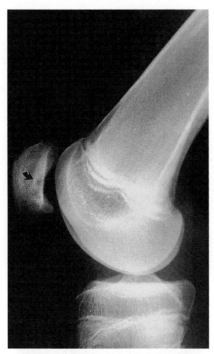

Figure 10-50 CHONDROMALACIA PATELLAE. Lateral Knee. Note the small localized area of radiolucency on the retropatellar surface (*arrow*). This lesion is infrequently seen in this disorder. (Courtesy of Stephen J. Bardsley, DC, Mornington, Australia.)

to chondromalacia. It is the angle formed by the line of the quadriceps muscle and the patellar ligament. Measurement is performed clinically by assessing the angle formed by these two lines: (*a*) from the anterosuperior iliac spine to the center of the patella and (*b*) from the tibial tubercle to the center of the patella. The normal range of this angle is 15–20°, with a measure > 20° being considered abnormal. (94)

Pathologic Features. *Chondromalacia* literally means "cartilage softening." The pathogenetic sequence is characteristic and parallels that seen in DJD. (95) Initial swelling and softening of the cartilage produces a blister-type of cartilage lesion. Subsequently, fissuring and fibrillation occur, predominantly involving the medial facet of the patella. (93) Involvement of the lateral facet has also been documented but rarely occurs. (94)

Radiologic Features. Specific radiographic findings are characteristically absent. MRI is the most accurate method of detecting focal cartilage defects. (96) Bone changes are limited to occasional underlying osteoporosis of the patellar articular surface, particularly the medial facet. (95) (Fig. 10-50) Loss of joint space denotes more advanced changes of DJD and is usually absent in chondromalacia. (97)

Malalignment of the patella can be assessed as a possible contributing factor to chondromalacia. A patella that is situated too high on the femur does not allow proper redirection of the quadriceps muscle action and is termed *patella alta*. (98) (See Chapter 2.)

Ankle and Tarsal Joints

The ankle is an uncommon site for DJD unless significant previous trauma has occurred. The most likely association with arthrosis of the ankle mortise is a previous tibiofibular diastasis that

results in chronic joint instability. An osteophyte from the dorsal aspect of the distal talus (talar beak) often is a sign of tarsal coalition. (99) In regard to the tarsal articulations, which are infrequently involved, only the first tarsometatarsal joint demonstrates visible radiographic changes. (Fig. 10-51) Degenerative changes at this articulation should arouse suspicion about the presence of a congenital talocalcaneal bar. Degenerative calcaneal spurs are common at the plantar and posterior surfaces but are not necessarily symptomatic. (Fig. 10-52) These bony excrescences are well defined and sharply marginated, in contrast to inflammatory new-bone proliferation, such as in ankylosing spondylitis, psoriasis, and Reiter's syndrome.

Foot

Of all forefoot articulations, the most commonly involved articulation is that of the first metatarsophalangeal joint. The radiographic signs are distinctive but on occasion may be identical to those seen in early gout. The most characteristic signs are osteophytes and deformity. (Fig. 10-53A) Osteophytes are usually at the dorsal and medial surfaces of the first metatarsal head. Osteo-

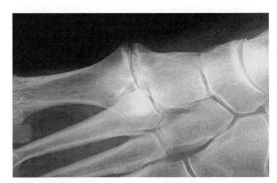

Figure 10-51 DEGENERATIVE JOINT DISEASE. First Tarsal-Metatarsal Joint: Oblique Foot. Note the loss of joint space, sclerosis, and osteophytes.

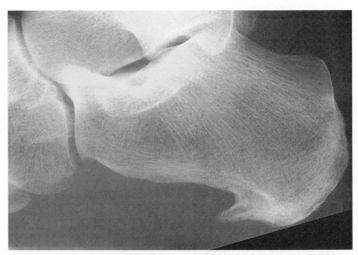

Figure 10-52 DEGENERATIVE CALCANEAL SPUR: LATERAL HEEL. Note the smooth bony excrescence at the plantar surface. *COMMENT:* The smooth surface connotes a degenerative, stress origin rather than an inflammatory one, such as in Reiter's syndrome or psoriasis.

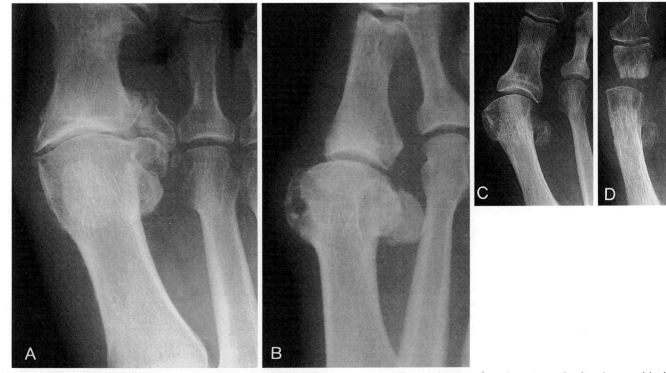

Figure 10-53 **DEGENERATIVE JOINT DISEASE: FIRST META-TARSOPHALANGEAL JOINT. A. Hallux Rigidus.** Note the loss of joint space, osteophytes, and loose bodies. **B. Bunion.** Note that the bony excrescence from the metatarsal head contains a degenerative cyst, simulating gouty changes.

C. Hallux Valgus Deformity. Note the bunion and hallux valgus deformity. **D. Bunionectomy and Keller Procedure.** Note that the site of bunionectomy is clearly seen. The hallux valgus deformity has been corrected by resection of the phalangeal base.

phytes are occasionally seen arising from the hallux sesamoids. Hyperostosis on the medial aspect of the metatarsal head may appear cystic and simulates the changes of gout. (Fig. 10-53*B*) Clinically, this bony outgrowth gives rise to a bunion. Valgus deformity with lateral displacement of the phalanx on the metatarsal head is frequently observed. (Fig. 10-53*C*) Additional signs apparent in varying degrees are loss of joint space, sclerosis, and small subchondral cysts.

Shoulder

Degenerative changes in the acromioclavicular joint are far more common than in the glenohumeral joint. Consequently, any signs of DJD in the glenohumeral joint should arouse suspicion of previous significant trauma or an underlying cartilage disease such as CPPD, crystal deposition disease, ochronosis, or acromegaly.

Acromioclavicular Joint. In the acromioclavicular joint, loss of joint space, sclerosis, and osteophyte formation are characteristic. Small subchondral cysts may be observed in the distal clavicle. (Fig. 10-54)

Glenohumeral Joint. Articular changes in the glenohumeral joint consist of a non-uniform loss of joint space, sclerosis, and osteophyte formation, particularly at the inferior humeral head. (Fig. 10-55*A*) Associated subchondral cysts may be seen at the articular surface, although these are usually small.

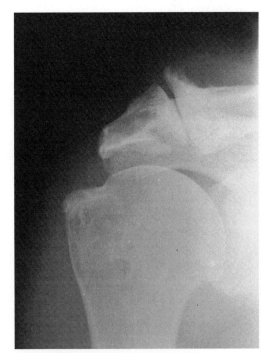

Figure 10-54 **DEGENERATIVE JOINT DISEASE: ACROMIOCLAVICULAR JOINT.** Note the loss of joint space, sclerosis, and osteophytes. Note the cystic changes in the greater tuberosity owing to degenerative tendinitis.

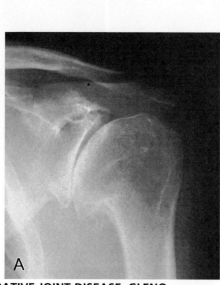

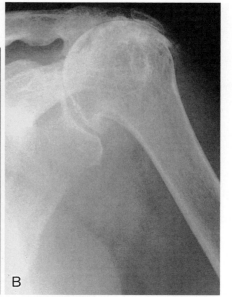

Figure 10-55 DEGENERATIVE JOINT DISEASE: GLENO-HUMERAL JOINT. A. AP Shoulder, Primary Disease. Note the deformity of the articular surface, non-uniform loss of joint space, and osteophytes, which are characteristic. **B. AP Shoulder, Primary Disease with Rotator Cuff Tear.** Note the rotator cuff tear with erosion of the clavicle and acromion. Observe the superior position of the humerus, which is diagnostic for rotator cuff tear owing to the unopposed action of the deltoid. *COMMENT:* Degenerative joint disease is uncommon in the glenohumeral joint and should suggest another underlying cause, such as previous trauma or cartilage disease such as calcium pyrophosphate dihydrate crystal deposition.

Rotator cuff degeneration may manifest as small cyst formation in the tuberosities. Rotator cuff disruption is characterized by a superior migration of the humerus in relation to the glenoid cavity, owing to the unopposed action of the deltoid muscle. Erosion with sclerosis of the inferior surface of the acromion usually accompanies this superior humeral displacement. (Fig. 10-55*B*) Diagnosis of a torn rotator cuff can be achieved with arthrography, ultrasound, or MRI.

Calcific Tendinitis and Bursitis. Commonly, calcific tendinitis and bursitis are seen radiographically in both symptomatic and asymptomatic shoulders. Calcification is the sequela of degenerative tendinitis at the bony attachments of the tendon. Frequently, there is bilateral involvement simultaneously.

The most common location for calcification is the supraspinatus tendon insertion at the greater tuberosity, best seen on the external rotation view. The second most common site is calcification in the subacromial bursa, which is seen below the acromion and above the humeral head. Other tendons that may develop calcification are the infraspinatus, teres minor, and subscapularis. (See "Hydroxyapatite Deposition Disease.")

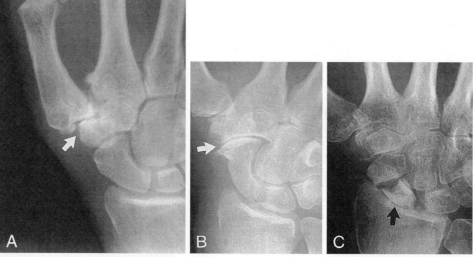

Figure 10-56 DEGENERATIVE JOINT DISEASE: WRIST.
A. First Metacarpal Trapezium Joint. Note the loss of joint space, sclerosis, and lateral displacement of the metacarpal (*arrow*). **B. Scaphoid–Trapezium Joint.** Note the osteophytes and a small subchondral cyst (*arrow*). **C. Radiocarpal Joint.** Observe the narrowing of the joint space secondary to avascular necrosis from a scaphoid fracture (*arrow*). Radiocarpal arthrosis is usually secondary to trauma or pseudo-gout. (Panel B courtesy of Paul W. Thielen, DC, Hamilton, Montana.)

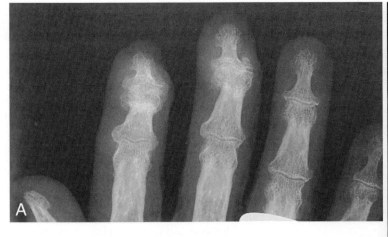

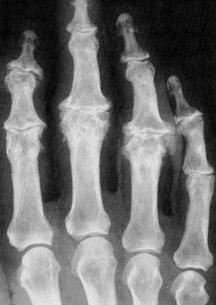

Figure 10-57 **DEGENERATIVE JOINT DISEASE: FINGERS. A. Distal interphalangeal joints (Heberden's nodes). B. Proximal interphalangeal joints (Bouchard's nodes).**

Elbow

Involvement of the elbow is invariably secondary to previous trauma, occupation, or other abnormality. Signs consist predominantly of loose body formation and osteophytes. A common finding is an olecranon spur at the triceps tendon insertion.

Wrist

Primary degenerative changes in the wrist are usually limited to the first metacarpal-trapezium joint. Degenerative joint disease in any other wrist articulation is invariably secondary in origin. (Fig. 10-56)

First Metacarpal–Trapezium Joint. Radiographic signs in the first metacarpal–trapezium joint are distinctive and consist of radial subluxation of the first metacarpal base, sclerosis, osteophytes, and occasional loose bodies. (Fig. 10-56A)

Radiocarpal Joint. The most common predisposing conditions to degeneration of the radiocarpal joint are radial and scaph-oid fractures, carpal ischemic necrosis (scaphoid and lunate), and CPPD crystal deposition disease. (Fig. 10-56C) Characteristically, there is diminution of the radiocarpal joint space, sclerosis, and osteophytes. Subchondral cysts are often seen in the carpal bones. Calcification of the triangular cartilage in the radioulnar joint space may provide the clue for the diagnosis of CPPD.

Hand

Involvement of the interphalangeal joints of the hand is a distinctive feature of DJD. Clinically, visible enlargement of the degenerating joints has been termed various eponyms according to location—Heberden's nodes for DIP joints and Bouchard's nodes for proximal interphalangeal joints (PIP). (Fig. 10-57) Radiographic changes consist of lateral osteophytes, sclerosis, loss of joint space, and malalignment, especially in the distal interphalangeal joints.

CAPSULE SUMMARY   Degenerative Joint Disease

General Considerations

- Non-inflammatory degeneration of joint cartilage with secondary effects on adjacent bone.
- This is the most common form of arthritis.
- Synonyms include osteoarthritis.

Clinical Features

- Pain, stiffness, crepitus, deformity, and swelling, with normal laboratory studies.

- Three types identified: primary, secondary, and erosive.
  Primary: unknown cause, 5th–6th decade, females 10:1, weight-bearing joints.
  Secondary: known cause, 2nd–6th decade, equal sex distribution, any joint.
  Erosive osteoarthritis: inflammatory cause, 4th–5th decade, females 3:1, interphalangeal joints.

Pathologic Features

- Begins focally and gradually increases in size.

(continued)

CAPSULE SUMMARY Degenerative Joint Disease (continued)

- Initial loss of chondroitin sulfate leads to fibrillation and flaking, with secondary stress effects on adjacent bone.
- Escape of synovial fluid into subchondral bone forms subchondral bone cysts (geodes).

Radiologic Features

- Asymmetric distribution, non-uniform loss of joint space, osteophytes, subchondral sclerosis, subchondral cysts, loose bodies, and subluxation.
- *Spine:* C5–C7, T9–T12, L4–L5.
  Cervical: osteophytes, loss of disc height, intervertebral foramen encroachment, occasionally related to vertebral artery syndromes and spinal stenosis (< 12 mm).
  Thoracic: osteophytes on right side, increasing kyphosis.
  Lumbar: osteophytes, loss of disc height, facet arthrosis, vacuum sign; anterolisthesis (L4), stenosis (< 12 mm), instability.

Associated Degenerative Syndromes

- *Degenerative spondylolisthesis:* occurs as a combination of loss of joint space, loss of disc height, remodeling of the facet surfaces to a more sagittal orientation and broadening of the pedicle facet angle. Most common at L4 and C7.
- *Instability:* comparing intersegmental movements at extremes of physiological motion; sagittal (flexion–extension), coronal (lateral bending), and axial (compression–distraction). Cervical spine sagittal intersegmental motion > 3.5 mm or > 11° considered unstable. In the lumbar spine anterior or posterior displacement, narrowed foramen, wide facet joint space, and offset spinous processes signs used.
- *Synovial (ganglion, juxta-articular) cysts:* in conjunction with degenerative facet arthropathy, most commonly at L4–L5;

rarely visible on plain film examination; an extradural mass on myelography; a soft tissue mass on CT sometimes with a low attenuation central zone containing gas or even eroding the lamina and facet surface; a mass with a central zone on MRI.
- *Hemispheric spondylosclerosis (HSS):* prominent subchondral sclerosis.
- *Baastrup's syndrome (kissing spine syndrome):* Impingement between adjacent spinous processes owing to excessive lordosis resulting in interspinous osteoarthrosis.
- *Sacroiliac:* unilateral, sclerosis, superior and inferior spurs.
- *Hip (malum coxae senilis):* femur migration superiorly and laterally, osteophytes, sclerosis, large cysts.
- *Knee:* medial compartment most common site, then lateral, and least frequently the patellofemoral compartment; loss of joint space, small osteophytes, sclerosis, and often loose bodies.
- *Chondromalacia patellae:* variant in young of DJD, patella alta.
- *Ankle and foot:* ankle involvement uncommon. First metatarsophalangeal joint–hallux valgus, bunion.
- *Shoulder:* acromioclavicular affected more frequently than glenohumeral joint; rotator cuff tear shows as a superior position of the humerus; rotator cuff calcifying tendinitis (supraspinatus).
- *Elbow:* uncommon and usually owing to previous fracture.
- *Wrist and hand:* first metacarpal trapezium. Radiocarpal arthritis usually secondary to radial or scaphoid fracture. Interphalangeal joints—DIP Heberden's nodes; PIP Bouchard's nodes.

EROSIVE OSTEOARTHRITIS

Erosive osteoarthritis is a distinctive clinical and radiographic variant of DJD first delineated by Crain in 1961. (1) The two most common terms applied to this arthropathy are erosive osteoarthritis and inflammatory osteoarthritis.

Clinical Features

In contrast to primary degenerative joint disease, the onset of erosive osteoarthritis is characterized by episodic and acute inflammation of the DIP and PIP joints of both hands in a symmetric manner. (2) (Table 10-13) Pain, edema, redness, nodules, and restricted motion are found at the involved articulations of the hands. This arthropathy is most commonly found in middle-aged females in the 4th or 5th decades of life and a familial tendency has been suggested. Laboratory investigations are inconclusive, with normal to slightly elevated erythrocyte sedimentation rate (ESR) and negative rheumatoid factor. (3) Chronic progression of the disease is to be expected with nodular, unstable, and malaligned finger joints. The intensity of symptoms with each inflammatory episode may continue to be severe for many years. Approximately 15% of cases may develop rheumatoid arthritis, with an average onset of 12 years after the initial episode of erosive osteoarthritis. (3)

Table 10-13	Clinical Fractures of Erosive Osteoarthritis
	Middle-aged females
	Symmetric
	Distal and proximal interphalangeal joints
	Normal laboratory findings
	Pain, edema, redness
	Residual deformities

Treatment is currently of a conservative nature (2) and the use of the nutriceutical, chondroitin sulfate, has been shown to limit the increase in the number of joints involved. (4)

Pathologic Features

Variable tissue changes are found, ranging from proliferative rheumatoid-like synovial abnormalities to cartilage degeneration and bony proliferation, as seen in primary degenerative joint disease.

Radiologic Features

Essentially, the radiographic changes are that of DJD with superimposed bone erosions predominantly involving the distal and proximal interphalangeal joints. (Table 10-14) (Fig. 10-58) Occasional involvement of the thumb at the metacarpophalangeal and carpometacarpal joints may occur, as well as between the trapezium and scaphoid articulations. (3,5) (Fig. 10-59) Involvement of the ulnar compartment of the carpus is significantly spared, differentiating involvement from rheumatoid arthritis. (6) All other joints of the body are generally uninvolved.

Radiographic changes are characterized by osteophytes, loss of joint space, and sclerosis. Osteophytes are identical to those seen in DJD. They are marginal in origin, taper distally, and are often larger at the distal articular component. Loss of joint space is usually non-uniform, with adjacent subchondral sclerosis. Superimposed changes of erosions, periostitis, and ankylosis on these degenerative features are characteristic of erosive osteoarthritis. Bone erosions are distinctively centrally located on the proximal articular surface and more peripherally at the distal articular surface. The resultant altered joint surface contour has been called the *gull wings sign*. (7) (Fig. 10-60) Adjacent linear periostitis is occasionally seen. Bony ankylosis is an uncommon but not unexpected sequela of one or more interphalangeal joints.

The main differential considerations are rheumatoid arthritis, psoriasis, and non-inflammatory degenerative joint disease. Rheumatoid arthritis rarely involves the distal interphalangeal joints and has a positive latex test. Psoriatic arthropathy is characterized by discrete marginal erosions with adjacent fluffy periostitis (*mouse ears sign*). (7) Non-inflammatory DJD will show no erosions but will otherwise appear identical to erosive osteoarthritis.

Table 10-14	Radiologic Manifestations of Erosive Osteoarthritis
	Ankylosis
	Central articular erosions (gull wings)
	Non-uniform joint space loss
	Osteophytes
	Periostitis
	Sclerosis

CAPSULE SUMMARY
Erosive Osteoarthritis

General Considerations
- Inflammatory variant of DJD involving the interphalangeal joints of the hands.

Clinical Features
- Common in females 40–50 years old.
- Acute pain, swelling, redness, and residual deformity.
- Often confused with rheumatoid arthritis but is seronegative.

Pathologic Features
- Cartilage degeneration and synovial proliferation.

Radiologic Features
- At DIP and PIP joints of hands.
- Erosions (gull wings sign), sclerosis, osteophytes, periostitis (mouse ears sign), ankylosis, and non-uniform loss of joint space.

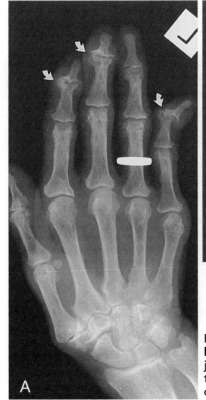

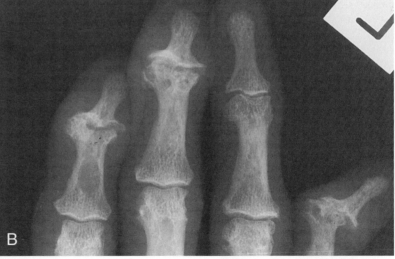

Figure 10-58 **EROSIVE OSTEOARTHRITIS: HANDS. A. Target Distribution.** Note the selective involvement of the distal interphalangeal joints (*arrows*). **B. Radiologic Features.** Note that closer inspection of these involved joints reveals osteophytes, sclerosis, loss of joint space, cystic erosions, and deformity.

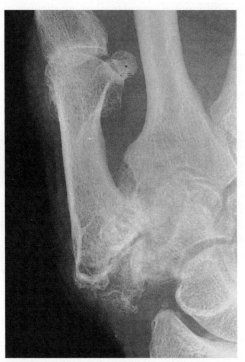

Figure 10-59 EROSIVE OSTEOARTHRITIS: THUMB. Note that the exhibited changes are identical to degenerative joint disease, although more severe. Note the osteophytes, loose bodies, and deformity.

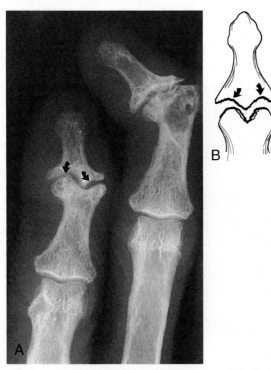

Figure 10-60 EROSIVE OSTEOARTHRITIS. A and B. Gull Wings Sign. Note the characteristic biconcave articular contour (*arrows*).

DIFFUSE IDIOPATHIC SKELETAL HYPEROSTOSIS

Diffuse idiopathic skeletal hyperostosis (DISH) is a generalized spinal and extraspinal articular disorder that is characterized by ligamentous calcification and ossification. The most prominent radiographic expressions of this disease are encountered in the spine, involving predominantly the anterior longitudinal ligament (ALL). It is a distinct entity and does not represent ankylosing spondylitis or DJD. An incidence of 12% of middle-aged and elderly individuals in the United States has been estimated. (1) DISH has been labeled by various terms, including spondylosis hyperostotica, spondylitis ossificans ligamentosa, senile ankylosing hyperostosis, and Forestier's disease. (2–3) (Table 10-15) The most universally accepted term of DISH was first introduced by Resnick et al. (5) to emphasize the frequent separate or co-existent involvement of the extraspinal structures.

Clinical Features

DISH is characterized clinically by its broad spectrum of presentations. Despite a radiographic diagnosis of DISH, the patient may be asymptomatic, highlighting the clinical variability of the disorder.

Complaints by the patient are similar to those of degenerative joint disease, during the 5th or 6th decade of life, with morning stiffness and low-grade musculoskeletal pain, especially of the spine and its related articulations. (Fig. 10-61) An additional complaint in approximately 20% of DISH patients may be dysphagia owing to anterior proliferative bone growths from the cervical spine or esophageal obstruction in the thoracic spine compressing the adjacent esophagus. (1,6) Hoarseness of the voice, stridor, and dyspnea have also been recorded (7–8). Extraspinal symptomatology consists of localized pain, occasional swelling, and ossific masses, especially of the Achilles and quadriceps tendons.

Table 10-15	Synonyms of Diffuse Idiopathic Skeletal Hyperostosis
Term	
Common	
(Senile) ankylosing	
hyperostosis	
Forestier's disease	
Diffuse idiopathic	
skeletal hyperostosis	
Uncommon	
First descriptions	
Spondylosis hyperostotica	
Moniliform hyperostosis	
Spondylitis ossificans	
ligamentosa	
Vertebral melorheostosis	
Spondylorheostosis	
Physiologic vertebral	
ligamentous calcification	
Generalized juxta-articular	
ossification of ligaments (5)	
of the vertebral column	

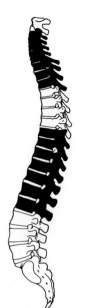

Figure 10-61 **SPINAL DISTRIBUTION OF DIFFUSE IDIOPATHIC SKELETAL HYPEROSTOSIS.**

Table 10-16	Clinical Features of Diffuse Idiopathic Skeletal Hyperostosis

General
    Usually > 50 years of age
    Predominantly males
    Up to 20% have diabetes mellitus
Spine
    Most common site of involvement
    Pain and stiffness, especially in the morning
    Loss of cervical and lumbar lordoses
    Increased thoracic kyphosis
    Dysphagia
    Rarely signs of spinal stenosis
Extraspinal
    Joint pain
    Tendon pain—Achilles, olecranon, quadriceps
    Synovitis
    Nodular masses in tendons

Despite the radiographic evidence of segmental ankylosis, paradoxically, the vertebral motion may be remarkably unaffected. This most likely is relative to the articular sparing of the apophyseal joints in this disorder. Slight to moderate flattening of the lumbar and cervical lordoses is common, as well as an increase in the thoracic kyphosis. (Table 10-16) Complicating fractures can occur through the ankylosing new bone similar to carrot-stick fractures seen in ankylosing spondylitis with severe neurological sequelae, including quadriplegia. (8,10,11) The cervical spine is the most common site for these fractures, especially at C5–C7, which accounts for 90% of cases; the rest are found in the thoracolumbar spine. (12) These are most often precipitated by low-energy, seemingly trivial injuries. (12) In cases of fused lower segments, atlantoaxial instability may rarely occur. (13) Additionally, fractures of adjacent uninvolved segments, such as the odontoid, may be seen with no effect on those segments involved with DISH. (14)

A predisposition to developing heterotopic new bone at the site of a joint prosthesis has been documented. (15) Spinal stenosis owing to DISH is uncommon unless associated with ossification of the posterior longitudinal ligament, hypertrophic posterior osteophytes, or ligamentum flavum hypertrophy. (16–18) In most cases, conservative care and non-steroidal anti-inflammatory drugs (NSAIDs) are the treatments of choice, whereas surgical resection may be warranted in patients with severe dysphagia. (19–21)

Laboratory investigations are generally unrewarding; however, numerous authors have outlined an association with adult onset of diabetes mellitus in up to 50% of patients with DISH. (18,22–24) Later reports have since delineated a lesser incidence of association in the realm of 13–32%, which would appear to be more accurate. (25–27) Patients with DISH show hyperinsulinemia after glucose challenge tests. Specialized evaluation for HLA-B8 antigen may be positive in approximately 40% of patients with DISH. (25)

Pathologic Features

The pathologic stigmata of DISH revolves around the apparent exaggerated response of some patients to form bone to an as yet un-

identified stimulus. This predisposition to bone forming has led DISH to be referred to as an ossifying diathesis. Distinctively, this predisposition to produce extraosseous bone occurs in ligamentous and tendinous attachments, particularly in the spine. It has been suggested that an increased output of the pituitary growth hormone may assist the production of these hyperostotic bone formations. (28) In addition, growth hormone exerts a diabetogenic action systemically by inducing hyperglycemia, glycosuria, and ketonuria and would appear to correlate with the increased frequency of diabetes mellitus in DISH. (29) Laboratory investigations evaluating levels of growth hormone, however, have been unrewarding. (30)

Pathologic examination of involved vertebral columns reveal initial calcification followed by subsequent ossification of the ALL. (Figs. 10-62 and 10-63) This process typically begins in the midportion of the vertebral body and extends to bridge the adjacent intervertebral disc. (31) Notably, the deep fibers of the ALL, adjacent to the anterior vertebral body margins may be uninvolved initially, resulting in a vertical intervening radiolucent shadow that is radiographically visible. (Fig. 10-64) Later, the ligamentous ossification may blend imperceptibly into the adjacent vertebral body, obliterating this lucency.

Frequently, at the level of the intervertebral disc a horizontal or oblique line of unossified tissue occurs in the ossifying ALL. This is owing to anterolateral fibrous discal extensions originating from the outer annulus, which grow in and around the fibers of the ALL and inhibit the calcification-ossification process. (32) This may isolate islands of calcification, creating T- and Y-shaped radiolucencies on a radiograph adjacent to the involved disc, simulating but not representing fractures or apparent pseudoarthroses. (Fig. 10-65)

Radiologic Features

The definitive criteria for the diagnosis of DISH are as follows (5):

- The presence of flowing calcification and ossification along the anterolateral aspect of at least four contiguous vertebral bodies.
- Relative preservation of intervertebral disc height of the involved segments and lack of other associated signs of disc degeneration.

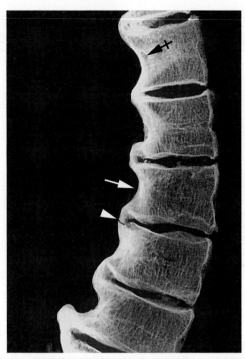

Figure 10-62 DIFFUSE IDIOPATHIC SKELETAL HYPEROSTOSIS: SPECIMEN RADIOGRAPH. Note that this sagittal specimen of the thoracic spine demonstrates the characteristic features: hyperostosis of the anterior longitudinal ligament extending into the midvertebral body (*arrow*), clefts through the hyperostosis at the disc level (*arrowhead*), and residual unossified deep ligamentous fibers (*crossed arrow*). (Courtesy of Donald Resnick, MD, San Diego, California.)

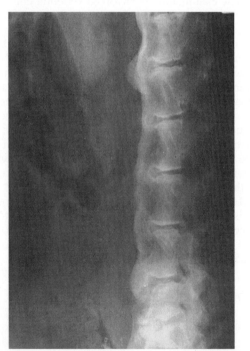

Figure 10-63 DIFFUSE IDIOPATHIC SKELETAL HYPEROSTOSIS: CANINE INVOLVEMENT (DOGGY DISH). The exuberant anterior hyperostosis is dramatically visible. Note the relatively "tall" vertebrae owing to the quadruped stance and lack of axial loading, a common finding in humans who have never become upright.

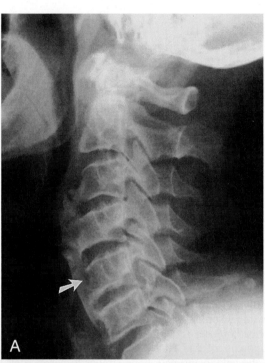

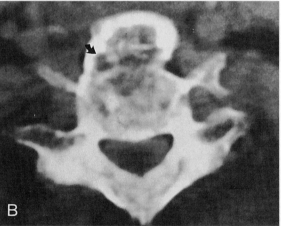

Figure 10-64 DIFFUSE IDIOPATHIC SKELETAL HYPEROSTOSIS: ANTERIOR LUCENCY. A. Lateral Cervical. Note the discrete radiolucency below the ossified anterior bony shield (*arrow*). **B. Axial CT: C5.** Note the location of the lucency is confirmed at the anterior longitudinal ligament–vertebral body interface (*arrow*). *COMMENT:* The lack of ossification in the deep fibers of the anterior longitudinal ligament produces this lucency and is a consistent sign of the disorder. (Courtesy of Lawrence A. Cooperstein, MD, Pittsburgh, Pennsylvania.)

• Absence of apophyseal joint ankylosis and sacroiliac joint erosion, sclerosis, or intra-articular osseous fusion.

The purpose of using these criteria is to exclude on radiologic grounds the diagnoses of DJD and ankylosing spondylitis.

Target Sites of Involvement

Spine. Involvement of the spine is characterized by its multisegmental distribution, resulting in more than one spinal region being involved simultaneously. Statistically, the most common spinal region affected is the thoracic spine, particularly the lower segments. (32)

Cervical Spine. Bony hyperostosis is most frequent and most exuberant in the lower segments (C4–C7). Typically, the hyperostosis begins from the anteroinferior vertebral body margin and extends downward, tapering at its distal extent. Eventually, complete intervertebral discal bridging is present, with a flowing, bumpy anterior contour. (Tables 10-17 and 10-18) The thickness of this anterior hyperostosis may be > 1 cm. (Fig. 10-66) At discs where fusion is evident, the thickness of the anterior hyperostosis does not increase in contrast to mobile segments where broadening of the ossification advances. (33) Horizontal radiolucent linear clefts owing to anterior discal extrusions are most frequently seen in this region of the spine and should not be confused with fractures or pseudoarthroses. (Fig. 10-65) Complicating dysphagia can occur secondary to these exuberant anterior bony outgrowths, as evidenced on the lateral film by adjacent displacement of the pharyngeal air shadow. (22,33)

Additional ossification may be present posteriorly in the form of body hyperostosis and osteophytes and within the posterior longitudinal ligament and nuchal ligament. Ossification within the posterior longitudinal ligament (PLL) can be associated with myelopathy. (34) Significantly, the intervertebral discs and apophyseal joints remain relatively normal, although minor degenerative changes may be superimposed.

Thoracic Spine. The thoracic spine is the most common site of spinal involvement, especially between T7 and T11. Typically, the majority of the hyperostosis is found on the right side of the spine owing to the pulsation–inhibition effect of the adjacent left-sided aorta. (32) (Fig. 10-67) In situs inversus this distribution is reversed, with hyperostosis on the left side. (35) Thickness of the hyperostosis is variable, but can be up to 2 cm and can rarely obstruct the esophagus as low as T9–T10. (6) A vertical radiolucent cleft separating the ossified ligament and anterior vertebral body is often apparent. (Fig. 10-67, *C* and *D*) Characteristically, the apophyseal joints are unaffected. The costovertebral and costotransverse articulations may be bridged with the hyperostotic process in up to 20% of patients. (36)

Lumbar Spine. Lumbar involvement is most common and most prominent in the upper three segments and closely resembles those changes observed in the cervical spine. Initially, the hyperostosis begins from the middle and anterosuperior vertebral body margin, extending upward and tapering at its distal extent, simulating a candle flame. (3) (Fig. 10-68) Eventual complete continuity across the intervertebral disc may occur, but it often is interrupted with horizontal linear radiolucent clefts owing to anterior discal extrusions. Occasionally, the adjacent aorta may appear displaced. Ossification posteriorly is less prominent than in the cervical spine, but may be seen in the interspinous ligaments.

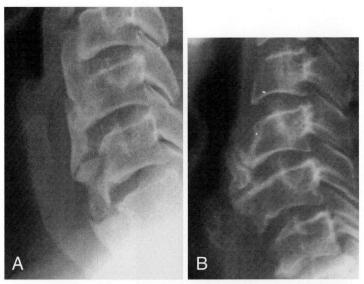

Figure 10-65 **DIFFUSE IDIOPATHIC SKELETAL HYPEROSTOSIS: LINEAR RADIOLUCENCIES. A. T-Shaped (C5–C6). B. Y-Shaped (C4–C5).** Note that these lucencies should not be confused with fractures. (Courtesy of Randolph F. Baca, DC, DACBR, Denver, Colorado.)

Table 10-18	Descriptive Synonyms for Spinal Hyperostosis
	Dripping candle wax
	Flame-shaped osteophytes
	Flowing hyperostosis
	Undulating (bumpy) contour

Table 10-17	Radiologic Features of DISH in the Spine	
Pathologic Features		**Radiographic Features**
Calcification and later ossification of ALL involving four or more segments		Anterior flowing hyperostosis (exuberant hyperostosis)
Increased ossification thickness of ALL at the level of the intervertebral disc		Bumpy anterior spinal contour
Unossified ALL owing to fibrous tissue extensions originating from annulus fibers		Radiolucent horizontal or oblique cleft through hyperostosis
Incomplete ossification of deep layers of ALL		Radiolucent vertical shadow between ossified ligament and vertebral body
Normal to mildly diminished nuclear hydration		Disc preservation

ALL, anterior longitudinal ligament.

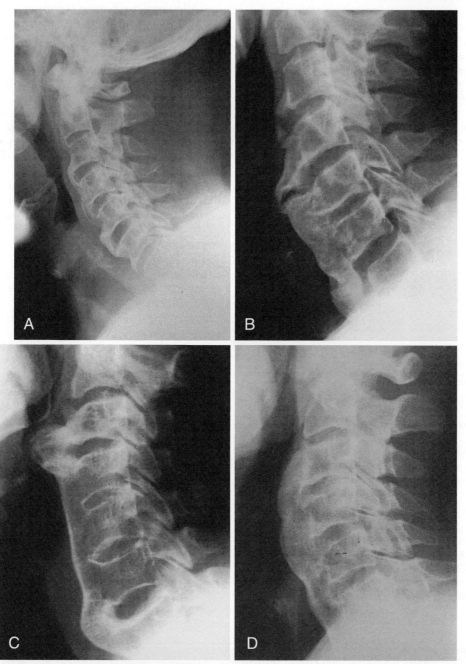

Figure 10-66 **DIFFUSE IDIOPATHIC SKELETAL HYPEROSTOSIS: CERVICAL SPINE. A–D. Various Manifestations.** Note that the anterior ossification can conform to a multitude of configura-tions from thin to thick ossifications, bumpy to smooth contours, and solid or incomplete bridging. (Panel D courtesy of Barry Kinge, DC, Bellflower, California.)

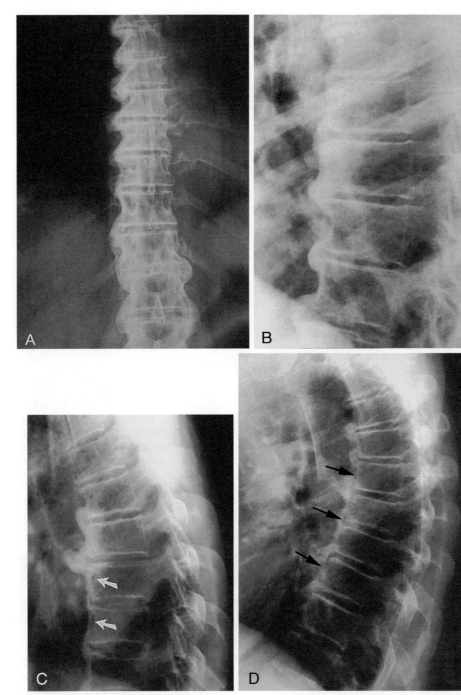

Figure 10-67 **DIFFUSE IDIOPATHIC SKELETAL HYPER-OSTOSIS: THORACIC SPINE. A. AP Thoracic.** Note the lack of left-sided hyperostosis owing to the inhibitive effect of the aortic pulsations. **B. Bumpy Contour.** Note the continuous uneven anterior contour. **C. Isolated Hyperostosis.** Observe the exuberant hyperostosis limited to a few levels. Note the prominent anterior lucency beneath the hyperostosis (*arrows*). **D. Linear Form.** Note the anterior bony shield involves contiguous levels, separated from the vertebral bodies by a radiolucent zone (*arrows*).

Sacroiliac Joint. Involvement of the sacroiliac joint in DISH is usually seen when signs are already apparent in the spine. Typically, there is a lack of involvement of the synovial portion of the joint, as evidenced by smooth articular margins and normal adjacent bone density. Ossification, however, is observed to involve the sacroiliac ligaments at the extreme superior and inferior joint margins. (Fig. 10-69)

Extraspinal Sites. Extraspinal sites of DISH can virtually occur at any ligamentous or tendinous insertion. The most common sites are the pelvis, patella, calcaneus, foot, and elbow (5,37), and these sites may be involved in approximately 30% of patients with DISH of the spine. (5) (Fig. 10-70) The characteristic radiographic manifestations are roughening of bony attachments (*whiskering*), ossification within a ligament or tendon, and normal adjacent joint space.

Differential Diagnosis

A number of spinal disorders are characterized by bony outgrowths that may simulate the appearance of DISH. The most difficult differential exclusions include DJD, ankylosing spondylitis, psoriasis, and Reiter's syndrome. Other less-common considerations may include acromegaly, fluorosis, and axial neuropathic arthropathy. Non-involvement of the lower sacroiliac joint is a good indicator that ankylosing spondylitis is not present. In addition, the presence of hyperostoses from the pelvis, including the iliac crests, iliolumbar ligament, supra-acetabular region, trochanters, ischial tuberosity, and symphysis pubis, are also excellent features for differentiating from ankylosing spondylitis. (38)

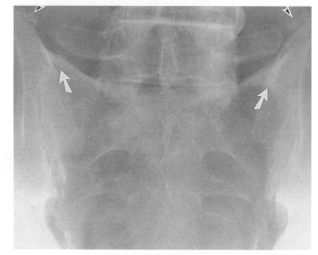

Figure 10-69   DIFFUSE IDIOPATHIC SKELETAL HYPEROSTOSIS: SACROILIAC JOINTS. Note the ossification of the superior sacroiliac ligaments, visible as the increased densities at the sacral ala (*arrows*). Notably, the lower (synovial) joint space and joint margins are unaffected, excluding a diagnosis of ankylosing spondylitis. Partial ossification of the iliolumbar ligaments bilaterally is also visible (*arrowheads*).

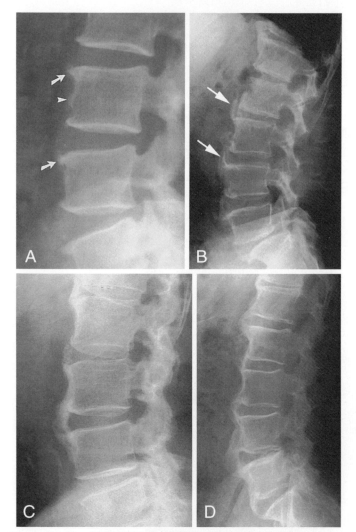

Figure 10-68   DIFFUSE IDIOPATHIC SKELETAL HYPEROSTOSIS: LUMBAR SPINE. A. Early Changes. Note the beginnings of hyperostosis at the body margins (*arrows*) and midbody (*arrowhead*). **B. Candle Flame Hyperostosis.** Note the bulk of the ossification is in an upward direction (*arrows*). **C. Complete Anterior Bridging.** Observe the thickness and midbody distribution of the hyperostosis. These are characteristic and aid in the differentiation of ankylosing spondylitis. **D. Advanced Changes.** Note complete anterior bridging has occurred at every disc level. Observe the residual bumpy anterior contour. (Courtesy of Robert J. Longenecker, DC, DACBR, Dallas, Texas.)

CAPSULE SUMMARY
Diffuse Idiopathic Skeletal Hyperostosis

General Considerations

- Generalized articular disorder, with an axial predilection characterized by ligamentous ossification, especially of the anterior longitudinal ligament.
- Synonyms include ankylosing hyperostosis and Forestier's disease.

Pathologic Features

- Predisposition to form bone owing to unknown factors (ossifying diathesis).
- Calcification and ossification of anterior longitudinal ligament, interrupted by discal extensions.

(*continued on pg. 998*)

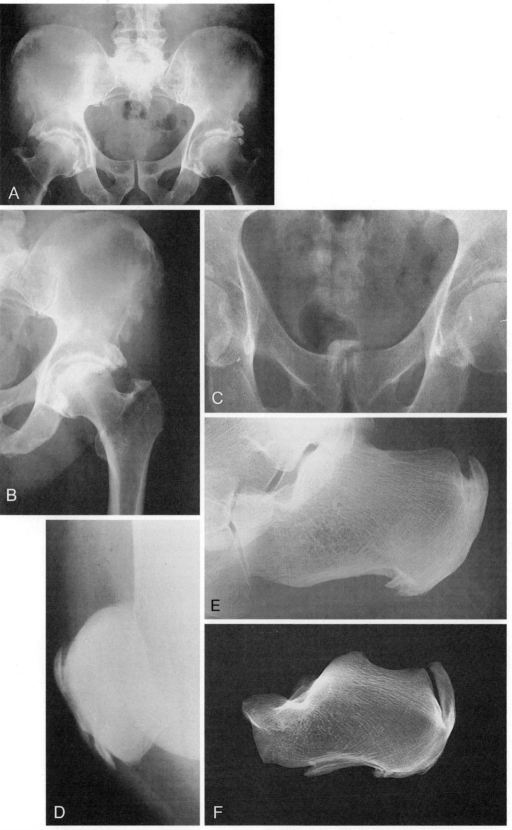

Figure 10-70   **DIFFUSE IDIOPATHIC SKELETAL HYPER-OSTOSIS: EXTRASPINAL MANIFESTATIONS. A. AP Pelvis.** Note the typical distribution and bilateral symmetry of hyperostosis involving the iliac crests, iliac spines, and acetabulum. **B. Hip.** Note that the close-up view clearly demonstrates entheseal hyperostosis from the anterosuperior iliac spine, anteroinferior iliac spine, supra-acetabulum, and trochanters. **C. Symphysis Pubis.** Observe the large bony spur partially bridging the joint. **D. Patella.** Note the ossification of the quadriceps tendons at their patellar attachments. **E and F. Calcaneus.** Note the hypostotic bone formation within the Achilles tendon attachment and plantar aponeurosis.

CAPSULE SUMMARY
Diffuse Idiopathic Skeletal Hyperostosis (continued)

Clinical Features

- Male predilection, usually after 5th decade of life.
- Variable symptomatology, though chronic and low grade, with joint motion relatively unaffected.
- Approximately 30% of cases have peripheral joint manifestations.
- Adult onset diabetes mellitus in 13–32% of cases.
- Dysphagia in 20% of patients.
- No predisposition to spinal fractures, but may develop spinal stenosis owing to ossification of the PLL.

Radiologic Features

- *Spine:* diagnostic criteria include flowing ossification of at least four contiguous segments, disc height relatively normal, apophyseal and sacroiliac joints normal.
- Hyperostosis is usually anterior to the spine and can be 1–20 mm thick, continuous or flame configuration.
- About 50% of cases have ossification of the PLL, which is separated from the posterior vertebral body by a vertical lucent area and is most common in the cervical spine; conservative care unless severe, then laminectomy.
- *Extraspinal sites:* roughened bony attachments, ligament or tendon ossification.

OSSIFIED POSTERIOR LONGITUDINAL LIGAMENT SYNDROME

Ossification of the posterior longitudinal ligament (OPLL) is a condition that may result in compression myelopathy of the spinal cord. The first recorded case was in 1960 by Tsukimato, an autopsy of a 47-year-old male with progressive myelopathy that revealed ossification in a thickened posterior longitudinal ligament. (1) The actual term of ossification of the posterior longitudinal ligament was introduced in 1964 by Terayama et al. (2)

Since the publication of these original works, numerous reports of OPLL syndrome have been published. Evaluation of these reports demonstrates a definite association between the simultaneous presence of diffuse idiopathic skeletal hyperostosis and an inherent predisposition for such to occur in the Japanese population (*Japanese disease*). (3,4) It has been suggested that the traditional high-salt, low-meat Japanese diet may influence the prevalence of OPLL in this population. (5) Other sources believe that OPLL is far more common in Europe and North America than documented but is less symptomatic owing to a relative decrease in the narrowing of the spinal canal when compared with the Japanese population. (6) The first reported involvement in non-Japanese patients was by Minagiand Gronner in 1969. (7) The most common location for OPLL to occur is in the cervical spine, followed by the thoracic and lumbar spines. (4)

Clinical Features

OPLL may or may not be symptomatic. (3,8,9) The most common symptom-producing region when involved with OPLL is the cervical spine. Conversely, the least symptom-producing region is the thoracic spine. (10) Abnormalities, when seen, are generally insidious in onset, with motor and sensory disturbances predominantly involving the legs. A common initial complaint is progressive difficulty in walking as cord myelopathy progresses. Sensory changes consist of paresthesias and diminished tactile sensations over gradually increasing regions. Pain in the spine is often absent but, when present, is identical to pain of musculoskeletal origin. These aberrations are particularly prominent when the ossified posterior longitudinal ligament occupies > 60% of the sagittal diameter of the cervical canal. Laboratory evaluations are typically unrewarding. Laminectomy should be performed on patients displaying signs of myelopathy. (11)

Pathologic Features

Examination of the ossified ligament reveals some unique findings that correlate closely with the observed radiographic depiction. Macroscopically, the PLL is thicker and broader than normal. Usually, ossification is present as a continuous band over three to four segments traversing the intervening disc spaces. Occasionally, it may be localized to a single segment. (12) (Fig. 10-71) The ossified ligamentous tissue is distinctively hard and non-deforming.

Microscopically, the involved ligament shows a cortical bone appearance composed of lamellar bone, well-developed Haversian canals, and poorly developed marrow cavities. This ossification occurs predominantly in the superficial layers of the ligament, leaving the underlying deep layers relatively unaffected. (13) Adjacent hyperostosis of the posterior vertebral body is also often seen. (3) There is usually a distinct absence of posterior disc protrusion, although it can occur. (12)

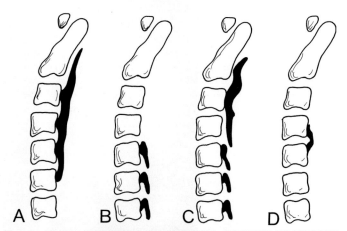

Figure 10-71 PATTERNS OF CERVICAL OSSIFIED POSTERIOR LONGITUDINAL LIGAMENT. These range from isolated to contiguous forms, but note the tendency to remain separated from the posterior vertebral bodies. (Adapted from **Hirabayashi K, Miyakawa J, Satomi K, et al.:** *Operative results and postoperative progression of ossification among patients with ossification of cervical posterior longitudinal ligament.* Spine 6(4):354, 1981.)

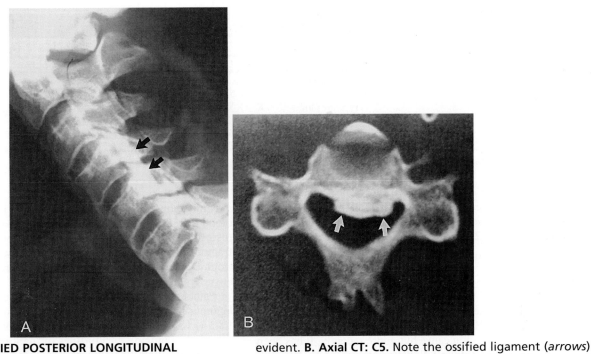

Figure 10-72 **OSSIFIED POSTERIOR LONGITUDINAL LIGAMENT: CERVICAL SPINE. A. Lateral Cervical.** Note the thick band of ossification posterior to the C3 and C4 segments (*arrows*). Exuberant anterior body hyperostosis is also evident. **B. Axial CT: C5.** Note the ossified ligament (*arrows*) with a decreased central canal size. (Courtesy of Lawrence A. Cooperstein, MD, Pittsburgh, Pennsylvania.)

Spinal cord changes in OPLL are well documented and consist of compression-related abnormalities, such as flattening, gray matter infarction, and demyelination of the posterior and lateral white columns. (14)

Radiologic Features

Radiographic examination is the most dependable diagnostic method for identifying OPLL. Irrespective of what spinal region is involved, the roentgen signs are distinctive and best portrayed on the lateral radiograph. Characteristically, the most common location for OPLL is in the cervical spine, particularly the middle and upper regions. Less commonly, involvement of the thoracic (T4–T7) and lumbar spines (L1–L3) will be seen. (4)

The most reliable diagnostic sign is the characteristic dense, linear radiopaque strip of 1–5 mm thickness, paralleling the posterior vertebral body margins. (Fig. 10-72) Commonly, a radiolucent zone is interspaced between the ossified ligament and vertebral body, corresponding to the unossified deeper ligamentous layers. This is well shown on axial CT sections. MRI may show OPLL as a high signal intensity (fatty marrow) or hypointense band (fibrous replacement of fatty marrow). (15) The length of this ossification may be only one vertebral body width or traverse a number of contiguous segments.

Usually, the adjacent intervertebral discs and apophyseal joints are normal, although minor degenerative changes may be apparent. The most commonly associated abnormal radiographic findings seen in up to 85% of cases are those seen in DISH, with exuberant anterior hyperostosis and lesser posterior body hyperostosis. (13) OPLL is reported as occurring in 50% of patients with DISH. (3)

Subsequent follow-up studies using either CT or MRI are necessary to delineate the degree of encroachment present. MRI has the advantage of examining the integrity of the cord for changes of myelopathy. (15) The usual method of treatment is conservative, unless the myelopathy is progressive, where decompressive laminectomy may be necessary. (2) Prognosis after surgery is unpredictable, but up to 70% of patients will show improvement. (14)

NEUROTROPHIC ARTHROPATHY

Neurotrophic arthropathy is a destructive articular disease that occurs secondary to a loss or impairment in joint proprioception. Subsequently, the involved joint undergoes premature and excessive traumatic degenerative changes that lead to severe destruction and instability. Other terms descriptive of this condition are neurogenic arthropathy, neuroarthropathy, neurogenic osteoarthropathy, and the classic term of Charcot's joints. (1) Charcot, a French physi-

Table 10-19	Causes of Neurotrophic Arthropathy
Congenital	Acquired
Congenital indifference to pain	Alcoholism
Dysautonomia	Amyloidosis
Spina bifida vera (meningocele, etc.)	Charcot-Marie-Tooth disease
Iatrogenic	Diabetes mellitus
Indomethacin	Leprosy, yaws
Phenylbutazone	Multiple sclerosis
Steroids	Neurosyphilis
	Syringomyelia
	Trauma
	Tumor

Disease	Incidence Ranking	Percent Disease	Predominant Type	Spine			Lower Extremity				Upper Extremity			
				C	T	L	Hip	Knee	Ankle	Foot	Shoulder	Elbow	Wrist	Hand
Diabetic neuropathy	1	35	Hypertrophic			XX	X	X	XXX	XX				
Syringomyelia	3	25	Atrophic	X		X					XXX	XX	XXX	X
Syphilitic tabes	2	20	Hypertrophic		X	XXX	X	XXX	XX	X				
Myelomeningocele	4	Variable	Both				X	XXX	XX	X				
Others	5	Variable	Both						Involvement variable					

Table 10-20 Sites of Involvement in Neurotrophic Joint Disease

C, cervical; *T*, thoracic; *L*, lumbar; *X*, uncommon; *XX*, common; *XXX*, very common.

cian, in 1868 first noted a cause-and-effect association between destructive joint disease and lesions of the nervous system, specifically tabes dorsalis. (2)

Clinical Features

Neurotrophic joint disease may occur secondary to a number of conditions (Table 10-19). In the past, syphilitic neuroarthropathy had been the most common cause but, more recently, it has been replaced by diabetes. (3) Of all diabetic patients, up to 35% will develop neurotrophic arthropathy, (1) usually involving the ankle, subtalar joints, and feet, known as *Charcot's foot*. (4,5) Of syphilis patients, approximately 20% will show changes, especially in the lumbar spine, knee, and ankle. Alcoholism can produce the same hypertrophic joint destruction as diabetes in the tarsal and metatarsal articulations. (6) After traumatic paraplegia of the lumbar spine, neuropathic arthropathy below the lesion is not uncommon. (7) Up to 25% of syringomyelia patients will suffer neurotrophic arthropathy of the upper extremity, involving the shoulder, elbow, and wrist. (8) (Table 10-20) (Fig. 10-73)

Charcot's arthropathy is often a misdiagnosis (9) and neurological signs such as altered gait patterns, loss of deep reflexes, and pain insensitivity should alert the physician to the possibility of the underlying condition. Evaluation of the involved joint will reveal relatively painless instability, enlargement, and crepitus, all of which may be extreme (*bag of bones*). (10) In the early phases, recurrent, painless effusions may be the only sign. A neurotrophic joint may develop over a period of weeks, months, or years, depending on the cause, location, and severity of the underlying disease. (11) Laboratory findings will be negative for the joint disease but positive when applicable to the causative disease, such as syphilis or diabetes.

Pathologic Features

No uniform consensus exists on the exact pathogenetic sequence of events in neuroarthropathy. (10,12) Charcot in 1868 ascribed the bone and joint changes to a lack of nutrition from the central nervous system trophic centers (*French theory*). (10) Volkmann and Virchow perceived the resultant joint destruction as the cumulative effects of multiple unprotected mechanical microtraumatic events (*German theory*). (12)

Currently, there is general agreement on the neurotraumatic theory whereby destructive joint changes occur as the sequela to an ineffective protective neurological mechanism. (Fig. 10-74) However, a neurovascular theory has been proposed to explain the cyclic progression of radiographic changes. (12) This mech-

anism is thought to be owing to an initial increased intraosseous blood flow that is neurologically initiated, stimulating osteoclastic resorption. Consequently, as bone is resorbed (atrophic phase), fractures and joint damage occur. With weight bearing, hypertrophic changes such as osteophytes, sclerosis, and loose bodies ensue (hypertrophic phase).

Pathologic examination of an involved joint demonstrates cartilaginous fibrillation, flaking, and denudation of the articular cortex. Intra-articular osseous and cartilaginous debris may be extreme and found even outside the confines of the joint capsule. (13) Bony alterations consist of fragmentation, sclerosis, and osteophytes of variable size.

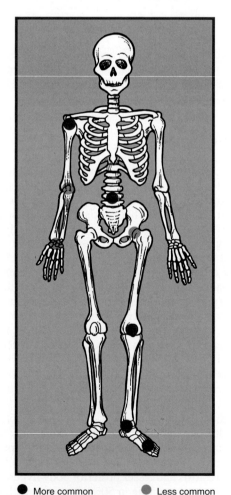

● More common   ● Less common

Figure 10-73 **SKELETAL DISTRIBUTION OF NEUROTROPHIC ARTHROPATHY.**

Altered neurological status
(sensation, proprioception)

↓

Supporting structure relaxation
(muscles, ligaments)

Physiological
activity →

↓

Misalignment

↓

Progressive joint destruction
(cartilage disruption, bone fragmentation, sclerosis)

↓

Disorganization
(Charcot's joint)

Figure 10-74 **PATHOGENETIC SEQUENCE OF EVENTS IN NEUROTROPHIC JOINT DISEASE.**

Table 10-21	Radiologic Features in Neurotrophic Arthropathy	
Hypertrophic		**Atrophic**
Distended joint		Resorbed articular surface
Density increase		Tapered bone ends
Debris production		
Dislocation		
Disorganization		
Destruction		

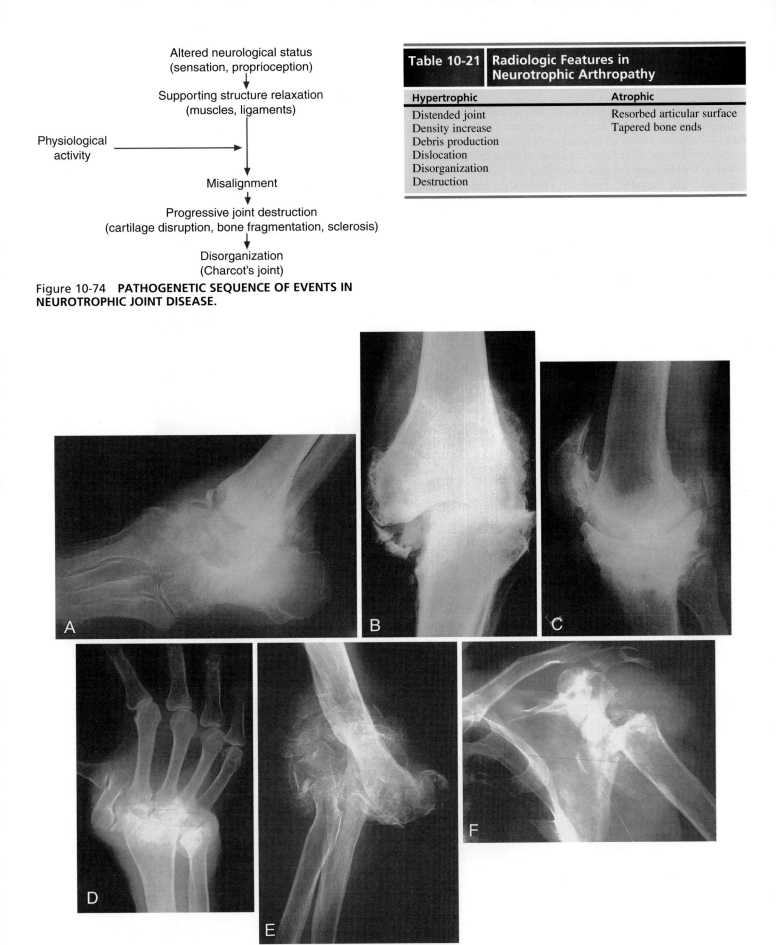

Figure 10-75 **NEUROTROPHIC ARTHROPATHY: HYPER-TROPHIC FEATURES. A. Ankle. B and C. Knee.** Syphilis. **D. Wrist. E. Elbow. F. Shoulder.** Syringomyelia. *COMMENT:* Hypertrophic neurotrophic arthropathy is characterized by the *six Ds:*—**d**istension, **d**ensity increase, **d**ebris, **d**islocation, **d**isorganization, and **d**estruction.

Radiologic Features

Distinctive radiographic changes in the early phases of the developing arthropathy are usually absent, except for a chronic, painless effusion, signs of degenerative joint disease, and spontaneous fractures. (14) Over a period of months to years, the changes will become more advanced as the joint becomes disorganized and unstable; however, observable and often rapid destruction may occur within a number of weeks. (11) Two essential radiographic appearances of a joint occur, according to the degree of bony proliferation or resorption: hypertrophic and atrophic. (Table 10-21)

Hypertrophic Pattern. The hypertrophic pattern characterized by the *six Ds:* joint **d**istension, increased subchondral den-

sity, **d**ebris, **d**islocation, **d**isorganization, and bone **d**estruction. This is most commonly found and more pronounced in the weight-bearing joints of the lumbar spine, hips, knees, and ankles. (Figs. 10-75 and 10-76)

Atrophic Pattern. Conversely, the atrophic pattern shows a distinct lack of the "hypertrophic" features. It may occur as a secondary change in a previously hypertrophic joint or arise in an otherwise normal joint. This type is seen most commonly in the non-weight-bearing joints of the upper extremity, especially the shoulder, elbow, and wrist, as well as the hip and foot. (15) The appearance may simulate a sharp transverse surgical amputation of the articular end of the bone. At other times the bone will taper gradually toward the joint space and has been likened to a *licked candy stick.* (Fig. 10-77)

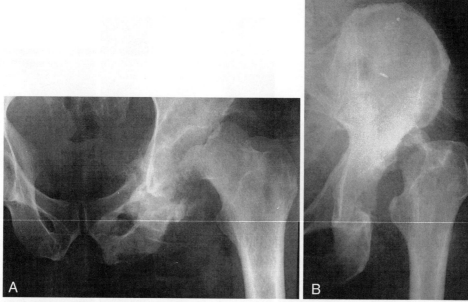

Figure 10-76   NEUROTROPHIC ARTHROPATHY: SYPHILIS.
A. Hypertrophic Pattern, AP Hip. Observe the density, debris, destruction, and dislocation of the joint. **B. Atrophic Pattern,** **AP Hip.** In contrast, observe that the femoral head has been resorbed, with a distinct lack of debris. (Panel A courtesy of Lawrence A. Cooperstein, MD, Pittsburgh, Pennsylvania.)

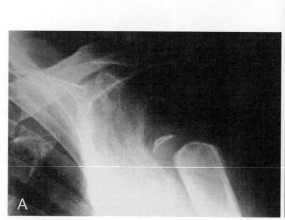

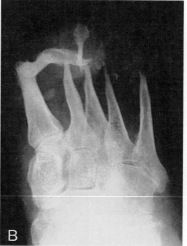

Figure 10-77   NEUROTROPHIC ARTHROPATHY: ATROPHIC **FEATURES. A. Syringomyelia, Shoulder.** Note the amputated appearance to the humerus. **B. Diabetes, Foot.** Note that the distal metatarsals are tapered, producing a licked candy stick configuration.

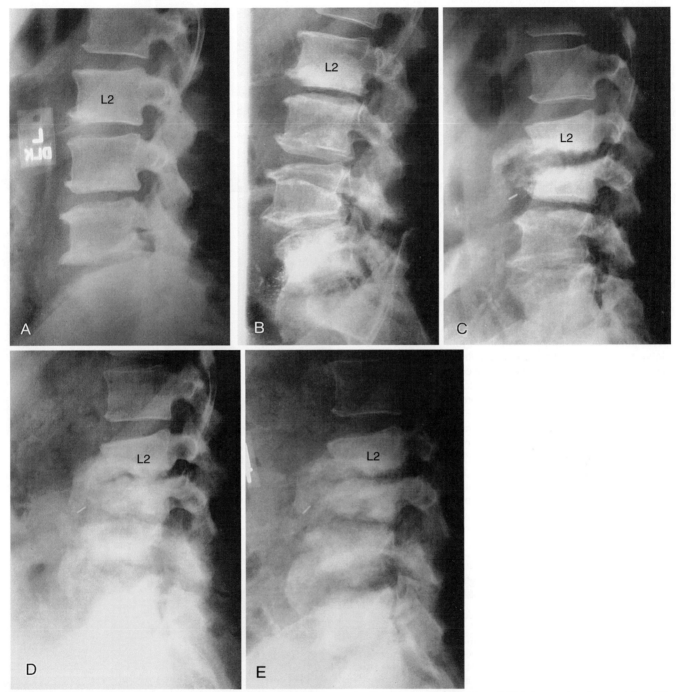

Figure 10-78 **NEUROTROPHIC ARTHROPATHY: PROGRESSIVE CHANGES WITH SYPHILIS. LUMBAR SPINE. A. Initial Study.** Note that degenerative changes are visible with osteophytes and loss of disc height. **B. 3-Year Follow-Up.** Note that advancement of the degenerative changes is most prominent at L2 and L5. **C. 6-Year Follow-Up.** Observe the severe discovertebral joint destruction with sclerosis and bony debris at the L2–L3 level. **D. 9-Year Follow-Up.** Note that the process has extended to the remaining lower lumbar levels with progressive collapse of the lumbar vertebral bodies. **E. 10-Year Follow-Up.** Observe the complete destruction of vertebral bodies and intervertebral disc spaces with exuberant bone formation and debris, completing the process (tumbling building-block spine, jigsaw vertebra). (Courtesy of Lawrence T. Sellers, DC, DACBR, Portland, Oregon.)

Target Sites Involvement

Spine. The most common location is in the lumbar spine. The pattern is distinctively hypertrophic in character, with prominent loss of disc height, sclerosis, osteophytes, and vacuum phenomena. (16) (Fig. 10-78) In addition, there may be fragmentation of the vertebral body, which may be extensive (*jigsaw vertebra*). (17) Vertebral malalignment with anterior, posterior, and lateral displacements (*tumbling building-block spine*) denotes the underlying ligamentous instability. (17) (Table 10-22) These spinal changes are most frequent in syphilitic neuroarthropathy and may be the only site of involvement at the time of first presentation. (8)

Knee. Neurotrophic arthropathy of the knee is distinctively hypertrophic in nature. (Figs. 10-75, *B* and *C,* and 10-79) In the earliest phases joint effusion and degenerative changes can be the only observable changes. An early finding may be a fracture, especially through the medial tibial plateau. Generally, localization of changes to the medial compartment of the joint in the early phases is common. More advanced changes exhibit features of the hypertrophic variety. Subchondral sclerosis may extend a considerable distance along the femoral and tibial epiphyses and metaphyses. Debris is often prominent. Destruction of the articular surface is a key sign, especially of the tibial plateau. Malalignment can be severe, with lateral displacement of the tibia and fibula in relation to the femur. The patella also may be dislocated laterally.

Foot. At the ankle, the characteristic early site of involvement is the subtalar joints. (Figs. 10-75*A* and 10-80) This is demonstrated by hypertrophic changes at the talocalcaneal junction and collapse of the lowest portions of the talus. Later, with more widespread involvement, the entire talus may be destroyed. In addition, at the ankle mortise, malleolar fractures and destructive alterations at the tibia and talar articulating surfaces can be prominent, with sclerosis, fragmentation, and malalignment. In the forefoot there is frequently isolation of changes to the metatarsal head region. Fractures through the shafts and necks are frequent and occasionally are found at the tarsometatarsal region. There is a tendency toward an atrophic pattern, as evidenced by a tapered configuration of the metatarsal bones and adjacent phalanges. (Fig. 10-81) Frequently, the metatarsals appear spread apart owing to the disrupted support in the soft tissue. Resnick described this process as radiographically resembling "osteoarthritis with a vengeance." (8)

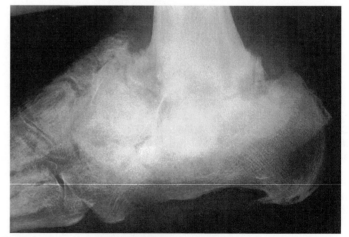

Figure 10-79 NEUROTROPHIC ARTHROPATHY: SYPHILIS. A–D. AP Knee. Observe the rapidity of the progressive changes over a 4-month period. Note the characteristic early collapse of the medial tibial plateau and the relative sparing of the femoral condyles, even in the most advanced film.

Table 10-22	Summary of Terms Used in Neurotrophic Joint Disease
Term	**Definition**
Bag of bones	Clinical term to describe the palpable signs of an advanced neuropathic joint
Charcot's joints	Physical appearance of a neuropathic joint of any cause owing to disorganization, debris, and distension
Clutton's joints	Physical appearance of bilateral nonpainful swelling, usually in the knees, owing to congenital syphilis
Jigsaw vertebra	Fragmented appearance of a vertebral body owing to multiple fractures
Licked candy stick	Generalized pencil-like tapering of a long bone toward a joint owing to atrophic resorption
Surgical amputation	Abrupt end to a long bone some distance from its articulation with complete absence of the epiphysis and often the entire metaphysis
Tumbling building-block spine	Multisegmental subluxated vertebral bodies simulating falling building blocks

Figure 10-80 NEUROTROPHIC ARTHROPATHY: SYPHILIS. Lateral Ankle. Note that the total collapse and fragmentation of the talus have produced the classic signs of hypertrophic neuroarthropathy in this location.

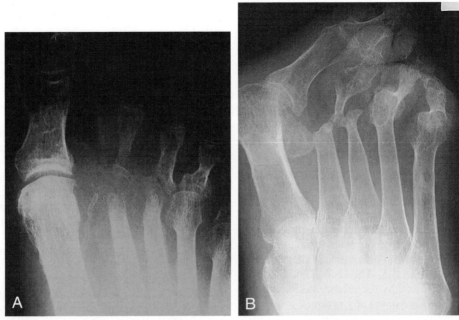

Figure 10-81   **NEUROTROPHIC ARTHROPATHY: DIABETES. FOREFOOT. A. Early Atrophic Changes.** Note the tapered contour of the second and third metatarsal heads. Note the vascular calcification frequently seen in diabetic patients.

B. Later Changes. Observe that the tapered configuration is easily identified in association with osteolysis of adjacent bones.

CAPSULE SUMMARY   Neurotrophic Arthropathy

General Considerations

- Occurs in any joint where there is a loss of or impairment in the sensory and proprioceptive pathways.
- This results in abnormal joint stresses, which eventually produce excessive, premature articular degeneration and instability.

Clinical Features

- Distinct lack of objective and subjective pain despite joint swelling, instability, and crepitation.
- Absent deep reflexes, analgesia, ataxia, and serology (possibly) positive for underlying pathological cause.

Pathologic Features

- Loss of the normal protective nervous reflexes leads to lax ligaments and muscles.
- Abnormal joint mechanics result in rapid and excessive degeneration of articular cartilage, hypertrophic spurs and bone formation, fractures, and complete joint disorganization.
- Later, bone may be resorbed at the articular surfaces, especially in the upper extremity and when weightbearing is no longer possible.

Radiologic Features

- *Two basic types:* hypertrophic and atrophic.
- *Hypertrophic:* classic type in which bone production is the dominant feature and summarized as the six Ds:
  Distension: earliest finding owing to effusion.
  Density: increase in subchondral bone sclerosis.
  Debris: bony intra-articular fragments.
  Dislocation: joint surfaces often malaligned.
  Disorganization: joint components usually disrupted (bag of bones).
  Destruction: articular bone shows loss of bone substance.
- Usually predominates in the weight-bearing joints such as the lumbar spine, hips, knees, ankle, and tarsus.
- *Atrophic:* may follow hypertrophic phase or occur as an isolated finding, and is especially more common in the shoulder, hip, and foot.
- Articular ends of bone may appear surgically amputated or tapered like a licked candy stick; absence of six Ds.
- *Spine:* usually lumbar region, with large osteophytes, prominent sclerosis, advanced discopathy, severe subluxations, and body fragmentation.
- *Knee:* hypertrophic features—sclerosis, debris, destruction, and dislocation.
- *Foot:* hypertrophic, especially in subtalar joints. Atrophic in forefoot, especially in metatarsophalangeal joint region.

SYNOVIOCHONDROMETAPLASIA

Synoviochondrometaplasia is a benign arthropathy characterized by synovial tissue undergoing metaplastic transformation to produce foci of cartilage. (1,2) This results in multiple loose bodies within the joint and ensuing clinical findings ranging from the complete absence of symptoms to acute joint locking and pain. The condition has otherwise been referred to as synovial chondromatosis, osteochondromatosis, osteochondral loose bodies, and joint mice. This condition is not owing to osteochondritis dissecans but is a separate and distinct entity.

Clinical Features

Synoviochondrometaplasia is most frequently encountered in the 3rd–5th decades, occurring in males approximately three times more commonly. (3) It is often precipitated by trauma and the knee is the most common site of involvement, being affected in approximately 70% of cases. (1,4,5) The second most common site is the hip (20%), followed by the elbow, ankle, shoulder, and wrist. (4–6) (Fig. 10-82) Almost any synovial joint can be involved, but it is distinctively uncommon outside these locations. (7,8) It is rare in the spine but when present may be a

source of compressive myelopathy. (9) Extra-articular synovial tissues of bursae and tendon sheaths are also infrequently involved. Although formation in popliteal cysts is well recognized, they may move between examinations (*migrating mouse sign*). (10–13)

The onset is usually insidious with often no antecedent history of direct trauma. Clinical manifestations are generally mild and chronic, with intermittent swelling, low-grade dull pain, reduced motion, and crepitus. Usually only a single joint is involved. (4) Intermittent acute exacerbations of pain, swelling, and joint locking can occur as sequelae to the osteochondral fragment being entrapped between opposing joint surfaces. Generally, there is a paucity of interference in joint function, despite the size of the cartilage masses. There is a gradual tendency of a progressive intensification of these symptoms over a period of years. They seem to promote early DJD of the involved joint. (4,14) Occasionally, spontaneous regression may occur but, usually, surgical removal is indicated. (15,16) Once removed, recurrence may occur in up to 15% of cases within a variable period. (4,14) In the absence of recurrence, surgical intervention has a good prognostic outcome. (17,18) A tenuous link to degeneration to chondrosarcoma has been described at an approximate incidence of 5%. (4,19) Malignant change has not been correlated with the age of the patient, the age of the lesion, or the site of the lesion. (4)

Pathologic Features

Two types of synoviochondrometaplasia are evident: primary and secondary. In the primary form no single causal factor can be isolated. This form apparently arises spontaneously, although recurrent microtrauma has been strongly implicated. The more common secondary form occurs as a sequela to degenerative and neuropathic joint disease, osteochondritis dissecans, osteochondral fractures, and joint dislocations.

The pathologic alterations in the two types are essentially identical. There is evidence to suggest that the formation of these

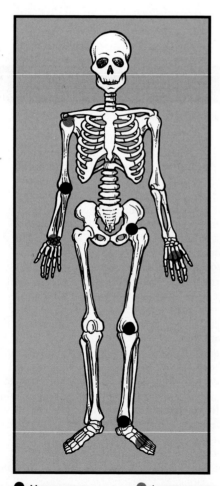

● More common   ● Less common

Figure 10-82 **SKELETAL DISTRIBUTION OF SYNOVIOCHONDROMETAPLASIA.**

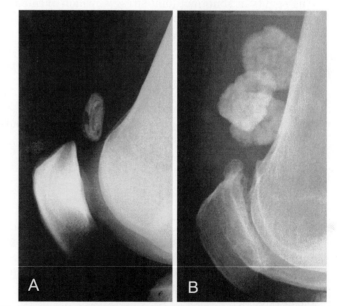

Figure 10-83 **RADIOGRAPHIC APPEARANCE OF LOOSE BODIES: KNEE. A. Laminated.** Note the alternating opaque and lucent layers. **B. Stippled.** Observe the circular lucent areas in the opaque matrix.

osteochondral bodies is an expression of benign neoplasia. (5) The pathologic changes consist of the synovial cells beneath the surface lining of the synovium transforming to produce discrete foci of cartilage cells and cartilage matrix. This involves at least 2 cm of synovium. These cartilaginous clusters enlarge and eventually protrude beyond the synovial surface. Some remain attached to the synovium, while others ultimately break free and result in freely mobile intra-articular loose bodies. Each loose body maintains nutrition from the surrounding synovial fluid, allowing further growth. The cartilage cells may eventually become more metaplastic, producing calcification and ossification within the loose body, giving the distinctive radi-

ographic appearance of laminated and stippled radiolucencies within the opaque matrix. (11,16) (Fig. 10-83)

Malignant transformation has been documented, but is rare. Repeated trauma to the articular surfaces by these loose bodies will predispose the patient to premature degenerative joint disease.

Radiologic Features

Radiologic evaluations will be unrewarding if the loose bodies lack calcification or ossification and may be visible only as indistinct soft tissue masses. Arthrograms and arthroscopy will be

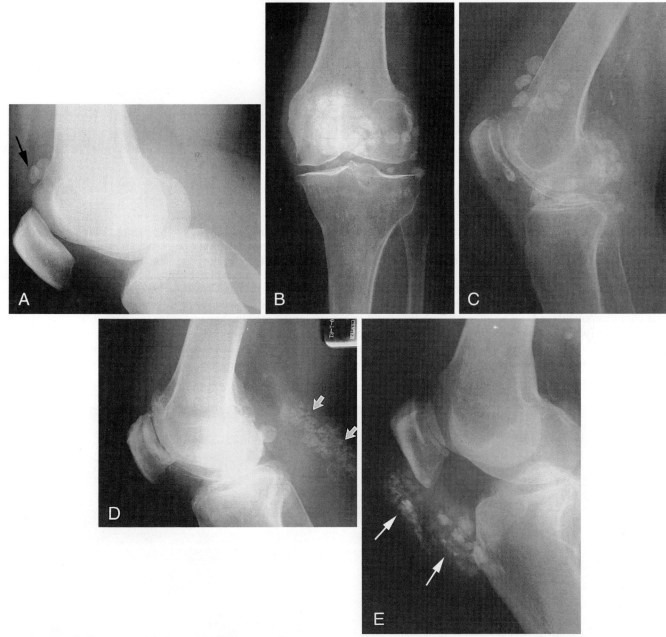

Figure 10-84   **SYNOVIOCHONDROMETAPLASIA: KNEE.**
A. Suprapatellar Pouch. Note the two loose bodies above the patella (*arrow*). **B and C. Intra-articular.** Note the multiple loose bodies throughout the entire joint. Of incidental notation is atherosclerotic plaquing of the distal femoral artery. **D. Baker's Cyst.** Observe the loose bodies extending far posteriorly, beyond the normal capsular boundaries (*arrows*). **E. Prepatellar Bursa.** Note the multiple densities anterior to the patellar ligament (*arrows*). (Panel A courtesy of Debra J. Proechel, DC, Waseca, Minnesota. Panel E courtesy of Tyrone Wei, DC, DACBR, Portland, Oregon.)

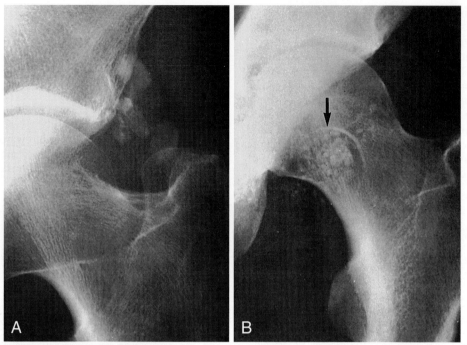

Figure 10-85 SYNOVIOCHONDROMETAPLASIA. A and B. AP Hip. Note the multiple loose bodies. Also observe the associated extrinsic pressure erosion of the femoral neck (*arrow*).

necessary for the diagnosis to be established (20); however, when opacified, as in up to 85% of cases, their appearance is virtually diagnostic. (21) (Figs. 10-84 to 10-90; Table 10-23) CT is useful in identifying small ossicles and extrinsic intra-articular pressure erosions, if present. (22) (Fig. 10-86)

Each individual loose body varies in size from 1 to 20 mm; however, large concretions up to 20 cm have been recorded (giant synovial chondromatosis). (23) The shape is usually round to ovoid, but a flat, faceted contour may be present where another loose body or adjacent bone comes into contact. The margins are distinctively sharp and well defined, especially in larger loose

bodies. The internal matrix characteristically demonstrates evidence of concentric opaque and lucent laminations or stippled, isolated lucencies within a homogenous opacity. Occasionally, the loose body may be homogeneously sclerotic and structureless, while at other times individual trabecular patterns are identifiable. MRI will reveal focal low signal intensities on all pulse sequences, with areas of isointensity on T1-weighted images and hyperintensity on T2-weighted images. (24)

Extrinsic intra-articular pressure erosions of bone may be visible, especially in joints with a tight joint capsule such as the hip. (25) (Fig. 10-85B) These are seen as concave indentations of the

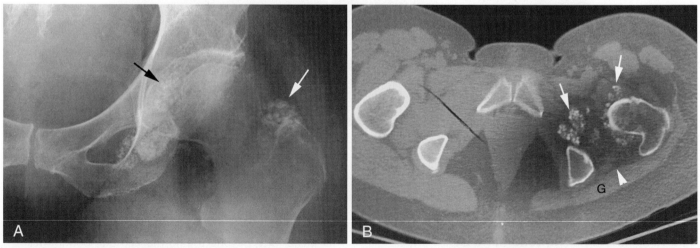

Figure 10-86 SYNOVIOCHONDROMETAPLASIA: HIP. A. AP Hip. Note the multiple punctate opacities throughout the hip joint (*arrows*). No extrinsic bone erosions are present. **B. Bone Window Axial CT: Hip.** Observe the calcified loose bodies around the hip (*arrows*). Also carefully observe, by comparing with the contralateral normal side, the increased fat separating muscle planes (*arrowhead*) and the diminished muscle mass of the gluteus maximus (*G*) owing to disuse atrophy from long-standing hip dysfunction. (Courtesy of Lawrence A. Cooperstein, MD, Pittsburgh, Pennsylvania.)

cortex within the confines of the joint capsule and distinctively display a sclerotic margin with no associated periosteal new bone formation. The concentric erosion of the femoral neck produces an *apple core deformity*. (26,27) MRI is useful in the identification of bone erosions, being identified in 80% of cases. (21) Following removal of the loose bodies, the erosions resolve within 12 months. (27) Varying degrees of DJD are also frequently visible.

The differential diagnosis of synoviochondrometaplasia includes pseudo-gout, synovioma, chondrosarcoma, pigmented villonodular synovitis, tuberculous arthritis, and normal sesamoid bones. (3,28) (Fig. 10-91) The most commonly confused normal variant at the knee is the fabella, a sesamoid bone in the lateral head of the gastrocnemius tendon. Radiographically, the fabella is seen in the popliteal fossa; on the AP view, it appears in the lateral joint compartment and lacks the typical laminated appearance of an osteochondral loose body.

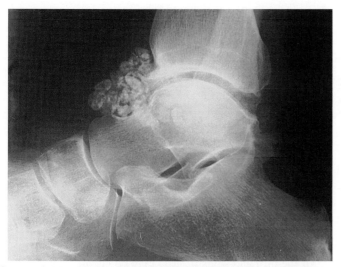

Figure 10-87 **SYNOVIOCHONDROMETAPLASIA: ANKLE.** Note the loss of joint space and the anterior collection of calcified loose bodies with evidence of an anterior osteophyte from the tibia.

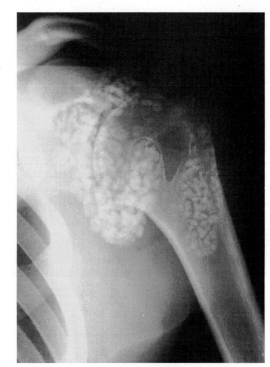

Figure 10-88 **SYNOVIOCHONDROMETAPLASIA: SHOULDER.** Observe the large number of opacified loose bodies outlining the extent of the synovial joint and bursae.

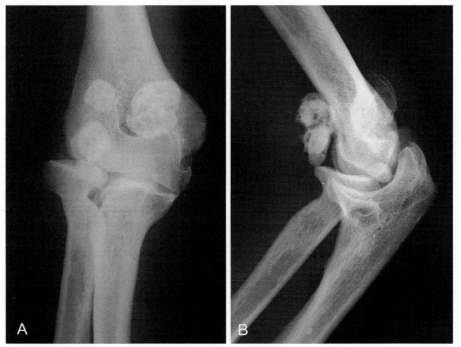

Figure 10-89 **SYNOVIOCHONDROMETAPLASIA. A and B. Elbow.** Observe the lucent stippling of the loose bodies. Note the old fracture deformity of the radial head.

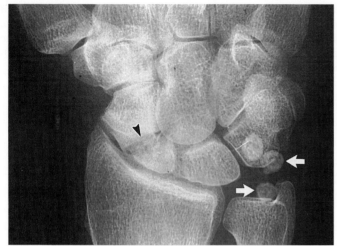

Figure 10-90   SYNOVIOCHONDROMETAPLASIA: WRIST.
Note the stippled osteochondral loose bodies in the ulnar compartment of the wrist (*arrows*). Observe the un-united and avascular scaphoid fracture (*arrowhead*).

Table 10-23	Radiologic Features of Synoviochondrometaplasia	
Feature	**Common**	**Uncommon**
Locations	Knee, hip, ankle, elbow, wrist	Shoulder, hand, foot, extra-articular (esp. popliteal cysts)
Appearance	Soft tissue masses Single or multiple Opacities—round ovoid, 1–20 mm laminated or stippled Faceted Degenerative joint disease Mobile	Intracapsular extrinsic bone erosion Multiple joint involvement
Differential diagnosis	Sesamoid bones Osteochondritis dissecans	Pigmented villonodular, synovitis, pseudo-gout, chondrosarcoma, synovioma, tuberculosis

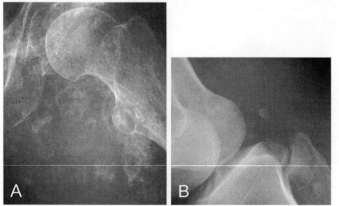

Figure 10-91   DIFFERENTIAL DIAGNOSIS: SYNOVIOCHONDRO-METAPLASIA. A. Chondrosarcoma. Note the multiple, thin, curvilinear calcifications. **B. Fabella.** Note its characteristic location in the popliteal space.

CAPSULE SUMMARY
Synoviochondrometaplasia

General Considerations
- Benign arthropathy characterized by formation of intra-articular loose bodies with variable symptomatology.
- Synonyms include osteochondromatosis, osteochondral loose bodies, and joint mice.

Clinical Features
- Appears at 30–50 years, males 3:1.
- Insidious but intensifying pain and swelling; crepitus with locking.
- *Most common joints:* knee, hip, ankle, elbow, wrist.

Pathologic Features
- Synovial metaplasia to form cartilage, which detaches and may calcify or ossify, resulting in multiple intra-articular loose bodies.
- Primary and secondary forms.

Radiologic Features
- May be normal if the loose bodies are not calcified or ossified.
- *Loose bodies:* round to ovoid, smooth faceted, laminated, or stippled, may have internal trabeculae.
- Occasional extrinsic bone erosion (apple core deformity of the hip) and signs of DJD may be visible.
- Simulated by sesamoid bones, pseudo-gout, synovioma, chondrosarcoma, pigmented villonodular synovitis, and tuberculosis.

INFLAMMATORY DISORDERS

RHEUMATOID ARTHRITIS

Rheumatoid arthritis is a generalized connective tissue disorder of unknown cause that selectively targets synovial tissue, particularly in the peripheral joints of the hands and feet, as well as larger joints and the cervical spine. The synovium of tendon sheaths and bursae may also be affected. The disease is characterized by the bilateral symmetry and progressive nature of the joint disease, ultimately leading to deformity. Abnormalities of the cartilaginous joints are uncommon, except in the cervical spine intervertebral discs. Involvement of bone–tendon or bone–ligament junctions (enthesopathy) is an infrequent manifestation. Other body systems may be involved, including the heart, lungs, small blood vessels, nervous system, eyes, and reticulo-endothelial system.

Clinical Features

The diagnosis of classic rheumatoid arthritis requires the presence of a number of basic criteria. Early in the disease process findings may be less apparent and are, therefore, given a less definite diagnosis. (1,2) (Table 10-24) However, the clinical manifestations are often distinctive, especially when correlated with the radiographic and laboratory changes.

The onset occurs typically between the ages of 20 and 60 years, with a peak between 40 and 50 years. The disease is more prevalent in women, especially in the 20- to 40-year age group, with a 3:1 predominance over men. After 40 years, the gender predeliction approximates to 1:1. (3) There are no differences between the sexes in terms of severity, clinical signs, or radiographic features. (4) An onset before the age of 16 is classified as juvenile rheumatoid arthritis.

Signs and symptoms usually begin in an insidious manner and may be preceded by physical or emotional stress. The most prominent complaints usually are articular in nature, with pain, tenderness, swelling, and stiffness, particularly in the morning (*jelling phenomenon*). Redness of the periarticular skin is notably absent. The disease hallmark is often the bilateral and symmetric peripheral joint involvement, particularly of the hands and feet. Occasionally, limited expressions of the disease such as a monoarthritis or tenosynovitis occur initially. A paralyzed limb will notably not develop rheumatoid changes.

Most commonly, articular symptoms begin in the interphalangeal and metacarpophalangeal joints and progress proximally toward the trunk. The spine is rarely affected early, but later the cervical region will become involved in up to 80% of patients. (5) (Fig. 10-92) Joint abnormalities may have distinctive physical manifestations and have been labeled by various terms. (Table 10-25)

In addition to the articular manifestations, constitutional symptoms such as fatigue, malaise, generalized muscle weakness, and fever may be present. A variety of other clinical abnormalities can also be found, including tendon rupture, bursal extensions, Raynaud's phenomenon, osteopenia, and cervical spine subluxations or dislocations. Firm, non-tender rheumatoid nodules may be

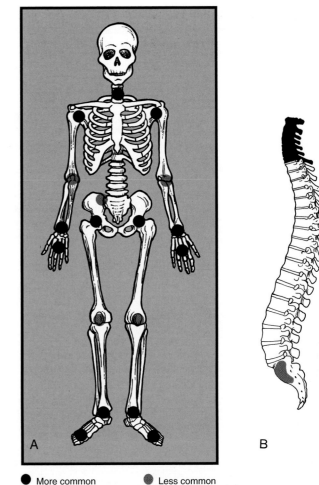

● More common   ● Less common

Figure 10-92 **SKELETAL DISTRIBUTION OF RHEUMATOID ARTHRITIS. A. Whole body. B. Spine.**

Table 10-24	Diagnostic Criteria for Rheumatoid Arthritis

Physical
   Morning stiffness
   Pain on motion or tenderness in at least one joint
   Soft tissue swelling or joint effusion in at least one joint
   Swelling of at least one other joint (within 3 months)
   Bilateral, symmetrical, and simultaneous joint swelling (except distal interphalangeal joints)
   Subcutaneous nodules—bony protuberances (extensor surfaces), juxta-articular
Laboratory
   Positive sheep agglutination test (rheumatoid factor)
   Poor mucin precipitate from synovial fluid
   Synovium—at least three of
      Marked villous hypertrophy
      Superficial synovial cell proliferation
      Marked inflammatory cell infiltrate fibrin deposition
      Foci of cell necrosis
   Nodules—granulomas with central necrosis, proliferated fixed cells, peripheral fibrosis, and chronic inflammatory cell infiltrate
   Typical changes—uniform joint space loss, marginal erosions, etc.
Classification
   Classic: > 7 criteria (with swelling for > 6 months)
   Definite: > 5 criteria (with continuous joint symptoms > 6 weeks)
   Probable: > 3 criteria (with continuous joint symptoms for 4–6 weeks)
   Possible: at least two of stiffness, pain, swelling, nodules, elevated erythrocyte sedimentation rate or C-reactive protein, or iritis, with joint symptoms for at least 3 weeks.

Data from **Ropes MW, Cobb S, Jacox R, et al.:** *Proposed diagnostic criteria for rheumatoid arthritis.* Ann Rheum Diss 16: 118, 1957; and **Ropes MW, Bennett GA, Cobb S, et al.:** *Diagnostic criteria for rheumatoid arthritis* (1958 revision). Ann Rheum Dis 18:49, 1959.

Table 10-25	Nomenclature Used in Rheumatoid Arthritis
Term	**Description**
Arthritis mutilans	Severe, polyarticular joint deformity characterized by severe articular destruction
Baker's cyst	Enlargement of the gastrocnemius–semimembranosus bursa is common and may be large in rheumatoid arthritis
Boutonniere deformity	Flexion of PIP; extension of DIP joint owing to rupture (buttonhole) of central slip of extensor digitorum communis at the PIP joint
Caplan's syndrome	Combination of pneumoconiosis and rheumatoid arthritis
Felty's syndrome	Combination of leukopenia, splenomegaly, and rheumatoid arthritis
Fibular deviation	Lateral orientation of the toes toward the fibula compartment
Haygarth's nodes	Soft tissue periarticular swellings at the dorsal surfaces of the metacarpophalangeal joints
Hitchhiker's thumb	Boutonniere deformity of the thumb; flexion of the PIP, extension of the DIP
Jelling's phenomenon	Joint is notably stiff after periods of inactivity and rest
Lanois' deformity	Fibular deviation of the digits and dorsal subluxation at the metatarsal phalangeal joints
Mallet finger	Persistent flexion of the DIP occasionally seen owing to rupture of the extensor digitorum communis tendon at the base of the distal phalanx
Rheumatoid nodule	Soft tissue accumulation of inflammatory cells with a central zone of necrosis, middle pallisaded zone, and outer zone of fibrosis; seen on extensor surfaces
Spindle digit	Fusiform appearance of a digit owing to localized PIP joint swelling
Swan-neck deformity	Flexion of DIP, extension of PIP
Ulnar deviation	Orientation of the fingers from the metacarpophalangeal joints toward the ulnar side of the wrist (ulnar drift)
Atlantoaxial instability	Excessive nonphysiologic movement of the atlas, most commonly in an anterior direction, owing to a ruptured or stretched transverse ligament
Carpal rotation	Displacement of proximal carpal bones toward the radius
Dot–dash appearance	Intermittent absence of the articular cortex owing to erosion and subchondral bone resorption
Marginal erosion	Rat bite, pocket erosion; localized loss of intra-articular cortex adjacent to the capsular insertion owing to pannus erosion at the anatomic bare area
Norgaard's projection	Ball catcher's, AP radiograph with the hands obliqued to 45°, as if to catch a ball, specifically to evaluate for erosions of the metacarpal head
Pencil-sharpened spinous processes	Appearance of tapered spinous processes most commonly seen in the cervical spine
Protrusio acetabuli	Medial migration of the acetabulum
Rheumatoid discitis	Combination of loss of disc height and endplate erosions
Summation effect	Decrease in neck length owing to the combination of loss of disc height, osteolysis, and upward migration of the odontoid
Terry Thomas sign	Separation of the scaphoid and lunate owing to disruption of the interosseous ligament
Zigzag deformity	Configuration of the hand in the combination of ulnar deviation and carpal radial rotation

DIP, distal interphalangeal, *PIP*, proximal interphalangeal.

palpable in approximately 20% of patients on the forearms, knees, ankles, hands, and over the sacrum. These range in size from 5 mm to 3 cm and most commonly are found immediately distal to the olecranon. (6) When present, rheumatoid nodules often denote that the course of the disease is more severe. The soft tissue swellings adjacent to the metacarpal phalangeal joints are called Haygarth's nodes.

Extra-articular manifestations may result in long nerve tract changes and peripheral compression syndromes, especially of the carpal tunnel. In the eyes, perforation of the sclera (scleromalacia perforans) can precipitate ocular complications. Atrophy of the lacrimal glands may be associated, leading to dry eyes (keratoconjunctivitis sicca—Sjögren's syndrome). Vasculitis subsequently will produce skin ulceration and gangrenous sequelae, especially of the periphery.

Laboratory evaluations are usually supportive. Anemia (normochromic, normocytic), elevated or normal leukocyte count, and elevated ESR and C-reactive protein (CRP), paralleling the levels of disease activity are typical. Demonstration of the rheumatoid factor in up to 70% of patients is a useful determinant but is not specific for rheumatoid arthritis. (7) A small percentage of patients will have false positives for syphilis and lupus erythematosus. An unusual combination of rheumatoid arthritis, leukopenia, and splenomegaly has been called Felty's syndrome. (8)

The course and prognosis of the disease is unpredictable but recent research has found that markers such a CRP and rheumatoid factor may be of benefit. (9) The identification of structural damage through imaging is also of use in determining outcome. (10) The average patient can expect periods of remission and exacerbations with gradual progression of deformity and disability. The minority will experience complete remission. Features associated with a poor prognosis include (*a*) presence of subcutaneous nodules and high levels of rheumatoid factor; (*b*) exacerbation of disease for more than 1 year's duration; (*c*) onset earlier than the age of 30; and (*d*) extra-articular manifestations.

Pathologic Features

Synovial Articulations

The sequential pathologic changes in synovial tissue of joints, bursae, and tendon sheaths are distinctive and correlate closely with observable radiographic alterations. (Table 10-26) (Fig. 10-93) ***General Pathologic Process.*** The initial abnormalities consist of acute synovitis with edema and congestion in the synovial membrane, effusion, periarticular edema, and juxta-articular hyperemia. (11) Subsequent synovial proliferation forms pannus,

Table 10-26	Pathologic–Radiologic Correlation in Rheumatoid Arthritis
Pathologic Features	**Radiologic Features**
Synovial edema and effusion	Periarticular soft tissue swelling
Rheumatoid nodule	Subcutaneous soft tissue mass
Cartilage destruction by pannus	Uniform loss of joint space
Pannus eroding in the bare area	Marginal erosion
Intraosseous pannus and synovial fluid intrusions	Subchondral bone cysts
Inflammatory hyperemia	Juxta-articular osteoporosis
Periostitis	Juxta-articular periosteal new bone (linear)
Fibrous tissue metaplasia	Ankylosis
Capsule and ligamentous laxity, tendon rupture	Deformity

a vascular granulation tissue that spreads over the intra-articular surfaces of bone and cartilage. At the anatomic bare area, where intra-articular bone is in direct contact with this proliferating synovium, marginal bone erosions are found. (12) Intrusion of the pannus into the marrow spaces of the subchondral bone produces cyst-like cavities. The hyaline cartilage erodes and narrows as the overlying adherent pannus releases chondrolytic collagenase enzymes and interferes with its nutrition. Eventually, the whole joint cavity is filled with proliferating pannus, which undergoes progressive fibrosis, precipitating fibrous ankylosis, and, less commonly, bony ankylosis.

Atlantoaxial Joint. The conspicuous pathologic changes that occur at the synovial atlantoaxial joint warrant special evaluation. The unique anatomy of this articulation allows for frequent and often serious pathologic changes to occur. Synovial tissue is normally present between the anterior tubercle and the anterior odontoid surface as well as between the transverse ligament and posterior odontoid surface. Occasionally, synovial tissue may be present adjacent to the apex of the odontoid. Pannus formation in these sites of synovial tissue often precipitates odontoid erosion, even to the extent of complete odontoid dissolution. (13) (Fig. 10-94) In addition, the transverse ligament becomes stretched from the combined action of the adjacent distended synovium and tissue

changes, as well as the associated hyperemia, promoting loosening of the ligamentous attachments by decalcification.

The resultant sequela is atlantoaxial instability, which may progress to subluxation or complete dislocation with cord compression and vertebrobasilar insufficiency. (14) This sequence of events is the common pathophysiologic pathway by which all of the inflammatory spondyloarthropathies produce atlantoaxial instability. (Table 10-27).

Cartilaginous Articulations

The pathologic mechanisms involved in the development of cartilaginous joint changes at the intervertebral disc and other sites are poorly understood. At the discovertebral junction, loss of disc height and endplate erosions are common, particularly in the cervical spine. They may represent erosions from invading pannus at the adjacent von Luschka's (neurocentral) joints or from Schmorl's node formation precipitated by apophyseal joint instability. (15,16)

Entheses

Inflammatory changes at bone–ligament or bone–tendon junctions (enthesopathy) is uncommon in rheumatoid arthritis, in contrast to the seronegative arthropathies of ankylosing spondylitis, psoriasis, Reiter's syndrome, and enteropathic arthritis. The most apparent entheseal change occurs at the tips of the spinous processes of the cervical vertebrae, with erosions, sclerosis, and an eventual overall *tapered appearance;* however, inflammatory changes and pannus formation within interspinous bursae may be additionally implicated.

Rheumatoid Nodules

Nodules occur in up to 20% of individuals with rheumatoid arthritis. Three distinct zones are apparent: a central focus of necrosis, a middle layer of palisaded histiocytes, and an outer layer of fibrous tissue with plasma cell and lymphocytic infiltrate. Most commonly, these are subcutaneous in location but can occur in visceral organs, serous linings, and within bone. (Fig. 10-95)

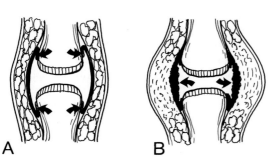
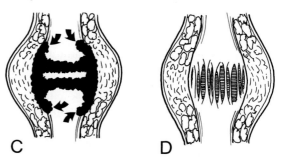

Figure 10-93 **GENERAL PATHOLOGIC PROCESS OF RHEUMATOID ARTHRITIS. A. Normal Joint.** Note the exposed bone not covered with cartilage—bare area (*arrows*). **B. Initial Changes.** Synovial proliferation (pannus) (*arrows*) with periarticular edema. **C. Bone and Joint Destruction.** Cartilage is destroyed, narrowing the joint space, while bone erosion produces radiologic changes, especially at the joint margins—marginal erosions (*arrows*). **D. Ankylosis.** This may be fibrous or bony. (Adapted from **Resnick D, Niwayama G:** *Diagnosis of Bone and Joint Disorders,* ed 2. Philadelphia, WB Saunders, 1988.)

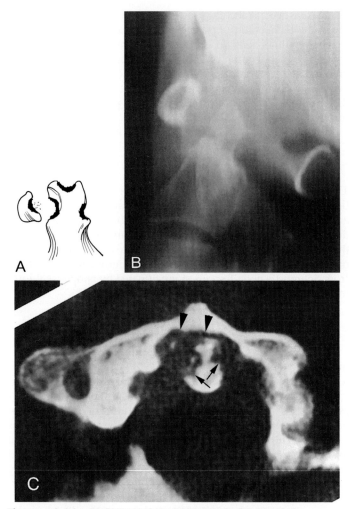

Figure 10-94 **RHEUMATOID ARTHRITIS: ODONTOID PROCESS EROSIONS. A. Diagram.** The target sites for synovial erosion of the odontoid are shown. **B. Tomogram: C1–C2.** Note the erosions at the target sites, which have diminished the size of the odontoid (whittled), eroded the anterior arch, and compromised the transverse ligament as evidenced by a widened predental interspace. **C. Axial CT: C1–C2.** Note that the odontoid is eroded as evidenced by the multiple cortical excavations (*arrows*). The anterior atlas arch is similarly eroded (*arrowheads*). (Courtesy of Steven P. Brownstein, MD, Springfield, New Jersey.)

Radiologic Features

Common radiographic expressions of rheumatoid arthritis in any joint consist of a number of well-recognized abnormalities. (Fig. 10-96; Table 10-28)

Bilateral Symmetry. Invariably, parallel changes will be seen on both sides of the body simultaneously and to a similar degree of involvement.

Periarticular Soft Tissue Swelling. Owing to soft tissue edema and intra-articular effusion, displacement of fat lines and peripheral skin contours will be visible. The density of the periarticular soft tissues is usually increased. These are typically the first radiographic signs of rheumatoid arthritis.

Juxta-Articular Osteoporosis. Early in the disease, owing to inflammatory hyperemia, there is a localized loss of bone density of the epiphysis and metaphysis adjacent to the involved joint.

Table 10-27	Inflammatory Spondyloarthropathies Associated with Atlantoaxial Instability
	Rheumatoid arthritis (most common)
	Ankylosing spondylitis
	Psoriatic arthritis
	Reiter's syndrome
	Systemic lupus erythematosus

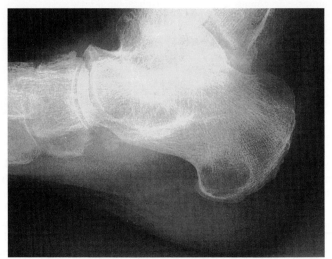

Figure 10-95 **INTRAOSSEOUS RHEUMATOID CYST: LATERAL HEEL.** The geographic loss of bone density in the calcaneus in this patient with long-standing rheumatoid arthritis was diagnosed as a Brodie's abscess. On biopsy, however, the diagnosis of an intraosseous rheumatoid nodule was made. (Courtesy of David M. Walker, DPM, Melbourne, Australia.)

Later, following disuse and steroid therapy, a more generalized osteopenia may ensue that predisposes the patient to acute and stress-type fractures. (17) Care should be taken in the evaluation of patients with long-term arthritis because the diagnosis of insufficiency fractures is often delayed or missed by simply accrediting the pain to an arthritic exacerbation. (17)

Uniform Loss of Joint Space. The entire joint space is diminished, with no isolated intra-articular compartmentalization as seen in degenerative joint disease. (Fig. 10-97)

Marginal Erosions (Rat Bite Erosions). A localized loss of articular cortex at the bare area of the joint margin with no definite sclerotic border at its edge is characteristic.

Juxta-Articular Periostitis. Not a frequent sign but, when present, juxta-articular periostitis consists of either a solid or single lamination in the metaphyseal-proximal diaphyseal region adjacent to the involved joint.

Large Pseudo-Cysts. These are analogous to subchondral bone cysts of DJD and are owing to the combination of synovial fluid and intraosseous extension of synovial pannus. Frequently, they will become large, up to 4–6 cm, and simulate a subarticular neoplasm or infection. (Fig. 10-98)

Deformity. Owing to a combination of joint destruction, ligamentous laxity, and altered muscular action, subluxations, dislocations, and osseous misalignments are common and predictable.

Owing to its availability and low cost, plain film radiography is the most common imaging modality used to assess the

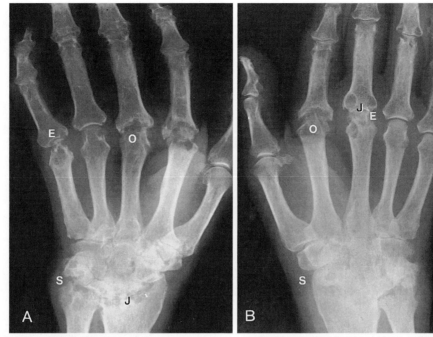

Figure 10-96 RHEUMATOID ARTHRITIS, GENERAL FEATURES. A and B. Bilateral Hands. Note the bilateral symmetry and soft tissue swelling (*S*), juxta-articular osteoporosis (*O*), uniform loss of joint space (*J*), and marginal erosions (*E*).

Table 10-28	General Radiologic Features in Rheumatoid Arthritis
	Bilateral symmetry
	Periarticular soft tissue swelling
	Uniform loss of joint space
	Marginal erosions
	Juxta-articular osteoporosis
	Juxta-articular periostitis
	Large pseudo-cysts
	Joint deformity

early suspicion of rheumatoid arthritis. (18) However, concern regarding delayed diagnosis due to the insensitivity of plain film imaging during the early stages of rheumatoid arthritis is challenging its use. (19) It is believed that the introduction of MRI to assess patients suspected of showing signs of early rheumatoid arthritis may allow for an early diagnosis, quicker treatment, and better prognosis. (20)

Target Sites of Involvement

The most common regions involved in rheumatoid arthritis are the hand, wrist, foot, knee, hip, and cervical spine.
Hand. The targeted articulations are those of the PIP and metacarpophalangeal joints. (Table 10-29) There is a distinct absence of DIP joint involvement, in contrast to psoriasis, degenerative joint disease, and erosive osteoarthritis. Radiographic diagnosis frequently precedes the clinical diagnosis, emphasizing the role of recognition of early abnormalities. This is facilitated with specialized projections and technique. In general, a minimum of 3–6 months from the time of onset is necessary for irreversible radiographic changes to occur, such as loss of joint space and marginal erosions. (12)

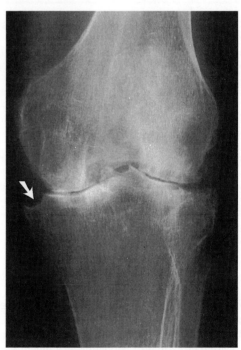

Figure 10-97 RHEUMATOID ARTHRITIS: UNIFORM LOSS OF JOINT SPACE. AP Knee. Observe the uniform decreased medial and lateral joint spaces characteristic of rheumatoid arthritis. Observe the marginal erosion of the medial tibial plateau (*arrow*).

Soft Tissue Changes. The earliest signs are those of soft tissue swelling. This is often difficult to perceive, but may be visible as displaced skin contours (spindle digit) and fascial planes or a slight increase in periarticular soft tissue density. (21) (Fig. 10-99
Articular Changes. The earliest articular change is the demonstration of a marginal erosion. The most common locations for

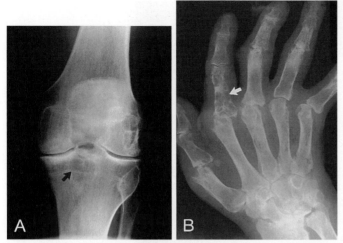

Figure 10-98 RHEUMATOID ARTHRITIS: LARGE PSEUDO-CYSTS. A. AP Knee. Note the localized subarticular loss in bone density (*arrow*). **B. PA Hand.** Note the complete loss of normal internal architecture (*arrow*).

Table 10-29	Radiologic Manifestations of Rheumatoid Arthritis in the Hand and Wrist	
Feature	**Hand**	**Wrist**
Early		
Soft tissue swelling	PIP, MCP	Radial ulnar styloid
Marginal erosions	PIP, MCP	Ulnar styloid
Osteoporosis	Juxta-articular	Juxta-articular
Loss of joint space	PIP, MCP	Middle and proximal joints
Periostitis	Proximal phalanx	Absent, proximal metacarpal, radius, ulna
Late		
Ankylosis	Rare	Common
Deformities	Ulnar deviation	Radial rotation
	Boutonniere	Scapholunate
	Swan neck	separation
	Arthritis mutilans	Zigzag deformity

MCP, metacarpal–phalangeal; *PIP,* proximal interphalangeal.

early marginal erosions are at the radial margins of the second and third metacarpal heads and the radial margins of the distal and proximal ends of the proximal phalanges. (12) (Fig. 10-100) Specialized views as described by Brewerton (22) and Norgaard (23) may be necessary to delineate these difficult to see bony defects. A marginal erosion will be visible as a lucent defect in the lateral extent of the articular cortex. Its boundaries are typically irregular, are poorly defined, and will have no sclerotic border. Varying degrees and rapidity in progression of uniform joint space loss will often be present in the same articulations.

Bone Changes. Within the adjacent bone, osteoporosis is frequently prominent early in the epiphyses and metaphyses. (Fig. 10-101A) Often, the articular cortex may appear intermittently interrupted owing to this acute diminution in bone mass (*dot–dash appearance*). Later, the osteopenia becomes more generalized and involves the diaphysis. Periosteal new bone is occasionally visible adjacent to the metaphysis and proximal diaphysis

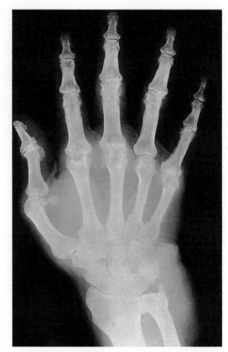

Figure 10-99 RHEUMATOID ARTHRITIS: SOFT TISSUE SWELLING. PA Hand. Note that this can be best recognized at the ulnar styloid, metacarpophalangeal, and proximal interphalangeal joints.

as a solid or single lamination. Homogenous sclerosis of the terminal phalanx (ivory phalanx) may be seen, but is a non-specific sign also seen in normal individuals and others with collagen disease. (Table 10-30) (Fig. 10-101B)

Deformities. With progression of the disease a number of characteristic digital deformities occur. These include the boutonniere, swan-neck, and ulnar deviation (ulnar drift) deformities. (24) (Fig. 10-102) Following joint dislocation, pressure erosions can occur at the site of bone compression. (25)

The boutonniere (buttonhole) deformity is characterized by extension of the DIP joint and flexion at the PIP joint. (Fig. 10-102A) It is owing to avulsion or stretching of the central slip of the extensor tendon at the base of the middle phalanx. Subsequently, the lateral extensions of the tendon act as the buttonhole as unopposed flexion at the PIP joint displaces the joint (the button) through it. At the thumb this is the most common deformity. The swan-neck deformity is flexion at the DIP and extension at the PIP joint and has a more complex pathogenesis. (Fig. 10-102B) Essentially, there is reduced ability of flexion owing to synovitis of the flexor tendon sheaths followed by shortening of the intrinsic muscles pulling on the extensor tendon at the PIP and loosening of the flexor tendon and capsular ligament on its palmar surface.

At the metacarpophalangeal joints palmar subluxation of the proximal phalanx and flexion may occur. In addition, there may be deviation of the digits toward the ulnar side from the metacarpal joints distally (ulnar deviation). (Fig. 10-102, C and D) The cause is not fully understood, but appears to be the result of metacarpophalangeal joint swelling, loss of ligamentous integrity, and the action of the long flexor tendons crossing at an angle across the joints. Associated with ulnar drift there is radial deviation of the carpal bones. The combination of digital ulnar deviation and carpal radial deviation is called the *zigzag deformity*. (26)

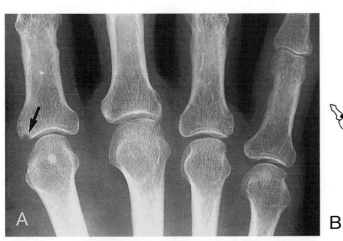

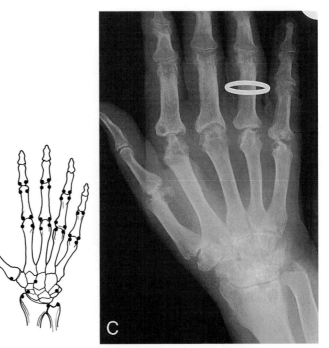

Figure 10-100   **RHEUMATOID ARTHRITIS: MARGINAL EROSIONS. A. Proximal Phalanx.** Note the erosion at the second digit (*arrow*). **B. Target Sites.** The principal sites for marginal erosions in the hand are shown. **C. PA Hand.**

Radiographic appearance of target site marginal erosions. (Panel C adapted from **Martel W:** *The pattern of rheumatoid arthritis in the hand and wrist.* Radiol Clin North Am 2:221, 1964.)

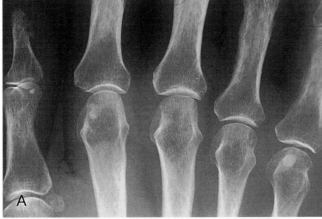

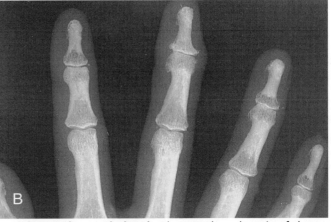

Figure 10-101   **RHEUMATOID ARTHRITIS: BONE DENSITY CHANGES. A. Juxta-Articular Osteoporosis.** Note the distinct demineralization of the metacarpal heads and phalangeal bases owing to inflammatory hyperemia. **B. Phalangeal**

Sclerosis (Ivory Phalanx). Observe the sclerosis of the terminal phalanges. This is not a specific sign of rheumatoid arthritis, and the cause is unclear.

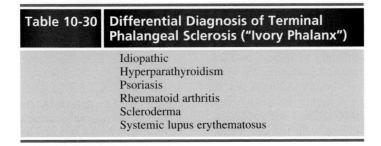

Table 10-30	Differential Diagnosis of Terminal Phalangeal Sclerosis ("Ivory Phalanx")
	Idiopathic
	Hyperparathyroidism
	Psoriasis
	Rheumatoid arthritis
	Scleroderma
	Systemic lupus erythematosus

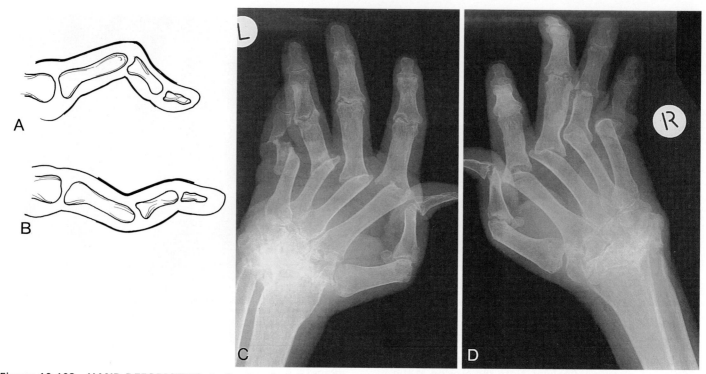

Figure 10-102 HAND DEFORMITIES. A. Boutonniere Deformity. B. Swan-Neck Deformity. C and D. Ulnar Phalangeal Deviation and Arthritis Mutilans.

The end-stage deformity of the hand may be arthritis mutilans, in which the degree of joint destruction and resultant deformities allow complete disorganization of anatomic relationships. (Fig. 10-102, *C* and *D*)

Wrist. Radiographic findings of rheumatoid arthritis frequently are first visible at the wrist, with 60% being more severe than hand changes and at least 20% of cases showing no hand changes at all. (27) These findings have a predilection to occur in distinctive locations and produce characteristic radiographic abnormalities. (Fig. 10-100, *B* and *C; Table 10-29) Isotopic bone scan shows increased uptake in episodes of inflammation (28) (Fig. 10-103), and tenosynovitis can be identified in > 50% of patients using MRI. (29) The extensor carpi ulnaris tendon is most commonly involved. (29)

Distal Ulna. Frequently, soft tissue swelling is first visible at this location as a manifestation of synovitis within the joint or adjacent tendons. Erosions of the ulnar styloid occur secondary to subperiosteal resorption and pannus from the radioulnar joint, prestyloid recess, or overlying tendon sheath of the extensor carpi ulnaris. (30) (Fig. 10-104) The origin of the pannus corresponds to the anatomic site of the ulnar erosion.

Distal Radius. Marginal erosions are often visible at the radial styloid and adjacent scaphoid. Not infrequently, there is a uniform loss of radiocarpal joint space with no reactive subchondral sclerosis. MRI will often demonstrate synovial thickening. (29)

Carpus. Marginal erosions are frequently visible in multiple carpal bones, especially the triquetrum and pisiform. (28) When multiple marginal erosions are present throughout the carpus, the radiographic appearance of the wrist is distinctive and has been called the *spotty carpal sign.* (Fig. 10-96A) The same appearance may be encountered in gout, tuberculous arthritis, and Sudeck atrophy.

The midcarpal joint space invariably will narrow in a uniform manner, and this is usually co-existent with identical narrowing in the radiocarpal joint. This pancompartmental distribution is distinctive and is in contrast to the selective compartmentalization seen in degenerative joint disease and CPPD crystal deposition disease of the wrist. As a sequela complete midcarpal ankylosis may occur but will rarely fuse the radiocarpal joint. (Fig. 10-105)

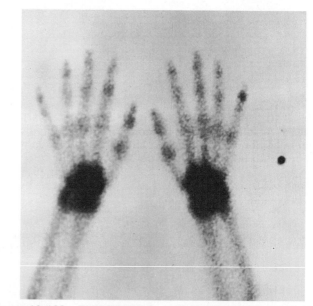

Figure 10-103 RHEUMATOID ARTHRITIS: BONE SCAN. Note that despite normal-appearing radiographs, a bilateral, symmetric uptake has occurred in both wrists owing to inflammatory synovitis and hyperemia.

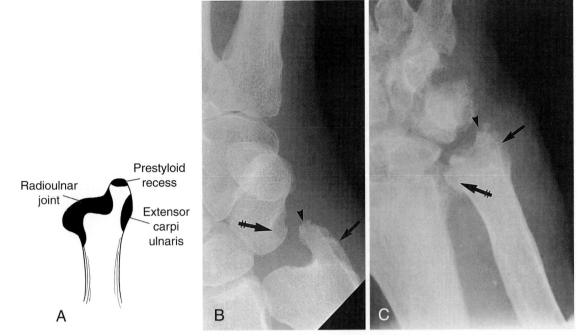

Figure 10-104   RHEUMATOID ARTHRITIS: ULNAR EROSIONS.
A. Diagram. Three sites for potential erosions to occur are shown. **B. Erosions.** Note the erosion from the extensor carpi ulnaris (rat bite lesion) (*arrow*) and prestyloid recess (*arrow-head*). Note the adjacent erosion on the triquetral bone (*crossed arrow*). **C. Erosions.** Note the three sites of ulnar erosion: extensor carpi ulnaris (*arrow*), prestyloid recess (*arrow-head*), and radioulnar articulation (*crossed arrow*). Observe the adjacent soft tissue swelling.

Malalignment at the carpus is common. Radial rotation of the proximal carpal row often occurs, with the digital ulnar drift at the metacarpal phalangeal joints producing the zigzag deformity. Separation of the scaphoid and lunate owing to disruption of the interosseous ligament is frequent in long-standing disease (*Terry Thomas' sign*) (31) and may be seen in association with palmar subluxation of the two bones. (32) Evaluation for this separation is best performed with the wrist in ulnar deviation. In addition, diastasis at the radioulnar joint may displace the ulna dorsally and may precipitate extensor tendon rupture (*caput ulnae syndrome*). (32)

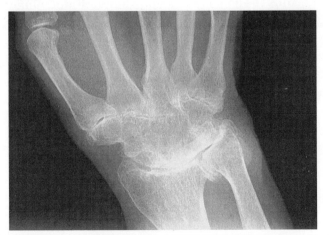

Figure 10-105   RHEUMATOID ANKYLOSIS: WRIST. Note that midcarpal fusion has occurred but has conspicuously not affected the radiocarpal joint.

Foot. The foot is a common target site for rheumatoid arthritis. Abnormalities in the feet generally parallel those encountered in the hands in distribution and radiographic features; however, in approximately 15% of patients the feet may be the initial site of involvement. (33,34)

The most characteristic articulations affected are the interphalangeal joint of the big toe and the metatarsal phalangeal joints. The most common metatarsophalangeal joint affected is the fifth, decreasing in incidence toward the great toe. (34) Radiographic changes at these sites include soft tissue swelling, marginal erosions, juxta-articular osteoporosis, uniform loss of joint space, occasional linear periostitis, and deformities.

Erosions are usually marginal, appearing earlier and remaining more prominent on the medial surface of each metatarsal head. (Fig. 10-106) The fifth metatarsal head is the exception, where the earliest erosions usually are visible on its lateral margin. At the big toe metatarsal–phalangeal joint, the erosions are more prominent on the medial aspect of the metatarsal head, with occasional erosions visible on the adjacent hallux sesamoid bones. At the calcaneus, on the plantar and posterior surfaces, poorly defined erosions may be visible.

Deformities are common and include digital fibular deviation at the metatarsal–phalangeal joints, except at the fifth digit, and flexion deformities of the toes often associated with subluxation and even dislocation at these same joints (*Lanois' deformity*). (Fig. 10-107) A prominent hallux valgus is frequent. The metatarsal bones often appear spread apart and the longitudinal arch flattened.

Soft tissue callus formation is often prominent in the advanced rheumatoid foot at the metatarsophalangeal joints on the plantar surface and medial aspect of the great toe (bunion). Occasionally,

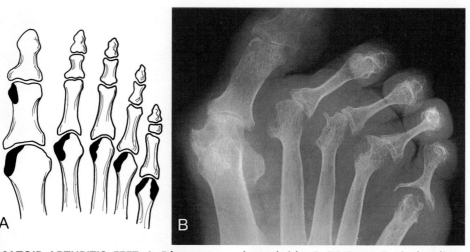

Figure 10-106 RHEUMATOID ARTHRITIS: FEET. A. Diagram, Marginal Erosions. Target sites for marginal erosions lie on the medial surfaces of the metatarsal heads, except for the fifth metatarsal where early erosions can occur on the lateral side. **B. PA Foot.** Typical radiographic depiction of the locational predominance on the medial metatarsal surfaces, except at the fifth. Note the phalangeal fibular deviation.

subcutaneous nodules are present over the skin adjacent to the Achilles tendon.

Spine. Rheumatoid arthritis most commonly involves the cervical spine in 50–80% of individuals. (35) (Table 10-31) Up to 5% of patients may demonstrate discovertebral alterations at the thoracolumbar region, consisting of opposing endplate irregularities, sclerosis, and loss of disc height, resembling advanced degenerative spondylosis or even infection. (36) Pathologic fracture owing to osteopenia or avascular necrosis secondary to corticosteroid therapy with an intravertebral collection of gas in the vertebral body (*intravertebral vacuum cleft sign*) may also be seen. (Fig. 10-108)

Clinically, cervical involvement usually follows as a sequel to the peripheral manifestations but may antedate these changes in exceptional instances. Radiographic evaluation of the cervical spine in patients with rheumatoid arthritis, in addition to standard projections, must include the open-mouth frontal view and a lateral view with the neck in flexion. These views are especially useful in the evaluation of rheumatoid changes involving the upper cervical joint complexes. CT and MRI are also particularly useful in this location. (37) The most common changes in patients with disease of < 10 years' duration are odontoid erosions, subaxial subluxations, facet erosions and sclerosis, and loss of disc height. (38)

Atlanto-Occipital Articulation. Changes within the atlantooccipital joints are common and consist of erosion, sclerosis, and loss of joint space. They may eventually ankylose. Progressive destruction and remodeling of the bony architecture may precipitate vertical translocation of the odontoid, which can be fatal (*pseudo-basilar invagination*). (11,39) (Fig. 10-109) Evaluation of the normal relationship between the odontoid tip and skull base is accomplished by Chamberlain's or McGregor's line. (See Chapter 2.) The combination of upward migration of the odontoid process, decrease in multiple intervertebral disc heights, and

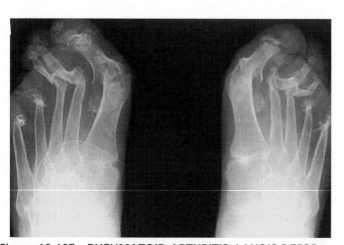

Figure 10-107 RHEUMATOID ARTHRITIS: LANOIS DEFORMITY. Bilateral PA Feet. Observe the advanced joint destruction, dislocation, and fibular deviation.

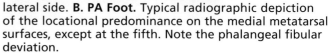 Table 10-31	Radiologic Manifestations of Rheumatoid Arthritis in the Cervical Spine

Atlanto-occipital joint
   Loss of joint space and erosions
   Ankylosis
   Upward odontoid translocation (pseudo-basilar invagination)
Atlantoaxial joint
   Apophyseal joint erosions and ankylosis
   Atlas instability, subluxation, dislocation (ADI > 3 mm)
   Odontoid erosion and destruction
Subaxial joints (C3–C7)
   Apophyseal joints: erosions, sclerosis, subluxation, ankylosis
   Decreased neck length (summation effect)
   Intervertebral discs: narrowed
   Spinous processes: tapered contour and erosions
     (pencil sharpened)
   Vertebral bodies: osteoporotic, subluxation (stairstepping),
     end-plate erosions

ADI, atlantodental interspace.

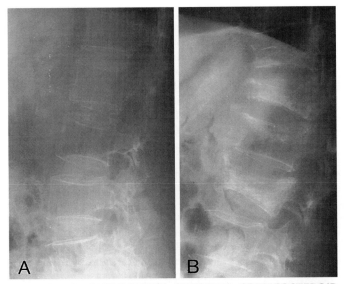

Figure 10-108 **RHEUMATOID ARTHRITIS: CORTICOSTEROID COMPLICATIONS. A. Lateral Lumbar Osteoporosis.** Note that the initial film demonstrates severe osteoporosis. **B. Lateral Lumbar Pathologic Fracture.** Note that 3 months after the administration of corticosteroids, multiple compression fractures are visible. Note the prominent callus at the fracture sites typical of corticosteroid-induced changes. (Courtesy of Bryan Hartley, MD, Melbourne, Australia.)

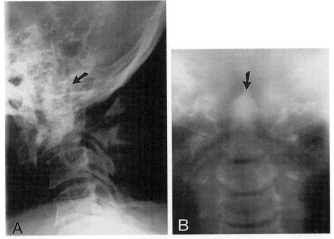

Figure 10-109 **RHEUMATOID ARTHRITIS: PSEUDO-BASILAR INVAGINATION. A. Lateral Cervical. B. AP Tomogram: C1–C2.** Note the translocation of odontoid into and beyond the foramen magnum (*arrows*) owing to erosion and destruction of the upper two cervical vertebrae.

vertebral osteolysis produces a decrease in neck length of up to 50% (*summation effect*).

Atlantoaxial Articulation. Involvement of this articular complex in rheumatoid arthritis is a frequent manifestation. The most important clinical and radiographic conspicuous signs focus on changes at the atlanto-odontoid joint. The consensus on the frequency of involvement in rheumatoid patients is approximately 30%; however, this frequency may increase up to 50% with disease severity and progression. (40–42)

Table 10-32	Causes of Atlantoaxial Joint Instability

Congenital
  Occipitalization
  Odontoid agenesis
  Os odontoideum
  Syndromes: Down's syndrome, Morquio's disease, chondro-
    dystrophia calcificans congenita, spondyloepiphyseal dysplasia
Arthritis
  Rheumatoid arthritis
  Ankylosing spondylitis
  Psoriatic arthritis
  Reiter's syndrome
  Systemic lupus erythematosus
Infection
  Osteomyelitis
  Postpharyngeal infection (Grisel's disease)
Tumor
  Primary or secondary
Trauma
  Ruptured transverse ligament
  Fractured, ununited odontoid

Table 10-33	Pathologic Radiologic Correlation at the Atlantoaxial Joint

Pathologic Features	Radiologic Features
Atlanto-odontoid joint	
Insufficient transverse ligament	C1, C2 instability
Pannus	Erosions, dissolution
Hyperemia	Osteoporosis
Apophyseal joint	
Pannus	Erosions of joint surface
Cartilage loss	Loss of joint space
Ligamentous laxity	Instability

It is the unique articular anatomy of the upper cervical complex that predisposes to distinct pathologic, radiographic, and clinical expressions of rheumatoid involvement in this area. Similar changes may be noted in other inflammatory spondyloarthropathies such as ankylosing spondylitis, psoriatic arthritis, and Reiter's syndrome. (Table 10-27) Other entities may also predispose the patient to atlantoaxial instability. (Table 10-32) The combined sequelae of inflammation, pannus, and ligamentous weakening leads to atlantoaxial instability and varying degrees of odontoid erosion. (Table 10-33)

- *Instability.* Loss of ligamentous integrity, particularly of the transverse ligament, may result in displacement of the atlas anteriorly, laterally, or anteroinferiorly. The most common displacement is in an anterior direction, seen in up to 35% of patients. (43) This is best visualized on a lateral projection, with the neck in flexion, with the atlanto-dental interspace > 3 mm. (Fig. 10-110) MRI can depict inflammatory tissue within the joint and effects of the displacement on the adjacent spinal cord. (Fig. 10-111) It is especially useful, when it too is performed in flexion and extension. (37,44) With greater degrees of displacement, the spinal canal will be encroached by the posterior arch, which may be apparent as a disruption in the posterior cervical (spinolaminar junction) line. Clinically, an atlantodental interspace up to 12 mm may be asymptomatic owing to the physiologic space surrounding the spinal cord (*Steele's rule of thirds*). (45) Atlantoaxial instability most commonly occurs in the 2nd to 3rd decades of the disease. (38)

- *Erosion.* The sites of bony erosion are intimately related to the locations of adjacent synovial tissue from which invading pannus originates and are analogous to the peripheral joint marginal erosion. (43) Consequently, erosions occur on the odontoid predominantly at the base in a circumferential manner, but they are most prominent on the posterior and anterior surfaces. Additional erosions may

be visible on the posterior surface of the C1 anterior tubercle. The shape of the odontoid is altered, with a narrowed base and normal upper portion. (Figs. 10-94 and 10-112) Occasionally, an erosion may be visible at the odontoid apex. With progressive erosions, complete dissolution of the odontoid may occur. (Fig. 10-113) The odontoid subsequently appears as an attenuated, osseous stump. It should also be noted that the odontoid is increasingly susceptible to fracture in rheumatoid arthritis.

Subaxial Articulations (C3–C7). Alterations in joint complexes below the axis vertebra are common and associated with distinctive radiographic signs.

- *Subluxations.* Most commonly, these are present at the C2–C4 levels and are invariably anterior displacements. (13,43) A single level of anterolisthesis is most frequent at the C3 or C4 segment. Simultaneous multilevel anterolistheses are more distinctive and produce a *stepladder or doorstep appearance* on the lateral radiograph. A lateral view in flexion is the most diagnostic in the evaluation of these intersegmental derangements. The pathogenesis of anterolisthesis in rheumatoid arthritis is the combination of loss in disc height, apophyseal joint disease, and ligamentous laxity.
- *Apophyseal joints.* Erosions, loss of joint space, instability, and infrequent bony ankylosis characterize apophyseal involvement. Instability is best demonstrated in flexion, in which widening of the joint and interspinous spaces will be visible as will forward displacement of the inferior articulating process of the vertebra above.
- *Intervertebral disc and discovertebral junction.* Narrowing of the disc space is frequent. Additional changes at the vertebral endplates result in erosions and loss of the cortical contours, particularly in the posterior aspect of the vertebral body (rheumatoid discitis). (15,16) Multisegmental involvement is more frequent. A distinctive but not invariable finding is the lack of osteophytes and sclerosis at the involved level.
- *Bone abnormalities.* Generalized osteoporosis is a prominent and common finding, especially in individuals treated

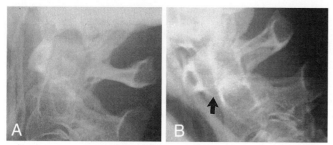

Figure 10-110 RHEUMATOID ARTHRITIS: ATLANTOAXIAL INSTABILITY. A. Neutral Lateral Cervical. B. Flexion Lateral Cervical. Observe the atlantodental interspace increased to 5 mm (*arrow*). *COMMENT:* Demonstration of this instability is frequently only shown on the flexion study.

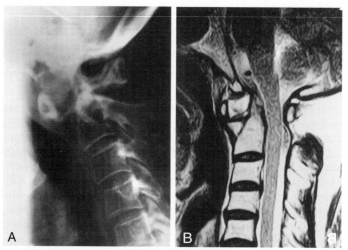

Figure 10-111 RHEUMATOID ARTHRITIS: INSTABILITY OF THE UPPER CERVICAL SPINE. A. Lateral Cervical Flexion Radiograph. B. T1-Weighted MRI: Sagittal Cervical. Observe the increase of the atlanto-dental interspace and resorption (whittling) of the odontoid peg. With anterior atlantoaxial subluxation, the posterior tubercle of the atlas compresses the posterior surface of the spinal cord with resultant narrowing of the sagittal dimensions of the spinal canal at this level. *COMMENT:* Patients with rheumatoid arthritis often develop rupture of the transverse ligament with an increase in the atlantodental interspace. This is seen in approximately 35% of patients with long-standing rheumatoid arthritis. Demonstration of atlantoaxial instability as a result of rupture of the transverse ligament is often shown only on the flexion radiograph. (Courtesy of Jonathan H. Griffiths, DC, DABCO, Birmingham, Alabama.)

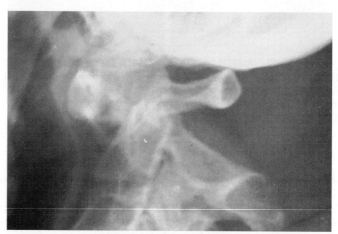

Figure 10-112 RHEUMATOID ARTHRITIS: ODONTOID DESTRUCTION AND ATLANTOAXIAL INSTABILITY. Lateral Cervical. Note that the atlas has dislocated anteriorly with a predental interspace of at least 12 mm. Note the odontoid is small and attenuated (whittled) owing to synovial erosion.

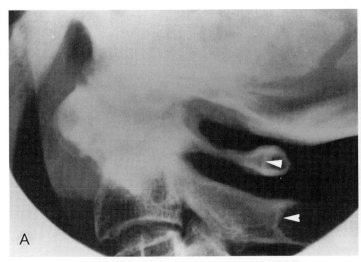

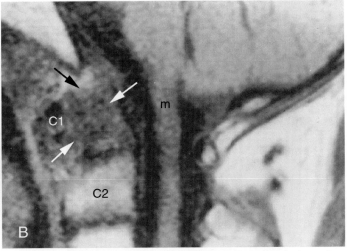

Figure 10-113 **RHEUMATOID ARTHRITIS: ODONTOID DESTRUCTION AND ATLANTOAXIAL INSTABILITY. A. Lateral Cervical.** Note that the atlas is displaced forward as identified by the disruption of the spinolaminar line (*arrowheads*). The odontoid is not visible. **B. T1-Weighted MRI: Cranio-Vertebral Junction.** Observe that the vertebral body of the axis shows the normal high signal from the marrow cavity (C2). The anterior arch of the atlas can also be determined (C1). The entire odontoid region is replaced with a low signal intensity tissue representing pannus and eroded bone (*arrows*). *COMMENT:* Anterior translation of the posterior arch can be seen to produce a guillotine-type mechanism on the adjacent medulla (*m*). MRI is the imaging method of choice in the evaluation for abnormalities of the craniovertebral junction.

with corticosteroids for > 5 years. This may rarely predispose patients to compression fractures of the vertebral bodies. A peculiar manifestation of rheumatoid involvement in the cervical spine is the early erosion and subsequent altered tapered contour of the lower spinous processes (*sharpened pencil*). (46) The cause is unclear, but may be related to supraspinous ligament enthesopathy, pannus erosions from adjacent nuchal bursae, or mechanical pressure resorption from approximated spinous processes.

Hip. Abnormalities of the hip are usually seen in long-standing and severe peripheral joint disease in approximately 35% of patients. The radiographic features are generally distributed bilaterally and symmetrically.

Soft tissue abnormalities are notably infrequent. Within the joint cavity there is a uniform diminution in the interosseous space, resulting in migration of the femoral head superior and medial in the plane of the femoral neck (axial migration). (47) (Table 10-34) With weight bearing, approximation of the joint surfaces, and intraosseous hyperemia, the acetabulum is displaced medially (protrusio acetabuli, arthrokatadysis, Otto's pelvis). This occurs in approximately 15% of patients. (48,49) Rheumatoid arthritis is the most common cause for bilateral protrusio acetabuli, which is more common in those who are treated with steroids. The combination of bilateral protrusio acetabuli and small, eroded femoral heads is characteristic. (Fig. 10-114) Additional causes for protrusio acetabuli include Paget's disease, degenerative joint disease, and other disorders. (Table 10-35)

With time, secondary degenerative changes will become evident as subchondral sclerosis and osteophytes complicate the radiographic picture. Bone abnormalities consist of erosions, cysts, osteoporosis, and frequently osteonecrosis of the femoral head. Erosions are usually small and may appear as cyst-like lesions

Table 10-34	Patterns of Hip Migration		
Factor	**Superior**	**Medial**	**Axial**
Disease association	Degenerative joint disease Pseudo-gout (CPPD)[a] Old slipped epiphysis	Paget's disease Degenerative joint disease	Rheumatoid arthritis Infection
Radiologic features			
Compartments involved	Superior	Medial	All
Osteophytes	Prominent	Minimal	Absent
Subchondral cysts	Prominent	Prominent	Minimal to absent
Neck buttress	Prominent	Prominent	Minimal to absent
Protrusio acetabuli	Absent	Mild	Moderate to prominent
Tilt deformity	Present	Absent	Absent

[a] Suspect if the degenerative process is severe or bilateral.
CPPD, calcium pyrophosphate dihydrate.

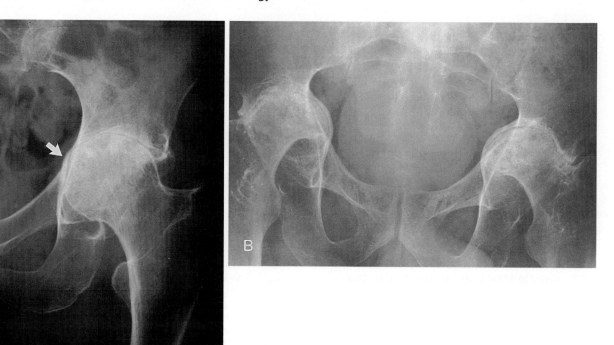

Figure 10-114 RHEUMATOID ARTHRITIS: PROTRUSIO ACETABULI. A. AP Hip Unilateral. Observe the symmetric loss of joint space and axial migration of the femoral head, creating a protrusio acetabuli (*arrow*). **B. AP Pelvis Bilateral.** Note the uniform loss of joint space, small femoral heads, and protrusio acetabuli, characteristic of long-standing rheumatoid arthritis. *COMMENT:* The most common cause for bilateral protrusio acetabuli in the adult is rheumatoid arthritis.

Table 10-35	Diseases Associated with Protrusio Acetabuli		
Disease	**Unilateral**	**Bilateral**	**Incidence**
Idiopathic		X	U
Congenital			
Osteogenesis imperfecta		X	U
Mucopolysaccharidoses		X	U
Arthritides			
Degenerative	X		C
Rheumatoid arthritis		X	C
Juvenile rheumatoid arthritis		X	U
Psoriasis	X	X	U
Ankylosing spondylitis		X	U
Reiter's	X	X	U
Gout	X	X	U
Ochronosis		X	U
Metabolic			
Paget's disease	X	X	U
Osteomalacia		X	U
Rickets		X	U
Osteoporosis		X	U
Hyperparathyroidism		X	U
Steroids		X	U
Trauma			
Acetabular fracture	X		C
Infection			
Pyogenic, tuberculosis	X		U
Neoplasm			
Primary, secondary	X		U

C, common; U, uncommon.

just below the articular margin of the femoral head. Cysts may be large and numerous. Osteoporosis is distinctively generalized and prominent. Complicating osteonecrosis (avascular necrosis) of the femoral head, especially in those being treated with corticosteroids, will be apparent by collapse of the articular cortex and disruption of the smooth surface by a *step-like defect,* usually at the superior weight-bearing surface.

Insufficiency fractures secondary to osteopenia most commonly involve the sacrum and pubis. (50) In the sacrum, these may involve the sacral ala. Frequently, they follow hip replacement. (See Chapter 14.)

Other Joints

Sacroiliac Joint. The sacroiliac joint is an uncommon site of involvement in contrast to ankylosing spondylitis. (Fig. 10-115) Fewer than 25–35% of rheumatoid arthritis patients, even of those with long-standing or severe peripheral joint changes, have sacroiliac disease. (51) Features of rheumatoid sacroiliitis include mild loss of joint space, iliac erosions, and minimal or absent sclerosis. (52) Ankylosis may occur but is infrequent. Distinctively, it may be unilateral or, if bilateral, asymmetric in severity and distribution. Osteoporosis of the pelvis is a frequent accessory finding.

Shoulder. Prominent bilateral and symmetric findings are frequent in both the glenohumeral and acromioclavicular joints. (53) (Fig. 10-116) Soft tissue swelling over the shoulder may be large, owing to bursal involvement, with extension into adjacent regions.

At the glenohumeral joint, loss of joint space is not prominent. Early and frequent rotator cuff rupture subsequently elevates the humeral head as the deltoid acts unopposed. In this

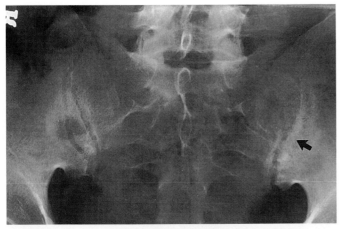

Figure 10-115 RHEUMATOID ARTHRITIS: SACROILIAC JOINT. Note the unilateral erosive changes (*arrow*) but no sclerosis, which is often seen in other inflammatory sacroiliac arthropathies such as ankylosing spondylitis.

displacement, the distance between the acromion and the humeral head is diminished, and there may be a concavity on the inferior surface of the acromion with sclerosis and cyst formation on both opposing surfaces. Inflammatory synovial erosions are most apparent on the humeral head and initially originate near the greater tubercle, simulating a posterior dislocation impaction deformity (*Hill-Sachs lesion*). With time, the erosions will deform and may even appear to resorb the entire humeral head as in atrophic neuroarthropathy.

At the acromioclavicular articulation, clavicular erosions predominate, which in long-standing disease precipitate a tapered, resorbed distal clavicle. These changes are usually a bilateral phenomenon and should be differentiated from other causes, especially hyperparathyroidism. (Table 10-36) An additional concave defect may be apparent on the inferior surface of the distal clavicle 2–4 cm from the acromioclavicular joint. (54) The cortical margin of the adjacent coracoid process is often irregular in combination with the clavicular erosion.

Elbow. The extensor surface of the forearm is a common region for the development of rheumatoid nodules, radiographically visible as protruding soft tissue masses. (Fig. 10-117) Enlargement of the olecranon bursa may produce a similar localized density. Intra-articular effusion is visible on the lateral view as the anterior and posterior fat-pads are displaced (*fat-pad sign*), a sign seen in up to 90% of rheumatoid elbows. (55) At the joint, uniform loss of interosseous space, osteoporosis, and erosions are initially minimal. An early erosion may be visible on AP and oblique radiographs in the proximal ulna opposing the neck of the adjacent radius (*supinator notch sign*). (56) With progression, osteolysis of all the joint components occurs, simulating atrophic neuroarthropathy. Rarely, adjacent subcutaneous rheumatoid nodules may result in extrinsic pressure erosions of the ulna and radius.

Knee. The knee is a frequent site of involvement. Soft tissue swelling is often prominent from synovial effusion in the suprapatellar and popliteal regions. (Figs. 10-97 and 10-118) Large Baker's cysts are a frequent complication and may be visible in the popliteal space. (57)

At the joint, a uniform bicompartmental loss of joint space is the radiographic hallmark. Inclusion of the patellofemoral joint in the disease process may also occur. Before this loss of joint space, marginal erosions are usually visible at the peripheral as-

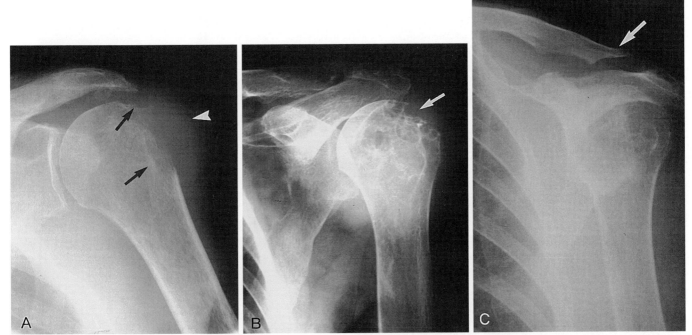

Figure 10-116 RHEUMATOID ARTHRITIS: SHOULDER.
A. Humerus. Note the marginal erosions at the humeral head (*arrows*). Note the adjacent soft tissue swelling (*arrowhead*). **B. Humerus.** Observe the large marginal erosion of the greater tuberosity (*arrow*). Also note the multiple rheumatoid interosseous cysts scattered throughout the humeral head. **C. Glenohumeral Subluxation.** Observe that as a result of inflammatory rupture of the rotator cuff tendons, the now-unopposed action of the deltoid leads to cephalic migration of the humeral head. An additional sign of rheumatoid arthritis is the pencil-like tapering of the distal clavicle (*arrow*).

Table 10-36	Differential Diagnosis of Distal Clavicle Erosion or Defect
Common	**Uncommon**
Hyperparathyroidism	Cleidocranial dysplasia
Lytic metastasis	Gout
Multiple myeloma	Histiocytosis "X"
Post-traumatic osteolysis	Osteogenesis imperfecta
Rheumatoid arthritis	Osteomyelitis
	Scleroderma
	Surgery

pects of the femur and especially the tibia. In addition, subchondral cysts of large proportions are commonly demonstrated. Ankylosis is rare at this joint.

Ankle. Involvement of the tarsal joints and ankle mortise is relatively frequent but more difficult to visualize than in the wrist. Abnormalities most commonly consist of soft tissue swelling, erosions, and osteoporosis; and it may eventually ankylose. Uniform loss of joint space and occasional linear periostitis is most notable at the ankle mortise.

Chest. The pathologic sites of involvement in the chest are the heart, pleura, lungs, and ribs, which may show radiographically visible changes. (58)

- *Heart.* The radiographic findings are non-specific and consist of mild to moderate cardiomegaly, occasional signs of valvular insufficiency, and pericarditis.
- *Lungs.* Two patterns of involvement may occur separately or simultaneously. The first pattern is the formation of

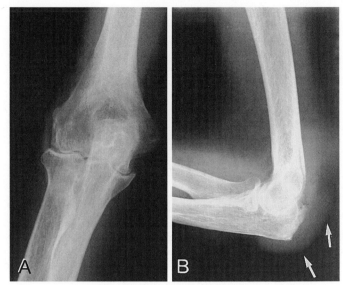

Figure 10-117 RHEUMATOID ARTHRITIS. A. AP Elbow. Observe the uniform loss of joint space. **B. Lateral Elbow.** Observe the subcutaneous nodules (*arrows*).

nodular densities, which may cavitate (*necrobiotic nodules*) and represent pulmonary rheumatoid nodules. (58) This appearance may simulate bloodborne pulmonary metastases. The second pattern is the formation of diffuse interstitial fibrosis initially basilar in distribution but eventually involving the entire lung (*honeycomb lung*). A unique combination of rheumatoid arthritis and pneumoconiosis is referred to as *Caplan's syndrome.*

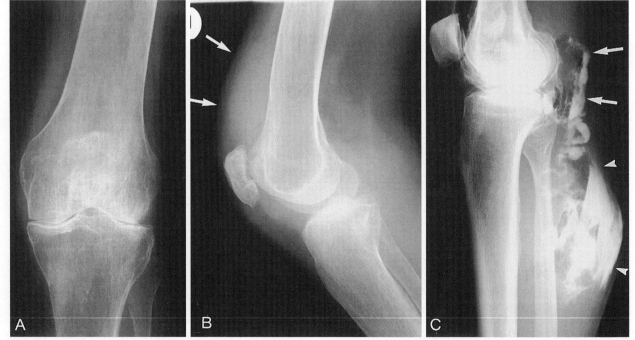

Figure 10-118 RHEUMATOID ARTHRITIS: KNEE. A. Uniform Loss of Joint Space. Despite the loss of joint space, note the distinct absence of subchondral sclerosis and diffuse osteopenia. **B. Suprapatellar Effusion.** Observe the bulging soft tissue density owing to effusion (*arrows*). A patellar erosion can also be appreciated. **C. Baker's Cyst.** Note that on arthrography the extent of the cyst is defined extending into the popliteal space (*arrows*). Observe the rupture and dissection of the rheumatoid cyst into the posterior calf (*arrowheads*).

(59) The pneumoconiosis may be caused by inhalation of coal, asbestos, gold, chalk, or other industrial substances. (60)

- *Pleura.* Although predominantly asymptomatic, small to moderate pleural effusions may be visible at any stage of the disease and have a tendency to be chronic. Radiographically, blunting of the lateral and posterior costophrenic sulci and the sweeping concave lung fluid interface (*meniscus sign*) on upright chest films will be visible. Localized pleural adhesions may be evident.
- *Rib cage.* In patients with rheumatoid arthritis of > 14 years' duration, asymptomatic erosions of the superior margins of the third, fourth, and fifth posterior ribs may be visible. (61) These erosions can be short based, discrete excavations < 1 cm, or broader, shallow concave defects up to 6 cm in length. At times these defects simulate malignant bone destruction.

CAPSULE SUMMARY   Rheumatoid Arthritis

General Considerations

- A systemic connective tissue disease that selectively targets synovial tissue, resulting in a widespread inflammatory polyarticular process.

Clinical Features

- Onset is usually between 20 and 60 years of age, with the highest incidence among the 40- to 50-year-old group.
- Under 40, females 3:1; over 40, equal, 1:1.
- Signs and symptoms are variable and may be episodic or persistent.
- Low-grade fever, fatigue, weight loss, muscle soreness, and atrophy.
- Symmetric peripheral joint pain and swelling, particularly of the hands.
- Later deformities may ensue—ulnar deviation, boutonniere, swan neck, Lanois, and arthritis mutilans.
- Rheumatoid arthritis latex positive in 70% of cases, anemia, and elevated ESR.

Pathologic Features

- Initial synovial inflammation within joints, bursae, and tendon sheaths, with cellular infiltrate, hyperemia, edema, and increased synovial fluid.
- Synovium becomes hypertrophied to form granulation tissue (pannus), which spreads over cartilage surface.
- At the bare areas pannus directly invades into the bone, resulting in marginal erosions and cartilage destruction.
- Eventually, fibrous and bony ankylosis ensues.
- A rheumatoid nodule is diagnostic and consists of three distinct zones: fibrinoid degeneration and necrosis (central), radial palisading of fibroblasts (middle), and fibrous tissue with small cell infiltrate (outer).

Radiologic Features

- Early radiographic changes are most commonly seen in the hands and feet.
- Bilateral and symmetric distribution, periarticular soft tissue swelling, juxta-articular osteoporosis, juxta-articular solid or laminated periostitis, marginal erosions and cysts, and uniform loss of joint space.
- Later, radiographic changes may be seen, including marked deformities with subluxation, dislocation, articular bony destruction, bony fusion, and complete destruction of joint space.
- The most commonly involved areas are the hands and feet, with a tendency to progress proximally.
- *Hand:* earliest changes are seen at the metacarpophalangeal and PIP joints. Evaluation should include the semisupination view of the hands (Norgaard projection) for marginal erosions on metacarpal heads; deformities—ulnar deviation, boutonniere, swan neck, spindle digit.
- *Wrist:* earliest change is erosion of ulnar styloid, multiple carpal erosions (spotty carpal sign), most common location for bony ankylosis, carpal radial rotation, zigzag deformity, Terry Thomas' sign.
- *Feet:* earliest changes seen at the fourth and fifth metatarsal phalangeal joints. Changes parallel and are identical to that seen in the hands; Lanois deformity—dorsal subluxation of the metatarsal–phalangeal joints, with fibular deviation.
- *Cervical spine:* most commonly affected area of the spine; involved in up to 70% of rheumatoid patients. Increased atlantodental interspace > 3 mm (especially in flexion), odontoid erosions, subluxations (especially C3, C4, and C5). Narrowed intervertebral discs, apophyseal joints show erosions and narrowed joint space and may ankylose. Tapered spinous processes and generalized osteoporosis.
- *Hips:* uniform loss of joint space (axial migration), minimal erosions, protrusio acetabuli (most common cause), particularly bilaterally.
- *Knees:* uniform loss of joint space, marginal erosions (particularly at the tibial condyles), and osteoporosis; often associated with large Baker's cysts.
- *Shoulders:* uniform loss of glenohumeral joint space, marginal erosions (particularly at the superior lateral portion of the humerus), humerus often subluxated superiorly, tapered distal clavicle, seemingly widened acromioclavicular joint space.
- *Sacroiliac:* usually unilateral and involving the lower two thirds of the joint; erosions present but no sclerosis; rarely, ankylosis.
- *Chest:* small pleural effusions with blunting of the costophrenic sulci. Occasional rheumatoid nodules that simulate neoplasms and often cavitate (necrobiotic nodules). Diffuse or basilar interstitial fibrosis, resulting in an irregular cardiac silhouette or honeycomb lung.

JUVENILE RHEUMATOID ARTHRITIS

Childhood onset of rheumatic disease is not uncommon, representing the most frequent systemic autoimmune inflammatory disease affecting children. (1) This group of disorders is often given the label of juvenile chronic polyarthritis, which constitutes a heterogeneous but well-defined number of disease entities. (2) (Table 10-37) Of these the most common is Still's disease, the seronegative form characterized by three distinct modes of involvement. The term Still's disease arises from the original documentation in 1897 by George Frederick Still (3) of a systemic disease that involves visceral organs and large joints and produces muscular wasting, fatigue, and fever. However, this designation has since been used to describe rheumatoid arthritis in children, as has the term juvenile rheumatoid arthritis (JRA). (4,5) This form of arthritis affects about 250,000 American children. (6)

Essentially, juvenile rheumatoid arthritis is a disease of unknown cause similar to the adult form of rheumatoid arthritis, occurring under the age of 16 years. (2,7) However, there are distinct differences in terms of patterns of articular and systemic involvement, as well as in prognosis. (Table 10-38) Attempts to standardize diagnostic criteria have resulted in generalized criteria such as persistent arthritis of at least 6 weeks in one or more joints with the exclusion of other causes. (8,9)

Clinical Features

Categories of JRA have been made based on the presence of rheumatoid factor, articular distribution, and visceral involvement. (2,10) (Table 10-38) (Fig. 10-119)

Seropositive Juvenile Onset, Adult Type

In the presence of rheumatoid factor (seropositive) the articular disease resembles and behaves similar to the adult form. This type of JRA occurs in approximately 10% of individuals and has the poorest prognosis. (11)

Seronegative Chronic Arthritis (Still's Disease)

Absence of rheumatoid factor is characteristic of seronegative chronic arthritis. This type is by far the most frequently encountered. (12) In addition, subcutaneous rheumatoid nodules are rarely found. Based on the number of joints involved and the degree of systemic manifestations, three forms are identified—classic systemic disease, polyarticular disease, and pauciarticular or monoarticular disease. (Table 10-39)

Classic Systemic Disease. The classic variety is distinguished by the pronounced systemic involvement of organ systems and

Table 10-37	Classification of Juvenile Chronic Arthritis

Juvenile onset, adult-type rheumatoid arthritis (seropositive)
Seronegative chronic arthritis (Still's disease)
   Classic systemic form
   Polyarticular
   Pauciarticular or monoarticular
Juvenile onset, ankylosing spondylitis
Psoriatic arthritis
Enteropathic arthritis
Miscellaneous (systemic lupus erythematosus, etc.)

Adapted from: **Ansell BM, Kent PA:** *Radiologic changes in juvenile chronic polyarthritis.* Skeletal Radiol 1: 129, 1977.

Table 10-38	Differential Features of Juvenile and Adult Rheumatoid Arthritis	
Features	**Juvenile**	**Adult**
Age	< 16	> 16
Systemic		
Fever	+++	+
Rash	+++	+
Chronic iridocyclitis	+++	+
Articular		
Monoarticular	++	+
Large joints	+++	+
Symmetry	+	+++
Nonarticular		
Subcutaneous nodules	+	+++
Growth abnormalities	+++	—
Laboratory		
Leukocytosis	+++	—
Rheumatoid factor	—	+++

+++, very common; ++, common; +, uncommon; —, rare.

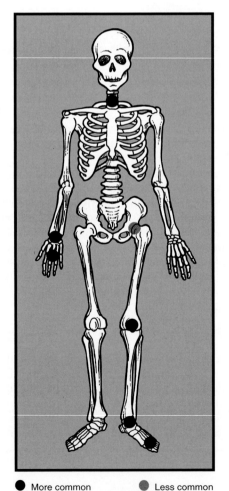

● More common   ● Less common

Figure 10-119 **SKELETAL DISTRIBUTION OF JUVENILE RHEUMATOID ARTHRITIS.** (Polyarticular Disease).

Table 10-39	Forms of Seronegative Juvenile Rheumatoid Arthritis		
Features	Systemic	Polyarticular	Pauciarticular–Monoarticular
Incidence	20%	50%	30%
Sex (male to female)	1:1	1:2	1:3
Major systemic findings	High fever, rash, carditis	Low-grade fever, carditis	Uncommon, iridocyclitis
Articular findings			
Joints	Any	Knee, ankle, feet, wrist, hand	Knee, hip, ankle, elbow, wrist
Symmetry	Variable	Present	Absent
Cervical spine	Rare	Common	Rare
X-ray findings	Rare	Common	Uncommon
Prognosis			
Majority	Recurrence common	Variable	Resolution
Complications	Heart disease	Growth disturbances	Chronic polyarthritis
	Polyarthritis	Amyloidosis	

general body function. About 20% of all JRA patients present with this onset. (5,7,10) There is an equal sex distribution. The onset is usually heralded by a high, acute, intermittent fever; lymphadenopathy; hepatosplenomegaly; polyserositis; carditis; leukocytosis; and anemia. (12) A common finding is the appearance of a pale erythematous rash over the trunk, face, or extremities that is fleeting and migratory, occurring primarily in the afternoon or early evening. (7,13) The rash can be precipitated by scratching the skin surface, and within several minutes to hours isolated macules appear along the site of irritation. Joint manifestations are generally mild and lack radiographic changes.

Polyarticular Disease. Polyarticular disease is the most common variety, affecting up to 50% of JRA individuals, females twice as frequently. (5) It is characterized by bilateral, symmetric involvement, with pain and swelling of the metacarpophalangeal, wrist, foot, ankle, and knee articulations as well as the cervical spine. This is the most common form of JRA to demonstrate definite radiographic changes. It can occur as the initial and only manifestation or be a sequela of the classic systemic form of the disease. Systemic signs such as fever, lymphadenopathy, and rash may be present but are generally mild to moderate in severity. Persistence of systemic symptoms for > 6 months often denotes a poorer prognosis. (14) The entire clinical spectrum closely simulates rheumatic fever. Following a chronic course the physical appearance has been described as *bird-like,* owing to the frail and delicate features of the limbs and face in combination with a small, receded jaw.

Pauciarticular–Monoarticular Disease. Involvement of four or less joints is seen in approximately 30% of JRA individuals, affecting females three times more frequently. (5) The most common sites affected are the larger joints of the knee, ankle, hip, elbow, or wrist. (4) It is rare in the small joints of the hand or foot. The most common monoarticular site is the knee. Onset is usually insidious, with mild swelling, stiffness, and pain. Systemic manifestations are distinctly infrequent. In all JRA patients the monoarticular onset most commonly is complicated with iridocyclitis, which, if untreated, may result in blindness. (4,12) Radiographic changes are also commonly observed in this form of JRA.

Generally, the prognosis in JRA is good. Fewer than 20% of cases have progressive destructive disease, with the majority entering into long periods of remission without significant joint damage. (10) Laboratory investigations are not diagnostic. The presence of rheumatoid factor is a poor prognostic sign and is found in < 10% of JRA patients. (2) In the active acute phases elevated ESR and a positive CRP are to be expected. Anemia

and leukocytosis are also common findings. Numerous histocompatibility antigens, including HLA-B27, may be present, especially with spinal involvement. (10)

Pathologic Features

The pathologic characteristics in JRA are virtually identical to the adult form; however, discrete differences exist in the synovium, where there is a lower degree of inflammatory changes as evidenced by less fibrinous exudate and cellular proliferation. (15) Pannus is less extensive but still produces significant cartilage and osseous destruction. Articular bony ankylosis is a frequent sequela, especially of the carpus, tarsus, and cervical apophyseal joints. Growth disturbances of bone owing to either accelerated growth plate activity or its premature fusion are common. The pathogenesis is most likely related to increased blood flow at the growth plate, as well as inactivity, steroids, and neurogenic factors. (16) Owing to looser attachment of periosteum to bone in a child, periostitis is a common response to adjacent articular, periarticular, and intraosseous inflammatory hyperemia.

Radiologic Features

Radiographic manifestations of JRA depend on age, severity, and variety of the disease, but diagnosis is still primarily based on the plain film findings. (17)

Table 10-40	General Radiologic Features of Juvenile Rheumatoid Arthritis
Early
Soft tissue swelling
Osteoporosis
Periostitis
Late
Uniform loss of joint space
Articular erosions
Growth disturbances
Intra-articular bony ankylosis
Joint subluxation
Epiphyseal compression fractures

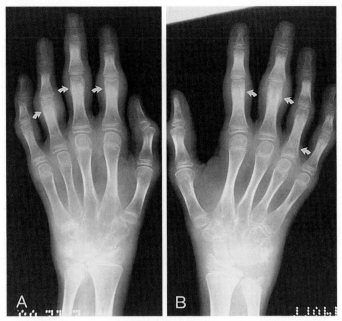

Figure 10-120 **JUVENILE RHEUMATOID ARTHRITIS. A and B. Bilateral PA Hands.** Note the periarticular soft tissue swelling and periostitis (*arrows*).

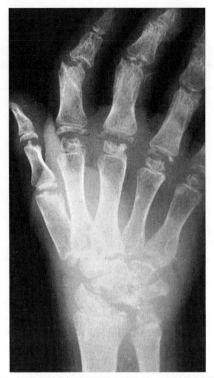

Figure 10-121 **JUVENILE RHEUMATOID ARTHRITIS: EROSIONS. Oblique Hand.** Observe the irregular articular contours of the epiphyses.

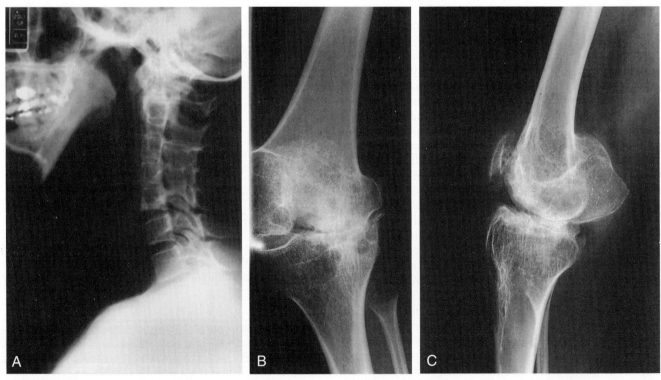

Figure 10-122 **JUVENILE RHEUMATOID ARTHRITIS: SPINAL AND KNEE ABNORMALITIES. A. Lateral Cervical.** Observe the posterior facet ankylosis at C2–C5, which is associated with hypoplastic vertebral bodies and discs. This occurs secondary to the lack of mechanical stimulus from bone deposition during the growth period. Also note the shortening in the vertical ramus and body of the angle of the mandible (antegonial notching). This hypoplastic appearance of the angle of the mandible and vertebral bodies of the cervical spine is classic for juvenile rheumatoid arthritis. **B. AP Knee.**

C. Lateral Knee. Observe the megacondyle as a result of overgrowth of the epiphyses (ballooned epiphyses). Squaring of the inferior surface of the patella is a frequent finding when juvenile rheumatoid arthritis is demonstrated. The overgrowth of the condyle has produced premature stress on the lateral weight-bearing compartment of the knee, and inflammatory joint changes of juvenile rheumatoid have deteriorated the articular cartilage. (Courtesy of Ronald Baxter, MD, Department of Radiology, University Hospital, Denver, Colorado.)

General Radiologic Features

A number of radiographic changes may be visible either singly or in combination with each other. (16) (Table 10-40)

Soft Tissue Swelling. A non-specific sign is soft tissue swelling, but it is generally present as a combination of intra-articular and periarticular soft tissue swelling. (Fig. 10-120)

Osteoporosis. Juxta-articular or diffuse loss of bone density may be present. The presence of transverse, linear growth arrest lines may also be evident.

Periostitis. Frequently, linear periostitis will be visible at the metaphyses of the involved articulation, especially in the hands and feet. (Fig. 10-120)

Uniform Loss of Joint Space. Late in the course of the disease a uniform diminution of joint space may be evident; but it is not a prominent feature.

Articular Erosions. Articular erosions are also relatively late findings. Both marginal and central erosions may be visible. (Fig. 10-121)

Growth Disturbances. The most distinctive radiographic findings are seen as the result of altered growth patterns. Alterations in long bones may be in their length or diameter. Enchondral bones may become too long or too short. Epiphyses are often large and expansile (*ballooned epiphyses*), while the adjacent metaphysis and diaphyses appear constricted. (Fig. 10-122)

Intra-Articular Bony Ankylosis. A common sign of resolution is complete bony ankylosis of the involved joint. This is a most common sequela in the hands, feet, and apophyseal joints of the cervical spine. (Fig. 10-123)

Joint Subluxations. Joint subluxations are varied in their appearance and occur secondary to effusions and to ligament and muscle fibrosis.

Epiphyseal Fractures. Compression fractures of weight-bearing epiphyses may be visible, especially in the lower extremities.

Additional Features. Infrequent associated findings include radiolucent submetaphyseal bands, growth arrest lines, and soft tissue and arterial calcification.

Target Sites of Involvement

The most common sites involved are the knees, ankles, hands, feet, hips, and cervical spine.

Hand and Foot. Involvement of the small articulations of the hands and feet is common, but tends to spare the distal joints. (Figs. 10-120 and 10-121) Tarsal and carpal involvement is characteristic. Isolated and multiple digital length changes may be observed, especially brachydactyly. Ankylosis is most commonly observed in the interphalangeal joints, carpus, and tarsus. The combination of tarsal and carpal ankylosis in a single patient is strongly suggestive of JRA. Because of carpal ankylosis in childhood the ossific carpal mass remains small with adult growth and gives the appearance of an absent or small carpal compartment (*squashed carpi*). At the ankle a tibiotalar slant deformity may occur.

Cervical Spine. Spinal involvement outside the cervical region is unusual except for the occurrence of steroid-induced osteopenia with subsequent thoracic and lumbar compression deformities. (2,16) (Fig. 10-124A) The most conspicuous findings occur in the

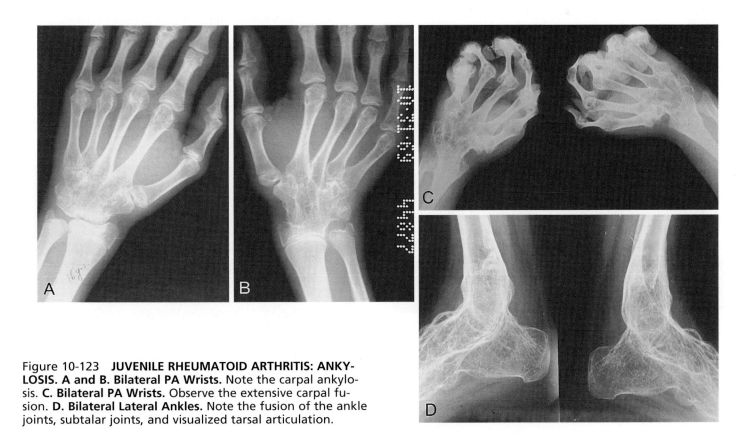

Figure 10-123 **JUVENILE RHEUMATOID ARTHRITIS: ANKY-LOSIS. A and B. Bilateral PA Wrists.** Note the carpal ankylosis. **C. Bilateral PA Wrists.** Observe the extensive carpal fusion. **D. Bilateral Lateral Ankles.** Note the fusion of the ankle joints, subtalar joints, and visualized tarsal articulation.

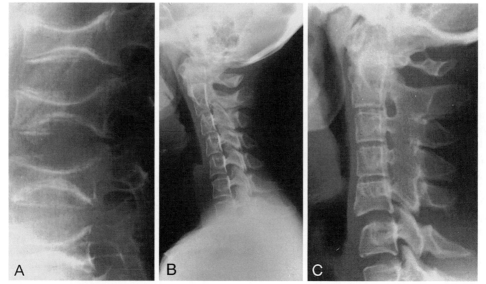

Figure 10-124 JUVENILE RHEUMATOID ARTHRITIS: SPINAL ABNORMALITIES. A. Lateral Lumbar Corticosteroid Complications. Note that osteoporosis and compression fractures have produced a biconcave appearance of the endplates. **B. Lateral Cervical.** Observe the vertebral body hypoplasia of the second, third, fourth, and fifth segments. The odontoid appears enlarged. **C. Lateral Cervical.** Note that the vertebral bodies are hypoplastic in combination with posterior joint ankylosis. These are characteristic cervical spine changes.

upper cervical segments, specifically C1–C4 (18,19), and may be the initial site of involvement. (Table 10-41) About 20% of JRA patients will have radiographic changes in the upper cervical spine. (16) At the atlantoaxial joint, instability of the atlas is present in approximately 30% of these patients owing to secondary disruption of the transverse ligament. (16,18) Additionally, the odontoid may show erosions and at times a generalized increase in length. (20) Abnormalities of this articulation are best evaluated in flexion, where the ADI should be < 5 mm in a child. (21)

The apophyseal joints between the C2 and C4 segments may ankylose. The vertebral bodies, intervertebral discs, and spinous processes also at the same segments will be hypoplastic, similar to congenital block vertebrae. (Fig. 10-124, *B* and *C*) Notably, the spinal canal and intervertebral foramina are unaffected. It is most likely that the attenuated growth of the vertebral bodies and intervening discs is secondary to the apophyseal joint fusion, which eliminates the mechanical stimulus for bone deposition during the growth period. (16)

Other Sites
- *Spine.* Vertebral compression fractures and osteoporosis may occur following steroid therapy. (19)
- *Sacroiliac joint.* Involvement is infrequent but is usually unilateral with erosions, resolving in bony ankylosis. (20–23)

Table 10-41	Radiologic Features of Spinal Involvement in Juvenile Rheumatoid Arthritis

Cervical spine
  Atlantoaxial instability (subluxation, dislocation)
    Apophyseal joint fusion, C2–C4
    Hypoplastic vertebral bodies
    Hypoplastic intervertebral discs
Thoracic and lumbar spine
  Steroid-induced osteoporosis and fractures

- *Knee.* The epiphyses often appear large. The patella is squared at its inferior pole owing to retarded growth of the secondary growth center, similar to that of hemophilia; however, a squared inferior patella configuration is more frequent in JRA. (24) The intercondylar notch may be enlarged. Early depiction of synovial hypertrophy and effusion can be identified on MRI. (25)
- *Hip.* The femoral head can be enlarged and flattened, with the trochanters appearing larger than normal. (Fig. 10-125)
- *Pelvis.* The obturator size appears greater than it should for the size of the pubis and ischia.
- *Mandible.* There will be shortening in the vertical rami and body with a concave notch anterior to the angle of the mandible (*antegonial notching*). (26) This is owing to inhibition of growth from the condylar growth plate. (16)

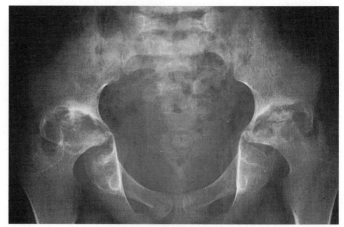

Figure 10-125 JUVENILE RHEUMATOID ARTHRITIS: HIPS. AP Pelvis. Note the combination of large, eroded femoral heads bilaterally. This is characteristic in a young patient.

CAPSULE SUMMARY   Juvenile Rheumatoid Arthritis

General Considerations
- Chronic polyarthritis resembling rheumatoid arthritis clinically and histologically beginning before 16 years of age.
- Tendency for JRA to have more systemic involvement.
- Synonyms include Still's disease and juvenile chronic arthritis.

Clinical Features
- More common in females < 16 years, with peak incidence at 2–5 and 9–12 years.
- *Basic types:* Adult form (seropositive)
  - Poorest prognosis
  - Seronegative form
  - Classic systemic
  - Polyarticular
  - Pauciarticular–monoarticular
    - Distinct lack of rheumatoid factor
    - Symptoms include fever, characteristic rash, lymphadenopathy, iridocyclitis (especially in monoartic-

ular forms), no subcutaneous nodules, and growth disturbance.
- Distinct lack of rheumatoid arthritis

Pathologic Features
- Essentially same as adult form but less fibrosis and proliferation.
- Profound effects on bone growth owing to hyperemia.

Radiologic Features
- General features include soft tissue swelling, osteoporosis, periostitis, growth disturbances, ankylosis, loss of joint space, erosions, subluxations, and epiphyseal compression fractures.
- Target sites include cervical spine, hands, feet, knees, and hips.
- *Cervical spine:* atlantoaxial dislocations, hypoplastic C2–C4 vertebral bodies and discs with ankylosed apophyseal joints.
- Tarsal and carpal ankylosis common.
- *Growth deformities:* brachydactyly, ballooned epiphyses, squashed carpi, and squared patellae.

ANKYLOSING SPONDYLITIS

Ankylosing spondylitis is a chronic inflammatory disorder, predominantly affecting younger adult males, which distinctively involves the axial skeleton. It is characterized by the sequelae of articular bony ankylosis, ligamentous ossification, and manifestations of enthesopathy. Its cause remains unknown.

A plethora of synonyms and eponyms have appeared in the literature. (Table 10-42) An Irish physician, Bernard Connor, in 1691 published the first comprehensive account of an exhumed skeleton afflicted with ankylosing spondylitis. Toward the end of the nineteenth century Bechterew, Strumpell, and Marie published separate and precise clinical observations of ankylosing spondylitis. (1–4) Subsequently, the use of their names as eponyms has become commonplace and at times confusing. Bechterew's descriptions were so vague that it is not clear if the unique pattern he described of a progressive ankylosis and kyphosis beginning in the cervical region and descending the spine was in fact owing to ankylosing spondylitis. Instead it would appear that the entity he

Table 10-42	Synonyms Applied to Ankylosing Spondylitis
Common	
Marie Strumpell's disease	
Bechterew's disease	
Uncommon	
Pelvospondylitis ossificans	
Rheumatic spondylitis	
Rhizomelic spondylitis	
Spondylitis ankylopoietica	
Spondylitis ossificans ligamentosa	
Rheumatoid arthritis of the spine	
Rheumatoid spondylitis	

described was DISH or senile kyphosis, and therefore the term Bechterew's disease as a synonym for ankylosing spondylitis should not be used.

Various other descriptive terms were used in an attempt to characterize the axial predilection and ossifying features. The root derivations of the two terms are from the Greek words *ankylos,* meaning "stiffening of a joint," and *spondylos,* meaning "vertebra."

Clinical Features

Ankylosing spondylitis is a common cause of chronic low back pain in young men, which often evades diagnosis over a protracted period. It is not unexpected that a patient with ankylosing spondylitis may be subjected to various diagnostic evaluations and may receive numerous consultations within a wide variety of health disciplines before the condition is diagnosed. (5) Once identified, appropriate pain control, careful and judicial joint mobilization, and exercise can be implemented, with the aim of maintaining joint mobility and preventing deformity. (6)

The clinical age of onset is usually between 15 and 35 years of age, with an average of 26–27 years; however, it has been suggested that the disease process begins many years before the onset of the first symptoms. (7,8) A juvenile onset has been documented, as has a delayed onset beyond the 4th decade of life. (9,10) Attempts to accurately determine the male to female ratio have shown wide variations from 4 to 15:1, but clearly there is a distinctly male preponderance. (1,11,12) More recent studies have indicated a higher incidence in females than previously shown. (13) Blacks appear to be involved less commonly than whites by a ratio of 1:4. (14) Standardized criteria for ankylosing spondylitis were proposed in 1961 and revised in 1966, but diagnostic accuracy varies considerably. (15–17)

Axial symptoms typically originate in the low back, with aching and stiffness of variable intensity localized to the sacrum, buttocks, and thighs. (18) (Fig. 10-126) The pattern of pain distribution often changes and may alternate from side to side or may be bilateral. Sciatica, if present, usually does not extend beyond the knee. Pain intensity is maximal in the morning, evening, and night hours. Periods of complete remission are not uncommon in the early stages, but studies have suggested that the overall progression of the disease is still the most rapid during the first 10 years after onset. (19) Initial localization of pain may occasionally be encountered in the cervical and thoracic spine or the hips and shoulders. (12,9) An increased mortality rate of up to 50% can be expected in patients with ankylosing spondylitis. (19)

The cauda equina syndrome is occasionally encountered in long-standing ankylosing spondylitis. (20,21) Its development is usually slow but progressive and is often associated with dural ectasia in the lumbosacral spine. (22) Patients with cauda equina may benefit from surgical intervention to improve or halt neurological symptoms. (22) Paraspinal muscle spasm and atrophy, flattened spinal curvatures, percussion tenderness, and reduced mobility are observed. Diminished chest expansion occurs early as a manifestation of costovertebral ankylosis. Advanced deformities, where the chin is virtually fixed onto the chest, are not to be expected if therapeutic regimens are adequate and properly performed. (6) Anterior chest pain owing to costochondral and manubriosternal involvement may mimic cardiac or pleuritic conditions.

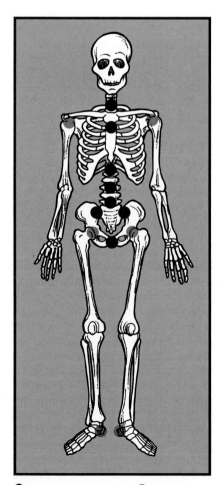

● More common   ● Less common

Figure 10-126 **SKELETAL DISTRIBUTION OF ANKYLOSING SPONDYLITIS.**

Peripheral involvement of the large joints occurs in up to 50% of patients, while up to 30% will have involvement of the smaller joints. The most common peripheral sites are the hips, shoulders, knees, and heels. Typical findings include regional pain, limitation of motion, muscle atrophy, and contractures. Recent studies have correlated a worse prognosis for those patients with early involvement of the hip. (19) Approximately 25% of patients have involvement of the hip. (8) Pain and tenderness over bony protuberances may be present as a manifestation of enthesopathy. This is most frequently observed at the calcaneus, pubic symphysis, iliac crest, trochanters, ischial tuberosities, and costal cartilages.

The most significant extraskeletal manifestations of ankylosing spondylitis involve the eyes, heart, and great vessels and the pulmonary, gastrointestinal, and genitourinary systems.

Ocular involvement is usually manifested as iritis, which is recurrent and unilateral and rarely results in visual impairment. (11) Approximately 25% of ankylosing spondylitis patients will develop iritis, which may precede the spinal involvement by months or years. (10,11) Cardiac involvement consists of tachycardia conduction defects, aortic insufficiency, myocardial fibrosis aortitis, and complicating aortic aneurysms. (23–25) Pulmonary manifestations include upper lung fibrosis with evidence of cavitation simulating tuberculosis. (26,27) These manifestations are more common in long-standing disease.

Gastrointestinal involvement is typically of an inflammatory nature, especially ulcerative colitis and Crohn's disease. (28–30) Up to 18% of these patients may develop ankylosing spondylitis, a 20 times greater incidence than in the general population. (29,30) Chronic prostatitis is associated in 80% of male patients. (31) Up to 8% may develop renal failure secondary to amyloidosis. (32) In previous years, when irradiation was used as a treatment modality, complicating blood dyscrasias and iatrogenic sarcomas were frequently encountered. (33)

Clinical laboratory studies, with the exception of the ESR, are generally not helpful in the diagnostic evaluation of ankylosing spondylitis. The ESR is frequently increased in the active phase of the disease but normalizes once the disease process has resolved or enters into remission. (10) The histocompatibility antigen HLA-B27 is found in up to 90% of the male and female patients with ankylosing spondylitis. (13,16,34,35) This antigen is found in only 6–8% of the normal population and is the most helpful laboratory finding. The distinctive absence of a rheumatoid factor designates this disorder as a *seronegative spondyloarthropathy,* along with enteropathic arthritis, psoriatic arthritis, Reiter's syndrome, and Behçet's syndrome.

Pathologic Features

Little is known concerning the causes of ankylosing spondylitis; however, genetics seems to play a role in determining the susceptibility and severity of the disease process. (36–38) Knowledge of the pathogenetic sequence of events, especially during the early and active phases, is also relatively limited because of the difficulty in obtaining biopsy material and infrequent autopsies. (32) However, lesions of ankylosing spondylitis tend to localize in the axial skeleton at junctions of fibrous and bone tissue (entheses), as well as affecting the synovium. (32,39)

Synovial Articulations

Initial changes consist of synovial proliferation and inflammatory cell infiltrate, producing pannus. (Fig. 10-127) This prolif-

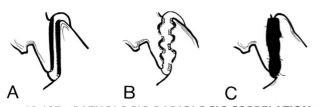

Figure 10-127 **PATHOLOGIC–RADIOLOGIC CORRELATION AT A SYNOVIAL JOINT. A. Normal Joint. B. Inflammatory Erosions with Pseudo-Widening. C. Ankylosis with Obliteration of the Joint Space.** This sequence of changes can occur in any synovial joint, especially those of the spine and pelvis.

erative synovial tissue forms a layer over the articular cartilage, resulting in its destruction and subchondral erosion of bone. Later, this same synovial tissue undergoes fibrosis and cellular transformation to cartilage and bone-producing tissue, leading to intra-articular osseous ankylosis. The joint capsule undergoes the same changes from inflammation to ossification. (32)

Cartilage Articulations

The initial changes occur in the subchondral bone as an osteitis, with an infiltration of chronic inflammatory cells and granulation tissue. (32) Subsequently, there is extensive replacement of the involved bone and intra-articular fibrocartilage by fibrous tissue, which is seen radiographically as joint surface erosions. Eventually, the fibrous tissue undergoes ossification, resulting in os-

seous trabeculae traversing the entire joint space and creating bony ankylosis.

Entheses

An *enthesis* is an anatomic term for a bone–ligament or bone–tendon junction. A normal enthesis is characterized by the gradual transition of fibrous tissue to cartilage, calcified cartilage, and bone. Mechanical stress, blood flow, and metabolic activity at entheses is high and may explain the predilection to be involved in inflammatory connective tissue diseases. (10,39,40) The sequence of entheseal changes begins at the bone–ligament junction, when an inflammatory cell infiltrate replaces the chondrified and calcified parts of the ligament, resulting in bone erosion. (40) (Fig. 10-128) Repair of the erosion is characterized by deposition of woven bone, which projects away from the original surface, producing spur-like bony spicules. Later, this is remodeled and replaced by lamellar bone. (39) The process of enthesopathy is not limited to ankylosing spondylitis; it is also seen in psoriasis, Reiter's syndrome, and enteropathic spondylitis.

Radiologic Features

Radiographic findings in ankylosing spondylitis are distinctive in their appearance and location. The most characteristic articular sites of involvement are the sacroiliac, apophyseal, costovertebral, pubic symphysis, discovertebral, and manubriosternal joints. (41–43) The sequence of articular involvement

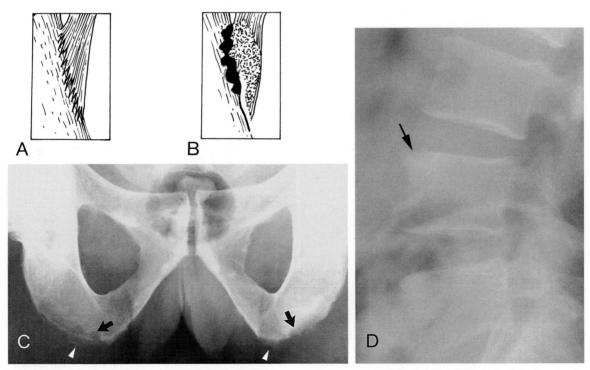

Figure 10-128 **PATHOLOGIC–RADIOLOGIC CORRELATION AT ENTHESES. A. Normal Enthesis.** Note the smooth blending of the tendon into the bony surface. **B. Enthesopathy.** Inflammatory cellular infiltrates erode the adjacent bone. **C. Ischium (whiskering).** Note that erosions create an irregular appearance of the cortex (*arrows*). Reactive periosteal new bone formation can be seen as a veil-like density extending away from the cortex (*arrowheads*). **D. Discovertebral Junction (Romanus lesion).** Note the erosive defect localized to the anterosuperior margin of L4 (*arrow*).

is distinctive, with early bilateral sacroiliac changes and an ascending progression of spinal alterations. Approximately 60% of patients will demonstrate the first spinal radiographic abnormalities at the thoracolumbar area and, less commonly, the lumbosacral region. (44) In women the pattern of involvement is often different, being less severe in intensity, demonstrating peripheral joint involvement more frequently and having a tendency to exhibit sacroiliac changes with minimal to no spinal involvement. (45)

General Features

Essentially, the radiographic features of ankylosing spondylitis relate to the inflammatory, erosive, and ankylosing nature of the disease. The basic changes consist of osteoporosis, erosions, and surrounding reactive sclerosis, followed by bony ankylosis. Notably, these changes are bilateral and symmetric in nature.

Target Sites of Involvement

Sacroiliac Joint. Sacroiliac involvement is the hallmark of ankylosing spondylitis. The identification of sacroiliitis in association with an appropriate clinical presentation is virtually diagnostic for ankylosing spondylitis. (46) Roentgen changes in this joint are usually visible on the initial evaluation of the patient but are often difficult to interpret. (47) In equivocal circumstances, immediate MRI evaluation or radiographic re-evaluation in 3–6 months should show definitive alterations. (47–49) Even radionuclide imaging of sacroiliac joint disease is not definitive and emphasizes the role of plain film radiography in early detection. (50) Upright films will not allow optimum visualization of the joint margins owing to the sacral base inclination. (Fig. 10-129) The most diagnostic projections of the sacroiliac joints are on AP or PA angulated spot views, which visualize the entire joint margin not seen

on routine AP views. The use of oblique projections is not usually necessary if this view is obtained. (Fig. 10-130)

Characteristically, the sacroiliac joints are involved bilaterally and symmetrically, although early in the disease this is not invariable. (51) The major radiographic abnormalities are more apparent on the iliac side owing to the protective sacral hyaline cartilage, which is three times thicker than the iliac hyaline cartilage. (52) The changes also are more prevalent in the lower two thirds of the joint corresponding to the synovial portion, where the pathologic process predominates. (53)

Radiographic findings reflect the sequence of inflammation, bone destruction, and ossification. (Tables 10-43 and 10-44) Forestier classified these sequential changes into three stages. (54) (Fig. 10-131)

Stage 1. Pseudo-Widening of the Joint Space. Loss of the articular cortical bone margin simulates widening of the joint cavity. This is the result of subchondral osteoporosis and produces hazy joint definition.

Stage 2. Erosive and Sclerotic Changes. Superimposed on the widened joint space discrete erosive areas will be seen in the subarticular bone, resulting in an irregular joint margin that has been called the *rosary bead appearance*. (55) Reactive sclerosis, particularly in the adjacent ilium, usually accompanies these erosions. This is the most common stage encountered when the diagnosis is first made. CT scan delineates the erosive osteoarticular lesions. (Fig. 10-132)

Stage 3. Ankylosis. Narrowing and eventual obliteration of the joint space follows the appearance of the erosions. Reactive sclerosis gradually dissipates, to be replaced by generalized osteoporosis. Occasionally, the anterior sacroiliac joint marginal cortex will remain visible through the ankylosis and is referred to as a *ghost joint*. (56) The upper ligamentous portion of the joint will also demonstrate bridging ossification. When prominent, it will be seen on an AP film as a triangular radiopacity (*star sign*). (56) (Fig. 10-133) The time required for ankylosis to occur from the onset of the first radiologic abnormality varies from 7 to 23 years,

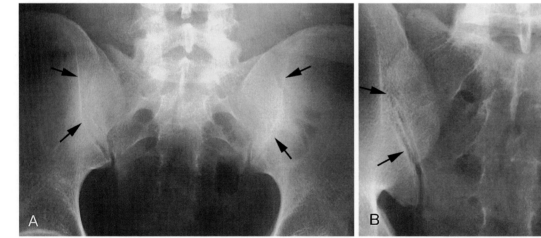
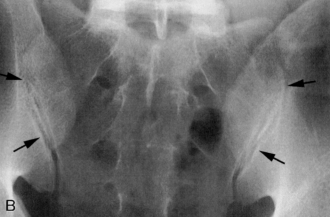

Figure 10-129 **PSEUDO-SACROILIITIS. A. Non-Angulated AP Lumbosacral Spot.** Note the iliac margins bilaterally are blurred and indistinct (*arrows*). There is also the suggestion of iliac sclerosis simulating active sacroiliitis. **B. Tilt-Up View Lumbosacral Spot.** Observe that with the tube tilted cephalad the effects of the angled sacral base are removed and the joint margin comes into clear view. Note the smooth, continuous articular margins and normal subchondral bone density (*arrows*). *COMMENT:* Non-angulated films will not allow optimum visualization of the joint margins owing to the sacral base inclination. The most diagnostic projections of the sacroiliac joints are on AP or PA tilt views, to visualize the entire joint margin not seen on routine AP views. The use of oblique projections is not usually necessary if this view is obtained.

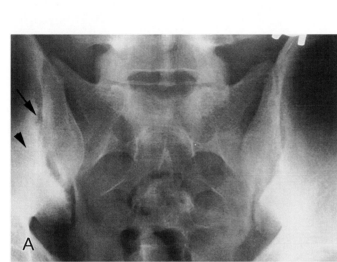
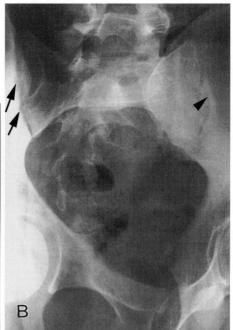

Figure 10-130 **ANKYLOSING SPONDYLITIS: SACROILIAC JOINTS. A. Tilt-Up View Lumbosacral Spot.** Note the characteristic signs of bilateral sacroiliitis: iliac erosions (*arrow*) and sclerosis (*arrowhead*). **B. Oblique Sacroiliac.** Observe that the joint is shown in profile, isolating the erosive defects (*arrows*). On the contralateral side the opposite joint can be seen, although no definite sign can be determined (*arrowhead*). *COMMENT:* AP or PA tilt views optimally show sacroiliac detail. The use of oblique projections is not usually necessary if this view is obtained. (Courtesy of Donald M. Kuppe, DC, Denver, Colorado.)

Table 10-43	Radiologic Changes in the Sacroiliac Joints in Ankylosing Spondylitis

General
   Bilateral, symmetric
   Iliac side more extensively involved
   Initially involves lower two-thirds of joint
Early (sacroiliitis)
   Articular erosions (rosary bead)
   Diminished joint space
   Loss of articular cortex definition (pseudo-widening)
   Patchy reactive sclerosis
   Subchondral osteoporosis
Late
   Bony ankylosis
   Generalized osteoporosis—disappearance of reactive sclerosis
   Ghost joint margin
   Star sign

Table 10-44	Radiologic Differential Diagnosis of Sacroiliac Disease

Disease	Bilateral Symmetric	Bilateral Asymmetric	Uni-Lateral
Ankylosing spondylitis	+++	+ (early)	+ (early)
DISH	+ (upper joint)	—	—
Enteropathic sacroiliitis	+++	—	—
Gouty arthritis	+	+	+
Hyperparathyroidism	+++	—	—
Infection	—	—	+++
Osteitis condensans ilii	+++	+	+
Osteoarthritis (DJD)	—	+	++
Psoriatic spondylitis	+	+++	++
Reiter's syndrome	++	++	+++
Rheumatoid arthritis	—	+	+++

DISH, diffuse idiopathic skeletal hyperostosis; *DJD*, degenerative joint disease; —, absent; +, rare; ++, common; +++, very common.

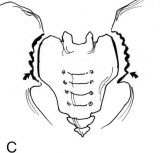

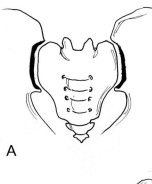

A

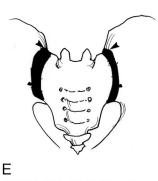

C

E

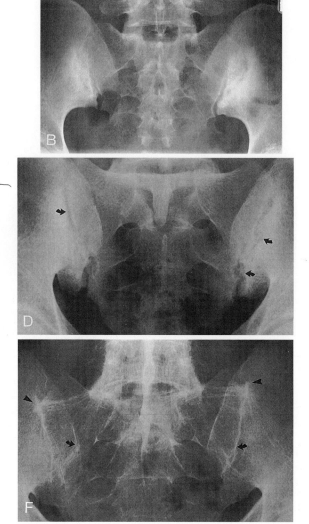

Figure 10-131 **ANKYLOSING SPONDYLITIS: SACROILIAC JOINTS. A and B. Stage 1.** Note that the joint margins appear hazy and frayed, and the joint cavity is widened. **C and D. Stage 2.** Observe that erosions (*arrows*) and adjacent reactive sclerosis are evident. This is the most frequent appearance found on the initial examination. **E. Stage 3.** On the detail, note the obliterated joint space (*arrows*) and the fused upper joint space (*arrowheads*). **F. Stage 3.** Observe the obliterated joint space, ghost joint (*arrows*), and star sign (*arrowheads*).

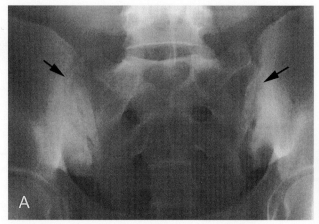

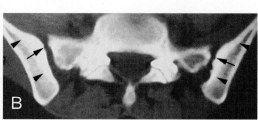

Figure 10-132 **ANKYLOSING SPONDYLITIS: SACROILIAC JOINTS. A. AP Sacrum.** Note that bilateral sacroiliitis is clearly seen with erosions, hazy joint margin, and subchondral iliac sclerosis (*arrows*). **B. Axial CT: Sacroiliac Joints.** Observe the erosive iliac lesions (arrows) and the subchondral sclerosis (*arrowheads*). (Courtesy of Gary L. Boog, DC, Lancaster, New Hampshire.)

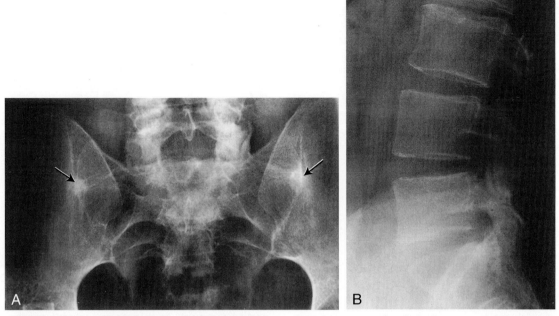

Figure 10-133   **ANKYLOSING SPONDYLITIS: STAR SIGN AND SQUARED VERTEBRA. A. AP Tilt-Up View, Sacroiliac Joints.** Note the bilateral ankylosis of the lower two thirds of the sacroiliac joint. Observe the area of bony density at the junction of the fibrous and synovial portion of the joint, known as the star sign (*arrows*). Note that the upper third (fibrous portion) of the sacroiliac joint is uninvolved. A char-acteristic trait of ankylosing spondylitis is to involve only the synovial portion of the sacroiliac joints. **B. Lateral Lumbar.** Observe the squared-off appearance of the verte-bral bodies, characteristic of end-stage ankylosing spondyli-tis of the spine. (Courtesy of Joel G. Green, DC, Salem, Massachusetts.)

with a mean of 14 years. (57) At least 50% of cases will develop complete and bilateral sacroiliac fusion, and approximately 40% will progress to stage 2 and resolve. (58) A similar parallel sequence of events and radiographic signs is often observed in the symphysis pubis.

This staging of sacroiliitis differs from the one formulated by the National Institute of Arthritis and Metabolic Diseases. (17) *Spine.* Localization of abnormalities in the spine occurs at the discovertebral junction, apophyseal, and costovertebral joints as well as at the atlantoaxial joint and spinous process entheses, each of which requires specific views for adequate evaluation. (59) (Tables 10-45 and 10-46) The earliest spinal manifestations are usually found first at the thoracolumbar and second at the lumbosacral regions. (44) (Figs. 10-134 and 10-135) With progression of the spinal involvement, an ascending phenomenon is generally observed that may result in complete vertebral column ankylosis.

Discovertebral Junction (Syndesmophyte Formation). The pathogenetic sequence of events that occurs involving the outer fibers of the annulus fibrosus and its attachment to the vertebral body rim eventually results in segmental ankylosis by the formation of syndesmophytes. (54) The process of syndesmophyte formation follows a distinct pattern, characterized by inflammation, destruction, and ossification within ligamentous tissue.

The initial alteration at the outer annulus enthesis is a focal destruction of the vertebral body rim. This results in a discrete radiolucent corner erosion termed a *Romanus lesion*. (60) (Fig. 10-136) This decreases the anterior vertebral body concavity, creating a *squared contour*. (55) (Fig. 10-137A) Occasionally, the reparative process may be exuberant and create an anterior convexity of the vertebral body, termed a *barrel-shaped ver-*

tebra. (61) (Fig. 10-137B) As the corner erosions heal, a transient reactive sclerosis will occur in the subadjacent bone, which radiographically is termed the *shiny corner sign.* (Figs. 10-136 and 10-138) All of these early radiographic signs are relatively transient and not easily recognized.

After these peripheral discovertebral changes, ossification of the outer annulus fibers and the tissue directly beneath the ante-

Table 10-45	Radiologic Diagnostic Technologic Correlation in Ankylosing Spondylitis			
Location	AP Routine	AP Angulated	Lateral	Oblique
Cervical spine				
C1–C2	+	—	+++	+
Syndesmophytes	—	—	+++	+++
Apophyseal joints	—	+	+++	+++
Thoracic spine				
Squaring	+	—	+++	+++
Syndesmophytes	+++	—	+++	+
Costovertebral	+++	—	—	+
Lumbar spine				
Squaring	+	—	+++ (T10–L2)	++
Syndesmophytes	++	—	+++ (T10–L2)	+++
Corner erosions	+	—	+++ (T10–L2)	++
Sclerosis	+	—	+++ (T10–L2)	++
Apophyseal	+	—	+	+++
Sacroiliac	+	+++	—	+

—; will not be visible; +, difficult visualization; ++, good visualization; +++, most optimum visualization.

Table 10-46	Radiologic Manifestations of Ankylosing Spondylitis in the Spine

Early
Locations: sacroiliac, thoracolumbar, lumbosacral, atlantoaxial
  Apophyseal joint erosions and ankylosis
  Atlantoaxial instability
  Lumbar hyperlordosis
  Marginal syndesmophytes
  Vertebral body corner erosions (Romanus lesion)
  Vertebral body corner sclerosis (shiny corner)
  Vertebral body squaring
Late
  Discovertebral instability (Andersson's lesion)
  Endplate concavity (ballooning)
  Facet fusion (trolley track)
  Fractures (carrot stick)
  Ligamentous ossification (dagger sign)
  Marginal syndesmophytes (bamboo spine)
  Osteoporosis
  Peripheral joint involvement
  Posture changes (kyphosis, chin on chest)
  Vertebral body atrophy (cervical spine)

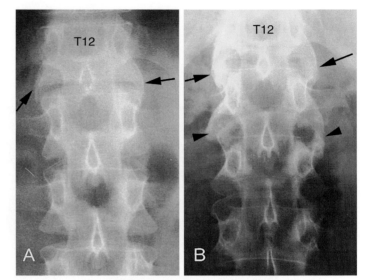

Figure 10-135 ANKYLOSING SPONDYLITIS: THORACO-LUMBAR PROGRESSION. A. Initial Study. Note that early bilateral marginal syndesmophytes extend between T12 and L1 (*arrows*). At this stage early bilateral sacroiliitis was evident with no other evidence of spinal involvement. **B. 5-Year Follow-Up.** Note the T12–L1 syndesmophytes have completely bridged the interspace (*arrows*). There is now extension of syndesmophyte formation between L1 and L2 (*arrowheads*). (Courtesy of John C. Slizeski, DC, Denver, Colorado.)

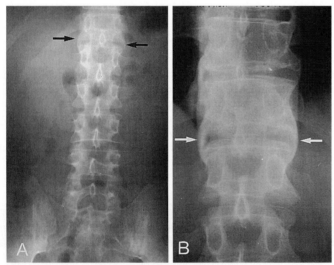

Figure 10-134 ANKYLOSING SPONDYLITIS: EARLY SPINAL INVOLVEMENT. A. Bilateral Sacroiliitis. In conjunction with the evidence of bilateral sacroiliitis, observe the early syndesmophyte formation at the thoracolumbar junction (*arrows*). **B. Marginal Syndesmophytes.** Note the syndesmophytes (*arrows*). *COMMENT:* This is a common site for the earliest spinal changes to occur. Whenever an equivocal diagnosis of sacroiliitis is suspected, the thoracolumbar region should be carefully evaluated for additional radiologic signs such as syndesmophytes. (Panel A courtesy of John C. Slizeski, DC, Denver, Colorado. Panel B reprinted with permission from **Yochum TR:** *Ankylosing spondylitis (shiny corner sign).* ACA J Chiro December, 1980.)

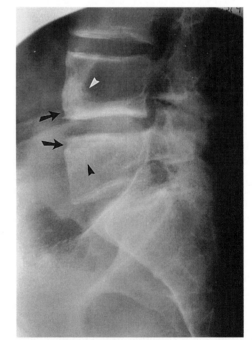

Figure 10-136 ANKYLOSING SPONDYLITIS: ROMANUS LESION. Lateral Lumbar. Note the early anterior body margin erosions (*arrows*). This is an infrequently observed sign before the formation of syndesmophytes. A localized surrounding reactive sclerosis (shiny corner sign) is also present (*arrowheads*).

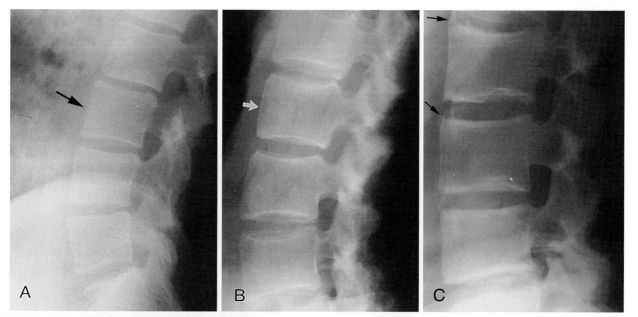

Figure 10-137 **ANKYLOSING SPONDYLITIS: LUMBAR VERTEBRAL BODY CHANGES. A. Squared Vertebrae.** Observe that the anterior concavity of the vertebral bodies has been obliterated at all levels (*arrow*). **B. Barrel-Shaped Vertebra.** Note that the anterior body contour is convex owing to cor-ner erosions and subligamentous new bone formation (*arrow*). **C. Early Syndesmophyte Formation.** Note the small, thin, vertical ossification of the outer annulus fibers extending from the vertebral body margins (*arrows*). (Panel B courtesy of Gerald A. Fitzgerald, MD, Sydney, Australia.)

rior longitudinal ligament occurs. Contrary to popular belief, the ALL does not ossify, except late in the disease and only in its deepest fibers. (58) This inflammatory ossification of spinal ligamentous tissue is called a *syndesmophyte* and has morphologic features that distinguish it from other spinal outgrowths. (Fig. 10-139) Radiographically, this syndesmophyte is seen as a fine, vertical bridging ossification at the outer disc limit, which originates at

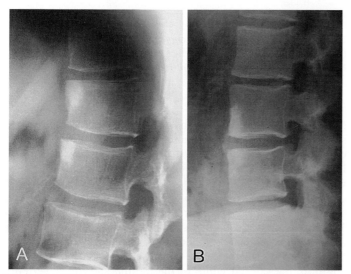

Figure 10-138 **ANKYLOSING SPONDYLITIS: SHINY CORNER SIGN. A. L1–L2. B. L3–L4.** Note the dense reactive sclerosis, which signifies inflammatory osteitis at the body margins before syndesmophyte formation. This is a transient phenomenon and will disappear when interbody fusion is achieved. (Reprinted with permission from **Yochum TR:** *Ankylosing spondylitis (shiny corner sign).* ACA J Chiro December, 1980. Courtesy of Miriam E. Minty, DC, Perth, Australia.)

the extreme of adjacent vertebral body margins. The correct terminology is *marginal syndesmophyte,* to emphasize its point of bony attachment. Early in their formation, these syndesmophytes are best seen on oblique and lateral projections, although later they will also be visible on frontal views. When multiple segments are ankylosed by symmetric, marginal syndesmophytes, the continuous undulating spinal contour is termed the *bamboo spine* or *poker spine.* (Fig. 10-140)

Other destructive foci may appear along the endplate area and may or may not be symptomatic. (62,63) (Fig. 10-141) When localized, these most likely represent pathologic Schmorl's node herniations through adjacent osteoporotic bone. If the entire endplate is irregular and poorly defined, this is usually the sequela of hypermobility through a fractured, previously ankylosed segment and is termed an *Andersson lesion* (64), which is radiographically identical to intervertebral disc infection or neuropathic arthropathy.

The internal contents of the intervertebral disc, including the nucleus pulposus and inner layers of the annulus fibrosus, will also ossify later in the disease, once syndesmophytes are present. The bone within the disc will contain organized trabeculae and hematopoietic marrow. (31) The height of the involved intervertebral discs is variable; however, if a change is present, it will usually be uniform throughout the involved region, except in instances of late onset of ankylosing spondylitis, where isolated segmental degenerative changes may be superimposed. Occasionally, in combination with osteoporosis, the endplates may demonstrate an exaggerated concavity, resulting in a *ballooning phenomenon* of the disc.

Vertebral osteoporosis is often prominent and frequently seen early in the disease process. (Figs. 10-140 and 10-142) The osteoporosis is caused by a combination of the inflammatory process, resultant immobility following ankylosis, and drug therapy. Compression fractures of the spine may occur with a slightly greater frequency.

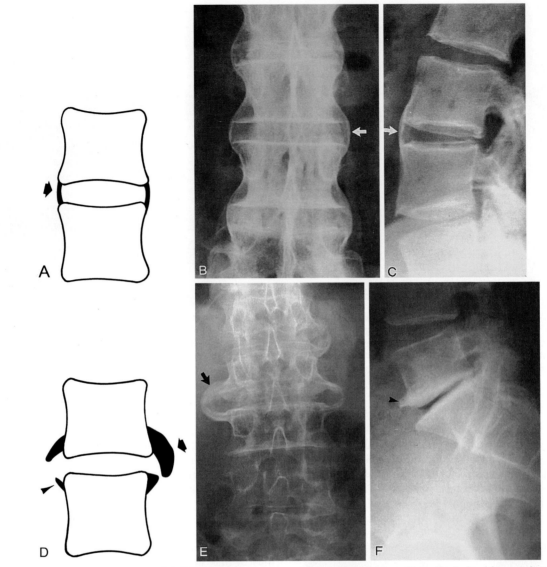

Figure 10-139 **SYNDESMOPHYTES AND OSTEOPHYTES: RADIOLOGIC DIFFERENTIATION. A–C. Marginal Syndesmophyte.** Observe the vertical orientation and thin nature of the ossification (*arrows*) typical of ankylosing spondylitis.

D–F. Osteophytes. Note that claw (*arrows*) and traction (*arrowheads*) spurs are more horizontally oriented, thicker, and more distinctive in degenerative joint disease.

Apophyseal and Costovertebral Joints. The earliest signs are erosions, sclerosis, and loss of joint space. To optimally observe these changes, oblique views in the lumbar spine and the lateral view of the cervical spine are necessary. Thoracic spine apophyseal joint involvement is difficult to assess. Similar changes will be seen in the costovertebral joints. An initial site of involvement that is readily visible is the upper costotransverse articulations, as seen on the AP projection. (65) Erosions and blurring of the joint margins are the most prominent early signs, followed by ankylosis. Once articular ankylosis has occurred, the bony trabeculae will be continuous across the previous joint cavity. (Fig. 10-143) In the lumbar spine, ossification of the joint capsule, ligamentum flavum, and interspinous ligaments produces three parallel linear densities on an AP film and is referred to as the *trolley track sign*. (Fig. 10-144)

If only the interspinous and supraspinous ligaments ossify and show as a single but central radiodense vertical stripe connecting the lumbar spinous processes, this is referred to as the *dagger sign*.

(Fig. 10-145) Entheseal erosions of the spinous processes may result in new bone formation and tapering, especially in the cervical spine. The lumbar lordosis is usually flattened, with complete loss of intersegmental motion on flexion–extension films.

Cervical Spine. Radiographic abnormalities consist of a decreased lordosis, often in association with the head being considerably anterior to the normal weight-bearing position. (Fig. 10-146A) Anterior squaring, syndesmophytes, and osteoporosis are evident at the vertebral bodies. Early syndesmophyte formation is often seen between the C2–C3 and C6–C7 interspaces. In addition, the sagittal width of the middle and lower vertebral bodies may appear decreased owing to disuse atrophy in more chronic cases. (Fig. 10-146B) Posteriorly, the apophyseal joints show varying degrees of erosions, sclerosis, loss of joint space, and ankylosis. Entheseal erosions of the spinous processes in the lower segments results in a tapered contour similar to rheumatoid arthritis. Periostitis at the sites of these erosions is an associated feature. The overall diameter of the intervertebral foramen may

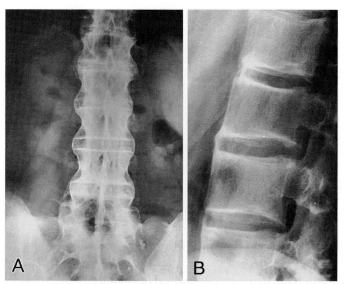

Figure 10-140 **ANKYLOSING SPONDYLITIS: LUMBAR SPINE. A and B. Bamboo Spine.** Note that complete interbody ankylosis by marginal syndesmophytes produces this distinctive undulating spinal contour.

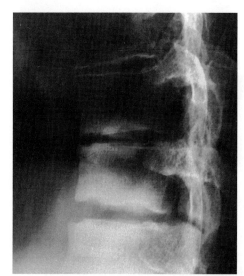

Figure 10-141 **ANKYLOSING SPONDYLITIS: ENDPLATE EROSIONS. Lateral Thoracic.** Observe the irregular contour of the endplates owing to Schmorl's nodes.

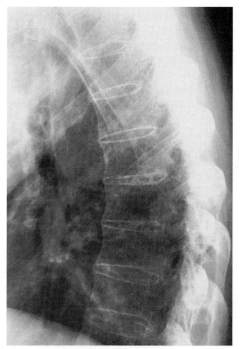

Figure 10-142 **ANKYLOSING SPONDYLITIS: LATERAL THORACIC.** Note the anterior syndesmophytes and osteoporotic nature of the vertebral bodies.

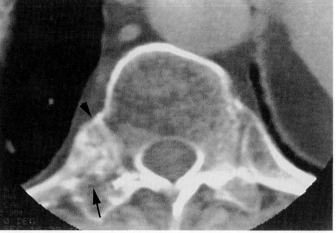

Figure 10-143 **ANKYLOSING SPONDYLITIS: COSTOVERTEBRAL ANKYLOSIS. Axial CT: T11.** Note that the CT scan through the T11 level shows ankylosis of the costotransverse (*arrow*) and costovertebral (*arrowhead*) joints.

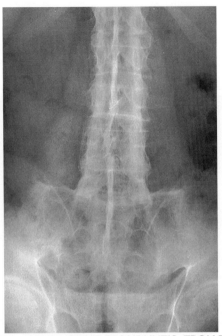

Figure 10-144 ANKYLOSING SPONDYLITIS: TROLLEY TRACK APPEARANCE. AP Lumbar. Note that ossification within the facet joint capsules and ligamentum flavum bilaterally produces two vertical linear densities at the lateral aspects of the vertebral bodies. There is co-existent ossification within the interspinous–supraspinous ligaments, creating the midline linear opacity.

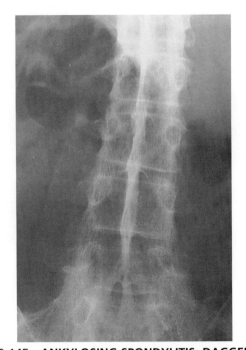

Figure 10-145 ANKYLOSING SPONDYLITIS: DAGGER SIGN. AP Lumbar. Observe that isolated ossification of the interspinous and supraspinous ligament produces this central, linear opacity. (Courtesy of Lawrence A. Cooperstein, MD, Pittsburgh, Pennsylvania.)

appear increased in advanced cases owing to arachnoid dilation. Temporomandibular joint involvement often parallels the appearance of changes in the cervical spine.

Involvement at the atlantoaxial joint in ankylosing spondylitis is less common and less severe than in rheumatoid arthritis, with an incidence between 2% and 15%. (66–68) Development of atlantoaxial changes is usually a late phenomenon but may be an early complication. (69) This is frequently asymptomatic but is potentially life threatening. (70) Manifestations of involvement include an increased ADI (> 3 mm, especially in flexion), odontoid erosions, and increased density of the odontoid (*shiny odontoid sign*). The earliest change is usually an increased ADI secondary to transverse ligament instability. (Figs. 10-146*C* and 10-147) Reankylosis in the subluxated position may occur.

Peripheral Joints. Peripheral involvement is variable but most frequently involves the hips, shoulders, and heel, usually in a bilateral symmetric manner. (Fig. 10-148) Approximately 50% of all patients with ankylosing spondylitis will develop peripheral joint disease. (71)

Hip. Changes in the hip consist of a uniform loss of joint space with axial migration of the head, which may produce protrusio acetabuli. In addition, small osteophytes and subchondral cysts in the femoral head can be apparent, with eventual ankylosis. Entheseal changes of erosion and periostitis may be visible at the trochanters and adjacent ischial tuberosity. (Fig. 10-149)

Shoulder. Erosive lesions will be visible at the lateral aspect of the humerus. Often, signs of rotator cuff tear will be evident, with humeral head elevation. Erosions and eventual resorption of the distal clavicle may occur, with evidence of enthesopathy at the coracoclavicular ligaments and humeral tuberosities.

Calcaneus. Radiologic changes involve the posterior Achilles and plantar aponeurosis insertions. The abnormalities at these locations consist of erosions, localized osteoporosis, and periostitis. (34)

Enthesopathy. Involvement of bone–ligament junctions is most prominent at the iliac crests, ischial tuberosities, femoral trochanters, spinous processes, and peripherally at the calcaneal plantar surface. Radiographic signs of enthesopathy include a bilateral and symmetric distribution of cortical erosions; sclerosis; and fine, periosteal new bone formation termed *whiskering*. (72,73) (Fig. 10-149) These periosteal whiskers initially are very fine and extend away from the bone of origin in the direction of the ligament or tendon and usually correspond to sites of pain. Differentiation should be made between ankylosing spondylitis and the more common degenerative changes, especially at the ischial tuberosities, as well as enthesopathy of other inflammatory arthropathies. (73) (Table 10-47)

Complications

Carrot-Stick Fractures. A fracture caused by the brittle nature of the ankylosed vertebral column is called a *carrot-stick fracture*. (Fig. 10-150*A*) The risk of fracture in patients with ankylosing spondylitis tends to increase during the duration of the disease process. (74) Fractures through ankylosed segments most frequently occur in the lower cervical and thoracolumbar regions and may follow relatively trivial trauma. (75–77) Cervical fractures are often disabling and can be lethal. Associated epidural hematoma occurs in about 20% of carrot stick fractures. (78) Thoracic and lumbar fractures may be relatively asymptomatic, though aortic injuries can occur. (75,77,79) The use of MRI should be considered during the assessment of spinal fractures to assess for further complications. (80) Progressive and increasing disability may require orthopedic fixation. (81,82)

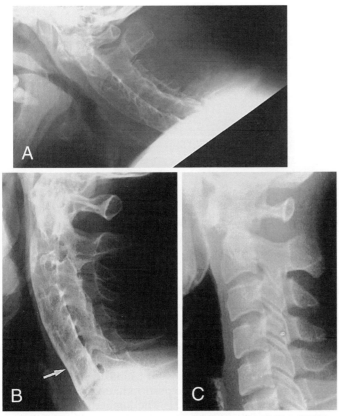

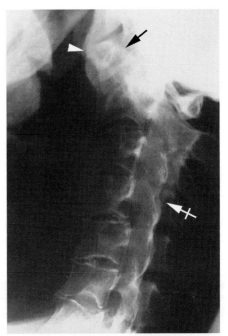

Figure 10-147 **ANKYLOSING SPONDYLITIS: ATLANTOAXIAL INSTABILITY. Lateral Cervical.** Note that the atlantoaxial joint space is 7 mm (*arrow*). Note the displacement of the prevertebral soft tissues from the advancing anterior arch (*arrowhead*). There is extensive involvement of the entire cervical spine with ankylosis of all facet joints (*crossed arrow*).

Figure 10-146 **ANKYLOSING SPONDYLITIS: CERVICAL SPINE. A. Altered Posture.** Note that the anterior carriage of the head with fusion of the apophyseal joints and bodies characterizes sequelae in this part of the spine. **B. Ankylosis and Vertebral Body Atrophy.** Observe that loss of normal mechanical forces has produced disuse osteopenia and resorption of the anterior vertebral body (*arrow*). **C. Atlantoaxial Instability.** Note that the atlantodental interspace is widened in this 20-year-old man who presented with bilateral sacroiliitis.

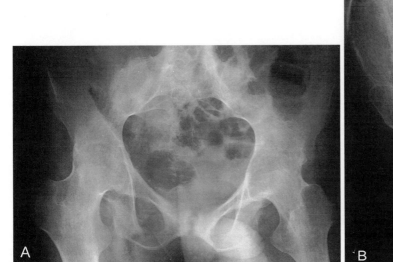

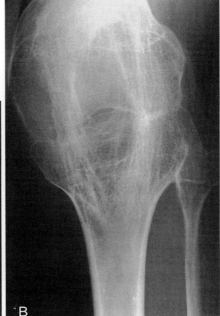

Figure 10-148 **ANKYLOSING SPONDYLITIS: PERIPHERAL JOINTS. A. AP Pelvis: Ankylosis.** Note the bilaterally symmetric ankylosis of the hips, the associated sacroiliac fusion, and the erosive changes at the symphysis pubis. **B. AP Knee: Ankylosis.** Observe the fusion of the tibiofemoral and tibiofibular articulations.

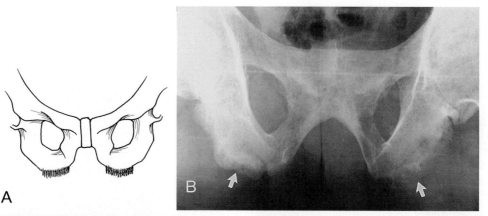

Figure 10-149 **ANKYLOSING SPONDYLITIS. A and B. Enthesopathy.** Observe the periosteal new bone formation at the ischial tuberosities bilaterally (whiskering) (*arrows*). The symphysis pubis is ankylosed.

Table 10-47	Inflammatory Arthropathies Associated with Enthesopathy and Periostitis	
Fluffy, Irregular (Spiculated)	**Sharp, Well-Defined (Laminated, Solid)**	
Ankylosing spondylitis	Rheumatoid arthritis	
Psoriasis	Juvenile rheumatoid arthritis	
Reiter's disease	Hypertrophic osteoarthropathy	
	Septic arthritis	

Andersson's Lesion. Following fractures through an ankylosed segment, there is often a failure to reankylose. (Fig. 10-150, *B* and *C;* Table 10-48) The sequela to this non-union is the development of pseudo-arthrosis through the intervertebral disc. (64) Radiographically, there is a rapid loss of the adjacent endplates, sclerosis, and fragmentation of the underlying vertebral body. The appearance is identical to an active infection or a neurotrophic process involving the intervertebral disc space. Surgical fusion is the treatment of choice.

Arachnoid Diverticula. Generalized dural ectasia in association with diverticula formation has been described and appears closely linked to the development of cauda equina syndrome. (21) (Fig. 10-151) Other causes for cauda equina syndrome in ankylosing spondylitis include postirradiation ischemia, demyelination, and arachnoiditis. (21) The lumbar spine is the most common site for diverticular formation, followed by the thoracic spine. It is rare in the cervical spine. Most diverticula are directed posteriorly and can erode the pedicles, lamina, and spinous process. They are best shown by CT. Scalloping of the posterior vertebral body can be also seen. (83) Myelography should not be attempted in the ankylosed spine because it may lead to deterioration of the patient's condition. (84)

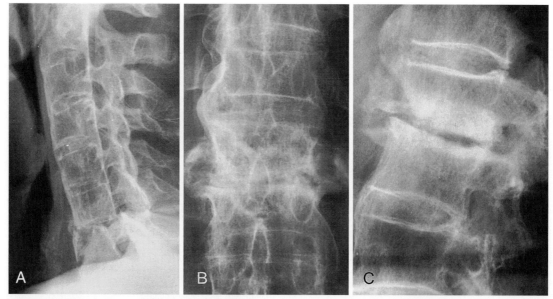

Figure 10-150 **ANKYLOSING SPONDYLITIS: DISCOVERTEBRAL COMPLICATIONS. A. Lateral Cervical, Carrot-Stick Fracture.** Note that a fracture has occurred at the C6 interspace following trivial trauma to this completely ankylosed spine. **B and C. Lumbar Spine, Andersson's Lesion.** Observe that a fracture has occurred through an ankylosed segment, producing hypermobility, sclerosis, and body destruction, simulating an infection or a neurotrophic process. These severe degenerative changes occurred within 1 year after trauma. (Panel A courtesy of David P. Thomas, MD, Melbourne, Australia. Panels A–C reprinted with permission from **Yochum TR:** *Discovertebral destruction associated with ankylosing spondylitis (the Andersson lesion).* ACA J Chiro, August, 1981.)

Table 10-48	Miscellaneous Terminology Applied to Ankylosing Spondylitis
Term	**Definition**
Andersson's lesion (pseudo-arthrosis)	Usually in advanced cases in which a single level becomes mobile, resulting in instability and adjacent destruction that simulates infection or neuropathy
Bamboo spine (poker spine)	Undulating and segmented appearance of the spine owing to uniform and symmetric bridging syndesmophytes
Barrel vertebra	Accentuated convexity of anterior vertebral body
Carrot-stick fracture	Term applied to a fracture that occurs through an ankylosed segment to amplify the brittleness of the spine
Dagger sign	Ossification of supraspinous and interspinous ligaments appears on the AP lumbar film as a midline vertical linear radiopacity
Discal ballooning	Endplate biconcavity owing to mechanical effect of the nucleus pulposus on osteoporotic vertebral bodies
Enthesopathy	Inflammatory infiltration at a bone–ligament junction, resulting in bone erosion followed by new bone formation
Ghost joint	Visualization of articular cortex through an ankylosed joint
Romanus lesion	Erosion at the anterior vertebral body margin at annulus insertion as a precursor to syndesmophyte formation
Rosary bead	Undulating appearance of sacroiliac articular margins owing to joint erosions
Seronegative	Lack of rheumatoid factor in the blood and applied to ankylosing spondylitis, psoriasis, Reiter's syndrome, and enteropathic arthritis
Shiny corner sign	Transient reactive sclerosis adjacent to a Romanus lesion as a precursor to syndesmophyte formation
Star sign	Ossification of superior sacroiliac ligaments, creating a triangular radiopacity
Squaring	Loss of normal anterior vertebral body concavity owing to a Romanus lesion and anterior periostitis
Syndesmophyte	Inflammatory ossification of a spinal ligament
Trolley track spine	Three vertical lines seen in advanced case on the AP lumbar film owing to ossification in the apophyseal joints and interspinous and supraspinous ligaments
Whiskering	Seen at entheses as fine to coarse spicules of bone extending away from the bone owing to periostitis

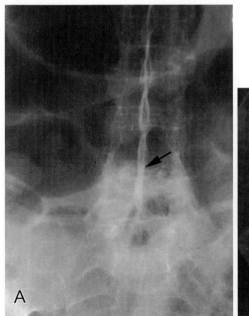
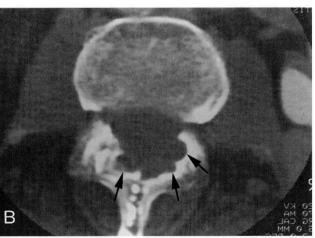

Figure 10-151   **ANKYLOSING SPONDYLITIS: ARACHNOID DIVERTICULA. A. AP Lumbar.** Note that no evidence of pedicle or other destruction can be seen. Observe the features of advanced ankylosing spondylitis with bilateral fusion of the sacroiliac joints and ossification of the interspinous and supraspinous ligament producing the dagger sign (*arrow*). **B. Axial CT: L5.** Note the extensive erosive lesions of the inner aspects of the lamina bilaterally (*arrows*). Each erosion is demarcated by a sclerotic margin denoting the slow and extrinsic nature of the defects from the adjacent arachnoid diverticula. *COMMENT:* This finding is frequently associated with neurological complications. (Courtesy of Lawrence A. Cooperstein, MD, Pittsburgh, Pennsylvania.)

Ankylosis of Joint Prostheses. The hip is the most common joint to be replaced, which can dramatically restore mobility and function. However, studies have revealed that bony ankylosis of the prosthesis can occur in 30–60% of patients within 6 months. (85,86)

Atlantoaxial Rotary Subluxation. Unilateral displacement of the atlantoaxial joint, which then fixates in the position, may complicate < 1% of patients. (87)

CAPSULE SUMMARY   Ankylosing Spondylitis

General Considerations

- A chronic inflammatory disorder principally affecting the articulations, ligaments, and tendons of the spine and pelvis, often resulting in complete polyarticular ankylosis.
- Synonyms include Marie-Strumpell disease, rhizomelic spondylitis, pelvospondylitis ossificans, and rheumatoid spondylitis.

Clinical Features

- Onset is usually between 15 and 35 years and involves males 10:1.
- Initially at the sacroiliac joints bilaterally, then ascends the spine.
- Skip involvement, particularly to the thoracolumbar spine; costal articulations and cervical spine are not uncommon.
- Pain and tenderness, especially over bony protuberances, and increasing stiffness.
- Sciatica is often bilateral or may alternate from side to side.
- Heel pain, muscle spasm, and atrophy may be prominent.
- Complications include iritis, aortitis, valvular incompetence, aneurysms, conduction blocks, upper lobe pulmonary fibrosis, inflammatory bowel disease, renal failure owing to secondary amyloidosis, carrot-stick fractures, Andersson's lesion, and prosthesis ankylosis.
- Laboratory findings will show ESR elevation, depending on disease activity, mild anemia, positive HLA-B27 (90%; 6% false positive), and negative rheumatoid arthritis latex (seronegative).

Pathologic Features

- In synovial joints, the initial change is that of a non-specific synovitis similar to rheumatoid arthritis, except that it is less extensive and of lower intensity (pannus formation), with subsequent fibroplasia and cartilaginous metaplasia, leading to resultant ossification.
- In cartilage joints, the initial subchondral osteitis is replaced by fibrous tissue that subsequently ossifies. In the outer annulus fibers this forms syndesmophytes.
- At entheses, inflammatory changes at ligamentous attachments (enthesopathy) result in bony erosions, sclerosis, and periostitis.

Radiologic Features

- Initial changes occur in the sacroiliac joints, then at the thoracolumbar and lumbosacral junctions; the remainder of the spine shows progressive changes, generally in an ascending manner.
- Up to 50% of cases have rhizomelic involvement (hips, shoulders).
- Major signs are osteoporosis, erosions with surrounding sclerosis, and bony ankylosis. Enthesopathy is usually evident when sacroiliac changes are seen, especially in the pelvis.

- The most commonly involved areas are the sacroiliac joints, spine, and proximal large joints of the shoulder, hip, and rib cage.
- *Sacroiliac joint:* involvement is usually bilateral and symmetric, with iliac involvement early owing to thinner iliac cartilage, especially in the lower two thirds of joint.
- Stages of involvement are pseudo-widening (stage 1), erosions and sclerosis (stage 2), and ankylosis (stage 3).
- *Spine:* affects the discovertebral junction and apophyseal and costal articulations.
- Discovertebral junction changes lead to syndesmophyte formation. Initial osteitis owing to enthesopathy at the anterior vertebral bodies results in erosions (Romanus lesion) and anterior squaring. Erosion often surrounded by reactive sclerosis (shiny corner sign) and most prominent in thoracolumbar region. Both erosions and sclerosis will disappear once ankylosis occurs.
- Marginal syndesmophytes appear as fine vertical ossifications in the outer annulus fibers and lateral vertebral body margins. When multiple contiguous segments are involved, the result is the bamboo spine appearance.
- Apophyseal joints show erosions, sclerosis, and ankylosis.
- *Cervical spine:* findings include decreased lordosis, body and facet fusion, atlantoaxial instability and odontoid erosions, decreased vertebral body size in lower levels, tapered spinous processes, and intervertebral foramen enlargement and is the most common area for carrot-stick fractures (C5–T1).
- *Thoracic spine:* changes include syndesmophytes, facet and costal fusion, increased kyphosis, and osteoporosis.
- *Lumbar spine:* changes include decreased lordosis and sacral angle, facet fusion, (trolley track sign), bamboo spine; early involvement (Romanus lesion, shiny corner) common at thoracolumbar junction.
- *Pelvis:* abnormalities include symphysis pubis changes, similar and parallel sacroiliac involvement.
- Most prominent areas for whiskering at iliac crests, ischial tuberosities, and trochanters.
- *Hip:* involvement is usually bilateral and reasonably symmetric. Signs include small osteophytes, subchondral cysts, and uniform loss of joint space, with axial migration of the femoral head. May eventually ankylose and not uncommon following prosthesis.
- *Shoulder:* involved in 30% of cases and is usually bilateral. Signs include surface erosions and, occasionally, a hatchet erosion at the superolateral aspect of the humerus and uniform loss of joint space. Enthesopathy at coracoclavicular ligamentous attachments at inferior clavicular surface.
- *Foot:* manifestations localize to the calcaneus, with enthesopathy, especially at Achilles and plantar insertions. Spurs usually fluffy and irregular compared with degenerative spurs.

ENTEROPATHIC ARTHRITIS

Enteropathic arthritis is an all-encompassing term used to group together diseases of gastrointestinal origin that produce articular abnormalities. (1) The most common diseases include ulcerative colitis and regional enteritis (Crohn's disease). (2) Less common conditions are collagenous colitis, (3) Whipple's disease and certain intestinal infections such as *Salmonella, Shigella,* and *Yersinia.* (Table 10-49) Synonyms used include colitic arthritis, enteropathic arthropathy, and enteropathic spondylitis (to denote the spinal involvement). (4)

Clinical Features

The most common causes for enteropathic arthritis are ulcerative colitis and regional enteritis. (5) Distinctively, these two disorders have an onset in younger adults characterized by malaise, anorexia, weight loss, abdominal pain, and an alteration in stool characteristics. Definitive diagnosis is dependent on appropriate barium examination and appropriate pathologic studies to demonstrate the intestinal alterations. Extraintestinal manifestations, especially those of the musculoskeletal system, usually occur after the onset of the enteric disorder and increase in incidence and severity, with chronicity of the bowel disorder. (4)

Musculoskeletal involvement is typified by arthralgias, joint effusions, and erythema and is encountered in approximately 15% of patients with inflammatory bowel disease. (4) The most common joints involved are the knees, ankles, elbows, and wrists. (5,6) Generally, exacerbation of articular symptoms closely parallels the clinical status of the intestinal disease. (6) The attacks are usually self-resolving, within 1–3 months, with no permanent peripheral joint damage. (4,6)

Involvement of the axial skeleton is invariably identical to that of ankylosing spondylitis, with bilateral sacroiliac disease and spondylitis. (Fig. 10-152) The full clinical picture of ankylosing spondylitis may occur in up to 10% of patients with ulcerative colitis (7,8) and, to a lesser extent, regional enteritis. (9,10) This represents a 20 times greater incidence of ankylosing spondylitis than in the general population. (11) Both ulcerative colitis and ankylosing spondylitis show a slight familial predilection. (12) Isolated bilateral sacroiliac disease without spinal involvement is seen in both ulcerative colitis and regional enteritis up to 4 times more commonly than the combined sacroiliac and spinal disease of ankylosing spondylitis. (9,10,13,14)

Laboratory studies will show an approximate incidence of 10–12% of HLA-B27. Patients with the HLA-B27 antigen often

Table 10-49	Causes for Enteropathic Arthritis
Common	
Ulcerative colitis	
Regional enteritis (Crohn's disease)	
Uncommon	
Whipple's disease	
Salmonella gastroenteritis	
Shigella gastroenteritis	
Yersinia gastroenteritis	
Post-bypass operations	
Collagenous colitis	

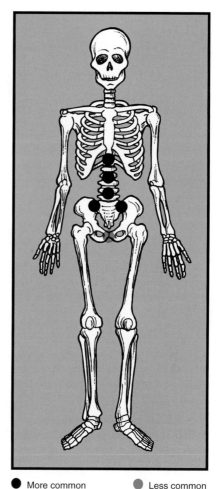

● More common   ● Less common

Figure 10-152 SKELETAL DISTRIBUTION OF ENTEROPATHIC ARTHRITIS.

endure a worse prognosis for the disease. (15) No rheumatoid factor is found, designating it as one of the *seronegative spondyloarthropathies,* along with ankylosing spondylitis, psoriatic arthropathy, Reiter's disease, and Behçet's syndrome. (16)

Pathologic Features

The cause and pathogenesis of articular involvement in inflammatory bowel disease is unclear. The transmission of unidentified toxic substances via the pelvic and vertebral venous systems has been suggested; however, antigen release from the bowel with formation of inflammation-producing antigen–antibody complexes is the most accepted explanation. (17,18) The changes within the spinal articulations are identical to those of ankylosing spondylitis.

Radiologic Features

Sacroiliac Joints

Radiographic abnormalities of the spine and pelvis are indistinguishable from those in classic ankylosing spondylitis. (19) (Fig. 10-153) Involvement is distinctively bilateral and symmetric, with erosions, sclerosis, and altered joint space, particularly at the iliac margin. Bony ankylosis is a characteristic sequela. Isolated sacroiliitis may occur, without spinal alterations, especially

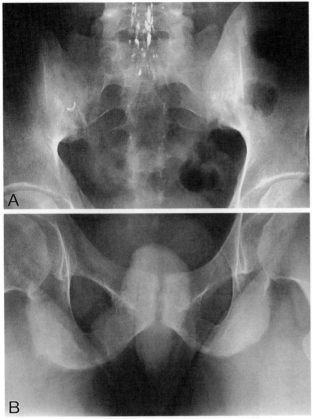

Figure 10-153 **ENTEROPATHIC ARTHRITIS: BILATERAL SACROILIITIS IN A CROHN'S PATIENT. A. AP Sacrum. B. AP Pubes.** Of incidental note is remnant myelographic contrast media and a metallic artifact overlying the sacroiliac joint. Observe also symphyseal erosions with ischial tuberosity enthesopathy and whiskering. *COMMENT:* The patient was a 22-year-old man with known Crohn's disease. These changes are indistinguishable from ankylosing spondylitis.

in regional enteritis patients. (13,14) In equivocal cases, high-resolution CT will better delineate the presence of sacroiliitis and erosions. (20)

Spine

Discovertebral abnormalities occur, with erosions, sclerosis, vertebral body squaring, and formation of thin, bilateral, marginal syndesmophytes. A bamboo spine configuration may occur in long-standing cases. The spinal apophyseal and costovertebral joints undergo a sequence of erosive changes, with sclerosis, loss of joint space, and eventual ankylosis. There is a distinct tendency for continuous cephalad progression of these spinal changes, as seen in ankylosing spondylitis.

Peripheral Joints

In the peripheral joints radiographic signs are non-specific, with often only soft tissue swelling and periarticular osteoporosis being evident. Occasionally, erosive disease may occur, especially in the hip. (21) Findings of hypertrophic osteoarthropathy may occasionally be seen, with bilateral, linear, periosteal new bone formation along the metaphyses and diaphyses of long bones, especially in the radius, ulna, tibia, and fibula. (22,23)

CAPSULE SUMMARY
Enteropathic Arthritis

General Considerations

- Arthritis is associated with diseases of gastrointestinal origin, especially ulcerative colitis and regional enteritis (Crohn's disease).
- Synonyms include colitic arthritis, enteropathic arthropathy and spondylitis.

Clinical Features

- Usually begins in young adults.
- Peripheral arthralgias, with rapid resolution and no residual sequelae common, especially knee, ankle, elbows, and wrists.
- Spinal involvement identical to ankylosing spondylitis seen in up to 10% of ulcerative colitis and, to a lesser extent, regional enteritis and may precede onset of intestinal disease.
- Increased incidence of HLA-B27.

Pathologic Features

- Pathogenesis unknown, but most likely related to formation of immune complexes, resulting in inflammatory joint involvement.

Radiologic Features

- Identical to ankylosing spondylitis—bilateral sacroiliitis, leading to ankylosis.
- Syndesmophytes and apophyseal ankylosis in the spine.
- Occasional peripheral long-bone periostitis (hypertrophic osteoarthropathy).

PSORIATIC ARTHRITIS

Psoriasis is a common skin disorder that is associated with an erosive and at times deforming arthropathy. (1) Psoriatic arthritis accounts for approximately 15% of patients suffering from arthritic conditions resulting from synovitis. (2) Following rheumatoid arthritis, psoriatic arthritis represents the second most common diagnosis within this population. (3) The predominant distribution of arthritic changes is in the peripheral joints of the hands and feet, but it may also affect the sacroiliac joints and spine. (4) There is no entirely satisfactory single definition of psoriatic arthropathy because of the spectrum of its clinical and radiologic features. In particular, there may be great similarities with rheumatoid arthritis, except for the absence of the rheumatoid factor, designating psoriasis as one of the *seronegative spondyloarthropathies*. (4) (Table 10-50) In addition, the differentiation from Reiter's syndrome both clinically and radiographically, may be on occasion almost impossible. (5)

Clinical Features

The physical manifestations of psoriasis are usually easily discernible on the extensor surfaces of the forearm, knee, back, scalp,

Table 10-50	Seronegative Arthropathies[a]
	Ankylosing spondylitis
	Behçet's syndrome
	Enteropathic arthritis
	Psoriatic arthritis
	Reiter's syndrome

[a] This designation can be used interchangeably with *seronegative spondyloarthropathies* when they involve the spine.

and pubic regions. The individual skin lesion is sharply demarcated, non-elevated, erythematous, and is covered by dry, silvery scales that, when removed, result in punctate bleeding from the exposed skin surface. At times these lesions may undergo remission, and a careful search must be made in the "hidden" regions of the scalp, ear, umbilicus, lower abdomen, perineum, and gluteal crease. (5,6)

The onset of arthritis is usually between 20 and 50 years of age, with no sex predilection. Hereditary factors may play a role. Generally, there is no relationship between the predisposition in developing arthritis and the duration or extensiveness of the skin disease; however, up to 42% of patients with psoriasis will develop arthritis. (4,6) There appears to be a greater possibility for developing arthritis within 5 years of the onset of the skin disease. (7) With the development of skin lesions and arthritis within the same year, the severity of arthritic symptoms may directly correlate to the severity of the skin condition. (8) Remissions of arthritic symptoms may occur and is more common in patients with an initial presentation involving fewer joints. (9) Males also appear to display an increased rate of remission. (9) Exacerbations of arthritic symptoms may occur synchronously with an increase of apparent psoriasis. (8) Infrequently, the arthritis may antedate the skin lesions by months or years. (10) The most significant physical correlation is the presence of nail involvement. (11) Up to 80% of patients exhibiting pitting, ridging, discoloration, loss of the nail, or thickening of the skin under the nail tip (subungual hyperkeratosis) will develop joint disease, especially of the distal interphalangeal articulations. (7,11–13)

Early involvement is characterized by DIP joint redness, swelling, and pain. (Fig. 10-154) At times the entire digit may be swollen owing to tenosynovitis and is termed a *cocktail sausage digit*. More advanced deformities may include *arthritis mutilans* as joint destruction progresses. Female patients tend to have an increased predilection toward progression (14) as do patients with involvement of five or more joints upon presentation. (15) Sacroiliac involvement manifests as low back pain that may or may not radiate. Spinal involvement most commonly is in the lower thoracic and upper lumbar regions and is usually associated with chronic, low-grade pain. Current treatments include anti-inflammatory medications, with only marginal results. (4,16)

There is no gold standard for the diagnosis of psoriatic arthritis (17) and laboratory findings are relatively non-specific. Expected findings usually include an elevated ESR in the acute phase, negative rheumatoid factor, and occasional hyperuricemia. The presence of the HLA-B27 antigen seems to correlate with the susceptibility of developing psoriatic arthritis, and up to 75% of patients with sacroiliac involvement will have this antigen. (18,19) In those with peripheral joint disease only, this prevalence is reduced to 30%. (20) The incidence of HLA-B27 in the normal population is approximately 6–8%. (19,20)

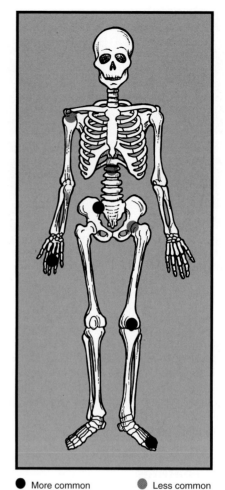

● More common   ● Less common

Figure 10-154   **SKELETAL DISTRIBUTION OF PSORIATIC ARTHRITIS.**

Pathologic Features

Psoriatic arthritis is believed to be an immune reaction similar to rheumatoid arthritis, but distinctive differences are apparent in its pathological process. (4,10,21,22) In the synovial joint, an initial proliferative synovitis results in pannus formation with prominent fibrosis. Superficial cartilage and marginal bone erosions occur secondary to the invading pannus, which narrows the joint space. Adjacent to the erosions periostitis results in new bone formation.

At bone–ligament junctions similar erosive and proliferative changes may occur (*enthesopathy*), especially at the calcaneus, hand, and foot. Prominent fibrous tissue production within the joint cavity may widen the joint and eventually undergo metaplasia to produce bony ankylosis. In contrast to rheumatoid arthritis, psoriatic arthritis shows a distinct lack of intense synovial hyperemia, maintaining normal bone mineralization adjacent to the involved joint.

In the spine, the precise pathologic process, resulting in *nonmarginal syndesmophyte* formation, has not been clearly delineated; however, paravertebral ossification occurring within loose areolar tissue outside the periosteum of the vertebral body has been documented and may be the result of inflammation or periosteal new bone from the spine at bone–ligament or muscle attachments.

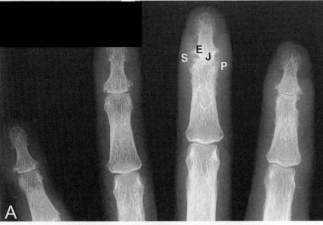

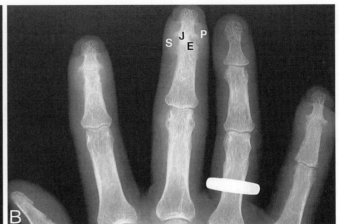

Figure 10-155 PSORIATIC ARTHRITIS: CHARACTERISTIC FEATURES. A and B. PA Hand. Note the asymmetrical but predominantly distal distribution. Prominent periarticular swelling (*S*), uniform loss of joint space (*J*), marginal erosions (*E*), and fluffy periostitis (*P*) complete the radiologic picture.

(23,24) This ossification is initially in the form of woven bone, eventually remodeling to become lamellar bone. With time, the ossification progresses to involve the fibers of the annulus and longitudinal ligament in a localized manner, potentially precipitating fusion to the adjacent vertebral body.

Involvement of the atlantoaxial and sacroiliac joints demonstrates pathologic changes that are in no way different from the peripheral articular changes.

Radiologic Features

Psoriatic arthritis demonstrates distinct features in distribution and appearance. The most common locations are the small joints of the hands, especially the DIP joints. (25) Other target sites for involvement include the small joints of the feet, the sacroiliac joint, and spine. Occasional involvement of the larger joints such as the knee, hip, and shoulder may also occur.

General Features

The most prominent and diagnostic signs are an asymmetric distribution, soft tissue swelling, normal bone mineralization, erosions, fluffy periostitis, and a narrowed or widened joint space. Residual sequelae include ankylosis and joint deformities. (Fig. 10-155; Table 10-51)

Soft Tissue Swelling. Soft tissue swelling may be the earliest and only radiographic sign. Swelling can be observed in the peri-articular tissues as a fusiform soft tissue displacement (*spindle digit*) or involve the entire digit (*cocktail sausage digit*).

Bone Density. Normal bone density is usually evident, despite destructive changes, and is a useful differential feature from rheumatoid arthritis. (7)

Joint Space. Most commonly, in large joints there is a uniform narrowing of the joint cavity. In small joints of the fingers and toes the joint space may appear widened owing to bone erosion and/or fibrous tissue deposition.

Erosions. Distinctively, early erosions are marginal in origin. With progression these erosions result in an increasingly tapered bony end. Central articular erosions are less prominent.

Periostitis. Adjacent to these marginal erosions, as well as at tendinous and ligamentous insertions, fluffy and spiculated new bone is deposited. (26) The external surface of this periostitis is typically frayed and hazy. It is seen in 30% of cases and not seen in rheumatoid arthritis. Farther away from the joint a linear, well-defined periosteal new bone formation may be evident. (Fig. 10-156A) Internally, endosteal periostitis may create a sclerotic bone, especially of the terminal phalanges (*ivory phalanx*). (Fig. 10-156B)

Ankylosis. Complete osseous ankylosis is a frequent sequela, especially in the interphalangeal joints of the hands and feet. Ankylosis in psoriasis is more common than in rheumatoid arthritis.

Deformity. Joint destruction may precipitate various deformities such as the *pencil-in-cup telescoping deformity,* leading to the *opera glass hand* and *arthritis mutilans.* Ulnar and fibular digital deviation, boutonniere, and swan-neck deformities are far less common than in rheumatoid arthritis. (7)

Target Sites of Involvement

Hand

Distribution. The most common joints of the hand involved are the DIP and PIP joints. (Fig. 10-154) It is distinctly uncommon for the metacarpophalangeal joints and wrist to be involved. (7) Occasionally, all three articulations of a single digital ray, including the metacarpophalangeal, proximal, and distal interphalangeal joints, will be involved, which is virtually a diagnostic sign of psoriasis (*ray pattern*). (27) (Fig. 10-157) An asymmet-

Table 10-51	General Radiologic Features of Psoriatic Arthritis
	Asymmetric
	Soft tissue swelling
	Normal bone density
	Marginal erosions and tapered bone ends
	Fluffy juxta-articular periostitis
	Widened joint space

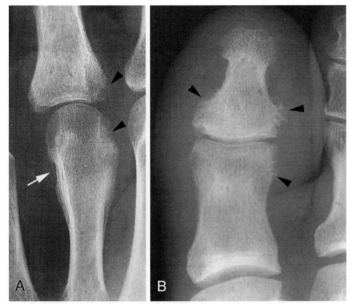

Figure 10-156 **PSORIATIC ARTHRITIS: PERIOSTITIS. A. PA Hand. Fluffy and Linear.** Note that close to the joint near the site of articular erosion, the periosteal new bone is typically fluffy (*arrowheads*). Farther down the shaft a linear pattern may be seen (*arrow*). **B. Great Toe: Fluffy.** Note that adjacent to the erosions a fluffy and irregular type of periostitis can be seen (*arrowheads*). The entire distal phalanx is sclerotic, a reliable sign of psoriatic arthritis involving the great toe. COMMENT: This fluffy type of periostitis is typical of seronegative spondyloarthropathies rather than rheumatoid arthritis. (Courtesy of Lawrence A. Cooperstein, MD, Pittsburgh, Pennsylvania.)

ric distribution from side to side and digit to digit is also to be expected.

Erosions. Erosions are common at the joint margins. Adjacent to these erosions there is frequently fluffy periosteal new bone formation, which has been called the *mouse ears sign*. (27) (Figs. 10-158 and 10-159) Progression of the erosions results in a whittling effect of the distal articular end of the phalanx. Eventually, with associated muscle action this tapered bony end will mechanically erode into the adjacent articular surface, creating the *pencil-in-cup deformity* (*pestle and mortar, mushroom and stem, balancing pagoda, cup and saucer*). (Fig. 10-160) Subsequent overall shortening of the digit owing to a telescoping phenomenon creates the *opera glass hand*. Severe articular deformity may result in *arthritis mutilans*, but rarely in ulnar deviation. (4) (Fig. 10-161) Accompanying resorption of the tuft of the distal phalanx (*acro-osteolysis*) is also infrequently observed. (7)

Joint Space. At the joint space, changes are common. Initial widening is owing to bone erosion and intraarticular fibrous tissue deposition. (Fig. 10-157) In up to 15% of patients intra-articular osseous ankylosis may ensue, which is a useful diagnostic feature. (28) (Fig. 10-162) Differential diagnosis includes rheumatoid arthritis, DJD, and erosive osteoarthritis.

Foot. The alterations in the feet parallel those in the hand by involving predominantly the distal articulations. (28) (Fig. 10-163) A characteristic location for early and more advanced changes is at the interphalangeal joint of the great toe. (7) (Fig. 10-164) Soft tissue swelling, normal bone density, erosions, fluffy periostitis, and joint-space widening are the most common signs. Osteolysis is most prominent in the metatarsal heads and distal tufts. (Figs. 10-165 and 10-166) A dense sclerotic first distal phalanx is occasionally encountered (*ivory phalanx*). (29) (Fig. 10-164) Calcaneal erosions and periostitis may be present at the Achilles and plantar ligament insertions. (Fig. 10-167) Ankylosis of the intertarsal joints is an uncommon sequelae. (Fig. 10-168)

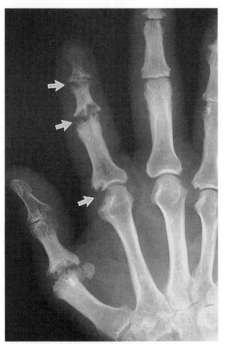

Figure 10-157 **PSORIATIC ARTHRITIS: RAY PATTERN. PA Hand.** Note the erosive changes are present at the three joints of the second digit (*arrows*). This pattern of arthritis is virtually diagnostic of psoriasis. Also note the involvement of the first ray.

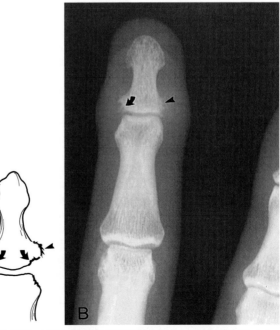

Figure 10-158 **PSORIATIC ARTHRITIS. A and B. PA Hand. Early Distal Interphalangeal Joint Changes.** Note that erosions (*arrows*), periostitis (*arrowheads*), and soft tissue swelling characterize the earliest abnormalities.

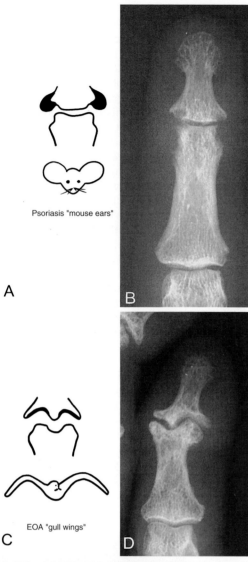

Psoriasis "mouse ears"

A

B

EOA "gull wings"

C

D

Figure 10-159 **PSORIATIC ARTHRITIS VERSUS EROSIVE OSTEOARTHRITIS. A and B. Mouse Ears.** Note the combination of erosions and fluffy periostitis produces the mouse ears appearance in psoriasis. **C and D. Gull Wings.** Observe that the biconcave articular contour produces the gull wings appearance of erosive osteoarthritis.

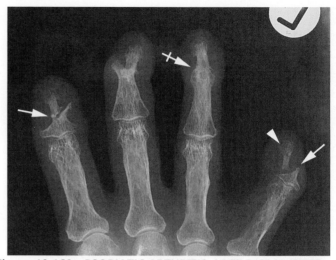

Figure 10-160 **PSORIATIC ARTHRITIS: LATE DISTAL INTER-PHALANGEAL JOINT CHANGES. PA Hand.** Note that progression of the erosions results in a whittling effect, creating the pencil-in-cup deformity (*arrows*). Subsequently there is an overall shortening of the digit owing to a telescoping phenomenon. Some resorption of the tuft of the distal phalanx (acroosteolysis) can be observed (*arrowhead*). Ankylosis of the distal joint is a strong sign of psoriatic arthritis (*crossed arrow*).

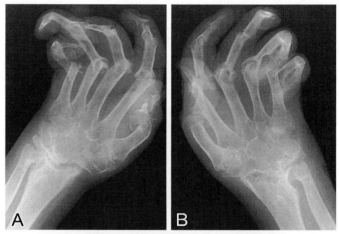

A

B

Figure 10-161 **PSORIATIC ARTHRITIS. A and B. Bilateral Hands, Arthritis Mutilans.** Observe the severe destruction of all joints with carpal ankylosis.

Sacroiliac Joint. Between 30% and 50% of individuals with psoriatic arthritis will have involvement of the sacroiliac joint. (30–32) Bilateral asymmetric sacroiliitis is the most common type of manifestation. (31,33,34) (Fig. 10-169) Occasionally, a purely unilateral pattern may be encountered. (Table 10-52)

The specific roentgen signs of psoriatic sacroiliitis include erosions, hazy joint margin, and sclerosis, predominantly along the entire length of the iliac surface. (35) Narrowing of the joint space and ankylosis are infrequent findings. (31) Isotopic bone scans may show active joint disease in the absence of specific plain film radiographic changes. (32) In addition, enthesopathy with erosions and periostitis may be visible at the iliac crests, ischial tuberosities, and femoral trochanters. Occasionally in severe psoriatic arthritis, erosion of the femoral head and associated protrusio acetabuli may simulate rheumatoid arthritis, although bone density remains relatively preserved. (Fig. 10-170)

Spine. Manifestations of psoriatic spondylitis may occur in approximately 60% of individuals with the skin disease. (34) Radiographic signs of spinal involvement include coarse, asymmetric *non-marginal syndesmophytes (paravertebral ossifications)*; atlantoaxial subluxation; and discovertebral erosions with sparing of the apophyseal joints, except in the cervical spine. (28,35–37)

Non-Marginal Syndesmophytes. The most frequent location for non-marginal syndesmophytes to occur are in the upper three lumbar and lower two thoracic segments; however, any part of the spine may be affected. (23,24) Initially, ossification appears lateral and separate from the vertebral body as a thick and fluffy or thin and well-defined unilateral curvilinear radiopacity. Eventually, the

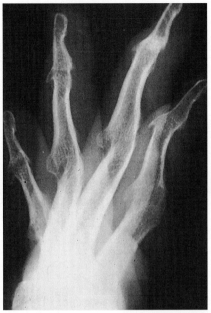

Figure 10-162   **PSORIATIC ARTHRITIS: JOINT ANKYLOSIS. Lateral Hand.** Note that complete osseous ankylosis is evident at all of the finger articulations. Such a finding is an important sign of long-standing psoriatic arthritis and excludes the diagnosis of degenerative joint disease or rheumatoid arthritis. (Reprinted with permission from **The Learning File:** *Skeletal Section, SK-313.* The Center for Devices and Radiological Health, FDA, and the American College of Radiology.)

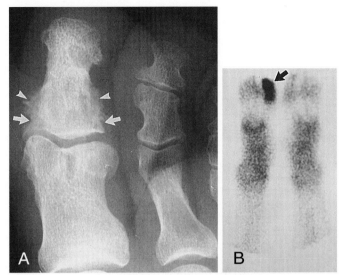

Figure 10-164   **PSORIATIC ARTHRITIS: GREAT TOE. A. Plain Film.** Note that early involvement is seen at the interphalangeal joint of the great toe characterized by marginal erosions (*arrows*), fluffy periostitis seen in only 30% of cases (*arrowheads*), and soft tissue swelling. The density of the entire distal phalanx is slightly increased (ivory phalanx).
B. Bone Scan. Observe that the bone scan demonstrates the inflammatory nature of the joint changes with increased isotopic uptake in the big toe (*arrow*). *COMMENT:* The interphalangeal joint of the great toe is a frequent site for early and advanced psoriatic changes.

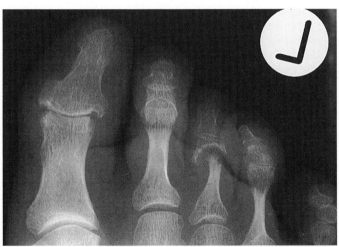

Figure 10-163   **PSORIATIC ARTHRITIS: FOOT.** Note the interphalangeal joint of the big toe where erosions and soft tissue swelling are present. A pencil-in-cup deformity is seen at the third digit.

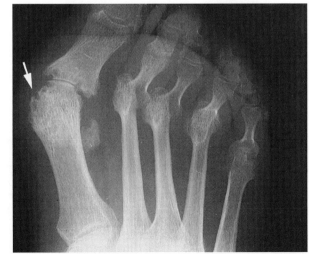

Figure 10-165   **PSORIATIC ARTHRITIS: FOOT.** Note that prominent erosions can be identified at the first metatarsophalangeal joint (*arrow*). There is also subluxation of the remaining metatarsophalangeal joints with fibular deviation. The normal bone density is in contradistinction to the osteopenia of rheumatoid arthritis.

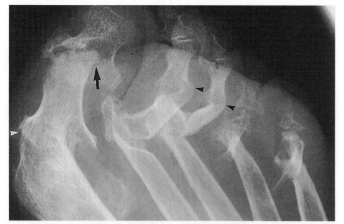

Figure 10-166 **PSORIATIC ARTHRITIS: ARTHRITIS MUTILANS. PA Foot.** Note severe joint destruction, especially at the metatarsophalangeal articulations, has resulted in fibular deviation and dorsal dislocation of the digits (Lanois' deformity). The presence of a pencil-in-cup deformity (*arrow*) at the interphalangeal joint of the big toe and osseous ankylosis of the first metatarsophalangeal and second and third proximal interphalangeal articulations (*arrowheads*) makes the diagnosis of psoriatic arthritis most likely. (Courtesy of David M. Walker, DPM, Melbourne, Australia.)

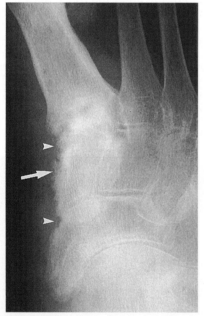

Figure 10-167 **PSORIATIC ARTHRITIS: ENTHESOPATHY. PA Hand.** Observe the irregular, poorly defined periosteal new bone formation at the medial cuneiform and navicular bones (*arrow*). This is a manifestation of enthesopathy and is a relatively important sign of psoriatic arthritis, seen in 30% of cases and not present in rheumatoid arthritis. Erosive changes are evident at the first metatarsal–cuneiform joint and at the medial cuneiform–navicular joint (*arrowheads*).

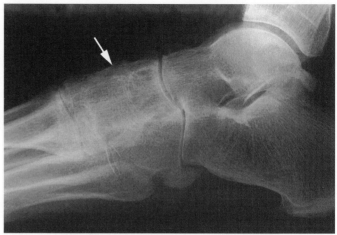

Figure 10-168 **PSORIATIC ARTHRITIS: TARSAL ANKYLOSIS. Lateral Foot.** Observe the fusion of the tarsus (*arrow*), which is a relatively uncommon finding in psoriatic arthritis.

ossification process extends to involve the adjacent vertebral body and annulus fibers, resulting in a thicker, well-defined bony excrescence from the midportion of the vertebral body. These are called *non-marginal syndesmophytes or parasyndesmophytes*. (23,24,38) (Fig. 10-171) Characteristically, these involve the spine

in an asymmetric or unilateral manner. (31) Their configuration is variable, sometimes completely or incompletely bridging the intervertebral disc, but nearly always unilateral. The following morphologic shapes may be apparent radiographically, particularly on the AP film: (23,30,34) (Fig. 10-172)

- *Complete, non-marginal.* This is attached to the midportion of two contiguous vertebral bodies with a thick base and may taper as it extends across the intervertebral disc.
- *Incomplete non-marginal.* Three types may occur:
  Comma shaped, inverted comma (teardrop). This originates and is contiguous with the midportion of the vertebral body, tapering at its distal extent as it begins to bridge the intervertebral disc.
  Bagpipe. This is similar to the comma shape except it is larger and bulkier at its base (*the bag*) and has a tapered protuberance over the disc region (*the pipe*).
  Bywaters-Dixon (floating). This designation is applied to the paravertebral ossification that bridges the disc space and approximates but does not unite with the contiguous vertebral bodies.
- *Marginal.* These are usually seen in ankylosing spondylitis and, infrequently, in psoriasis and Reiter's disease as thin, vertical ossifications in the outer annulus fibers. They originate and insert at contiguous vertebral body margins at the peripheral body–endplate junction. They may be complete or incomplete and usually bilateral. An additional distinction from ankylosing spondylitis is the decreased frequency of corner erosions, anterior squaring, and apophyseal joint involvement. (34)

The non-marginal syndesmophytes of psoriatic arthritis are identical to those seen in Reiter's disease and should be differentiated from the marginal syndesmophytes of ankylosing spondylitis. (24) (Table 10-53) Additional differentiation must be made between the osteophytes of degenerative joint disease and the hyperostosis of DISH. (Table 10-52)

Cervical Spine. Cervical involvement occurs in 35–75% of patients with psoriatic arthritis. (39) The major features include nar-

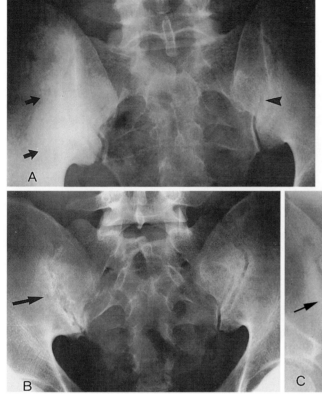

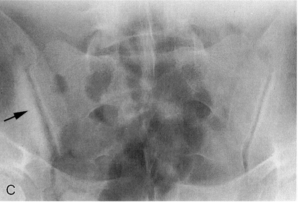

Figure 10-169   PSORIATIC SACROILIITIS. A. Bilateral, Asymmetric Pattern. Observe the dense reactive subchondral sclerosis and blurred sacroiliac joint margins (*arrows*). On the opposite joint early erosive changes have also obliterated the joint margin (*arrowhead*). This is the most common sacroiliac presentation of psoriasis. **B. Unilateral Erosive Pattern.** Note the erosions, sclerosis, and loss of joint space (*arrow*). **C. Unilateral Pseudo-Widening Form.** Note the blurring of the iliac articular margin with underlying subchondral sclerosis (*arrow*).

Table 10-52	Radiologic Differential Diagnosis of Sacroiliac Disease		
Disease	**Bilateral Symmetric**	**Bilateral Asymmetric**	**Unilateral**
Ankylosing spondylitis	+++	+ (early)	+ (early)
DISH	+ (upper joint)	—	—
Enteropathic sacroiliitis	+++	—	—
Gouty arthritis	+	+	+
Hyperparathyroidism	+++	—	—
Infection	—	—	+++
Osteitis condensans ilii	+++	+	+
Osteoarthritis	—	+	++
Psoriatic spondylitis	+	+++	++
Reiter's syndrome	++	++	+++
Rheumatoid arthritis	—	+	+++

DISH, diffuse idiopathic skeletal hyperostosis; —, absent; +, rare; ++, common; +++, very common.

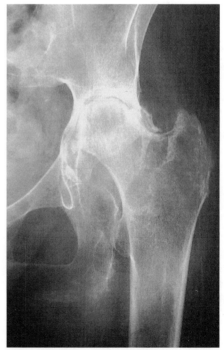

Figure 10-170   PSORIATIC ARTHRITIS: HIP. AP Hip. Note that the femoral head is eroded and small, with an associated protrusio acetabuli. Enthesopathy is visible at the ischial tuberosity.

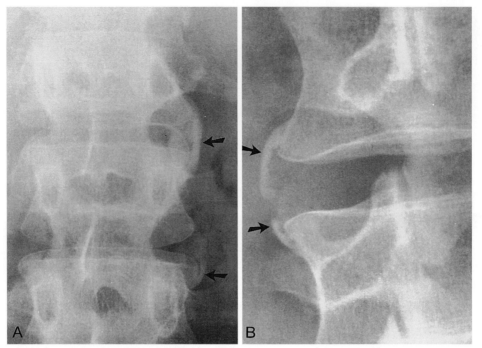

Figure 10-171   **PSORIATIC ARTHRITIS: LUMBAR SPINE. A and B. Non-Marginal Syndesmophyte.** Note the thick, vertical ossifications that arise just beyond the vertebral body margins (*arrows*).

rowing or fusion of the apophyseal joints and anterior atlantoaxial subluxation. (40) Syndesmophytes (marginal and non-marginal) may also be present.

Atlantoaxial Joint. Involvement of the upper cervical complex, resulting in atlantoaxial instability, may be present in up to 45% of psoriatic arthritis patients. (31) (Fig. 10-173) Manifestations of instability are evaluated in flexion of the cervical spine, with an ADI > 3 mm. Accompanying sclerotic and erosive changes may be visible on the odontoid at the anterior, posterior, and lateral surfaces.

Table 10-53 | Differential Diagnosis of Psoriatic Arthritis

Feature	Psoriatic Arthritis	Reiter's Syndrome	Rheumatoid Arthritis	Ankylosing Spondylitis
Distribution		—		
Upper extremity hand	+++	—	+++	+
	DIP/PIP		MCP/wrist	—
Lower extremity	+++	+++	+++	+
Sacroiliac	++	++	+	+++
Bilateral	++	++ (asymmetric)	+	+++
Unilateral	++	+++	+++	+
Spine	++	+	++ (cervical)	+++
Key signs				
Osteoporosis	—	+	+++	+++
Joint space	++ (widening)	+ (narrowing)	+++ (narrowing)	++ (narrowing)
Ankylosis	++	—	+	+++
Periostitis	+++ (fluffy)	+++ (fluffy)	+ (linear)	+++ (fluffy)
Tuft resorption	+++	—	—	—
Soft tissue swelling	++	++	+++	+
Laboratory				
ESR	+	++	+++	+++
RA factor	—	—	+++	—
HLA-B27	30–75%	75%	6–8% (normal)	90%

DIP, distal interphalangeal; *ESR*, erythrocyte sedimentation rate; *MCP*, metacarpal–phalangeal; *PIP*, proximal interphalangeal; *RA*, rheumatic arthritis; —, rare; +, uncommon; ++, common; +++, very common.

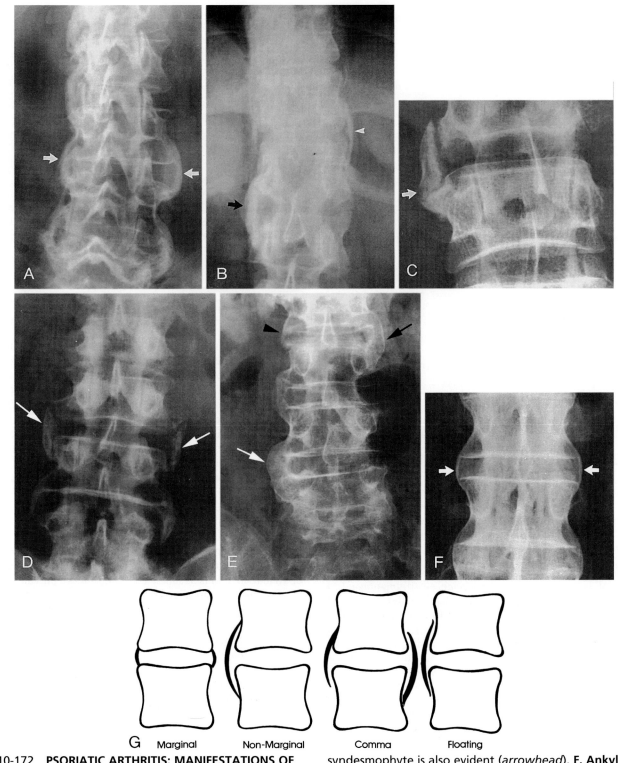

Figure 10-172 **PSORIATIC ARTHRITIS: MANIFESTATIONS OF LUMBAR SYNDESMOPHYTES. A. Complete Non-Marginal.** Note the syndesmophytes (*arrows*). **B. Incomplete Non-Marginal.** Note the comma-shaped (*arrow*) and floating (*arrowhead*) configurations. **C. Incomplete Non-Marginal.** Observe the bagpipe variety (*arrow*). **D. Incomplete Non-Marginal.** Note the floating type (Bywaters-Dixon) (*arrows*). **E. Complete Non-Marginal.** Note the coarse bridging syndesmophytes at multiple levels (*arrows*). A single marginal syndesmophyte is also evident (*arrowhead*). **F. Ankylosing Spondylitis.** For comparison, observe the classic marginal syndesmophytes (*arrows*). **G. Marginal Versus Non-Marginal Syndesmophytes.** (Panel A courtesy of Friedrich H. W. Heuck, MD, Stuttgart, West Germany. Panel C courtesy of David P. Thomas, MD, Melbourne, Australia. Panel D courtesy of John A. M. Taylor, DC, DACBR, Seneca Falls, New York. Panel E courtesy of Lawrence A. Cooperstein, MD, Pittsburgh, Pennsylvania.)

CAPSULE SUMMARY   Psoriatic Arthritis

General Considerations

- Psoriasis is a common skin disorder associated with joint disease and characterized by peripheral joint destruction and deformity: sacroiliitis and non-marginal syndesmophyte formation.

Clinical Features

- Age 20–50 years; equal sex ratio.
- Skin lesions characteristic, usually on extensor surface (knees, elbows, back), also scalp, abdomen, and genital region. Lesions are well-defined, dry, raised, red and silvery, scaly patches.
- Severity and duration of skin disease show no relationship to the onset of arthritis.
- Presence of nail changes seen in 80% of arthritis patients.
- Arthritis is usually in peripheral joints, especially DIP joints.
- Whole finger or toe may show soft tissue swelling (sausage digit).
- Rarely results in severe arthritis mutilans.
- ESR normal (except in acute phase), negative rheumatoid arthritis latex, positive HLA-B27 in 75% of patients with sacroiliac involvement and 30% in peripheral arthritis.

Pathologic Features

- Fundamentally similar to rheumatoid arthritis, but pannus affects cartilage less and erosions are smaller and slower in their development.
- Adjacent to erosions, there is often prominent periosteal new bone that is typically fluffy.
- Erosions often will progressively taper the end of an entire bone.
- Large amount of intra-articular fibrous tissue widens the joint and results in eventual bony ankylosis.
- No subcutaneous nodules or rheumatoid factor.

Radiologic Features

- General features include soft tissue swelling, normal bone mineralization, erosions, and tapered bone ends, prominent juxta-articular fluffy periostitis, and joint-space widening or bony ankylosis.
- *Hands and feet:* asymmetric involvement, ray pattern, most commonly involves DIP joints, no osteoporosis, mouse ears sign, widened joint space owing to fibrous tissue deposition and bone resorption, pencil-in-cup deformity, opera glass hand deformity, no ulnar deviation.
- *Sacroiliac joint:* involved in up to 50% of psoriatic arthritis patients, usually bilateral but asymmetric and unusual to be narrowed and ankylosed.
- *Spine:* atlantoaxial subluxation and dislocation, normal apophyseal joints (except in the cervical spine), syndesmophytes of two types—non-marginal, marginal (non-marginal are the most common)—broad-based and tapered, asymmetric, unilateral, and most common in the upper lumbar and lower thoracic spine.

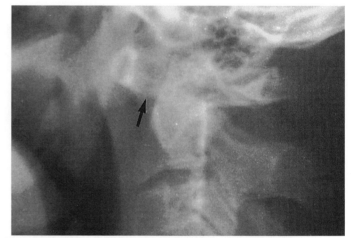

Figure 10-173   PSORIATIC ARTHRITIS: ATLANTOAXIAL INSTABILITY. Lateral Cervical. Observe the increased atlanto-dental interspace (*arrow*).

REITER'S SYNDROME

Reiter's syndrome, also called *reactive arthritis* owing to its association with infection, is defined as a triad of urethritis, conjunctivitis, and polyarthritis. (1–3) The recognition of this triad dates well before Hans Reiter's original description in 1916 when he linked it to the onset of acute dysentery in a cavalry officer serving at the Balkan front. (4) Presently, the most common cause appears to be venereal in origin, and it is a male-dominated disease. Disorders of the bowel are also causally linked. Joint involvement is usually peripheral and self-limiting, particularly of the lower extremity, although axial involvement is frequently observed.

Clinical Features

Reiter's syndrome is the most common inflammatory polyarthritis affecting young men. (2) It typically occurs between the ages of 18 and 40, and is as much as 50 times more prevalent in males. (5) The classic triad of urethritis, conjunctivitis, and polyarthritis may not be present simultaneously but, alternatively, may occur at irregular intervals. (6) Less commonly, patients may not experience all three aspects of the triad and the term *incomplete Reiter's syndrome* may be used to describe these cases. (7)

Two modes of onset are apparent: venereal and enteric. The majority of cases are venereal in origin and manifested by urethritis appearing shortly after sexual intercourse. The urethritis is non-specific, often with no organism being isolated. Dysuria, discharge, and prostatitis may be the only symptoms. (8,9) This is soon followed by arthritis, iritis, and occasionally characteristic skin lesions. Reiter's syndrome may also be the initial symptoms of HIV infection. (2) The other less common type of onset follows within 1–3 weeks of an acute dysenteric illness from *Shigella flexneri, Yersinia enterocolitica,* or *Salmonella.* (10–13) Conjunctivitis often occurs early, being frequently bilateral, with prominent itchiness and burning sensations. Less commonly, iritis may ensue, particularly in recurrent episodes. (8) In up to 30% of patients a distinctive skin lesion almost identical to pustular psoriasis may develop (*keratoderma blenorrhagica*). (14) This is most commonly seen on the soles of the feet and palms of the hands.

Additional mucocutaneous lesions may be seen on the penis (*balanitis circinata*), oral mucosa, tongue, and hard palate. (6)

Joint symptoms typically consist of an asymmetric painful effusion, especially of the lower extremity. The knee, ankle, forefoot, calcaneus, low back, shoulder, and wrist are the most likely sites of involvement, in descending order of frequency. (Fig. 10-174) Pain at the plantar or Achilles calcaneal attachment (*lover's heels*) in a young male patient should suggest the diagnosis. These joint symptoms are of short duration and self-limiting within 2–3 months, but recurrences are common. (8,15) Patients with multiple recurrences are prone to develop residual joint damage, particularly in the feet, sacroiliac joints, and vertebral column. (16) More severe complications include urinary tract obstructions, iritis, retrobulbar neuritis, corneal ulceration, aortitis, atrioventricular blocks, and cranial nerve palsy. (8, 17,18) Reiter's syndrome is rarely fatal. (5)

Laboratory findings consist of anemia, elevated ESR, and leukocytosis, and 75% or more cases will be positive for the HLA-B27 antigen. (10,19,20) There is no rheumatoid factor present, designating it with ankylosing spondylitis, enteropathic arthritis, and psoriatic arthritis as a *seronegative spondyloarthropathy*.

Pathologic Features

The exact cause and pathogenesis of the disease are unknown, although a reaction to an infectious agent seems likely. In view of the direct relationship with genitourinary and gastrointestinal infections, no single specific infective agent has been isolated. Venereally, *Chlamydia trachomatis* is most commonly identified, (2) while other organisms such as *Mycoplasma, Bedsonia, Shigella, Salmonella,* and viruses have been implicated enterically. (2, 21) Once the infectious agent is removed, the immune system of these genetically susceptible individuals will continue to "react," therefore rendering antimicrobial or antibiotic therapy virtually unsuccessful. (2,7) It is suggested that the spinal and sacroiliac involvement is secondary to hematogenous diffusion via the venous plexuses of Batson. (9) An immunologic basis for the disease may also be operative in view of the high incidence of HLA-B27 antigen. (22–24)

Pathologic changes at the involved joint consist of synovitis and fibrous proliferation with associated periostitis. At bone–ligament junctions (entheses) erosions and periostitis are commonly observed, especially at the plantar and posterior Achilles surface of the calcaneus, ankle malleoli, and metatarsals. (25,26)

In the spine the precise pathologic process resulting in *nonmarginal syndesmophyte* formation has not been clearly delineated; however, paravertebral ossification occurring within loose areolar tissue outside the periosteum of the vertebral body has been demonstrated. (6,27,28) The cause for this ossification is unknown, but may be owing to inflammation or periosteal new bone from the spine bone–ligament or muscle junctions (enthesopathy). (29,30) The initial osseous tissue is composed of woven bone eventually remodeling to lamellar bone. From the beginning, these paravertebral ossifications are unattached to the vertebral body but, with time they may unite to be contiguous. The histopathologic changes appear to be identical to psoriatic syndesmophyte formation. (17,30)

Radiologic Features

Articular involvement in Reiter's syndrome is characterized by articular and periarticular soft tissue swelling, osteoporosis, uniform loss of joint space, marginal erosions, and periostitis. (26,31) (Table 10-54) These changes are most apparent in the lower extremity and distributed asymmetrically. (32) Arthritic changes are most commonly seen at the metatarsophalangeal and interphalangeal joints of the foot, calcaneus, ankle, and knee. (27,28,33) Less commonly, the hand, shoulder, elbow, C1–C2 articulation and temporomandibular joint are affected. (34) (Table 10-55)

Target Sites of Involvement

Foot and Ankle. Soft tissue swelling in the foot and ankle is often prominent, especially in the toes. Erosions are best seen at the metatarsophalangeal and interphalangeal joints. Usually,

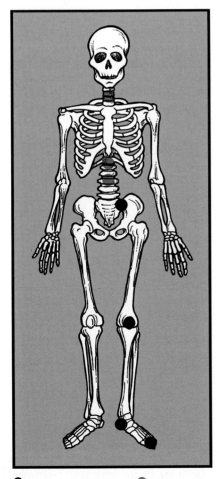

● More common   ● Less common

Figure 10-174 **SKELETAL DISTRIBUTION OF REITER'S SYNDROME.**

Table 10-54	General Radiologic Features of Reiter's Syndrome
	Predilection for lower extremity
	Soft tissue swelling
	Osteoporosis
	Uniform loss of joint space
	Marginal erosions
	Periostitis (linear/fluffy)
	Deformity

Table 10-55	Articular Distribution in Reiter's Syndrome

Common
    Lower Extremity
        Feet: metatarsophalangeal, interphalangeal joints
        Calcaneus: Achilles, plantar insertion
        Ankle
        Knee
    Sacroiliac
        Bilateral, asymmetric
    Spine
        Thoracolumbar region
Uncommon
    Hand
    C1–C2
    Shoulder
    Elbow
    Temporomandibular

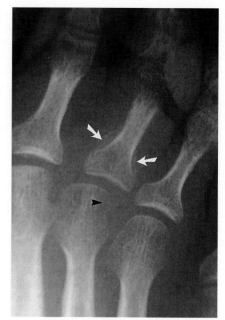

Figure 10-176 REITER'S SYNDROME: PERIOSTITIS. PA Foot. Observe the thin layer of periosteal new bone at the phalangeal base at the third metatarsophalangeal joint (*arrows*). There is also a notable diminished density in the metatarsal head (*arrowhead*). These features are indicative of an acutely inflamed joint such as in Reiter's syndrome and rheumatoid arthritis.

there is associated osteoporosis and linear or fluffy periostitis. (Figs. 10-175 to 10-177) These changes are often most prominent at the interphalangeal joint of the big toe. (27) Dorsal subluxation of the proximal phalanges and fibular deviation of the digits results in the *Lanois deformity*. At the calcaneus, erosions, fluffy periostitis, and soft tissue swelling are visible in up to 50% of patients at the Achilles and plantar insertions (*lover's heels*). (8, 25,27,35) (Figs. 10-178 and 10-179) At the ankle, prominent swelling and periostitis at the malleoli may be evident.

Knee. The only change usually visible at the knee is effusion and, occasionally, periostitis of the distal femoral metaphysis. A Pellegrini-Stieda type calcification of the medial collateral ligament may be seen in up to 10% of long-standing Reiter's patients. (26) (Fig. 10-180)

Sacroiliac Joint. Sacroiliac involvement is common and may be seen in up to 50% of patients on plain film examination. (25,28) Isotopic bone scans have demonstrated up to 70% of all patients with the disease to have sacroiliac joint involvement, but many resolve without visible plain film changes. (15). Patterns of

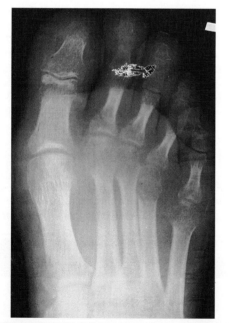

Figure 10-175 REITER'S SYNDROME: ACUTE EPISODE. PA Foot. Note the prominent juxta-articular osteoporosis about all metatarsophalangeal joints owing to inflammatory hyperemia. Although not a specific finding, such a presentation in this location of a young adult male should suggest the diagnosis.

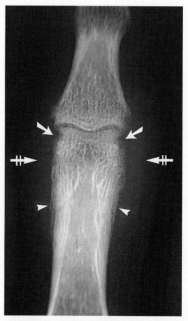

Figure 10-177 REITER'S SYNDROME: FINGER. Note the marginal erosions (*arrows*), linear periostitis (*arrowheads*), and soft tissue swelling (*crossed arrows*) at the proximal interphalangeal joint. Although an uncommon site for such articular abnormalities, these are frequent findings in Reiter's syndrome.

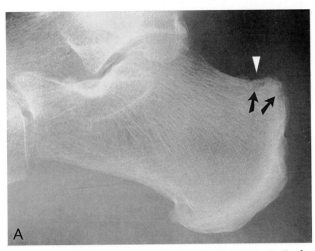
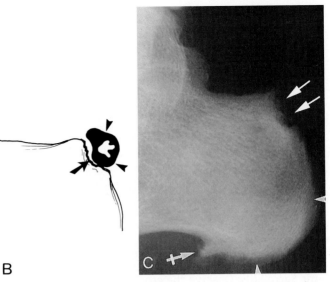

Figure 10-178 **REITER'S SYNDROME: CALCANEUS. A. Early Erosive Changes: Achilles Tendon.** Note the small lucent defects (*arrows*) and adjacent periostitis (*arrowhead*). **B. Pathophysiology.** The inflamed pre-Achilles bursa (*arrowheads*) becomes the site for pannus formation and sub- sequent subperiosteal resorption of the adjacent calcaneus (*arrow*). **C. Advanced Erosive Changes.** Note that the lucent defects are larger (*arrows*), with prominent periostitis (*arrowheads*). Note the fluffy calcaneal spur owing to inflammatory enthesopathy (*crossed arrow*).

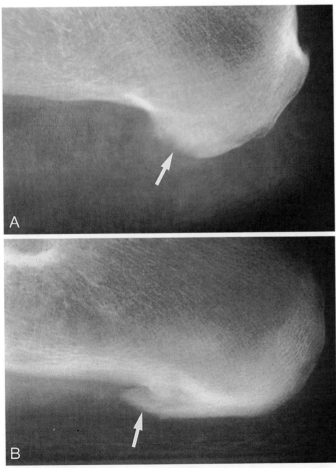

Figure 10-179 **REITER'S SYNDROME: CALCANEAL PLANTAR SURFACE ABNORMALITIES. A. Initial Study.** Note that initially the radiographic abnormality consists of irregular cortical erosions (*arrow*). **B. Later Study.** Observe that later periostitis ensues, producing irregular, fluffy, new bone formation (*arrow*).

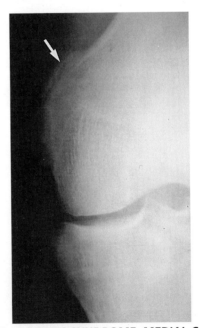

Figure 10-180 **REITER'S SYNDROME: MEDIAL COLLATERAL LIGAMENT CALCIFICATION.** Note the irregular linear density adjacent to the medial epicondyle (*arrow*). This is a Pellegrini-Stieda type of calcification within the medial collateral ligament and may be seen in approximately 10% of Reiter's syndrome patients.

involvement are variable, being unilateral or bilateral, symmetric or asymmetric; however, there is a tendency toward a bilateral but asymmetrical pattern in contrast to the symmetry seen in ankylosing spondylitis. (15,27,28) (Fig. 10-181)

Radiographic signs of sacroiliac disease consist of erosions, hazy joint margin, variable sclerosis, and altered joint space. These changes are especially prominent on the iliac margin of

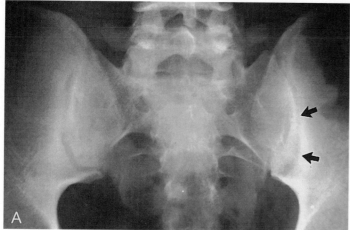
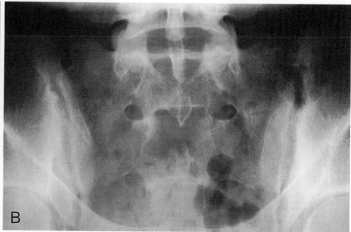

Figure 10-181 **REITER'S SYNDROME: SACROILIITIS.**
A. Bilateral Asymmetric Sacroiliitis. Note the disparity in the appearance of the sacroiliac joints, with the right joint showing more apparent sclerosis and erosions (*arrows*). This is the most common form of Reiter's sacroiliitis. **B. Bilateral Symmetric Sacroiliitis.** Observe the erosions, sclerosis, and hazy joint margins bilaterally. The majority of these changes are present on the iliac margin owing to the thicker protective articular cartilage on the sacrum. This presentation of Reiter's syndrome is relatively infrequent and is indistinguishable from ankylosing spondylitis.

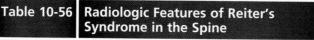

Table 10-56	Radiologic Features of Reiter's Syndrome in the Spine
Common	Uncommon
Non-marginal syndesmophytes	Atlantoaxial instability
Thoracolumbar region	Identical to ankylosing spondylitis
Asymmetric	Marginal syndesmophytes (bamboo spine)
Skip type of distribution	Apophyseal joint fusion
Complete or incomplete	
Vertical	
Thick, tapered	
Fluffy or well-defined	

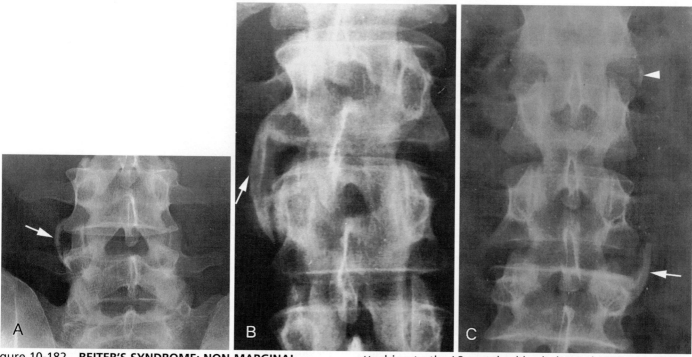

Figure 10-182 **REITER'S SYNDROME: NON-MARGINAL LUMBAR SYNDESMOPHYTES. A. Complete Non-Marginal.** Note that a thin ossification bridges the L4–L5 interspace (*arrow*) **B. Incomplete Non-Marginal.** Observe the thick ossification (comma syndesmophyte) extending down to but not attaching to the L2 vertebral body (*arrow*). **C. Incomplete Non-Marginal.** Observe that a small ossification is unconnected to either of the adjacent vertebral bodies (floating syndesmophyte) (*arrowhead*). Lower down a tapered excrescence can be seen (comma syndesmophyte) (*arrow*).

the joint. Progression to articular osseous ankylosis is less frequent than in ankylosing spondylitis. (28)

Spine. Involvement of the spine is most commonly isolated to the lower thoracic and upper lumbar regions. Occasional involvement of the atlantoaxial joint may result in instability and dislocation of the atlas in < 2% of cases. (36,37) (Table 10-56)

Thoracolumbar manifestations predominantly consist of the formation of paravertebral ossifications in the connective tissues external to the annulus and ALL. They are identical in appearance to those seen in psoriatic spondyloarthropathy and are seen in up to 15% of patients with Reiter's syndrome. (30) The sacroiliac and peripheral joints may concurrently be radiographically normal. Initially, these paravertebral ossifications are fluffy and poorly defined; later, they may become more clearly defined. (30) Characteristically, these ossifications are vertically oriented and relatively thick and may or may not attach to a vertebral body. If bony continuity is present, it will typically be toward the midportion of the vertebral body, away from the peripheral body endplate margin. As such these ossifications are called *non-marginal* or *coarse syndesmophytes.* (38) (Fig. 10-182) Distinctively, these syndesmophytes are distributed asymmetrically and unilaterally in the vertebral column, often skipping numerous segments. (33) Various radiographic morphologic appearances may be visible, especially on an AP film. (29,39)

- *Complete non-marginal.* This is attached to the midportion of two contiguous vertebral bodies, thick at its base, and tapering as it extends across the intervertebral disc space.
- *Incomplete non-marginal.* Three types may be apparent:
  Comma-shaped (inverted comma, teardrop). This originates and is continuous with the midportion of a single vertebral body, tapering at its distal extent as it begins to bridge the disc space.
  Bagpipe shaped. This is similar to the comma shape, except it is larger and bulkier at its base (*the bag*) and has a thin protuberance over the disc region (*the pipe*).
  Bywaters-Dixon (floating). This eponym is used to describe the paravertebral ossification that bridges the disc space but does not unite with the vertebral bodies. (29)
- *Marginal.* Distinctively, these are found almost exclusively in ankylosing spondylitis but, infrequently, may be apparent in psoriasis and may complicate Reiter's syndrome in up to 20% of cases. (16) These syndesmophytes represent ossification in the outer annular fibers and areolar tissue under the longitudinal ligament. Radiographically, they characteristically are bilateral and symmetric, thin, vertical, and originate at the peripheral vertebral body endplate margin. (Table 10-57)

Table 10-57	Differential Diagnosis between Marginal and Non-Marginal Syndesmophytes	
Feature	**Marginal**	**Non-Marginal**
Disease	Ankylosing spondylitis	Psoriasis or Reiter's
Origin	Vertebral body corner	Midvertebral body
Attachment	Attached	Attached or separated
Size	Small	Large
Thickness	Thin	Thick, tapered
Symmetry	Symmetric	Asymmetric
Distribution	Continuous	Skips
Definition	Sharp	Fluffy
Bridging	Complete	Incomplete

CAPSULE SUMMARY   Reiter's Syndrome

General Considerations

- A triad of urethritis, conjunctivitis, and polyarthritis, usually following sexual exposure or, less commonly, certain types of dysentery.

Clinical Features

- Affects males 50:1, 18–40 years of age.
- Arthritis predominantly of lower extremity, especially foot, calcaneus (lover's heels), ankle, knee, sacroiliac, and thoracolumbar spine; residual deformities if chronic.
- Bilateral conjunctivitis, non-specific urethritis, mucocutaneous lesions (keratodermia blenorrhagicum).
- Laboratory signs of inflammation; positive HLA-B27 in 75% of cases.

Pathologic Features

- No organism isolated; inflammatory joint changes.

Radiologic Features

- Swelling, osteoporosis, uniform loss of joint space, erosions, periostitis.
- *Specific target sites:* forefoot, calcaneus, ankle, knee, sacroiliac, spine.
- *Foot:* metatarsophalangeal and interphalangeal joints.
- *Calcaneus:* plantar and Achilles insertions.
- *Ankle:* loss of joint space, swelling, periostitis.
- *Sacroiliac:* erosions, sclerosis, loss of joint margin, asymmetric and often unilateral.
- *Spine:* thoracolumbar, asymmetric, skip non-marginal syndesmophytes and, rarely, atlantoaxial instability.

SYSTEMIC LUPUS ERYTHEMATOSUS

Systemic lupus erythematosus (SLE) is a relatively common disorder, affecting up to 48/100,000 people in the world. (1) The disease is characterized as a generalized connective tissue disorder involving multiple organ systems and demonstrating significant immunologic abnormalities. (2) SLE is typically a chronic disease interspersed with periods of acute exacerbation and exhibits a variable prognosis. (3) The most characteristic radiographic findings occur in the hands. The term *lupus* is Latin for "wolf" and is used to describe the malar erythema seen in SLE, which is similar to the facial markings of a wolf.

Clinical Features

SLE is distinctively more frequent in women, particularly in the 2nd–4th decades of life. The onset is often dismissed clinically as a transient self-limited rheumatic disorder. Certain drugs may precipitate onset of a lupus-like illness. Signs and symptoms of SLE are generally initially constitutional, with malaise, fever, anorexia, weight loss, polyarthralgia, and a skin rash. (4) Spontaneous tendon rupture can be a presenting feature. (5)

It is the skin rash that is the most characteristic physical feature and is often brought on by exposure to sunlight. The rash is erythematous and symmetric, involving the face, neck, elbows, and dorsum of the hands. Up to 40% of patients will show the classic *butterfly rash* over the bridge of the nose and malar eminences. (1) Alopecia is an accompanying symptom occurring in 24% of cases, (1) and may precede the onset of the other typical symptoms. (6) Ulcerations of the oral mucosa will be present in approximately 19% of individuals. (1)

The most frequent and serious feature of SLE is involvement of the kidney, which leads to nephropathy and renal failure. Investigation of renal involvement is warranted in all SLE patients. Up to 98% of patients without signs of kidney involvement will show abnormal histopathologic findings indicating *silent lupus nephritis*. (7) Other organs affected include heart, lungs, and nervous system. Pericarditis is the most frequent cardiac manifestation, occurring in 60% of cases. (8) Raynaud's phenomenon may also occur.

Articular signs and symptoms occur in up to 90% of SLE patients. Arthritis and skin disease are usually the most common presenting complaints. (1,4) It is usually bilateral, symmetric, and most frequently involves the hand, knee, wrist, and shoulder. Manifestations of swelling, pain, and stiffness are usually seen, simulating rheumatoid arthritis. A characteristic physical sign later in the disorder is the easy transient reversibility of deformities commonly seen in the hand such as the swan-neck, boutonniere, and ulnar drift configurations. Hypermobility of the joints is a common association with SLE patients. (9) Spine-related features are often lacking and, when present, are non-specific in nature.

The administration of steroids in the treatment of SLE may lead to osteoporosis, avascular necrosis, spinal fractures, and large gastric or duodenal ulcerations. (10–12) Complications such as osteonecrosis, may occur as quickly as 1 month after high-dose corticosteroid treatment. (13) Laboratory evaluations reveal a normochromic, normocytic anemia, thrombocytopenia, leukopenia, elevated ESR, and abnormal plasma proteins such as antinuclear factor (ANF). The demonstration of lupus erythematosus cells and/or antinuclear antibodies (ANAs) is used to confirm the diagnosis; however, lupus erythematosus cell preparation is subjective and costly, leading many authorities to advocate the isolated use of antinuclear antibody screening. (14,15)

Pathologic Features

Pathologically, SLE is characterized by deposition of immune complexes and fibrinoid material in body tissues. This is particularly prevalent in blood vessels, synovium, and serous membranes. The resultant tissue changes are those of a vasculitis (especially of small caliber vessels), synovitis, pleuritis, and pericarditis. (4,16) Other changes include skin edema and necrosis, myocarditis, and, most commonly, glomerulitis, leading to diffuse membranous glomerulonephritis and eventual renal failure.

In the bone marrow the lupus erythematosus cell is commonly seen. This cell is a mature neutrophil that contains a vacuole filled with nuclear chromatin material in varying stages of breakdown. (14)

Radiologic Features

The most distinctive features of SLE involving the musculoskeletal structures in a bilateral, symmetric fashion are the reversible deformities, osteoporosis, minimal arthropathy, soft tissue atrophy,

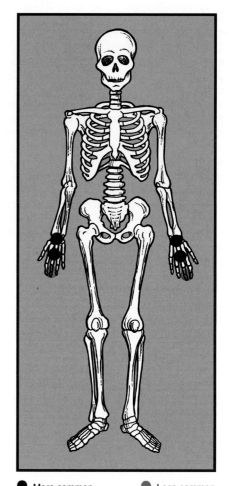

● More common ● Less common

Figure 10-183 **SKELETAL DISTRIBUTION OF SYSTEMIC LUPUS ERYTHEMATOSUS.**

Table 10-58	Radiologic Manifestations of Systemic Lupus Erythematosus
Common	
Hands	
Bilateral symmetry	
Ulnar deviation (reversible)	
Boutonniere and swan-neck deformities (reversible)	
Osteoporosis	
Normal joint space	
Soft tissue atrophy	
Long bones	
Osteonecrosis (hips, shoulders, knees, hands, feet)	
Osteoporosis	
Spontaneous fractures	
Chest	
Pleural effusions and thickening	
Cardiomegaly	
Uncommon	
Atlantoaxial instability	
Calcinosis universalis, cutis	
Tendon rupture	
Tuft resorption	

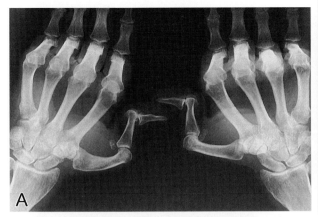
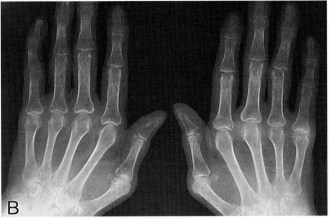

Figure 10-184   **SYSTEMIC LUPUS ERYTHEMATOSUS: DEFORMITIES. A. PA Hands.** Note the complete dislocation of the metacarpophalangeal joints, swan-neck deformities of the fingers, and boutonniere configuration of the thumbs bilaterally. **B. Hands.** Same patient with hands placed firmly on the cassette. Note the reversibility of all deformities.

calcification, and an increased incidence of osteonecrosis. (17) The majority of these features are most prominent in the hands. (Fig. 10-183; Table 10-58)

Target Sites of Involvement

Hands

Deformities. Digital ulnar deviation, boutonniere, and swan-neck deformities of the hands are characteristic but not usually permanent in nature. These deformities are reversible owing to the tendinous and ligamentous laxity, but will reappear immediately once the hand is moved. (Fig. 10-184) Ulnar deviation is also seen in rheumatoid arthritis and Jaccoud's arthropathy.

Arthropathy. Changes in the joint space and subchondral bone are unusual and are useful differential features from rheumatoid arthritis. (18) Generalized osteoporosis of the osseous structures, however, may be prominent. Small degrees of tuftal resorption may be seen in patients with accompanying Raynaud's phenomenon identical to those seen in scleroderma. (19)

Soft Tissue. Atrophy of the overlying musculature may be striking. Occasionally, sheet-like or punctate calcifications within myofascial planes and subcutaneous tissues may be seen. (20–23) (Fig. 10-185) Premature peripheral vascular calcifications can also be observed. (20–23)

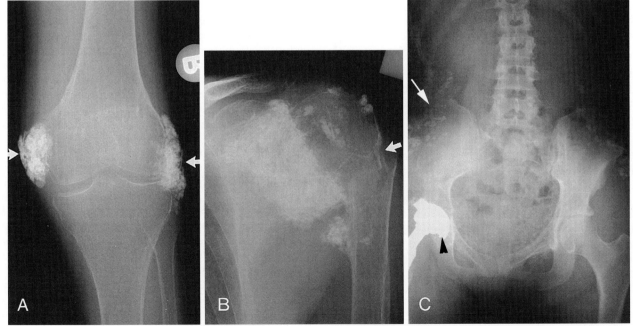

Figure 10-185   **SYSTEMIC LUPUS ERYTHEMATOSUS: CALCINOSIS CIRCUMSCRIPTA. A. AP Knee.** Observe the soft tissue calcifications (*arrows*). **B. AP Shoulder.** Note the generalized osteoporosis and fracture of the humerus (*arrow*). **C. Abdomen.** Note the diffuse soft tissue calcification (*arrow*). A hip prosthesis has been performed for corticosteroid-induced osteonecrosis (*arrowhead*). *COMMENT:* Even though soft tissue calcification is found in systemic lupus erythematosus, the diagnosis cannot be made from this single finding alone. Additional clinical data and further radiographs are needed to confirm the diagnosis. (Panel C courtesy of D. B. Drozdov, DC, Baton Rouge, Louisiana.)

Other Sites

Spine. Spinal changes are distinctly unusual. The only complication may be atlantoaxial instability, encountered in < 5% of SLE patients. (24,25) This is delineated by an increased ADI of > 3 mm, especially in flexion. Compression fractures may complicate corticosteroid therapy.

Long Bones. Osteonecrosis is seen in 5–10% of adults and in up to 40% of younger SLE patients. (12,25–27) (Fig. 10-186) The most common sites are the femoral and humeral heads, often simultaneously and bilaterally. (26) Other locations include the femoral condyles, talus, wrist, tarsus, and metacarpal and metatarsal heads. (28–30) The signs of SLE-related ischemic necrosis are identical to those of people who do not have the disease, except for SLE involving multiple and often unusual sites. The onset of osteonecrosis still can occur without the administration of steroid therapy. (11,16,31) Generalized osteoporosis is often severe, especially in those treated with large doses of corticosteroids, and may predispose to fracture.

Chest. The most frequently observed abnormalities in the chest are small, bilateral pleural effusions, pleural thickening, mild to moderate cardiomegaly, and pericardial effusion. (32)

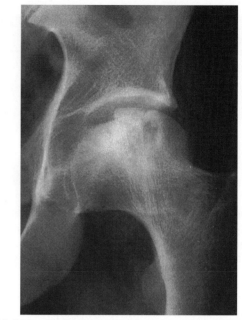

Figure 10-186 SYSTEMIC LUPUS ERYTHEMATOSUS: AVASCULAR NECROSIS OF THE FEMORAL HEAD. AP Hip. Note the collapse of the articular cortex. *COMMENT:* This is a common complication of steroid therapy for lupus.

CAPSULE SUMMARY   Systemic Lupus Erythematosus

General Considerations

- Generalized connective tissue disorder involving multiple organ systems.

Clinical Features

- Women of childbearing age.
- Onset with fever, malaise, skin rash, and arthralgias.
- Laboratory findings show elevated ESR, ANF, and lupus erythematosus cell.

Pathologic Features

- Immune complexes and fibrinoid material are deposited in body tissues, resulting in inflammatory changes in blood vessels, synovium, and serous membranes.

Radiologic Features

- Most prominent features visible in the hands.
- Reversible subluxations, dislocations and deformities, normal joint spaces, osteoporosis, osteonecrosis, soft tissue atrophy, and calcification.
- *Hand:* ulnar deviation, boutonniere, and swan-neck deformities; normal joints; osteoporosis.
- *Spine:* atlantoaxial instability; steroid-induced compression fractures.
- *Chest:* pleural effusions and thickening, cardiomegaly, pericardial effusion.

JACCOUD'S ARTHRITIS

An infrequent consequence of rheumatic fever consisting of predominantly hand and, to a lesser extent, foot deformities was first described by Jaccoud. (1) These deformities are similar to rheumatoid arthritis and SLE, but lack the deforming, erosive joint changes. The hallmarks of the disorder are ulnar deviation and flexion of the metacarpophalangeal joints. (2) As rheumatic fever and its recurrences disappear with earlier diagnosis and prophylaxis, this chronic but harmless condition will become more infrequent. Various terms have been applied to this disorder, including Jaccoud's syndrome, Jaccoud's arthritis, Jaccoud's arthropathy, and chronic postrheumatic fever arthropathy.

Clinical Features

The manifestations of rheumatic fever are well described in the literature. Criteria for guidance in the diagnosis of rheumatic fever have been formulated. (3) However, the most prominent findings include an antecedent streptococcal pharyngitis, transitory migratory peripheral myalgias and arthralgias, skin rash (*erythema marginatum*), fever, sweating, pallor, fatigue, and weight loss. The patient may be diagnosed as having rheumatoid arthritis.

Following numerous attacks of joint involvement in the hands and feet, more definitive changes will be apparent. (Fig. 10-187) It is these resultant articular abnormalities that are designated as Jaccoud's arthropathy, in association with additional clinical criteria. (4) (Table 10-59) In the hands, ulnar drift and finger deformities are evident, such as the boutonniere and swan-neck configurations. (5) In addition, palmar subluxation at the metacarpophalangeal joints is common, especially at the fourth and fifth digits. As in SLE, these deformities are reversible but will re-

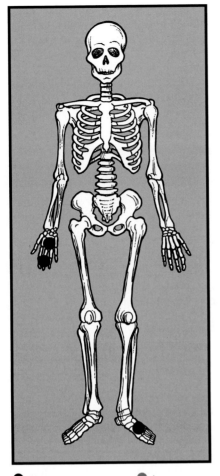

● More common   ● Less common

Figure 10-187   **SKELETAL DISTRIBUTION OF JACCOUD'S ARTHRITIS.**

Table 10-60	Radiologic Features of Jaccoud's Arthritis

Predilected locations
   Hand: metacarpophalangeal
   Foot: metatarsophalangeal (especially fourth and fifth digits)
Acute phase
   Joint effusion
   Juxta-articular osteoporosis
Chronic phase
   Reversibly deforming nonerosive arthropathy
   Hand
      Ulnar deviation
      Palmar-flexion subluxation of metacarpophalangeal joints
      Boutonniere deformity
      Normal joint spaces
      Rarely metacarpal head radial hook erosions
   Foot
      Fibular deviation
      Dorsiflexion subluxation at metatarsophalangeal joints
      Normal joint spaces

lagen fibers undergo a fibrinous change. Distinctively, there is no alteration in joint cartilage or subchondral bone. As the acute episode recedes, these synovial and capsular changes may completely regress with no permanent residual sequelae.

In instances of chronic recurrence, progressive fibrosis of the capsular and periarticular tendons and fascia results in the characteristic digital ulnar deviation and deformities. (2,8,9) Rarely, there may be loss of the joint cartilage in a uniform manner, especially at the metacarpophalangeal joints.

Radiologic Features

The essential radiologic features of Jaccoud's arthritis are those of a peripheral deforming, non-erosive arthropathy. (Table 10-60) The most common sites of involvement are the metacarpophalangeal and PIP joints of the hands as well as the metatarsophalangeal joints of the feet. (5) In the acute episode, radiographic evaluations of these locations are frequently unrewarding and non-specific. Acute manifestations are joint swelling and preservation of normal joint space and contour. (2)

cur on normal physiologic movements. (5,6) Parallel foot changes are seen less frequently with digital fibular deviation and metatarsophalangeal subluxations. (7)

Pathologic Features

The articular and periarticular pathologic manifestations closely parallel the acute and chronic phases of the arthropathy. (8) The acute episode is characterized by a mild synovitis with minimal edema and cellular infiltrate of the superficial synovial layers only. Within the deeper synovial strata and joint capsule, the col-

Table 10-59	Definitive Criteria for the Diagnosis of Jaccoud's Arthritis

- Recurrent attacks of acute rheumatic fever
- Slow resolution of joint inflammation followed by stiffness and deformity, especially at the metacarpophalangeal joints
- Characteristic hand deformity (ulnar deviation, flexed metacarpophalangeal joint), soft tissue swelling, and associated periarticular, fascial, and tendon fibrosis
- Tendon crepitus
- Asymptomatic joint disease with no active synovitis and good functional capacity

Adapted from **Zvaifler NJ:** *Chronic post rheumatic fever (Jaccoud's Arthritis).* N Engl J Med 267:10, 1962.

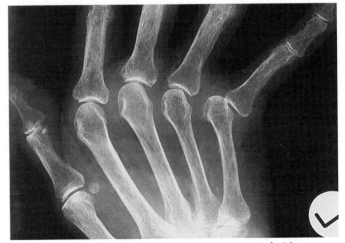

Figure 10-188   **JACCOUD'S ARTHRITIS. PA Hand. Observe the ulnar deviation and lack of articular changes identical to those of systemic lupus erythematosus.**

In the chronic stage the most definitive findings in the hands are ulnar deviation, especially at the fourth and fifth digits; flexion–palmar subluxations at the metacarpophalangeal joints; and boutonniere and swan-neck configurations at the interphalangeal joints. (2) (Fig. 10-188) These are easily corrected, but will resume the deformed configuration with normal physiologic movements. Notably, the articular cavity of all these involved joints is usually of normal thickness, although occasionally a mild uniform diminu-

tion may be observed. (9) No subchondral marginal erosions should be visible, an important differential sign from rheumatoid arthritis. Occasionally, the appearance of a cystic lucency on the radial side of a metacarpal head produces a hook-like protuberance of the articular cortex that may simulate a marginal erosion. (5,9) In the feet, analogous findings such as fibular deviation and dorsiflexion of the digits are seen.

CAPSULE SUMMARY   Jaccoud's Arthritis

General Considerations

- Jaccoud's arthritis is an infrequent, deforming, non-erosive, peripheral arthropathy affecting the hands and feet after rheumatic fever.

Clinical Features

- *Manifestations of previous rheumatic fever:* antecedent streptococcal pharyngitis, fever, transitory and migratory arthralgias, myalgia, fatigue, and weight loss, and residual mitral valve disease.
- Articular involvement initially episodic with swelling and pain.

- If recurrent, results in deformities such as ulnar and fibular deviation, boutonniere and swan-neck configurations.

Pathologic Features

- Initial mild synovitis with associated fibrosis of joint capsule, tendons, and fascia resulting in instability, especially at the metacarpophalangeal joints.
- Joint cartilage notably unaffected.

Radiologic Features

- Ulnar and fibular deviation deformities; subluxations, normal joint spaces, no erosions, and normal bone density.

IDIOPATHIC CHONDROLYSIS OF THE HIP

Clinical Features

Idiopathic chondrolysis of the hip (ICH) was first recognized in 1971 by Jones. (1) ICH is an uncommon crippling articular disorder predominantly of adolescent females. There is approximately a 6:1 female predominance. (2) It most frequently begins at 11–12 years of age up until age 20. (2) It is far more common bilaterally than unilaterally.

The typical presentation is that of an adolescent girl with hip pain, stiffness, and restriction of motion. This can rapidly progress within months to a crippling flexion contracture of the hip, increased lumbar lordosis, and an inability to stand. (3) Complete blood count, ESR, rheumatoid factor, ANA, HLA-B27, blood proteins, and urinalysis are all normal. (4–7)

The process of chondrolysis can be primary (idiopathic) or secondary. Secondary chondrolysis of the hip may occur as a sequel to slipped capital femoral epiphysis, extended immobilization, paraplegia, septic arthritis, rheumatoid arthritis, and trauma. (8,9) The most common cause for secondary chondrolysis of the hip is slipped femoral capital epiphysis. (10)

The long-term prognosis is unpredictable. (2) The condition may resolve spontaneously, progress to ankylosis, develop avascular necrosis, or deform the hip. (9) Approximately 20% of cases go on to fusion, and 30% regain good mobility. (2) Mild cases can resolve with physical measures, analgesia, and non-weight bearing. (5,10) Regular swimming has been advocated. (2)

Pathologic Features

Chondrolysis of the hip is of unknown origin. (11) It is characterized by an extensive loss of articular cartilage of the femoral head

and acetabulum. (12) Pathologic findings are non-specific, allowing for the exclusion of other diagnostic possibilities. (2,5,13) Synovial fluid aspirations are unrewarding. The articular cartilage changes include loss and thinning of the superficial areas. (13) The synovium lacks inflammatory changes, although some degree of villous formation; nodular lymphoid hyperplasia of the subsynovium; and perivascular infiltrates of lymphocytes, plasma cells, and monocytes can be observed. (13) Immunofluorescent studies for deposition of immune complexes within the synovium should be normal. (14) No fibrinoid necrosis or granuloma formation is seen. Thickening of the joint capsule is common. (13,15) The adjacent bone is osteoporotic with cysts filled with synovium. Later stages can be associated with cysts, osteophytes, obliteration of the joint cavity, and deformity. Underlying osteonecrosis has been described. (9)

Radiologic Features

Imaging findings consist of diminished joint space, protrusio acetabuli, localized periarticular osteopenia, subchondral cysts, erosion or blurring of the articular cortex, premature closure of the epiphysis, lateral overgrowth of the femoral head, and broadening of the femoral neck. (2,4,13,16) The hallmark of the condition is narrowing of the hip joint space without frank osteophyte formation in conjunction with periarticular osteopenia in a young female. (13) (Fig. 10-189) Isotopic bone scans are normal in the flow and blood pool phases but demonstrate a periarticular increased uptake within the femoral head and acetabulum on delayed scans. (6,16) Arthrography demonstrates the patchy loss of articular cartilage with a *dappled pattern* of contrast over the femoral head. (13) MRI shows loss of cartilage in a patchy distribution.

The differential diagnosis at its acute adolescent presentation includes idiopathic protrusio acetabuli, trauma, slipped femoral

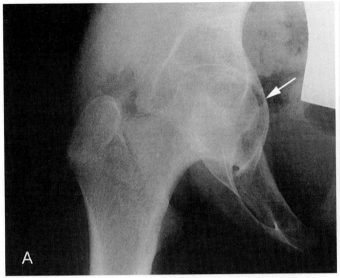 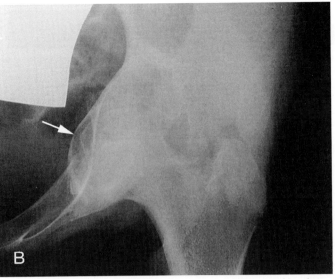

Figure 10-189   **IDIOPATHIC CHONDROLYSIS OF THE HIP. A and B. Bilateral Joint Disease.** Note the concentric and uniform narrowing of the joint space bilaterally. Also observe the bilateral protrusio acetabuli (*arrows*) and periarticular

osteopenia. Both of these hips were active on nuclear bone scan. *COMMENT:* The hallmark of the condition is narrowing of the hip joint space without frank osteophyte formation in conjunction with periarticular osteopenia in a young female.

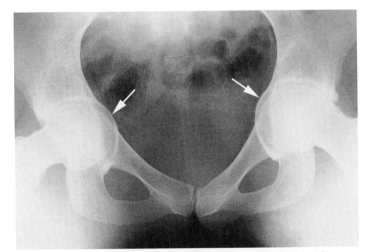

Figure 10-190   **IDIOPATHIC PROTRUSIO ACETABULI. AP Pelvis.** Note that in this young female the bilateral protrusio acetabuli deformity is well developed with no evidence of articular disease (*arrows*). There were no peripheral signs of rheumatoid arthritis. *COMMENT:* It is likely that these patients are asymptomatic through adolescence until they develop secondary osteoarthritis after 40 years of age. The cause is unknown. (Courtesy of Wesley E. Wilvert, DC, Parker, Colorado.)

capital epiphysis, septic arthritis, tuberculosis, migratory or transitory osteoporosis, reflex sympathetic dystrophy, Perthes disease, pigmented villonodular synovitis, synovioma, and rheumatoid arthritis. (3,5,6,16)

Idiopathic protrusio acetabuli is a difficult entity to exclude and has been confused in the literature. (17) It is likely that these patients are asymptomatic through adolescence until they develop secondary osteoarthritis after 40 years of age. (18) (Fig. 10-190) The major exclusion criteria is the finding of protrusio acetabuli in an asymptomatic individual.

SCLERODERMA

Scleroderma is a generalized systemic inflammatory connective tissue disease of unknown cause involving the skin, lungs, gastrointestinal tract, heart, kidneys, and musculoskeletal system. (1,2) Radiographic manifestations of scleroderma affecting the musculoskeletal system principally depend on adjacent skin changes and, therefore, are usually seen once the disease has become well developed. Spinal involvement is distinctly lacking, with the most characteristic alterations occurring in the appendicular skeleton.

A variety of descriptive terms has been applied to scleroderma. (2) (Table 10-61) Synonyms include progressive systemic sclerosis (PSS), CREST syndrome, and acrosclerosis. The combination of soft tissue calcinosis, scleroderma, Raynaud's phenomenon, and generalized telangiectasia has been called the Thibierge-Weissenbach syndrome. (3,4) Others have generalized the combination of calcinosis and scleroderma as constituting this syndrome. (5)

Clinical Features

The onset typically is between 30 and 50 years of age and is more frequent in females with a ratio of at least 3:1; (5,6) childhood onset is rare. The appearance of the skin is the most unique feature; however, gastrointestinal complaints are frequently the initial symptom and often treated in isolation for months to years before the appropriate diagnosis is made based on skin appearance. (7) Progression of the skin disorder is through three stages: edema, induration, and atrophy. (5) The initial symptoms are insidious and consist of rheumatoid-like changes with puffy, painful swelling of the extremities. (8,9) In > 90% of patients, exposure to cold or even emotional upset may precipitate peripheral vasoconstrictive changes of pallor followed by a painful vasodilation producing exquisite pain and swelling (Raynaud's phenomenon). (6,10) This vasomotor abnormality often antedates the onset of the skin changes. (5,11)

Table 10-61	Terms Used in Association with Scleroderma
Acrosclerosis	Peripheral predilection for changes in the skin
Calcinosis cutis	Calcification within the skin
Calcinosis circumscripta	Localized calcifications in soft tissue often seen in collagen diseases
Calcinosis universalis	Generalized calcifications in soft tissue often seen in collagen diseases
CREST syndrome	Acronym for identifying the major associations in scleroderma: calcinosis, Raynaud's phenomenon, esophageal abnormality, scleroderma, telangiectasia
Raynaud's phenomenon	Sympathetic nervous system dysfunction characterized by cyclic vascular changes usually of the hands; precipitated by cold or emotional upset; an initial vasoconstriction is followed by vasodilation with severe pain and swelling
Thibierge-Weissenbach syndrome	Combination of soft tissue calcification, scleroderma, Raynaud's phenomenon, and generalized telangiectasia

With advancement of the disease, skin edema is replaced by gradual thickening, induration, and adherence to underlying structures, becoming *hidebound*. Typically, this involves the face, producing a *mouselike facies* (*mauskopff*); fingers; and dorsums of the hands and feet. Later, atrophy of the underlying tissues and skin occurs. Other skin changes of telangiectasia, vitiligo, and hyperpigmentation may be seen. (2) Nodular subcutaneous calcific masses occasionally ulcerate through the overlying skin, particularly in pressure areas such as the fingers, ulnar aspect of the forearm, and ischial regions. Muscle weakness and atrophy are often prominent. (12)

The most apparent clinical systemic effects will be related to the mobility of the gastrointestinal tract. (1,7) Dysphagia and heartburn owing to decreased motility and dilation of the esophagus will be seen in up to 90% of individuals. (3,6) The acid reflux associated with scleroderma is usually of a more severe nature than its idiopathic counterpart and infrequently resolves completely. (3,6,13) Generally, the bowel is sluggish and dilated, resulting in distension, constipation, and reduced absorptive capacity. Later, involvement of the lungs and heart is common. (6) Pulmonary arterial hypertension (14,15) and pericardial effusions (16) are the most common associations, with pleural effusion found less frequently. (16) Owing to current medications, the association of mortality as a result of kidney involvement is rarely seen. (1,13)

Pathologic Features

The pathologic changes observed are predominately vascular in nature, consisting of a low-grade inflammatory reaction in the perivascular tissue, with atrophy and fibrosis of adjacent collagen. (8,17) The smaller diameter arterioles show progressive intimal thickening and a medial fibrosis with eventual thrombosis. The net result on tissue is inflammation, decreased vascularity, and promotion of fibrous tissue deposition and induration. (6) Muscle

tissue reveals inflammatory myositis and degeneration. (8,12) Examination of synovium reveals inflammatory cellular infiltration with fibrin internally and externally. (8)

Radiologic Features

The most prominent changes are characteristically in the hand, although other areas may be involved. (Fig. 10-191; Table 10-62) The spine, pelvis, and large joints of the periphery are generally spared.

Hand and Wrist

Soft Tissue. Usually, the earliest signs appear in the overlying skin contour, especially of the distal fingertips. Resorption of the soft tissue results in a tapered, conical configuration of the fingertip with retraction of the tip in a proximal manner. (Fig. 10-192) Soft tissue retraction at the fingertip is present when the vertical thickness of the soft tissue is < 20% of the width at the base of the distal phalanx. (18) The normal periarticular skinfolds also may be obliterated.

Soft tissue calcification is seen in up to 20% of patients. Approximately 75% of these patients will show soft tissue calcification in the hands. (19,20) The pattern of calcification is variable, from punctate to sheet-like. (Fig. 10-193) The location of these calcifications seems related to areas of trauma such as the radial surface of the second digit and ulnar aspect of the forearm, (9,10) especially in the dominant hand. (20) (Fig. 10-194) The tissue site

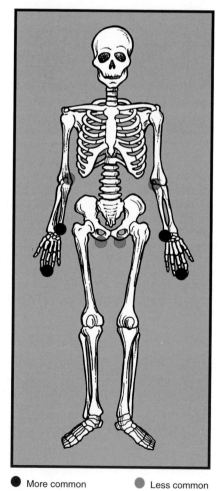

● More common ● Less common

Figure 10-191 **SKELETAL DISTRIBUTION OF SCLERODERMA.**

Table 10-62	Radiologic Features of Scleroderma in the Hands

Soft tissue
  Tapered, conical fingertips
  Retraction of fingertip
  Loss of overlying skin folds
  Calcification: skin (calcinosis cutis) intra-articular
Bone
  Resorption—distal tufts
Joints
  Normal
  Manifestations of rheumatoid arthritis, erosive osteoarthritis, or psoriasis
  Erosive arthropathy at first metacarpal-carpal joint

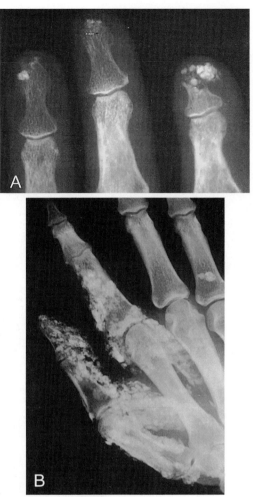

Figure 10-193 **SCLERODERMA: DIGITAL PATTERNS OF CALCINOSIS CUTIS. A. Punctate. B. Sheet-Like.**

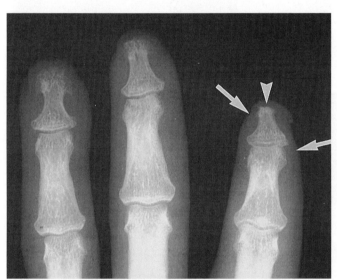

Figure 10-192 **SCLERODERMA WITH DIGITAL SKIN RETRACTION AND EARLY ACROOSTEOLYSIS.** Note the atrophy and retraction of the soft tissues of the fingertip at the fourth digit (*arrows*). Resorption of the distal tuft is also seen (*arrowhead*). The combination of these two findings is highly indicative of scleroderma.

of calcification is predominately subcutaneous (*calcinosis cutis*), although it may occur along myofascial planes (*sheet-like*) and joint capsules and may even be intra-articular. (21)

Bones. The most commonly involved osseous structures are the distal phalanges, particularly the terminal tufts. (18) Changes consist of a resorbing osteolysis initially at the tip, lateral, and palmar aspects of the tuft, leading to a sharpened, tapered, distal phalanx. (19,22) (Figs. 10-195 and 10-196) These changes may be seen in up to 80% of cases. (8) Eventually, complete osteolysis of the phalanx may be evident. These bony changes closely parallel the tapering phenomenon observed in the overlying skin. Localized osteolysis may also be observed adjacent to sites of soft tissue calcification. (Fig. 10-197) Generalized osteoporosis is usually the result of disuse and immobilization. Rarely, scleroderma-induced vasculitis of the femoral head may result in avascular necrosis, which is radiographically indistinguishable from the idiopathic form. (23)

Joints. Articular alterations are variable. Bilateral selective involvement of the first carpometacarpal joint of the wrist with resorption of the opposing first metacarpal base and trapezium is distinctive. (24) Occasionally, intra-articular calcification may be visible. (21) Other manifestations may include those seen in rheumatoid arthritis, erosive osteoarthritis, and psoriatic arthritis. (25,26)

Other Sites of Involvement

Soft Tissue. Calcifications in varied forms may be seen in areas of mechanical stress such as the wrist, elbow, ischial tuberosities, hip, and knee. (20)

A specific dental sign is thickening of the radiolucent periodontal membrane three to four times the normal. (27) Pulmonary changes are non-specific with variable degrees of interstitial fibrosis, particularly at the lung bases. (28) Gastrointestinal abnormalities seen on barium studies consist of dilation and decreased peristaltic activity, particularly of the esophagus and small bowel. (5,19,28) Distinctive broad-based, wide-mouthed pseudo-diverticula are sometimes seen on the antimesenteric surface of the colon. (19)

Bone. Osteolysis of bone closely adjacent to overlying skin may be seen at the distal clavicles, mandible, and posterior ribs. In regard to the spine, a single case report has been recorded of a cervical spine with marked kyphosis, atrophic neural arches, and soft tissue calcification. (29) No sacroiliac alterations have been documented.

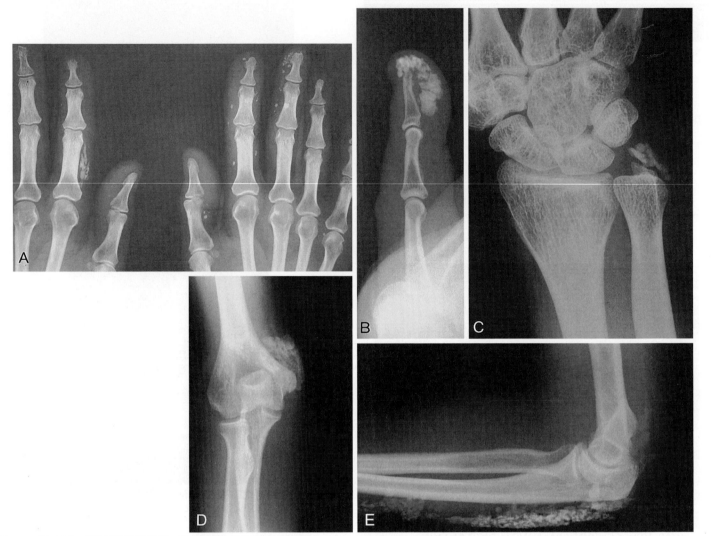

Figure 10-194 **SCLERODERMA: CHARACTERISTIC SITES OF CALCIFICATION. A. Radial Side.** Second and third digits. **B. Palmar Surface.** Fingertips. **C. Ulnar Side.** Forearm. **D. Extensor Surface.** Ulna. **E. Medial Epicondyle.** Distal humerus. (Courtesy of Maggie Craw, DC, DACBR, Sacramento, California.)

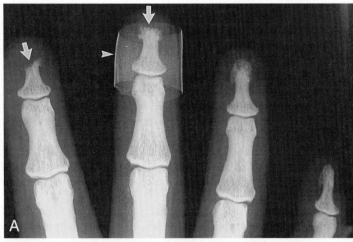

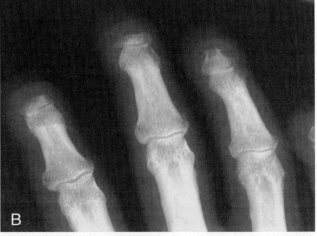

Figure 10-195 **SCLERODERMA: ACROOSTEOLYSIS. A. PA Hand.** Note the early resorption of the distal tufts (*arrows*). Incidentally noted is a bandage (*arrowhead*). **B. PA Hand.** Observe the advanced resorption of the distal tufts.

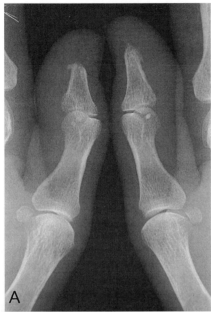

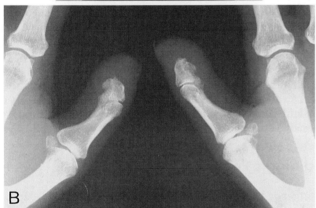

Figure 10-196 **SCLERODERMA: ACROOSTEOLYSIS OF THE THUMB. A. Early Resorption.** Note the tapered, conical shape of the distal tufts of the thumbs. **B. Advanced Resorption.** Note the extensive resorption of the distal tufts of the thumbs.

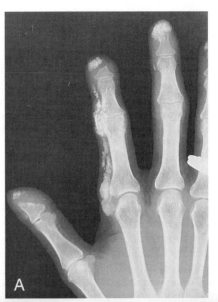

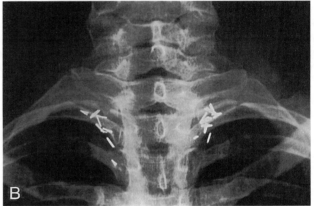

Figure 10-197 **SCLERODERMA: CHARACTERISTIC MANIFES-TATIONS. A. Diagnostic Finger Changes.** Note that the combination of calcinosis cutis and acroosteolysis is virtually diagnostic of scleroderma. **B. Surgery: Raynaud's Phenomenon.** Observe the surgical clips in the lung apices bilaterally, suggesting previous sympathectomy for Raynaud's disease, a frequent association in scleroderma.

CAPSULE SUMMARY   Scleroderma

General Considerations

- Systemic inflammatory connective tissue disease affecting the skin, lungs, gastrointestinal tract, heart, kidneys, and musculoskeletal system.
- Synonyms include progressive systemic sclerosis and CREST syndrome.

Clinical Features

- More common in females 30–50 years of age.
- Initial peripheral pain and swelling, with high incidence of Raynaud's phenomenon.
- Skin becomes thick, taut, and hidebound, involving hands and face. Involvement of the esophagus with dysphagia is common.

Pathologic Features

- Low-grade perivascular inflammation with atrophy and fibrosis of adjacent collagen.

Radiologic Features

- Hand most commonly involved.
- *Soft tissue:* retraction, tapered fingers, and calcification.
- *Bone:* resorption, especially distal phalanges.
- *Joints:* first carpometacarpal joint—signs of rheumatoid, erosive, or psoriatic arthritis.

OSTEITIS CONDENSANS ILII

Osteitis condensans ilii is an isolated sacroiliac arthropathy of controversial origin and significance. It is a joint affliction predominantly found in women of childbearing age named after the characteristic radiologic depiction of a well-defined triangular region of sclerosis localized in the subchondral bone of the ilium. (1,2) (Fig. 10-198)

Clinical Features

A great disparity often exists in the physical and radiologic presentation of osteitis condensans ilii. (3,4) The symptomatic patient is typically a multiparous woman between 20 and 40 years of age with chronic low back pain and stiffness. The female predominance of this condition may exceed 9:1. (2,4)

Examination of a symptomatic patient reveals lack of or excessive sacroiliac motion. (5,6) Pain and tenderness are elicited directly over the joint with positive orthopedic tests. Radiation of pain into the lower extremity and groin may also occur. Adjacent paraspinal muscle spasm in the lumbar spine is present in varying degrees. When acute, misdiagnosis of intervertebral disc or posterior joint syndrome is often made. (1,6) Exclusion of other low

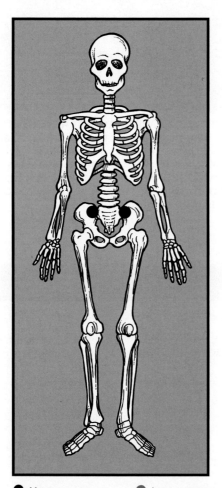

● More common   ● Less common

Figure 10-198 **SKELETAL DISTRIBUTION OF OSTEITIS CONDENSANS ILII.**

back arthropathies should include ankylosing spondylitis, psoriatic spondylitis, and DJD. (7–10) (Table 10-63) Specific chiropractic manipulative therapy to the sacroiliac joints may initially increase symptoms, but it quickly resolves them with almost complete resolution of the pain syndrome. (6)

Laboratory investigations are notably unrewarding. (11) The ESR, cell differential, and serum analysis will all be within normal limits. The incidence of the HLA-B27 antigen will be no greater than in the general population, serving as a useful differential point from ankylosing spondylitis. (8,12)

Pathologic Features

The cause of osteitis condensans ilii is unknown, and there is a distinct lack of pathologic delineation. Implicated factors include hormonal, mechanical, infectious, inflammatory, and degenerative factors. (4,7,11,13–16) The predominant theory focuses on the combination of hormonal and secondary mechanical stresses in producing the increase in iliac bone density. (11,17,18) It is postulated that the reversible ligamentous laxity of pregnancy and even within the normal menstrual cycle may ultimately result in permanent ligamentous damage. The mechanical sequela of this pelvic ligamentous laxity is increased physical forces through the subchondral bone, particularly the ilium, where the cartilage is substantially thinner than on the sacrum. Subsequently, physiologic thickening of the supporting trabeculae occur. Pathologic evaluation of an involved sacro-iliac joint demonstrates increased osseous vascularity, thickened trabeculae, mild inflammatory cellular infiltrate, marrow changes, and usually normal to mild degenerative changes of the joint cartilage. (3,16,17)

Radiologic Features

Osteitis condensans ilii is best depicted on an AP 30° cephalad tube angulated view (*tilt-up view*). (11) The characteristic finding is bilateral, symmetric, triangle-shaped areas of sclerosis involving only the lower half of the ilium (*hyperostosis triangularis ilii*). (3,4,17) (Fig. 10-199) There is usually no abnormality of the joint margins or joint space, which aids in differentiating inflammatory sacroiliitis such as in ankylosing spondylitis and psoriasis. (9,11) (Table 10-64) CT is especially useful in delineating the presence of erosive lesions of inflammatory sacroiliitis. (11) If erosive changes are seen at these locations, the exclusion of ankylosing spondylitis as the cause must be done by laboratory evaluations. Unilateral changes with osteophytes and an altered joint space indicate DJD. Complete regression of the iliac sclerosis has been documented over periods of 3– 20 years. (4)

Osteitis Condensans of the Clavicle

Osteitis condensans can be seen in the medial clavicle, exhibiting similar bone changes to that in osteitis condensans ilii, but is unrelated to pregnancy. (19) Clinically, a history of localized mechanical stress in the sternoclavicular region, with pain and swelling, is present. Radiographically, the medial portion of the clavicle demonstrates increased density with a normal adjacent joint space. (Figs. 10-200 and 10-201) Occasionally, an intraosseous air-filled cyst (*intraosseous pneumatocyst*) may be seen on CT. (20) The differential diagnosis includes low-grade osteomyelitis, Paget's disease, osteosarcoma, and degenerative arthritis.

Table 10-63	Differential Diagnosis of Osteitis Condensans Ilii			
Features	Osteitis Condensans Ilii	Ankylosing Spondylitis	Psoriasis	Degenerative Joint Disease
Clinical				
Age	20–40	15–35	20–50	20–50
Sex	Female > male	Male > female	Female > male	Female > male
Symptoms	None to mild	Mild to severe	Mild to severe	None to severe
Laboratory	Normal	ESR	ESR	Normal
		HLA-B27	HLA-B27	Normal
Radiologic				
Sacroiliac joint				
Distribution	Usually bilateral, symmetric	Bilateral, symmetric	Unilateral to bilateral, asymmetric	Unilateral
Location	Ilium	Ilium, sacrum	Ilium, sacrum	Ilium
Sclerosis	Triangular, sharp	Hazy margin	Hazy, minimal	Small, hazy
Erosions	Absent	Common	Common	Absent
Ankylosis	Absent	Present	Absent or present	Absent
Spine	Normal	Marginal syndesmophytes	Non-marginal syndesmophytes	Osteophytes
Peripheral joints	Normal	Hips, shoulders	Common—hands, feet	Common—multiple

ESR, erythrocyte sedimentation rate.

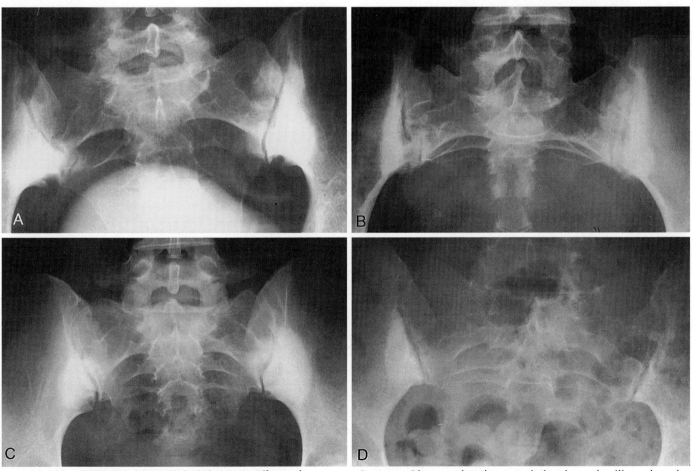

Figure 10-199   **OSTEITIS CONDENSANS ILII. A. Bilateral Symmetric Pattern (Prominent). B. Bilateral Symmetric Pattern. C. Bilateral Asymmetric Pattern. D. Unilateral Pattern.** Observe the characteristic triangular iliac sclerosis (hyperostosis triangularis ilii). (Courtesy of John K. Hyland, DC, DACBR, DABCO, Denver, Colorado.)

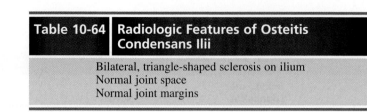

Table 10-64	Radiologic Features of Osteitis Condensans Ilii
	Bilateral, triangle-shaped sclerosis on ilium
	Normal joint space
	Normal joint margins

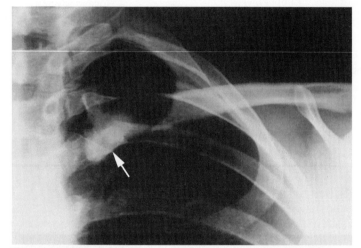

Figure 10-200 **OSTEITIS CONDENSANS OF CLAVICLE. PA Clavicle.** Note that the medial end of the clavicle is increased in density (*arrow*). Note that the middle and distal portions of the clavicle are normal. (Courtesy of Constant Boshoff, DC, Rapid City, South Dakota.)

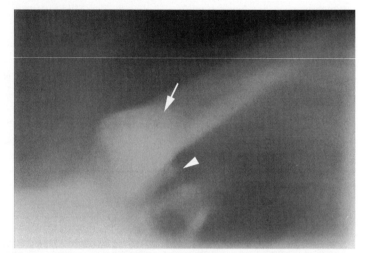

Figure 10-201 **OSTEITIS CONDENSANS OF CLAVICLE. AP Tomogram.** Note that on tomography the extent of the sclerosis can be appreciated (*arrow*). Note the presence of a degenerative spur at the sternoclavicular joint, which is a frequent additional finding (*arrowhead*).

CAPSULE SUMMARY   Osteitis Condensans Ilii

General Considerations

- A bilateral, symmetric sacroiliac disorder predominantly found in multiparous females.

Clinical Features

- Women 20–40 years, 9:1 predominance, and usually multiparous.
- Wide variation from asymptomatic to chronic low back and leg pain.
- Usually self-limiting over a protracted period.
- No positive laboratory findings.

Pathologic Features

- Combination of hormone-induced ligamentous laxity and increased mechanical joint stresses results in low-grade inflammatory and sclerotic changes of the iliac subchondral bone.

Radiologic Features

- Bilateral, dense, triangle shaped iliac subchondral sclerosis involving the lower half of the joint margin.
- Joint space and joint margins are normal.
- The most important differential exclusion is ankylosing spondylitis.

OSTEITIS PUBIS

Osteitis pubis is a painful condition of the pubic symphysis articulation characterized by bony resorption and spontaneous reossification. Although the pathogenesis is uncertain, the most common related antecedent event is surgery within close proximity to the symphysis. (1) The first report of the condition was in 1924 by Beer, who described these changes as a common sequela to bladder surgery. (2)

Clinical Features

Onset of signs and symptoms is usually within 1–3 months after surgery in the locality of the symphysis pubis articulation. The frequency of this postsurgical complication is between 1% and 3%. (3–5) The most common types of surgery are for the prostate, bladder, urethra, uterus, and cervix. Statistically, prostate surgery is the most commonly associated surgical procedure. (6) Additional causes include pregnancy, trauma, and, often, unknown factors. (7–10)

Symptomology may be localized or referred and is usually described as *groin burning*. (11) Pain is often excruciating on direct palpation. Exercise or activities involving thigh adduction, trunk flexion or even walking may refer pain to the perineal, testicular, suprapubic or inguinal area. (11) In addition, an audible click in the area of the pubic symphysis may be heard during these activities. (12) Postejaculatory pain referral to the scrotum and perineum has been noted in males. (11) The symptoms are generally relieved by rest. (11) Redness or heat is usually not present. The gait is antalgic, with trunk flexion and waddling to prevent symphyseal stress.

Pain typically subsides over an indefinite period up to 1–2 years, but may require arthrodesis. (4,5) With persistent pain and biomechanical alterations in gait, early sacroiliac degenerative changes could ensue. (13) Therapies used with varying degrees of success include immobilization; vitamin B; antibiotics; radiation; diathermy; and injections of cortisone, local anesthetic, and other anti-inflammatory drugs. (9) Laboratory investigations are generally unrewarding, except in the acute phase, when the ESR may be elevated.

Pathologic Features

The exact cause, pathogenesis, and morphologic changes are poorly understood. (6,12) The most prominent theory relates to localized venous stasis creating intraosseous venous engorgement and thus promoting the localized osteoporosis. (5,12) Similarities to Sudeck's atrophy have been speculated. (8,14) Others implicate an isolated inflammatory condition, especially when present in athletes, whereas a low-grade infection as the primary cause is usually suspected after pelvic surgery. (1,15) Biopsy-proven acute and chronic inflammatory changes of the pubic symphysis have been associated with cultured bacteria. When an infective agent is isolated, the most common organisms are Gram-negative bacilli, especially *Pseudomonas aeruginosa* and *Escherichia coli*. (3,16)

Radiologic Features

There is a radiographic latent period after the onset of symptoms of 1–3 weeks; however, some patients will never manifest definitive radiologic changes. (3,6,12) When present, the findings may simulate joint infection. (7)

The most characteristic radiographic appearance is a bilateral and usually symmetric involvement of the pubic bone and adjacent rami. (Fig. 10-202; Table 10-65) Irregularity of the joint margin, subchondral sclerosis, and a moth-eaten type of osteoporosis, with widening of the joint space, can be striking. (6,12,16) (Fig. 10-203) With resolution, there is reconstitution of normal

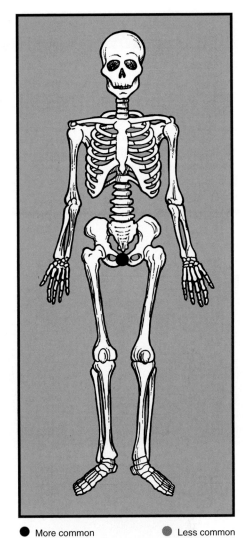

● More common   ● Less common

Figure 10-202 SKELETAL DISTRIBUTION OF OSTEITIS PUBIS.

Table 10-65	Radiologic Features of Osteitis Pubis

Acute
   Bilateral, symmetric abnormalities
   Hazy joint margin
   Osteoporosis
   Sclerosis
   Widened joint space
Sequelae
   Ankylosis
   Joint surface irregularity
   Residual instability

bone density, but the joint margin frequently remains irregular and may even be ankylosed. (6) Residual instability at the articulation with offset of the opposing pubic bones is often visible and may be an indication for surgical fusion if pain and instability persists. (5,17)

CAPSULE SUMMARY   Osteitis Pubis

General Considerations

- An uncommon non-suppurative inflammation of the symphysis pubis following pelvic surgery or childbirth, particularly when complicated by infection.

Clinical Features

- Previous history of childbirth, pelvic surgery, or trauma, with pain and restricted motion.
- Requires drug therapy for inflammation and may require arthrodesis if conservative measures fail.

Pathologic Features

- Controversial but most likely owing to intraosseous venous engorgement.
- Occasionally the result of bacterial infection.

Radiologic Features

- Joint surfaces show erosions, subchondral sclerosis, moth-eaten localized osteoporosis, and widening of the joint space.
- Looks identical to infection.
- Sequelae include joint irregularity, instability, and ankylosis.

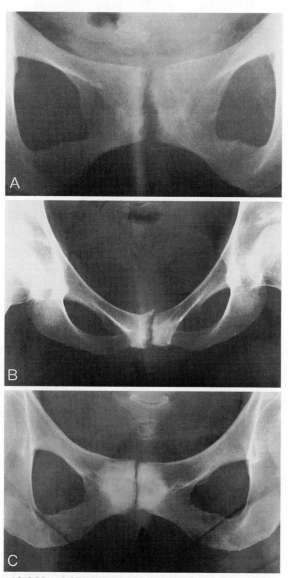

Figure 10-203   OSTEITIS PUBIS. A. Erosive Stage. Note the erosions and irregularity of the joint margin. **B and C. Sclerotic Stage.** Observe the sclerosis and instability, which occur in later progression, in these other two patients. (Courtesy of Donald M. Kuppe, DC, Denver, Colorado.)

HYPERTROPHIC OSTEOARTHROPATHY

Hypertrophic osteoarthropathy (HOA) was first described independently by Marie and Bamberger in the late nineteenth century. (1) The disease is composed of a triad of digital clubbing, symmetric arthritis, and periostitis, occurring as a sequel to a major visceral disorder, usually intrathoracic in location. Evidence suggests that the formation of peripheral symptomatology is intimately related to abnormal neurovascular reflexes, especially of the vagus nerve. (2,3)

Clinical Features

Clinical manifestations of hypertrophic osteoarthropathy are often non-specific and may simulate various rheumatologic diseases, especially rheumatoid arthritis. There is a male predominance of the condition, and it is most frequently encountered in the 4th–6th decades. (1) Signs of the disease develop gradually and may take up to 20 years to completely evolve. (4) The classic triad of findings includes digital clubbing, arthritis, and periostitis. (5) The complete triad is not necessarily present in each and every case. The most common cause of hypertrophic osteoarthropathy is bronchogenic carcinoma, although other causes have been documented. (1,6–9) (Table 10-66) Up to 10% of all bronchogenic carcinomas will produce the classic triad. (10)

Digital clubbing is identified as a bulbous enlargement of the distal fingertips owing to soft tissue thickening. Other signs include an increased curvature of the nail contour. Clubbing is a physical manifestation seen in association with thoracic and abdominal disease, as well as in heroin addicts. (11) Only in rare cases will clubbing of the digits not be associated with hypertrophic osteoarthropathy. (12) Arthritis is objectively verified as a synovitis with effusion, warmth, and redness, most commonly seen in the knees, ankles, elbows, wrists, and proximal fingers. Periostitis is suggested clinically by vague diffuse pain along the diaphyses of long bones, especially of the leg and forearm. (Fig. 10-204)

All of these findings may precede manifestations of the primary causative disease. Careful evaluation of the chest should be performed in any patient suspected of having this disorder.

Table 10-66	Causes of Hypertrophic Osteoarthropathy

Thoracic
  Neoplasms
    Bronchogenic carcinoma (most common)
    Hodgkin's disease
    Metastasis
    Mesothelioma
    Esophageal carcinoma
  Obstructions
    Cystic fibrosis
    Bronchiectasis
    Emphysema
  Infections
    Abscess
  Cardiac
    Cyanotic heart disease
Extrathoracic
  Abdominal
  Heroin addicts
  Liver cirrhosis
  Regional enteritis
  Ulcerative colitis

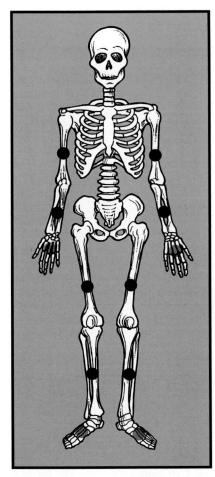

● More common   ● Less common

Figure 10-204   **SKELETAL DISTRIBUTION OF HYPERTROPHIC OSTEOARTHROPATHY.**

Laboratory investigations depend on cause, but generally the ESR will be elevated.

Symptoms of hypertrophic osteoarthropathy secondary to an intrathoracic abnormality rapidly regress after removal of the primary lung lesion with vagal resection and occasionally just with thoracotomy. (3,13) The radiographic features resolve more slowly over a number of months, but their persistence does not indicate surgical failure. (14)

Pathologic Features

Examination of the sites of periosteal response reveal round cell infiltration in the outer fibrous layer followed by cambium new bone proliferations. Adjacent to the cortex is coarse fibrous tissue, which may be seen radiographically as a linear interspaced radiolucency. (15) Later this lucency may be obliterated, creating an overall thickened cortex. (7) Clubbed digits show dilated vessels and neovascularity, as well as thickening of collagen and cellular infiltration. (7) Capillary blood flow studies in acquired clubbed digits have shown increased circulation that appears to be responsible for tissue hypertrophy and hyperplasia. (16)

The exact pathogenesis of the condition is unknown. Notably, the periosteal new bone formation does not represent a metastatic manifestation; however, two theories have been proposed to result in the increased peripheral blood flow: humoral and neurogenic. The less accepted humoral theory proposes that the production of an unidentified substance from the visceral abnormality results in increased peripheral blood flow. The neurogenic theory is more formally accepted, based on the reports of regression of the triad following vagotomy or removal of the neoplasm. (3,13) Afferent neural impulses from the abnormal viscus are thought to result in vagal efferent reflex vasodilation at the periphery, leading to stimulation of periosteal new bone formation. (2,9)

Radiologic Features

Bone. The most apparent and consistent radiographic sign is periostitis. (Figs. 10-205 and 10-206; Table 10-67) This is seen radiographically as a solid or single lamination of new bone adjacent to the bone cortex. The outer surface of this new bone formation is often undulating and is initially separated from the underlying bone by a radiolucent layer. Later, this lucent zone is obliterated as the periosteal new bone eventually merges into the adjacent cortical bone. Characteristically, periosteal new bone is limited to the metaphyses and diaphyses of long bones and is invariably bilateral and symmetric. The changes are more apparent distal to the knees and elbows and most pronounced in the lower extremities. (17)

The most common bones involved, in order of frequency, are the tibia and fibula, radius and ulna, metacarpals and metatarsals, and femur and humerus. Radionuclide uptake studies are highly sensitive in the detection of periostitis and show the increased diaphyseal periosteal uptake as the *double stripe sign* as the two opposing cortices are highlighted. (17)

Joints. The only radiographic sign that may be apparent is that of joint effusion. There is no specific sign of joint disease.

Soft Tissue. Digital clubbing may be visible as a bulbous enlargement of the distal fingertips. Radiographs of the chest may isolate the pulmonary mass or abnormality.

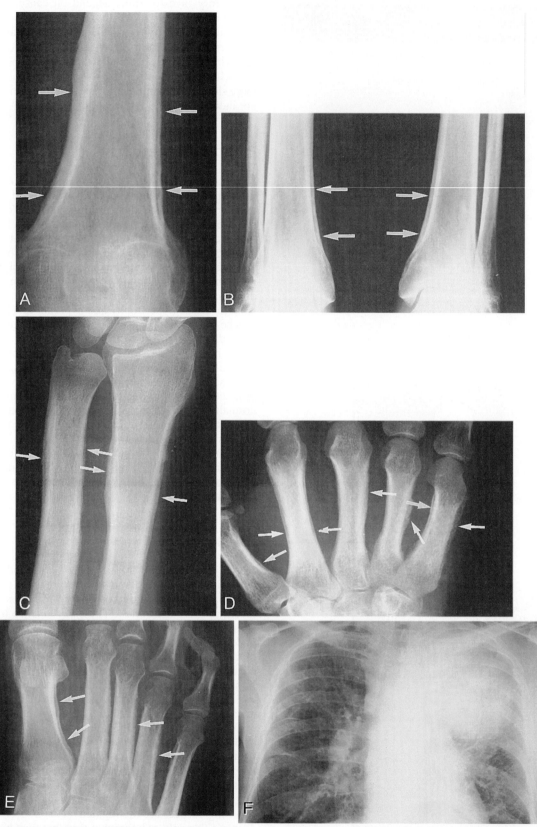

Figure 10-205   **HYPERTROPHIC OSTEOARTHROPATHY SECONDARY TO BRONCHOGENIC CARCINOMA. A. Distal Femur. B. Distal Tibia and Fibula. C. Distal Radius and Ulna. D. Metacarpals. E. Metatarsals.** Manifestations of periostitis can be identified as a single lamination of new bone con- fined to the diaphysis and metadiaphysis (*arrows*). **F. Bronchogenic Carcinoma.** Observe the large left upper lobe neoplasm, which caused the changes of hypertrophic osteoarthropathy in this patient.

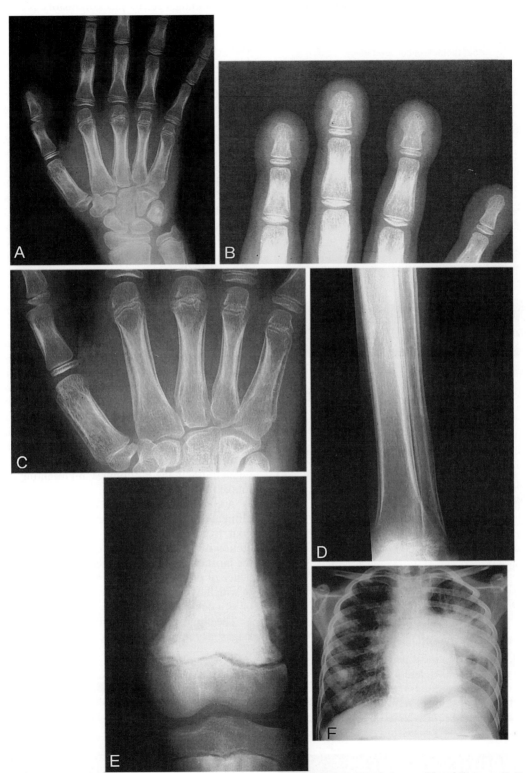

Figure 10-206   **HYPERTROPHIC OSTEOARTHROPATHY SECONDARY TO METASTATIC OSTEOSARCOMA. A. PA Hand. B. Close-Up of Fingertips.** Observe the bulbous soft tissues of the fingertips (*digital clubbing*). **C. Close-Up of Metacarpal Periostitis. D. Tibia and Fibula Periostitis.**

E. Primary Osteosarcoma: Distal Femur. F. Pulmonary Metastases. *COMMENT:* The periostitis is secondary to the pulmonary metastases, creating a reflex disturbance in peripheral blood flow. (Courtesy of Bryan Hartley, MD, Melbourne, Australia.)

Table 10-67	Radiologic Features of Hypertrophic Osteoarthropathy

Bone
    Long-bone periostitis
        Tibia/fibula, radius/ulna, metacarpals/metatarsals
        Bilateral and symmetric
        Diaphyseal and metaphyseal
        Solid or thin laminated periosteal new bone
        Normal bone structure
Joints
    Peripheral joint swelling
        Knees, ankles, elbows, wrists, fingers
        Intra-articular effusion
        Normal joint spaces
Soft tissue
    Digits
        Clubbing of fingertips
    Chest
        Mass
        Interstitial disease

CAPSULE SUMMARY
Hypertrophic Osteoarthropathy

General Considerations

- Triad of peripheral arthritis, digital clubbing, and long-bone periostitis secondary to a thoracic or abdominal abnormality.
- The most common cause is bronchogenic carcinoma.
- Synonyms include Marie-Bamberger syndrome and hypertrophic pulmonary osteoarthropathy.

Clinical Features

- Most common in males in the 4th–6th decades.
- Triad of clubbing, arthritis, and periostitis diagnostic.
- Findings of lung carcinoma—cough, hematemesis, etc.
- Laboratory studies reveal elevated ESR only.

Pathologic Features

- Pathophysiology uncertain but related to neurovascular disturbance involving the vagus nerve with resultant increase in peripheral blood flow.

Radiologic Features

- *Bone:* bilateral, symmetric, linear periostitis; most common in the tibia, fibula, radius, and ulna.
- *Joints:* effusion.
- *Soft tissue:* clubbing, chest abnormality.

METABOLIC DISORDERS

GOUT

Gout is a common arthritide and (1) has been known throughout history, often afflicting famous and influential people who sub-sequently have become favorite subjects of caricature and satire. (2–4) Gout is often seen as a symbol of retribution of excessive human indulgence. Its place in history is a long and fascinating one, encompassing the use of many medicines and virtually all of the healing arts. (5) The disease is varied in cause and is manifested by hyperuricemia in combination with a characteristic acute inflammatory arthritis that tends to be recurrent. (6) The arthritis is induced by intra-articular deposits of sodium monourate. Some patients develop aggregations of these crystals (*tophi*), which may lead to a destructive and deforming arthropathy.

The term *gout,* derived from the Latin word *gutta* ("a drop"), reflected the Hippocratic belief that the disease was caused by a poison falling drop by drop into the joint. (7) The term *podagra* was used to describe the predilection to involvement of the foot (Greek: *pous,* "foot"; *agra,* "attack"); *tophus* (Greek: "chalk stone") described the chalky, white deposits of urate found in articular and periarticular tissues. The most common manifestations are predominantly musculoskeletal in nature, especially affecting the feet. The spine, although often clinically involved, shows radiographic changes only in advanced, long-standing disease. (8,9)

Clinical Features

Onset of the disease is usually in a male patient > 40 years of age with peaks in the 4th and 5th decades. (10) Males suffer from this disease approximately 20 times more commonly than women; however, postmenopausal women using diuretics show a significantly higher incidence. (11,12) A family history for gout is frequent, especially in females. (12,13) Certain racial predilections have been demonstrated, particularly in Polynesian and New Zealand natives. (14,15) Filipinos living in the United States have significantly higher mean serum levels of uric acid than when living in the Philippines, highlighting the effects of dietary intake. (16,17)

A classification based on cause has traditionally been used in clinical descriptions: primary and secondary. (6,18) In primary gout, hyperuricemia is owing to an overproduction or lack of excretion of uric acid because of an inborn enzymatic defect and is the most common type. A recent study revealed a rise in the incidence of primary gout. (19) Secondary gout refers to those cases in which hyperuricemia develops in the course of another disease or as a consequence of drug action. (Table 10-68)

The clinical manifestations of gout have been divided into four stages: asymptomatic, acute, polyarticular, and chronic. (20)

Table 10-68	Secondary Causes of Gout
Blood dyscrasia	Leukemia, hemolytic anemia, multiple myeloma, pernicious anemia, lymphoma
Drugs	Salicylates, diuretics
Endocrine	Thyroid and parathyroid disease, calcium imbalance, diabetes mellitus and insipidus
Heart and kidney disease	Myocardial infarction, hypertension, chronic renal disease
Hereditary diseases	Down's syndrome, glycogen storage
Miscellaneous	Obesity, starvation, psoriasis, sprue, lead poisoning

Asymptomatic Hyperuricemia

In many individuals, despite hyperuricemia, no signs or symptoms of articular gout develop. These individuals generally do not require any treatment; however, they should be questioned as to atherosclerotic risk factors as well as their familial predisposition to renal calculi and acute gouty arthritis. (21,22)

Acute Gouty Arthritis

The onset is characterized by acute inflammatory monoarticular or oligoarticular arthritis, usually in the early hours of the morning. The most common sites of involvement are in the lower extremity, especially at the first metatarsophalangeal and intertarsal joints, and knees. (Fig. 10-207) Up to 60% of the initial attacks will occur at the first metatarsophalangeal joint. (23)

Distinctively, the affected joint is swollen and hot, but dry, in contrast to other arthritides, which are usually moist. Rapid recovery within days of the attack is the rule, but recurrence may occur within a short period. A proportion of individuals will remain asymptomatic for many years. Renal uric acid calculi are encountered with increasing frequency after the onset of articular attacks. (24)

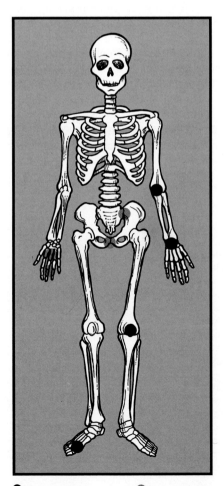

● More common ● Less common

Figure 10-207 **SKELETAL DISTRIBUTION OF GOUT.**

Polyarticular Gouty Arthritis

Patients who experience multiple attacks of acute gouty arthritis are predisposed to involvement of more than one joint simultaneously, especially in the lower extremity. It is at this stage that radiographic changes are most frequently first encountered. In addition, the small joints of the hand, wrist, and elbow may be affected. In instances of prolonged disease, inflammatory articular changes may be seen in the hip, spine, and sacroiliac joints.

Chronic Tophaceous Gout

Once a common and expected sequel to long-standing gout, the localized accumulations of sodium monourate (*tophi*) are now an unusual feature, largely owing to the advent of long-term drug therapy. (25–27) The onset of tophaceous deposits follows numerous attacks over many years, with an average duration of 10–12 years. (24) Tophi characteristically have a predilection for relatively avascular tissues, including tendons and subcutaneous layers of the elbow, forearm, hand, knee, foot, helix of the ear, synovium, periarticular soft tissues, and subchondral bone. (24,28) Tophi close to the skin surface may ulcerate and extrude their contents to the exterior. The effects on bones and joints are often severely destructive and deforming and may require surgery (29). Rarely, tophi may deposit within the spinal canal and act as a space-occupying mass, resulting in various neurological complications. (30) Other complications of gout include renal damage, renal stones, hypertension, atherosclerosis, and thrombophlebitis. (31,32)

Laboratory evaluations in gout are especially helpful in the acute arthritis stage. Elevation of ESR, serum uric acid > 6 mg %, and a moderate leukocytosis are to be expected. (6,33) Occasionally, low-grade proteinuria may occur. The demonstration of sodium monourate crystals in the synovial fluid is diagnostic (34), as is the dramatic symptomatic remission within 48 hr of administration of colchicine. (26,35)

Management of gout focuses on reducing levels of serum uric acid. In the acute phase, NSAIDs, colchicine, ACTH, and phenylbutazone are used. (26,36,37) Regional ice application has been shown to be of benefit to aid in pain management. (38) Oral steroids are notably ineffective. Alcohol, aspirin, diuretics, and low-calorie diets should be avoided as they promote urate retention in the kidney. (26,36) In long-term management, the administration of drugs that promote uric acid excretion (uricosuric drugs) prevents tophaceous deposits and their deforming sequelae. Additionally, increased fluid intake, weight reduction, urine alkalization, reduced purine intake, and avoidance of salicylates will assist in maintaining normal uric acid concentrations. (26,36)

Lesch-Nyhan Syndrome

A rare hereditary clinical syndrome, Lesch-Nyhan syndrome, associated with hyperuricemia, mental retardation, and abnormal self-destructive aggressive behavior has been recognized. (39,40)

Pathologic Features

The inciting inflammatory agent is the crystal of sodium monourate. (34) Hyperuricemia is the necessary precursor to the deposition of these crystals. Uric acid is derived predominantly from the breakdown of the purine nucleic acids adenine and guanine. (26) (Fig. 10-208) Dietary sources of purine also contribute, but to a lesser extent. (6) In the biochemical cascade from purine to uric acid the enzyme xanthine oxidase is crucial and is the specific site for inhibition by the commonly used drug Allopurinol (xyloprim). (27) Chronic lead intoxication impairs uric acid clearance in the kidney and can also precipitate gout (*saturnine gout*). Aspirin, diuretics, alcohol, and nicotinic acid also reduce uric acid excretion. (6)

In the presence of uric acid crystals, the body tissues demonstrate acute inflammatory changes. (35) The anatomic sites of deposition are the synovium, cartilage, joint capsule, periarticular tissues, and subchondral bone. (31) Initially, these deposits are usually microscopic, but with time will become macroscopically apparent. The marked predilection of acute gout for peripheral joints may partially relate to their lower temperature, especially the great toe, which decreases uric acid solubility and promotes tissue deposition. (6) Other mechanisms that may be active include levels of tissue proteoglycan turnover, microtrauma, and serum globulin abnormalities. (41) The immediate effect on the joint is to cause an initial acute synovitis.

In recurrent attacks, as chronicity predominates, synovial hyperplasia and pannus formation occur, with subsequent degradation of articular cartilage and the appearance of marginal erosions. (24) Cartilage additionally is degraded by the action of urate crystal depositions in its superficial layers.

Foci of urate crystal deposition are also apparent within the subchondral bone (intraosseous tophi) and periarticular soft tissues. In the subchondral bone, trabeculae are resorbed owing to pressure from the enlarging intraosseous tophus and may predispose the patient to collapse of the subchondral bone. Periarticular tissues such as bursae, tendon sheaths, ligaments, and subcutaneous elements may be additional sites for tophi to develop.

The histopathology of a tophus consists of layers of urate crystals within a mineralized crystalline matrix. Surrounding the tophus is a low-grade granulomatous reaction within the host tissue. (24) A long-standing tophus may develop calcification or ossification usually at its periphery.

Radiologic Features

Distinctively, radiographic findings lag behind clinical manifestations with a latent period of 5–10 years. (42) However, when present, they are frequently quite specific. (23) (Table 10-69)

General Features

Soft Tissue Changes. In acute attacks evidence of joint effusion may be visible; however, the most important and readily identifiable finding is the presence of tophi. Tophi are manifested as a localized increase in soft tissue density from 5 mm up to as large as 5 cm in size. Distinctively, they are eccentric; are usually, but not always, periarticular; and occur in predictable locations such as the forearm, elbow, dorsum of the hand, knee, ankle, and forefoot. (23) Occasionally, peripheral calcification within the tophus may be apparent. (Fig. 10-209)

Joint Space. A distinctive and consistent finding is the preservation of the articular space despite co-existent soft tissue and bony changes. Later in the disease a uniform loss of joint space may be seen as the entire joint cartilage diminishes in thickness. Contrary to rheumatoid or psoriatic arthritis, bony ankylosis is an infrequent consequence. (23,43)

Bone Erosions. Three types of bone erosions are encountered: marginal, periarticular, and intraosseous. (Fig. 10-210)

Marginal. Owing to synovial pannus within the joint acting on the exposed bare area, intra-articular loss of the cortex and underlying bone up to 2–3 mm in size may be apparent. These may further enlarge and spread to involve the central articular region.

Periarticular. Distant to the joint capsule, extrinsic pressure erosions of bone are often visible, especially in the presence of a soft tissue tophus. Characteristically, these types of erosions

Table 10-69	General Radiologic Features of Gout
Avascular necrosis	
Medullary infarcts	
Femoral and humeral heads	
Bone density	
Normal	
Bone erosions	
Marginal	
Periarticular (overhanging margin sign)	
Intraosseous	
Chondrocalcinosis	
Uncommon	
Wrist (triangular cartilage)	
Knee (menisci)	
Symphysis pubis	
Joint space	
Usually normal	
Uniform loss late	
Periosteal new bone	
Uncommon	
Solid pattern	
Secondary degenerative joint changes	
Subchondral sclerosis	
Osteophytes	
Misalignment	
Soft tissue	
Effusion	
Tophi (occasionally calcify)	

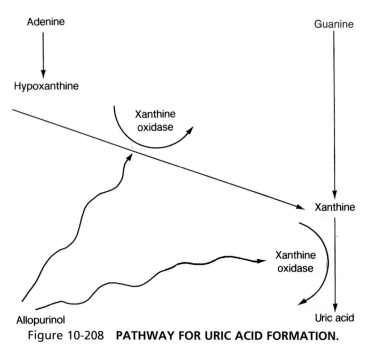

Figure 10-208 **PATHWAY FOR URIC ACID FORMATION.**

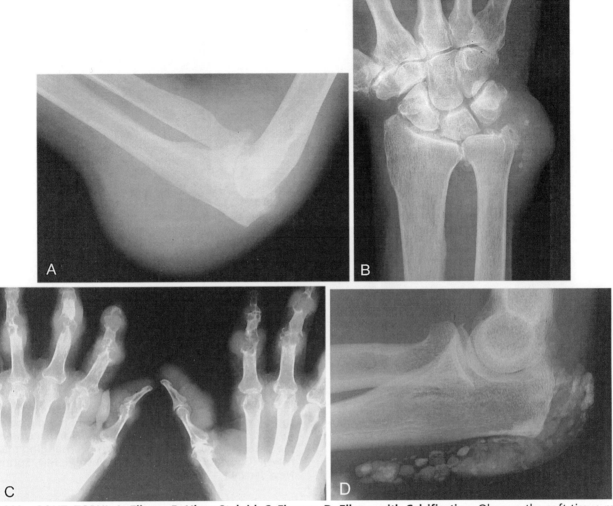

Figure 10-209   **GOUT: TOPHI. A. Elbow. B. Ulnar Styloid. C. Fingers. D. Elbow with Calcification.** Observe the soft tissue masses.

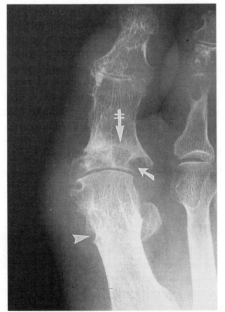

Figure 10-210   **GOUT: BONE EROSIONS. PA Foot.** Observe the marginal erosion, demonstrating a classic overhanging margin sign (*arrow*), periarticular erosion (*arrowhead*), and intraosseous erosion (*crossed arrow*).

occur within the metaphysis or diaphysis; are eccentric; have a dense, sclerotic margin; and often have a protruding lip of bone extending away from the bone into the soft tissues (*overhanging margin sign*). (44) (Fig. 10-211) Occasionally, extension of a marginal erosion may have this overhanging edge of bone at its periphery.

Intraosseous. Accumulations of tophi within bone will be visible as well-circumscribed, oval, or round punched out radiolucencies usually within the medullary cavity. (23) The most common location for these lesions to occur is in the subchondral bone adjacent to the involved joint. These may predispose the patient to collapse of the articular cortex. (42)

Bone Density. Osteoporosis either localized or generalized is notably unusual. Mild rarefaction of subchondral bone may be visible in acute articular attacks.

Periosteal New Bone. Linear periosteal new bone may sometimes appear to have thickened the cortex and reduced the metaphyseal–diaphyseal constricted contour.

Secondary Degenerative Joint Changes. Subchondral sclerosis, osteophytes, and articular misalignment are common and complicate the radiographic picture.

Chondrocalcinosis. Calcification within the triangular cartilage of the wrist, menisci of the knee, and symphysis pubis is observed in up to 5% of gout patients. (42,45,46)

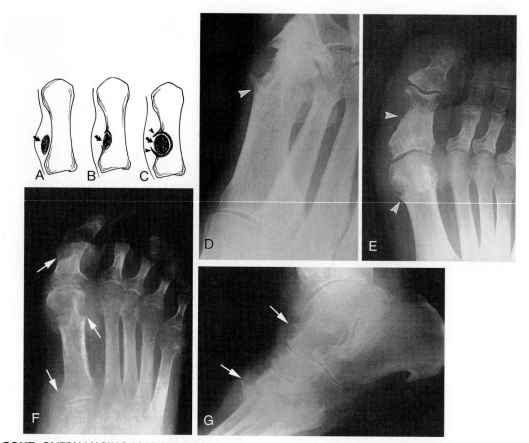

Figure 10-211   GOUT: OVERHANGING MARGIN SIGN.
A–C. Diagram: Pathogenesis. A tophus (*arrows*) may gradually erode an adjacent bone, producing a protruding lip of
bone (*arrowheads*). **D. Metatarsal Head.** Observe the sharp,
excavated defect flanked by a distinctive bony projection,
referred to as the overhanging margin sign (*arrowhead*).

E. Great Toe. Note that two sites of erosion from adjacent
tophi can be seen with an overhanging margin peripherally
(*arrowheads*). **F and G. Great Toe and Tarsus.** Observe multiple defects in multiple bones, with overhanging margins (*arrows*). (Courtesy of Steven P. Brownstein, MD, Springfield,
New Jersey.)

Avascular Necrosis. Medullary infarcts and epiphyseal necrosis of the femoral and humeral heads are infrequently associated
abnormalities. (47–49)

Target Sites of Involvement

There is a definite predilection for the lower extremity, especially
the foot, to be targeted. (50) In addition, the hands and wrists may
show radiographic abnormalities. The spine, sacroiliac, and hip
joints are rarely involved.

Foot. The most distinctive location for gouty articular changes is
the first metatarsophalangeal joint. (51) (Figs. 10-210 and 10-211;
Table 10-70) At this site the earliest changes are erosions of the
metatarsal head, particularly of the medial and dorsal aspects.
Additional erosions may also be visible on the adjacent phalanx,
at other metatarsophalangeal joints (especially the fifth), and at
the first PIP joint. Only late in the disease will the joint space
show uniform diminution. (Fig. 10-212) Soft tissue tophi and
swelling are most prominent at these joints, as well as at the dorsum of the feet.

With MRI, gouty tophi characteristically reveal a low signal
intensity on both T1- and T2-weighted images. (Fig. 10-213) In
more advanced cases the appearance of periarticular erosions may

result in prominent overhanging margins adjacent to these tophi.
(44,52) Intraosseous tophi produce discrete, well-circumscribed,
punched out, lytic defects that may coalesce and destroy the bone
and joint. (23,52) Distinctively, there is a lack of osteoporosis
except in the acute phase.

Hand. Asymmetric joint involvement of any articulation may
be seen in the hand. Erosions, soft tissue swelling, and misalignments are the main features. (Fig. 10-214) At the wrist, erosions of the carpus may lead to the *spotty carpal sign* which is
also seen in rheumatoid arthritis and tuberculosis. Similarly, the
ulnar styloid may show erosion. Notably, bone density is normal
and ulnar drift of the digits is lacking. Tophi have been known
to be a cause of carpal tunnel syndrome when gout affects the
wrist. (53)

Table 10-70	Radiologic Features of Gout at the Great Toe
Soft tissue swelling	
Marginal erosions—medial, dorsal surface metatarsal head	
Periarticular erosions—head, shaft (overhanging margin)	
Hallux valgus	
Normal joint space	
Normal mineralization	

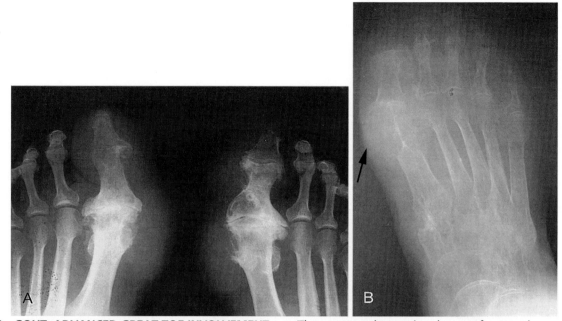

Figure 10-212 **GOUT: ADVANCED GREAT TOE INVOLVEMENT.**
A. Bilateral Joint Disease. Note the severe erosive changes,
loss of joint space, and large tophi. **B. Severe Tophaceous
Destruction.** Note that at the first metatarsal head there is significant destruction from adjacent tophi (*arrow*). *COMMENT:*

These severe destructive changes from tophaceous gout are
less commonly encountered in recent times owing to the use
of prophylactic uricosuric agents. (Panel A courtesy of Bryan
Hartley, MD, Melbourne, Australia.)

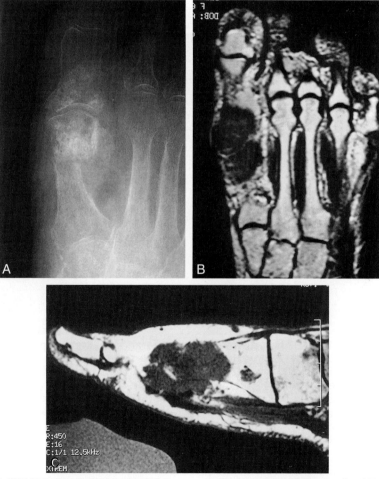

Figure 10-213 **GOUT OF THE GREAT TOE: SIGNAL CHARAC-
TERISTICS. A. PA Foot.** Observe the soft tissue swelling in a
juxta-articular position about the great toe. The tophi have
calcified with juxta-articular erosions and relative preservation of the joint space. This is the characteristic plain film
finding of gouty arthritis. **B. T1-Weighted MRI, Coronal Foot.**

C. T1-Weighted MRI, Sagittal Foot. Note the low signal intensity in the area of the tophi erosion of the bony structures,
which correlates with the plain film findings. The signal intensity in gouty tophi is low on T1- and T2-weighted images.
(Courtesy of Garin M. Tomaszewski, MD, Department of
Radiology, University Hospital, Denver, Colorado.)

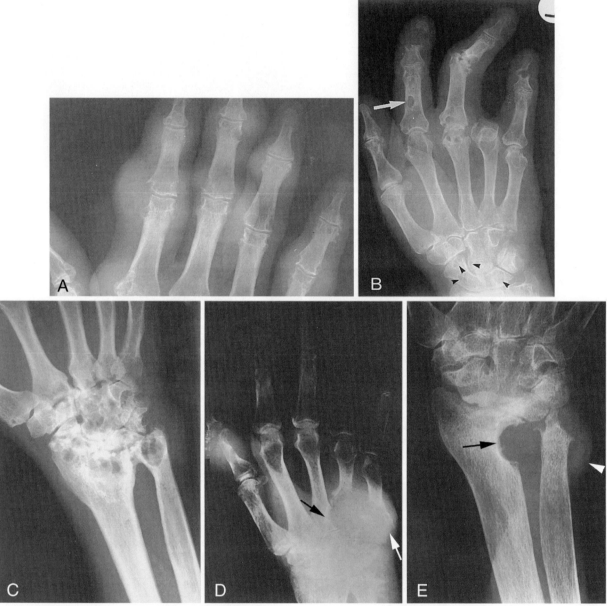

Figure 10-214 **GOUT: HAND AND WRIST. A. Fingers.** Note the large tophi and erosive changes. **B. Hand.** Observe the multiple areas of bone destruction owing to the presence of tophi. A large intraosseous tophus is seen in the second digit (*arrow*). Numerous erosions are also visible in the carpal bones, creating the spotty carpal sign (*arrowheads*). The fourth digit was surgically removed. **C. Spotty Carpal Sign.** Note that multiple carpal erosions have resulted in this appearance. **D. Metacarpal Destruction.** Observe that at the base of the metacarpals extensive bony destruction has occurred from adjacent tophi (*arrows*). **E. Radioulnar Erosion.** Note the large erosive excavations at the distal radius and ulna (*arrow*). The outline of the adjacent tophus can be seen (*arrowhead*). (Courtesy of Scott A. Sole, DC, Denver, Colorado.)

Others

Knee. Erosions are seen at the medial and lateral condyles. Tophi may be visible in the prepatellar region (*pseudo-tumor of gout*). Erosion of the superolateral pole of the patella in the presence of a soft tissue mass, which often contains calcium, is a strong diagnostic sign of gout. (54)

Elbow. Erosions of the olecranon and adjacent ulna are frequent and usually are co-existent with soft tissue swelling of the adjacent forearm. (Fig. 10-215) Tophaceous involvement of the olecranon bursa leads to a prominent mass that, on a lateral view, has been called the *rising sun sign.* (52) (Fig. 10-209A)

Sacroiliac. In approximately 15% of individuals the sacroiliac joint will be affected, as evidenced by articular erosions and adjacent sclerosis. (8,55,56) (Fig. 10-216) There appears to be a predominance of bilateral but asymmetric sacroiliac disease although unilateral sacroiliac involvement does occur. (57) A rare pathologic fracture through an intraosseous tophus in the pubic rami has been reported. (16)

Spine. Specific radiographic abnormalities are exceptional, though 75% of patients with gout report back pain. (58) The most-recorded radiologic signs have been made in the cervical spine, such as odontoid erosions, atlantoaxial and subaxial instability, and endplate erosions. (9,30,31) However, endplate erosions and posterior apophyseal degeneration in the lumbar spine have been demonstrated. (16,59,60) Osteophytes and annulus calcification have been associated with spinal gout, but are not specific roentgen signs. (8,16,23,58) Epidural tophi have been documented to precipitate compression myelopathy, leading to paresis most commonly of the thoracic and lumbar spines. (61–63) MRI may be a useful modality when assessing for spinal tophaceous gout. Periarticular deposits of tophi characteristically reveal a low signal intensity on all MRI sequences. (64) Gouty arthritis of the spine will usually benefit from surgical decompression and appropriate pharmaceutical therapy. (61,65)

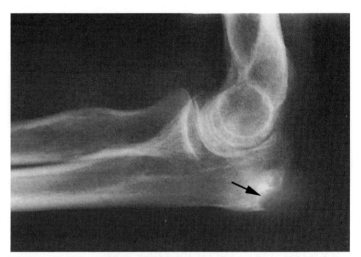

Figure 10-215 **GOUT: ELBOW.** Note the tophus within the olecranon bursa, which has created an extrinsic erosion of the olecranon process (*arrow*).

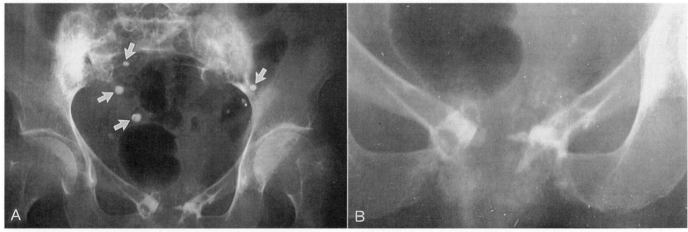

Figure 10-216 **GOUT: SACROILIAC AND PUBIC ARTICULATIONS. A and B.** Observe the severe erosive and destructive changes at both sacroiliac and pubic articulations. Of incidental note is the radiopaque contrast material present in colonic diverticulae (*arrows*). (Courtesy of Paul E. Siebert, MD, Denver, Colorado.)

CAPSULE SUMMARY   Gout

General Considerations

- Disorder of purine metabolism in which hyperuricemia leads to deposition of sodium monourate crystals into cartilage, synovium, periarticular, and subcutaneous tissues.
- These crystals evoke a strong inflammatory arthritis usually in the lower extremity.

Clinical Features

- Affects males 20:1, usually in the 4th and 5th decades.
- May be primary or less commonly secondary.
- *Four stages apparent:* asymptomatic hyperuricemia, acute gouty arthritis (especially at the first metatarsophalangeal joint), polyarticular gouty arthritis (chronic, long-standing disease), and chronic tophaceous gout (soft tissue accumulations of sodium monourate).
- Laboratory studies show elevated ESR, leukocytosis, and hyperuricemia.

Pathologic Features

- Accumulation of these crystals (tophi) results in synovial pannus, bony marginal erosions, cartilage degradation, and bone destruction.

Radiologic Features

- General features include dense soft tissue tophi, preservation of joint space, bone erosions (marginal, periarticular overhanging margin sign, intraosseous) normal bone density, periosteal new bone, secondary degenerative joint changes, chondrocalcinosis, and avascular necrosis.
- The most frequently targeted areas of involvement are the first metatarsophalangeal joint, other metatarsophalangeal joints, the hands, and wrists.
- Spine and sacroiliac articulations show infrequent erosions. Occasional epidural tophi occur leading to compression myelopathy.

CALCIUM PYROPHOSPHATE DIHYDRATE CRYSTAL DEPOSITION DISEASE

Calcium pyrophosphate dihydrate (CPPD) crystal deposition disease is an articular disease characterized by the production of gout-like symptoms (*pseudo-gout*) in the presence of these crystals. (1,2) A common radiologic association, though not specific, is chondrocalcinosis, which may precipitate premature and often advanced DJD (*pyrophosphate arthropathy*). Involvement of the spine is limited to degenerative changes, especially in the lumbar segments, but peripherally it may be severe enough to simulate neurotrophic joint disease.

Clinical Features

A number of different clinical presentations may occur in an individual with CPPD crystal deposition disease that may simulate a number of arthropathies, including gout, rheumatoid arthritis, degenerative joint disease, and even neurotrophic arthropathy. (3,4) (Table 10-71) Onset is usually after 30 years of age, with a peak at 60 years. (2) The most common form of presentation is similar to DJD, with chronic progressive joint pain, intermittent swelling, reduced range of motion, and crepitus. Acute attacks may intersperse an otherwise chronic course and may occur after acute immobility. (5,6) CPPD crystal deposition disease involves predominantly the peripheral joints, especially the knees, wrists, hands, ankles, hips, and elbows, in approximate order of decreasing frequency. (2) (Fig. 10-217) Rare cases have been reported of calcium pyrophosphate crystal deposition affecting the atlanto-axial joint and the periodontal area. (7,8) Involvement of this space with CPPD crystal deposition disease is often termed the *crowned dens syndrome* and may precipitate cervical cord compression. (9) Reports have also been made of temporomandibular joint involvement. (10) In the wrist it may be associated with carpal tunnel syndrome. (11) Occasionally, pain and reduced mobility may be exhibited in the cervical and lumbar spine. (3,12)

A number of other diseases often have CPPD crystal deposition disease associated, including diabetes mellitus, degenerative joint disease, gout, hyperparathyroidism, hemochromatosis, Wilson's disease, neuroarthropathy, and ochronosis. In addition, there is a hereditary factor in Czechoslovakian, Chilean, and Dutch populations. (13)

Table 10-71	Patterns of Clinical Presentation of CPPD Crystal Deposition Disease	
Pattern	Incidence (%)	Manifestations
Type A: Pseudo-gout	10–20	Acute or subacute, self-limited, knee, hip, shoulder, elbow, forefoot
Type B: Pseudo-rheumatoid	2–6	Continuous acute attacks of weeks to months, stiffness, fatigue, hypomobility, elevated ESR
Type C: Pseudo-osteoarthritis	35–60	Chronic and progressive, acute episodes, bilateral and symmetric, all peripheral joints, knee and elbow contractures
Type D: Pseudo-osteoarthritis	10–35	Chronic and progressive; no acute episodes
Type E: Asymptomatic	10–20	Chondrocalcinosis only
Type F: Pseudo-neuropathy	0–2	Relatively asymptomatic, unstable, destructive joint disease
Type G: Miscellaneous	0–1	Variable

Adapted from **Resnick D, Niwayama G, Georgen TG, et al.:** *Clinical, radiographic and pathologic abnormalities in calcium pyrophosphate dihydrate crystal deposition disease (CPPD). Pseudogout.* Radiology 122:1, 1977.
CPPD, calcium pyrophosphate dihydrate; *ESR,* erythrocyte sedimentation rate.

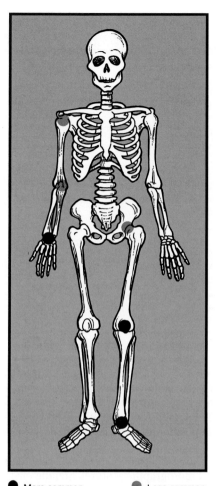

Figure 10-217 **SKELETAL DISTRIBUTION OF CALCIUM PYROPHOSPHATE DIHYDRATE CRYSTAL DEPOSITION DISEASE.**

● More common   ● Less common

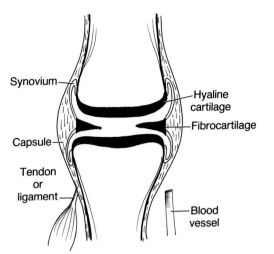

Figure 10-218 **POTENTIAL SITES OF CALCIFICATION IN CALCIUM PYROPHOSPHATE DIHYDRATE CRYSTAL DEPOSITION DISEASE.**

As a pathogenetic sequel to cartilage degeneration, structural articular alterations occur (*pyrophosphate arthropathy*). Essentially, these changes bear a striking resemblance to DJD and often approach the advanced destructive findings of neurotrophic joint disease. Morphologic changes include loss of and fibrillation of joint cartilage, thickened subchondral trabeculae, multiple subchondral cysts (*geodes*), intra-articular loose bodies, osteophytes, and often fragmentation, with collapse of the articular cortex. (Table 10-72)

Radiologic Features

The general and specific radiographic features of CPPD crystal deposition disease have been clearly delineated. (3) Generally, the two essential features are calcification within or around the joint and findings of pyrophosphate arthropathy. (Table 10-72)

Calcification

Cartilage (Chondrocalcinosis). Chondrocalcinosis is the most common and characteristic form of calcification, involving either hyaline or fibrocartilage. (19) Hyaline calcification is visible as a thin, linear, continuous or interrupted calcification

Laboratory evaluations other than the demonstration of pyrophosphate crystals in the synovial fluid are unrewarding. Serum levels of calcium, phosphorus, alkaline phosphatase, and uric acid are invariably within normal ranges. (1)

Pathologic Features

The mechanism of CPPD crystals depositing into cartilage, synovium, tendons, and ligaments is unknown. (14,15) (Fig. 10-218) Injection of the crystals into a normal joint of a human or animal produces an acute synovitis resembling the naturally occurring disease. Factors operative in precipitating tissue deposition are related to age, genetics, and the presence of co-existing disease, including diabetes, gout, and hyperparathyroidism. (16)

In cartilage, crystal deposition is found in both hyaline and fibrous types adjacent to chondrocytes. (14) The crystals are usually located in the intermediate layer of the cartilage and never on its surface. (17) Variable degrees of associated cartilage degeneration may be present. Within the synovium and synovial fluid CPPD crystals will be apparent, particularly by polarized light microscopy, and are usually found within phagocytes. (18) Tendinous deposits are most common in the Achilles, triceps, quadriceps, and supraspinatus tendons. The capsular ligament is also a common site of accumulations of CPPD crystals.

Table 10-72	Pathologic Radiologic Correlation in Pyrophosphate Arthropathy
Pathologic Features	**Radiologic Features**
Bone proliferation	Osteophytes
Calcification in cartilage, synovium, and periarticular structures	Linear intra-articular and extra-articular radiopacities
Cartilage degeneration	Loss of joint space
Fractured, collapsed articular surface	Articular cortex deformed and fragmented
Intra-articular debris	Loose bodies
Subchondral cysts	Geographic, subarticular lucencies
Trabecular thickening	Subchondral sclerosis

Table 10-73	Radiologic Patterns of Chondrocalcinosis	
Hyaline Cartilage	**Fibrocartilage**	
Locations		
Elbow	Acromio/sternoclavicular	
Glenohumeral	Annulus fibrosus	
Hip	Hip and shoulder labrum	
Knee	Knee menisci	
Wrist	Symphysis pubis	
	Wrist triangular cartilage	
Appearance		
Thin	Thick	
Linear	Irregular and shaggy	
Separated from cortex		
Parallel to joint cortex		

Table 10-74	Diseases Associated with Chondrocalcinosis (the 3 Cs)
Cartilage degeneration	
Degenerative joint disease	
Neurotrophic joint disease	
Acromegaly	
Cation disease	
Ca^{++}—hyperparathyroidism	
Fe^{++}—hemochromatosis	
Cu^{++}—Wilson's disease	
Crystal deposition	
CPPD—pseudo-gout, diabetes	
Sodium monourate—gout	
Homogentisic acid—ochronosis	
Others	
Idiopathic	
Paget's disease	
Systemic lupus erythematosus	
Osteochondritis dissecans	

Adapted from **Forrester DM, Brown JC, Nesson JW:** *The Radiology of Joint Disease,* ed 2. Philadelphia, WB Saunders, 1978.
CPPD, calcium pyrophosphate dihydrate.

separated from but parallel to the articular cortex. This is most commonly seen in the wrist, knee, elbow, hip, and shoulder. Fibrocartilage calcifications are thick, irregular, and have a shaggy, poorly defined margin. The most frequent locations include the knee menisci, triangular cartilage of the wrist, symphysis pubis, and annulus fibrosus. (3,20) (Table 10-73) Arthropathy is more common when chondrocalcinosis is present. (21) The phenomenon of chondrocalcinosis may be encountered in a number of other diseases and is not necessarily symptomatic. (4,12, 22–24) (Table 10-74) The high incidence in pseudo-gout of chondrocalcinosis at the wrist, knee, and pubic symphysis, where it approaches 100%, allows for a screening procedure of suspected individuals by performing collimated spot views of those articulations. (3,5)

Hemochromatosis. Hemochromatosis is a rare metabolic disorder, characterized by deposition of iron into all body tissues, which may result in severe bodily dysfunction involving the liver (cirrhosis), pancreas (diabetes), skin (brown discoloration) and the heart (cardiomyopathy). A diagnostic triad includes cirrhosis, diabetes, and a bronze colored skin (*bronze diabetes*).

The primary form is a genetic defect of gastrointestinal absorption; the secondary form arises from alcoholic cirrhosis, multiple transfusions, anemia, and overingestion. Men are most affected by a ratio of 20:1, manifesting between 40 and 60 years. Arthropathy is the result of deposition of iron and CPPD crystals into cartilage and synovium, especially of the second and third metacarpophalangeal joints of the hand, knees, hips, and shoulders.

Generalized radiographic features include osteopenia, chondrocalcinosis and periarticular calcifications. Radiographic evidence of arthropathy includes uniform diminished joint space, osteophytes (*beak* or *hook*), subchondral cysts, and sclerosis. (Fig. 10-219)

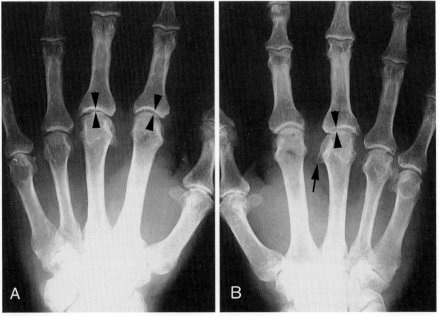

Figure 10-219   **HEMOCHROMATOSIS. A and B. Bilateral Hands.** Note the second and third metacarpals are the characteristic site for arthropathy to manifest (*arrowheads*). Key features include diminished joint space, osteophytes (beak or hook) (*arrow*), subchondral cysts, and sclerosis.

Wilson's disease. A rare, autosomal recessive, inherited disorder, Wilson's disease is characterized by the deposition of copper into the basal ganglia (*hepatolenticular degeneration*), liver (*cirrhosis*), and cornea (*Kayser-Fleischer ring*). Copper deposits into synovium and cartilage. Key signs of arthropathy include osteopenia, chondrocalcinosis, cysts, and irregular cortex, osteophytes, ossicles); in the spine, squaring of the vertebral bodies and Schmorl's nodes occur. (Fig. 10-220)

Synovial Calcification. Synovial calcifications are poorly defined calcifications at the joint margins.

Capsule Calcification. Capsule calcifications are also found at the joint margins. However, they are more linear and tend to bridge across the joint space.

Other Soft Tissue Calcification. Tendon and ligament calcifications are visible as thin linear calcifications extending away from the joint for a variable, but often considerable, distance. Vascular calcification is visible as two linear parallel lines and may relate to co-existent diabetes. Massive deposition may produce a localized soft tissue mass (*tumorous CPPD*) that is near a single joint, shows calcification, and is usually associated with adjacent extrinsic bone erosions. (25)

Pyrophosphate Arthropathy

Pyrophosphate arthropathy refers to the structural joint changes that occur as a sequel to the presence of CPPD crystals within a joint. The radiographic features are similar to degenerative joint disease (osteoarthritis), with loss of joint space, subchondral sclerosis, cyst formation, osteophytes, loose bodies, and joint deformity. Chondrocalcinosis may or may not be visible despite these changes.

CPPD crystal deposition disease may be distinguished from DJD, however, by five recognizable features: (3)

- *Unusual articular distribution.* Features of degenerative joint disease without history of previous trauma or surgery may be the result of CPPD crystal deposition; for example, at the wrist, elbow, and glenohumeral joints.
- *Unusual intra-articular distribution.* Involvement of selective joint compartments within an articular complex suggests pyrophosphate arthropathy. The most common sites include degenerative changes in the radiocarpal, trapezioscaphoid, talocalcaneal, and patellofemoral compartments.
- *Prominent subchondral cysts (geodes).* Intraosseous synovial fluid extrusions often result in numerous and large subchondral cysts.
- *Severe, destructive subchondral bone changes.* Rapidly progressive subchondral fragmentation and collapse, with loose body formation, may simulate neuropathic joint disease. (4)
- *Variable osteophyte formation.* Osteophytes may be large or absent, despite severe joint space changes.

Target Sites of Involvement

Table 10-75 provides a summary of sites affected by CPPD crystal deposition.

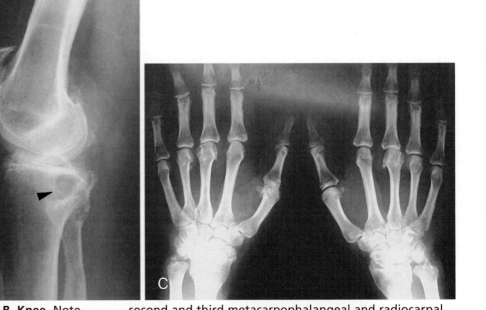

Figure 10-220   **WILSON'S DISEASE. A and B. Knee.** Note that key signs of arthropathy include osteopenia, chondrocalcinosis (*arrow*), cysts (*arrowheads*), irregular cortex, osteophytes, and ossicles. Note the patellofemoral joint narrowing, a key indication of an underlying crystal-induced arthropathy. **C. Bilateral Hands.** Observe arthropathy in the second and third metacarpophalangeal and radiocarpal joints. *COMMENT:* These changes are similar to both hemochromatosis and calcium pyrophosphate dihydrate crystal deposition disease. (Courtesy of John Duda, MD, Denver, Colorado.)

Table 10-75	Summary of Major Articulations Involved in CPPD Crystal Deposition		
Location	Compartments	Chondrocalcinosis	Pyrophosphate Arthropathy
Knee	Medial > patella > lateral	Hyaline, menisci	Medial, patella
Wrist	Ulnacarpal	Triangular cartilage, hyaline	Absent
	Radiocarpal	Hyaline	Stepladder, Terry Thomas' sign
	Trapezoscaphoid	Absent	Moderate
Hand	2–3 metacarpophalangeal	Hyaline, capsular	Metacarpal head
Hip	Superior	Hyaline, labrum	Femoral head
Shoulder	Glenohumeral	Hyaline, labrum	Glenohumeral
	Acromioclavicular	Hyaline, bursae, fibrocartilage	Minimal
Elbow	Medial, lateral	Hyaline	Radius, ulna
Foot	Talonavicular	Absent	Foot dorsum
Pelvis	Symphysis pubis	Fibrocartilage	Pubic
Spine	Lumbar discs	Annulus fibrosus	Disc space, bodies

CPPD, calcium pyrophosphate dihydrate.

Knee. The knee is the most frequent joint for both clinical and radiologic changes to be visible. (20) The most distinctive radiographic features are chondrocalcinosis and co-existing or isolated unusual compartmental involvement. (Fig. 10-221)

Chondrocalcinosis of the hyaline cartilage and menisci is characteristic. Up to 7% of asymptomatic individuals over the age of 60 years, however, may have chondrocalcinosis. (22) Hyaline chondrocalcinosis is most visible on the femoral condyles and posterior surface of the patella. Meniscal fibrocartilage chondrocalcinosis is seen on the AP projection as triangular calcifications with the apices directed medially in the medial and lateral compartment. (14,26) The lateral meniscus may be slightly denser than the medial.

Intra-articular compartmental involvement most commonly is found in the medial femorotibial region, followed by patellofemoral and lateral femorotibial portions of the joint. Isolated patellofemoral compartmental changes have been stressed as an important sign of CPPD crystal deposition disease. (3) Other accompanying features include subchondral sclerosis and cysts, articular fragmentation, and loose body formation.

Wrist. As in the knee, the wrist is a frequently affected articulation, with characteristic sites of calcification and arthropathy. Calcification of the triangular cartilage in the ulnocarpal joint space is frequently visible. (3) (Fig. 10-222) Hyaline chondrocalcinosis may be seen adjacent to any bones within the carpus. Other structures that may calcify include the synovium and various ligaments of the wrist, especially between the scaphoid and the lunate bones.

Arthropathy distinctly has a predilection for the radiocarpal joint. (27) Signs of involvement include loss of joint space between the scaphoid and distal radius, subchondral sclerosis, cysts, and osteophytes. Disruption of the intervening ligament between the scaphoid and the lunate results in a widened scaphoid–lunate articular space (*Terry Thomas' sign, scapholunate dissociation*). (3,28) (Figs. 10-222D and 9.206A) In addition, the scaphoid may move proximally and alter the articular contour of the radius, while the lunate moves distally toward the capitate, creating a *stepladder appearance* in the radiocarpal joint alignment. (3,29) The combination of diminished radiocarpal joint space, scapholunate dissociation, and rotary subluxation of the scaphoid allows the capitate to migrate proximally, producing the scapholunate advanced collapse (SLAC) deformity. (30) (Fig. 10-222E) Severe

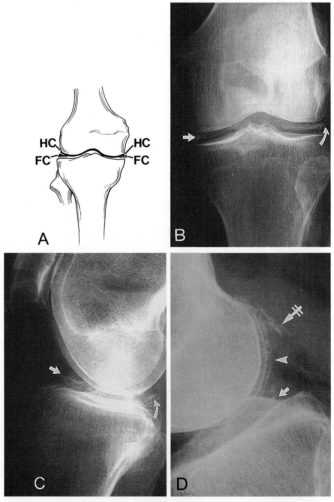

Figure 10-221 CALCIUM PYROPHOSPHATE DIHYDRATE CRYSTAL DEPOSITION DISEASE: KNEE. A. Diagram. Chondrocalcinosis can be seen in either the fibrocartilage (*FC*) or hyaline cartilage (*HC*). **B and C. Meniscal Chondrocalcinosis.** Note the chondrocalcinosis (*arrows*). **D. Calcification.** Note the calcification in the meniscus (*arrow*), hyaline cartilage (*arrowhead*), and synovial membrane (*crossed arrow*).

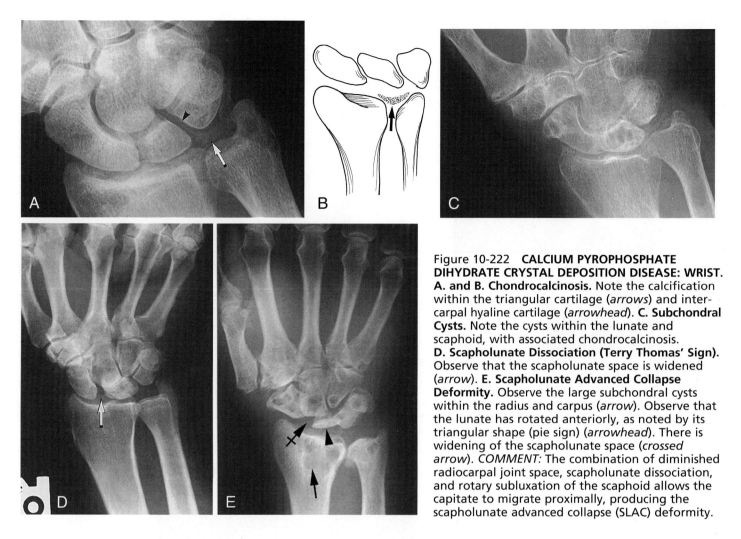

Figure 10-222   **CALCIUM PYROPHOSPHATE DIHYDRATE CRYSTAL DEPOSITION DISEASE: WRIST. A. and B. Chondrocalcinosis.** Note the calcification within the triangular cartilage (*arrows*) and intercarpal hyaline cartilage (*arrowhead*). **C. Subchondral Cysts.** Note the cysts within the lunate and scaphoid, with associated chondrocalcinosis. **D. Scapholunate Dissociation (Terry Thomas' Sign).** Observe that the scapholunate space is widened (*arrow*). **E. Scapholunate Advanced Collapse Deformity.** Observe the large subchondral cysts within the radius and carpus (*arrow*). Observe that the lunate has rotated anteriorly, as noted by its triangular shape (pie sign) (*arrowhead*). There is widening of the scapholunate space (*crossed arrow*). *COMMENT:* The combination of diminished radiocarpal joint space, scapholunate dissociation, and rotary subluxation of the scaphoid allows the capitate to migrate proximally, producing the scapholunate advanced collapse (SLAC) deformity.

degenerative signs are also common in the trapezioscaphoid joint. There is always a lack of articular alterations in the radioulnar compartment, unlike rheumatoid arthritis.

Spine. Manifestations in the vertebral column are relatively infrequent, often non-specific, and usually asymptomatic. (31) The predominant changes are seen in the lumbar spine and to a lesser extent in the cervical spine. (3,27)

The most common findings include loss of disc height, vacuum phenomena, considerable vertebral body sclerosis, osteophytes, and facet arthropathy. Calcification within the annulus may simulate marginal syndesmophyte formation of ankylosing spondylitis, with fine, slender, vertical, and peripheral discal calcification. The nucleus pulposus is infrequently opacified. (26) An epidural deposit of crystals within the canal may simulate the imaging appearances of a disc herniation. (31) Ligamentum flavum calcification may occasionally be visible, which on MRI shows a thickened, bulging ligament of low signal intensity. (32) Additional destructive phenomena may manifest as angular deformities and vertebral displacement, even at the atlantoaxial joint. (27,33)

Other Sites. Any site can be affected with characteristic manifestations of arthropathy, chondrocalcinosis, and soft tissue calcification. (3,5)

Hands. There is a predilection to involve the second and third metacarpophalangeal joints, with loss of joint space, sclerosis, and metacarpal head fragmentation. (Fig. 10-223)

Shoulder. Selective degenerative changes in the glenohumeral joint with hyaline chondrocalcinosis is characteristic. (29) (Fig. 10-224) In up to 35% of patients, calcification of the intraarticular fibrocartilage of the acromioclavicular joint may be visible. (34)

Hip. Chondrocalcinosis of the hyaline cartilage on the femoral head and acetabular labrum is visible, with degenerative changes either in the superolateral compartment or of the entire joint. (29) Protrusio acetabuli may occur with time.

Foot. Involvement of the foot dorsum at the talonavicular joint is distinctive, with osteophytes, sclerosis, and fragmentation.

Symphysis Pubis. A vertical linear calcification in the joint fibrocartilage with associated degenerative changes in the adjacent pubic joint margin is characteristic. (Fig. 10-225)

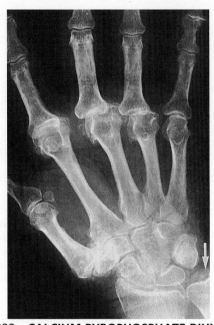

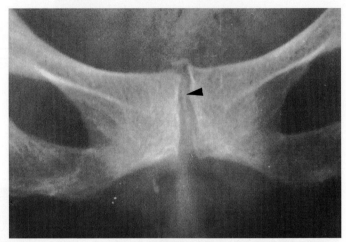

Figure 10-225 **CALCIUM PYROPHOSPHATE DIHYDRATE CRYSTAL DEPOSITION DISEASE: SYMPHYSIS PUBIS.** Note the chondrocalcinosis within the fibrocartilage disc of the pubic symphysis (*arrowhead*). (Courtesy of Donald Resnick, MD, San Diego, California.)

Figure 10-223 **CALCIUM PYROPHOSPHATE DIHYDRATE CRYSTAL DEPOSITION DISEASE: HAND.** Note the articular changes at the metacarpophalangeal joints. Calcification of the triangular cartilage is evident in the ulnar compartment of the wrist (*arrow*). Also noted is exuberant degenerative change in the first carpometacarpal joint, secondary to crystal deposition.

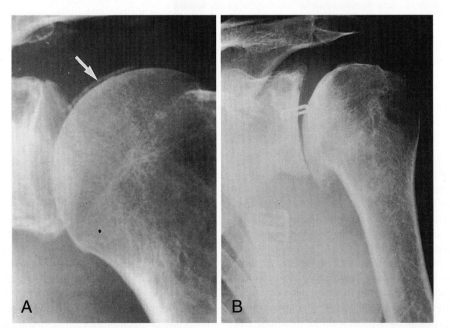

Figure 10-224 **CALCIUM PYROPHOSPHATE DIHYDRATE CRYSTAL DEPOSITION DISEASE: SHOULDER. A. Chondrocalcinosis.** Note the curvilinear calcification paralleling the articular surface of the humeral head (*arrow*). **B. Degenerative Joint Disease.** Note the changes secondary to CPPD are typical of degenerative change, including non-uniform loss of joint space, osteophytes, and sclerosis. *COMMENT:* Calcium pyrophosphate dihydrate crystal deposition disease is considered a cause for this appearance because this is an uncommon site for primary degenerative joint disease.

CAPSULE SUMMARY Calcium Pyrophosphate Dihydrate Crystal Deposition Disease

General Considerations

- An inflammatory joint disease caused by deposition of CPPD into the synovial fluid, linings, and articular cartilage.
- Synonyms include pseudo-gout, chondrocalcinosis, and pyrophosphate arthropathy.

Clinical Features

- Usually > 30 years of age, with a peak at 60 years; equal sex distribution.
- Can be acute or chronic and may be asymptomatic.
- Acute presentations (20%) may simulate gout or rheumatoid arthritis with swollen, hot, tender joints; usually affects knees, wrists, and hands, with attacks lasting 1–7 days.
- Chronic presentations (60%) simulate DJD, with bony swelling, crepitus, and stiffness.
- Asymptomatic cases (20%) exist in which the only sign is radiographic chondrocalcinosis.
- Other diseases are associated with CPPD deposition (*three Cs*).
- Laboratory signs include a raised ESR with synovial fluid crystal evaluation diagnostic.

Pathologic Features

- CPPD crystals are deposited into the chondrocyte lacunae within articular cartilage (hyaline or fibrous).
- Chondrocytes subsequently die, resulting in impaired cartilage replacement and maintenance, followed by thinning and cracking, simulating DJD.
- Crystals are shed into the joint as the cartilage degenerates, inciting an inflammatory response in the synovial tissues.

Radiologic Features

- Basic radiographic signs are soft tissue calcification and pyrophosphate arthropathy.

- Cartilage calcification (chondrocalcinosis) is the most common radiographic sign of CPPD crystal disease in the knees, wrists, symphysis pubis, elbows, and hips.
- Fibrocartilage is shaggy and irregular (knee menisci, wrist triangular cartilage, symphysis pubis).
- Hyaline is thin, linear, and parallel to and separated from the adjacent subchondral bone (wrist, elbow, shoulder, knee, hip); additional calcification in capsule, synovium, ligaments, tendons, and blood vessels.
- Pyrophosphate arthropathy is most common in the knee, wrist, and metacarpophalangeal joints.
- Articular changes simulate DJD, except unusual articular distribution, unusual intra-articular distribution, prominent subchondral cysts, bone destruction, and variable osteophyte size.
- The knee is the most commonly involved joint radiographically and clinically. Chondrocalcinosis of menisci. Intra-articular osseous and calcific bodies are common. Diagnosis strongly suggested if patellofemoral joint is selectively and/or severely involved.
- In the wrist, chondrocalcinosis of the triangular fibrocartilage and the hyaline cartilages of the entire carpus. Advanced and exuberant degenerative changes in the radiocarpal compartment. Scaphoid moves proximally and the lunate distally (stepladder appearance).
- In the spine, ligamentous calcification of the outer annulus fibers resembles syndesmophytes of ankylosing spondylitis. The ligamentum flavum may also calcify, but not the nucleus pulposus. Advanced discopathy and osteophytic changes with secondary instability.
- Hip and shoulders show hyaline chondrocalcinosis and signs of DJD.

HYDROXYAPATITE DEPOSITION DISEASE

Commonly encountered clinical findings with hydroxyapatite deposition disease are tendinitis, bursitis, and joint pain. Radiographic correlation with the clinical presentation often is remarkably inconsistent. A frequent radiographic finding is deposition of calcium within the tissue involved, especially in the shoulder, elbow, wrist, hip, ankle, and spine. Nomenclature associated with this entity is diverse and includes such terms as calcifying tendinitis and bursitis, peritendinitis calcarea, periarthritis calcarea, and hydroxyapatite rheumatism. Because of the delineation of the crystal present, some have advocated the term hydroxyapatite crystal deposition disease (HADD). (1–3) This entity should not be confused with CPPD crystal deposition disease, which has different clinical, pathologic, and radiographic features.

Clinical Features

The disease affects both men and women, particularly in the 40- to 70-year age group. Distinctively, signs and symptoms are localized in proximity to a single joint with no evidence of systemic or constitutional disease. The most frequent pattern of presentation is a single site involvement; less commonly, two simultaneous locations; and, rarely, three or more. (3,4) The most common joint involved is the shoulder. Other joints afflicted include elbow, wrist, fingers, hip, knee, ankle, foot, and cervical and lumbar spine. (Fig. 10-226)

Acute clinical features include pain, tenderness, localized swelling, and reduced range of motion. Chronic cases demonstrate the same findings but less extreme in nature. Laboratory investigations are invariably unrewarding. The most definitive method of diagnosis is radiographic depiction of the characteristic pattern and location of calcification.

Pathologic Features

The exact cause and pathogenesis of the disorder is unknown. Various causes have been implicated, including an apparent genetic basis, physiologic aging, biomechanical, traumatic, vascular, and neurological factors. The most universally accepted pathogenetic sequence is that following a focus of degeneration within tissue in which calcium hydroxyapatite crystals are deposited. (5–7) These crystals have also been identified in the synovial fluid. (3,8)

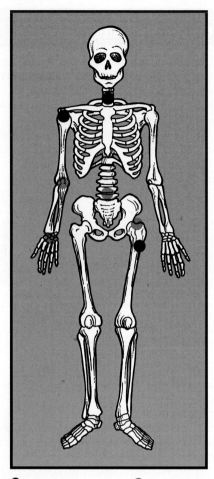

More common   Less common

Figure 10-226 **SKELETAL DISTRIBUTION OF HYDROXY-APATITE DEPOSITION DISEASE.**

Histopathologic examinations of diseased tissue are based mainly on observations made at the shoulder. These evaluations reveal necrosis, fibrosis, inflammatory cell infiltrate, and granular deposits of hydroxyapatite. (7) The persistent localization of the hydroxyapatite crystals within the supraspinatus tendon occurs in an area labeled *the critical zone*. (9) This represents an area of anatomically vascular compromised tissue where there is a poor anastomosis between tendinous and osseous vessels. (Fig. 10-227) The disappearance of calcifications within tendons or bursae may occur after the application of local physiotherapy (e.g., ultrasound). (Fig. 10-228)

Radiologic Features

The radiologic features are determined by the joint and anatomic components that are involved. The tendon is the most common structure affected; the clinician must have knowledge of insertion locations to make the diagnosis. Bursal calcifications are less frequently encountered.

General Features

Tendon Calcification. Distinctively, the site of calcification in the involved tendon occurs within a short distance of the in-

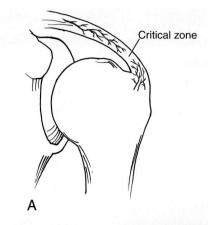

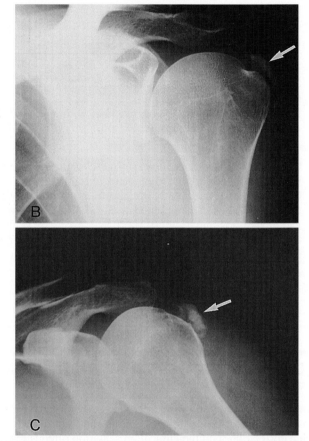

Figure 10-227 **HYDROXYAPATITE DEPOSITION DISEASE: SHOULDER. A. Diagram.** Within the tendon, a relatively poor zone of arterial anastomosis and perfusion between muscular and osseous vessels occurs (critical zone). **B and C. AP Shoulder.** This corresponds closely to the site of calcium deposition (*arrows*). COMMENT: The supraspinatus tendon is the most common site for hydroxyapatite deposition disease.

sertion and does not blend into the cortex of the adjacent bone. The density of the calcification initially may be veil-like and poorly defined. Later the calcification usually becomes more homogenous and well defined. The shape is variable, but tends to be round to oval with sharp margins. Additionally, a linear pattern may be apparent. Variations in density, size, and shape with sequential examinations are not unusual. Complete disappearance

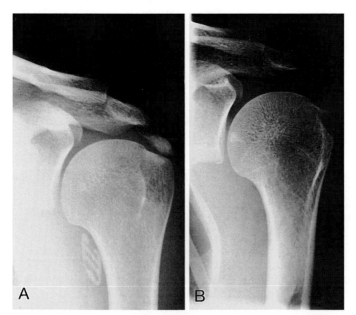

Figure 10-228   HYDROXYAPATITE DEPOSITION DISEASE: SUPRASPINATUS TENDINITIS WITH DISAPPEARANCE. A. Initial Film. Note the distinctive calcific density adjacent to the greater tuberosity within the supraspinatus tendon. **B. 3-Year Follow-Up.** Observe that there has been complete resorption of the calcification following the use of ultrasound and active mobilization.

Table 10-76	Anatomic Sites of Hydroxyapatite Deposition Disease	
Shoulder		Hip
Supraspinatus		Gluteus maximus
Infraspinatus		Gluteus medius
Teres minor		Rectus femoris
Subscapularis		Piriformis
Biceps—long, short heads		Gluteal, ischial bursa
Elbow		Knee
Extensor tendon		Patella tendon
Flexor tendon		Biceps femoris
Triceps		Collateral ligaments
Olecranon bursa		Ankle/Foot
Collateral ligaments		Flexor hallicus brevis
Wrist/Hand		Flexor hallicus longus
Flexor carpi ulnaris		Peroneus longus
Flexor carpi radialis		Flexor digitorum longus
Flexor digitorum		Extensor digitorum
Extensor carpi ulnaris		
Metacarpophalangeal joints		
Spine		
Longus colli		
Nucleus pulposus		
Annulus fibrosus		

of the calcification may also occur. The most commonly calcified tendons are those of the shoulder rotator cuff, hip, and upper cervical spine.

Bursal Calcification. Bursal calcifications are similar in appearance to a calcified tendon, and differentiation is often impossible on plain film examination. However, usually the calcification conforms to a known bursal location, is homogeneously dense, and is always round or oval. The most frequent sites for bursal calcification are in the subacromial, subdeltoid, and ischial bursae.

Target Sites of Involvement

The most common site is the shoulder, followed by the hip, spine, fingers, elbow, wrists, knees, and ankles. (1) (Table 10-76)
Shoulder. The most common site for calcification within tendons and bursae is the shoulder. A population frequency of shoulder calcifications may be expected of approximately 3% of individuals. (10) More than half of these calcifications will be bilateral. If unilateral, the right side is involved twice as often as the left. The most common sites for calcification, in order of frequency, are tendons at the humeral head of the supraspinatus, infraspinatus, teres minor, and subscapularis (***SITS*** *tendons*). Less common sites are the long and short heads of the biceps and the subacromial and subdeltoid bursae. Spontaneous resolution, reappearance, and movement of the calcification may occur. (10) Radiographic examination must be performed in both external and internal rotation to identify and locate the calcification. (5,11)
Supraspinatus. Distinctively, the supraspinatus is the most common tendon to demonstrate deposition of hydroxyapatite. The optimum view is external rotation, in which the calcification will appear in profile adjacent to but not superimposed on the promontory of the greater tuberosity. (Figs. 10-227 to 10-229) On internal

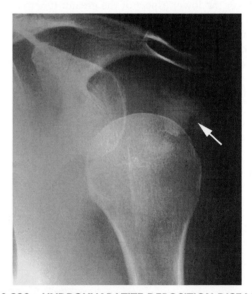

Figure 10-229   HYDROXYAPATITE DEPOSITION DISEASE: SUPRASPINATUS CALCIFIC TENDINITIS, GLENOHUMERAL SUB-LUXATION. AP Shoulder. Note the calcification within the tendon (*arrow*). The humerus is displaced inferiorly as evidenced by the widened acromiohumeral distance (*drooping shoulder sign*). *COMMENT:* The drooping shoulder sign is often associated with lesions of the brachial plexus, Pancoast's tumor, cerebrovascular accidents, and infections of the glenohumeral joint.

rotation the calcification tends to be projected over the humeral head, but may remain in profile. On all MRI sequences the area of calcification exhibits low signal intensity.
Infraspinatus. The infraspinatus inserts more posteriorly and lower on the greater tuberosity. On external rotation, a contained calcification will overlie the middle third of the greater tuberosity and come into profile on internal rotation.

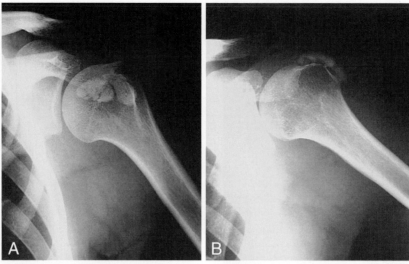

Figure 10-230   **HYDROXYAPATITE DEPOSITION DISEASE: BURSAL CALCIFICATION. A. External Rotation, Shoulder.**   **B. Internal Rotation, Shoulder.** Observe the large, smooth, calcific, oval-shaped densities.

Teres Minor.   The teres minor also inserts posteriorly, but onto the lower third of the greater tuberosity below the infraspinatus attachment. External rotation will show the calcification superimposed over the lower aspect of the greater tuberosity. Internal rotation will project the density away from the tuberosity.

Subscapularis.   Attaching to the middle third of the lesser tuberosity, the calcified subscapularis is seen in the external rotation view projected over the humeral head. On internal rotation the calcification moves medially to project in profile adjacent to the inner cortex of the humerus.

Biceps.   Calcification within the long head of the biceps is visible adjacent to the superior margin of the glenoid fossa. The short head tendon will show as a density adjacent to the coracoid process. These do not move with internal or external rotation.

Bursae.   Subacromial bursal calcification is visible medial to the greater tuberosity beneath the acromion process as a homogenous, sharply defined opacity. Subdeltoid bursal calcification extends more laterally adjacent to the greater tuberosity. (Fig. 10-230)

Hip.   A common site for tendinous calcification in and around the hip is the femoral insertion of the gluteus maximus into the linea aspera. (12,13) (Fig. 10-231). The lesions are locally painful, especially on deep pressure, and may simulate referred sciatic pain. Radiographic examinations are virtually diagnostic. On the frontal radiograph, the calcification is inferior to the trochanteric

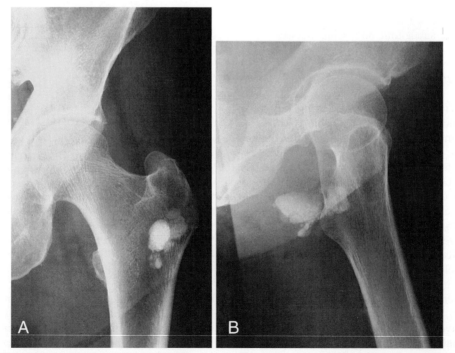

Figure 10-231   **HYDROXYAPATITE DEPOSITION DISEASE: GLUTEUS MAXIMUS TENDON. A and B. AP Frog-Leg Hip.** Observe the amorphous calcification within the insertion of the gluteus maximus tendon. (Reprinted with permission from **Yochum TR:** *Calcifying peritendinitis of the gluteus maximus tendon.* ACA J Chiro April, 1982.)

region and superimposed over the lateral portion of the femoral shaft. The lateral (frog-leg) radiograph will demonstrate the calcification outside the cortex on the medial surface of the lesser trochanter. The calcification is dense and homogenous and may be multiple. The underlying cortex of bone may be irregular, simulating a malignant transformation of an osteochondroma. (13) Additional differential considerations should include a calcified lymph node, a calcified tuberculous infection, liposarcoma, synovioma, synoviochondrometaplasia, and scleroderma. Without the frog-leg projection it may also be confused with a bone island.

An additional site for calcification in the hip region is adjacent to the greater and lesser trochanter, within the gluteal and piriformis muscle insertions and adjacent bursae. (14) Additional calcifications may be seen at the anterior inferior iliac spine, acetabular margin, and ischial tuberosity.

Spine. Two anatomic sites in the spine for hydroxyapatite deposition have been identified: the longus colli muscle and the intervertebral disc.

Longus Colli. A self-limiting, transient, and acutely symptomatic hydroxyapatite deposition occurs at the superolateral group of tendons as they insert anterior to the C1 and C2 vertebral bodies. (15,16) (Fig. 10-232) Symptomatically, the patient complains of a painful and stiff neck, muscle spasm, painful dysphagia, and a sense of globus hystericus. (17) These symptoms typically arise abruptly, reaching a maximum within 2–5 days, and then gradually resolve over the following 1–2 weeks. The lateral radiograph is diagnostic in the symptomatic phase, demonstrating an amorphous calcification up to 2 cm in diameter anterior and inferior to the anterior tubercle of the atlas within the retropharyngeal soft tissues. (15,17) (Fig. 10-233) Occasionally, the calcification may occur lower between C2 and C6. (18) The retropharyngeal interspace is often increased locally to > 7 mm.

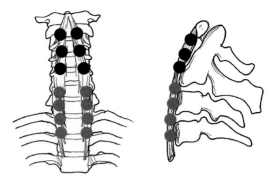

Figure 10-232   HYDROXYAPATITE DEPOSITION DISEASE: SITES OF CALCIFICATION WITHIN THE LONGUS COLLI.

On T2-weighted MRI, the superior portion of the longus colli is of high signal intensity corresponding to edema. (19) In addition, the lordosis is often diminished owing to the associated muscle spasm. As the symptoms subside, resorption of the prevertebral calcification and swelling occurs. Subsequent complete resolution of the soft tissue abnormality occurs coinciding with the involution of the clinical picture. No permanent sequelae are to be expected. (20,21)

Intervertebral Disc. Original anatomic descriptions of discal calcification were first noted in 1858 by von Luschka and delineated radiographically in 1922 by Calve and Galland. (22,23) Various disease entities may result in opacification of the intervertebral disc, including DJD, block vertebra, spinal fusion, ochronosis, and others. (24) (Table 10-77)

The location, appearance, and pathophysiologic mechanisms will vary according to the disease process. Calcium is most com-

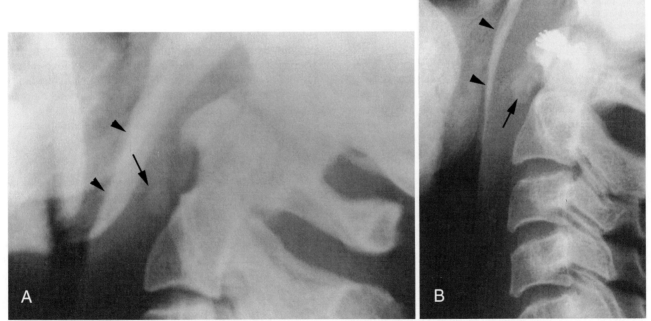

Figure 10-233   HYDROXYAPATITE DEPOSITION DISEASE: LONGUS COLLI. A. Lateral Cervical Subtle Calcification. Note the thin veil-like calcification immediately inferior to the odontoid region (*arrow*). Also note the anteriorly displaced retropharyngeal space owing to edema (*arrowheads*).
B. Lateral Cervical Dense Calcification. Note the discrete circular concretion outlined in the prevertebral soft tissues (*arrow*). Characteristically, the retropharyngeal soft tissues are displaced anteriorly (*arrowheads*). (Panel A courtesy of Carsten Hviid, DC, Arhus, Denmark. Panel B courtesy of Edwardo Seda, MD, Denver, Colorado.)

Table 10-77	Calcification within the Intervertebral Disc		
Condition	Mechanism	Crystal	Location
Common			
Congenital block vertebra	Immobilization	HA	NP
Degenerative disc disease	Dystrophic	HA	NP, AF
Idiopathic (child, adult)	Unknown	HA	NP
Sequestered disc protrusion	Dystrophic	HA	NP (ectopic)
Uncommon			
Acromegaly	Degeneration-dystrophic	HA	NP, AF
Amyloidosis	Amyloid-dystrophic	?	NP, AF
Ankylosing spondylitis	Immobilization, inflammation	HA	NP, AF
Gout	Uric acid-dystrophic	HA, urate, ?	AF
Hemochromatosis	Iron-dystrophic	CPPD	NP, AF
Herpes zoster	Unknown	?	NP
Hyperparathyroidism	Subchondral bone injury	CPPD	NP, AF
Hypervitaminosis D	Hypercalcemia	?	AF
Juvenile rheumatoid arthritis	Immobilization	?	NP
Ochronosis	Homogentisic acid-dystrophic	HA	NP, AF
Poliomyelitis	Immobilization	?	NP, AF
Pseudo-gout	CPPD crystals	CPPD	AF
Spinal fusion	Immobilization	?, HA	NP

Adapted from **Weinberger A, Myers AR:** *Intervertebral disc calcification in adults. A review.* Semin Arthritis Rheum 8(1):69, 1978.

AF, annulus fibrosus; *CPPD,* calcium pyrophosphate dihydrate; *HA,* hydroxyapatite; *NP,* nucleus pulposus; *?,* unknown.

monly deposited as hydroxyapatite or pyrophosphate crystals. (24) In general, the nucleus pulposus will be visible as a homogenous round to oval radiopacity located centrally but slightly posterior in the disc space, simulating the appearance seen on a normal discogram. (Fig. 10-234) Histopathologic examination reveals the calcium to be deposited within crevices of the nucleus pulposus. (25) Annulus fibrosus calcification is statistically more common than nuclear calcifications, being present in > 70% of all autopsies. (25,26) The radiographic appearance of annular calcification is distinctively located at the disc periphery, with a thin, curvilinear configuration that is orientated toward the vertebral body margin. As in the nucleus pulposus, calcium is deposited into annular fissures and necrotic fibers. (25) Calcification within the vertebral body endplate cartilage will appear as a thin linear density separated from but parallel to the bony cortex.

The most commonly encountered causes for discal calcification are degenerative disc disease, sequestered disc prolapse (non-contained discs), congenital block vertebra, and two peculiar idiopathic forms (childhood and adult).

Degenerative Disc Disease. In association with disc degeneration, calcification within the nucleus pulposus and annulus fibrosus is a commonly identified radiologic finding. These discal calcifications are visible in association with the other signs of DJD, including loss of disc height, endplate sclerosis, and osteophytes. Nuclear calcification may assume a round to flattened oval configuration or be fragmented and even linear. Most commonly, the oval contour is apparent with evidence of fragmentation. Calcification within the annulus fibers is a far more frequently observed finding in degenerative disc disease. These are usually visible at the anterior aspect of the disc, especially in the lower cervical spine. Less commonly, they may be apparent at the lateral margins of the disc space. The calcification characteristically is < 2 mm thick, vertical, slightly curvilinear, and usually not continuous with the adjacent vertebral body margin. These annular calcifications have been called intercalary bones; they sometimes simulate syndesmophytes seen in ankylosing spondylitis. (27) (Fig. 10-234C)

Sequestered Disc Prolapse (Non-Contained Disc). Occasionally, discal disruption leads to escape of the nuclear material from the confines of the intervertebral disc. This may be in an anterior, lateral, or posterior direction as well as through the vertebral body endplate (Schmorl's nodes). All of these discal extrusions may subsequently calcify, rendering them radiographically visible. Anterior and lateral prolapses do not commonly calcify and are invariably asymptomatic. In contrast, posterior prolapses may precipitate formations of loose fragments within the spinal canal, which can be symptomatic and visible on radiographic examination. Infrequently, intrabody discal herniations (Schmorl's nodes) may show calcification. (25,28)

Congenital Block Vertebrae. Calcification of the vestigial nucleus pulposus between two synostosed vertebral bodies is a common radiologic association in congenital block vertebrae. (29) The calcified nucleus will appear as a small, rounded, homogenous opacity interposed between the two fused vertebral bodies. (Fig. 10-235) Calcification within the discal material between the normally fused sacral and sacrococcygeal segments is also common. (30) It appears that loss of intersegmental physiologic motion impairs discal nutrition and results in dystrophic deposition of calcium hydroxyapatite within the nucleus. The same dystrophic phenomenon can be seen in any situation in which intersegmental fusion occurs, including Klippel-Feil syndrome, ankylosing spondylitis, juvenile rheumatoid arthritis, myositis ossificans progressiva, and surgical fusion. (29)

Idiopathic. Two forms of idiopathic calcifications are apparent based on age: childhood and adult.

- *Childhood.* Childhood idiopathic intervertebral disc calcification is a peculiar clinical and radiologic phenomenon. (Table 10-78) The age of onset is usually between 6 and 12 years of age, with males being involved twice as commonly. (31,32) The cause is unknown, but trauma, infection, inflammation, and other factors have all been implicated. (31,33–35) The most common site affected is the cervical spine, followed by the thoracic spine and, least commonly, the lumbar spine. (31,32) (Figs. 10-236 and 10-237) Usually, only one disc is involved, but there may be multiple involvement in up to 30% of cases. (34) The calcification is distinctively located within the nucleus pulposus and not the annulus fibrosus. (33,36) Prolapse of the calcified nucleus may occur but is usually not associated with neurological symptoms. (31,37,38)

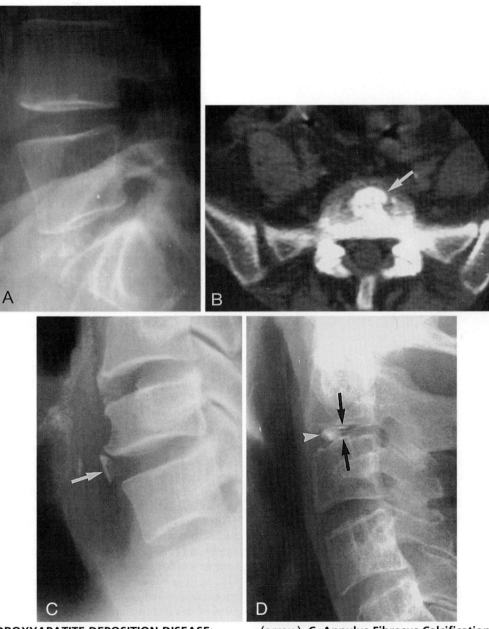

Figure 10-234 **HYDROXYAPATITE DEPOSITION DISEASE: INTERVERTEBRAL DISC. A. Nucleus Pulposus Calcification.** Note the faint amorphous nuclear calcification at the L5 interspace. **B. Axial CT: L5/S1.** Note the nuclear calcification (*arrow*). **C. Annulus Fibrosus Calcification.** Note the intercalary bone (*arrow*). **D. Endplate Cartilage Calcification.** Note the linear calcification (*arrows*) surrounding the nuclear calcification (*arrowhead*).

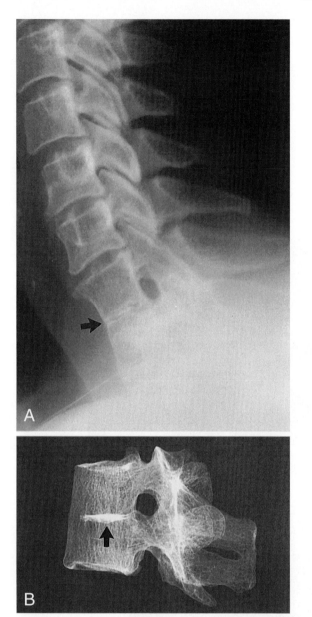

Figure 10-235 **HYDROXYAPATITE DEPOSITION DISEASE: CONGENITAL BLOCK VERTEBRAE. A. Lateral Cervical. B. Specimen Radiograph.** Note the central dense nuclear calcification (*arrows*).

Table 10-78	Summary of Childhood Idiopathic Intervertebral Disc Calcification
Clinical Features	**Radiologic Features**
6–10 years old, males 2:1	Cervical spine, C4–C6
Equal sex distribution	Nucleus pulposus calcification
Most common in cervical	Mild increase in disc height spine
Unknown cause	Moderate flattening of adjacent bodies
Acute onset—pain, stiffness, fever	Progressive dissolution and fragmentation of calcification
Self-limiting in 2 weeks to 2 months	Persistent localized vertebral body flattening
Supportive therapy only	Premature disc degeneration

CT does not usually add significant supplementary information, though it should be obtained if neurological complications are present. (39)

Clinically, a spectrum of presentations occur. Approximately 70% of these patients will have pain, 30% an associated fever, and 4% neurological symptoms. (33) Up to 15% of cases will remain totally asymptomatic. Other associated findings include neck stiffness simulating meningitis, localized tenderness, scoliosis, elevated ESR, and leukocytosis. (26)

The radiographic features are distinctive. The calcified nucleus pulposus appears as a flattened oval or rounded opacity within a mildly widened intervertebral disc space. The opposing surfaces of the contiguous vertebral bodies are flattened in contour. (31,33) (Fig. 10-236)

The unique features of this syndrome are the self-limiting nature of the symptoms and the close temporal relationship with the appearance and disappearance of the discal calcification. (31) Usually, the symptoms subside within several weeks to months with only supportive pain control methods. (34,40) Observation of the discal calcification will also demonstrate gradual resorption and fragmentation over the same coinciding period. No serious residual deformity or impairment is to be expected; however, persistence of isolated vertebral body flattening and premature loss of disc height with osteophytic formation, coinciding with the level of previous calcification, may be expected. (26,31)

• *Adult.* Adult idiopathic intervertebral disc calcification is most likely degenerative in nature, but it lacks the associated radiographic features of osteophytosis, endplate sclerosis, and loss of disc height. (35) (Fig. 10-238) Clinically, these patients are asymptomatic, unless associated discal herniation is present. (24)

Others. Biochemical disorders such as gout, pseudo-gout, hemochromatosis, ochronosis, hyperparathyroidism, and hypervitaminosis D may predispose individuals to disc calcification of the nucleus pulposus, endplate cartilage, or the annulus fibrosus. Other miscellaneous related disorders include acromegaly, ankylosing spondylitis, herpes zoster, and poliomyelitis. (24–26)

Other Sites. Any periarticular tissue can be involved with painful and non-painful deposits of calcium hydroxyapatite. Generally, these tend to localize at points of greatest stress within the most mobile joints. (5) (Fig. 10-239)

Elbow. The most common location at the elbow is at the common extensor tendon at the lateral epicondyle. (5,41) Additional sites of calcification are within the common flexor tendon at the medial epicondyle, the triceps tendon at the olecranon process, and the olecranon bursa.

Wrist. The flexor carpi ulnaris tendon insertion at the pisiform is the most common site of involvement in the wrist. (5,42) This is best seen on the oblique view as an amorphous, poorly marginated opacity in proximity to the pisiform. (43,44) The second most common site is within the abductor pollicis longus and extensor pollicis brevis adjacent to the radial styloid and may be related to stenosing tenosynovitis of these same tendons (*de Quervain's disease*). (5) In the absence of calcification, displacement of the overlying skin and increased thickness of the soft tissue in the same region is usually visible. (45) Immediately

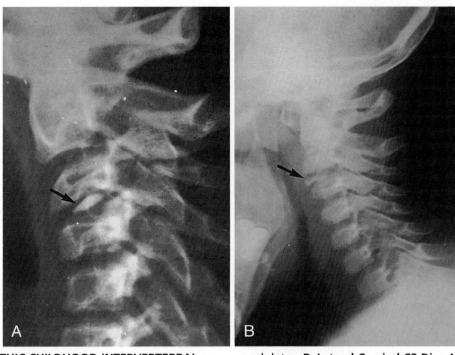

Figure 10-236 **IDIOPATHIC CHILDHOOD INTERVERTEBRAL DISC CALCIFICATION. A. Lateral Cervical C3 Disc.** Note the dense central calcification (*arrow*) and flattened adjacent endplates. **B. Lateral Cervical C3 Disc.** Note that the calcified nucleus has extruded anteriorly (*arrow*).

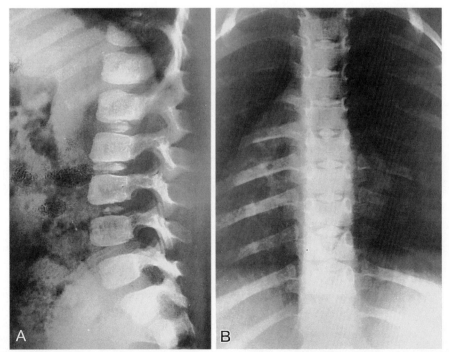

Figure 10-237 **IDIOPATHIC CHILDHOOD INTERVERTEBRAL DISC CALCIFICATION. A. Lateral Lumbar. B. AP Thoracic.** Note the multiple calcified discs throughout the thoracic and lumbar spine. (Reprinted with permission from **Yochum TR:** *Childhood idiopathic disc calcification—A case study.* ACA J Chiro February, 1981.)

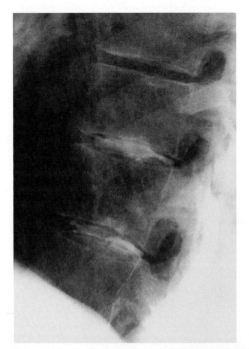

Figure 10-238 **IDIOPATHIC ADULT NUCLEUS PULPOSUS CALCIFICATION: LOWER THORACIC SPINE.** Note the central ovoid intradiscal density, typical of nuclear calcification. These are usually asymptomatic and of no clinical significance.

distal, adjacent to the first metacarpal trapezium joint, a similar calcification within the flexor carpi radialis may occur. (42) Additional sites at the wrist are within the common flexor tendons and extensor carpi ulnaris. (5)

Hand. Involvement is infrequent within the hand, but most commonly is seen at the metacarpophalangeal joints on the flexor surface of the metacarpal head either at the ligamentous or musculotendinous insertions. (42)

Knee. Rarely, calcification may be evident within the insertion of the quadriceps tendon to the patella and the biceps femoris insertion at the fibular head. Medial and lateral epicondylar calcifications are occasionally encountered. Following trauma, calcification within the medial collateral ligament may be visible (*Pellegrini-Stieda disease*). (Fig. 10-239*D*)

Ankle and Foot. The most common tendons demonstrating calcification in the ankle and foot are the flexor hallucis brevis and longus tendons at the metatarsophalangeal joint and within the peroneal tendons near the base of the fifth metatarsal. (46) (Fig. 10-239*E*) Occasionally, a painful calcification may be found on the dorsum of the foot in proximity to the base of the second metatarsal. (47)

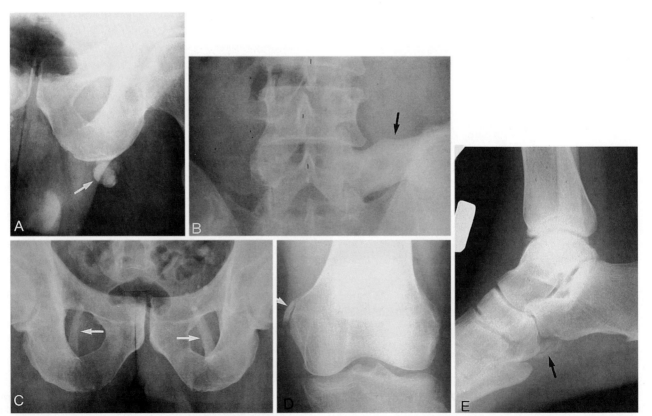

Figure 10-239 **HYDROXYAPATITE DEPOSITION DISEASE: MISCELLANEOUS SITES. A. Ischial Bursa. B. Iliolumbar Ligament. C. Sacrotuberous Ligament. D. Medial Collateral Ligament (Pellegrini-Stieda Disease). E. Peroneus Tendon.** Note the evidence of pathology at each site (*arrows*). (Panel B courtesy of David J. Byrnes, DC, Coffs Harbour, New South Wales, Australia.)

CAPSULE SUMMARY
Hydroxyapatite Deposition Disease

General Considerations

- Calcification within a tendon, bursa, or other periarticular soft tissue is a common radiographic finding.
- Various terms have been used, including calcifying tendinitis and peritendinitis calcarea.

Clinical Features

- Usually occurs in the 40- to 70-year age group, most commonly at the shoulder, hip, and cervical spine.
- Acute pain, tenderness, and swelling of the involved joint is found.
- Chronic cases have similar findings but are lower grade in nature.
- There is often a lack of correlation between clinical and radiographic findings.

Pathologic Features

- The origin and pathogenesis are unknown.
- Necrosis, fibrosis, inflammatory cell infiltrate, and deposits of hydroxyapatite characterize the involved tissue.

Radiologic Features

- Most common sites demonstrating depositions of hydroxyapatite are the shoulder, hip, and spine.
- *Shoulder:* supraspinatus most common, seen in profile on external rotation.
- Infraspinatus, teres minor in profile on internal rotation adjacent to greater tuberosity.
- Subscapularis in profile on internal rotation adjacent to lesser tuberosity.
- *Hip:* gluteus maximus most common below lesser trochanter.
- Additional sites include the trochanters, acetabuli, and anterior inferior iliac spines.
- *Spine:* longus colli anterior to C1 and C2.
- Transient, acutely symptomatic calcification with retropharyngeal swelling.
- Self-limiting within 1–2 weeks.
- *Nucleus pulposus:* calcification either in child or adult; idiopathic or secondary.
  Round to oval.
  Childhood idiopathic calcification is most common in cervical spine, acutely symptomatic, with fever, pain, and restricted motion.
  Calcification associated with widened disc space and flattened adjacent vertebral bodies in acute phase resolving within 2 months.
  Adult idiopathic calcification, common and asymptomatic.
- Secondary causes include degenerative joint disease, sequestered disc fragments, block vertebrae, and metabolic diseases.
- Annulus fibrosus calcification is far more common than nucleus pulposus and is usually degenerative. Intercalary bone is thin, curvilinear, and most commonly in the anterior aspect of the cervical disc.
- *Others:* wrist, elbow, knee, ankle, and foot.

OCHRONOSIS

Ochronosis is a rare autosomal recessive metabolic disorder of amino acid metabolism characterized by an absence of homogentisic acid oxidase. [1,2] This results in homogentisic acid being excreted in the urine (*alkaptonuria*) and deposited in tissues (*ochronosis*), causing joint disease (*ochronotic arthropathy*). [3] The historic aspects in this unique disorder trace back to early history, and examination of paleopathologic materials has demonstrated the disease. [3,4]

Clinical Features

A familial history of the disorder is often obtained. [5] It is two times more frequent in males and generally is asymptomatic until adult life, although childhood detection may occur owing to the identification of the characteristic urinary discoloration. [3] Clinical manifestations consist of bluish brown pigmentations of the skin, sclera, cornea, nose, and ear cartilages. [6] Joint symptoms closely resemble ankylosing spondylitis, although the pain is generally less severe. Progressive stiffness and pain of the spine, hips, knees, and shoulders is frequent, especially by the 4th decade of life. (Fig. 10-240) Occasionally, the initial presentation may be from acute disc herniation. [7] Large cartilaginous joints surfaces are pri-

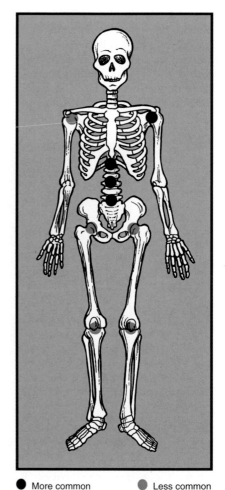

● More common   ● Less common

Figure 10-240 **SKELETAL DISTRIBUTION OF OCHRONOSIS.**

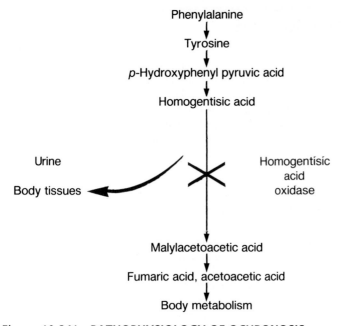

Phenylalanine

↓

Tyrosine

↓

p-Hydroxyphenyl pyruvic acid

↓

Homogentisic acid

Urine

Body tissues ◄

Homogentisic
acid
oxidase

Malylacetoacetic acid

↓

Fumaric acid, acetoacetic acid

↓

Body metabolism

Figure 10-241 **PATHOPHYSIOLOGY OF OCHRONOSIS.**
(Adapted from **LaDu BN, Sonnoni G, Laster L, et al.:** *The
nature of the defect in tyrosine metabolism in alcaptonuria.*
J Biol Chem 230:251, 1958.)

Table 10-79	Radiologic Features of Ochronosis

Spine
    Multiple contiguous disc calcifications
    Multiple loss of contiguous disc heights
    Multiple vacuum phenomena
    Small osteophytes
    Eventual ankylosis
Osteoporosis
    Reduced lordosis, increased kyphosis
Peripheral joints
    Advanced degenerative changes
    Chondrocalcinosis

urinary sugar test by copper reduction methods, such as Benedict or Clinitest, may be obtained, leading to the misdiagnosis of diabetes. (5,9) Owing to the lack of any truly effective or curative therapies (10,11) treatment is usually of a conservative nature unless the joints are severely affected. (12) Chiropractic manipulation in conjunction with passive modalities and active care has been successful in the reduction of symptomology in patients with ochronosis. (13)

Pathologic Features

The fundamental aberration is a genetic mutation occurring in about 1/1 million people. (14) This mutation of the HGO gene (10) ultimately results in the failure of tyrosine and phenylalanine to be metabolized to fumaric and acetoacetic acid, owing to the absence of homogentisic acid oxidase. (15) (Fig. 10-241) Subsequently, homogentisic acid is excreted in the urine and sweat and turns black when exposed to air or alkali. Deposition into body tissues, especially cartilage, sclerae, and skin, also results in yellow, blue, or

marily affected (8) with involvement of the spine in > 95% of cases, the knee in 30%, the shoulder in 20%, and the hip in 20%. (3) Posturally, there is progressive flattening of the lumbar lordosis and increasing thoracic kyphosis.

Laboratory urinary evaluations will demonstrate homogentisic acid, which is diagnostic. This is demonstrated by paper chromatography and by the urine becoming black on standing or by the addition of 10% sodium hydroxide. (9) In addition, a false-positive

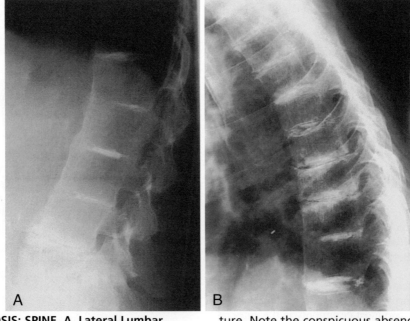

Figure 10-242 **OCHRONOSIS: SPINE. A. Lateral Lumbar Spine.** Note the multilevel discal calcification. **B. Lateral Thoracic Spine.** Note the universal discal calcification and vacuum phenomena, which characterize the radiological picture. Note the conspicuous absence of osteophytes despite the severe discal alterations. (Courtesy of David P. Thomas, MD, Melbourne, Australia.)

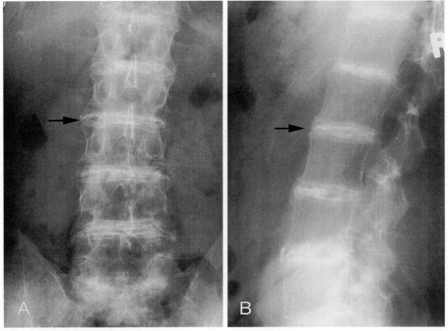

Figure 10-243 **OCHRONOSIS: LUMBAR SPINE. A. AP Lumbar.** Note that each intervertebral disc is calcified (*arrow*). **B. Lateral Lumbar.** Observe the universal intradiscal calcifica-tion at each level (*arrow*). Note also the prominent osteo-penia of the vertebrae. (Courtesy of Carr Chiropractic Clinic, Huron, South Dakota.)

black discoloration, which is macroscopically and often externally visible. (5) Microscopically, the pigment appears yellow (ochre), from which Virchow coined the term ochronosis. (3)

Accumulation in cartilage renders it brittle, and it rapidly de-generates, with advanced cracking, fibrillation, erosion, and calci-fication or ossification. In the spine the most commonly affected tissue is the intervertebral disc. Prominent pigmentation is espe-cially found in the hyaline cartilage covering the endplate, decreas-ing through the annulus to the nucleus pulposus. Characteristically, the most heavily calcified area within the disc is on the inner layers of the annulus fibrosus and is composed of apatite. (16) Fissuring and fragmentation within the disc are prominent, allowing for the formation of multiple vacuum phenomena.

Radiologic Features

Radiologic manifestations of ochronosis are most characteristic in the spine. (Table 10-79) These changes are especially apparent in the lumbar and thoracic spines and to a lesser extent in the cervi-cal spine. (16) (Figs. 10-242 and 10-243) The most distinctive abnormality is at the intervertebral disc, where loss of disc height, vacuum phenomenon, and thin, horizontal, wafer-like calcifica-tions are seen parallel to the body endplates. (17,18) These discal alterations are seen at multiple levels simultaneously. There is notably a low level of marginal bony proliferation, with only small osteophytes visible. As the disease progresses eventual osseous ankylosis across the disc space may occur, similar to ankylosing spondylitis, except the disc spaces are markedly diminished. There is no syndesmophyte formation, and the sacroiliac joints are un-fused. (18,19) The apophyseal joints will show advanced arthrosis and may also eventually ankylose. Osteoporosis is usually promi-nent, as is the loss of lumbar lordosis and increased thoracic kypho-sis. Ligamentous ossification may be apparent.

At other peripheral locations the radiographic features are iden-tical to DJD. (18) The exception is the hip, where similarity with rheumatoid arthritis is owing to uniform loss of joint space and rel-atively little osteophytes. (20) The most common peripheral joints involved are the hip, shoulder, and knee. Findings include loss of joint space, sclerosis, cysts, osteophytes, and chondrocalci-nosis. Flattening of articular surfaces is also seen. (21,22) Visceral involvement may be manifested by calculus formation in the kid-ney and prostate. The key to the radiographic diagnosis is the char-acteristic intervertebral disc changes and an early age of onset of advanced degenerative arthritis in often unexpected locations.

CAPSULE SUMMARY
Ochronosis

General Considerations

- Hereditary degenerative arthritis affecting large joints and the spine owing to a disorder in tyrosine metabo-lism.
- Synonyms include alkaptonuria, ochronotic arthropathy, and alkaptonuric arthritis.

Clinical Features

- Males 2:1; 20–40 years old; usually a family history of ochronosis.
- *Arthritis:* insidious onset of back pain and joint stiffness; minor trauma often precipitates acute episodes of joint pain, and predisposed to discal herniation before calcifi-cation.
- *Alkaptonuria:* urine turns black on standing owing to ox-idation of homogentisic acid (alkapton).

(continued)

CAPSULE SUMMARY
Ochronosis (continued)

- *Cartilage:* ears, nose, and costal cartilage appears brown, but blue on transillumination. Sclerae show brown patches adjacent to the corneal limbus.
- Skin may also be brown, especially in sweat areas.
- Renal and prostatic calculi are common.

Pathologic Features

- Failure of homogentisic acid oxidase to catalyze degradation of homogentisic acid (from tyrosine) to acetoacetic and fumaric acids.
- Homogentisic acid then accumulates and is oxidized to form a black pigment in cartilage and soft tissues. This weakens cartilage and leads to premature and advanced DJD.

Radiologic Features

- Advanced and premature DJD, chondrocalcinosis, and ligament calcification.
- *Spine:* increased kyphosis and lordosis; universal discal calcification, multilevel vacuum phenomena; universal disc thinning and degenerative change; and calcification in interspinous ligament and eventual vertebral fusion.
- Begins in the lumbar region, then ascends the spine. In the peripheral joints, advanced DJD, and chondrocalcinosis, especially in the hips, shoulders, and knees.

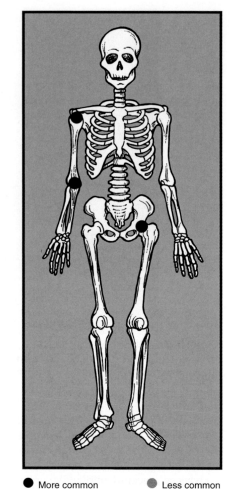

● More common   ● Less common

Figure 10-244 SKELETAL DISTRIBUTION OF TUMORAL CALCINOSIS.

TUMORAL CALCINOSIS

Tumoral calcinosis is a rare condition characterized by localized extracapsular accumulations of calcium. (1) The cause is unknown, but the condition is frequently associated with patients undergoing renal dialysis or suffering from hereditary conditions affecting calcium metabolism. (2,3)

Clinical Features

Children and adolescents most commonly are affected, usually between the ages of 6 and 25 years. Black individuals appear to be more frequently involved. (4) Distinctively, the developing soft tissue masses are discovered not because of pain but because of the presence of a palpable mass near a joint. (5) These masses progressively enlarge and may ulcerate the overlying skin. The most common locations for the lesions to occur are in proximity to the shoulder, hips, and elbows. (6) (Fig. 10-244) Rare incidences of tumoral calcinosis have been reported in the spine, fingers and wrist. (3,7–9) Laboratory evaluation usually reveals normal serum calcium levels with hyperphosphatemia. (10) Rarely, serum phosphate and alkaline phosphatase levels may be elevated. Treatment entails normalization of serum phosphate levels and resection of the lesion. (10) Complete surgical excision

is fundamentally curative of the lesion, whereas incomplete excision will invariably allow recurrence. (11)

Pathologic Features

The abnormal masses are multiloculated cysts filled with a viscous semifluid suspension of calcium triphosphate or carbonate salts in albumin. The walls of the cysts are composed of dense fibrous tissue lined with epithelioid and giant cells. (12)

Radiologic Features

Imaging is the best means of diagnosis (13), and the most notable radiographic feature is the dense calcific density near a joint. (6,14) (Fig. 10-245) Initially, the calcification begins as small, discrete nodules, which gradually enlarge and increase in density. They vary in size from 1 to 20 cm. The margins of the mass are lobulated and well defined. Rarely, a fluid level may be seen on upright films. (15) The adjacent bony and articular structures are usually unaffected, although extrinsic bone erosion has been documented, especially at the posterior distal humerus. (6) Isotopic bone scans show increased uptake within the calcific masses.

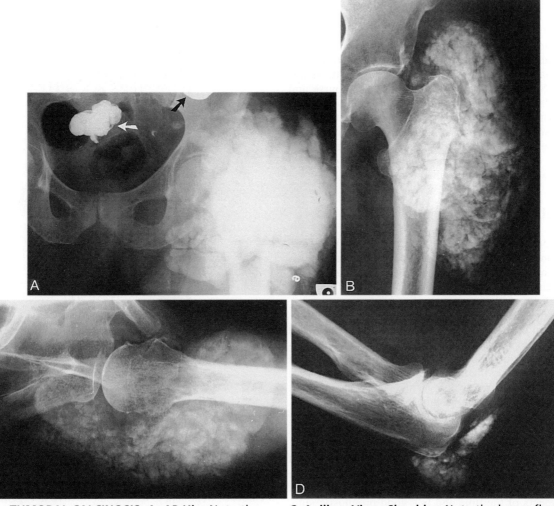

Figure 10-245   **TUMORAL CALCINOSIS. A. AP Hip.** Note the large, dense, lobulated, calcified soft tissue mass, which obscures the proximal femur. Of incidental notation is residual barium in the colon (*arrows*) **B. AP Hip.** Note that the flocculent calcification overlies the proximal third of the femur.

C. Axillary View, Shoulder. Note the large, flocculent calcification in the soft tissues. **D. Lateral Elbow.** Note the small area of dense soft tissue calcification adjacent to the olecranon and posterior humeral surface. (Panel C courtesy of Klaus W. Weber, MD, Fort Wayne, Indiana.)

CAPSULE SUMMARY   Tumoral Calcinosis

General Considerations
- A disorder of unknown cause characterized by localized accumulations of calcific masses.

Clinical Features
- Children and adolescents of 6–25 years.
- Blacks more commonly involved.
- Painless, enlarging periarticular soft tissue masses.
- Most common around the shoulders, hips, and elbows.

Pathologic Features
- Semifluid calcium suspension in albumin encapsulated by a fibrous lining.

Radiologic Features
- Dense, lobulated, well-marginated soft tissue masses.
- Adjacent bones and joints usually normal.
- Bone scans show localized increased uptake.

SARCOIDOSIS

Sarcoidosis is a disease of unknown cause affecting multiple organ systems. (1) Characteristic of the disorder is the formation of non-caseating granulomas, simultaneous involvement of many body tissues, and the predilection for young adults. (2) Skeletal manifestations are infrequent and may be present in up to 15% of cases, predominantly affecting the peripheral bones of the hands and feet. (1,3) Spinal involvement is rare. (4) The course and prognosis correlate with the mode of onset: An acute onset with erythema nodosum usually heralds a self-limiting course, with spontaneous resolution, whereas an insidious onset may be followed by relentless progressive fibrosis. (1) A common eponym is Boeck's sarcoid, after the Norwegian dermatologist who described the association with skin lesions.

Clinical Features

The initial diagnosis is usually made between the ages of 20 and 40 years, with an equal sex distribution. Black individuals are affected 10 times more commonly than whites in the United States. (1,2) Scandinavian individuals also have an increased frequency of the disease.

A wide spectrum of clinical presentations is encountered in sarcoidosis. (5) Often the disease is mild and incidentally diagnosed on routine chest radiographs. Any patient suspected of having sarcoidosis should have a radiographic examination of the chest because this is commonly the first site to show abnormality. (2) Systemic symptoms, particularly of fever and persistent coughing, are frequent findings. Anorexia, weight loss, lymphadenopathy, and hepatosplenomegaly can be additional findings. Ocular abnormalities most commonly manifest as uveitis (6); however, iritis and iridocyclitis can occur.

A skin rash over the face, neck, and shoulders, consisting of discrete red nodules, or purple in hue (*lupus pernio*), may also be evident (7). Occasionally erythema nodosum is evident over the anterior aspects of the tibia and is a good prognostic sign. (1) An acute onset of sarcoidosis may be heralded by high fever, arthralgia, lymphadenopathy, and erythema nodosum (*Löfgren's syndrome*). (8)

Acute sarcoidosis has a spontaneous rate of remission of approximately 66% (5) and is infrequently associated with bone lesions. (1) Conversely, an insidious onset of sarcoidosis usually occurs in patients > 40 years of age and results in debilitating and often fatal systemic fibrosis, especially in the lungs. Bone lesions appear more commonly in this chronic form and often parallel the presence of skin lesions. (1) Skeletal involvement is manifested in up to 15% of patients (9,10) and is characterized by arthralgia, swelling, and deformity, especially in the hands and feet (1,11); however, almost 50% of these lesions may be asymptomatic. (1) (Fig. 10-246) Although the prognosis generally is excellent, the outcome is fatal in up to 4% of patients. (5)

Laboratory investigations are usually supportive, with anemia, leucopenia, eosinophilia, reversed albumin to globulin (A:G) ratio, and often hypercalcemia. (1) A diagnostic antigen test is the Kveim test involving an intradermal injection of sarcoid tissue suspension and observation for the formation of superficial granulomas. (1) Abnormal calcium metabolism is often an associated finding in sarcoidosis, resulting in osteoporosis (40–55%), hypercalcuria (40–62%) and hypercalcemia (5–10%). (12) Elevated levels of angiotensin-converting enzyme (ACE) is also frequently

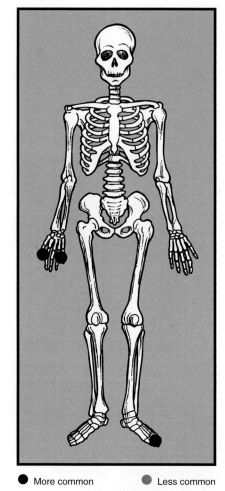

● More common   ● Less common

Figure 10-246   SKELETAL DISTRIBUTION OF SARCOIDOSIS.

present. The definitive diagnosis is made on the basis of histologic examination of a scalene node or liver biopsy. With osseous sarcoidosis, treatment is usually ineffective in regard to disease progression but should be provided for pain and swelling reduction. (13) Steroidal treatment is currently the treatment of choice. (14)

Pathologic Features

The pathologic appearances of sarcoidosis may be variable; (15) however the histopathologic hallmark of sarcoidosis is the presence of a non-caseating granuloma. (3,10) The lesion is identical to that of tuberculosis, except there is no evidence of caseous necrosis or *Mycobacterium*. (2) Examination of the granuloma reveals a compact focus of predominantly epithelioid cells in association with lymphocytes, giant cells, and plasma cells. The lesion acts primarily as a space-occupying mass that within bone results in a surrounding pressure atrophy of trabeculae. (3) The most common tissues in which these granulomas occur are within the lymph nodes, spleen, and liver. Resolution of the granulomatous foci leads to fibrous tissue replacement that, if extensive, may permanently inhibit the function of the affected organ.

Radiologic Features

The most common sites for radiographic depiction of distinctive manifestations of sarcoidosis are the chest (16) and small bones of the hands and feet. (9) (Table 10-80) Skeletal involvement has been estimated to occur in up to 15% of cases, especially in long-standing chronic disease. (1,3)

Target Sites of Involvement

Hands, Wrists, Feet. The hand is the most common site of osseous sarcoidosis, especially the middle and distal phalanges. (1,3,17) To a lesser extent lesions may be encountered in the proximal phalanges and metacarpals. Wrist and foot involvement is less frequent. Lesions are often bilateral but invariably asymmetric. (Fig. 10-247) Bone lesions are caused by the effects of sarcoid granulomas within the bone marrow spaces or per-osseous tissues. (3) A broad spectrum of radiographic abnormalities may be evident. (3) (Table 10-81) The most common presentations are the diffuse reticular and well-circumscribed types that may be superimposed on each other. (1,3,17) (Fig. 10-248)
Diffuse Reticular Pattern. The diffuse pattern is a manifestation of diffuse intraosseous perivascular granulomas infiltrating the Haversian canals and eroding the adjacent fine trabeculae. (Fig. 10-248A) Radiographically, the trabecular pattern in the medullary cavity appears coarse, prominent, and mildly osteoporotic. (3) As the infiltrates enlarge a distinct *lace-like trabecular pattern* emerges with more prominent areas of radiolucency. (17)

Table 10-80	Sites of Predilection in Sarcoidosis

Common
  Chest
    Lymph nodes (bronchopulmonary and paratracheal)
    Interstitium
  Hands
    Middle and distal phalanges
  Wrists
  Feet
    Middle and distal phalanges
Uncommon
  Spine
  Pelvis, skull
  Long bones

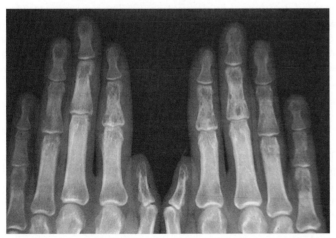

Figure 10-247 **SARCOIDOSIS: BILATERAL AND ASYMMETRIC DISTRIBUTION. PA Hands.** Note that well-circumscribed radiolucent osseous lesions are seen in multiple phalanges.

Well-Circumscribed Pattern. Localized rarefactions may occur simultaneously with a well-circumscribed pattern or as isolated expressions of the disorder. (Fig. 10-248, *B* and *C*) Distinctively, these cystic lucencies are round to ovoid, central or eccentric,

Table 10-81	Radiologic Patterns of Osseous Sarcoidosis

Common
  Circumscribed, lytic medullary defects
  Diffuse reticular pattern (lace-like)
Uncommon
  Mutilating form
  Bone resorption (especially distal phalanx)
  Sclerotic—diffuse or localized
  Periostitis
  Soft tissue nodules

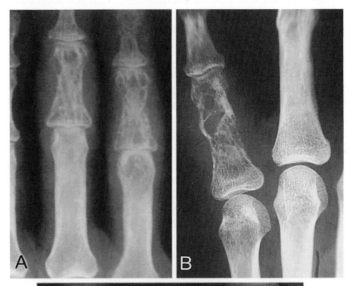

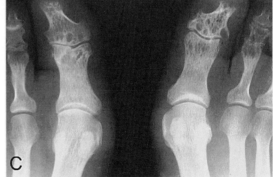

Figure 10-248 **SARCOIDOSIS: GENERAL CHARACTERISTICS. A. Hand: Infiltrative (Lace-Like) Variety.** Observe the coarsened trabeculae and the numerous interspersed small areas of loss in bone density. This appearance is owing to a perivascular granulomatous infiltration into the marrow cavity. **B. Hand: Combined Infiltrative and Well-Circumscribed Lesions.** Note the proximal aspect of the fifth phalanx shows the small, regular lesions of the early infiltrative type; distally, larger, more well-circumscribed defects are evident. **C. Toes.** Note the multiple, well-circumscribed cystic radiolucencies in the great toes bilaterally. Additional lesions are evident in the second right toe. The bilateral distribution and pattern of destruction are distinctive for foot involvement in sarcoidosis.

and well marginated. (1,2,17) Endosteal scalloping but no periosteal response are additional features. Rarely, progressive enlargement of these lesions may lead to crippling and grossly deforming bone destruction. Other findings may include resorption or sclerosis of the distal phalanx. (18)

Joints of the hands, wrists, and feet are often completely normal, but infrequently may exhibit mild loss of joint space, joint effusion, and subchondral collapse. (3)

Other Skeletal Sites. Involvement of other skeletal structures is distinctly uncommon. In long bones, a reticular or well-circumscribed destructive pattern within bone may occur, and periosteal response is rarely encountered. (19) Skull lesions are also uncommon, being lytic and non-specific in appearance. (20) Involvement of muscle with tumor-like masses can be difficult to differentiate from neoplasms, although marked uptake of gallium and technetium isotopes is characteristic in sarcoid masses. (21)

Vertebral sarcoidosis is rare. (22) Up to 75% of cases involve the lumbar spine and 25% the cervical spine. (23) It is most commonly limited to the vertebral body, especially at the thoracolumbar junction. (4) Notably, the intervertebral discs remain unaffected. Individual vertebral lesions can be lytic, surrounded by marginal reactive sclerosis. (24) Rarely, diffuse or solitary blastic lesions may simulate metastatic carcinoma. (20,25–27) MRI can show leptomeningeal and bone lesions, when plain films are normal, as low signal on T1- and high signal on T2-weighted images. (23)

Chest. Radiographic examination of the chest is frequently the method for initial diagnosis. (2) (Fig. 10-249) Diagnostic findings as seen on the PA view are bilateral bronchopulmonary and right paratracheal lymphadenopathy (*1-2-3 sign*). Bronchopulmonary lymph node enlargement (*potato nodes*) is identified as a fusiform opaque enlargement immediately lateral to the hilus, separated from the heart by a lucent layer of interposed lung. At various stages of the disease, additional findings include alveolar infiltrates, interstitial nodules, and fibrosis (*honeycomb lung*). (2,17)

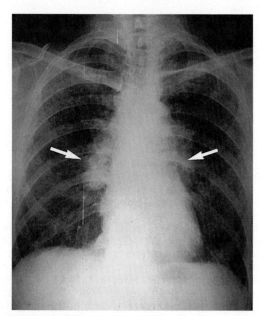

Figure 10-249   SARCOIDOSIS: CHEST. Observe the bronchopulmonary lymphadenopathy (potato nodes) (*arrows*) and the diffuse interstitial lung-field opacities.

CAPSULE SUMMARY   Sarcoidosis

General Considerations

- Systemic disease of young adults characterized by disseminated non-caseating granulomas, especially in the reticuloendothelial system.

Clinical Features

- At 20–40 years; equal sex distribution.
- More common in black and Scandinavian individuals.
- Symptoms include rash, fever, lymphadenopathy, fatigue, weight loss, arthralgia, and iritis.
- Laboratory shows elevated ESR, reversed A:G ratio, hypercalcemia, and positive Kveim test.
- *Löfgren's syndrome:* fever, arthralgia, erythema nodosum, and lymphadenopathy.

Pathologic Features

- Disseminated non-caseating granulomas, which resolve with fibrosis.

Radiologic Features

- Skeletal involvement in 15% of sarcoid patients.
- Most commonly in hands, wrists, and feet.
- Reticular and/or circumscribed lytic intraosseous lesions.
- Joints usually normal.
- Spine, pelvis, skull, and long bones rarely involved. Occasionally blastic lesions observed particularly in the axial skeleton. MRI may show lesions when plain films are normal.
- Pulmonary signs include lymphadenopathy (1-2-3 sign, potato nodes), infiltrates, and fibrosis.

PIGMENTED VILLONODULAR SYNOVITIS

Pigmented villonodular synovitis (PVNS) is an uncommon inflammatory lesion of the synovial tissue lining the joints and tendon sheaths. (1) Its cause is unknown. The first documented case was made in 1852 by Chassaignac (2) and in 1891, Hertaux again recorded its presence by description. (3) The term *pigmented villonodular synovitis* was not used until 1941, when named by Jaffe. (2) The incidence of this condition is rare, accounting for only 1–3 cases per million people. (2) Its classification as an inflammatory arthritic condition is doubted by many who believe it to be a benign synovial neoplasm. (4)

Clinical Features

The majority of patients are young to middle-aged adults. Males are slightly more affected. Any location where synovial tissue is found can be affected; however, the most common sites involve the lower extremities, particularly the knee (2,5) and hip. (5,6) Other joints, which account for < 5% of the cases, involve the ankle, wrist, hand, and foot. (6) (Fig. 10-250) It rarely presents in the elbow, shoulder, and spine but may originate from a lumbar facet joint similar to a synovial cyst, causing extradural compression symptoms such as radicular pain. (2,7–10) Polyarticular involvement is extremely uncommon. (11,12) The usual findings include

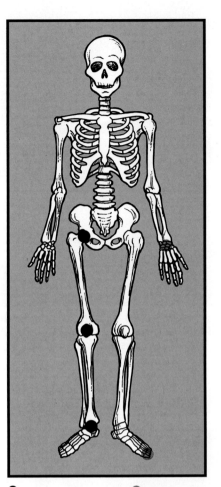

● More common   ● Less common

Figure 10-250 **SKELETAL DISTRIBUTION OF PIGMENTED VILLONODULAR SYNOVITIS.**

insidious and slowly progressive joint swelling, stiffness, and locking. Within the knee the initial presumptive diagnosis is often a meniscal injury, although a history of trauma is frequently lacking.

Arthroscopy may be a useful tool in the diagnosis, but should be confirmed on histologic evaluation by the presence of a brown or serosanguineous synovial fluid aspirate. (13) No other laboratory tests will be positive. Steroidal injections have been employed as a means of treatment but is often of limited benefit. (14) Arthroscopic complete synovectomy is the treatment of choice; however, on excision recurrence is common, ranging between 25% and 45%. (15–18) Radiation therapy may be of benefit in the reduction of recurrence postsurgically. (19) Patients who received radiation therapy had a recurrence rate of only 4%. (18) Malignant degeneration is extremely rare. (5,15)

Pathologic Features

Histologic evaluations are often misinterpreted as being a sarcoma or benign neoplasm. The lesion may be termed localized or diffuse, depending on the amount of synovial tissue involved. The pathogenesis of the synovitis is undefined; however, connective tissue hyperplasia, phagocytic cellular infiltrations, and the deposition of hemosiderin characterize the microscopic appearance. (20) Gross examination reveals large, folded masses that appear red

and brown in color. Notably, these masses, when in close opposition to a bony surface, will cause an extrinsic pressure erosion. These bony defects are far more prevalent in tightly constricted or compartmentalized joints, such as the hip, ankle, and wrist.

Radiologic Features

Both soft tissue and bone abnormalities occur in pigmented villonodular synovitis. (21,22) (Table 10-82)

Soft Tissue

Abnormalities in the soft tissues consist of intra-articular effusions, dense lobulated masses, and displacement of overlying fascial planes. (Fig. 10-251) The soft tissue masses are best evaluated by arthrography, CT, or MRI scan. Angiograms demonstrate a vascular lesion, indistinguishable from a malignant soft tissue tumor with neovascularity, *puddling,* and a *tumor blush.* (23) Despite this vascularity, PVNS does not enhance with contrast on CT. Arthrography reveals a nodular intrinsic filling defect of the joint cavity. MR imaging is the modality of choice (14,24) and will characteristically reveal the synovial lining as a low signal intensity on T1 and T2 images. (25) This finding is characteristic of the hemosiderin deposition seen in PVNS. (25,26) Other MRI findings are joint edema, as a low signal on T1- and high signal on T2-weighted images. (23) (Fig. 10-252) Ultrasound shows a soft tissue mass with some solid and cystic areas. (23)

Bone

In articulations where there is room for intra-articular expansion, such as the knee and shoulder, bone lesions are infrequent. (27) Conversely, "tight" joints such as the hip, ankle, elbow, wrist, and hand often demonstrate associated bone defects. In the hip, concentric erosion of the femoral neck produces an *apple core deformity.* (28,29) (Figs. 10-253 and 10-254) Bony lesions that reveal marginal erosions and smooth, well-defined cortical excavations, which may give the bone a *bubbly appearance,* are suggestive of the diagnosis. (Fig. 10-254) When present, these bone abnormalities usually occur on all bony joint components. These may also simulate other synovial lesions, such as rheumatoid arthritis and gout. (Figs. 10-255 and 10-256) CT defines clearly the extrinsic bone erosions, which usually exhibit a sclerotic margin. MRI of bone lesions shows the adjacent marrow to be of low signal intensity. (23) (See Chapter 6.)

Table 10-82	Radiologic Features of Pigmented Villonodular Synovitis
Lower extremity: knee most common	
Bone	
Marginal erosions	
Pressure erosions	
Opposing bone surfaces	
Soft tissue	
Effusion	
Dense, lobulated soft tissue masses	
Arthrographic filling defects	

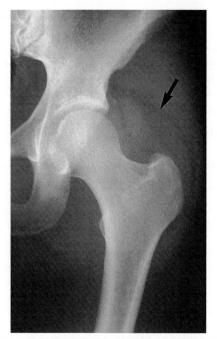

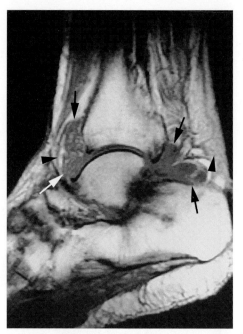

Figure 10-251   **PIGMENTED VILLONODULAR SYNOVITIS: HIP.** Note the distended gluteus medius fascial plane, indicating capsular distension (*arrow*). No bone erosions are present.

Figure 10-252   **PIGMENTED VILLONODULAR SYNOVITIS: T1-Weighted MRI. Sagittal Ankle.** Note that on MRI, low signal intensity soft tissue masses are demonstrated (*arrows*).

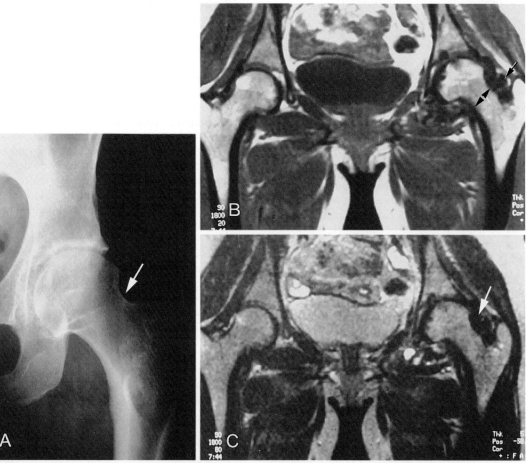

Figure 10-253   **PIGMENTED VILLONODULAR SYNOVITIS.**
A. AP Hip. Note that no overt changes are evident, though there is a suggestion of an apple core deformity on the lateral margin (*arrow*). **B. T1-Weighted MRI: Coronal Hip.** Observe the low signal intensity soft tissue mass within the joint capsule (*arrow*). The concentric narrowing of the femoral neck (apple core deformity) is more apparent (*arrowheads*). **C. T2-Weighted MRI: Coronal Hip.** Note the soft tissue mass remains of low signal intensity (*arrow*). The marrow signal from the proximal femur is generally diminished. (Courtesy of Joseph N. Fiore, DC, Pasadena, Maryland.)

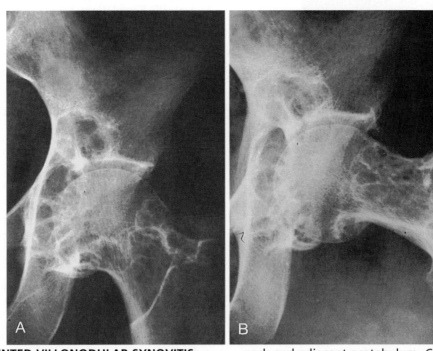

Figure 10-254   **PIGMENTED VILLONODULAR SYNOVITIS: HIP. A. AP Hip.** Note the multiple intra-articular erosions within the acetabulum and femoral neck. **B. Frog-Leg Hip.** Observe the multiple extrinsic bone erosions at the femoral neck and adjacent acetabulum. *COMMENT:* The femoral neck is concentrically narrowed, producing an apple core deformity, characteristic of a synovial-based disease. (Courtesy of Paul E. Siebert, MD, Denver, Colorado.)

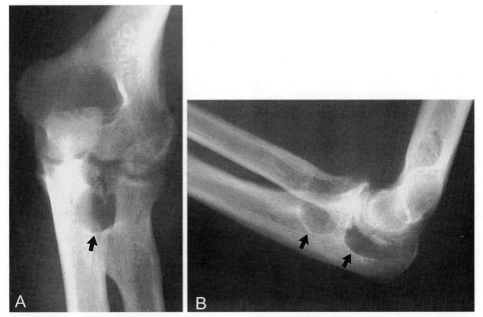

Figure 10-255   **PIGMENTED VILLONODULAR SYNOVITIS: ELBOW. A. Oblique Elbow. B. Lateral Elbow.** Note the extrinsic bone erosions, which are prominent on the ulna (*arrows*). (Courtesy of Steven P. Brownstein, MD, Springfield, New Jersey.)

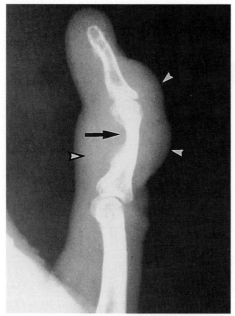

Figure 10-256 PIGMENTED VILLONODULAR SYNOVITIS: FINGER. Note the extrinsic bone erosion on the palmar surface of the middle phalanx (*arrow*) in association with the soft tissue mass (*arrowheads*). (Courtesy of Bryan Hartley, MD, Melbourne, Australia.)

CAPSULE SUMMARY
Pigmented Villonodular Synovitis

General Considerations

- Inflammatory synovial lesion of unknown cause.

Clinical Features

- Young to middle-aged adults, especially males.
- Lower extremities, monoarticular, especially in the knee.
- Joint swelling, stiffness, and locking.
- Brown or serosanguineous synovial aspirate.
- Tend to recur.

Pathologic Features

- Connective tissue hyperplasia, phagocytes, and hemosiderin deposition.
- Results in large, lobulated, intraarticular, soft tissue masses.

Radiologic Features

- *Soft tissue:* dense, lobulated masses and effusion.
- Ultrasound shows a mixture of solid and cystic matrix.
- CT demonstrates a mass that does not enhance. MRI shows a heterogeneous mass with intermediate and hypointense signal areas. Angiography shows neovascularity identical to soft tissue sarcoma.
- *Bone:* marginal erosions and extrinsic defects on opposing articular surfaces. Apple core deformity of the proximal femur.

■ References

INTRODUCTION TO RADIOLOGIC INTERPRETATION IN JOINT DISEASE

1. **Arthritis Foundation: Arthritis: A Serious Look at the Facts** [Pamphlet 5785/1-82]. Atlanta, Arthritis Foundation, 1982.
2. **Forrester DM, Brown JC:** *The radiographic assessment of arthritis. The plain film.* Clin Rheum Dis 9(2):291, 1983.

PERSPECTIVES IN INTERPRETATION OF JOINT DISEASE

1. **Edeiken J:** *Radiologic approach to arthritis.* Semin Roentgenol 28(1):8, 1982.
2. **Robinson WD:** *The problem of diagnosis in arthritis.* Med Clin North Am 45(5):1117, 1961.
3. **Wood PHN:** *Age of the rheumatic diseases. Population studies of the rheumatic diseases.* Int Congress ser. 148:26, 1968.

RADIOLOGIC CONSIDERATIONS

1. **Forrester DM, Brown JC, Nesson JW:** *The Radiology of Joint Disease,* ed 2. Philadelphia, WB Saunders, 1978.

DIFFERENTIAL DIAGNOSIS OF ARTHRITIS

1. **Forrester DM, Brown JC:** *The radiographic assessment of arthritis. The plain film.* Clin Rheum Dis 9(2):291, 1983.
2. **Robinson WD:** *The problem of diagnosis in arthritis.* Med Clin North Am 45(5):1117, 1961.
3. **Wiesel SW, Tsourmas N, Feffer HL, et al.:** *A study of computer-assisted tomography. I. The incidence of positive CAT scans in an asymptomatic group of patients.* Spine 9:549, 1984.
4. **Jensen MC, Brant-Zawadzki MN, Obuchowski N, et al.:** *Magnetic resonance imaging of the lumbar spine in people without back pain.* N Engl J Med 331:69, 1994.
5. **Boden SD, McGowan PR, Davis DO, et al.:** *Abnormal magnetic-resonance scans of the cervical spine in asymptomatic subjects.* J Bone Joint Surg 72A:1178, 1990.
6. **Yochum TR, Rowe LJ:** *Arthritides of the Upper Cervical Complex.* In: *Aspects of Manipulative Therapy,* ed 2. Melbourne, Australia, Churchill Livingstone, 1985.

DEGENERATIVE DISORDERS

DEGENERATIVE JOINT DISEASE

1. **Tarnopolsky S:** *Revision de la nomenclature rhumatologique I. Les nomes de l'arthrose.* Rev Rhum 17:497, 1950.
2. **Oppenheimer A:** *Calcification and ossification of vertebral ligaments (spondylitis ossificans ligamentosa).* Radiology 38:160, 1942.
3. **Kellgren JH, Moore R:** *Generalised osteoarthritis and Heberden's nodes.* Br Med J 1:181, 1952.
4. **Kellgren JH, Lawrence JS, Bier F:** *Genetic factors in generalized osteo-arthrosis.* Ann Rheum Dis 22:237, 1963.
5. **Kellgren JH, Lawrence JS:** *Osteoarthrosis and disc degeneration in an urban population.* Ann Rheum Dis 17:388, 1958.
6. **Nesterov AI:** *The clinical course of Kashin-Beck disease.* Arthritis Rheum 7(1):29, 1964.
7. **McRae DL:** *The significance of abnormalities of the cervical spine.* AJR 84:3, 1960.
8. **Phoon S, Manolios N:** *Glucosamine. A nutraceutical in osteoarthritis.* Aust Fam Physician 31(6):539, 2002.
9. **Sheehan S, Bauer R, Meyer J:** *Vertebral artery compression in cervical spondylosis.* Neurology 10:968, 1960.
10. **Rowe LJ:** *The radiology of ageing. Geriatric Symposium Proceedings: Quality Health Care of the Elderly.* Minneapolis, Northwestern College of Chiropractic, 1986.
11. **Aigner T, Kurz B, Fukui N, Sandell L:** *Roles of chondrocytes in the pathogenesis of osteoarthritis.* Curr Opin Rheumatol 14(5):578, 2002.
12. **Farfan HF, Gracovetsky S:** *The nature of instability.* Spine 9:714, 1984.
13. **Bogduk N, Twomey LT:** *Clinical Anatomy of the Lumbar Spine,* ed 2. Melbourne, Churchill Livingstone, 1991.
14. **Aoki J, Yamamoto I, Kitamura N, et al.:** *End plate of the discovertebral joint: Degenerative change in the elderly adult.* Radiology 164:411, 1987.

15. **Kauppila LI, Penttila A, Karhunen P, et al.:** *Lumbar disc degeneration and atherosclerosis of the abdominal aorta.* Spine 19:923, 1994.
16. **Unger K, Rahimi F, Bareither D, Muehleman C:** *The relationship between articular cartilage degeneration and bone changes of the first metatarsophalangeal joint.* J Foot Ankle Surg 39(1);24, 2000.
17. **Nathan H:** *Osteophytes of the vertebral column. An anatomic study of their development according to age, race and sex, with consideration to their etiology and significance.* J Bone Joint Surg 31A:619, 1962.
18. **Resnick D, Niwayama G, Coults RD:** *Subchondral cysts (geodes) in arthritic disorders. Pathologic and radiographic appearance of the hip joint.* AJR 128:799, 1977.
19. **Bolton PS, Ware AE:** *Degenerative joint disease in the cervical spine of chiropractic patients.* J Austral Chiro Assoc 18:51, 1988.
20. **Gore DR, Sepic SR, Gardner GM:** *Roentgenographic findings of the cervical spine in asymptomatic people.* Spine 11:521, 1986.
21. **Berlemann U, Laubli R, Moore RJ:** *Degeneration of the atlanto-axial joints: A histological study of 9 cases.* Acta Orthop Scand 73(2):130, 2002.
22. **Star MJ, Curd JG, Thorne RP:** *Atlantoaxial lateral mass osteoarthritis. A frequently overlooked cause of severe occipitocervical pain.* Spine 17:S71, 1992.
23. **Benitah S, Raftopoulos C, Baleriaux D, et al.:** *Upper cervical spinal cord compression due to bony stenosis of the spinal canal.* Neuroradiology 36:231, 1994.
24. **Genez BM, Willis JJ, Lowrey CE, et al.:** *CT findings of degenerative arthritis of the atlantoodontoid joint.* AJR 154:315, 1990.
25. **Rowe LJ:** *The split vertebral body: A pseudofracture.* J Austral Chiro Assoc 29:5, 1990.
26. **Daffner RH, Deeb ZL, Rothfis WE:** *Pseudofractures of the cervical vertebral body.* Skeletal Radiol 15:295, 1986.
27. **Constantin P, Lucretia C:** *Relations between the cervical spine and the vertebral arteries.* Acta Radiol 11:91, 1971.
28. **Macnab I:** *Cervical spondylosis.* Clin Orthop 109:69, 1975.
29. **Yousem DM, Atlas SW, Goldberg HI:** *Degenerative narrowing of the cervical foramina: Evaluation with high-resolution 3DFT gradient-echo MR imaging.* AJNR 12:229, 1991.
30. **Reymond RD, Wheeler PS, Perovie M, et al.:** *The lucent cleft, a new radiographic sign of cervical disc injury or disease.* Clin Radiol 23:188, 1972.
31. **Facer MJC:** *Osteophytes of the cervical spine causing dysphagia.* Arch Otolaryngol 86:117, 1967.
32. **Ogino H, Tada K, Okada K, et al.:** *Canal diameter, anteroposterior compression ratio and spondylotic myelopathy of the cervical spine.* Spine 8(1):1, 1983.
33. **Proctor D, Dupuis P, Cassidy JD:** *Thoracolumbar syndrome as a cause of low-back pain: A report of two cases.* J Can Chiro Assoc 29:71, 1985.
34. **Dreyfus P, Tibliletti C, Dreyer SJ:** *Thoracic zygapophyseal joint pain patterns.* Spine 19:807, 1994.
35. **Robert FW:** *Costotransverse arthrosis of the tenth dorsal vertebra (D10).* AJR 134:423, 1980.
36. **Yochum TR:** *Robert's syndrome.* ACA J Chiro November, 1982.
37. **Benhamou CL, Roux C, Tourliere D, et al.:** *Pseudovisceral pain referred from costovertebral arthropathies.* Spine 18:790, 1993.
38. **Culver GJ, Pirson HS:** *Preventative effect of aortic pulsations on osteophytic formation in the thoracic spine.* AJR 84(5):937, 1960.
39. **Shapiro R, Balt H:** *Unilateral thoracic spondylosis.* AJR 83(4):660, 1960.
40. **Nathan HA, Schwartz A:** *Inverted pattern of development of thoracic vertebral osteophytosis in situs inversus and in other instances of right sided aorta.* Radiol Clin (Basel) 31:150, 1962.
41. **Schmorl G, Junghanns H:** *The Human Spine in Health and Disease,* ed 2, trans EF Besemann. New York, Grune & Stratton, 1971.
42. **Fujiwara A, Tamai K, An HS, et al.:** *Orientation and osteoarthritis of the lumbar facet joint.* Clin Orthop Apr(385):88, 2001.
43. **Pathria M, Sartoris DJ, Resnick D:** *Osteoarthritis of the facet joints: Accuracy of oblique radiographic assessment.* Radiology 164:227, 1987.
44. **Abel MS:** *The unstable apophyseal joint: An early sign of lumbar disc disease.* Skeletal Radiol 2:31, 1977.
45. **Pate D, Goobar J, Resnick D, et al.:** *Traction osteophytes of the lumbar spine: Radiographic-pathologic correlation.* Radiology 166:843, 1988.
46. **Macnab I:** *The traction spur: An indicator of segmental instability.* J Bone Joint Surg 33A:663, 1971.
47. **Frymoyer JW, Newberg A, Pope MH, et al.:** *Spine radiographs in patients with low-back pain.* J Bone Joint Surg 66A:1048, 1984.
48. **Knuttson F:** *The vacuum phenomenon in the intervertebral discs.* Acta Radiol 23:173, 1942.
49. **Ford LT, Gilula LA, Murphy WA, et al.:** *Analysis of gas in vacuum lumbar disc.* AJR 128:1056, 1977.
50. **Marr JT:** *Gas in intervertebral discs.* AJR 70:804, 1953.
51. **Gershon-Cohen J:** *The phantom nucleus pulposus.* AJR 56(1):43, 1946.
52. **Rowe LJ:** *Vacuum phenomenon.* J Austral Chiro Assoc 18:125, 1988.
53. **Resnick D, Niwayama G, Guerra, J et al.:** *Spinal vacuum phenomena: Anatomical study and review.* Radiology 139:341, 1981.
54. **Fuiks DM, Grayson CE:** *Vacuum pneumarthrography and the spontaneous occurrence of gas in the joint spaces.* J Bone Joint Surg 32A:933, 1950.
55. **Williams JL:** *Gas in the symphysis pubis during and following pregnancy.* AJR 73(3):403, 1955.
56. **Rowe LJ:** *Degenerative disc space narrowing—Differential considerations.* J Austral Chiro Assoc 19:60, 1989.
57. **Rosenburg NJ:** *Degenerative spondylolisthesis. Predisposing factors.* J Bone Joint Surg 57A:467, 1975.
58. **Rowe LJ, Steiman I:** *Anterolisthesis in the cervical spine—Spondylolysis.* J Manipulative Physiol Ther 10:11, 1987.
59. **Lee C, Woodring JH, Rogers LF, et al.:** *The radiographic distinction of degenerative slippage (spondylolisthesis and retrolisthesis) from traumatic slippage of the cervical spine.* Skeletal Radiol 15:439, 1986.
60. **Pope MH, Frymoyer JW, Krag MH:** *Diagnosing instability.* Clin Orthop 279:60, 1992.
61. **Friberg O:** *Lumbar instability: A dynamic approach by traction-compression radiography.* Spine 12:119, 1987.
62. **Dupuis PR, Yong-Hing K, Cassidy JD, et al.:** *Radiologic diagnosis of degenerative spinal instability.* Spine 10:262, 1985.
63. **Pearcy MJ:** *Stereoradiography of lumbar spine motion.* Acta Orthop Scand (Suppl) 212:1, 1985.
64. **White AA, Johnson RM, Panjabi MM:** *Biomechanical analysis of clinical stability in the cervical spine.* Clin Orthop 109:85, 1975.
65. **Kirkaldy-Willis WH, Hill RJ:** *A more precise diagnosis of low back pain.* Spine 4(2):102, 1979.
66. **Cassidy JD, Mior S:** *Lateral nerve entrapment: Pathological, clinical and manipulative considerations.* J Can Chiro Assoc 26(1):13, 1982.
67. **Ben-Elijahu D, Rutili M, Przybysz J:** *Lateral recess syndrome; Diagnosis and chiropractic management.* J Manipulative Physiol Ther 6(1):25, 1983.
68. **Gorey MT, Hyman RA, Black KS, et al.:** *Lumbar synovial cysts eroding bone.* AJNR 13:161, 1992.
69. **Quaghebeur G, Jeffree M:** *Synovial cyst of the high cervical spine causing myelopathy.* AJNR 13:981, 1992.
70. **Schulz EE, West WL, Hinshaw DB, et al.:** *Gas in a lumbar extradural juxtaarticular cyst: A sign of synovial origin.* AJR: 143, 875, 1984.
71. **Jackson DE, Atlas SW, Mani JR, et al.:** *Intraspinal synovial cysts: MR imaging.* Radiology 170:527, 1990.
72. **Dilhmann W:** *Hemispherical spondylosclerosis—A polyetiologic syndrome.* Skeletal Radiol 7:99, 1981.
73. **Rowe LJ:** *Hemispherical spondylosclerosis: A case report.* J Austral Chiro Assoc 18:55, 1988.

74. **Baastrup CI:** *On the spinous processes of the lumbar vertebrae and the soft tissues between them, and on pathological changes in that region.* Acta Radiol (Stockh) 14:52, 1933.

75. **Franck S:** *Surgical treatment of interspinal osteoarthrosis ("kissing spine").* Acta Orthop Scand 14:127, 1943.

76. **Sartoris DJ, Resnick D, Tyson R, et al.:** *Age-related alterations in vertebral spinous processes and intervening soft tissues: Radiologic-pathologic correlation.* AJR 145:1025, 1985.

77. **Bowen V, Cassidy JD:** *Macroscopic and microscopic anatomy of the sacroiliac joint from embryonic life until the eighth decade.* Spine 6(6):620, 1981.

78. **Resnick D, Niwayama G, Georgen TG:** *Comparison of radiographic abnormalities of the sacroiliac joint in degenerative disease and ankylosing spondylitis.* AJR 128:189, 1977.

79. **Kumar B, Sriram KG, George C:** *Osteophyte at the sacroiliac joint as a cause of sciatica: a report of four cases.* J Orthop Surg (Hong Kong) 10(1):73, 2002.

80. **Healy JH, Vigorita VJ, Lane JM:** *The coexistence and characteristics of osteoarthritis and osteoporosis.* J Bone Joint Surg 67A:586, 1985.

81. **Resnick D:** *Patterns of migration of the femoral head in osteoarthritis of the hip. Roentgenographic-pathologic correlation and comparison with rheumatoid arthritis.* AJR 124:62, 1975.

82. **Haywood I, Bjorkengren AG, Pathria M, et al.:** *Patterns of femoral head migration in osteoarthritis of the hip: A reappraisal with CT and pathologic correlation.* Radiology 166:857, 1988.

83. **Pessis E, Chevrot A, Grape JL, et al.:** *Study of the joints space of the hip on supine and weight-bearing digital radiographs.* Clin Radiol 54(8):528, 1999.

84. **Yoshida M, Konishi N:** *Subchondral cysts arise in the anterior acetabulum in dysplastic osteoarthritic hips.* Clin Orthop Nov(404): 291, 2002.

85. **Resnick D:** *The "tilt deformity" of the femoral head in osteoarthritis of the hip: A poor indicator of previous epiphysiolysis.* Clin Radiol 27:355, 1976.

86. **Mont MA, Radjadhyaksha AD, Low K, et al.:** *Anatomy of the knee extensor mechanism: correlation with patellofemoral arthrosis.* J South Orthop Assoc 10(1):24, 2001.

87. **Kerrigan DC, Lelas JL, Karvosky ME:** *Women's shoes and knee osteoarthritis.* Lancet 357(9262):1097, 2001.

88. **Bergman AG, Willen HK, Lindstrand AL, et al.:** *Osteoarthritis of the knee: Correlation of subchondral MR signal abnormalities with histopathologic and radiographic features.* Skeletal Radiol 23:445, 1994.

89. **Ahlback S:** *Osteoarthritis of the knee. A radiographic examination.* Acta Radiol (Suppl) 277, 1968.

90. **Ostlere SJ, Seeger LL, Eckardt JJ:** *Subchondral cysts of the knee.* Skeletal Radiol 19:287, 1990.

91. **Greenspan A, Norman A, Tchang FK:** *"Tooth" sign in patella degenerative disease.* J Bone Joint Surg 59A:483, 1977.

92. **Budinger K:** *Uber auosung von gelenksteilen und verwandte prozesse.* Deutsche Z Chir 84:311, 1906.

93. **Outerbridge RE, Dunlop JA:** *The problem of chondromalacia patellae.* Clin Orthop 110:177, 1975.

94. **Insall J, Falvo KA, Wise DW:** *Chondromalacia patellae. A prospective study.* J Bone Joint Surg 58A:1, 1976.

95. **Wiles P, Andrews PS, Bremner RA:** *Chondromalacia of the patella. A study of later results of excision of articular cartilage.* J Bone Joint Surg 42B:65, 1960.

96. **McCauley TR, Kier R, Lynch KJ, et al.:** *Chondromalacia patellae: Diagnosis with MR imaging.* AJR 158:101, 1992.

97. **Abernathy PJ, Townsend PR, Rose RM, et al.:** *Is chondromalacia patellae a separate clinical entity?* J Bone Joint Surg 60B:205, 1978.

98. **Insall J, Salvati E:** *Patella position in the normal knee joint.* Radiology 101:101, 1971.

99. **Resnick D:** *Talar ridges, osteophytes and beaks: A radiologic commentary.* Radiology 151:329, 1984.

EROSIVE OSTEOARTHRITIS

1. **Crain DC:** *Interphalangeal osteoarthritis characterized by painful inflammatory episodes resulting in deformity of the proximal and distal articulations.* JAMA 175:1049, 1961.

2. **Ehrlich GE:** *Erosive osteoarthritis: Presentation, clinical pearls, and therapy.* Curr Rheumatol Rep 3(6):484, 2001.

3. **Ehrlich GE:** *Osteoarthritis beginning with inflammation. Definitions and correlations.* JAMA 232:157, 1975.

4. **Rovetta G, Monteforte P, Molfetta D, Balestra V:** *Chondroitin sulfate in erosive osteoarthritis of the hands.* Int J Tissue React 24(1):29, 2002

5. **Greenway G, Resnick D, Weisman M, et al.:** *Carpal involvement in inflammatory (erosive) osteoarthritis.* J Can Assoc Radiol 30:95, 1979.

6. **Marmor L, Peter JB:** *Osteoarthritis of the hand.* Clin Orthop 64:164, 1969.

7. **Martel W, Stuck KJ, Dworin AM, et al.:** *Erosive osteoarthritis and psoriatic arthritis: A radiologic comparison in the hand, wrist and foot.* AJR 134:125, 1980.

DIFFUSE IDIOPATHIC SKELETAL HYPEROSTOSIS

1. **Resnick D, Shapiro RF, Wiesner KB, et al.:** *Diffuse idiopathic skeletal hyperostosis (DISH). Ankylosing hyperostosis of Forestier and Rotes-Querol.* Semin Arthritis Rheum 7:153, 1978.

2. **Oppenheimer A:** *Calcification and ossification of vertebral ligaments (spondylitis ossificans ligamentosa). Roentgen study of pathogenesis and clinical significance.* Radiology 38:160, 1942.

3. **Forestier J, Rotes-Querol J:** *Senile ankylosing hyperostosis of the spine.* Ann Rheum Dis 9:321, 1950.

4. **Akhtar S, O'Flynn PE, Kelly A, Valentine PM:** *The management of dysphasia in skeletal hyperostosis.* J Laryngol Otol 114(2):154, 2000.

5. **Resnick D, Shaul SR, Robins JM:** *Diffuse idiopathic skeletal hyperostosis (DISH): Forestier's Disease with extraspinal manifestations.* Radiology 115:513, 1975.

6. **Underberg-Davis S, Levine MS:** *Giant thoracic osteophyte causing esophageal food impaction.* AJR 157:319, 1991.

7. **Karlins NL, Yagan R:** *Dyspnea and hoarseness. A complication of diffuse idiopathic skeletal hyperostosis.* Spine 16:235, 1991.

8. **Mader R:** *Clinical manifestations of diffuse idiopathic skeletal hyperostosis of the cervical spine.* Semin Arthritis Rheum 32(2):130, 2002.

9. **Marks B, Schober E, Swoboda H:** *Diffuse idiopathic skeletal hyperostosis causing obstructing laryngeal edema.* Eur Arch Otorhinolaryngol 225(5):256, 1998.

10. **Yagan R, Karlins N:** *Quadriplegia in diffuse idiopathic skeletal hyperostosis after minor trauma.* AJR 147:858, 1986.

11. **Burkus K, Denis F:** *Hyperextension injuries to the thoracic spine in diffuse idiopathic skeletal hyperostosis.* J Bone Joint Surg 76A:237, 1994.

12. **Hendrix RW, Melany M, Miller F, et al.:** *Fracture of the spine in patients with ankylosis due to diffuse skeletal hyperostosis: Clinical and imaging findings.* AJR 162:899, 1994.

13. **Chiba H, Annen S, Shimada T, et al.:** *Atlantoaxial subluxation complicated by diffuse idiopathic skeletal hyperostosis.* Spine 17:1414, 1992.

14. **Fardon DF:** *Odontoid fracture complicating ankylosing hyperostosis of the spine.* Spine 3(2):108, 1978.

15. **Resnick D, Linovitz RJ, Feingold ML:** *Postoperative heterotopic ossification in patients with ankylosing hyperostosis of the spine (Forestier's disease).* J Rheumatol 3:313, 1976.

16. **Ono K, Ota H, Tada K, et al.:** *Ossified posterior longitudinal ligament.* Spine 2:126, 1977.

17. **Alengat J, Hallet M, Kido D:** *Spinal cord compression in diffuse idiopathic skeletal hyperostosis.* Radiology 142:119, 1982.

18. **Kopman R, Weinstein P, Gall E, et al.:** *Lumbar spinal stenosis in a patient with diffuse idiopathic skeletal hypertrophy syndrome.* Spine 7(6):598, 1982.

19. **Foshang TH, Mestan MA, Riggs LJ:** *Diffuse idiopathic skeletal hyperostosis: a case of dysphagia.* J Manipulative Physiol Ther 25(1):71, 2002.

20. **Ozgocmen S, Kiris A, Kocakoc E, Ardicoglu O:** *Osteophyte-induced dysphagia: Report of three cases.* Joint Bone Spine 69(2):226, 2002.
21. **Epstein NE:** *Simultaneous cervical diffuse idiopathic skeletal hyperostosis and ossification of the posterior longitudinal ligament resulting in dysphagia or myelopathy in two geriatric North Americans.* Surg Neurol 53:427, 2000. [Discussion 53:431, 2000.]
22. **Forestier J, Lagier R:** *Ankylosing hyperostosis of the spine.* Clin Orthrop 74:65, 1971.
23. **Hajkova Z, Streda A, Skrha F:** *Hyperostotic spondylosis and diabetes mellitus.* Ann Rheum Dis 24:536, 1965.
24. **Ott VR, Schwenkenbecher H, Iser H:** *Die spondylose bei diabetes mellitus.* Z Rheumaforsch 22:278, 1963.
25. **Rosenthal M, Bahaus I, Muller W:** *Increased frequency of HLA-B8 in hyperostotic spondylosis.* J Rheumatol 4(3):94, 1977.
26. **Julkunen H, Karava R, Biljannen V:** *Hyperostosis of the spine in diabetes mellitus and acromegaly.* Diabetologia 2:123, 1966.
27. **Julkunen H, Heinonen O, Pyorala K:** *Hyperostosis of the spine in an adult population. Its relation to hyperglycemia and obesity.* Ann Rheum Dis 30:605, 1971.
28. **Boulet P, Serre H, Mirouze J:** *Le rachis diabetique.* Semin Hop Paris 30:2392, 1954.
29. **Coaccioli S, Fatati G, Di Cato L, et al.:** *Diffuse idiopathic skeletal hyperostosis in diabetes mellitus, impaired glucose tolerance and obesity.* Panminerva Med 42(4):247, 2000.
30. **Harris J, Carter AR, Glick EN, et al.:** *Ankylosing hyperostosis. I. Clinical and radiological features.* Ann Rheum Dis 33:210, 1974.
31. **Fornasier V, Littlejohn G, Urowitz M, et al.:** *Spinal entheseal new bone formation: The early changes of spinal diffuse idiopathic skeletal hyperostosis.* J Rheumatol 10(6):939, 1983.
32. **Resnick D, Niwayama G:** *Radiographic and pathologic features of spinal involvement in diffuse idiopathic skeletal hyperostosis (DISH).* Radiology 119:559, 1976.
33. **Suzuki K, Ishida Y, Ohmori K:** *Long-term follow-up of diffuse idiopathic skeletal hyperostosis in the cervical spine.* Neuroradiology 33:427, 1991.
34. **Goldwin RL:** *Calcified plaque in the cervical spine with pain and paresthesia.* JAMA 241(6):601, 1979.
35. **Bahrt K, Nashel D, Haber G:** *Diffuse idiopathic skeletal hyperostosis in a patient with situs inversus.* Arthritis Rheum 26(6):811, 1983.
36. **Huang GS, Park YH, Taylor JAM, et al.:** *Hyperostosis of ribs: Association with vertebral ossification.* J Rheumatol 20:2073, 1993.
37. **Littlejohn G, Urowitz M:** *Peripheral enthesopathy in diffuse idiopathic skeletal hyperostosis (DISH). A radiologic study.* J Rheumatol 10(5):784, 1983.
38. **Haller J, Resnick D, Miller CW, et al.:** *Diffuse idiopathic skeletal hyperostosis: Diagnostic significance of radiographic abnormalities of the pelvis.* Radiology 172:835, 1989.

OSSIFIED POSTERIOR LONGITUDINAL LIGAMENT SYNDROME

1. **Tsukimoto H:** *An autopsy report of syndrome of compression of spinal cord owing to ossification within the spinal canal of cervical spine.* Arch Jpn Chiro 29:1, 1960.
2. **Terayama K, Maruyama S, Miyashita R, et al.:** *Ossification of the posterior longitudinal ligament in the cervical spine.* Orthop Surg 15:1083, 1964.
3. **Resnick D, Guerra J, Robinson CA, et al.:** *Association of diffuse idiopathic skeletal hyperostosis (DISH) and calcification and ossification of the posterior longitudinal ligament.* AJR 131:1049, 1978.
4. **Hiramatsu Y, Nobechi T:** *Calcification of the posterior longitudinal ligament of the spine among the Japanese.* Radiology 100:307, 1971.
5. **Wang PN, Chen SS, Liu HC, et al.:** *Ossification of the posterior longitudinal ligament of the spine. A case-control risk factor study.* Spine 24(2):142, 1999. [Discussion 24:145, 1999.]
6. **Ehara S, Shimamura T, Nakamura R, Yamazaki K:** *Paravertebral ligamentous ossification: DISH, OPLL, and OLF.* Eur J Radiol 27(3):196, 1998.

7. **Minagi H, Gronner AT:** *Calcification of the posterior longitudinal ligament: A cause of cervical myelopathy.* AJR 105:365, 1969.
8. **Nakanishi C, Mannen T, Toyokura Y:** *Asymptomatic ossification of the posterior longitudinal ligament of the cervical spine.* J Neurol Sci 19:375, 1973.
9. **Onji Y, Akiyama H, Shimomura Y, et al.:** *Posterior paravertebral ossification causing cervical myelopathy.* J Bone Joint Surg 49A:1314, 1967.
10. **Ono M, Russell W, Kudo, S et al.:** *Ossification of the thoracic posterior longitudinal ligament in a fixed population. Radiological and neurological manifestations.* Radiology 143(2):469, 1982.
11. **Epstein NE:** *Simultaneous cervical diffuse idiopathic skeletal hyperostosis and ossification of the posterior longitudinal ligament resulting in dysphagia or myelopathy in two geriatric North Americans.* Surg Neurol 53:427, 2000. [Discussion 453:31, 2000.]
12. **Palacios E, Brackett CE, Leary DJ:** *Ossification of the posterior longitudinal ligament associated with a herniated intervertebral disc.* Radiology 100:313, 1971.
13. **Hakuda S, Mochizuki T, Ogata M, et al.:** *The pattern of spinal and extraspinal hyperostosis in patients with ossification of the longitudinal ligament and the ligamentum flavum causing myelopathy.* Skeletal Radiol 10(2):79, 1983.
14. **Hirabayashi K, Miyakawa J, Satomi K, et al.:** *Operative results and postoperative progression of ossification among patients with ossification of cervical posterior longitudinal ligament.* Spine 6(4):354, 1981.
15. **Yoshino MT, Seeger JF, Carmody RF:** *MRI diagnosis of thoracic ossification of posterior longitudinal ligament with concomitant disc herniation.* Neuroradiology 33:455, 1991.

NEUROTROPHIC ARTHROPATHY

1. **Shah MK, Hugghins SY:** *Charcot's joint: An overlooked diagnosis.* J La State Med Soc 154:246, 2002.
2. **Sanders LJ:** *Jean-Martin Charcot (1825–1893). The man hehing the joint disease.* J Am Podiatr Med Assoc 92(7):375, 2002.
3. **Martin MM:** *Diabetic neuropathy. A clinical study of 150 cases.* Brain 76:594, 1953.
4. **Sommer TC, Lee TH:** *Charcot foot: The diagnostic dilemma.* Am Fam Physician 64(9):1591, 2001.
5. **Reinhardt K:** *The radiological residua of healed diabetic arthropathies.* Skeletal Radiol 7:167, 1981.
6. **Bjorkengren AG, Weisman M, Pathria MN, et al.:** *Neuroarthropathy associated with chronic alcoholism.* AJR 151:743, 1988.
7. **Brown CW, Jones B, Donaldson DH, et al.:** *Neuropathic (Charcot) arthropathy of the spine after traumatic spinal paraplegia.* Spine 17:S103, 1992.
8. **Cleveland M, Wilson HJ:** *Charcot disease of the spine. Report of two cases treated by spine fusion.* J Bone Joint Surg 41A(2):336, 1959.
9. **Osterhouse MD, Kettner NW:** *Neuropathic osteoarthropathy in the diabetic foot.* J Manipulative Physiol Ther 25(6):416, 2002.
10. **Delano PJ:** *The pathogenesis of Charcot's joint.* AJR 56(2)189:200, 1946.
11. **Norman A, Robbins H, Milgram JE:** *The acute neuropathic arthropathy—A rapid, severely disorganizing form of arthritis.* Radiology 90:1159, 1968.
12. **Brower AC, Allman RM:** *Pathogenesis of the neurotrophic joint: Neurotraumatic vs. neurovascular.* Radiology 139:349, 1981.
13. **Harrison RB:** *Charcot's joint: Two new observations.* AJR 128:807, 1977.
14. **Katz I, Rabinowitz JG, Dziadiw R:** *Early changes in Charcot's joints.* AJR 86(5):965, 1961.
15. **Schwartz GS, Berenyi MR, Siegel MW:** *Atrophic arthropathy of diabetic neuritis.* AJR 106(3):523, 1969.
16. **Feldman F, Johnson AM, Walter JF:** *Acute axial neuroarthropathy.* Radiology 3:1, 1974.
17. **Forrester DM, Brown JC, Nesson JW:** *The Radiology of Joint Disease,* ed 2. Philadelphia, WB Saunders, 1978.

SYNOVIOCHONDROMETAPLASIA

1. **Yu GV, Zema RL, Johnson RW:** *Synovial osteochondromatosis. A case report and review of the literature.* J Am Podiatr Med Assoc 92(4):247, 2002.
2. **Nogueira A, Alcelay O, Pena C, et al.:** *Synovial osteochondromatosis at the elbow producing ulnar and median nerve palsy. Case report and review of the literature.* Chiro Manipulation 18(2):108, 1999.
3. **Zimmerman C, Sayegh V:** *Roentgen manifestations of synovial osteochondromatosis.* AJR 83:680, 1960.
4. **Davis RI, Hamilton A, Biggart JD:** *Primary synovial chondromatosis: A clinicopathological review and assessment of malignant potential.* Jum Pathol 29(7):683, 1998.
5. **Mussey RD, Henderson MS:** *Osteochondromatosis.* J Bone Joint Surg 31A:619, 1949.
6. **Giustra PE, Furman RS, Roberts L, et al.:** *Synovial osteochondromatosis involving the elbow.* AJR 127:347, 1976.
7. **Lewis MM, Marshall JL, Mirra J:** *Synovial chondromatosis of the thumb.* J Bone Joint Surg 56A:180, 1974.
8. **Akhtar M, Mahajan S, Kott E:** *Synovial chondromatosis of the temporomandibular joint.* J Bone Joint Surg 59A:266, 1977.
9. **Birchall D, Khangure MS, Spagnolo DV:** *Vertebral synovial osteochondromatosis with compressive myelopathy.* Spine 24:921, 1999.
10. **Goldberg RP, Genant HK:** *Calcified bodies in popliteal cysts: A characteristic radiographic appearance.* AJR 131:857, 1978.
11. **Milgram JW:** *The development of loose bodies in human joints.* Clin Orthop 124:292, 1977.
12. **Wilson AJ, Ford LT, Gilula LA:** *Migrating mouse: A sign of dissecting popliteal cyst.* AJR 150:867, 1988.
13. **Pope TL, Keats TE, de Lange EE, et al.:** *Idiopathic synovial chondromatosis in two unusual sites: Inferior radioulnar joint and ischial bursa.* Skeletal Radiol 16:205, 1987.
14. **Lagier R:** *Primary synovial osteochondromatosis of the knee with extensive bone formation observed over a period of 13 years. Case report 451.* Skeletal Radiol 16:660, 1987.
15. **Knoeller SM:** *Synovial osteochondromatosis of the hip joint. Etiology, diagnostic investigation and therapy.* Acta Orthop Belg 67(3):201, 2001.
16. **Milgram JW:** *Synovial osteochondromatosis.* J Bone Joint Surg 59A:792, 1977.
17. **Mueller T, Barthel T, Cramer A, et al.:** *Primary synovial chondromatosis of the elbow.* J Shoulder Elbow Surg 9:319, 2000.
18. **Giordano V, Giordano M, Knackfuss IG, Giordano J:** *Synovial osteochondromatosis of the retrocalcaneal bursa: A case study.* Foot Ankle Int 20(8):534, 1999.
19. **Perry BE, Mcqueen DA, Lin JJ:** *Synovial chondromatosis with malignant degeneration to chondrosarcoma.* J Bone Joint Surg 70A:1259, 1988.
20. **Critteraden JJ, Jones DM, Santarelli AG:** *Knee arthrogram in synovial chondromatosis.* Radiology 94:133, 1970.
21. **Wittkop B, Davies AM, Mangham DC:** *Primary synovial chondromatosis and synovial chondrosarcoma: A pictorial review.* Eur Radiol 12:2112, 2002.
22. **Ginaldi S:** *Computed tomography feature of synovial osteochondromatosis.* Skeletal Radiol 5:219, 1980.
23. **Edeiken J, Edeiken BS, Ayala AG, et al.:** *Giant solitary synovial chondromatosis.* Skeletal Radiol 23:23, 1994.
24. **Kim SH, Hong SJ, Park JS, et al.:** *Idiopathic synovial osteochondromatosis of the hip: Radiographic and MR appearances in 15 patients.* Korean J Radiol 3(4):254, 2002.
25. **Goldman AB:** *Some miscellaneous joint diseases.* Semin Roentgenol 17(1):60, 1982.
26. **Goldberg RP, Weissman BN, Naimark A:** *Femoral neck erosion: A sign of hip synovial disease.* AJR 41:107, 1983.
27. **Freidman B, Nerubay J, Blankstein A, et al.:** *Synovial chondromatosis (osteochondromatosis) of the right hip: "Hidden" radiological manifestations. Case report 439.* Skeletal Radiol 16:504, 1987.
28. **Ellman MH, Krieger MI, Brown N:** *Pseudogout mimicking synovial chondromatosis.* J Bone Joint Surg 57A:863, 1975.

INFLAMMATORY DISORDERS
RHEUMATOID ARTHRITIS

1. **Ropes MW, Cobb S, Jacox R, et al.:** *Proposed diagnostic criteria for rheumatoid arthritis.* Ann Rheum Dis 16:118, 1957.
2. **Ropes MW, Bennett GA, Cobb S, et al.:** *Diagnostic criteria for rheumatoid arthritis (1958 Revision).* Ann Rheum Dis 18:49, 1959.
3. **Fletcher DE, Rowley KA:** *Radiographic enlargements in diagnostic radiology.* Br J Radiol 24:598, 1951.
4. **Pathria M, Bjorkengren AG, Jacob J, et al.:** *Rheumatoid arthritis: Similarity of radiographic abnormalities in men and women.* Radiology 167:793, 1988.
5. **Bouchaud-Chabot A, Liote F:** *Cervical spine involvement in rheumatoid arthritis. A review.* Joint Bone Spine 69(2):141, 2002.
6. **Moore CP, Wilkens RF:** *The subcutaneous nodule: Its significance in the diagnosis of rheumatic disease.* Semin Arthritis Rheum 7:63, 1977.
7. **Rodnan GP, Schumacher HR:** *Primer on the Rheumatic Diseases,* ed 8. Atlanta, Arthritis Foundation, 1983.
8. **Felty AR:** *Chronic arthritis in the adult associated with splenomegaly and leukopenia. A report of 5 cases of an unusual clinical syndrome.* Johns Hopkins Hosp Bull 35:16, 1924.
9. **Conaghan PG, Green MJ, Emery P:** *Established rheumatoid arthritis.* Baillieres Best Pract Res Clin Rheumatol 13(4):561, 1999.
10. **van der Heijde D:** *Radiographic progression in rheumatoid arthritis: Does it reflect outcome? Does it reflect treatment?* Ann Rheum Dis 60(Suppl 3):47, 2001.
11. **Harris ED, DiBona DR, Krane SM:** *A mechanism for cartilage destruction in rheumatoid arthritis.* Trans Assoc Am Physicians 83:167, 1970.
12. **Martel W:** *The pattern of rheumatoid arthritis in the hand and wrist.* Radiol Clin North Am 2:221, 1964.
13. **Lipson SJ:** *Rheumatoid arthritis of the cervical spine.* Clin Orthop 182:143, 1984.
14. **Jones MW, Kaufman JCF:** *Vertebrobasilar artery insufficiency in rheumatoid atlantoaxial subluxation.* J Neurol Neurosurg Psychiatry 39:122, 1976.
15. **Ball J:** *Pathology of the rheumatoid cervical spine.* Lancet 1:86, 1958.
16. **Martel W:** *Pathogenesis of cervical discovertebral destruction in rheumatoid arthritis.* Arthritis Rheum 20:1217, 1977.
17. **Elkayam O, Paran D, Flusser G, et al.:** *Insufficiency fractures in rheumatic patients: misdiagnosis and underlying characteristics.* Clin Exp Rheumatol 18(3):369, 2000.
18. **McGonagle D, Conaghan PG, Wakefield R, Emery P:** *Imaging the joints in early rheumatoid arthritis.* Best Pract Res Clin Rheumatol 15(1):91, 2001.
19. **Devauchelle-Pensec V, Saraux A, Alapetite S, et al.:** *Diagnostic value of radiographs of the hands and feet in early rheumatoid arthritis.* Joint Bone Spine 69(5):434, 2002.
20. **Sugimoto J, Takeda A, Hyodoh K:** *Early-stage rheumatoid arthritis: Prospective study of the effectiveness of MR imaging for diagnosis.* Radiology 216(2):569, 2000.
21. **Makela P, Virtama P:** *The pre-erosive radiologic signs of rheumatoid arthritis in soft tissue radiography of the hands.* Skeletal Radiol 2:213, 1978.
22. **Brewerton DA:** *A tangential radiographic projection for demonstrating involvement of metacarpal heads in rheumatoid arthritis.* Br J Radiol 40:233, 1967.
23. **Norgaard F:** *Earliest roentgen changes in polyarthritis of the rheumatoid type. Continued investigations.* Radiology 92:299, 1969.
24. **Swanson AB:** *Pathogenesis and pathomechanics of rheumatoid deformities in the hand and wrist.* Orthop Clin North Am 4:1039, 1973.
25. **Monsees B, Destouet JM, Murphy WA, et al.:** *Pressure erosions of bone in rheumatoid arthritis: A subject review.* Radiology 155:53, 1985.
26. **Stack HG, Vaughn-Jackson OJ:** *The zig-zag deformity in the rheumatoid hand.* Hand 3:62, 1971.

27. **Hendrix RW, Urban MA, Schroeder JL, et al.:** *Carpal predominance in rheumatoid arthritis.* Radiology 164:219, 1987.

28. **Resnick D:** *Rheumatoid arthritis of the wrist. The compartmental approach.* Med Radiogr Photogr 52:50, 1976.

29. **Stewart NR, McQueen FM, Crabbe JPL:** *Magnetic resonance imaging of the wrist in early rheumatoid arthritis: A pictorial essay.* Austral Radiol 45(3):268, 2001.

30. **Resnick D:** *Rheumatoid arthritis of the wrist. Why the ulnar styloid?* Radiology 112:29, 1974.

31. **Frankel VH:** *The Terry Thomas sign.* Clin Orthop 129:321, 1977.

32. **Collins LC, Lidsky MD, Sharp JT, et al.:** *Malposition of carpal bones in rheumatoid arthritis.* Radiology 103:95, 1972.

33. **Calabro JJ:** *A critical evaluation of the diagnostic features of the feet in rheumatoid arthritis.* Arthritis Rheum 5(1):19, 1962.

34. **Thould AK, Simon G:** *Assessment of radiological changes in the hands and feet in rheumatoid arthritis. Their correlation with prognosis.* Ann Rheum Dis 25:220, 1966.

35. **Bland JH, Buskirk FW, Davis PH, et al.:** *Rheumatoid arthritis of the cervical spine.* Arthritis Rheum 5:637, 1967.

36. **Matsumine A, Shichikawa K, Yamashita K, et al.:** *Rheumatoid arthritis causing paraplegia.* J Bone Joint Surg 70A:1410, 1988.

37. **Reynolds H, Carter SW, Murtagh FR, et al.:** *Cervical rheumatoid arthritis: Value of flexion and extension views in imaging.* Radiology 164:215, 1987.

38. **Wolfe BK, O'Keefe D, Mitchell DM, et al.:** *Rheumatoid arthritis of the cervical spine: Early and progressive radiographic features.* Radiology 165:145, 1987.

39. **Swinson DR, Hamilton EBD, Mathews JA, et al.:** *Vertical subluxation of the axis in rheumatoid arthritis.* Ann Rheum Dis 31:359, 1972.

40. **Mathews JA:** *Atlanto-axial subluxation in rheumatoid arthritis.* Ann Rheum Dis 28:260, 1969.

41. **McGuire RA:** *The rheumatoid cervical spine.* Curr Opin Orthop 5:91, 1994.

42. **Isdale IC, Conlon PW:** *Atlanto-axial subluxation. A six-year follow-up report.* Ann Rheum Dis 30:387, 1971.

43. **Cabot A, Becker A:** *The cervical spine in rheumatoid arthritis.* Clin Orthop 131:130, 1978.

44. **Reijnierse M, Breedveld FC, Kroon HM, et al.:** *Are magnetic resonance flexion views useful in evaluating the cervical spine of patients with rheumatoid arthritis?* Skeletal Radiol 29:85, 2000.

45. **Steele HH:** *Anatomical and mechanical considerations of the atlantoaxial articulation.* J Bone Joint Surg 50A:1481, 1968.

46. **Park WM, O'Neill M, McCall IW:** *The radiology of rheumatoid involvement of the cervical spine.* Skeletal Radiol 4:1, 1979.

47. **Resnick D:** *Patterns of migration of the femoral head in osteoarthritis of the hip: Roentgenographic-pathologic correlation and comparison with rheumatoid arthritis.* AJR 124:62, 1975.

48. **Hastings DE, Parker SM:** *Protrusio acetabuli in rheumatoid arthritis.* Clin Orthop 108:76, 1975.

49. **Edelstein G, Murphy WA:** *Protrusio acetabuli. Radiographic appearance in arthritis and other conditions.* Arthritis Rheum 26(12):1511, 1983.

50. **West SG, Troutner JL, Baker MR, et al.:** *Sacral insufficiency fractures in rheumatoid arthritis.* Spine 19:2117, 1994.

51. **Dixon AS, Lience E:** *Sacroiliac joint in adult rheumatoid arthritis and psoriatic arthropathy.* Ann Rheum Dis 20:247, 1961.

52. **Elhabali M, Scherak O, Seidl G, et al.:** *Tomographic examinations of sacroiliac joints in adult patients with rheumatoid arthritis.* J Rheumatol 6:417, 1979.

53. **Sbarbaro JL:** *The rheumatoid shoulder.* Orthop Clin North Am 6:593, 1975.

54. **Resnick D, Niwayama G:** *Resorption of the undersurface of the distal clavicle in rheumatoid arthritis.* Radiology 120:75, 1976.

55. **Jackman RJ, Pugh DG:** *The positive elbow fat pad sign in rheumatoid arthritis.* AJR 108:812, 1970.

56. **Foster DR, Park WM, McCall IW, et al.:** *The supinator notch sign in rheumatoid arthritis.* Clin Radiol 31:195, 1980.

57. **Perri JA, Rodnan GP, Mankin HJ:** *Giant synovial cysts of the calf in patients with rheumatoid arthritis.* J Bone Joint Surg 50A:709, 1968.

58. **Martel W, Abell M, Mikkelsen W, et al.:** *Pulmonary and pleural lesions in rheumatoid disease.* Radiology 90:641, 1968.

59. **Caplan A:** *Certain unusual radiological appearances in the chests of coal miners suffering from rheumatoid arthritis.* Thorax 8:29, 1953.

60. **Hurd ER:** *Extra-articular manifestations of rheumatoid arthritis.* Semin Arthritis Rheum 8(3):151, 1979.

61. **Alpert M, Feldman F:** *The rib lesions of rheumatoid arthritis.* Radiology 82:872, 1964.

JUVENILE RHEUMATOID ARTHRITIS

1. **Chikanza IC:** *Juvenile rheumatoid arthritis: Therapeutic perspectives.* Paediatr Drugs 4(5):335, 2002.

2. **Ansell BM, Kent PA:** *Radiological changes in juvenile chronic polyarthritis.* Skeletal Radiol 1:129, 1977.

3. **Still GF:** *On a form of chronic joint disease in children.* Med Chiro Trans 80:47, 1897.

4. **Bywaters EGL, Ansell BM:** *Monoarticular arthritis in children.* Ann Rheum Dis 24:116, 1965.

5. **Calabro JJ, Marchesano JM:** *The early natural history of juvenile rheumatoid arthritis.* Med Clin North Am 52:567, 1968.

6. **Arthritis Foundation:** *Arthritis: A Serious Look at the Facts* [Pamphlet 5785/1-82]. Atlanta, Arthritis Foundation, 1982.

7. **Calabro JJ, Katz RM, Maltz BA:** *A critical reappraisal of juvenile rheumatoid arthritis.* Clin Orthop 74:101, 1971.

8. **Bywaters EGL:** *Diagnostic Criteria for Still's Disease (Juvenile RA). Population Studies of the Rheumatic Diseases.* Int Congress ser. 148:235, 1968.

9. **Rodnan GP, Schumacher HR:** *Criteria for the Diagnosis of Juvenile Rheumatoid Arthritis. Primer on Rheumatic Diseases,* ed 8. Atlanta, Arthritis Foundation, 1983.

10. **Schaller JG:** *Chronic arthritis in children.* Clin Orthop 182:79, 1983.

11. **Ansell BM:** *Chronic arthritis in childhood.* Ann Rheum Dis 37:107, 1978.

12. **Schaller J, Wedgwood RJ:** *Juvenile rheumatoid arthritis: A review.* Pediatrics 50:940, 1972.

13. **Isdale IC, Bywaters EGL:** *The rash of rheumatoid arthritis and Still's disease.* Q J Med 25(99):377, 1956.

14. **Howite NT:** *Current treatment of juvenile rheumatoid arthritis.* Pediatrics 109:109, 2002.

15. **Wynn-Roberts CR, Anderson CH, Turano AM, et al.:** *Light and electron microscopic findings of juvenile rheumatoid arthritis synovium: Comparison with normal juvenile synovium.* Semin Arthritis Rheum 7(4):287, 1978.

16. **Martell W, Holt JF, Cassidy JT:** *Roentgenologic manifestations of juvenile rheumatoid arthritis.* AJR 88:400, 1962.

17. **Cohen PA, Job-Desiandre CH, Lalande G, Adamsbaum C:** *Overview of the radiology of juvenile idiopathic arthritis (JIA).* Eur J Radiol 33(2):94, 2000.

18. **Nathan FF, Bickel WH:** *Spontaneous axial subluxation in a child as the first sign of juvenile rheumatoid arthritis.* J Bone Joint Surg 50A(8):1675, 1968.

19. **Salliere D, Clerc D, Bisson M, et al.:** *Involvement of the cervical spine in chronic juvenile arthritis. 29 cases followed for more than 5 years.* Sem Hop Paris 60(2):97, 1984.

20. **Epstein B:** *The Spine. A Radiologic Text and Atlas,* ed 4. Philadelphia, Lea & Febiger, 1976.

21. **Locke GR, van Epps EF:** *Atlas-dens interval (ADI) in children. A survey based on 200 normal cervical spines.* AJR 97(1):135, 1966.

22. **Badley BWD, Ansell BM:** *Fractures in Still's disease.* Ann Rheum Dis 19:135, 1960.

23. **Carter ME, Loewi G:** *Anatomical changes in normal sacroiliac joints during childhood and comparison with the changes in Still's disease.* Ann Rheum Dis 21:121, 1962.

24. **Chosta EM, Kuhns LR, Holt JF:** *The "patella ratio" in hemophilia and juvenile rheumatoid arthritis.* Radiology 116:137, 1975.

25. **Gylys-Morin VM, Graham TB, Blebea JS, et al.:** *Knee in early juvenile rheumatoid arthritis: MR imaging findings.* Radiology 220:696, 2001.
26. **Becker MH, Coccaro PJ, Converse JM:** *Antegonial notching of the mandible. An often overlooked mandibular deformity in congenital and acquired disorders.* Radiology 121:149, 1976.

ANKYLOSING SPONDYLITIS

1. **Blumberg B, Ragan C:** *The natural history of rheumatoid spondylitis.* Medicine 35:1, 1956.
2. **Bechterew VM:** *Stiffening of the spine in flexion: A special form of disease* [Trans.] Clin Orthop 143:4, 1979.
3. **Marie P:** *Sur la spondylose rhizomelique.* Rev de Med 18:285, 1898.
4. **Strumpell A:** *Observations on chronic-ankylosing inflammation of the vertebrae and hip joints* [Trans.] Clin Orthop 74:4, 1971.
5. **Chou LW, Lo SF Kao MJ, et al.:** *Ankylosing spondylitis manifested by spontaneous anterior atlantoaxial subluxation.* Am J Phys Med Rehabil 81(12):952, 2002.
6. **Smythe H:** *Therapy of the spondyloarthropathies.* Clin Orthop 143:84, 1979.
7. **Polley HF, Slocumb CH:** *Rheumatoid spondylitis—A study of 1035 cases.* Ann Intern Med 26:240, 1947.
8. **Brophy S, Mackay K, Al-Saidi A, et al.:** *The natural history of ankylosing spondylitis as defined by radiological progression.* J Rheumatol 29(6):1236, 2002.
9. **Schaller J, Bitnum S, Wedgewood RJ:** *Ankylosing spondylitis with childhood onset.* J Pediatr 74(4):505, 1969.
10. **Wilkinson M, Bywaters EGL:** *Clinical features and course of ankylosing spondylitis as seen in a follow-up of 222 hospital referred cases.* Ann Rheum Dis 17:209, 1958.
11. **Ogryzlo MA, Rosen PS:** *Ankylosing (Marie-Strumpell) spondylitis.* Postgrad Med J 45:182, 1969.
12. **Sigler JW, Bluhm GB, Duncan H, et al.:** *Clinical features of ankylosing spondylitis.* Clin Orthop 74:14, 1971.
13. **Hill HFH, Hill AGS, Bodmer JG:** *Clinical diagnosis of ankylosing spondylitis in women and relation to presence of HLA-B27.* Ann Rheum Dis 35:267, 1976.
14. **Baum J, Ziff M:** *The rarity of ankylosing spondylitis in the black race.* Arthritis Rheum 14:12, 1971.
15. **Bennett PH, Burch TA:** *New York symposium on population studies in rheumatic diseases: New diagnostic criteria.* Bull Rheum Dis 17:453, 1967.
16. **Masi AT, Medsger TA:** *A new look at the epidemiology of ankylosing spondylitis and related syndromes.* Clin Orthop 143:15, 1979.
17. **Moll JMH, Wright V:** *New York clinical criteria for ankylosing spondylitis: A statistical evaluation.* Ann Rheum Dis 32:354, 1973.
18. **Forouzesh S, Bluestone R:** *The clinical spectrum of ankylosing spondylitis.* Clin Orthop 143:53, 1979.
19. **Braun J, Pincus T:** *Mortality, course of disease and prognosis of patients with ankylosing spondylitis.* Clin Exp Rheumatol 20(Suppl 28):S16, 2002.
20. **Bowie EA, Glasgow GL:** *Cauda equina lesions associated with ankylosing spondylitis. Report of three cases.* Br Med J 2:24, 1961.
21. **Mitchell MJ, Sartoris DJ, Moody D, et al.:** *Cauda equina syndrome complicating ankylosing spondylitis.* Radiology 175:521, 1990.
22. **Ahn NU, Ahn UM, Nallamshetty L, et al.:** *Cauda equina syndrome in ankylosing spondylitis (the CES-AS syndrome): Meta-analysis of outcomes after medical and surgical treatments.* J Spinal Disord 14(5):427, 2001.
23. **Yildirir A, Aksoyek S, Calguneri M, et al.:** *Echocardiographic evidence of cardiac involvement in ankylosing spondylitis.* Clin Rheumatol 21(2):129, 2002.
24. **Graham DC, Smythe H:** *The carditis and aortitis of ankylosing spondylitis.* Bull Rheum Dis 9(3):171, 1958.
25. **Lautermann D, Braun J:** *Ankylosing spondylitis—Cardiac manifestations.* Clin Exp Theumatol 20(Suppl 28):S11, 2002.
26. **Davies D:** *Ankylosing spondylitis and lung fibrosis.* Q J Med 41:395, 1972.
27. **Jessamine AG:** *Upper lung lobe fibrosis in ankylosing spondylitis.* Can Med Assoc J 98:25, 1968.
28. **Baeten D, De Keyser F, Mielants H, Veys EM:** *Ankylosing spondylitis and bower disease.* Best Pract Res Clin Rheumatol 16(4):537, 2002.
29. **Jayson MIV, Bouchier IAD:** *Ulcerative colitis with ankylosing spondylitis.* Ann Rheum Dis 27:219, 1968.
30. **Mueller CE, Seeger JF, Martell W:** *Ankylosing spondylitis and regional enteritis.* Radiology 112:579, 1974.
31. **Mason RM, Murray RS, Oates JK, et al.:** *Prostatitis and ankylosing spondylitis.* Br Med J 1:748, 1958.
32. **Cruickshank B:** *Pathology of ankylosing spondylitis.* Clin Orthop 74:43, 1971.
33. **Edgar MA, Robinson MP:** *Postradiation sarcoma in ankylosing spondylitis: A report of five cases.* J Bone Joint Surg 55B(91):183, 1973.
34. **Bluestone R, Pearson CM:** *Ankylosing spondylitis and Reiter's syndrome. Their interrelationship and association with HLA-B27.* Adv Intern Med 22:1, 1977.
35. **Schlosstein L, Teraski PI, Bluestone R, et al.:** *High association of HL-A antigen, B27, with ankylosing spondylitis.* N Engl J Med 288(14):704, 1973.
36. **Reveille JD, Ball EJ, Khan MA:** *HLA-B27 and genetic predisposing factors in spondyloarthropathies.* Curr Opin Rheumatol 13(4):265, 2001.
37. **Stafford L, Youssef PP:** *Spondyloarthropathies: An overview.* Intern Med J32(1):40, 2002.
38. **Hamersma J, Cardon LR, Bradbury L, et al.:** *Is disease severity in ankylosing spondylitis genetically determined?* Arthritis Rheum 44(6):1396, 2001.
39. **Ball J:** *Articular pathology of ankylosing spondylitis.* Clin Orthop Rel Res 143:30, 1979.
40. **Ball J:** *Enthesopathy of rheumatoid and ankylosing spondylitis.* Ann Rheum Dis 30:213, 1971.
41. **de Vlam K, Meilants H, Veys EM:** *Involvement of the zygapophyseal joint in ankylosing spondylitis relation to the bridging syndesmophyte.* J Rheumatol 26(8):1738, 1999.
42. **Le T, Biundo J, Aprill C, Deiparine E:** *Costovertebral joint erosion in ankylosing spondylitis.* Am J Phys Rehabil 80(1):62, 2001.
43. **Jajic Z, Jajic I, Grazio S:** *Radiological changes of the symphysis in ankylosing spondylitis.* Acta Radiol 41(4):307, 2000.
44. **Dihlmann W:** *Current radiodiagnostic concept of ankylosing spondylitis.* Skeletal Radiol 4:179, 1979.
45. **Braunstein EM, Martel W, Mordel R:** *Ankylosing spondylitis in men and women: a clinical and radiographic comparison.* Radiology 144(1):91, 1982.
46. **Sieper J, Braun J, Rudwaleit M, et al.:** *Ankylosing spondylitis: An overview.* Am Rheum Dis 61(Suppl 3):8, 2002.
47. **Macrae IF, Haslock DI, Wright V:** *Grading of films for sacroiliitis in population studies.* Ann Rheum Dis 30:58, 1971.
48. **Khan MA:** *Thoughts concerning the early diagnosis of ankylosing spondylitis and related diseases.* Clin Exp Rheumatol 20(Suppl 28):S6, 2002.
49. **Berens D:** *Roentgen features of ankylosing spondylitis.* Clin Orthop 74:20, 1971.
50. **Esdaile J, Hawkins D, Rosenthal L:** *Radionuclide joint imaging in seronegative spondyloarthropathies.* Clin Orthop 143:46, 1979.
51. **Resnick D, Niwayama G, Goergen T:** *Comparison of radiographic abnormalities of the sacroiliac joint in degenerative disease and ankylosing spondylitis.* AJR 128:189, 1977.
52. **Bowen V, Cassidy JD:** *Macroscopic and microscopic anatomy of the sacroiliac joint from embryonic life until the eighth decade.* Spine 6(6):620, 1981.
53. **Borak J:** *Significance of sacroiliac findings in Marie-Strumpell's spondylitis.* Radiology 47:128, 1946.
54. **Forestier J:** *The importance of sacroiliac changes in the early diagnosis of ankylosing spondyloarthritis.* Radiology 33:389, 1939.
55. **Boland E, Shebesta E:** *Rheumatoid spondylitis: Correlation of clinical and roentgenographic features.* Radiology 47:551, 1946.

56. **Hart FD, Robinson KD:** *Ankylosing spondylitis in women.* Ann Rheum Dis 18:15, 1959.
57. **Forestier J, Deslous P:** *Radiological study of sacroiliac joints in ankylosing spondylitis with reference to the evolution of the disease.* Ann Rheum Dis 16:31, 1957.
58. **Cruickshank B:** *Pathology of ankylosing spondylitis.* Bull Rheum Dis 10:211, 1960.
59. **Resnick D:** *Radiology of the seronegative spondyloarthropathies.* Clin Orthop 74:20, 1971.
60. **Romanus R, Yden S:** *Pelvospondylitis Ossificans, Rheumatoid or Ankylosing Spondylitis. A Roentgenological and Clinical Guide to Its Early Diagnosis (Especially Anterior Spondylitis).* Copenhagen, Munksgaard, 1955.
61. **Dilhmann W:** *Diagnostic Radiology of the Sacroiliac Joints,* trans LS Michaelis. Chicago: Yearbook Medical, 1980.
62. **Cawley MID, Chalmers MT, Kellgren JH, et al.:** *Destructive lesions of vertebral bodies in ankylosing spondylitis.* Ann Rheum Dis 31:345, 1972.
63. **Little H, Urowitz MB, Smythe HA, et al.:** *Asymptomatic spondylodiscitis. An unusual feature of ankylosing spondylitis.* Arthritis Rheum 17:487, 1974.
64. **Andersson O:** *Rontgenbilden vid spondyloarthritis ankylopoetica.* Nord Med Tidskr 14:2000, 1937.
65. **Rolleston GL:** *The early radiological diagnosis of ankylosing spondylitis.* Br J Radiol 20(235):288, 1947.
66. **Little H, Swinson DR, Cruickshank B:** *Upward subluxation of the axis in ankylosing spondylitis.* Am J Med 60:279, 1976.
67. **Meikle JAK, Wilkinson M:** *Rheumatoid involvement of the cervical spine: Radiological assessment.* Ann Rheum Dis 30(2):154, 1971.
68. **Sharp J, Purser DW:** *Spontaneous atlantoaxial dislocation in ankylosing spondylitis and rheumatoid arthritis.* Ann Rheum Dis 20:47, 1961.
69. **Sorin S, Askari A, Moskowitz RW:** *Atlantoaxial subluxation as a complication of early ankylosing spondylitis.* Arthritis Rheum 22(3):273, 1979.
70. **Martel W, Page JW:** *Cervical vertebral erosions and subluxations in rheumatoid arthritis and ankylosing spondylitis.* Arthritis Rheum 3:546, 1960.
71. **Resnick D:** *Patterns of peripheral joint disease in ankylosing spondylitis.* Radiology 110:523, 1974.
72. **Guest C, Jacobson H:** *Pelvic and extrapelvic osteopathy in rheumatoid spondylitis: A clinical and roentgenographic study of ninety cases.* AJR 65(5):760, 1951.
73. **Resnick D, Niwayama G:** *On the nature and significance of bony proliferation in "rheumatoid variant" disorders.* AJR 129:275, 1977.
74. **Mitra D, Elvins DM, Speden DJ, Collins AJ:** *The prevalence of vertebral fractures in mild ankylosing spondylitis and their relationship to bone mineral density.* Rheumatology (Oxford) 39(1):85, 2000.
75. **Gelman M, Umber JS:** *Fractures of the thoracolumbar spine in ankylosing spondylitis.* AJR 130:485, 1978.
76. **Woodruff F, Dewing S:** *Fracture of the cervical spine in patients with ankylosing spondylitis.* Radiology 80:17, 1963.
77. **Rinsky LA, Reynolds GG, Jameson RM, et al.:** *A cervical spinal cord injury following chiropractic manipulation.* Paraplegia 13:223, 1976.
78. **Brower AC:** *Arthritis in Black and White.* Philadelphia, WB Saunders, 1988.
79. **Schaberg FJ Jr:** *Aortic injury occurring after minor trauma in ankylosing spondylitis.* J Vasc Surg 4:410, 1986.
80. **Shih TT, Chen PQ, Li YW, Hsu CY:** *Spinal fractures and pseudoarthrosis complicating ankylosing spondylitis: MRI manifestation and clinical significance.* J Comput Assist Tomogr 25(2):164, 2001.
81. **Hitchon PW, From AM, Brenton MD, et al.:** *Fractures of the thoracolumbar spine complicating ankylosing spondylitis.* J Neurosurg 97(2 Suppl):218, 2002.

82. **Taggard DA, Traynelis VC:** *Management of cervical spinal fractures in ankylosing spondylitis with posterior fixation.* Spine 25(16):2035, 2000.
83. **Abello R, Rovira M, Sanz MP, et al.:** *MRI and CT of ankylosing spondylitis with vertebral scalloping.* Neuroradiology 30:272, 1988.
84. **Young A, Dixon A, Getty J, et al.:** *Cauda equina syndrome complicating ankylosing spondylitis: Use of electromyography and computed tomography in diagnosis.* Ann Rheum Dis 40:317, 1981.
85. **Bisla RS, Ranawat CS, Inglis AE:** *Total hip replacement in patients with ankylosing spondylitis with involvement of the hip.* J Bone Joint Surg 58A(2):233, 1976.
86. **Resnick D, Swosh IL, Goergen TG, et al.:** *Clinical and radiographic "reankylosis" following hip surgery in ankylosing spondylitis.* AJR 126:1181, 1976.
87. **Leventhal MR, Maguire JK, Christian CA:** *Atlantoaxial rotary subluxation in ankylosing spondylitis.* Spine 15:1374, 1990.

Enteropathic Arthritis

1. **Wollheim FA:** *Enteropathic arthritis: how do the joints talk with the gut?* Curr Opin Rheumatol 13(4):305, 2001.
2. **Zvaifler NJ, Martel W:** *Spondylitis in chronic ulcerative colitis.* Arthritis Rheum 3:76, 1960.
3. **Zunino A, Morera G, Main M, Paira S:** *Enteropathic arthritis in association with collagen colitis.* Clin Rheumatol 17(3):253, 1998.
4. **Wright V, Watkinson G:** *The arthritis of ulcerative colitis.* Br Med J 65(2):670, 1965.
5. **Ford DK, Vallis DG:** *The clinical course of arthritis associated with ulcerative colitis and regional ileitis.* Arthritis Rheum 2:526, 1959.
6. **Palumbo PJ, Ward LE, Sauer WG, et al.:** *Musculoskeletal manifestations of inflammatory bowel disease.* Mayo Clin Proc 48:411, 1973.
7. **Jayson MIV, Salmon PR, Harrison WJ:** *Inflammatory bowel disease in ankylosing spondylitis.* Gut 11:506, 1970.
8. **Jayson MIV, Boucher IA:** *Ulcerative colitis with ankylosing spondylitis.* Ann Rheum Dis 27:219, 1968.
9. **Wright V, Watkinson G:** *The arthritis of ulcerative colitis.* B Med J 2:675, 1965.
10. **Mueller CE, Seeger JF, Martel W:** *Ankylosing spondylitis and regional enteritis.* Radiology 112:579, 1974.
11. **Acheson ED:** *An association between ulcerative colitis, regional enteritis and ankylosing spondylitis.* Q Med J 29:489, 1960.
12. **Macrae I, Wright V:** *A family study of ulcerative colitis with particular reference to ankylosing spondylitis and sacroiliitis.* Ann Rheum Dis 32:16, 1973.
13. **Clark RL, Muhletaler CA, Margulies SI:** *Colitic arthritis: Clinical and radiographic manifestations.* Radiology 101:585, 1971.
14. **Haslock I, Wright V:** *The musculoskeletal complications of Crohn's disease.* Medicine 52(3):217, 1973.
15. **Leirisalo-Repo M:** *Enteropathic arthritis, Whipple's disease, juvenile spondyloarthropathy, uveitis, and SAPHO syndrome.* Curr Opin Rheumatol 7(4):284, 1995.
16. **Masi AT, Medsger TA:** *A new look at the epidemiology of ankylosing spondylitis and related syndromes.* Clin Orthop 143:15, 1979.
17. **McBride JA, King MJ, Baikie AG, et al.:** *Ankylosing spondylitis and chronic inflammatory diseases of the intestines.* Br Med J 2:483, 1963.
18. **Thayer WR:** *Are the inflammatory bowel diseases immune complex diseases?* Gastroenterology 70:136, 1976.
19. **McEwen C, Lingg C, Kirsner JB:** *Arthritis accompanying ulcerative colitis.* Am J Med 33:923, 1962.
20. **Mester AR, Mako EK, Karlinger K, et al.:** *Enteropathic arthritis in the sacroiliac joint. Imaging and differential diagnosis.* Eur J Radiol 35:199, 2000.
21. **Tibbles AC, Mierau DR, Sibley J:** *Destructive arthritis of the hip in a patient with Crohn's disease.* J Manipulative Physiol Ther 16:601, 1993.
22. **Arlat IP, Maier W, Leupold D, et al.:** *Massive periosteal new bone formation in ulcerative colitis.* Radiology 144:507, 1982.

23. **Oppenheimer DA, Jones HH:** *Hypertrophic osteoarthropathy of chronic inflammatory bowel disease.* Skeletal Radiol 9(2):109, 1982.

PSORIATIC ARTHRITIS

1. **Christophers E:** *Psoriasis-epidemiology and clinical spectrum.* Clin Exp Dermatol 26(4):314, 2001.
2. **Veale D, FitzGerald O:** *Psoriatic arthritis.* Best Pract Res Clin Rheumatol 16(4):523, 2002.
3. **Veale DJ, FetzGerald O:** *Psoriatic arthritis—Pathogenesis and epidemiology.* Clin Exp Rheumatol 20(Suppl 28):S27, 2002.
4. **Gladman DD, Brockbank J:** *Psoriatic arthritis.* Expert Opin Invest Drug 9:1511, 2000.
5. **Peterson CC Jr, Silbiger ML:** *Reiter's syndrome and psoriatic arthritis. Their roentgen spectra and some interesting similarities.* AJR 101:860, 1967.
6. **Moll JMH:** *The clinical spectrum of psoriatic arthritis.* Clin Orthop Rel Res 143:66, 1979.
7. **Avila R, Pugh D, Slocumb CH, et al.:** *Psoriatic arthritis: A roentgenologic study.* Radiology 75:691, 1968.
8. **Elkayam O, Ophir J, Yaron M, Caspi D:** *Psoriatic arthritis: Interrelationships between skin and joint manifestations related to onset, course and distribution.* Clin Rheumatol 19(4):301, 2000.
9. **Gladman DD, Hing EN, Schentag CT, Cook RJ:** *Remission in psoriatic arthritis.* J Rheumatol 28(5):1045, 2001.
10. **Loebl DH, Kirby S, Stephenson R, et al.:** *Psoriatic arthritis.* JAMA 242:2447, 1979.
11. **Wright V:** *Psoriasis and arthritis.* Ann Rheum Dis 15:348, 1956.
12. **Baker H, Golding DN, Thompson M:** *The nails in psoriatic arthritis.* Br J Dermatol 76:549, 1964.
13. **Zaias N:** *Psoriasis of the nail. A clinical-pathologic study.* Arch Derm 99:567, 1969.
14. **Gladman DD, Farewell VT:** *Progression in psoriatic arthritis: role of time varying clinical indicators.* J Rheumatol 26:2409, 1999.
15. **Queiro-Silva R, Torre-Alonso JC, Tinture-Eguren T, Lopez-Lagunas I:** *A polyarticular onset predicts erosive and deforming disease in psoriatic arthritis.* Ann Rheum Dis 62(1):68, 2003.
16. **Jones G, Crotty M, Brooks P:** *Interventions for psoriatic arthritis.* Cochrane Database Syst Rev 3:[CD000212] 2000.
17. **Taylor WJ:** *Epidemiology of psoriatic arthritis.* Curr Opin Rheumatol 14(2):98, 2002.
18. **Queiro R, Sarasqueta C, Belzunegui J, et al.:** *Psoriatic spondyloarthropathy: A comparative study between HLA-B27 positive and HLA-B27 negative disease.* Semin Arthritis Rheum Jun 31:413, 2002.
19. **Lambert JR, Wright V, Rajah SM, et al.:** *Histocompatibility antigens in psoriatic arthritis.* Ann Rheum Dis 35:526, 1976.
20. **Brewerton DA, Walters D, Caffrey MJ, et al.:** *HLA-B27 and the arthropathies associated with ulcerative colitis and psoriasis.* Lancet 1:956, 1974.
21. **Costello P, FitzGerald O:** *Disease mechanisms in psoriasis and psoriatic arthritis.* Curr Rheumatol Rep 3(5):419, 2001.
22. **Gladman DD:** *Psoriatic arthritis.* Rheum Dis Clin North Am 24:829, 1998.
23. **Bywaters EGL, Dixon AS:** *Paravertebral ossification in psoriatic arthritis.* Ann Rheum Dis 24:313, 1965.
24. **Sundaram M, Patton JT:** *Paravertebral ossification in psoriasis and Reiter's disease.* Br J Radiol 48:628, 1975.
25. **Meaney TF, Hays RA:** *Roentgen manifestations of psoriatic arthritis.* Radiology 68:403, 1957.
26. **Forrester DM, Kirkpatrick J:** *Periostitis and pseudoperiostitis.* Radiology 118:597, 1976.
27. **Martel W, Stuck KJ, Sworin AM, et al.:** *Erosive osteoarthritis and psoriatic arthritis: A radiologic comparison in the hand, wrist, and foot.* AJR 134:125, 1980.
28. **Gold, RH, Bassett LW, Theros EG:** *Radiologic comparison of erosive polyarthritides with prominent interphalangeal involvement.* Skeletal Radiol 8:89, 1982.
29. **Resnick D, Broderick RW:** *Bony proliferation of terminal phalanges in psoriasis. The "ivory" phalanx.* J Can Assoc Radiol 28:187, 1977.

30. **Harvie JN, Lester RS, Little AH:** *Sacroiliitis in severe psoriasis.* AJR 127:579, 1976.
31. **Killebrew K, Gold RH, Sholkoff SD:** *Psoriatic spondylitis.* Radiology 108:9, 1973.
32. **Barraclough D, Russell AS, Percy JS:** *Psoriatic spondylitis. A clinical, radiological and scintiscan survey.* J Rheumatol 4(3):282, 1977.
33. **Jajic I:** *Radiological changes in the sacroiliac joints and spine of patients with psoriatic arthritis and psoriasis.* Ann Rheum Dis 27:1, 1968.
34. **McEwen C, Ditata D, Lingg C, et al.:** *Ankylosing spondylitis and spondylitis accompanying ulcerative colitis, regional enteritis, psoriasis, and Reiter's disease.* Arthritis Rheum 14:291, 1971.
35. **Dixon AS, Lience E:** *Sacroiliac joint in adult rheumatoid arthritis and psoriatic arthropathy.* Ann Rheum Dis 20:247, 1961.
36. **Scarpa R:** *Discovertebral erosions and destruction in psoriatic arthritis.* J Rheumatol 27(4):975, 2000.
37. **Kaplan D, Plotz CM, Nathanson L, et al.:** *Cervical spine in psoriasis and Reiter's disease.* Br J Radiol 48:628, 1975.
38. **Dilhmann W:** *Diagnostic Radiology of the Sacroiliac Joints,* trans LS Michaelis. Chicago, Yearbook Medical, 1980.
39. **Jenkinson T, Armaas J, Evison G, et al.:** *The cervical spine in psoriatic arthritis: A clinical and radiological study.* Br J Rheumatol 33:255, 1994.
40. **Laiho K, Kauppi M:** *The cervical spine in patients with psoriatic arthritis.* Ann Rheum Dis 61(7):650, 2002.

REITER'S SYNDROME

1. **Amor B:** *Reiter's syndrome. Diagnosis and clinical features.* Rheum Dis Clin North Am 24(4):677, 1998.
2. **Barth WF, Segal K:** *Reactive arthritis (Reiter's syndrome).* Am Fam Physician 60(2):499, 1999.
3. **Toivanen P, Toivanen A:** *Two forms of reactive arthritis?* Ann Rheum Dis 58(12):737, 1999.
4. **Reiter H:** *Uber eine bisher unerkannte Spirochateninfektion (Spirochaetosis arthritica).* Dtsch Med Wochenschr 42:1535, 1916.
5. **Smith DL, Bennett RM, Regan MG:** *Reiter's disease in women.* Arthritis Rheum 23(3):335, 1980.
6. **Good AE:** *Reiter's disease.* Postgrad Med 61(1):153, 1977.
7. **Parker CT, Thomas D:** *Reiter's syndrome and reactive arthritis.* J Am Osteopath Assoc 100(2):101, 2000.
8. **Ford DK:** *The clinical spectrum of Reiter's syndrome and similar postenteric arthropathies.* Clin Orthop 143:59, 1979.
9. **Oates JK, Young AC:** *Sacroiliitis in Reiter's disease.* Br Med J 1:1013, 1959.
10. **Leirisalo M, Skylv G, Kousa M, et al.:** *Follow-up study on patients with Reiter's disease and reactive arthritis with special reference to HLA-B27.* Arthritis Rheum 25(3):249, 1982.
11. **Noer HR:** *An "experimenta" epidemic of Reiter's syndrome.* JAMA 197(7):693, 1966.
12. **Weiss JJ, Thompson GR, Good A:** *Reiter's disease after Salmonella typhimurium enteritis.* J Rheumatol 7 (2):211, 1980.
13. **Young RH, McEwen EG:** *Bacillary dysentery as the cause of Reiter's syndrome.* JAMA 134 (7):1456, 1947.
14. **Perry HO, Mayne JG:** *Psoriasis and Reiter's syndrome.* Arch Dermato 92(2):129, 1965.
15. **Russell AS, Davis P, Percy JS, et al.:** *The sacroiliitis of acute Reiter's syndrome.* J Rheumatol 4:293, 1977.
16. **Good AE:** *Involvement of the back in Reiter's syndrome. Follow-up study of thirty-four cases.* Ann Int Med 57:44, 1962.
17. **Cliff JM:** *Spinal bony bridging and carditis in Reiter's disease.* Ann Rheum Dis 30:171, 1971.
18. **Rodnan GP, Benedek TG, Shaver JA, et al.:** *Reiter's syndrome and aortic insufficiency.* JAMA 189(12):889, 1964.
19. **Brewerton DA, Nichols A, Oates JK, et al.:** *Reiter's disease and HL-A27.* Lancet 11:996, 1973.
20. **Morris R, Metzger AL, Bluestone R, et al.:** *HL-A W27—a clue to the diagnosis and pathogenesis of Reiter's syndrome.* N Eng J Med 290(10):554, 1974.

21. **Schachter J, Barnes MG, Jones JP, et al.:** *Isolation of bedsoniae from the joints of patients with Reiter's syndrome.* Proc Soc Exp Biol Med 122:283, 1966.

22. **Bluestone R, Pearson CM:** *Ankylosing spondylitis and Reiter's syndrome: Their interrelationship and association with HLA B27.* Adv Intern Med 22:1, 1977.

23. **Grimble A:** *Anti-prostate antibodies in arthritis.* Br Med J 2:263, 1965.

24. **Wakefield D, Robinson P, Penny R:** *Reiter's syndrome and reactive arthritis* [Letter]. N Eng J Med 310(23):1538, 1984.

25. **Mason RM, Murray RS, Oates JK, et al.:** *A comparative radiological study of Reiter's disease, rheumatoid arthritis, and ankylosing spondylitis.* J Bone Joint Surg 41B:137, 1959.

26. **Peterson CC, Silbiger ML:** *Reiter's syndrome and psoriatic arthritis; their roentgen spectra and some interesting similarities.* AJR 101(4):860, 1967.

27. **Sholkoff SD, Glickman MG, Steinbach HL:** *Roentgenology of Reiter's syndrome.* Radiology 97:497, 1970.

28. **Weldon WV, Scalettar R:** *Roentgen changes in Reiter's syndrome.* AJR 86(2):344, 1961.

29. **Bywaters EGL, Dixon ASJ:** *Paravertebral ossification in psoriatic arthritis.* Ann Rheum Dis 24:313, 1965.

30. **Sunduram M, Patton JJT:** *Paravertebral ossification in psoriasis and Reiter's disease.* Br J Radiol 48:628, 1975.

31. **Murray RS, Oates JK, Young AC:** *Radiological changes in Reiter's syndrome and arthritis associated with urethritis.* J Fac Radiol 9:37, 1958.

32. **Kim SH, Chung SK, Bahk YW, et al.:** *Whole-body and pinhole bone scintigraphic manifestations of Reiter's syndrome: Distribution patterns and early and characteristic signs.* Eur J Nucl Med 26(2):163, 1999.

33. **Martel W, Braunstein EM, Barlaza G, et al.:** *Radiologic features of Reiter's disease.* Radiology 132:1, 1979.

34. **Kononen M, Kovero O, Wenneberg B, Konttinen YT:** *Radiographic signs in the temporomandibular joint in Reiter's disease.* J Orofac Pain 16(2):143, 2002.

35. **Resnick D, Feingold ML, Curd J, et al.:** *Calcaneal abnormalities in articular disorders.* Radiology 125:355, 1977.

36. **Latchaw RE, Meyer GW:** *Reiter's disease with atlantoaxial subluxation.* Radiology 126:303, 1978.

37. **Kransdorf MJ, Maj MC, Whehrle A, et al.:** *Atlantoaxial subluxation in Reiter's syndrome.* Spine 13:12, 1988.

38. **Ball J:** *Articular pathology of ankylosing spondylitis.* Clin Orthop Rel Res 143:30, 1979.

39. **McEwan C, DiTata D, Lingg C, et al.:** *Ankylosing spondylitis and spondylitis accompanying ulcerative colitis, regional enteritis, psoriasis and Reiter's disease.* Arthritis Rheum 14:291, 1971.

SYSTEMIC LUPUS ERYTHEMATOSUS

1. **Patel P, Werth V:** *Cutaneous lupus erythematosus: A review.* Dermatol Clin 20(3):373, 2002.

2. **Wang DY:** *Diagnosis and management of lupus pleuritis.* Curr Opin Pulm Med 8(4):312, 2002.

3. **Haq I, Isenberg DA:** *How does one assess and monitor patients with systemic lupus erythematosus in daily clinical practice?* Best Pract Res Clin Rheumatol 16(2):181, 2002.

4. **Labowitz R, Schumacher HR:** *Articular manifestations of systemic lupus erythematosus.* Ann Intern Med 74:911, 1971.

5. **Twinning RH, Marcus WY, Gavey JL:** *Tendon rupture in systemic lupus erythematosus.* JAMA 189(5):337, 1964.

6. **Chaudhuri S, Basu K, Dhar MC, et al.:** *Alopeecia universalis in a case of systemic lupus erythematosus.* J Assoc Physicians India 50:1073, 2002.

7. **Zabaleta-Lanz M, Vargas-Arenas RE, Tapanes F, et al.:** *Silent nephritis in systemic lupus erythematosus.* Lupus 12:26, 2003.

8. **Bijl M, Brouwer J, Kallenberg GG:** *Cardiac abnormalities in SLE: Pancarditis.* Lupus 9(4):236, 2000.

9. **Guma M, Olive A, Roca J, et al.:** *Association of systemic lupus erythematosus and hypermobility.* Ann Rheum Dis 61(11):1024, 2002.

10. **LaPorte DM, Mont MA, Mohan V, et al.:** *Multifocal osteonecrosis.* J Rheumatol 25(10):1968, 1998.

11. **Dubois EL, Cozen L:** *Avascular (aseptic) bone necrosis associated with systemic lupus erythematosus.* JAMA 174(8):966, 1960.

12. **Bergstein JM, Wiens C, Fish AJ, et al.:** *Avascular necrosis of bone in systemic lupus erythematosus.* J Pediatr 85(1):31, 1974.

13. **Oinuma K, Harada Y, Nawata Y, et al.:** *Osteonecrosis in patients with systemic lupus erythematosus develops very early after starting high dose corticosteroid treatment.* Ann Rheum Dis 60(12):1145, 2001.

14. **Hargraves MM, Richmond H, Morton R:** *Presentation of two bone marrow elements: The "tart" cell and the "LE" cell.* Proc Mayo Clin 23(2):25, 1948.

15. **Keren DF:** *Antinuclear antibody testing.* Clin Lab Med 22:447, 2002.

16. **Siemsen JK, Brook J, Meister L:** *Lupus erythematosus and avascular bone necrosis. A clinical study of three cases and review of the literature.* Arthritis Rheum 5(5):492, 1962.

17. **Russell AS, Percy JS, Rigal WM, et al.:** *Deforming arthropathy in systemic lupus erythematosus.* Ann Rheum Dis 33:204, 1974.

18. **Kramer LS, Ruderman JE, Dubois EL, et al.:** *Deforming, nonerosive arthritis of the hands in chronic systemic lupus erythematosus* [Abstract]. Arthritis Rheum 13(3):329, 1970.

19. **Weissman BN, Rappaport AS, Sosman JL, et al.:** *Radiographic findings in the hands in patients with systemic lupus erythematosus.* Radiology 126:313, 1978.

20. **Bulgrin JG, Dubois EL, Jacobson G:** *Chest roentgenographic changes in systemic lupus erythematosus.* Radiology 74:42, 1960.

21. **Powell RJ:** *Systemic lupus erythematosus with widespread subcutaneous fat calcification.* Proc R Soc Med 67:215, 1974.

22. **Savin JA:** *Systemic lupus erythematosus with ectopic calcification.* Br J Dermatol 84:191, 1971.

23. **Weinberger A, Kaplan JG, Myers AR:** *Case report: Extensive soft tissue calcification (calcinosis universalis) in systemic lupus erythematosus.* Ann Rheum Dis 38:384, 1979.

24. **Klemp P, Meyers OL, Keyzer C:** *Atlantoaxial subluxation in systemic lupus erythematosus. A case report.* S Afr Med J 52:331, 1977.

25. **Noonan CD, Odone DT, Engeleman EP, et al.:** *Roentgenographic manifestations of joint disease in systemic lupus erythematosus.* Radiology 80:837, 1963.

26. **Klippel JH, Gerber LH, Pollak L, et al.:** *Avascular necrosis in systemic lupus erythematosus. Silent symmetric osteonecroses.* Am J Med 67:83, 1979.

27. **Aptekar RG, Klippel JH, Becker KE, et al.:** *Avascular necrosis of the talus, scaphoid and metatarsal head in systemic lupus erythematosus.* Clin Orthop 101:127, 1974.

28. **Smith FE, Sweet DE, Brunner CM, et al.:** *Avascular necrosis in SLE. An apparent predilection for young patients.* Ann Rheum Dis 34:227, 1976.

29. **Green N, Osmer JC:** *Small bone changes secondary to systemic lupus erythematosus.* Radiology 90:118, 1968.

30. **Ruderman M, McCarty DJ:** *Aseptic necrosis in systemic lupus erythematosus. Report of a case involving six joints.* Arthritis Rheum 7:42, 1960.

31. **Klipper AR, Stevens MB, Zizic TM, et al.:** *Ischemic necrosis of bone in systemic lupus erythematosus.* Medicine 55(3):251, 1976.

32. **Budin JA, Feldman F:** *Soft tissue calcifications in systemic lupus erythematosus.* Clin Orthop 101:127, 1974.

JACCOUD'S ARTHRITIS

1. **Jaccoud S:** *Lecons de Clinique Medicale Faites a l'Hopital de la Charite. Vingttroisieme Lecon sur une Forme de Rhumatisme Chronique.* Paris, Adrien Delahaye, 1867.

2. **Twigg H, Smith BF:** *Jaccoud's arthritis.* Radiology 80:417, 1963.

3. **Stollerman GH, Markowitz M, Taranta M, et al.:** *Jones criteria (revised) for guidance in the diagnosis of rheumatic fever.* Circulation. 32:664, 1965.

4. **Zvaifler NJ:** *Chronic postrheumatic fever (Jaccoud's) arthritis.* N Eng J Med 267:10, 1962.

5. **Murphy WA, Staple TW:** *Jaccoud's arthropathy reviewed.* AJR 118:300, 1973.
6. **Grahame R, Mitchell ABS, Scott JT:** *Chronic post rheumatic fever (Jaccoud's) arthropathy.* Ann Rheum Dis 29:622, 1970.
7. **Benjamin J, Chacko V:** *Chronic post rheumatic fever arthritis (Jaccoud's arthritis) involving the feet.* J Bone Joint Surg 66A(7): 1124, 1984.
8. **Bywaters EGL:** *The relation between heart and joint disease including "rheumatoid heart disease" and chronic post rheumatic arthritis (type Jaccoud).* Br Heart J 12:101, 1950.
9. **Girgis FL, Popple AW, Bruckner FE:** *Jaccoud's arthropathy. A case report and necropsy study.* Ann Rheum Dis 37:561, 1978.

IDIOPATHIC CHONDROLYSIS OF THE HIP

1. **Jones BS:** *Adolescent chondrolysis of the hip joint.* S Afr Med J 45:196, 1971.
2. **Daluga DJ, Millar EA:** *Idiopathic chondrolysis of the hip.* J Pediatr Orthop 9:405, 1989.
3. **Rowe LJ, Ho EK:** *Idiopathic chondrolysis of the hip.* Skeletal Radiol Feb: 25, 1996.
4. **Bleck EE:** *Idiopathic chondrolysis of the hip.* J Bone Joint Surg 65A:1266, 1983.
5. **Duncan JW, Nasca JR, Schrantz J:** *Idiopathic chondrolysis of the hip.* J Bone Joint Surg 61A:1024, 1979.
6. **Kozlowski K, Scougall J:** *Idiopathic chondrolysis—Diagnostic difficulties.* Pediatr Radiol 14:314, 1984.
7. **Roy DR, Crawford AH:** *Idiopathic chondrolysis of the hip: Management by subtotal capsulectomy and aggressive rehabilitation.* J Pediatr Orthop 8:203, 1988.
8. **Pellici PM, Wilson PD:** *Chondrolysis of the hips associated with severe burns.* J Bone Joint Surg 61A:592, 1979.
9. **Sivanantham M, Kannan Kutty M:** *Idiopathic chondrolysis of the hip: Case report with a review of the literature.* Aust NZ J Surg 47:229, 1977.
10. **Vrettos BC, Hoffman EB:** *Chondrolysis in slipped upper femoral epiphysis. Long term study of the etiology and natural history.* J Bone Joint Surg 75B:956, 1993.
11. **del Couz Garcia A, Fernandez PL, Gonzales MP, et al.:** *Idiopathic chondrolysis of the hip: long term evolution.* J Pediatr Orthop 19(4):449, 1999.
12. **Rachinsky I, Bogulavsky L, Cohen E, et al.:** *Bilateral idiopathic chondrolysis of the hip: A case report.* Clin Nucl Med 25:1007, 2000.
13. **Moule NJ, Golding JSR:** *Idiopathic chondrolysis of the hip.* Clin Radiol 25:47, 1974.
14. **van der Hoeven H, Keessen W, Kuis W:** *Idiopathic chondrolysis of the hip: A distinct clinical entity?* Acta Orthop Scand 60:661, 1991.
15. **Hughes AW:** *Idiopathic chondrolysis of the hip: A case report and review of the literature.* Ann Rheum Dis 44:268, 1985.
16. **Sartoris DJ, Resnick D:** *Radiologic vignette: Primary disorders of articular cartilage in childhood.* J Rheumatol 15:812, 1988.
17. **Shore A, Macauley D, Ansell BM:** *Idiopathic protrusio acetabuli in juveniles.* Rheumatol Rehab 20:1, 1981.
18. **Hooper JC, Jones EW:** *Primary protrusion of the acetabulum.* J Bone Joint Surg 53B:23, 1965.

SCLERODERMA

1. **Generini S, Fiori G, Moggi Pignoni A, et al.:** *Systemic sclerosis. A clinical overview.* Adv Exp Med Biol 1999;455:73–83
2. **Masi AT, Rodnam GP, Medsger TA, et al.:** *Preliminary criteria for the classification of systemic sclerosis (scleroderma).* Arthritis Rheum 23(5):581, 1980.
3. **Velayos EE, Masi AT, Stevens MB, et al.:** *The "CREST" syndrome. Comparison with systemic sclerosis (scleroderma).* Arch Int Med 139:1240, 1979.
4. **Thibierge G, Weissenbach RJ:** *Concretions calcaires sous-cutanees et sclerodermie.* Ann Dermatol Syph 2:129, 1911.
5. **Meszaros WT:** *The regional manifestations of scleroderma.* Radiology 70:313, 1958.

6. **Campbell PM, LeRoy EC:** *Pathogenesis of systemic sclerosis. A vascular hypothesis.* Semin Arthritis Rheum 4:351, 1975.
7. **Rose S, Young MA, Reynolds JC:** *Gastrointestinal manifestation of scleroderma.* Clin North Am 27(3):563, 1998.
8. **Rodnan GP, Medsger TA:** *Musculoskeletal involvement in progressive systemic sclerosis (scleroderma).* Bull Rheum Dis 17:419, 1966.
9. **Rodnan GP, Medsger TA Jr:** *The rheumatic manifestations of progressive systemic sclerosis (scleroderma).* Clin Orthop 57:81, 1968.
10. **Medsger T, Masi AT:** *Epidemiology of systemic sclerosis (scleroderma).* Ann Intern Med 74:714, 1971.
11. **Coffman JD, Cohen AS:** *Total and capillary fingertip blood flow in Raynaud's phenomenon.* N Engl J Med 285:259, 1971.
12. **Clements PJ, Furst DE, Campion DS, et al.:** *Muscle disease in progressive systemic sclerosis. Diagnostic and therapeutic considerations.* Arthritis Rheum 21(1):62, 1978.
13. **Steen VD:** *Treatment of systemic sclerosis.* Am J Clin Dermatol 2(5):315, 2001.
14. **Berends JC, Dompeling EC, van der Star JG, Hoorntje JC:** *Pulmonary hypertension with limited cutaneous scleroderma (CREST syndrome).* Neth J Med 57(6):229, 2000.
15. **Cossio M, Menon Y, Wilson W, deBoisblanc BP:** *Life-threatening complications of systemic sclerosis.* Crit Care Clin 18(4):819, 2002.
16. **Thompson AE, Pope JE:** *A study of the frequency of pericardial and pleural effusions in scleroderma.* Br J Rheumatol 37(12):1320, 1998.
17. **Fleischmajer R, Perlish JS, Reeves JRT:** *Cellular infiltrates in scleroderma skin.* Arthritis Rheum 20(4):975, 1977.
18. **Yune HY, Vix VA, Klatte EC:** *Early fingertip changes in scleroderma.* JAMA 215:1113, 1971.
19. **Fraser GM:** *The radiological manifestations of scleroderma (diffuse systemic sclerosis).* Br J Dermatol 78:1, 1966.
20. **Schlenker JD, Clark DD, Weckesscr EC:** *Calcinosis circumscripta of the hand in scleroderma.* J Bone Joint Surg 55A:1051, 1973.
21. **Resnick D, Scavulli JF, Goergen TG, et al.:** *Intra-articular calcification in scleroderma.* Radiology 124:685, 1977.
22. **Scarer L, Smith DW:** *Resorption of the terminal phalanges in scleroderma.* Arthritis Rheum 12(1):51, 1969.
23. **Wilde AH, Mankin HJ, Rodnan GP:** *Avascular necrosis of the femoral head in scleroderma.* Arthritis Rheum 13(4):445, 1970.
24. **Resnick D, Greenway G, Vint VC, et al.:** *Selective involvement of the first carpometacarpal joint in scleroderma.* AJR 131:283, 1978.
25. **Rabinowitz JG, Twersky J, Guttadauria M:** *Similar bone manifestations of scleroderma and rheumatoid arthritis.* AJR 121:35, 1974.
26. **Wild W, Beetham WP:** *Erosive arthropathy in systemic scleroderma.* JAMA 232:511, 1975.
27. **Stafne EC, Austin LT:** *A characteristic dental finding in acrosclerosis and diffuse scleroderma.* Am J Orthod 30:25, 1944.
28. **Gondos B:** *Roentgen manifestations in progressive systemic sclerosis (diffuse scleroderma).* AJR 84(2):235, 1960.
29. **Haverbush TJ, Wilde AH, Hawk WA Jr, et al.:** *Osteolysis of the ribs and cervical spine in progressive systemic sclerosis (scleroderma). A case report.* J Bone Joint Surg 56A:637, 1974.

OSTEITIS CONDENSANS ILII

1. **Hare HF, Haggart GE:** *Osteitis condensans ilii.* JAMA 128:723, 1945.
2. **Segal G, Kellog DS:** *Osteitis condensans ilii.* AJR 71:643, 1954.
3. **Gillespie HW, Lloyd-Roberts G:** *Osteitis condensans.* Br J Radiol 26(301):16, 1953.
4. **Numaguchi Y:** *Osteitis condensans ilii, including its resolution.* Radiology 98:1, 1971.
5. **McGregor M, Cassidy JD:** *Postsurgical sacroiliac joint syndrome.* J Manipulative Physiol Ther 6(1):1, 1983.
6. **Nykoliation J, Cassidy JD, Dupuis P:** *Osteitis condensans ilii—A sacroiliac stress phenomenon.* J Can Chiro Assoc 28(1):209, 1984.
7. **Jaqueline F, Arlet J:** *Osteitis condensans ilii. A comparison with the acetabular condensation observed in cases of osteoarthritis secondary to subluxation of the hip.* Arthritis Rheum 2:8, 1959.

8. **DeBosset P, Gordon DA, Smythe HA, et al.:** *Comparison of osteitis condensans ilii and ankylosing spondylitis in female patients: Clinical, radiological and HLA typing characteristics.* J Chron Dis 31:171, 1978.

9. **Resnick D, Niwayama G:** *Comparison of radiographic abnormalities of the sacroiliac joint in degenerative disease and ankylosing spondylitis.* AJR 128:189, 1977.

10. **Oliveri I, Gemignani G, Camerini E, et al.:** *Differential diagnosis between osteitis condensans ilii and sacroiliitis.* J Rheumatol 17:1504, 1990.

11. **Shipp FL, Haggart GE:** *Further experience in management of osteitis condensans ilii.* J Bone Joint Surg 32A:841, 1950.

12. **Singal DP, deBosset P, Gordon DA, et al.:** *HLA antigens in osteitis condensans ilii and ankylosing spondylitis.* J Rheumatol 4 (Suppl 3):105, 1977.

13. **Solonen KA:** *The sacroiliac joint in the light of anatomical, roentgenological and clinical studies.* Acta Orthop Scand (Suppl) 27:9, 1957.

14. **Szabados MD:** *Osteitis condensans ilii: Report of 3 cases associated with urinary tract infection.* J Fla Med Assoc 34:95, 1947.

15. **Ude WH:** *Osteitis condensans ilii: The possible relationship to juvenile epiphysitis.* Lancet 70:81, 1950.

16. **Wells J:** *Osteitis condensans ilii.* AJR 76 (6):1141, 1956.

17. **Dilhmann W:** *Diagnostic Radiology of the Sacroiliac Joints,* trans LS Michaelis. Chicago, Yearbook Medical, 1980.

18. **Borak J:** *Significance of the sacroiliac findings in Marie-Strumpell's spondylitis.* Radiology 47:128, 1946.

19. **Brower AC, Sweet DE, Keats TE:** *Condensing osteitis of the clavicle: A new entity.* AJR 121:17, 1974.

20. **Linker CS, Peterfy CG, Helms CA:** *Intraosseous pneumatocyst of the clavicle. Case 844.* Skeletal Radiol 23:315, 1994.

OSTEITIS PUBIS

1. **Combs JA:** *Bacterial osteitis pubis in a weight lifter without invasive trauma.* Med Sci Sports Exerc 30(11):1561, 1998.

2. **Beer E:** *(Osteitis pubis) periostitis of the symphysis and descending rami of the pubis following suprapubic operations.* Int J Med Surg 37:224, 1924.

3. **Burns JR, Gregory JG:** *Osteomyelitis of the pubic symphysis after urolic surgery.* J Urol 118:803, 1977.

4. **Cibert J:** *Post-operative osteitis pubis. Causes and treatment.* Br J Urol 24:213, 1952.

5. **Wiltse LL, Frantz CH:** *Non-suppurative osteitis pubis in the female.* J Bone Joint Surg 38A:500, 1956.

6. **Steinbach HL, Petrakis NL, Gillfillian RS, et al.:** *Pathogenesis of osteitis pubis.* J Urol 74:840, 1955.

7. **Bouza E, Winston DJ, Hewitt WL:** *Infectious osteitis pubis.* Urology 12(6):663, 1978.

8. **Schute WJ:** *Osteitis pubis.* Clin Orthop 20:187, 1961.

9. **Barnes, WC, Malament M:** *Osteitis pubis.* Surg Gynecol Obstet 117:277, 1963.

10. **Schneider R, Kaye JJ, Ghelman B:** *Adductor avulsive injuries near the symphysis pubis.* Radiology 120:567, 1976.

11. **Andrews SK, Carek PJ:** *Osteitis pubis: a diagnosis for the family physician.* J Am Board Fam Pract 11(4):291, 1998.

12. **Coventry MB, Mitchell WC:** *Osteitis pubis. Observations based on a study of 45 patients.* JAMA 178:898, 1961.

13. **Major NM, Helms CA:** *Pelvic stress injuries: the relationship between osteitis pubis (symphysis pubis stress injury) and sacroiliac abnormalities in athletes.* Skeletal Radiol 26(12):711, 1997.

14. **Wheeler WK:** *Periostitis pubes following suprapubic cystostomy.* J Urol 45:467, 1941.

15. **Pauli S, Willemsen P, Declerck K, et al.:** *Osteomyelitis pubis versus osteitis pubis: a case presentation and review of the literature.* Br J Sports Med 36(1):71, 2002.

16. **Gilbert DN, Azorr M, Gore R, et al.:** *The bacterial causation of postoperative osteitis pubis.* Surg Gynecol Obstet 141:195, 1975.

17. **Williams PR, Thomas DP, Downes EM:** *Osteitis pubis and instability of the pubic symphysis. When nonoperative measures fail.* Am J Sports Med 28(3):350, 2000.

HYPERTROPHIC OSTEOARTHROPATHY

1. **Segal AM, Mackenzie AH:** *Hypertrophic osteoarthropathy: A 10-year retrospective analysis.* Semin Arthritis Rheum 12(2):220, 1982.

2. **Caroll KB, Doyle L:** *A common factor in hypertrophic osteoarthropathy.* Thorax 29:262, 1974.

3. **Flavell G:** *Reversal of pulmonary hypertrophic osteoarthropathy by vagotomy.* Lancet 1:260, 1956.

4. **Jajic Z, Jajic I, Nemcic T:** *Primary hypertrophic osteoarthropathy: clinical, radiologic, and scintigraphic characteristics.* Arch Med Res 32:136, 2001.

5. **Kebudi R, Ayan I, Erseven G, et al.:** *Hypertrophic osteoarthropathy and intrathoracic Hodgkin disease of childhood.* Med Pediatr Oncol 29(6):578, 1997.

6. **Spruit S, Krijgsman AA, van den Broek JA, Tutein Nolthenius-Puylaer MC:** *Hypertrophic osteoarthropathy of one leg—a sign of aortic graft infection.* Skeletal Radiol 28(4):224, 1999.

7. **Gall E, Bennett GA, Bauer W:** *Generalized hypertrophic osteoarthropathy: Pathologic study of seven cases.* Am J Pathol 27:349, 1951.

8. **Oppenheimer DA, Jones HH:** *Hypertrophic osteoarthropathy of chronic inflammatory bowel disease.* Skeletal Radiol 9(2):109, 1982.

9. **Martinez-Lavin M, Bobadilla M, Casanova J, et al.:** *Hypertrophic osteoarthropathy in cyanotic congenital heart disease. Its prevalence and relationship to bypass of the lung.* Arthritis Rheum 25(10):1186, 1982.

10. **Holling HE, Brodey RS:** *Pulmonary hypertrophic osteoarthropathy.* JAMA 178:977, 1961.

11. **Chotkowski LA:** *Clubbing of the fingers in heroin addiction* [Letter]. N Engl J Med 311(4):262, 1984.

12. **Clarke S, Barnsley L, Peters M, et al.:** *Hypertrophic pulmonary osteoarthropathy without clubbing of the digits.* Skeletal Radiol 30(11):652, 2001.

13. **Holman CW:** *Osteoarthropathy in lung cancer: Disappearance after section of intercostal nerves.* J Thoracic Cardiovasc Surg 45(5):679, 1963.

14. **Orts D, Hernandez L, Barroso E, Romero S:** *Hypertrophic osteoarthropathy in lung cancer: are the radiographic bone changes reversible after curative resection?* Monaldi Arch Chest Dis 55(2):122, 2000

15. **Jaffe H:** *Metabolic, Degenerative and Inflammatory Diseases of Bones and Joints.* Philadelphia, Lea & Febiger, 1972.

16. **Racoceanu SN, Mendlowitz M, Suck AF, et al.:** *Digital capillary blood flow in clubbing. ^{85}Kr studies in hereditary and acquired cases.* Ann Int Med 75:933, 1971.

17. **Ali A, Tetalman MR, Fordham EW, et al.:** *Distribution of pulmonary osteoarthropathy.* AJR 134:771, 1980.

METABOLIC DISORDERS

GOUT

1. **Agudelo CA, Wise CM:** *Gout: diagnosis, pathogenesis, and clinical manifestations.* Curr Opin Rheumatol 13(3):234, 2001.

2. **Copeman WS:** *Historical aspects of gout.* Clin Orthop 71:14, 1970.

3. **Garrod AB:** *Treatise on gout.* Clin Orthop 71:3, 1970.

4. **Graham W, Graham KM:** *Martyrs to the gout.* Metabolism 6(3):209, 1957.

5. **Rodnan GP, Benedek TG:** *Ancient therapeutic arts in the gout.* Arthritis Rheum 6(4):317, 1963.

6. **Boss GR, Seegmiller JE:** *Hyperuricemia and gout. Classification, complications, and management.* N Engl J Med 300:1459, 1979.

7. **Hartung EF:** *Symposium on gout. Historical considerations.* Metabolism 6(3):196, 1959.

8. **Jajic I:** *Gout in the spine and sacroiliac joints. Radiologic manifestations.* Skeletal Radiol 8:209, 1982.

9. **Vinstein AL, Cockerill EM:** *Involvement of the spine in gout. A case report.* Radiology 103:311, 1972.

10. **Resnick D, Reinke RT, Taketa RM:** *Early onset gouty arthritis.* Radiology 114:67, 1975.

11. **Greenhut IJ, Silver RA, Campbell JA:** *Occurrence of gout in a female. Report of an unusual case.* Radiology 60:257, 1953.
12. **Yu T:** *Some unusual features of gouty arthritis in females.* Semin Arthritis Rheum 6(3):247, 1977.
13. **Becker MA, Seegmiller JE:** *Genetic aspects of gout.* Ann Rev Med 25:15, 1974.
14. **Prior IAM, Rose BS, Harvey HPB, et al.:** *Hyperuricemia, gout and diabetic abnormality in Polynesian people.* Lancet 1:333, 1966.
15. **Rose BS:** *Gout in Maoris.* Semin Arthritis Rheum 5(2):121, 1975.
16. **Burnham J, Fraker K, Steinbach H:** *Pathologic fracture in an unusual case of gout.* AJR 129:1116, 1977.
17. **Healey LA, Bayani-Sioson PS:** *A defect in the renal excretion of uric acid in Filipinos.* Arthritis Rheum 14 (6):721, 1971.
18. **Seegmiller JE:** *Metabolic aberrations in gout.* Clin Orthop 71:87, 1970.
19. **Arromdee E, Michet CJ, Crowson CS, et al.:** *Epidemiology of gout: is the incidence rising?* J Rheumatol 29(11):2403, 2002.
20. **Steinberg VL, Wenley WG, Mason RM:** *Gout: I. Pathogenesis and natural history; II. Treatment.* Br J Clin Pract 16:173, 1962.
21. **Dincer HE, Dincer AP, Levinson DJ:** *Asymptomatic hyperuricemia: to treat or not to treat.* Cleve Clin J Med 69(8):594, 2002
22. **van Doornum S, Ryan PF:** *Clinical manifestations of gout and their management.* Med J Aust 15;172(10):493, 2000.
23. **Watt I, Middlemiss H:** *The radiology of gout. Review article.* Clin Radiol 26:27, 1975.
24. **Rosenberg EF, Arens RA:** *Gout: Clinical, pathologic and roentgenographic observations.* Radiology 49:169, 1947.
25. **O'Duffy JD, Hunder GG, Kelly PJ:** *Decreasing prevalence of tophaceous gout.* Mayo Clin Proc 50:227, 1975.
26. **Seegmiller JE:** *The present day treatment of gout.* Med Clin North Am 45(5):1259, 1961.
27. **Yu T:** *Pathogenesis and medical management of chronic gouty arthritis.* Clin Orthop 72:40, 1970.
28. **Gelberman RH, Doty DH, Hamer ML:** *Tophaceous gout involving the proximal interphalangeal joint.* Clin Orthop 147:225, 1980.
29. **Larmon WA:** *Surgical management of tophaceous gout.* Clin Orthop 71:56, 1970.
30. **Koskoff YD, Morris LE, Lubic LG:** *Paraplegia as a complication of gout.* JAMA 152:37, 1953.
31. **Lichenstein L, Scott HW, Levin MH:** *Pathologic changes in gout.* Am J Pathol 32(5):871, 1956.
32. **Ogryzlo MA:** *Visceral (nonarticular) manifestations associated with gout.* Clin Orthop 71:46, 1970.
33. **Talbot JH:** *Diagnosis of gout.* Clin Orthop 71:23, 1970.
34. **McCarty DJ, Hollander JL:** *Identification of urate crystals in gouty synovial fluid.* Ann Intern Med 54:452, 1961.
35. **McCarty D:** *Pathogenesis and treatment of the acute attack of gout.* Clin Orthop 71:28, 1970.
36. **Pittman JR, Bross MH:** *Diagnosis and management of gout.* Am Fam Physician 59(7):1799, 1999.
37. **Molad Y:** *Update on colchicines and its mechanism of action.* Curr Rheumatol Rep 4(3):252, 2002.
38. **Schlesiger N, Detry MA, Holland BK, et al.:** *Local ice therapy during bouts of acute gouty arthritis.* J Rheumatol 29(2):331, 2002.
39. **Lesch M, Nyhan WL:** *A familial disorder of uric acid metabolism and central nervous system function.* Am J Med 36:561, 1964.
40. **Nyhan WL, James JA, Teberg AJ, et al.:** *A new disorder of purine metabolism with behavioral manifestations.* J Pediatr 74 (1):20, 1969.
41. **Spilberg I:** *Current concepts of the mechanism of acute inflammation in gouty arthritis.* Arthritis Rheum 18(2):129, 1975.
42. **Bloch C, Hermann G, Hu TF:** *A radiologic reevaluation of gout: A study of 2000 patients.* AJR 134:781, 1982.
43. **Good AE, Rapp R:** *Bony ankylosis. A rare manifestation in gout.* J Rheumatol 5:335, 1978.
44. **Martel W:** *The overhanging margin of bone: A roentgenologic manifestation of gout.* Radiology 91:755, 1968.
45. **Dodds WJ, Steinbach HL:** *Gout associated with calcification of cartilage.* N Engl J Med 275:745, 1966.

46. **Stockman A, Darlington LG, Scott JT:** *Frequency of chondrocalcinosis of the knees and avascular necrosis of the femoral heads in gout: A controlled study.* Ann Rheum Dis 39:7, 1980.
47. **Hunder GG, Worthington JW, Bickel WH:** *Avascular necrosis of the femoral head in a patient with gout.* JAMA 203:47, 1968.
48. **Miskew DBW, Goldflies ML:** *A traumatic avascular necrosis of the talus associated with hyperuricemia.* Clin Orthop 148:156, 1980.
49. **Schabel SI, Korn JH, Rittenberg GM, et al.:** *Bone infarction in gout.* Skeletal Radiol 3:42, 1978.
50. **Bailsford JF:** *The radiology of gout.* Clin Orthop 71:28, 1970.
51. **Egan R, Sartoris DJ, Resnick D:** *Radiographic features of gout in the foot.* J Foot Surg 26:434, 1987.
52. **Wright JT:** *Unusual manifestations of gout.* Aust Radiol 10:365, 1966.
53. **Chen CK, Chung CB, Yeh L, et al.:** *Carpal tunnel syndrome caused by tophaceous gout: CT and MR imaging features in 20 patients.* AJR Am J Roentgenol 175(3):655, 2000.
54. **Recht MP, Seragini F, Kramer J, et al.:** *Isolated or dominant lesions of the patella in gout: A report of seven patients.* Skeletal Radiol 23:113, 1994.
55. **Alarcon-Segovia D, Cetina JA, Diaz-Jouanen E:** *Sacroiliac joints in primary gout: Clinical and roentgenographic study of 143 patients.* AJR 118:438, 1973.
56. **Malawista SE, Seegmiller JE, Hathaway BE, et al.:** *Sacroiliac gout.* JAMA 194:954, 1965.
57. **Bastani B, Vemuri R, Gennis M:** *Acute gouty sacroilitis: A case report and review of the literature.* Mt Sinai J Med 64(6):383, 1997.
58. **Tkach S:** *Gouty arthritis of the spine.* Clin Orthop 71:81, 1970.
59. **Hall MC, Selin G:** *Spinal involvement in gout.* J Bone Joint Surg 42A(2):341, 1960.
60. **Lagier R, MacGee W:** *Spondylodiscal erosions due to gout: Anatomico-radiological study of a case.* Ann Rheum Dis 42(3):350, 1983.
61. **Yen HL, Cheng CH, Lin JW:** *Cervical myelopathy due to gouty tophi in the intervertebral disc space.* Acta Neurochir (Wien) 144:205, 2002.
62. **Sequira W, Bouffard A, Salgia K, et al.:** *Quadriparesis in tophaceous gout.* Arthritis Rheum 24:1428, 1981.
63. **Yasuhara K, Tomita Y, Takayama A, et al.:** *Thoracic myelopathy due to compression by the epidural tophus. A case report.* J Spinal Dis 7:82, 1994.
64. **Hsu CY, Shih TT, Huang KM, et al.:** *Tophaceous gout of the spine: MR imaging features.* Clin Radiol 57(10):919, 2002.
65. **Kao MC, Huang SC, Chiu CT, Yao YT:** *Thoracic cord compression due to gout: a case report and literature review.* J Formos Med Assoc 99(7):572, 2000.

CALCIUM PYROPHOSPHATE DIHYDRATE CRYSTAL DEPOSITION DISEASE

1. **McCarty DJ, Kohn NN, Fires JS:** *The significance of calcium phosphate crystals in synovial fluid of arthritic patients: The "pseudogout syndrome."* Ann Int Med 56 (5):711, 1962.
2. **McCarty DJ:** *Calcium pyrophosphate dihydrate crystal deposition disease: Nomenclature and diagnostic criteria.* Ann Int Med 87(2):240, 1977.
3. **Resnick D, Niwayama G, Goergen TG, et al.:** *Clinical, radiographic and pathologic abnormalities in calcium pyrophosphate dihydrate deposition disease (CPPD): Pseudogout.* Radiology 122:1, 1977.
4. **Helms CA, Chapman GS, Wild JH:** *Charcot-like joints in calcium pyrophosphate dihydrate deposition disease.* Skeletal Radiol 7:55, 1981.
5. **Moskowitz RW, Katz D:** *Chondrocalcinosis coincidental to other rheumatic disease.* Arch Intern Med 115:680, 1965.
6. **Taylor JAM, Resnick D:** *Acute wrist pain following hernia repair.* J Musculoskel Med Oct:79, 1992.
7. **Gerster JC, Doenz F:** *Unusual destructive and hypertrophic arthropathy of the atlanto-axial joint in calcium pyrophosphate dihydrate deposition disease.* Osteoarthritis Cartilage 2(4):275, 1994.

8. **Assaker R, Louis E, Boutry N, et al.:** *Foramen magnum syndrome secondary to calcium pyrophosphate crystal deposition in the transverse ligament of the atlas.* Spine 26:1396, 2001.
9. **Baysal T, Baysal O, Kutlu R, et al.:** *The crowned dens syndrome: A rare form of calcium pyrophosphate deposition disease.* Eur Radiol 10(6):1003, 2000.
10. **Greaves S, Fordyce A:** *Bilateral temporomandibular joint pseudogout.* Br Dent J 192(1):25, 2002.
11. **Lagier R, Boivin G, Gerster JC:** *Carpal tunnel syndrome associated with mixed calcium pyrophosphate dihydrate and apatite crystal deposition in tendon synovial sheath.* Arthritis Rheum 27:1190, 1984.
12. **Zitnan D, Sitaj S:** *Natural course of articular chondrocalcinosis.* Arthritis Rheum 19(3):363, 1976.
13. **Reginato AJ:** *Articular chondrocalcinosis in the Chiloe islanders.* Arthritis Rheum 19(3):395, 1976.
14. **McCarty DJ, Hogan JM, Galter RA, et al.:** *Studies in pathological calcifications in human cartilage.* J Bone Joint Surg 48A(2):309, 1966.
15. **Rubenstein J, Pritzker KPH:** *Crystal-associated arthropathies.* AJR 152:685, 1989.
16. **Currey HLF:** *Pyrophosphate arthropathy and calcific periarthritis.* Clin Orthop 71:70, 1971.
17. **Bjelle AO:** *Morphological study of articular cartilage in pyrophosphate arthropathy.* Ann Rheum Dis 31:449, 1972.
18. **Moskowitz RW, Harris BK, Schwartz A, et al.:** *Chronic synovitis as a manifestation of calcium crystal deposition disease.* Arthritis Rheum 14(1):109, 1971.
19. **Dalinka MK, Reginato AJ, Golden DA:** *Calcium deposition diseases.* Semin Roentgenol 17(1):39, 1982.
20. **Canhao H, Fonseca JE, Leandro MJ, et al.:** *Cross-sectional study of 50 patients with calcium pyrophosphate dihydrate crystal arthropathy.* Clin Rheumatol 20(2):119, 2001.
21. **Bundens WD, Brighton CT, Weitzman G:** *Primary articular cartilage calcification with arthritis (pseudogout syndrome).* J Bone Joint Surg 47A(1):111, 1965.
22. **Bocher J, Mankin HJ, Berk RN, et al.:** *Prevalence of calcified meniscal cartilage in elderly persons.* N Engl J Med 272(21):1093, 1965.
23. **Linden B, Nilsson BE:** *Chondrocalcinosis following osteochondritis dissecans in the femur condyles.* Clin Orthop 130:223, 1978.
24. **Stockman A, Darlington LG, Scott JT:** *Frequency of chondrocalcinosis of the knees and avascular necrosis of the femoral heads in gout: A controlled study.* Ann Rheum Dis 39:7, 1980.
25. **Sone M, Ehara S, Kashiwagi K, et al.:** *Massive calcium pyrophosphate dihydrate crystal deposition disease involving the wrist joint. Case 859.* Skeletal Radiol 23:475, 1994.
26. **McCarty DJ Jr, Haskin ME:** *The roentgenographic aspects of pseudogout (articular chondrocalcinosis): An analysis of 20 cases.* AJR 90:1248, 1963.
27. **Frankel VH:** *The Terry Thomas sign* [Letter]. Clin Orthop 129:321, 1977.
28. **Resnick D, Tusinger PD:** *The wrist arthropathy of "pseudogout" occurring with and without chondrocalcinosis.* Radiology 113:633, 1974.
29. **Resnick D, Pineda C:** *Vertebral involvement in calcium pyrophosphate dihydrate crystal deposition disease.* Radiology 153:55, 1984.
30. **Chen C, Chadnani VP, Kang HS, et al.:** *Scapholunate advanced collapse: A common wrist abnormality in calcium pyrophosphate dihydrate crystal deposition disease.* Radiology 177:459, 1990.
31. **Salcman M, Khan A, Symonds DA:** *Calcium pyrophosphate arthropathy of the spine: Case report and review of the literature.* Neurosurgery 34:915, 1994.
32. **Brown TR, Quinn SF, D'Agostino AN:** *Deposition of calcium pyrophosphate dihydrate crystals in the ligamentum flavum: Evaluation with MR imaging and CT.* Radiology 178:871, 1991.
33. **El-Khoury GY, Tozzi JE, Clark CR, et al.:** *Massive calcium pyrophosphate crystal deposition at the cranioverteberal junction.* AJR 145:777, 1985.
34. **Huang GS, Bachmann D, Taylor JAM, et al.:** *Calcium pyrophosphate dihydrate crystal deposition disease and pseudogout of the acromioclavicular joint: Radiographic and pathologic features.* J Rheumatol 20:2077, 1993.

HYDROXYAPATITE DEPOSITION DISEASE

1. **Bonavita JA, Dalinka MK, Schumacher HR Jr:** *Hydroxyapatite deposition disease.* Radiology 134:621, 1980.
2. **Fam AG, Pritzker KPH, Stein JL, et al.:** *Apatite-associated arthropathy: A clinical study of 14 cases and of 2 patients with calcific bursitis.* J Rheumatol 6:461, 1979.
3. **Pinals RS, Short CL:** *Calcific periarthritis involving multiple sites.* Arthritis Rheum 8:462, 1965.
4. **Friis J, Jensen EM, Karle AK:** *Calcified periarthritis at multiple sites including lumbar intervertebral discs.* Acta Radiologica 20:928, 1979.
5. **Gondos B:** *Observations on periarthritis calcarea.* AJR 77:93, 1957.
6. **Uhthoff HK, Sarkar K, Maynard JA:** *Calcifying tendinitis. A new concept of its pathogenesis.* Clin Orthop 118:164, 1976.
7. **McCarty DJ, Gatter RA:** *Recurrent acute inflammation associated with focal apatite crystal deposition.* Arthritis Rheum 9(6):804, 1966.
8. **Halverson PB, McCarty DJ:** *Identification of hydroxyapatite crystals in synovial fluid.* Arthritis Rheum 21:563, 1978.
9. **Greenway GD, Danzig LA, Resnick D, et al.:** *The painful shoulder.* Med Radiography Photography 58(2):61, 1982.
10. **Bosworth BM:** *Calcium deposits in the shoulder and subacromial bursitis: A survey of 12,122 shoulders.* JAMA 116:2477, 1941.
11. **ViGario DG, Keats TE:** *Localization of calcific deposits in the shoulder.* AJR 108:806.
12. **Yochum TR:** *Calcifying peritendinitis of the gluteus maximus tendon.* ACA J Chiro April, 1982.
13. **Berney JW:** *Calcifying peritendinitis of the gluteus maximus tendon.* Radiology 102:517, 1972.
14. **Callaghan BD:** *Unusual calcification in the region of the gluteus medius and minimus muscles.* Aust Radiol 21:362, 1977.
15. **Haun CL:** *Retropharyngeal tendinitis.* AJR 130:1137, 1978.
16. **Newmark H III, Forrester DM, Brown JC, et al.:** *Calcific tendinitis of the neck.* Radiology 128:355, 1978.
17. **Bernstein SA:** *Acute cervical pain associated with soft-tissue calcium deposition anterior to the interspace of the first and second cervical vertebrae.* J Bone Joint Surg 37A:426, 1975.
18. **Fahlgren H:** *Retropharyngeal tendinitis: Three probable cases with an unusually low epicentre.* Cephalgia 8:105, 1988.
19. **Artenian DJ, Lipman JK, Scidmore GK, et al.:** *Acute neck pain due to tendinitis of the longus colli: CT and MRI findings.* Neuroradiology 31:166, 1989.
20. **Hartley J:** *Acute cervical pain associated with retropharyngeal calcium deposit.* J Bone Joint Surg 46A(8):1753, 1964.
21. **Sutro CJ:** *Calcification of the anterior atlanto-axial ligament as the cause for painful swallowing and for painful neck.* Bull Hosp Joint Dis 28:1, 1967.
22. **von Lushka H:** *Die Halbgelenke des Menschichen Korpers.* Berlin, Reimer, 1858.
23. **Calve J, Galland M:** *Sur une affection particuliere de la colonne vertebrale simultant le mal de Pott.* J Radiol Electrol Med Nucl 6:21, 1922.
24. **Weinberger A, Meyers AR:** *Intervertebral disc calcification in adults. A review.* Semin Arthritis Rheum 8(1):69, 1978.
25. **Schmorl G, Junghanns H:** *The Human Spine in Health and Disease,* ed 2, trans EF Besemann. New York, Grune & Stratton, 1971.
26. **Lindberg T:** *Intervertebral calcinosis in childhood.* Ann Pediatr 201:173, 1963.
27. **Hadley LA:** *Anatomico-Roentgenographic Studies of the Spine,* ed 3. Springfield, Charles C Thomas, 1976.
28. **Smith DM:** *Acute back pain associated with a calcified Schmorl's node. A case report.* Clin Orthop 117:193, 1976.
29. **Dussault RG, Kaye JJ:** *Intervertebral disc calcification associated with spine fusion.* Radiology 125:57, 1977.

30. **Henry MJ, Grimes HA, Lane JW:** *Intervertebral disk calcification in childhood.* Radiology 89:81, 1967.
31. **Eyring EJ, Peterson CA, Bjornson DR:** *Intervertebral disc calcification in childhood. A distinct clinical syndrome.* J Bone Joint Surg 46A(7):1432, 1964.
32. **Silverman FN:** *Calcification of the intervertebral disks in childhood.* Radiology 62(6):801, 1954.
33. **von Blomquist HK, Lindqvist M, Mattson S:** *Calcification of intervertebral discs in childhood.* Pediatr Radiol 8:23, 1979.
34. **Melnick JC, Silverman FN:** *Intervertebral disc calcification in childhood.* Radiology 80:399, 1963.
35. **Rechtman AM, Hermel MB, Albert SM, et al.:** *Calcification of the intervertebral disk: Disappearing, dormant and silent.* Clin Orthop 7:218, 1956.
36. **Yochum TR:** *Childhood idiopathic disc calcification.* ACA J Chiro February, 1981.
37. **Ginalski JM, Landry M, Gudinchet F, et al.:** *Is tomography of intervertebral disc calcification useful in children?* Pediatr Radiol 22:59, 1992.
38. **Furukawa K, Hoshino R, Hasue M, et al.:** *Cervical intervertebral disc calcification in child. Case report with seven-year follow-up.* J Bone Joint Surg 59A:692, 1977.
39. **Mainzer F:** *Herniation of the nucleus pulposus. A rare complication of intervertebral disc calcification in children.* Pediatr Radiol 107:167, 1973.
40. **Sherman WD, Mulfinger GL, Garner JT, et al.:** *Calcified cervical intervertebral discs in childhood. Report of two cases.* Spine 1:155, 1976.
41. **Hughes ESR:** *Acute deposition of calcium near the elbow.* J Bone Joint Surg 32B(1):30, 1950.
42. **Seidenstein H:** *Acute pain in the wrist and hand associated with calcific deposits.* J Bone Joint Surg 32A(2):413, 1950.
43. **Gandee RW, Harrison RB, Dee PM:** *Peritendinitis calcarea of flexor carpi ulnaris.* AJR 133:1139, 1979.
44. **Martin JF, Brogdon BG:** *Peritendinitis calcarea of the hand and wrist.* AJR 78:74, 1957.
45. **Weston WJ:** *De Quervain's disease—Stenosing fibrous tendovaginitis at the radial styloid process.* Br J Radiol 40:446, 1967.
46. **deCarvalho A, Illum F, Jorgensen J:** *Calcifications simulating peroneus longus tendinitis.* Skeletal Radiol 12:37, 1984.
47. **Weston WJ:** *Tendinitis calcarea on the dorsum of the foot.* Br J Radiol 32:495, 1959.

OCHRONOSIS

1. **Dom K, Pittevils T:** *Ochronotic arthropathy: The black hip. Case report and review of the literature.* Acta Orthop Belg 63(2):122, 1997.
2. **Garcia SF, Egbert B, Swetter SM:** *Hereditary ochronosis: Hyperpigmented skin overlying cartilaginous structures.* Cutis 63(6):337, 1999.
3. **Obrien WM, LaDu BN, Bunim JJ:** *Biochemical, pathologic, and clinical aspects of alcaptonuria, ochronosis, and ochronotic arthropathy. Review of world literature (1584–1962).* Am J Med 34:813, 1963.
4. **Simon G, Zorab PA:** *The radiographic changes in alkaptonuric arthritis. A report on three cases (one an Egyptian mummy).* Br J Radiol 34(402):384, 1961.
5. **Thompson MM:** *Ochronosis.* AJR 78(1):46, 1957.
6. **Smith JW:** *Ochronosis of the sclera and cornea complicating alkaptonuria. Review of the literature and report of four cases.* JAMA 120(16):1282, 1942.
7. **McCollum DE, Odom GL:** *Alkaptonuria, ochronosis and low back pain.* J Bone Joint Surg 47A(7):1389, 1965.
8. **Nas K, Gur A, Akdeniz S, et al.:** *Ochronosis: A case of severe ochronotic arthropathy.* Clin Rheumatol 21:170, 2002.
9. **Ravel R:** *Clinical Laboratory Medicine: Clinical Application of Laboratory Data,* ed 3. Chicago, Year Book Medical, 1978.
10. **Phornphutkul C, Introne WJ, Perry MB, et al.:** *Natural history of alkaptonuria.* N Engl J Med 347(26):2111, 2002.

11. **Suzuki Y, Oda K, Yoshikawa Y, et al.:** *A novel therapeutic trial of homogentisic aciduria model of alkaptonuria.* J Hum Genet 44(2):79, 1999.
12. **Hamdi N, Cooke TD, Hassan B:** *Ochronotic Arthropathy: Case report and review of the literature.* Int Orthop 23(2):122, 1999.
13. **Mestan MA, Bustin GL, Wagner LA:** *Chiropractic care and ochronotic arthropathy.* J Manipulative Physiol Ther 22(7):473, 1999.
14. **Kocyigit H, Gurgan A, Terzioglu R, Gurgan U:** *Clinical, radiographic and echocardiographic findings in a patient with ochronosis.* Clin Rheumatol 17(5):403, 1998.
15. **LaDu BN, Zannoni VG, Laster L, et al.:** *The nature of the defect in tyrosine metabolism in alcaptonuria.* J Biol Chemistry 230:251, 1958.
16. **Lagier R, Sitaj S:** *Vertebral changes in ochronosis. Anatomical and radiological study of one case.* Ann Rheum Dis 33:86, 1974.
17. **Pomeranz MM, Friedman LJ, Tunick IS:** *Roentgen findings in alkaptonuric ochronosis.* Radiology 37:295, 1941.
18. **Pagan-Carlo J, Payzant AR:** *Roentgenographic manifestations in a severe case of alkaptonuric osteoarthritis.* AJR 80 (4):635, 1958.
19. **Harrold AJ:** *Alkaptonuric arthritis.* J Bone Joint Surg 38B(2):532, 1956.
20. **Lagier R, Steiger U:** *Hip arthropathy in ochronosis: Anatomical and radiological study.* Skeletal Radiol 5:91, 1980.
21. **Laskar FH, Sargison KD:** *Ochronotic arthropathy. A review with four case reports.* J Bone Joint Surg 52B(4):653, 1970.
22. **Mueller MN, Sorensen LB, Strandjord N, et al.:** *Alkaptonuria and ochronotic arthropathy.* Med Clin North Am 45:101, 1965.

TUMORAL CALCINOSIS

1. **Senol U, Karaal K, Cevikol C, Dincer A:** *MR imaging findings of recurrent tumoral calcinosis.* Clin Imaging 24(3):154, 2000.
2. **Harkess JW, Peters HJ:** *Tumoral calcinosis. A report of six cases.* J Bone Joint Surg 49A:721, 1967.
3. **Durant DM, Riley LH III, Burger PC, McCarthy EF:** *Tumoral calcinosis of the spine: A study of 21 cases.* Spine 26(15):1673, 2001.
4. **Agnew CH:** *Tumoral calcinosis. A radiologic teaching method.* J Kans Med Soc 62:100, 1961.
5. **Pakasa NM, Kalengayi RM:** *Tumoral calcinosis: A clinicopathological study of 111 cases with emphasis on the earliest changes.* Histopathology 31(1):18, 1997.
6. **Palmer PES:** *Tumoral calcinosis.* Br J Radiol 39:518, 1966.
7. **Murai S, Matsui M, Nakamura A:** *Tumoral calcinosis in both index fingers: A case report.* Scand J Plast Reconstr Surg Hand Surg 35(4):433, 2001.
8. **Sebesta A, Kamineni S, Dumont CE:** *Idiopathic tumoral calcinosis of the index finger. Case report.* Scand J Plast Reconstr Surg Hand Surg 34(4):405, 2000.
9. **Sanchez-Martin A, Proubasta-Renart I:** *Acute carpal tunnel syndrome caused by idiopathic tumoral calcinosis.* J South Orthop Assoc 10(2):92, 2001.
10. **Prahinski JR. Schaefer RA:** *Tumoral calcinosis of the foot.* Foot Ankle Int 22(11):911, 2001.
11. **Matsukado K, Amano T, Itou O, et al.:** *Tumoral calcinosis in the upper cervical spine causing progressive radiculomyelopathy—Case report.* Neurol Med Chir (Tokyo) 41(8):411, 2001.
12. **Hacihanefioglu V:** *Tumoral calcinosis: A clinical and pathologic study of eleven unreported cases in Turkey.* J Bone Joint Surg 60A:1131, 1978.
13. **Martinez S:** *Tumoral calcinosis: 12 years later.* Semin Musculoskelet Radiol 6(4):331, 2002.
14. **Barton DL, Reeves RJ:** *Tumoral calcinosis. Report of three cases and review of the literature.* AJR 86:351, 1961.
15. **Kolawole TM, Bohner SP:** *Tumoral calcinosis with "fluid levels" in the tumoral masses.* AJR 120:461, 1974.

SARCOIDOSIS

1. **James DG, Neville E, Carstairs LS:** *Bone and joint sarcoidosis.* Semin Arthritis Rheum 6:53, 1976.
2. **Longcope WT, Freiman DG:** *A study of sarcoidosis based on a combined investigation of 160 cases including 30 autopsies from Johns Hopkins and Massachusetts General Hospitals.* Medicine 31:1, 1952.

3. **Holt JF, Owens WI:** *The osseous lesions of sarcoidosis.* Radiology 53:11, 1949.
4. **Berk RN, Brower TD:** *Vertebral sarcoidosis.* Radiology 82:660, 1964.
5. **Lynch JP III, Sharma OP, Baughman RP:** *Extrapulmonary sarcoidosis.* Semin Respir Infect 13(3):229, 1998.
6. **Jones NP:** *Sarcoidosis and uveitis.* Ophthalmol Clin North Am 15(3):319, 2002.
7. **James DG:** *Dermatological aspects of sarcoidosis.* Q J Med 28:109, 1959.
8. **Lofgren S:** *Erythema nodosum. Studies on etiology and pathogenesis in 185 adult cases.* Acta Med Scand 124(Suppl 174):1, 1946.
9. **Poyanli A, Poyanli O, Sencer S, et al.:** *Vertebral sarcoidosis: Imaging findings.* Eur Radiol 10(1):92, 2000.
10. **Jelinek JS, Mark AS, Barth WF:** *Sclerotic lesions of the cervical spine in sarcoidosis.* Skeletal Radiol 37(12):702, 1998.
11. **Pierson DJ, Willet S:** *Sarcoidosis presenting with finger pain.* JAMA 239:2023, 1978.
12. **Conron M, Young C, Beynon HL:** *Calcium metabolism in sarcoidosis and its clinical implications.* Rheumatology (Oxford) 39(7):707, 2000.
13. **Wilcox A, Bharadwaj P, Sharma OP:** *Bone sarcoidosis.* Curr Opin Rheumatol 12(4):321, 2000.
14. **Giuffrida TJ, Kerdel FA:** *Sarcoidosis.* Dermatol Clin 20(3):435, 2002.
15. **Gal AA, Koss MN:** *The pathology of sarcoidosis.* Curr Opin Pulm Med 8(5):445, 2002.
16. **Ludwig V, Fordice S, Lamar R, et al.:** *Unsuspected skeletal sarcoidosis mimicking metastatic disease on FDG positron emission tomography and bone scintigraphy.* Clin Nucl Med 28(3):176, 2003.
17. **Stein GN, Israel HL, Sones M:** *A roentgenographic study of skeletal lesions in sarcoidosis.* Arch Intern Med 97:532, 1956.
18. **McBrine CS, Fisher MS:** *Acrosclerosis in sarcoidosis.* Radiology 115:279, 1975.
19. **Beasley EW III, Peterman SB, Hertzler GL:** *An unusual form of tibial sarcoidosis.* AJR 149:754, 1987.
20. **Lin S-R, Levy W, Go EB, et al.:** *Unusual osteosclerotic changes in sarcoidosis simulating osteoblastic metastases.* Radiology 106:311, 1973.
21. **Kobayashi H, Kotoura Y, Sakahara H, et al.:** *Solitary muscular sarcoidosis: CT, MRI, and scintigraphic characteristics.* Skeletal Radiol 23:293, 1994.
22. **Cohen NP, Gosset J, Staron RB, Levine WN:** *Vertebral sarxoidosis of the spine in a football player.* Am J Orthop 30(12):875, 2001.
23. **Le Breton C, Ferroir JP, Cadrenal J, et al.:** *Leptomeningeal and spinal-pelvic osseous sarcoidosis. Case 825.* Skeletal Radiol 23:297, 1994.
24. **Zimmerman R, Leeds NE:** *Calvarial and vertebral sarcoidosis. Case report and review of the literature.* Radiology 119:384, 1976.
25. **Young DA, Laman ML:** *Radiodense skeletal lesions in Boeck's sarcoid.* AJR 114:553, 1972.
26. **Abdelwahab IF, Norman A:** *Osteosclerotic sarcoidosis.* AJR 150:161, 1988.
27. **Golzarian J, Matos C, Golstein M, et al.:** *Case report: Osteosclerotic sarcoidosis of spine and pelvis: Plain film and magnetic resonance imaging findings.* Br J Radiol 67:401, 1994.

Pigmented Villonodular Synovitis

1. **Tatari H, Baran O, Lebe B, et al.:** *Pigmented villonodular synovitis of the knee presenting as a popliteal cyst.* Arthroscopy 16(6):13, 2000.
2. **Pimpalnerkar A, Barton E, Sibly TF:** *Pigmented villonodular synovitis of the elbow.* J Shoulder Elbow Surg 7(1):71, 1998.
3. **Hertaux A:** *Meylome des gaines tendineuses.* Arch Gen Med 27:40, 160, 1891.
4. **Stout AP, Lattes R:** *Tumors of the Soft Tissues. Atlas of Tumor Pathology,* ser 2, sasicle 1. Washington, DC, Armed Forces Institute of Pathology, 1967.
5. **Kalil RK, Unni KK:** *Malignancy in pigmented villonodular synovitis.* Skeletal Radiol 27(7):392, 1998.
6. **Ghert MA, Scully SP, Harrelson JM:** *Pigmented villonodular synovitis of the foot and ankle: A review of six cases.* Foot Ankle Int 20(5):326, 1999.
7. **Muller LP, Bitzer M, Degreif J, Rommens PM:** *Pigmented villonodular synovitis of the shoulder: Review and case report.* Knee Surg Sports Traumato Arthosc 7(4):249 1999.
8. **Sampathkumar K, Rajasekhar C, Robson MJ:** *Pigmented villonodular synovitis of lumbar facet joint: A rare cause of nerve root entrapment.* Spine 26(10):E213, 2001.
9. **Titlebaum DS, Rhodes CH, Brooks JSJ, et al.:** *Pigmented villonodular synovitis of a lumbar facet joint.* AJNR 13:164, 1992.
10. **Khoury GM, Shimkin PM, Kleinman GM, et al.:** *Computed tomography and magnetic resonance imaging findings of pigmented villonodular synovitis of the spine.* Spine 16:1236, 1991.
11. **Patkar D, Prasad S, Shah J, et al.:** *Pigmented villonodular synovitis: Magnetic resonance features of an unusual case of bilateral hip joint involvement.* Austral Radiol 44(4):458, 2000.
12. **Vedantam R, Strecker WB, Schoenecker PL, Salinas-Madrigal L:** *Polyarticular pigmented villonodular synovitis in a child.* Clin Orthop Mar(348):208, 1998.
13. **Mancini GB, Lazzeri S, Bruno G, Pucci G:** *Localized pigmented villonodular synovitis of the knee.* Arthropscopy 14(5):532, 1998.
14. **Durr HR, Stabler A, Maier M, Refior HJ:** *Pigmented villonodular synovitis. Review of 20 cases.* J Rheumatol 28(7):1620, 2001.
15. **Marberry K, Lowry K, Griffiths H, Kenter K:** *Radiologic case study. Pigmented villonodular synovitis.* Othopedics 24:647, 2001.
16. **Gonzalez Della Valle A, Piccaluga F, Potter HG, et al.:** *Pigmented villondular synovitis of the hip: 2- to 23-year followup study.* Clin Orthop July(388):187, 2001.
17. **Zvijac JE, Lau AC, Hechtman KS, et al.:** *Arthroscopic treatment of pigmented villonodular synovitis of the knee.* Arthroscopy 15(6):613, 1999.
18. **Kotwal PP, Gupta V, Malhotra R:** *Giant-cell tumour of the tendon sheath. Is radiotherapy indicated to prevent recurrence after surgery?* J Bone Joint Surg 82B:571, 2000.
19. **Cotton RE, Byers PD, Deacon OW, et al.:** *The diagnosis and treatment of pigmented villonodular synovitis.* J Bone Joint Surg 50B:290, 1968.
20. **Jaffe HL, Lichenstein L, Sutro CJ:** *Pigmented villonodular synovitis, bursitis, and tenosynovitis.* Arch Pathol 31:731, 1941.
21. **Breimer CW, Freiberger RH:** *Bone lesions associated with villonodular synovitis.* AJR 79:618, 1958.
22. **Smith JH, Pugh DG:** *Roentgenographic aspects of articular pigmented villonodular synovitis.* AJR 87:1146, 1962.
23. **Jelnik JS, Kransdorf MJ, Utz JA, et al.:** *Imaging of pigmented villonodular synovitis with emphasis on MR imaging.* AJR 152:337, 1989.
24. **Muscolo DL, Makino A, Costa-Paz M, Ayerza M:** *Magnetic resonance imaging evaluation and arthroscopic resection of localized pigmented villonodular synovitis of the knee.* Orthopedics 23(4):367, 2000.
25. **Bhimani MA, Wenz JF, Frassica FJ:** *Pigmented villonodular synovitis: Keys to early diagnosis.* Clin Orthop May(386):197, 2001.
26. **Frassica FJ, Bhimani MA, McCarthy EF, Wenz J:** *Pigmented villonodular synovitis of the hip and knee.* Am Fam Physician 60(5):1404, 1999.
27. **Farrokh D, Annaert JM, Fabeck L, et al.:** *Localized pigmented villonodular synovitis of the knee with bone involvement mimicking a benign bone tumor: CT and MR findings.* JBR-BTR 84(6):253, 2001.
28. **Goldberg RP, Weissman BN, Naimark A:** *Femoral neck erosion: A sign of hip synovial disease.* AJR 41:107, 1983.
29. **Freidman B, Nerubay J, Blankstein A, et al.:** *Synovial chondromatosis (osteochondromatosis) of the right hip: "Hidden" radiological manifestations. Case report 439.* Skeletal Radiol 16:504, 1987.

Tumors and Tumor-Like Processes

11

Terry R. Yochum and Lindsay J. Rowe

METASTATIC BONE TUMORS

GENERAL CONSIDERATIONS

Metastatic bone tumors are the most common malignant tumors of the skeleton. Approximately 70% of all malignant tumors are metastatic in origin, with only 30% being primary in nature. (Table 11-1) Most malignant tumors of bone are metastases from a primary extraskeletal focus, the majority are epithelial in origin. The most common primary sites are in the breast, lung, prostate, kidney, thyroid, and bowel. Occasionally, a primary sarcoma of bone, such as a Ewing's tumor, will metastasize to another osseous site. Apparently, with the exception of tumors of the central nervous system and basal cell carcinoma of the skin, almost all tumors have reported incidences of metastases to bone. The usual route is via tumor emboli carried by the vascular system. Those bones that are rich in red bone marrow are predisposed to develop osseous metastases; the target sites are the axial skeleton, skull, and proximal extremities; involvement distal to the knee and elbow is rare. Jaffe (1) states that metastasis to the skeleton may be just as common as it is to the lung or liver. Metastasis is the most sinister complication of any malignancy and often heralds relentless progression of the disease process, eventually leading to death.

Incidence

The true incidence of metastatic bone disease is difficult to ascertain. Autopsy findings are the most accurate means of assessment because bone scans and plain films have inherent limitations. The overall frequency of skeletal metastasis in several large autopsy series is estimated to be from 20 to 35% of all patients with malignancies. (2,3) In most cases the metastatic lesions are the cause of death in these patients. The validity of any autopsy incidence study depends on the number of bones examined and on the detailed nature of the examination.

The relative frequency of skeletal metastasis varies considerably with the organ of primary involvement. Metastasis to bone represents the third most common site of metastatic carcinoma. (4) Cancers of the breast, prostate, lung, and kidney account for 80% of all metastatic cancers to bone. (3) Metastases to bone tend to be multiple and affect primarily the axial skeleton. Solitary lesions occur in only 10% of patients. (5) In females, carcinoma of the breast is responsible for approximately 70% of all bony metastases, which places these women at an estimated fivefold increased risk for pathologic vertebral fracture. (6,7) The remaining 30% are owing primarily to carcinomas of the thyroid, kidney, and uterus. (6) In males, carcinoma of the prostate is responsible for about 60% of all skeletal metastases, whereas carcinoma of the lung causes an additional 25%. (6) (Table 11-2)

Table 11-1	Overview of Common Malignant Bone Lesions		
Primary (30%)	**Secondary (70%)**		
	Lytic (75%)	Blastic (15%)	Mixed (10%)
Multiple myeloma (most common)	Lung	Prostate	Prostate
Osteosarcoma (second most common)			
Chondrosarcoma (third most common)	Breast	Breast	Breast
Ewing's sarcoma (fourth most common)			

Table 11-2	Most Common Causes for Osseous Metastases	
Population	**Lytic**	**Blastic**
Female	Breast (80%)	Breast (10%)
Male	Lung (75%)	Prostate (80%)
Young (< 20 years)	Neuroblastoma (80%)	Hodgkin's (50%)

Clinical Features

Most patients presenting with skeletal metastases are in their second half of life, most commonly past the 4th decade. Metastatic osseous lesions occurring in children < 5 years of age usually are caused by neuroblastoma; between 10 and 20 years of age, Ewing's sarcoma and osteosarcoma are the most common causes; and between 20 and 35 years of age, Hodgkin's lymphoma is the most common source for skeletal metastases.

Most patients present with a history of recent weight loss, appear cachectic, and experience anemia and fever in advanced stages of the disease. Often, the secondary skeletal deposits create the first symptoms of the carcinomatous process. This is particularly common with carcinoma of the thyroid, liver, and kidney. The principal signs and symptoms of metastatic bone disease are pain and pathologic fracture. The pain is usually insidious in onset with bouts of remission and exacerbation. Classically, the pain, when present, is persistent and nocturnal, but these characteristics are often lacking. Patients frequently harbor bony metastases without any overt symptoms. The diagnosis of metastatic bone disease in most cases is radiologic and cannot be determined by physical examination or inspection of the patient. It is not unusual to find osseous metastases 10–15 years after treatment for the primary neoplasm. This is particularly common in patients who have had radical mastectomies for carcinoma of the breast.

Certain serologic findings may be present in patients with metastatic bone disease. An elevated erythrocyte sedimentation rate (ESR) is often present but is not pathognomonic of metastatic disease. Elevation of the serum calcium may occur in diffuse osteolytic metastatic carcinoma; however, in most cases the serum calcium levels are normal, even with diffuse lytic disease. Alkaline phosphatase is frequently elevated in blastic metastatic lesions of bone but overall is a relatively insensitive indicator of bone metastasis because liver disease and callus formation around a fracture will also raise the alkaline phosphatase enzyme. (8) The serum acid phosphatase or prostate specific antigen (PSA) is elevated > 10 ng/mL in patients with cancer of the prostate gland when the tumor has broken through the prostatic capsule and seeded Batson's venous plexus or has spread by direct extension. Recent research has suggested that patients with PSA values < 10 ng/mL should not undergo full body bone scans, as metastasis is rare in this stage (grade) of the disease. (9) However, it is still our opinion, as well as the opinions of many others, that to ensure the best prognostic outcome of patients with known prostatic carcinoma and bone pain, scintigraphy should still be done routinely irrespective of PSA value. (10,11)

Pathologic Features

Several events are involved in the development of a metastasis: (*a*) tumor cells or fragments capable of autonomous survival must be liberated, (*b*) a pathway of dissemination must be available, and (*c*) an appropriate environment for the establishment and growth of the implant must exist in the new site.

Pathways of Metastasis

Cancers metastasize through one of three routes: direct extension, lymphatic channels, or hematogenous dissemination.

Direct Extension. Direct invasion into a bone may occur from a soft tissue tumor lying adjacent to or near the bone. (Fig. 11-1) The tumors that most commonly do this are those that gain access to the peritoneal cavity and can seed anywhere within it. Carcinoma of the uterus is well known to cause direct extension to the iliac bones. Mechanical transport of tumor cells by instruments or gloves during surgery may produce implantation of uninvolved tissues and even of the incision itself. A much less common pathway of direct transplantation is the seeding of tumor along one of the natural pathways in the body, such as downstream seeding by an intestinal tumor or the seeding of the lower urinary tract from a higher lesion. Although this would seem at first to be a common and plausible mechanism, in actual fact it is rare.

Lymphatic Dissemination. Lymphatic channels uncommonly play a role in spreading tumor emboli to bone. It is thought that the absence of lymphatic channels in bone marrow is the reason for the relatively low incidence of lymphatic seeding of bone.

Hematogenous Dissemination. Spread through blood vessels, particularly the veins, is the most common pathway for tumor emboli. The arteries are thick walled and often resist tumor penetration, whereas the thin-walled veins offer little resistance to tumor penetration. The venous system, therefore, provides a frequent route for cancer cells that slough off to form tumor emboli. The three areas most commonly seeded in this manner are the lungs, liver, and axial skeleton.

In 1940, Batson (12) described a series of epidural vertebral veins that are valveless and function as a venous lake or pool, where the blood flow is sluggish and subject to arrest and even reversal. Changes in intra-abdominal or intrathoracic pressure may tend to reflux blood flow in the direction of the paravertebral plexus. Batson's plexus provides a series of venous passageways by which cancer cells can be directly seeded into the bones, bypassing the liver and lungs, whose extensive capillary beds normally create an efficient filtration of the venous circulation. (Fig. 11-2) Batson (12) demonstrated that the prostatic venous plexus can drain into the vertebral venous plexus, bypassing the caval system. This provides the pathophysiologic basis for early metas-

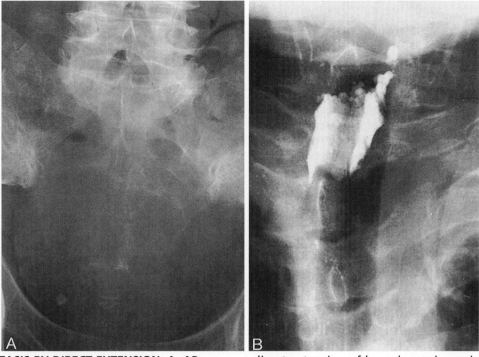

Figure 11-1 **METASTASIS BY DIRECT EXTENSION. A. AP Sacrum.** Observe the loss of trabecular patterns and destruction of the middle to lower portion of the sacrum because of direct extension of the tumor mass from carcinoma of the uterus. **B. AP Thoracic Spine.** Note the destruction of the pedicle, lamina, and half of the T2 vertebral body because of direct extension of bronchogenic carcinoma of the lung apex (Pancoast's tumor). *COMMENT:* The radiopaque material above the T2 level represents contrast material from a myelographic examination. (Courtesy of Bryan Hartley, MD, Melbourne, Australia.)

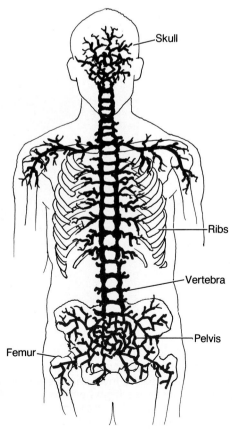

Figure 11-2 **THE VERTEBRAL VEIN SYSTEM (BATSON'S VENOUS PLEXUS).** This venous network is a common two-way avenue of metastatic spread of pelvic, abdominal, and thoracic tumors. A large portion of bony metastases results from dissemination of neoplastic cells through the vertebral vein system. (Adapted from **del Regato JA:** *Pathways of metastatic spread of malignant tumors.* Semin Oncol 4:33, 1977.)

tasis of prostate carcinoma to the pelvis, lumbar spine, and the remainder of the axial skeleton. (Figs. 11-3 and 11-4)

Lytic Versus Blastic Lesions

Lytic Destruction. In considering the pathogenesis of the lytic lesion, it is important to emphasize certain pathologic factors. The greatest majority of tumor emboli are deposited within the bone marrow. Most metastatic bone tumors are present for some time before they are recognized because a large amount of destruction must occur in the medullary canal before a perceptible alteration of bone density can be appreciated on plain film radiographs (at least 30% loss of bone density is necessary before detection). It is the pressure from the proliferating neoplasm on the surrounding trabecular structures and cortices that creates the so-called osteolytic lesion. These trabeculae may be partially or completely resorbed as the marrow is replaced by neoplastic tissue. It should be noted that the osteoclasts play little if any role in the pathogenesis of lytic metastases.

Notably, the majority of metastatic lesions begin within the medullary cavity and secondarily destroy the adjacent cortex. Metastasis to the cortex occurs uncommonly and is most frequently found in association with carcinoma of the lung, breast, and kidney. (13,14) (Fig. 11-5)

Blastic Metastases. The increased density in osteoblastic metastasis is owing to the laying down of new bone, which is nonneoplastic in nature but is actually a reactive response of the local osteoid tissue to the presence of the tumor. (Fig. 11-6) Therefore, progressive radiopacity of a cancer metastasis may be regarded as a reflection of increased new bone formation as a result of a futile attempt at bone repair. (15) However, as a patient's disease progresses, enlargement of existing blastic lesions, along with the pressure of additional lesions, is often a grave clinical sign.

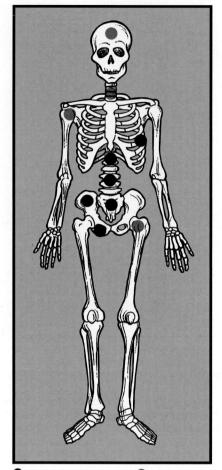

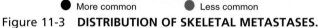

● More common   ● Less common

Figure 11-3   **DISTRIBUTION OF SKELETAL METASTASES.**

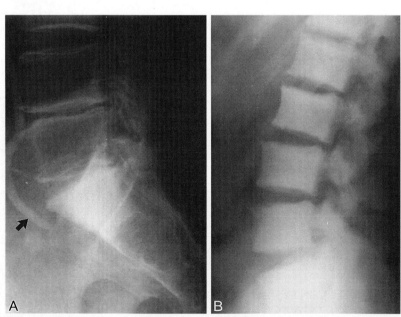

Figure 11-4   **HEMATOGENOUS METASTASIS. A. Localized.** Note that the focal radiopacity involving the sacral base represents osteoblastic metastasis from hematogenous dissemination of a previously diagnosed carcinoma of the bladder. The curvilinear radiopacity anterior to the L4 and L5 verte- brae (*arrow*) is owing to contrast media within the ureter. **B. Diffuse.** Observe the homogeneous areas of radiopacity throughout the T12–L5 vertebrae. This demonstrates the diffuse nature of osteoblastic metastatic carcinoma from the prostate gland.

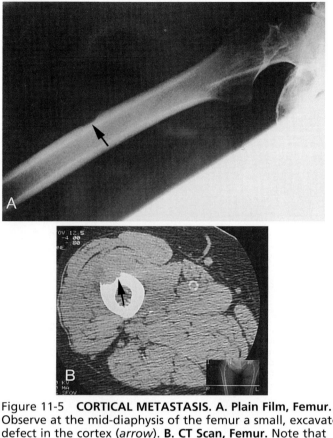

Figure 11-5 **CORTICAL METASTASIS. A. Plain Film, Femur.**
Observe at the mid-diaphysis of the femur a small, excavated
defect in the cortex (*arrow*). **B. CT Scan, Femur.** Note that
the cortical location of the defect is clearly demonstrated
(*arrow*). COMMENT: This type of lesion is considered an uncommon expression of metastatic carcinoma, most commonly seen from a primary tumor of the lung, followed by
the breast and kidney. It has been referred to as a *cookie-
bite lesion.* (Courtesy of John Duda, MD, Denver, Colorado.)

Certain benign conditions can simulate metastatic cancer.
(Table 11-3)

Radiologic Features

Radiographic Imaging

Nuclear Imaging (Bone Scans). Bone-seeking radiopharmaceuticals have greatly enhanced the early detection of metastatic
bone lesions. Whereas the early lesion is often not demonstrated
on plain film radiographs until the disease is well advanced, alterations of as little as 3–5% in the metabolic activity of bone may
be detected with bone scans. Technetium-99m–methylene diphosphonate (^{99m}Tc-MDP) is the agent of choice because it renders a low radiation dose; has a convenient half-life for clinical
use; and is a monoenergetic 140-keV photon, which is ideal for
current imaging devices. (16) The radiation-emitting substance
is taken up and concentrated in regions of high metabolic activity in bone.

Metastases result in a marked increase in osteoid production and
a disproportionate increase in immature woven bone and, therefore,
cause a *hot spot* on bone scans. (17) Animal experiments have
established that, after tumor implantation, there is new woven bone

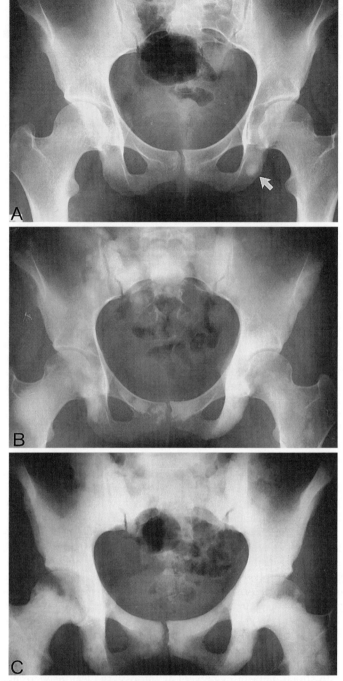

Figure 11-6 **BLASTIC METASTASIS: SERIAL PROGRESSION.
A. AP Pelvis.** Note the subtle circular radiopacities present
in the proximal femora and ischium (*arrow*). **B. 1-Year
Follow-Up.** Note the numerous diffuse blastic lesions scattered throughout the sacrum, pelvis, and proximal femora.
C. Diffuse Disease. Observe the complete opacification of
the bones of the pelvis and the proximal femora. This film
was taken approximately 2 years after panel A. COMMENT:
This is a relatively young female patient whose primary carcinoma was that of the parotid gland. The radiographic
presentation in this case is somewhat more typical of
prostate or breast metastases because parotid gland carcinoma with blastic lesions to bone is somewhat rare.
(Courtesy of Lawrence A. Cooperstein, MD, Pittsburgh,
Pennsylvania.)

Table 11-3	Benign Conditions Simulating Osseous Metastatic Cancer	
Osteolytic	**Osteoblastic**	
Neurofibromatosis	Melorheostosis	
Enchondromatosis	Osteopoikilosis	
Polyostotic fibrous dysplasia	Osteopathia striata	
Brown tumors (hyperparathyroidism)	Osteopetrosis	
	Paget's disease	
Gout	Sarcoidosis	
Osteomyelitis (fungal, tuberculosis)	Tuberous sclerosis	
Histiocytosis X	Secondary hyperparathyroidism (sclerotic form)	
Gorham's angiomatosis	Chronic osteomyelitis	
	Sickle cell anemia	
	Mastocytosis	
	Fluorosis	

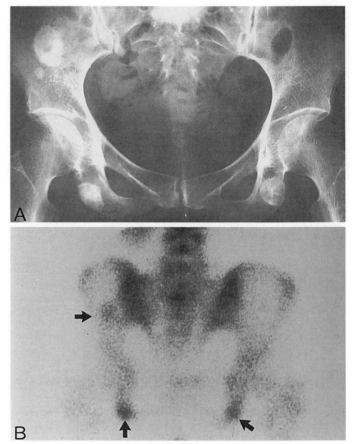

laid down about the tumor even before bone destruction occurs. (17) It is this osteoblastic response of new bone, which is a reaction to the underlying bone destruction, that renders the bone scan positive. (Fig. 11-7) A number of benign conditions can also render positive bone scans; examples are Paget's disease, fibrous dysplasia, fractures, osteomyelitis, osteoid osteoma, osteoblastoma, arthritides, and ischemic necroses. (Table 11-3) Thus the presence of a positive scan must be correlated with clinical data as well as plain film radiographs before a diagnosis of metastasis is offered. (18) In one study, 88% of solitary rib lesions found on bone scan in patients with proved extraskeletal cancers were benign and not metastatic in nature. (19)

Bone scanning is definitely a more accurate and sensitive indicator of the status of bone metastasis than conventional radiography. (20,21) In several large series it was found that up to 40% of cancer patients with abnormal scans have normal radiographs. (22,23) Bone scans may detect osseous metastases as early as 18 months before their detection on radiographs and have a reported sensitivity 50–80% greater than conventional radiographs. (24) It has been estimated that 30–50% of normal bone mineral must be lost before a bone metastasis is visible radiographically on plain film, whereas scans may be positive at 3–5% destruction of bone. (25) In the vertebrae the necessary mineral loss may be as high as 50–70%, and a lesion may need to be > 1.5 cm before it can be detected on plain film radiographs. (25) Furthermore, it has been found that in nearly 50% of patients with spinal metastases present at autopsy, the lesions were not detectable in premortem tomograms. (25)

Generally, abnormalities are shown on bone scans as either focal or diffuse regions of increased or decreased radionuclide accumulation compared with that of other skeletal areas. Both lytic and blastic lesions appear on the bone scan as hot spots (areas of increased radionuclide concentration). A positive scan is nonspecific, however, only in the sense that it reflects accelerated osteogenesis of any origin. Any positive scan must be correlated with the morphologic change on the plain film, which often allows appreciation of a characteristic pattern peculiar to a specific bone disorder other than metastases. About 5% of metastatic lesions may be missed by bone scanning, either because the tumor provokes little or no bone reaction (as in myeloma) or because of technical problems. Single-photon emission computed tomography (SPECT) scanning of the vertebral column will reveal meta-

Figure 11-7 POSITIVE BONE SCAN. A. AP Pelvis. Observe the blastic metastatic lesions in both ischia and in the midportion of one ilium. These lesions are secondary to carcinoma of the breast. **B. Bone Scan.** Note the areas of increased radionuclide uptake (*arrows*), which correspond directly to the skeletal lesions visualized in panel A. *COMMENT:* Early lesions in metastatic carcinoma are often not demonstrated on plain film radiographs until the disease is well advanced. Alterations of as little as 3–5% in the metabolic activity of bone may be detected with bone scans. These areas of increased radionuclide uptake have been referred to as hot spots. (Courtesy of Bryan Hartley, MD, Melbourne, Australia.)

static lesions with a higher diagnostic value than traditional planar scanning. (26)

Conventional Radiography. The usual radiologic skeletal survey consists of a lateral view of the skull, anteroposterior (AP) and lateral views of the cervical, thoracic, and lumbosacral spine, AP view of the pelvis, AP view of the ribs, and a posteroanterior (PA) view of the chest. The detection of a given metastatic lesion depends on a number of factors: the size of the lesion, its location in bone, and the effect of the bony lesion on the cortex or surrounding trabeculae. There must be at least 30–50% loss of bone density before it will be readily visible on a radiograph. In addition, the radiographs must be of optimum quality to adequately visualize the structures to be evaluated.

Approximately 80% of all osseous metastases are found in the central or axial skeleton. (27) The distribution is 28% in the ribs and sternum, 39% in the vertebrae, and 13% in the pelvis. (27) Only 10% are found in the skull, with a similar percentage in the proximal long bones. (27) Metastatic lesions distal to the knees and elbows are rare.

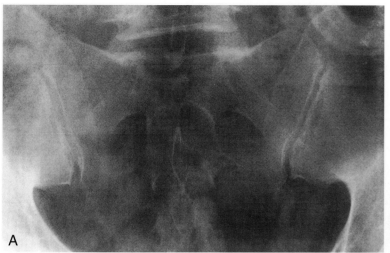
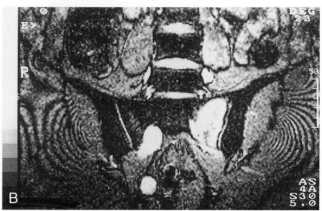

Figure 11-8 **OCCULT OSTEOLYTIC METASTATIC CARCINOMA: SACRAL ALA. A. AP Tilt-Up Lumbosacral.** Note that no bony pathology is seen in the sacroiliac joints or sacrum. **B. T2-Weighted Fat-Suppressed MRI, Lumbosacral.** Observe the large area of bright signal intensity in the left sacral ala, indicative of marrow replacement from metastatic tumor. *COMMENT:* This 44-year-old female patient was found to have an occult breast carcinoma with metastasis to the sacrum, which was not detected on conventional lumbosacral radiographs. MRI is the most sensitive imaging modality to determine marrow replacement. Approximately 50% loss of bone mass is necessary before the earliest signs of osteolytic destruction can be determined on conventional radiographs. (Courtesy of Wes Williams, DC, Gunnison, Colorado.)

CT. CT is far more sensitive than plain film studies and is particularly useful in the detection and evaluation of cortical bone involvement and the presence of a soft tissue mass. However, some subtle areas of marrow replacement by malignant tissues may be overlooked. It is especially useful for localizing biopsy sites.

MRI. MRI is superior to CT in both the detection of bone lesions and the assessment of adjacent soft tissue involvement. The infiltration of tumor cells into the fatty bone marrow results in loss of the normally bright signal intensity seen on T1-weighted spin echo images. The affected areas become heterogeneously hyperintense on T2-weighted pulse sequences. (Fig. 11-8) Subtle areas of abnormal tissue are best detected on short tau inversion recovery (STIR) images. This technique is heavily T1 weighted and results in suppression of the normally bright signal originating from marrow fat. Abnormal tissues are, therefore, more conspicuous, appearing quite hyperintense relative to the adjacent dark gray or black appearance of the normal marrow. Recent advances allowing whole-body bone marrow scans using these techniques (T1 weighting and STIR images) have been shown to detect up to 91% of metastatic lesions to bone, compared with approximately 85% detected by bone scintigraphy. (28) Of clinical note, it has been estimated that after the discovery of metastatic disease up to 21% of the primary sources will never be found, even after an extensive search. (29)

Fundamental Roentgen Signs

The roentgen signs of bone metastasis include alteration in bone density and architecture. They may be osteolytic, osteoblastic, or mixed. Osteolytic metastases are most common, representing approximately 75% of all metastatic lesions. A *moth-eaten* or *permeative pattern* of bone destruction is classic and occurs most frequently with breast and lung carcinoma. (Fig. 11-9) These lesions are not detectable on plain films until approximately 30% of a focal region of bone is destroyed. In lytic lesions, computed tomography may help when conventional radiography fails to demonstrate an abnormality in a region that is suspect for metastasis, either because of symptoms or because of radionuclide bone scanning. Osteoblastic metastases represent approximately 15% of all lesions and are most commonly produced by carcinoma of the prostate, breast, and cecum, as well as bronchial carcinoid tumors. These lesions are much easier to perceive because of their increased radiopacity, even though their margins are typically ill defined. (Fig. 11-10) The blastic lesions may assume a diffuse, scattered pattern, creating a multiple *snowball appearance*. Mixed lesions represent approximately 10% of all metastatic deposits. (Fig. 11-11) They are a combination of osteolytic and osteoblastic proliferation and occur most commonly with carcinoma of the breast and, occasionally, the lung. (Tables 11-4 and 11-5)

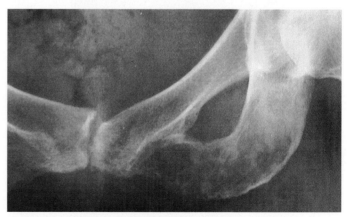

Figure 11-9 **ISCHIAL METASTASIS. AP Hip.** Observe the loss of bone density and a moth-eaten pattern of bone destruction scattered throughout the ischium. The poor zone of transition around the lytic lesion suggests an aggressive disorder of bone. This lytic metastasis is secondary to carcinoma of the breast. Of incidental notation are degenerative changes surrounding the pubic articulation.

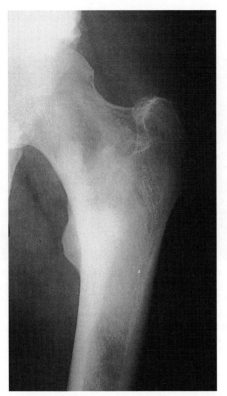

Figure 11-10 **BLASTIC METASTATIC DISEASE. AP Hip.** Note the ill-defined area of radiopacity in the intertrochanteric space and adjacent to the lesser trochanter. This represents blastic metastasis from carcinoma of the prostate gland. (Courtesy of Bryan Hartley, MD, Melbourne, Australia.)

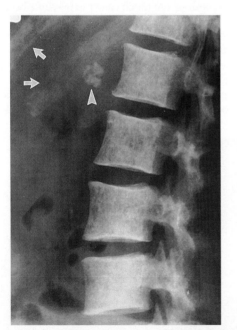

Figure 11-11 **MIXED METASTASIS: LATERAL LUMBAR SPINE.** Observe the diffuse osteolytic and osteoblastic lesions scattered throughout the entire lumbar spine. These lesions are secondary to carcinoma of the breast. Notice the mixed metastatic lesions in the visualized lower ribs (*arrows*). Of incidental notation is a calcified mesenteric lymph node (*arrowhead*).

Table 11-4	Radiologic Presentations of Metastatic Carcinoma		
Primary Organ Involvement	**Lytic (%)**	**Mixed (%)**	**Blastic (%)**
Breast	80	10	10
Lung	75	20	5
Renal	80	10	10
Wilms' tumor	80	20	—
Urinary bladder	90	10	—
Thyroid	90	10	—
Prostate	10	10	80
Salivary glands	100	—	—
Neuroblastoma	80	15	5
Esophagus	85	10	5
Stomach	90	10	—
Colon or rectum	75	5	20
Pancreas	80	10	10
Liver[a]	70	30	—
Gallbladder[a]	90	10	—
Uterine cervix	90	8	2
Uterine corpus	90	10	—
Ovary	90	7	3
Testis	75	5	20
Skin carcinoma	95	5	—
Malignant melanoma	90	10	—
Carcinoid	5	15	80
Hodgkin's lymphoma	40	10	50

[a]Cancer of these organs rarely metastasizes to bone.

Table 11-5	Radiologic Features of Metastatic Carcinoma to Bone

General
  Axial skeleton predilection
  Multiple sites
Osteolytic metastases (75%)
  Cortical and trabecular destruction
  Lack of periosteal response
  Moth-eaten, permeative destruction
  Small or absent soft tissue mass
  Multiple sites
Variants (lung, thyroid, kidney); solitary expansile soap bubble lesion
Osteoblastic metastases (15%)
  Localized or diffuse increased bone density
  Poorly defined margins
  Multiple sites
Mixed metastases (10%)
  Combination of blastic and lytic features

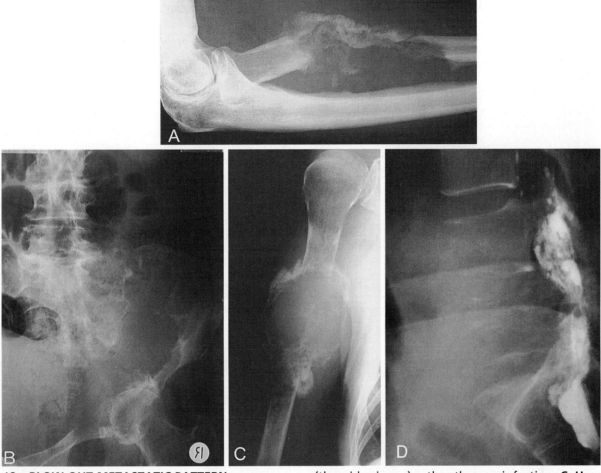

Figure 11-12 **BLOW-OUT METASTATIC PATTERN.**
A. Radius. Observe the extensive destruction of the proximal radius, which creates an altered angulation of the meta-diaphyseal portion of this bone (renal primary).
B. Ilium. Observe the extensive destruction of the iliac wing and supra-acetabular area. There is no destruction of the femoral head or disturbance of the joint space of the hip articulation. This presentation is consistent with a neoplasm (thyroid primary) rather than an infection. **C. Humerus.** Observe the grossly expansile mid-diaphyseal lesion of the humerus. There is a permeative pattern of bone destruction noted on both sides of the expanding lesion (renal primary). **D. Lumbar Spine.** Note the partial destruction of the L4 vertebral body and complete destruction of the L5 vertebral body.

Blow-Out Metastatic Lesions. Lesions that vary from the common roentgen patterns previously described or that are atypical in their presentation deserve special consideration. Although most metastatic lesions are multiple, as many as 10% may be solitary. (5) This more commonly occurs with carcinoma of the lung, thyroid, and kidney. Specific characteristics of the solitary lesion, such as a bubbly, highly expansile appearance, may suggest a renal or thyroid malignancy. This lesion is characteristically quite large and has been called the *blow-out metastatic pattern.* (Fig. 11-12) It is this type of metastasis that demonstrates bone expansion, a roentgen sign more frequently linked to primary tumors than to secondary ones. A solitary plasmacytoma or giant cell tumor may often give a similar appearance.

Primary Versus Secondary Tumors: Differential Diagnosis

It should be emphasized that the radiographic appearance of the osseous lesions of metastatic neoplasms does not permit a positive differentiation of metastatic neoplasm from primary malignant neoplasms of bone. A few helpful differential points do exist, however, allowing a fundamental differentiation of primary versus secondary malignant tumors. (Table 11-6) The presence of periosteal response is much more commonly found with primary malignant tumors than with secondary. The appearance of a soft tissue mass is rare in metastases but quite common in primary malignant tumors. Frequently, the length of the lesion is helpful, with the long lesions (> 6 cm) often representing a primary malignant tumor, and most metastatic tumors range between 2 and 4 cm in length. Most malignant tumors that expand bone are primary in nature, with the rare exception of the expansile metastatic tumors of renal and thyroid malignancies (blow-out lesions). Most primary tumors are solitary lesions, whereas metastatic lesions are usually multiple. These criteria should be used only as guidelines because occasional exceptions are seen. Definitive diagnosis of these lesions can be obtained only by biopsy.

Table 11-6	Malignant Bone Neoplasms: Differentiating Radiologic Features between Primary and Secondary Lesions	
Feature	**Primary**	**Secondary**
Incidence	30%	70%
Expansion of bone	+++	+
Joint involvement	—	—
Length of lesion	> 6 cm	2–4 cm
Periosteal response	+++	+
Solitary lesion	+++	+
Multiple lesions	+	+++
Soft tissue mass	+++	+

—, Does not occur; +, seldom occurs; ++, often occurs; +++, very commonly occurs.

Specific Anatomic Location

Spine

The spine is the most common osseous site for metastasis to occur, accounting for approximately 40% of all lesions. (27) The thoracic and lumbar spine are the regions most commonly affected. (Figs. 11-13 and 11-14) Cervical spine involvement does occur, but to a lesser extent. (Figs. 11-15 and 11-16) The atlas seems to be an infrequent site. (Fig. 11-17) The most frequently involved specific components of the spine in metastatic disease are the vertebral bodies and pedicles. One of the most difficult lesions to assess is a solitary vertebral metastasis.

Vertebral Body. The earliest and most subtle sign of osteolytic disease is a focal osteoporosis or radiolucency of a vertebral body, in contrast to the adjacent vertebral segments. (Fig. 11-18) This sign often occurs shortly before some trivial trauma induces a pathologic fracture. Bone scan may show increased uptake, and MRI reveals uniform marrow infiltration with decreased signal on T1-weighted studies and intermediate to increased signal intensity on T2-weighted images. (30) (Fig. 11-19)

Pathologic compression fractures exhibit both anterior and posterior loss of height (vertebra plana). (Fig. 11-20; Table 11-7) Close inspection of endplate integrity may show it to be destroyed, a feature also seen in infection, which usually has co-existing loss

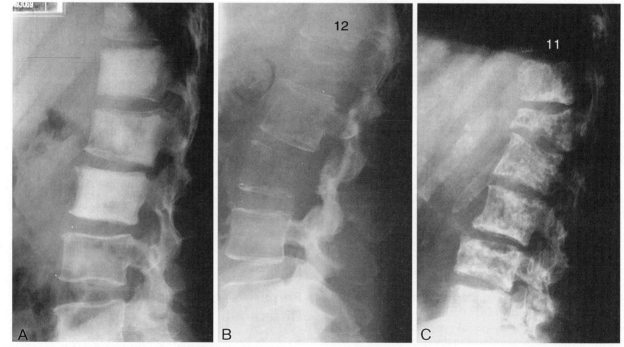

Figure 11-13 **DIFFUSE PATTERNS OF SPINAL METASTATIC DISEASE. A. Multiple Ivory Vertebrae.** Observe the diffuse radiopacity from metastatic disease of the prostate gland involving the upper lumbar vertebrae. **B. Grossly Lytic Vertebrae.** Note the extensive resorption of the L1 and L3 vertebral bodies and pedicles. Pathologic collapse of the L1 vertebral body has occurred. These represent blow-out lesions from carcinoma of the thyroid gland.

C. Diffuse Mixed Metastasis. Note the extensive lytic and blastic destruction scattered throughout the entire lumbar spine and lower thoracic vertebrae. There is a wedge-shaped pathologic compression fracture present at the L1 vertebra. Slight compression of the L4 vertebral body is also noted. (Reprinted with permission from **Yochum TR:** *A radiographic anthology of vertebral names.* J Manipulative Physiol Ther 8(2):4, 1985.)

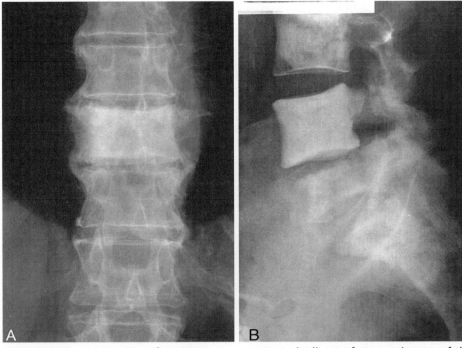

Figure 11-14   **SPINAL METASTASIS. A. Ivory Vertebra.** Note the diffuse, homogeneous radiopacity of the T10 vertebral body, representing blastic metastatic disease from carcinoma of the prostate gland. **B. Ivory Vertebra and Mixed Metastasis.** Observe the homogeneous radiopacity of the L4 vertebral body, without bone expansion. This represents blastic metastatic disease from carcinoma of the prostate gland. The visualized segments of L3, L5, and the sacrum demonstrate mixed lytic and blastic changes. A pathologic fracture is present in the L5 vertebral body. (Reprinted with permission from **Yochum TR:** *A radiographic anthology of vertebral names.* J Manipulative Physiol Ther 8(2):4, 1985.)

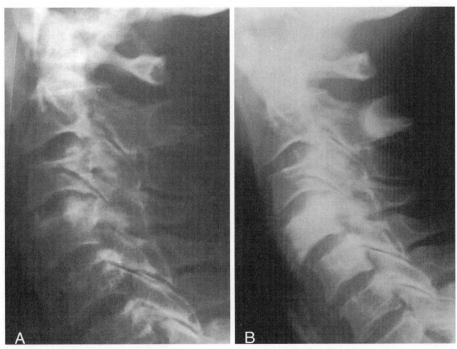

Figure 11-15   **CERVICAL SPINE METASTATIC DISEASE: SERIAL PROGRESSION. A. Initial Radiograph.** Observe that the initial radiographic examination of this patient demonstrates moderate osteoporosis with some spinal degenerative changes. No metastatic disease is evident at this time. **B. 1-Year Follow-Up.** Observe the homogeneous radiopacity (ivory vertebra) present at the C4 segment. A second blastic metastatic deposit is present in the spinous process of C2. These lesions are secondary to metastatic disease from carcinoma of the prostate gland. (Courtesy of Larry L. Sibley, DC, Plainview, Texas.)

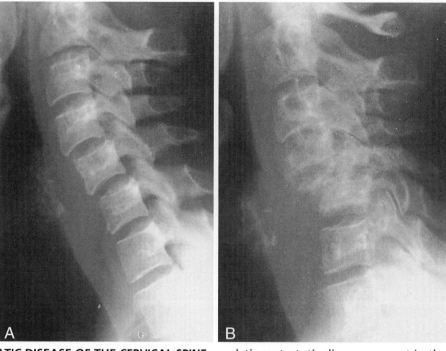

Figure 11-16 METASTATIC DISEASE OF THE CERVICAL SPINE: A SERIAL STUDY. A. Lateral Cervical Spine. This 30-year-old female presented with pain in the cervical area. A few years before this radiograph was taken she had a radical mastectomy for carcinoma. **B. 1-Year Follow-Up.** Note the diffuse lytic metastatic disease present in the vertebral body of C4. There is extensive collapse and vanishing of the vertebral body of C5, along with its articular pillars, lamina, and spinous process. (Courtesy of Raymond Roscioli, DC, DACBR, Easton, Pennsylvania.)

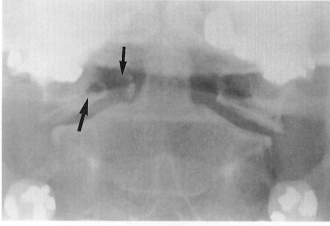

Figure 11-17 METASTASIS TO THE ATLAS. Observe the destruction of the most medial portion of the lateral mass of the atlas (*arrows*). *COMMENT:* This 30-year-old female presented with upper cervical pain. Two years before this radiograph was performed, she had a malignant pheochromocytoma removed from the adrenal gland. A total body bone scan revealed hot spots in two ribs and the L4 vertebral body, although plain films showed no abnormalities. Metastatic disease to the atlas is quite rare, as are primary tumors. (Courtesy of Teresa Shook, DC, Antioch, California.)

of disc height. (Fig. 11-21) MRI will characteristically delineate these ill-defined endplate irregularities and irregular nodular paravertebral soft tissue lesions as well as reveal abnormal signal involvement of the pedicles. (31) Wedge-shaped deformities can also occur. Pathological collapse of a vertebra is often a pain-ful event. Vertebroplasty and kyphoplasty have shown to be safe, effective, and long-lasting techniques to reduce deformity and pain in these patients. (32)

Bone weakening of the vertebral body may lead to disruption of the endplate either as an angular deformity or as Schmorl's nodes. (30,33) Smooth, curved endplate deformities are usually not associated with underlying malignancy. (30) Intrabody discal herniation owing to underlying malignant bone disease is referred to as a *malignant Schmorl's node*. This process is usually accentuated by significant or occult trauma. These defects within the vertebrae contain both tumor and disc material and predispose the disc to secondary degenerative changes. (33) Neoplasms can rarely locate within the intervertebral disc by direct or hematogenous spread. (33) Extensive involvement of the intervertebral disc or discal metastasis is indeed rare. (33) Invasion of any joint by any tumor is uncommon but is more likely in those joints that lack mobility, usually the sacroiliac joint and the disc and facet joint. (34,35)

Pedicle. The pedicle is an important, radiologically detectable site for osteolytic metastatic carcinoma. Any component of the neural arch can be involved, although the pedicle is by far the most common location. (Fig. 11-22) Destruction of the posterior vertebral body with contiguous involvement of the pedicle attachment results in loss of the cortical outline of the pedicle. (36) This has been referred to as the *one-eyed pedicle sign* or as the *winking owl sign* and is most commonly found in the lower thoracic and lumbar spine. (37,38) (Figs. 11-23 and 11-24) It is most easily visualized on the AP radiograph. (38) (Figs. 11-25 and 11-26) Most cases of pedicle destruction involve a single vertebra; however, multiple levels can be affected. (Fig. 11-27) Occasionally, bilateral pedicular destruction may occur and is referred to as the *blind vertebra*. (39) (Figs. 11-28 and 11-29; Table 11-8)

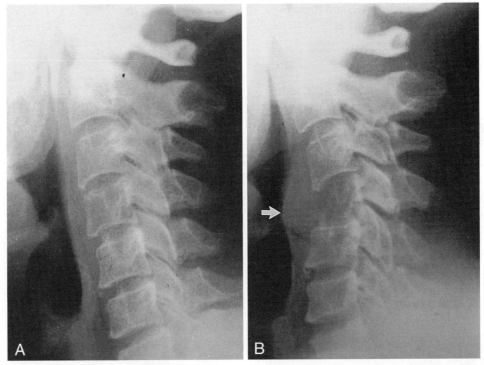

Figure 11-18 SUBTLE SIGNS OF EARLY LYTIC METASTATIC CARCINOMA. A. Lateral Cervical Spine. Observe the focal radiolucency of the vertebral body of C4 compared with the C3 and C5 vertebral segments. There is a subtle disruption in the superior vertebral cortical endplate of C4, representing early osteolytic change. **B. 6-Week Follow-Up.** Note the extensive osteolysis and collapse of the C4 vertebral body. Observe the increase in the retropharyngeal interspace anterior to C4 (*arrow*). This most likely represents hemorrhage and/or soft tissue tumor extension. *COMMENT:* This 55-year-old female had a history of carcinoma of the uterine cervix 5 years before the initial radiographs were taken. The early signs of carcinoma were detected by the initial radiologist, resulting in proper referral. It is unusual for a metastatic tumor to move so rapidly; most metastatic tumors would take 6 months to show such progressive changes. (Courtesy of James F. Winterstein, DC, DACBR, Chicago, Illinois.)

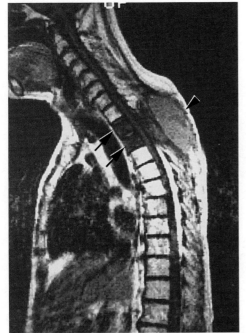

Figure 11-19 METASTATIC MARROW INFILTRATION. MRI. Note the low signal of the T2, T3 vertebral bodies due to neoplastic marrow infiltration (*arrows*). Note the overlying mass from a malignant melanoma (*arrowhead*). (Courtesy of Kenneth B. Reynard, MD, Denver, Colorado.)

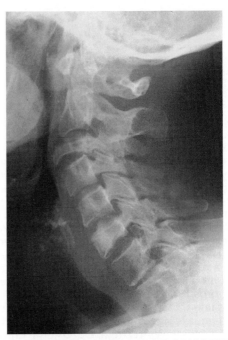

Figure 11-20 VERTEBRAL PATHOLOGIC COLLAPSE. Lateral Cervical Spine. Note the uniform collapse of the C3 vertebral body and, to a lesser extent, the C6 vertebral body. Compression of the posterior third of the vertebral body strongly suggests pathologic collapse, which is usually of neoplastic origin. This patient had carcinoma of the breast.

Table 11-7	Solitary Vertebral Collapse	
Common Causes	**Uncommon Causes**
Metastatic carcinoma	Chordoma
Myeloma (plasmacytoma)	Chondrosarcoma
Eosinophilic granuloma	Hemangioma
Traumatic fracture (healthy bone)	Hydatid cyst
Paget's disease	Ewing's sarcoma
Infection (any cause)	Osteosarcoma
Steroid abuse, Cushing's disease	Giant cell tumor
Malignant lymphoma	

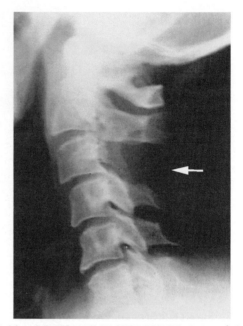

Figure 11-22   OSTEOLYTIC METASTASIS. Lateral Cervical Spine. Note that the spinous process, spinolaminar junction line, and the laminae have been destroyed at the C3 level (*arrow*). *COMMENT:* Congenital agenesis of an isolated neural arch is rare. Loss of the neural arch should be considered tumor induced until proven otherwise. (Courtesy of R. Scott Foster, DC, Memphis, Tennessee.)

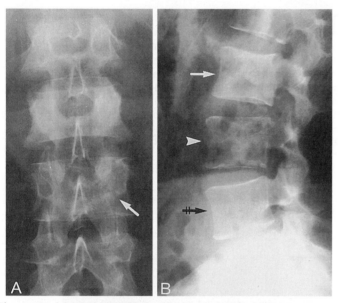

Figure 11-21   AN UNUSUAL PRESENTATION OF METASTATIC DISEASE. A. AP Lumbar Spine. Observe the destruction of one pedicle on L3 (*arrow*). Note the increase in bone density of the vertebral body of L2 and the generalized osteoporosis of the body of L3. **B. Lateral Lumbar Spine.** Observe the ivory vertebra at the L2 level (*arrow*). Note also the extreme loss of bone density at the L3 vertebral body with the destruction and loss of the cortical halo endplates on the superior and inferior surfaces of the L3 vertebral body (*arrowhead*). Observe the normal bone density and trabecular patterns of L4 (*crossed arrow*). *COMMENT:* This 60-year-old female had a previous history of primary carcinoma of the lung. It is quite unusual to have both an ivory vertebra and an adjacent grossly osteolytic vertebra from metastatic disease in the same spine. This patient had the additional classic one-eyed pedicle sign of osteolytic metastatic disease. (Courtesy of James F. Winterstein, DC, DACBR, Chicago, Illinois.)

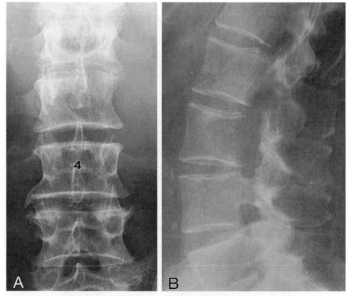

Figure 11-23   ONE-EYED PEDICLE SIGN. A. AP Lumbar Spine. Observe the unilateral destruction of the pedicle of L3, creating the one-eyed pedicle sign. The transverse process of L3 on the side of pedicle destruction has also been destroyed. **B. Lateral Lumbar Spine.** Observe the extensive destruction of the area of the pedicle of L3, with extension of the neoplasm into the posterior half of the vertebral body.

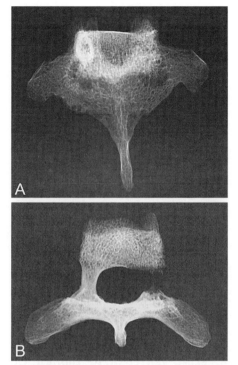

Figure 11-24 **ONE-EYED PEDICLE SIGN. A. AP Thoracic Specimen Radiograph. B. Axial Thoracic Specimen Radiograph.**

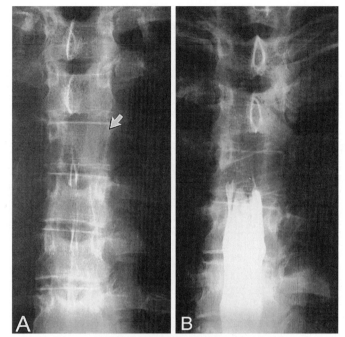

Figure 11-25 **ONE-EYED PEDICLE SIGN (WINKING OWL SIGN) OF LYTIC METASTATIC DISEASE. A. AP Thoracic Spine.** Observe the unilateral pedicle destruction at the T4 vertebra (*arrow*). **B. Myelographic Evaluation.** Note the block at the T4 level of the myelographic media as a result of extradural extension of the metastatic neoplasm. (Courtesy of David P. Thomas, MD, Melbourne, Australia.)

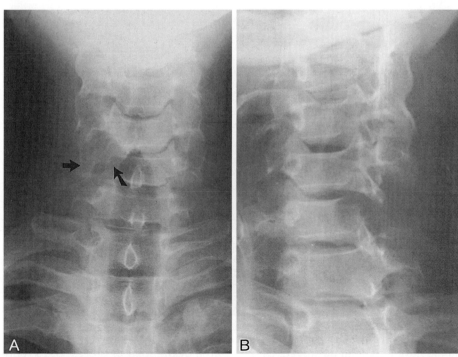

Figure 11-26 **OSTEOLYTIC METASTATIC DISEASE: ONE-EYED PEDICLE SIGN. A. AP Lower Cervical Spine.** Observe the unilateral destruction of the pedicle of C6 (*arrows*), along with a portion of its articular pillar. **B. Oblique Cervical Spine.** Note the massive osteolysis of the articular pillar and pedicle of C6.

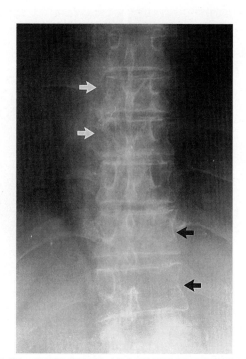

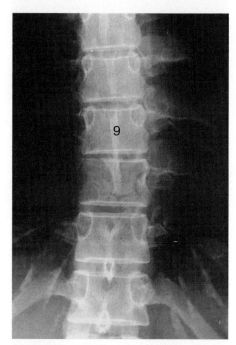

Figure 11-27 **METASTASIS AT MULTIPLE VERTEBRAL LEVELS. AP Thoracic.** Observe the one-eyed pedicle signs at T8, T9, T11, and T12 (*arrows*). (Courtesy of Bryan Hartley, MD, Melbourne, Australia.)

Figure 11-28 **BLIND VERTEBRA. AP Thoracic.** Observe the bilateral pedicular destruction at the T10 vertebral segment. This represents osteolytic metastasis from carcinoma of the breast.

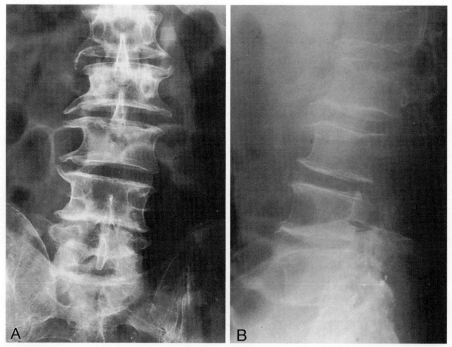

Figure 11-29 **BLIND VERTEBRA. A. AP Lumbar Spine.** Note the bilateral pedicular destruction at the L3 vertebra. The spinous process and laminae have also been destroyed. Of incidental notation are rather large spondylophytes scattered throughout the lumbar spine. **B. Lateral Lumbar Spine.**

Observe the complete destruction of the neural arch and pedicles of the L3 vertebra. The radiopaque densities in the area of the spinous process of L5 represent previous heavy-metal injections in the soft tissue structures.

Table 11-8	Radiologic Features of Spinal Metastasis

Location
  Lumbar and thoracic spine
  Vertebral body, pedicles
Signs
  Altered bone density
    Decreased: moth-eaten, permeative diffuse
    Increased: localized, ivory vertebra
  Cortical destruction
  Disc space unaffected
  Pathologic collapse
    Decreased posterior vertebral body height
    Endplate disruption (malignant Schmorl's node)
  Pedicle destruction
    One-eyed pedicle sign (winking owl sign)
    Blind vertebra (both pedicles destroyed)

Table 11-9	Differential Diagnosis of Pedicle Destruction

Congenital
  Agenesis (contralateral pedicular sclerosis)
  Hypoplasia
Neoplasm
  Benign
    Aneurysmal bone cyst
    Osteoblastoma
    Neurofibroma
    Osteoid osteoma
  Malignant
    Lytic metastasis
    Myeloma (rare)
Surgery
  Removal

The most common cause for a missing pedicle is osteolytic metastatic carcinoma; however, agenesis of a pedicle may also occur. (Fig. 11-30) The key to radiologic differentiation is to search for a stress-related reactive sclerosis and enlargement of the contralateral pedicle. (40,41) (Table 11-9) If this sign is present, it represents a firm assurance that osteolytic metastatic carcinoma has not occurred. Those cases of agenesis of the pedicle that create no stress hypertrophy of the opposite pedicle must be considered metastatic tumor until proven otherwise. (40,41) Previous radiographs in this circumstance will be helpful. Destruction of a pedi-

cle in a patient < 30 years of age is most commonly the result of aneurysmal bone cyst (ABC), osteoblastoma, metastases from neuroblastoma (< 3 years), or cord tumor.

Ivory Vertebra. Osteoblastic metastatic carcinoma may affect the vertebrae in either a diffuse or a localized form. (Figs. 11-31 to 11-33) When a singular vertebral body is involved exhibiting a diffuse homogeneous radiopacity, it has been called an *ivory vertebra.* (33,37) (Tables 11-10 and 11-11) The three most common causes for an ivory vertebra are osteoblastic metastatic carcinoma (usually from the prostate gland), Paget's

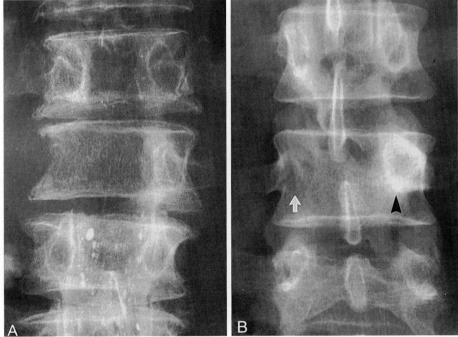

Figure 11-30 **MISSING PEDICLES: CONGENITAL VERSUS NEOPLASM. A. Metastatic Disease.** Observe the one-eyed pedicle sign present at the L1 segment as a result of diffuse osteolytic metastasis. There is also metastatic destruction of the lamina, spinous process, and a portion of the lateral body of L1. Note that the contralateral pedicle at L1 shows no evidence of sclerosis or enlargement. **B. Congenital Absence.** Note the agenesis of the pedicle of L4 (*arrow*), with compensatory sclerosis and hypertrophy of the contralateral pedicle (*arrowhead*). *COMMENT:* Sclerosis and enlargement of the pedicle adjacent to a missing pedicle are positive radiographic signs of congenital absence rather than of osteolytic metastatic disease.

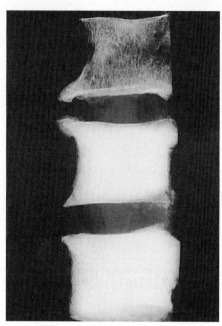

Figure 11-31 IVORY VERTEBRAE: SPECIMEN RADIOGRAPH. Note that two entire vertebral bodies exhibit homogeneous increase in density owing to metastatic carcinoma. Note the lack of expansion and normal anterior contours, helping exclude Paget's disease and Hodgkin's lymphoma, respectively. (Courtesy of Donald Resnick, MD, San Diego, California.)

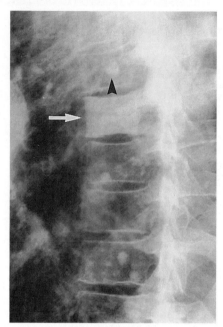

Figure 11-33 LOCALIZED IVORY VERTEBRA. Observe the localized osteoblastic response of a single thoracic vertebra (*arrow*). This represents osteoblastic metastasis from carcinoma of the breast. Of incidental notation are a number of circular radiopacities scattered throughout the lung field and superimposed on the spine, which represent calcified, healed tubercular granulomas (*arrowhead*).

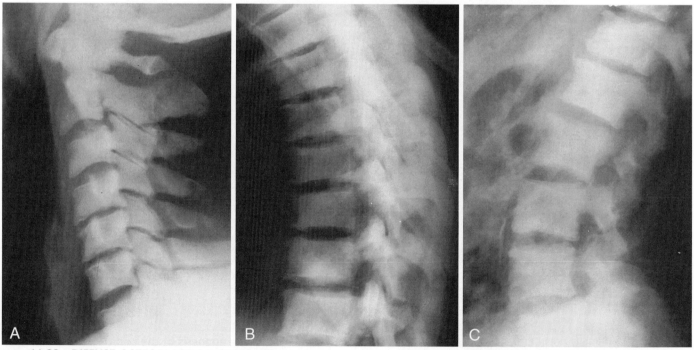

Figure 11-32 DIFFUSE OSTEOBLASTIC METASTASIS.
A. Lateral Cervical Spine. B. Lateral Thoracic Spine.
C. Lateral Lumbar Spine. Note that this 70-year-old male shows diffuse osteoblastic metastasis throughout the entire spine, secondary to primary carcinoma of the prostate gland. (Courtesy of Bryan Hartley, MD, Melbourne, Australia.)

Table 11-10 | Solitary Ivory Vertebra

Common Causes	Uncommon Causes
Osteoblastic metastasis	Sarcoidosis
Hodgkin's lymphoma	Chordoma
Paget's disease	Myeloma
Degenerative sclerosis	Osteosarcoma
Osteomyelitis (fungal or chronic)	Ewing's sarcoma
Idiopathic	Osteoid osteoma
	Osteoblastoma
	Bone island

Table 11-11 | Differential Diagnosis of an Ivory Vertebra

Factor	Blastic Metastases	Paget's Disease	Hodgkin's Disease
Age (years)	> 45	> 50	20–40
Increased density	+++	+++	+++
Expansion	—	+++	
Anterior scalloping	—	—	+++
Acid phosphatase	+++[a]	—	—
Alkaline phosphatase	++	+++	++

Males, prostate.

—, Does not occur; +, seldom occurs; ++, often occurs; +++, very commonly occurs.

disease (osteitis deformans), and Hodgkin's disease (lymphoma). (Figs. 11-34 and 11-35)

The radiographic differential diagnosis of a solitary ivory vertebra may be accomplished by inspecting the anterior aspect of the vertebra. The normal concavity of the vertebral body will be unaltered in patients with osteoblastic metastasis. Paget's disease usually creates a squaring off of the anterior surface of the vertebral body, as a result of the inherent cortical thickening and bone expansion. Rarely, Paget's disease may not expand the vertebral body, and if no other bony lesions are present, a biopsy may be required for final diagnosis.

In Hodgkin's lymphoma there is often anterior scalloping of the ivory vertebral body, thus accentuating the anterior vertebral concavity. The pathogenesis of this is thought to be from contiguous lymph node tissue pressing on the vertebral body as a result of transmitted aortic pulsations. The sclerotic changes of the vertebral body occur secondary to hematogenous metastases. Not all ivory vertebrae from Hodgkin's disease will demonstrate anterior scalloping; however, it is a classic sign when present and should always be searched for. Clinical differentiation is also helpful because most Hodgkin's patients are generally much younger (20–40 years), whereas Paget's disease and osteoblastic metastatic carcinoma both occur in the > 50-year age group. The alkaline phosphatase blood test is elevated in all three conditions, but the acid phosphatase and PSA should be elevated only when the blastic lesions are from the prostate gland as a primary source. (Fig. 11-36)

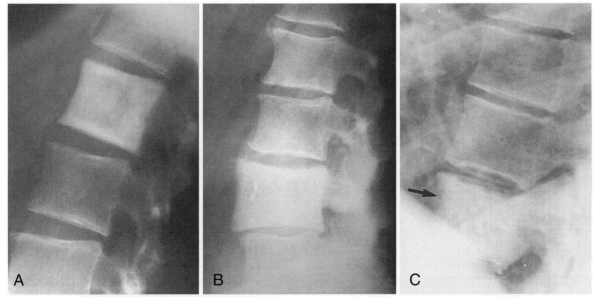

Figure 11-34 **A SOLITARY IVORY VERTEBRA: DIFFERENTIAL DIAGNOSIS. A. Osteoblastic Metastasis.** Note the homogeneous increase in density without cortical thickening or vertebral expansion at L2. **B. Paget's Disease.** Observe the gross expansion and squaring off of the anterior vertebral body margin of the L4 vertebra. These radiographic signs negate the possibility of osteoblastic metastasis and support Paget's disease. **C. Hodgkin's Lymphoma.** Note the solitary ivory vertebra at T12, with anterior vertebral body scalloping (*arrow*). This anterior vertebral body scalloping is classic for Hodgkin's lymphoma and is thought to be related to contiguous lymphoid tissue pressing on the anterior surface of the vertebral body. Not all ivory vertebrae from Hodgkin's disease will show anterior scalloping; however, it is a classic sign when present. (Panel A courtesy of Douglas B. Hart, DC, Carina, Queensland, Australia. Panel B courtesy of Joseph W. Howe, DC, DACBR, Fellow, ACCR, Los Angeles, California. Panel C courtesy of Paul E. Siebert, MD, Denver, Colorado.)

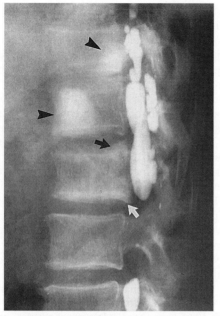

Figure 11-35 **PAGET'S DISEASE AND OSTEOBLASTIC META-STASIS WITHIN THE SAME PATIENT.** Observe the cortical thickening, the expansion of the posterior vertebral body margin (*arrows*), and the radiopacity of the L1 vertebral body. These changes are consistent with Paget's disease. Note also the nodular localized radiopacities in the vertebral bodies of T11 posteriorly and T12 anteriorly (*arrowheads*). These radio-pacities represent osteoblastic metastatic disease from carci-noma of the prostate gland. The radiopaque material in the spinal canal represents residual contrast media from a previous myelographic examination.

Pelvis

The sacrum and bones of the pelvis are involved in about 12% of skeletal metastases and may show either lytic or blastic lesions. (33) (Fig. 11-37) Seeding from the viscera via Batson's venous plexus explains this high incidence in the pelvis as well as in the lumbar spine. (Figs. 11-38 and 11-39) Blow-out lesions of renal and thyroid origin often affect the bony pelvis. Lesions located in the sacral ala or the posterior ilium are often difficult to perceive on standard radiographs. (Fig. 11-40) With the advent of CT scans, a wide variety of lesions involving the osseous pelvis can be more readily seen. (42) The ability of CT to provide accurate measurements of tissue attenuation coefficients and to provide a cross-sectional scan for three-dimensional viewing has made it a powerful tool in musculoskeletal diagnosis, with a profound in-fluence on patient management. (42) It provides information about the extent of the bony lesion, localization (for biopsy and radiation therapy), and relationships with other structures. (42) As equipment improves, it seems probable that CT will assume a more primary role in diagnostic evaluation, particularly of the pelvis, where the complexity of bones and the overlying bowel content prevent ideal evaluation with conventional radiographs. (42) (Fig. 11-41)

Occasionally, blastic lesions affecting the pelvic rim, especially from carcinoma of the prostate, exhibit an expansion of bone. (Fig. 11-42) This occurs as a result of cortical thickening from endosteal or periosteal apposition of bone. The bony enlarge-ment may mimic the appearance of Paget's disease. Usually, other skeletal lesions are present to assist in radiologic differen-tiation. Biopsy of the lesion may be necessary as a final step in diagnosis.

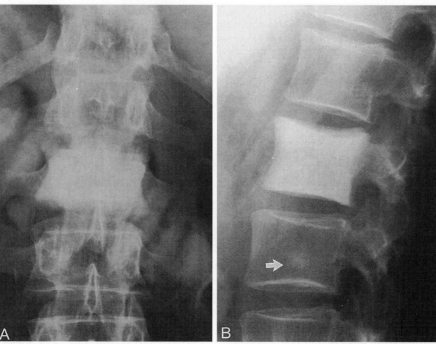

Figure 11-36 **IVORY VERTEBRA. A. AP Lumbar Spine.** Note the solitary ivory vertebra of L2. **B. Lateral Lumbar Spine.** Note the homogeneous radiopacity of the entire vertebral body of L2. There is no endplate thickening or vertebral body expansion, and the anterior concavity of the vertebral body is well maintained. These radiographic signs strongly support osteoblastic metastatic disease rather than Paget's disease. An additional supportive sign is a second lesion subtly present within the vertebral body of L3 (*arrow*).

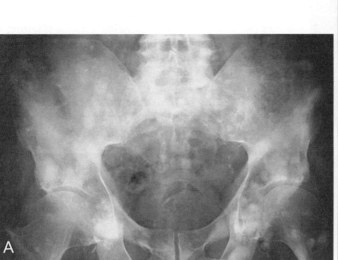

Figure 11-37 **BLASTIC VERSUS LYTIC METASTATIC LESIONS OF THE PELVIS. A. AP Pelvis.** Note the diffuse nodular snowball metastatic deposits throughout the entire pelvis, sacrum, and proximal femora. **B. AP Pelvis.** Observe the diffuse osteolytic metastasis throughout all the bones of the pelvis, sacrum, and proximal femora. (Courtesy of Felix G. Bauer, DC, DACBR(Hon), Sydney, Australia.)

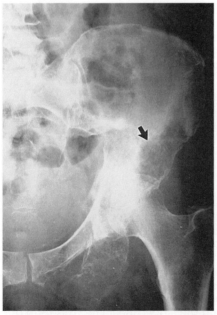

Figure 11-38 **METASTATIC DISEASE TO THE PELVIS. AP Hip.** Note the diffuse osteolytic metastatic destruction in the ischial tuberosity and the supra-acetabular area (*arrow*). These lesions are secondary to carcinoma of the breast.

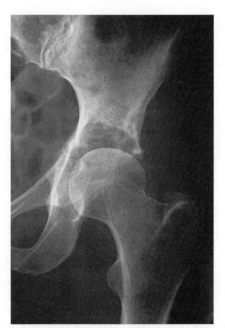

Figure 11-39 **METASTASIS ADJACENT TO THE HIP JOINT. AP Hip.** Observe the diffuse osteolytic destruction of the posterior superior surface of the acetabulum. Note the resorption of the cortical acetabular ridge above the femoral head. Observe the failure of this neoplasm to cross the joint space and affect the femoral head or attenuate the joint space, as might be expected if this were an infectious lesion. This metastatic lesion was secondary to carcinoma of the uterus.

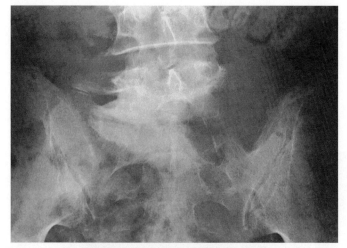

Figure 11-40   SACRAL ALA METASTASIS. AP Sacrum.
Observe the diffuse unilateral osteolytic destruction of the sacral ala. This lesion is secondary to carcinoma of the kidney and represents a blow-out lesion.

Skull

Approximately 10% of all metastatic lesions affect the calvaria. (27) Over 90% of the calvarial metastatic deposits will be lytic lesions, with blastic lesions representing < 10%. (27) (Fig. 11-43) The most common causes for calvarial lytic metastasis are thyroid and breast carcinoma, and prostate and carcinoid tumors create most blastic lesions. Skull lesions usually start as small foci, 1–3 cm in diameter, that gradually increase in size. There are multiple, well-defined holes without sclerotic borders. The lesions of both metastatic disease and myeloma may affect any or all bones of the skull. One means to differentiate myeloma from metastasis is to note the symmetry of the hole size affecting the calvarial vault. (Fig. 11-44) Myeloma lesions are permeative and usually similar in size throughout, whereas most cases of metastatic disease demonstrate both large and small lesions simulta-

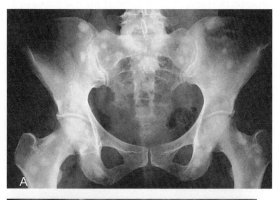

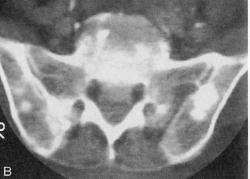

Figure 11-41   METASTATIC LESIONS. A. Plain Film, AP Hip.
Note the diffuse osteoblastic metastatic lesions scattered throughout the bones of the pelvis, sacrum, and proximal femora. These blastic lesions are secondary to carcinoma of the breast. **B. CT, Sacrum.** Note that the CT scan clearly demonstrates the nodular radiopacities scattered throughout both ilia and centrally in the sacrum. *COMMENT:* The majority of metastatic lesions from carcinoma of the breast are lytic (80%), with only 10% being blastic and 10% mixed. (Courtesy of Steven P. Brownstein, MD, Springfield, New Jersey.)

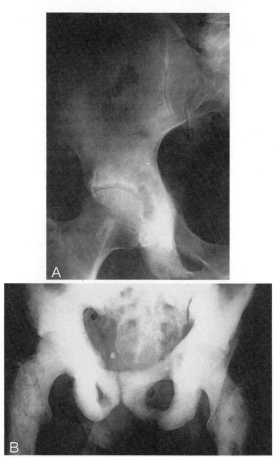

Figure 11-42   OSTEOBLASTIC METASTATIC DISEASE INVOLVING THE BRIM OF THE PELVIS. A. Obliteration of Köhler's Teardrop. Note the osteoblastic metastatic disease affecting the pelvic brim, obliterating Köhler's teardrop. There is a minimal degree of bony expansion of the ischial tuberosity and the iliopectineal line. This form of presentation of blastic metastasis may be difficult to differentiate from Paget's disease. Occasionally, biopsy is required for definitive evaluation. **B. Diffuse Osteoblastic Metastasis.** Observe the diffuse increase in bone density affecting the entire pelvis and proximal femora. These lesions are secondary to carcinoma of the prostate gland and may mimic the diffuse involvement of Paget's disease. Bone expansion and cortical thickening are the cardinal radiographic signs to differentiate Paget's disease from osteoblastic metastatic carcinoma.

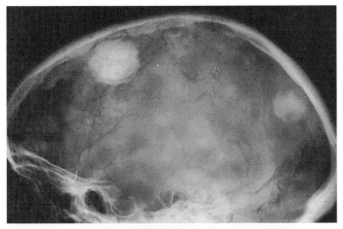

Figure 11-43 BLASTIC METASTASIS: LATERAL SKULL. Observe the numerous well-defined radiopacities scattered throughout the calvaria. These represent osteoblastic metastatic deposits secondary to carcinoma of the prostate gland. *COMMENT:* Approximately 10% of all metastatic lesions affect the calvaria, with > 90% of the calvarial metastatic deposits being lytic and only 10% being blastic.

neously. This is merely a guideline to differentiation because exceptions do occur.

Ribs and Sternum

Approximately 28% of metastatic bone lesions affect the ribs and sternum. (27) Rib metastasis is four times more common than sternal secondary involvement. (43) Both lytic and blastic lesions are encountered. (Fig. 11-45) The majority of the sternal cases have metastasized to the body rather than to the manubrium. (43) Routine chest roentgenograms can detect early metastasis when there is an observable, fortuitous cortical fracture and displacement. In widespread malignancy, metastasis to the skeletal chest

wall is a well-recognized occurrence. (43) Any portion of the rib may be destroyed, either partially or completely. (Fig. 11-46) Permeative holes are often observed, and pathologic fracture is common. Multiple ribs may be involved. Chest wall metastases may create a so-called *extrapleural sign* (43), and the most common cause for the extrapleural sign is metastasis to the ribs. (Fig. 11-47) Blow-out lesions from renal and thyroid carcinoma are not common in the rib cage. (43)

Extremities

Metastatic disease commonly affects the proximal femur and humerus. Typical patterns of lytic, blastic, and mixed lesions prevail, with the occasional pathologic fracture. Non-traumatic avulsion of the lesser trochanter can be a marker for unsuspected underlying metastatic disease. (44) Rarely does the metastatic process cross the joint space, which helps differentiate it from osteomyelitis. Approximately 10% of all metastatic lesions affect the long tubular bones (femur and humerus). (37) The scapula and clavicle are also involved in metastatic disease because shoulder lesions are not limited to the humerus. (Fig. 11-48)

Acral Metastasis. Metastatic lesions of bone rarely occur distal to the elbows and knees (*acral metastases*). (37) (Fig. 11-49) The most common site is the foot, with the hand following second in incidence. (37,45,46) The incidence of metastatic lesions to the foot and hand may be underestimated because asymptomatic lesions may never be recognized. These lesions may be missed because skeletal surveys for metastatic disease do not necessarily include radiographs of the foot and hand. The most frequent sources of these distant metastases are the lung, breast, and kidney, in decreasing order. (45,46) Most of these peripheral metastases are associated with disseminated disease, and in a few reported cases these were the cause of presenting signs and symptoms. (47) Besides routine radiographs, diagnostic modalities that are helpful in assessing these lesions include tomography and technetium bone scanning. CT may assist in determining the local extent of the osseous lesion, and a bone scan will help identify

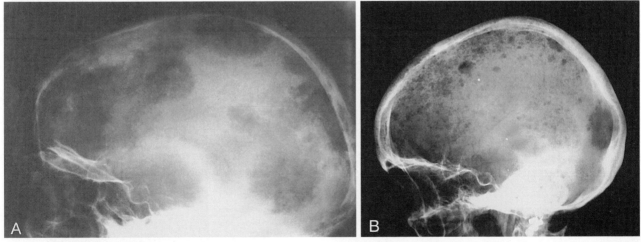

Figure 11-44 MYELOMA VERSUS METASTATIC DISEASE: SKULL. A. Lytic Metastasis. Note the diffuse osteolytic metastasis spread throughout the bony calvaria. Observe the poor zone of transition around these lytic lesions and their asymmetry in size. **B. Multiple Myeloma.** Note the diffuse permeative destructive lesions scattered throughout the entire calvaria. These permeative lesions are fairly sym-

metric in size. *COMMENT:* Multiple myeloma and lytic metastatic disease in the calvaria may look similar; however, one means of differentiation is to note the uniformity of the lesion size. Myeloma lesions are permeative, and they are usually similar in size throughout, whereas most cases of metastasis demonstrate both large and small lesions. (Courtesy of David P. Thomas, MD, Melbourne, Australia.)

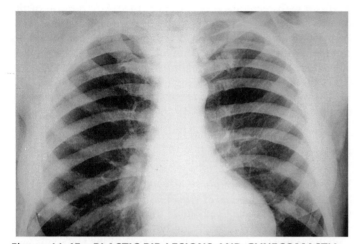

Figure 11-45 BLASTIC RIB LESIONS AND GYNECOMASTIA.
Note that this 59-year-old male demonstrates extensive bilateral metastases in nearly all the visualized rib structures. Because this patient has been on extensive estrogen therapy for his prostate carcinoma he has developed gynecomastia. (Courtesy of Bryan Hartley, MD, Melbourne, Australia.)

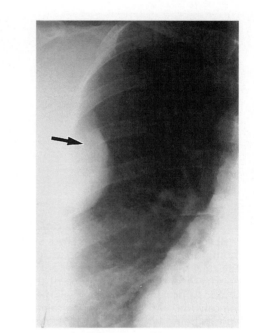

Figure 11-47 EXTRAPLEURAL SIGN: RIB METASTASIS.
Observe the nodular radiopacity at the lateral wall of the rib cage. This represents metastatic disease of a rib. Observe the sharp attenuation of the lateral margin of the sixth rib in the area of the extrapleural mass (*arrow*). *COMMENT:* The most common cause of an extrapleural sign is rib metastasis. This often presents as a radiopaque mass, with sharp borders convex to the lung field and with the peripheral margins gradually tapering to the chest wall. This patient's primary carcinoma was in the thyroid gland.

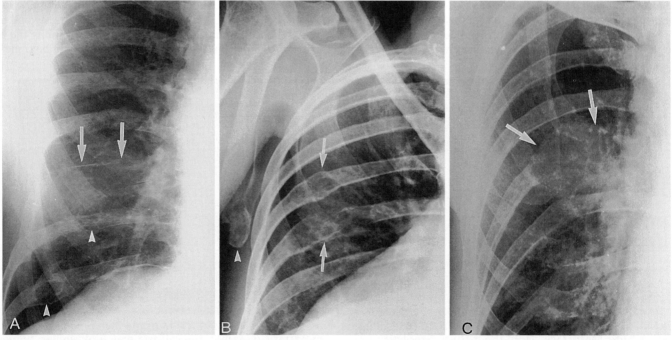

Figure 11-46 RIB METASTASIS. A. Ribs. Observe the near complete destruction of the posterior border of the eighth rib (*arrows*). Additional lytic lesions are also noted in the ninth and tenth lateral ribs (*arrowheads*). **B. Ribs.** Note the lytic destructive lesions of the posterior surfaces of the sixth and seventh ribs (*arrows*). In addition, there is a metastatic focus present at the inferior tip of the scapula (*arrowhead*). **C. Ribs.** Note the extensive destruction of the posterior sixth rib (*arrows*).

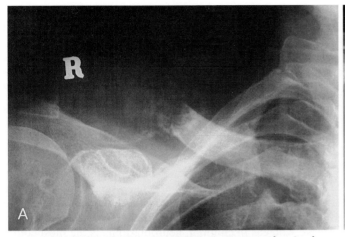

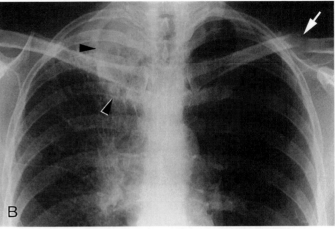

Figure 11-48 **METASTASIS: CLAVICLE. A. Destructive Lesion.** Note the extensive osteolytic metastasis to the distal clavicle. Observe the failure of the disease process to cross the joint space and involve the acromion process of the scapula. This 82-year-old patient has a previous history of carcinoma of the esophagus. **B. Pathologic Fracture.** Observe the patho- logic fracture through a subtle osteolytic metastatic lesion induced by a coughing bout (*arrow*). Also note the opacity in the right upper lobe owing to carcinoma (*arrowheads*). (Panel A courtesy of Bryan Hartley, MD, Melbourne, Australia. Panel B courtesy of Hardie B. Webb Jr., DC, Winter Garden, Florida.)

other metastatic lesions. Peripheral metastatic lesions are usually lytic and lack the periosteal reaction so common to an infectious process.

No obvious predilection for any particular bone exists in the foot. (45,46) In the hand, however, there is a great predilection for the distal phalanx, particularly from bronchogenic carcinoma. (Fig. 11-50) Extensive osteolysis of the distal phalanx, often with the presence of a soft tissue mass, is the usual mode of presentation. The articular space is usually uninvolved. Occurrences in other bones of the hand, such as the proximal and middle pha-

langes and the carpal and metacarpal bones, have been documented. (47) (Fig. 11-51)

It has been suggested that the only way cancer cells can reach the peripheral bones is by the arterial route. (38) This may explain why half of the metastatic lesions to the foot and hands originate in the lungs. (48) The tumor cell foci may enter the pulmonary vein, reach the arterial side of the circulation, and then be transported to the peripheral skeletal sites. (48) Other investigators suggest that the low rate of metastasis in the distal extremities is logically explained by the fact that the tumor cells do not find suitable soil in

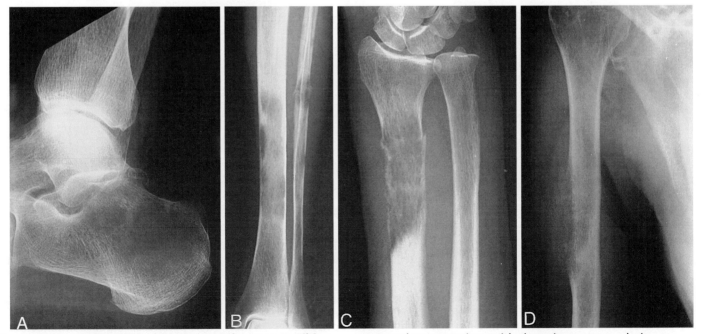

Figure 11-49 **ACRAL METASTASES. A. Calcaneus. B. Tibia and Fibula. C. Radius. D. Humerus.** Note that this patient presented with metastatic lesions in the calcaneus, tibia and fibula, distal radius, and diaphysis of the humerus. This is an unusual presentation, with the primary tumor being a bronchogenic carcinoma. *COMMENT:* Metastatic lesions of bone are rare distal to the elbows and knees (acral metastases).

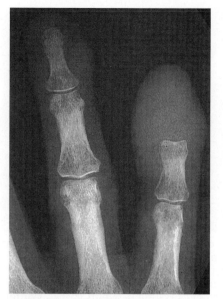

Figure 11-50 BRONCHOGENIC CARCINOMA METASTASIS TO THE DISTAL PHALANX OF THE HAND. Note the extensive destruction of the distal phalanx of the fifth finger. Soft tissue swelling indicates the possibility of hemorrhage and soft tissue tumor extension. Note the preservation of the joint space and the lack of tumor extension across the joint. *COMMENT:* Metastatic disease in the hand shows a great predilection for the distal phalanx, particularly when it is owing to bronchogenic carcinoma.

which to grow—that is, the tissue may not be warm enough because of a gradient of metabolic rate. (49) The sparse amount of red marrow in the extremities may suggest that the soil is not rich enough to allow growth. The exact explanation for the lesions of the terminal phalanx is not available. The prognosis upon discovery of metastasis to the hand is approximately 3 months, which represents the prognosis of bronchogenic carcinoma. (50)

Periosteal Response

The presence of periosteal new bone formation associated with a metastatic bone tumor in the absence of pathologic fracture is rare. (51) The primary organs most frequently causing a metastatic periosteal response in adults are the prostate, lung, and breast; whereas in children, neuroblastoma is the most common cause. (51) Periosteal new bone, which is usually of a *sunburst,* or spiculated, nature, is essentially a reaction to the tumor by the involved bone rather than an inherent property ascribable to the specific histologic type of metastatic tumor. (Fig. 11-52) Furthermore, the bone involvement often seems to precede the periosteal reaction, which is found with the more destructive and rapidly growing lesions. The new bone formation usually occurs on that portion or side of a bone that was farthest removed from the main concentration of tumor growth. (51) A striking, perpendicular spiculation may be seen along the inner rim of the pelvis, at the ischial tuberosity, or along the proximal femoral shaft, simulating a primary malignant bone tumor. This occurs

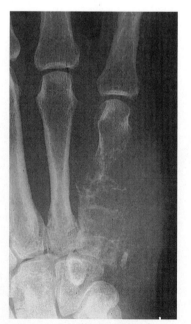

Figure 11-51 ACRAL METASTASES: HAND. Note the diffuse osteolytic destruction of nearly the entire portion of the fifth metacarpal. This patient had a hypernephroma 8 years before, having presented with pain in the hand. This lesion was confirmed as a metastatic tumor from the original primary carcinoma of the kidney.

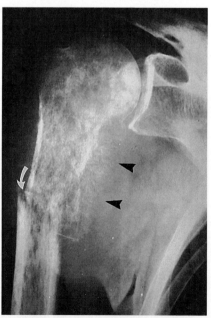

Figure 11-52 PERIOSTEAL RESPONSE WITH METASTATIC BONE TUMORS. Note the pathologic fracture in the proximal third of the humerus (*arrow*). A permeative pattern of bone destruction is scattered throughout the humeral head, metaphysis, and diaphysis. There is significant spiculated periosteal response present on the medial surface of the humerus (*arrowheads*). *COMMENT:* The periosteal response outlined in this case may be related to the associated pathologic fracture. In adults, the organs most frequently causing a metastatic periosteal response are the prostate, lung, and breast; in children, neuroblastoma is the most common cause.

in prostatic carcinoma in 5% of metastatic cases. (51) Involvement of the vertebrae with this florid, spiculated periosteal new bone is uncommon. (52) Sunburst periosteal reaction in the cranial vault is a feature of metastatic neuroblastoma and chronic hemolytic anemias (thalassemia major).

Complications

Pathologic Fracture. Pathologic fracture through a metastasis can be a distressing and painful event and is the most common complication of osseous metastasis. In a child this carries the further ramifications of potential effects on bone growth by damage to the physis from the tumor, the pathologic fracture, or the tumor treatment (chemotherapy, radiotherapy).

An extradural compression of the spinal cord may accompany a metastatic vertebral collapse, leaving the patient paraplegic. This complication is usually seen in the thoracic and lumbar spine, where vertebral body collapse is common. (Fig. 11-53) The humerus, ribs, cervical vertebrae (Fig. 11-54), and proximal femur are also documented sites of fracture. Pathologic fractures most commonly occur through lytic metastases and less frequently may develop in blastic lesions. (Fig. 11-55) One sixth of all fractures through skeletal metastases occur in the proximal fourth of the femur. (53) Fractures through this area of the proximal femur may produce an ischemic necrosis of the femoral head. A high proportion of the proximal femur pathologic fractures stem from breast carcinoma. (53) In the adult, pathologic fractures are highly unlikely when < 50% of the cortical bone is destroyed. (54) Fracture is much more likely when 50–5% of the cortex is destroyed, and most likely (an incidence of > 80%) when > 75% of the cortex is destroyed. (54) Such statistical analyses are undoubtedly less applicable in children.

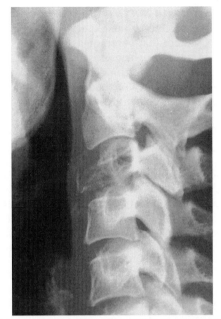

Figure 11-54 **PATHOLOGIC COLLAPSE: A COMPLICATION OF METASTATIC DISEASE. Lateral Cervical Spine.** Observe that the C3 vertebral body is severely collapsed, and underlying osteolytic destruction is apparent. This 26-year-old female had a 2-year history of pain in the foot and a recent episode of neck pain following trivial trauma. The primary tumor was a malignant synovioma in the foot, with the C3 vertebral lesion being a secondary metastatic focus.

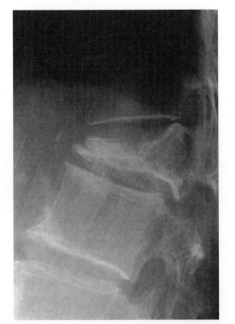

Figure 11-53 **PATHOLOGIC FRACTURE THROUGH A META-STATIC LESION.** Note the extensive collapse of the L1 vertebral body, with underlying osteolytic destruction. Note that there is collapse of the posterior portion of the vertebral body, which is an indication of a pathologic fracture. The primary lesion in this patient was carcinoma of the sigmoid colon.

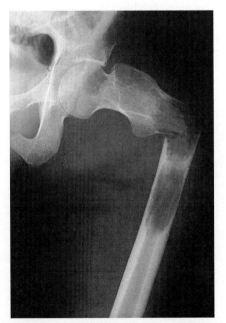

Figure 11-55 **PATHOLOGIC FRACTURE: PROXIMAL FEMUR.** Note the complete transverse fracture through a large lytic metastatic lesion in the metadiaphyseal area of the proximal femur. *COMMENT:* Pathologic fractures most commonly occur in lytic metastases and rarely develop in blastic lesions. One sixth of all fractures through skeletal metastases occur in the proximal femur. (Courtesy of David P. Thomas, MD, Melbourne, Australia.)

Bone Expansion and Soft Tissue Mass. Metastatic tumors on occasion will produce bone expansion. It is not a common roentgen sign, except that carcinomas frequently expand ribs. Although uncommon elsewhere, it is more likely to expand small tubular bones or the pelvic rim. The capacity to expand bone, however, is not a specific feature of a type of carcinoma but rather a secondary effect from other characteristics related to bone size and shape.

The presence of a soft tissue mass in association with a destructive osseous lesion usually denotes a primary malignant tumor, as a soft tissue mass is much less commonly associated with secondary neoplasm. (Fig. 11-56) The formation of an extraosseous soft tissue mass may occur in metastatic bone lesions, particularly when the skeletal site involves a small bone, such as a rib. Occasionally, a large component of the soft tissue mass is hemorrhage. CT and especially MRI are the best methods for demonstration because soft tissue extension is poorly seen on conventional radiographs. (42,55)

Response to Therapy

No definite means to accurately assess the response to therapy have yet been established. Many authors have found that pain relief is the most consistent indicator of response to treatment. (33,37,38,56) Palliative therapy is essential in patients with metastatic disease to ensure quality of life because morbidity and disability is usually high. (57) Bisphosphonates are common pharmaceutical agents currently used to treat lytic metastasis owing to their osteoclastic inhibiting effects. (58) They have shown to be effective in symptom relief as well as progression of the disease. (57) The demonstration of sclerosis in a previously lytic lesion is considered a sign of the healing process; however, this sign is somewhat unpredictable. (59) (Fig. 11-57) Bone scan seems to be the most reliable modality for assessing response to therapy. (56,60) A reduction in intensity of a lesion's uptake on serial bone scans is a sign of good response. On occasion, observer error is a

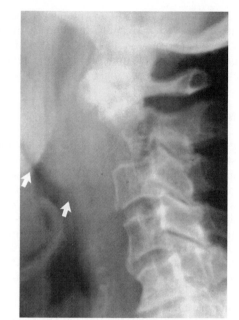

Figure 11-56 A METASTATIC LESION WITH SOFT TISSUE EXTENSION: LATERAL CERVICAL. Observe the grossly destructive lytic lesion in the vertebral body of C2. There is extension of the soft tissue tumor anterior to the C2 body, creating a large increase in the retropharyngeal interspace (*arrows*), which measured > 15 mm at C2. *COMMENT:* Most soft tissue masses are associated with primary malignant bone tumors rather than secondary neoplasms. On rare occasions metastatic tumors can produce soft tissue masses, and, often, a large component of the soft tissue mass is hemorrhage. The true incidence of this complication in metastases is not known. (Courtesy of Robert L. Mattin, DC, Perth, Western Australia, Australia.)

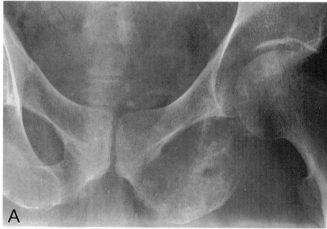
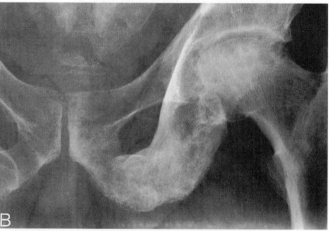

Figure 11-57 AVASCULAR NECROSIS AS A COMPLICATION OF RADIATION THERAPY. A. Ischium. Note that this male patient demonstrates a metastatic lesion of a mixed variety, secondary to carcinoma of the prostate gland. Observe the normal bone integrity of the femoral head at this time. **B. 2-Year Follow-Up.** Note that this study, made 2 years after radiation treatment of the ischial metastatic focus, demonstrates remarkable remodeling of bone in the ischium. There is deformity of the femoral head, with fragmentation and radiopacity present. The joint space of the hip is not affected. The radiographic changes in the femoral head are those of avascular necrosis, which was caused by the radiation therapy. (Courtesy of Richard W. Hooke, DC, Dalby, Queensland, Australia.)

problem. In patients with sclerotic metastases, further sclerosis can occur in response to either successful or unsuccessful systemic therapy; similarly, patients with mixed, sclerotic, and lytic disease are often difficult to assess. (56,60)

Failure to respond is often heralded by further osteolysis. It has been suggested that full assessment of the response of bone metastases to systemic treatment should include assessment of pain, blood tests, a full skeletal survey, and serial bone scans. On the basis of these four parameters, a rational decision as to continuation of treatment or change in regimen may be made. (56,60) It should be understood that when palliative irradiation is used during treatment, the therapeutic goal is for symptom control. (61) Irradiation generally needs to be provided for a period of 1 month before relief is noted. (61)

NEUROBLASTOMA

Neuroblastoma (sympathicoblastoma) is the second most common abdominal neoplasm in childhood, with Wilms' tumor being the most common. (1) This malignant tumor arises in the adrenal gland in approximately 75% of the patients; extra-adrenal sites are the posterior mediastinum (20%) and the paravertebral sympathetic ganglionated chain (5%). (1,2) There is some evidence that extra-adrenal tumors have a better prognosis than intra-adrenal tumors, which are highly fatal. One factor that might explain this is the earlier detection and treatment of tumors that are not buried deep within the abdomen. About 80% of neuroblastomas are found in children < 2.5 years of age, the remainder occurring before age 5. (1,3)

On plain films of the abdomen, a retroperitoneal mass may be seen displacing adjacent organs, particularly lowering the kidney. Approximately two thirds of the tumors demonstrate a granular pattern of calcification; this is seen both in adrenal and extra-adrenal sites. (Figs. 11-58 and 11-59)

The neuroblastoma metastasizes early, and the metastases are often multiple, diffuse, and fairly symmetric. Monostotic lesions rarely occur. Most lesions are osteolytic and may be indistinguishable from those produced by leukemia. Skeletal metastases occur in > 50% of cases. (4) The spine, pelvis, and ends of the long bones are common sites. (Fig. 11-58) The epiphysis is usually spared. Spinal involvement creates vertebral collapse and widening of the paravertebral stripe. (5) Skull metastases produce a characteristic roentgen appearance of lytic lesions and diffuse widening of the sutures. Occasionally, spreading of the sutures may occur without actual metastases to the calvaria. Metastatic deposits from neuroblastoma present as plaques on the brain surface, thus causing the wide separation of the sutures, which is so classic in this disease. A soft tissue mass and a striking *sunburst spiculation of the skull tables* is frequently encountered. These skull changes are unique and are virtually pathognomonic of metastatic neuroblastoma. (Fig. 11-60)

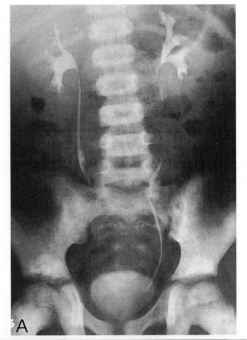

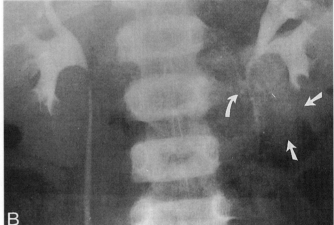

Figure 11-58 **NEUROBLASTOMA. A. Intravenous Pyelogram.** Observe the mottled, mixed radiolucency and radiopacity scattered throughout the lumbar spine, sacrum, pelvic bones, and visualized proximal femora. This radiographic appearance is consistent with malignant disease. There is no abnormality of the kidneys, ureters, or urinary bladder. **B. Close-Up of the Paraspinal Region.** Observe the granular calcification in the paraspinal region, just caudal to the inferior pole of the kidney (*arrows*). This punctate calcification is present within a paraspinal neuroblastoma (sympathicoblastoma) and is located within the paravertebral sympathetic ganglionated chain. *COMMENT:* Neuroblastoma is the second most common abdominal neoplasm in childhood, with Wilms' tumor being the most common. This malignant tumor arises in the adrenal gland in approximately 75% of patients; extra-adrenal sites are the posterior mediastinum (20%) and the paravertebral sympathetic ganglionated chain (5%). Neuroblastoma metastasizes early, and the metastases are often multiple, diffuse, and fairly symmetric. Most lesions are osteolytic and may be indistinguishable from those produced by leukemia. Skeletal metastases occur in > 50% of cases, with the spine, pelvis, and ends of the long bones being the most common sites.

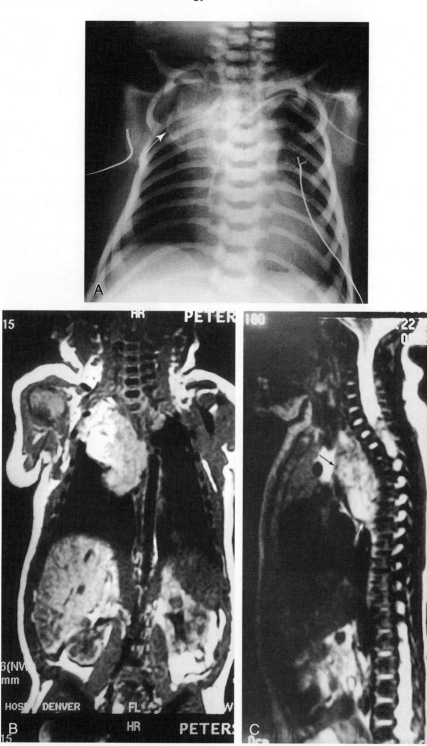

Figure 11-59 **NEUROBLASTOMA: HUGE POSTERIOR MEDI-ASTINAL MASS. A. AP Thoracic Spine.** Observe the diffuse sclerotic changes affecting nearly all bones visualized. There is destruction of the third rib on the right side. A calcified mass is seen in the posterior aspect of the right upper mediastinum (*arrow*). **B. T1-Weighted MRI, Coronal Thoracic Spine. C. T2-Weighted MRI, Sagittal Cervicothoracic Spine.** Observe the huge mediastinal mass engulfing the postero-superior aspect of the right upper mediastinum (*arrows*). *COMMENT:* This 3-day-old infant was born with a posterior mediastinal neuroblastoma with diffuse metastasis to the skeletal structures. MRI is the most sensitive imaging modality to evaluate the spinal cord and its neurological components. Approximately 20% of neuroblastomas occur in the posterior mediastinum, with the majority (75%) occurring in the adrenal gland. The remaining 5% occur in the paravertebral sympathetic ganglionated chain. (Courtesy of Loren Macey, MD, Department of Radiology, University Hospital, Denver, Colorado.)

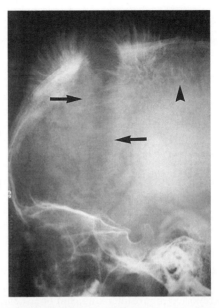

Figure 11-60   **METASTATIC NEUROBLASTOMA. Lateral Skull.** Observe the striking sunburst spiculation of the skull tables, along with gross widening of the sutures (*arrows*). Note the permeative destructive lesions affecting the calvaria (*arrowhead*). *COMMENT:* Skull metastases in neuroblastoma produce a characteristic roentgen appearance of lytic lesions and diffuse widening of the sutures. Metastatic deposits from neuroblastoma present as plaques on the brain surface, thus causing the wide separation of the sutures, which is so classic in this disease. A soft tissue mass and a striking sunburst spiculation on the skull tables are frequently encountered and virtually pathognomonic of metastatic neuroblastoma. (Courtesy of David P. Thomas, MD, Melbourne, Australia.)

CAPSULE SUMMARY   Metastatic Bone Tumors

General Considerations

- Metastatic bone tumors are the most common malignant tumors of the skeleton.
- Central nervous system tumors and basal cell carcinoma rarely spread to bone; all others have the potential.
- Metastasis is the most life-threatening complication of any malignancy.

Incidence

- 70% of all malignant tumors are metastatic; 30% are primary.
- Autopsy series reveal 20–35% of all patients with malignancies have osseous metastases.
- Cancers of the breast, prostate, lung, and kidney account for 80% of osseous metastases.
- In females, breast carcinoma accounts for 70% of all bony metastases; in males, the prostate is responsible for about 60% of metastatic lesions, and the lung accounts for 25%.

Clinical Features

- Most occur after the age of 40.
- Weight loss, cachexia, and bone pain, which is often worse at night, awakening the patient. Occasionally, pain is lacking in advanced disease.
- Metastatic lesions may occur 10–15 years after surgery or treatment for the primary neoplasm.
- Alkaline phosphatase enzyme may be elevated in blastic metastatic lesions; acid phosphatase is found elevated in prostatic carcinoma following rupture of the prostatic capsule.

Pathologic Features

- Cancers metastasize by three routes: direct extension, lymphatic channels, and hematogenous dissemination (most common pathway).

- Batson's venous plexus provides a rapid pathway for cancer cells to seed the bone, bypassing the liver and lungs.
- Lytic lesions occur as a result of pressure erosion from the medullary tumor deposits and are unrelated to osteoclastic activity.
- Blastic lesions represent a reactive repair response of local osteoid tissue to the presence of tumor.

Radiologic Features

- Technetium bone scans (^{99m}Tc-MDP) are more accurate in detecting early bone metastases than are conventional radiographs.
- 3–5% destruction of bone will render a positive, or hot scan, whereas plain films require at least 30% loss of bone before it can be detected visually.
- 80% of all metastases are located in the central or axial skeleton, with the spine and pelvis being the most common sites. Ribs, skull, humerus, and femur represent a lesser percentage.
- Metastatic tumors are rare below the elbows and knees.
- Fundamental roentgen signs are alteration in bone density and architecture.
- 75% of all metastatic lesions are osteolytic, creating a moth-eaten or permeative pattern of bone destruction.
- 15% of all metastatic lesions are osteoblastic in nature, creating a snowball pattern with diffuse lesions.
- 10% of all metastatic lesions are solitary.
- Blow-out lesions represent a bubbly, highly expansile appearance, usually found associated with renal or thyroid malignancy.
- Vertebral body and pedicles are the most common sites for metastatic deposits.
- Malignant Schmorl's node represents a neoplastic weakening of the vertebral endplate, allowing cartilaginous node formation.

(*continued*)

CAPSULE SUMMARY   Metastatic Bone Tumors (*continued*)

- Uniform vertebral collapse (vertebra plana) with compromise of the posterior third of the vertebral body can occur.
- One-eyed pedicle sign, or the winking owl sign, represents metastasis to one pedicle.
- Blind vertebra represents bilateral pedicular destruction from metastatic disease, leaving no eyes in the spine.
- Ivory vertebra may be caused by osteoblastic metastasis, Paget's disease, and Hodgkin's lymphoma.
- Rib metastases often create the extrapleural sign and represent its most common cause.
- Metastatic deposits in the hand are most commonly from bronchogenic carcinoma and affect the distal phalanges by extensive osteolysis.
- Periosteal response with metastatic tumors is rare in the absence of pathologic fracture; however, a sunburst pattern has been reported in prostate, lung, and breast carcinoma. A similar appearance is cited in the cranial vault in metastatic neuroblastoma.

Neuroblastoma (Sympathicoblastoma)

- Neuroblastoma represents the second most common abdominal neoplasm in childhood; Wilms' tumor is most common.
- 75% arise within the adrenal gland; 20% in the posterior mediastinum; and 5% in the sympathetic ganglionated chain.
- 80% are found in children < 2.5 years of age, the remainder before age 5.
- Two thirds of all neuroblastomas show granular calcification radiographically.
- Skeletal metastases are common (> 50% of cases) and are diffuse and fairly symmetric. They are seldom monostotic.
- The spine, pelvis, skull, and ends of the long bones are common sites.
- Skull deposits widen the sutures and create a classic sunburst spiculation of the skull tables, which is virtually pathognomonic of metastatic neuroblastoma.

PRIMARY MALIGNANT BONE TUMORS

MULTIPLE MYELOMA

General Considerations

Multiple myeloma occurs as a result of a malignant proliferation of plasma cells, which infiltrate the bone marrow. The first patient known to have multiple myeloma was seen in 1845, after severe recurrences of pain during a 17-month period. (1) His urine contained unusual "animal matter" that became soluble when boiled and formed again when cooled. (1) Although William MacIntyre recognized the effect of heat on the urine and outlined the clinical findings, it was the young physician and chemist Henry Bence Jones who described the protein in detail. (2) In 1873 von Rustizky named and outlined in detail the clinicopathologic features of this disease. (3) Multiple myeloma is occasionally referred to as Kahler's disease, after the clinician from Prague who lectured extensively on myeloma in the late nineteenth century. (4) In more recent times the diagnosis of myeloma was facilitated by Longsworth et al. (5) in 1939, with the development of electrophoretic techniques and with immunoelectrophoresis as described by Grabar and Williams. (6)

Incidence

Multiple myeloma is the most common primary malignant tumor of bone and accounts for 27% of biopsied bone tumors. Together, myeloma and osteosarcoma account for almost half (46%) of the primary malignant tumors of bone. (7) Multiple myeloma represents about 1% of all types of malignant disease and slightly > 10% of hematologic malignancies. In the

last 2 decades, the death rate from multiple myeloma has increased; however, it is likely that these increases are related to earlier and more improved diagnosis rather than representing an actual rise in incidence. (8)

Clinical Features

Age and Sex Distribution

Typically 75% of myeloma patients are between 50 and 70 years of age, with an average age of 60. It is rarely seen before the age of 40, but a few cases have been reported before the age of 30. (9) There is a male to female ratio of 2:1.

Signs and Symptoms

The clinical picture of the disease comprises four types of abnormalities: anemia owing to replacement or alteration of the hematopoietic tissues by proliferating plasma cells, deossification of bones that house red marrow, production of abnormal serum and urinary proteins, and renal disease. (10) Pain is the cardinal initial symptom, often suggesting arthritis or neuralgia.

Initially, the bone pain is intermittent; in later stages it becomes continuous. It is worse during the day and aggravated by exercise and weight bearing. The pain is often better at night with bedrest. Low back pain in myeloma patients is frequently misdiagnosed as disc or sciatic problems initially. A rapid onset of severe pain after slight strain or mild trauma usually indicates the development of a pathologic fracture. In the late stages of the disease, pathologic fractures occur in 20% of patients. (11) Paraplegia may occur with vertebral collapse and is more common with a solitary presentation (plasmacytoma). (7) As the disease progresses, the pain becomes more severe and prolonged, often requiring narcotics for relief.

Other common signs are weight loss, cachexia, anemia, and unexplained osteoporosis. Bacterial infections (particularly respiratory) occur in approximately 10% of cases, with Gram-negative organisms predominating. The impairment of antibody response, deficiency of the uninvolved immunoglobulins, reduction of delayed hypersensitivity in some instances, and depression of activity of the neutrophils all contribute to infection susceptibility in these patients.

Location

The spine is the most common site, with the lower thoracic and lumbar areas predominating. The marrow-rich flat bones of the pelvis, skull, ribs, clavicle, and scapula are also frequently involved. The diaphyses of the proximal long tubular bones (femur and humerus) are commonly affected. Skeletal involvement distal to the elbow and knee occurs in only 10% of cases. (10) (Fig. 11-61; Table 11-12)

Laboratory Findings

Blood Cytology. A normochromic normocytic anemia is common, along with rouleaux formation, thrombocytopenia, and an elevation in the ESR. Plasma cells in a peripheral blood smear are rare, except in patients with plasma cell leukemia.

Serum Calcium and Phosphorus. Hypercalcemia occurs in > 30% of cases and is secondary to the lytic destruction created by the myelomatoid tissue. Serum phosphorus is normal unless there is accompanying renal disease. (10)

Serum Proteins. Between 50% and 60% of patients with myeloma have elevated plasma proteins. Hyperglobulinemia with a reversal of the albumin to globulin (A:G) ratio is common. Other causes of A:G ratio reversal are sarcoidosis, chronic nephritis, chronic cirrhosis, and lymphogranuloma venereum. Serum electrophoresis confirms the abnormality in 80–90% of patients with multiple lesions and represents the definitive examination in establishing the diagnosis. The myeloma cells secrete a characteristic monoclonal globulin that varies in each patient. Approximately 50% of cases have G myeloma (IgG), 25% have A myeloma (IgA), and 1–2% have D myeloma (IgD), whereas IgE and IgM myelomas are rare. Protein electrophoresis demonstrates peaks between the β- and γ-globulin elevations or a characteristic M spike in 90% of patients. (12) Myeloma proteins are present in 90% of patients with disseminated plasma cell lesions. Kyle (8) showed the electrophoretic patterns to be diagnostic of myeloma protein in 75% of his study group. (Table 11-13)

Urine (Bence Jones' Proteoses). Bence Jones' protein is a light immunoglobulin representing a complete polypeptide chain. Its thermal behavior is peculiar in that it first coagulates and then dissolves at temperatures > 60°C. Approximately 40% of myeloma patients show detectable Bence Jones' proteinuria by the heating method, with a higher percentage being detected by electrophoresis. (8) Bence Jones' proteinuria may occur occasionally in other diseases, such as lymphoma, polycythemia vera, and metastatic disease (5% of cases).

Uric Acid in the Blood. Hyperuricemia frequently occurs because of accelerated nucleic acid metabolism. This finding is not specific for myeloma because it occurs in leukemia and gout as well.

Bone Marrow. Aspiration biopsy of the sternum or the iliac bone is the favored method to study smears of bone marrow and reveals columns of plasma cells at varying degrees of maturity. (10) This procedure is strongly diagnostic; however, it may not render accurate findings in each case. The presence of > 3% plasma cells is considered abnormal, and when the plasma cells are > 10%, the diagnosis of myeloma is histologically ensured. (10)

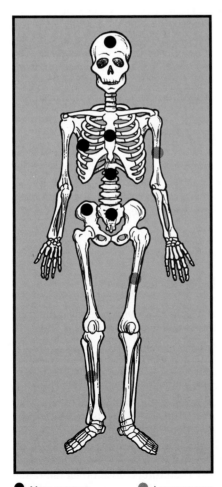

● More common   ● Less common

Figure 11-61 **SKELETAL DISTRIBUTION OF MULTIPLE MYELOMA.**

Table 11-12	Anatomic Sites of Multiple Myeloma in 320 Cases	
Site		**Percentage**
Vertebrae		69
Ribs		59
Skull		40
Pelvis		40
Femur		24
Humerus		20
Clavicle		15
Scapula		13

Reprinted with permission from **Wilner D:** *Radiology of Bone Tumors and Allied Disorders.* Philadelphia, WB Saunders, 1982.

Table 11-13	Laboratory Findings in Multiple Myeloma

Hematologic
    Anemia (60% of patients)
    Leukopenia (16% of patients)
    Thrombocytopenia (13% of patients)
    Lymphocytosis
    Neutropenia
    Eosinophilia
    Rare circulating plasma cells or plasma cell leukemia
    Elevated ESR
    Rouleaux's formation
Bone marrow abnormalities
    Focal areas with collections or sheets of plasma cells
    More than 15–20% plasma cells overall
    Abnormal plasma cells
        Flaming plasma cells
        Morula's cells
        Mott's cells
        Thesaurocytes
Biochemical abnormalities
    Hypercalcemia (30% of patients)
    Hyperuricemia (60% of patients)
    Azotemia with elevated BUN and serum creatinine (55% of patients)
    Alkaline phosphatase usually within normal limits
    Lowered anion gap (in IgG myeloma only)
    Rare hepatic dysfunction with hypophosphatemia
Immunoelectrophoretic abnormalities
    Monoclonal serum spike in relation to a region on cellulose acetate electrophoresis
    Immunoelectrophoresis of serum:
        IgG peak (50% of patients)
        IgA peak (25% of patients)
        IgD peak (1% of patients)
        IgE peak (peak usually not present)
    Immunoelectrophoresis of osmodialized urine:
        κ and λ light chains with serum peak (20% of patients)
        Light chains with no serum (20% of patients)
Urine abnormalities
    Bence Jones' proteinuria (40% of patients)

Courtesy of Alan H. Adams, DC, DACBN, Tallahassee, Florida.
BUN, blood urea nitrogen; ESR; erythrocyte sedimentation rate.

Pathologic Features

Osseous Involvement

The cause of this diffuse disorder remains unknown; however it is estimated that the initial oncogenic event occurs 10–15 years before disease symptomology. (13) In the classic form the skeleton contains multiple, permeative lesions, which are filled by gelatinous, red, soft masses of neoplastic plasma cells. These focal collections of plasma cells are surrounded by areas of increased osteoclastic activity. With increased cellular activity, extensive bone destruction, pathologic fractures, and hypercalcemia become evident. Myeloma has been classified as a round cell disorder, reflecting the microscopic appearance of the nuclei, which are round to oval. Often, the destructive lesions within the marrow may appear round, as well. Other round cell neoplasms include Ewing's sarcoma and non-Hodgkin's lymphoma of bone (reticulum cell sarcoma). (11)

Myeloma Kidney

Renal involvement may occur in all forms of the disease. Precipitation of protein in the tubules produces extensive and numerous hyaline casts. The tubular cells swell and become engorged with the Bence Jones' proteinaceous casts. These casts are accompanied by an inflammatory infiltrate in the surrounding interstitium, and permanent tubular damage will occur in up to 75% of patients, causing renal failure. (14) Signs of renal failure usually occurs within 2 months of diagnosis (14), representing the second most common cause of death in myeloma patients, with pneumonia and respiratory failure being first.

Amyloidosis

Approximately 15% of patients with classic multiple myeloma develop secondary amyloidosis. (15) The favorite target organs of amyloid are the kidney, heart, gastrointestinal tract, liver, and spleen. (15) Amyloid joint disease is a rare form of arthropathy. (16) The subcutaneous nodules, morning stiffness, weight loss, and symmetric involvement of diarthrodial joints may suggest rheumatoid arthritis initially; however, the non-inflammatory nature of amyloid arthropathy must be emphasized, and the severe early morning fatigue also helps distinguish it from rheumatoid disease. (15) Rarely, a circumscribed mass of amyloid around a joint is the first manifestation of myelomatosis. This presentation has been referred to as the *pad sign* of secondary amyloid arthropathy. (17) Amyloid deposits in the skeleton may undergo calcification, while infiltration of the kidney may lead to renal failure.

Extraosseous Plasmacytoma

The most common site for extramedullary plasmacytoma is the nasopharynx, with the nasal cavity, oral cavity, tonsils, sinuses, and larynx also affected. (10) Often these tumors will be locally invasive, eroding into adjacent bone.

Radiologic Features

Radionuclide Bone Scans

It has long been held that conventional radiography is the best way to visualize myelomatoid deposits. (18,19) Bone scans are relatively insensitive to the presence of myeloma lesions and frequently produce a normal (*cold*) scan, except at the sites of pathologic fracture, which will be focally hot. (18,19) (Fig. 11-62) A major reason for the negative scan or non-reactivity of the deposits is the release of an osteoclast activating factor (OAF) by the plasma cells. High OAF levels are found in patients with myeloma, causing an osteoclastic process to predominate. The uptake of radionuclide into lesions depends on osteoblastic activity, which is deficient in patients with non-fractured myeloma deposits. (18,19) Therefore, conventional radiography (a skeletal survey) continues to be the principal method of demonstrating skeletal involvement in the routine diagnostic workup of a patient with suspected multiple myeloma.

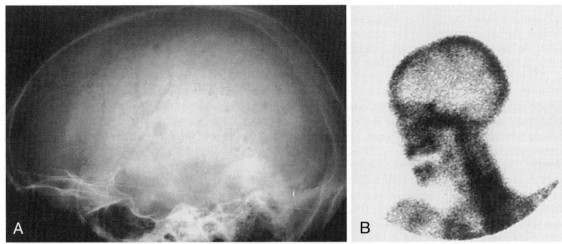

Figure 11-62   **MULTIPLE MYELOMA: COLD RADIONUCLIDE SCAN. A. Lateral Skull.** Note the multiple discrete osteolytic lesions distributed throughout the calvaria (raindrop skull). **B. Delayed Technetium Radionuclide Scan, Lateral Projection.** Note that this scan fails to demonstrate any coinciding tracer uptake corresponding to the osteolytic defects seen on the plain film. (Courtesy of William E. Litterer, DC, DACBR, Fellow, ACCR, Elizabeth, New Jersey.)

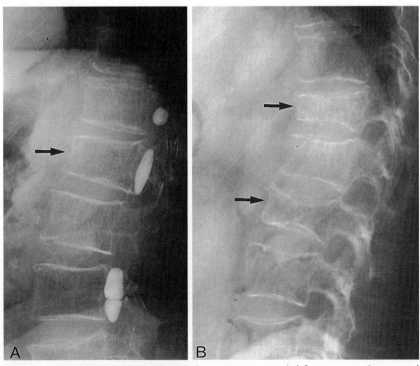

Figure 11-63   **OSTEOPOROSIS: THE EARLIEST RADIOGRAPHIC SIGN OF MYELOMA. A. Lateral Lumbar Spine.** Observe the gross osteoporosis throughout the lumbar spine. There is a compression fracture of the superior endplate of L2 (*arrow*). The radiopaque densities in the spinal canal represent con-trast material from a previous myelogram. **B. Lateral Lumbar Spine.** Note the diffuse osteoporosis throughout the entire lumbar spine. There are pathologic fractures of the T12 and L2 vertebral bodies (*arrows*).

Conventional Radiography

Osteoporosis. The mode of presentation controls the wide spectrum of roentgen findings in patients with multiple myeloma. Early in the disorder, the bones may appear normal, even though sternal biopsy and laboratory tests at this stage would be positive. Unless proper clinical workup is initiated, these patients may be labeled as neurotics. As the disease progresses, generalized and severe osteoporosis presents radiographically. This is usually most advanced within the spine, more frequently observed in the lower thoracic and lumbar regions. (20) The typical appearance is a diffuse loss of bone density with thinning of the cortex. In the spine the vertebral body may assume the same density as the intervertebral disc. At this stage, the bones are weak, and pathologic fracture is imminent. (Fig. 11-63)

Osteolytic Defects. The radiologic hallmark of multiple myeloma is the sharply circumscribed osteolytic defect. These radiolucent lesions have been historically referred to as *punched-out lesions.* They are multiple, round, and purely lytic. (Fig. 11-64) The most frequent sites are in bones with hematopoietic potential. This appearance is most common in the skull, pelvis, long bones, clavicles, and ribs. (Figs. 11-65 and 11-66) The pattern of widespread lytic lesions of the skull has been referred to as the *raindrop skull.* (21) (Figs. 11-67 and 11-68) Calvarial involvement may occasionally be differentiated from metastatic carcinoma by the more uniform size of the lytic lesions in myeloma. The co-existence of both large and small lesions is often the mode of presentation in metastatic disease.

Spine. The lower thoracic and lumbar spine are usual sites; however, no spinal region is exempt. Early osteoporosis may be the only radiographic sign. As the disease progresses, pathologic vertebral collapse is inevitable. This often takes the configuration of a vertebra plana, compromising the posterior third of the vertebral body as well as its anterior two thirds. (Fig. 11-69) Pathologic fracture in the spine may be singular or multiple and has been called the *wrinkled vertebra of myeloma.* (Figs. 11-70 and 11-71) Demonstration of punched-out lesions in the spine is rare. The vertebral pedicles are involved much less frequently than the body. Jacobson et al. (22) suggested that the paucity of red marrow in the pedicles may allow their preservation with vertebral involvement. This has been called the *pedicle sign of multiple myeloma.* (22) (Fig. 11-72) Since Jacobson et al.'s original paper in 1958, there have been numerous cases reported refuting this sign and demonstrating isolated pedicular or combined vertebral body and pedicular involvement in multiple myeloma. (23) Therefore, the usefulness of this pedicle sign to differentiate multiple myeloma from osteolytic metastatic carcinoma appears doubtful.

Pelvis and Long Bones. Diffuse osteolytic round or oval lesions predominate without any reactive sclerosis. Medullary bone destruction abuts the endosteal surface of the cortex. The diaphysis is an area frequently involved in the long bones, which is consistent with the anatomic distribution of active red bone marrow. The humerus and femur are favored sites. (Figs. 11-73 to 11-76) Widespread disease throughout the pelvis and sacrum creates diffuse lytic lesions, which are fairly symmetric. (Fig. 11-77)

Osteoblastic Lesions. Sclerotic forms of multiple myeloma before treatment with radiotherapy or drugs are rare. (24,25) Sclerotic lesions may occur as a solitary focus or as multiple foci. Solitary blastic lesions are most common in the ribs, sternum, and ilium; however, other sites include vertebrae, skull, and long bones. Less than 3% of patients present with sclerotic lesions. (24,25) A solitary ivory vertebra has been noted in some myeloma

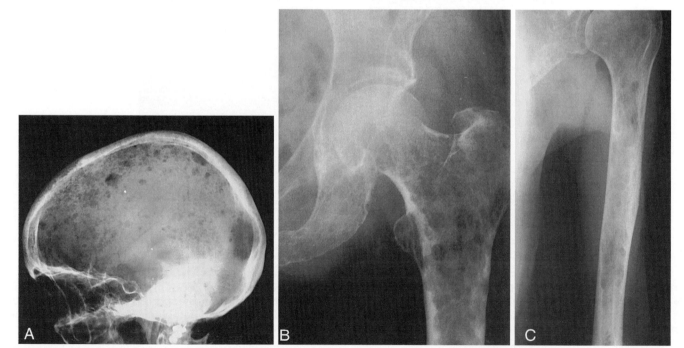

Figure 11-64 **PUNCHED-OUT LESIONS OF MULTIPLE MYELOMA. A. Skull. B. Proximal Femur. C. Humerus.** Note that the radiologic hallmark of multiple myeloma is the sharply circumscribed osteolytic defect that is clearly demonstrated on these radiographs. The lesions are multiple, round, and purely lytic. The most frequent sites are bones with hematopoietic potential. (Courtesy of David P. Thomas, MD, Melbourne, Australia.)

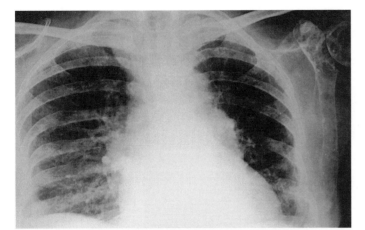

Figure 11-65 **MULTIPLE MYELOMA. Ribs.** Observe the diffuse osteolytic lesions involving nearly all the visualized rib structures. Similar osteolytic defects are present within the visualized scapula and humeral head.

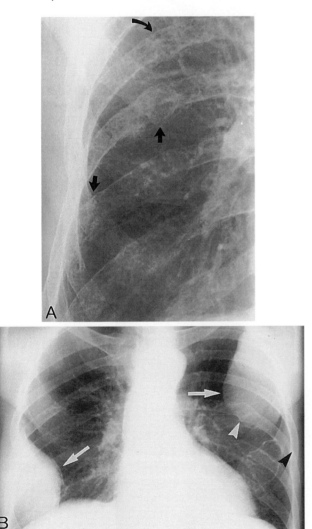

Figure 11-66 **MULTIPLE MYELOMA: RIBS. A. Pathologic Fractures.** Note the radiolucent defects scattered throughout the ribs, with numerous pathologic fractures (*arrows*). **B. Extrapleural Sign.** Observe the large, radiopaque, expansile lesions involving the ribs bilaterally (*arrows*). Smaller lytic expansile lesions are also noted involving the left rib cage (*arrowheads*). (Courtesy of Steven P. Brownstein, MD, Springfield, New Jersey.)

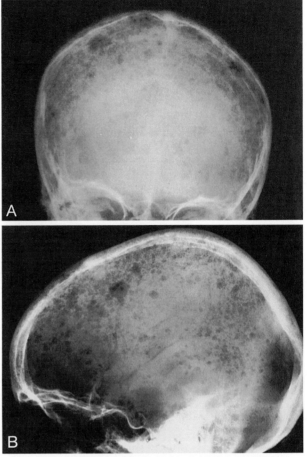

Figure 11-67 **MULTIPLE MYELOMA: RAINDROP SKULL.**
A. PA Skull. B. Lateral Skull. Observe the diffuse, permeative, or punched-out lesions throughout the calvaria. *COMMENT:* Multiple myeloma of the skull may be differentiated from metastatic carcinoma by the more uniform size of the lytic lesions in myeloma. The co-existence of both large and small lesions is often the mode of presentation of metastatic disease.

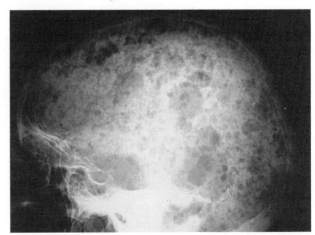

Figure 11-68 **MULTIPLE MYELOMA. Lateral Skull.** Observe the osteolytic lesions scattered throughout the bones of the skull. This is advanced multiple myeloma of the calvaria.

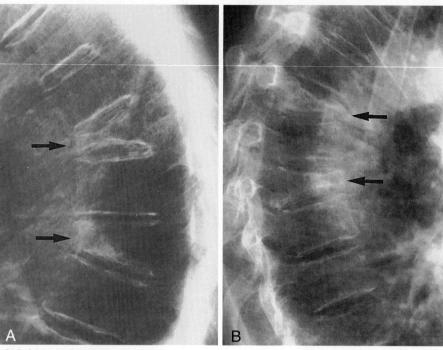

Figure 11-69 **PATHOLOGIC COLLAPSE, CREATING A VERTEBRA PLANA. A. Lateral Thoracic Spine.** Note the two pathologic fractures of the lower thoracic vertebrae secondary to multiple myeloma (*arrows*). Observe the gross osteoporosis and thinning of the cortical endplates of the remainder of the thoracic spine. **B. Lateral Thoracic Spine.** Observe two midthoracic vertebrae collapsed secondary to multiple myeloma (*arrows*). Observe the compromise of the posterior third of the vertebral body.

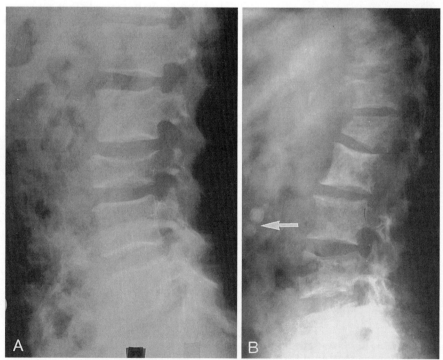

Figure 11-70 **MULTIPLE MYELOMA: LUMBAR SPINE. A. Localized Involvement.** Observe the uniform collapse of the vertebral body of L3, creating a vertebra plana. Note the overall loss of bone density within the matrix of the L3 vertebral body. **B. Diffuse Involvement.** Note the diffuse destructive lesions throughout the entire lumbar spine and lower thoracic vertebrae from multiple myeloma. Pathologic fractures are present in the upper lumbar and lower thoracic regions. Of incidental and unrelated notation are two calcified gallstones within the abdomen (*arrow*).

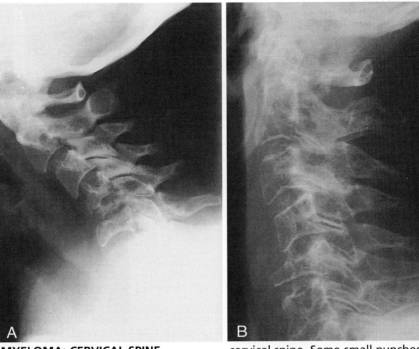

Figure 11-71 MULTIPLE MYELOMA: CERVICAL SPINE.
A. Lateral Cervical Spine. Observe the severe collapse of the C4 and C5 vertebral bodies as a result of multiple myeloma. A severe flexion deformity of the cervical spine, with a reversal of the cervical lordosis, is noted. **B. Lateral Spine.** Note the diffuse osteoporosis throughout the entire cervical spine. Some small punched-out lesions are present in the lamina and spinous processes of C2 and C3. There is a pathologic collapse of the C5 vertebral body, creating a vertebra plana secondary to multiple myeloma. (Courtesy of John A. Hinwood, DC, and Judy Hinwood, DC, Springwood, Queensland, Australia.)

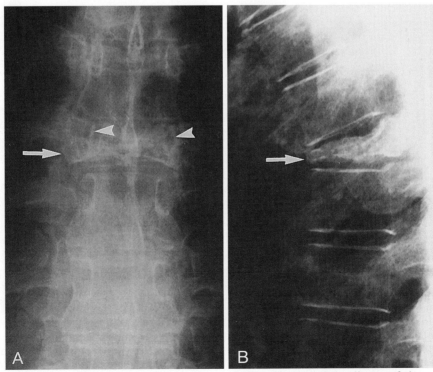

Figure 11-72 MULTIPLE MYELOMA: THE PEDICLE SIGN.
A. AP Thoracic. Observe the collapse of the T7 vertebral body (*arrow*). The pedicles have not been destroyed and are visualized on this frontal radiograph (*arrowheads*). **B. Lateral Thoracic.** Note the uniform collapse of the T7 vertebral body. Observe the collapse of the posterior third of the vertebral body, which strongly suggests a pathologic fracture, as was the case in this myeloma patient. This is a characteristic appearance for a vertebra plana or a wrinkled vertebra (*arrow*).

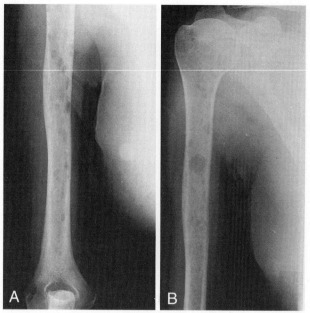

Figure 11-73 MULTIPLE MYELOMA: HUMERUS. A. and B. Humeral Diaphysis. Observe the well-defined, radiolucent, punched-out lesions in the diaphysis of these patients suffering from multiple myeloma. (Courtesy of David P. Thomas, MD, Melbourne, Australia.)

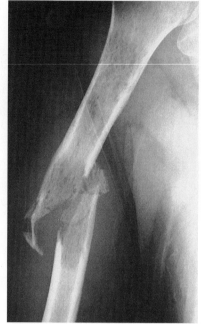

Figure 11-74 MULTIPLE MYELOMA, HUMERUS, WITH PATHOLOGIC FRACTURE. Observe the fine, permeative, punched-out lesions in the diaphysis of the humerus. This patient developed a pathologic fracture through the myelomatoid lesion after trivial trauma.

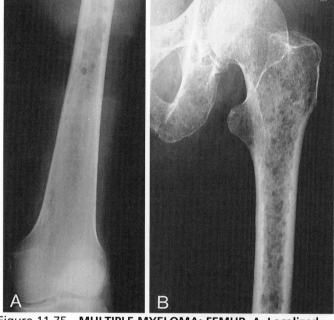

Figure 11-75 MULTIPLE MYELOMA: FEMUR. A. Localized Involvement. Observe the radiolucent destructive lesions within the diaphysis of the femur. **B. Diffuse Involvement.** Note the numerous radiolucent permeative lesions throughout the entire proximal femur and visualized ischium. *COMMENT:* There is a great predilection for multiple myeloma to affect the diaphysis of the long bones. Diaphyseal involvement in multiple myeloma is the result of this neoplasm developing in the red marrow within the shafts of the long bones. (Panel B reprinted with permission from **Yochum TR, Molyneux TP:** *Multiple myeloma.* ACA J Chiro June, 1983.)

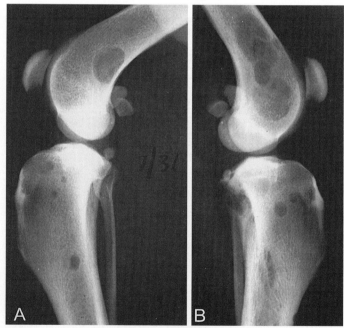

Figure 11-76 MULTIPLE MYELOMA IN A POODLE. A. Right Knee. B. Left Knee. Observe the multiple radiolucent destructive lesions in the distal femora and proximal tibiae. It is interesting to note that the pattern of bone destruction and radiographic presentation is no different in this poodle than it is in humans. (Courtesy of Steven P. Brownstein, MD, Springfield, New Jersey, and William E. Litterer, DC, DACBR, Fellow, ACCR, Elizabeth, New Jersey.)

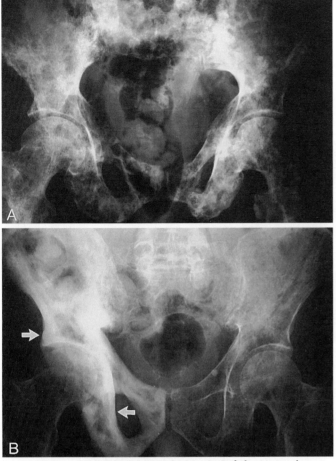

Figure 11-77 MULTIPLE MYELOMA. A. Pelvis. Note the diffuse lytic destruction of the entire pelvis and proximal femora. Pathologic fractures of both pubic rami are present. **B. Multiple Myeloma and Paget's Disease of the Pelvis.** Note the unilateral cortical thickening and expansion of the pelvis (*arrows*). The diffuse increase in bone density with scattered radiolucencies is a classic radiographic presentation of Paget's disease. Observe in the opposite hemipelvis a diffuse loss of bone density, with cortical thinning. The permeative destructive lesions that are seen in this side of the pelvis are characteristic of multiple myeloma.

patients. Differential diagnosis from osteoblastic metastasis, mastocytosis, lymphoma, and myelosclerosis may be difficult. (24,25) (Table 11-14)

Diagnostic Criteria. Diagnostic criteria are presented in Table 11-15.

Computed Tomography (CT)

CT is particularly useful in defining lesions that are visible on plain film, as well as those that are not seen. (26) By using varying window widths, soft tissue components can be defined. Bone lesions may be the characteristic punched-out type or more diffusely permeative. The marrow, when diffusely infiltrated, may exhibit higher attenuation values because of fatty marrow replacement. (26) (Fig. 11-78)

Table 11-14	Roentgen Signs of Multiple Myeloma

Early
   Normal radiographs
   Gross osteoporosis
Late
   Diffuse, punched-out lesions
   Uniform vertebral collapse (compromise of the posterior third of the body)
   Diaphyseal osteolytic lesions
   Rarely, sclerotic lesions (ivory vertebra)
   Pedicle sign (preservation of pedicles)

Table 11-15	Diagnostic Criteria

Require 10% of abnormal, atypical, or immature plasma cells in the bone marrow, plus one of the following:
- Serum M-protein spike
- Urine M-protein spike or Bence Jones' proteinuria
- Characteristic osteolytic lesions of bone
- Generalized osteoporosis—qualifies if the marrow contains 30% myeloma cells
- Biopsy-proven plasmacytoma

Courtesy of Alan H. Adams, DC, DACBN, Tallahassee, Florida.

Magnetic Resonance Imaging (MRI)

MRI is highly sensitive to marrow infiltration from myeloma. A broad spectrum of appearances arises, from discrete foci to diffuse lesions, which may involve the entire bone. On T1-weighted images, the affected areas are low in signal intensity. With T2 weighting a heterogeneous increase in signal intensity occurs. (27)

Treatment and Prognosis

In patients with multiple myeloma the overall prognosis is poor. (28) Over 90% die within 3 years, with the median survival rate being 33 months. (7,29) Survival rates generally increase when the patient's age is < 50. (30) Treatment is usually palliative, with the aim of minimizing the patient's suffering. (28) The two major forms of treatment are radiotherapy and chemotherapy. Plasma cells are characteristically radiosensitive, and radiotherapy is of established value in the control of localized symptomatic lesions, which typically transform to a blastic area. Of the chemotherapeutic agents presently available, melphalan and Cytoxan are the two drugs most useful in attempted long-term management, whereas melphalan combined with prednisone has become the standard of care. (31) The importance of ambulation and adequate hydration cannot be overemphasized. The constant threat of hypercalcemia, hypercalciuria, and hyperuricemia necessitates continual attention to these aspects of general care. Zoledronic acid has recently demonstrated to be of benefit in the treatment of related hypercalcemia seen in multiple myeloma. (32)

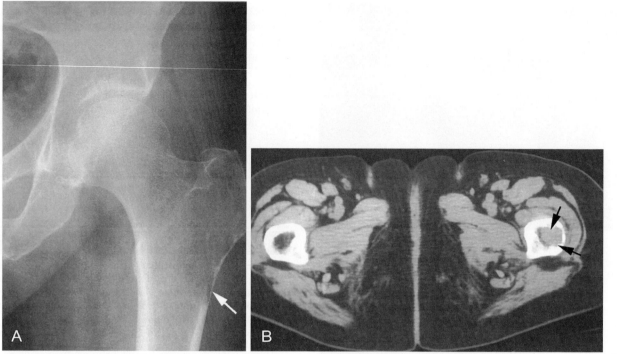

Figure 11-78 MULTIPLE MYELOMA: FEMUR. A. Plain film. Note the subtle endosteal scalloping in the region of the greater trochanter (*arrow*). **B. Soft Tissue Window CT Scan.** Note the increased density of the marrow space owing to tumor mass and the clear demonstration of endosteal scalloping (*arrows*). No extraosseous extension is present. (Courtesy of William E. Litterer, DC, DACBR, Fellow, ACCR, Elizabeth, New Jersey.)

SOLITARY PLASMACYTOMA

General Considerations

Solitary plasmacytoma represents a localized form of plasma cell proliferation. It is much less common than multiple myeloma. (1) Approximately 50% of patients present before age 50. (1) Most commonly, patients complain of localized pain. Laboratory findings are occasionally normal, or the abnormal serum electrophoresis may disappear after tumor excision. (2) The mandible, ilium, vertebrae, ribs, and proximal femur and scapula are the favored sites. (Figs. 11-79 to 11-87) Pathologic fracture is common. (Fig. 11-88) Isolated cases have been reported in extramedullary sites affecting the soft tissues of the upper respiratory tract. (3) Rarely, solitary plasmacytoma can present as an ivory vertebra. (4) The typical roentgen appearance is a geographic radiolucent lesion, often highly expansile, with a *soap bubble internal architecture.* (Fig. 11-89) The radiographic differential diagnosis includes pseudo-tumor of hemophilia, hydatid disease of bone, fibrous dysplasia, giant cell tumor, brown tumor of hyperparathyroidism, and blow-out metastases from renal or thyroid origin.

Often, these lesions initially appear benign; however, 70% of patients who have what seems to be a solitary focus develop diffuse multiple myeloma and die within 5 years. (1) Progression to multiple myeloma has been documented in cases up to 23 years after the initial presentation of solitary plasmacytoma (5), em-

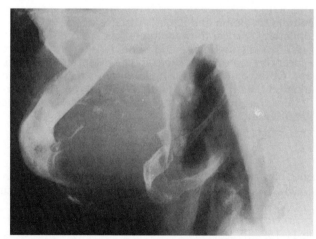

Figure 11-79 PLASMACYTOMA: MANDIBLE. Observe the grossly destructive, highly expansile lesion of the mandible. *COMMENT:* Plasmacytoma is a more localized form of multiple myeloma and is somewhat less aggressive than the diffuse form of multiple myeloma.

phasizing the importance of long-term follow-up with these patients. (6,7) The balance of the lesions remain localized and are treated quite successfully with local irradiation and/or surgical excision. (7–9) (Fig. 11-90)

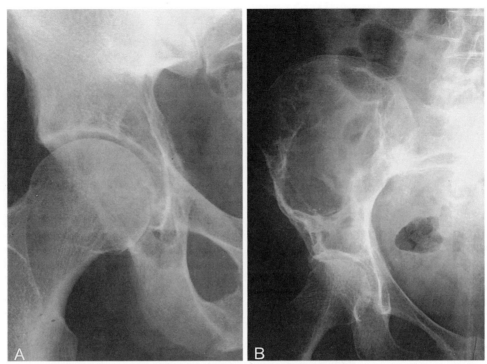

Figure 11-80   **PLASMACYTOMA: ILIUM. A. Localized Involvement. B. Diffuse Involvement.** Note the advanced osteolytic destruction of the ilium, the pattern of which assumes a soap bubble appearance.

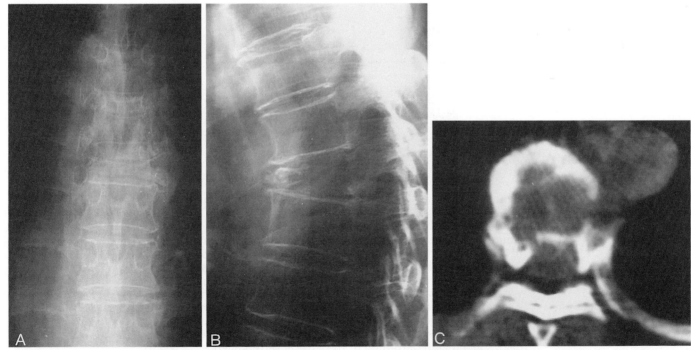

Figure 11-81   **PLASMACYTOMA: T8. A. AP Thoracic Spine. B. Lateral Thoracic Spine.** Note the diffuse collapse of the T8 vertebral body, creating a vertebra plana. This is the typical appearance of a pathologic fracture, with compromise of the posterior third of the vertebral body. **C. CT.** Observe the large, lytic destructive lesion present within the vertebral body of T8. (Courtesy of Steven P. Brownstein, MD, Springfield, New Jersey.)

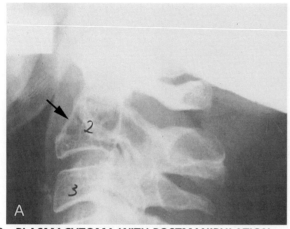

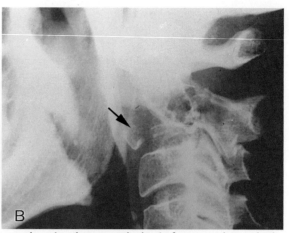

Figure 11-82 **PLASMACYTOMA WITH POSTMANIPULATION PATHOLOGIC FRACTURE: C2. A. Premanipulation.** Note a subtle decrease in density of the C2 vertebral body (*arrow*). This was overlooked on initial review, and manipulation was administered by a medical practitioner. **B. Postmanipulation.** Note that this film, taken 4 days later, after unremitting neck pain, shows pathologic fracture through the axis body (*arrow*). (Reprinted with permission from **Montileone M:** *Solitary Plasmacytoma* [Roentgenological Brief]. ACA Council Roentgenology, 1981. Case courtesy of Felix Bauer, DC, DACBR(Hon), Sydney, Australia.)

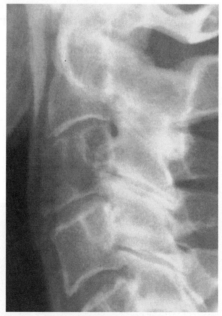

Figure 11-83 **PLASMACYTOMA: C3.** Observe the diffuse loss of bone density of the C3 vertebral body. Subtle destruction of the cortical vertebral endplate superiorly and, to a lesser extent, inferiorly is noted. There is minimal expansion of the C3 vertebral body as well. *COMMENT:* This 64-year-old male had a sacral plasmacytoma 2 years previously, which was treated with radiation therapy. The classic signs of diffuse loss of bone density, when compared with the vertebral bodies above and below, along with disruption of the cortical vertebral endplate, are the earliest radiographic signs of malignant disease within a vertebral body. A similar appearance is often found in a metastatic lesion of the vertebral body. (Courtesy of Ronald H. Collett, DC, DACBR, Winnipeg, Manitoba, Canada.)

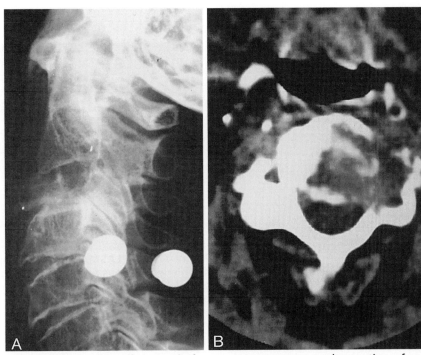

Figure 11-84 **PLASMACYTOMA: C3. A. Plain Film, Cervical Spine.** Note the extensive collapse of the C3 vertebral body, secondary to a solitary plasmacytoma. **B. Axial CT, C3.** Observe the lytic destruction of the vertebral body, trans- verse process, and a portion of one articular pillar. (Courtesy of William E. Litterer, DC, DACBR, Fellow, ACCR, Elizabeth, New Jersey.)

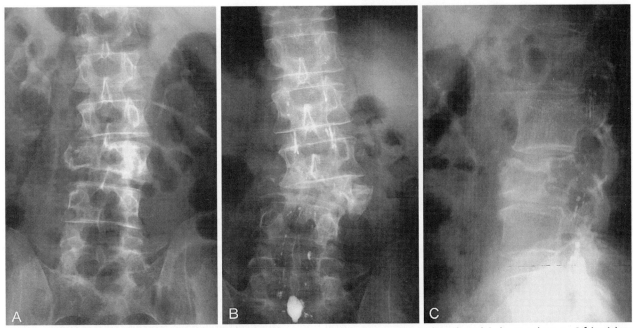

Figure 11-85 **PLASMACYTOMA: L3. A. AP Lumbar Spine.** Observe the osteolytic destruction and collapse of the L3 vertebral body unilaterally. **B. AP Lumbar Spine. C. Lateral Lumbar Spine.** Note that the 1-year follow-up radiographs demonstrate complete collapse of the L3 vertebral body, secondary to localized multiple myeloma. Of incidental notation is scattered radiopaque contrast material present within the spinal canal from previous myelographic investigation.

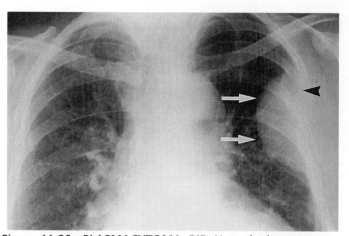

Figure 11-86 **PLASMACYTOMA: RIB.** Note the large extrapleural sign involving the left rib cage (*arrows*). This radiopacity represents bone destruction of the anterolateral surface of the left fourth rib, secondary to a solitary plasmacytoma (*arrowhead*). (Courtesy of Kenneth E. Yochum, DC, St. Louis, Missouri.)

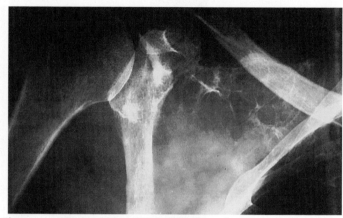

Figure 11-87 **PLASMACYTOMA. Scapula.** Observe the soap bubble lytic lesions present in the superior portion of the scapula. These lesions have the typical destructive appearance of plasmacytoma.

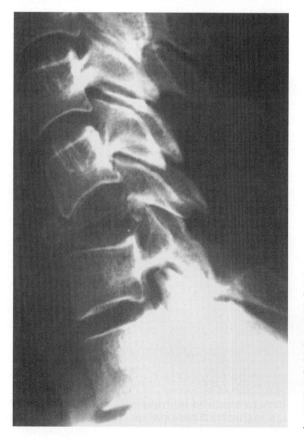

Figure 11-88 **MULTIPLE MYELOMA: C5 VERTEBRAL BODY AND NEURAL ARCH. Lateral Cervical Spine.** Observe the complete collapse and osteolytic destruction of the C5 vertebral body. The articular pillar, lamina, and spinous process of C5 are also destroyed. *COMMENT:* Neural arch involvement of multiple myeloma is somewhat unusual. This represented a solitary plasmacytoma. The lack of adjacent endplate destruction helps differentiate this from osteomyelitis. An infection that would have destroyed this much of the vertebral body would certainly have crossed the disc space and invaded the adjacent vertebral endplates. (Courtesy of Joel G. Green, DC, Salem, Massachusetts.)

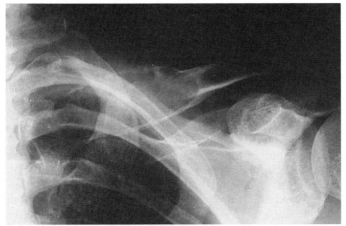

Figure 11-89 **PLASMACYTOMA. Clavicle.** Observe the expansile soap bubble lytic lesion present in the medial half of the clavicle. This is a typical appearance, but a somewhat unusual location for plasmacytoma. (Courtesy of David P. Thomas, MD, Melbourne, Australia.)

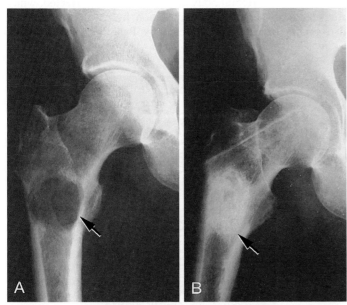

Figure 11-90 **PLASMACYTOMA: RADIOTHERAPY CHANGES. A. Initial Lesion.** Note that a well-demarcated lesion with endosteal scalloping is readily appreciated (*arrow*). **B. Postradiotherapy.** Observe that the lesion has become homogeneously sclerotic, characteristic of postradiation response.

CAPSULE SUMMARY
Multiple Myeloma

General Considerations
- First patient documented with the disease was in 1845.
- Henry Bence Jones described the proteinuria.
- May be called Kahler's disease.

Incidence
- The most common primary malignant bone tumor.
- Represents 10% of hematologic malignancies and 27% of biopsied bone tumors.

Clinical Features
- 75% of patients are between 50 and 70 years of age; 2:1 male preponderance.
- Pain is the cardinal initial symptom; the pain is relieved with bedrest and aggravated by weight bearing.
- Bacterial infections occur in 10% of cases, most of which are respiratory in nature.
- The spine, pelvis, skull, ribs, and scapula are the most frequently involved bones (the spine being the most common site).
- Pathologic fracture is a common complication.
- Laboratory findings reveal a normochromic normocytic anemia, thrombocytopenia, hypercalcemia, hyperglobulinemia with a reversed A:G ratio, hyperuricemia, and 40% show Bence Jones' proteinuria.
- Protein electrophoresis is helpful in diagnosis.
- Secondary amyloidosis is found in 15% of patients with myeloma.

Pathologic Features
- Myelogenous round cell proliferation of plasma cells is noted.
- Myeloma kidney occurs as a result of permanent tubular damage, leading to renal failure.
- The most common site for extramedullary plasmacytoma is the nasopharynx.

Radiologic Features
- Bone scans are cold.
- Gross osteoporosis may be the only early sign.
- Punched-out lesions are the radiologic hallmark of myeloma.
- Vertebra plana or wrinkled vertebra is characteristic.
- Raindrop skull (lytic myeloma defects) and pedicle sign of myeloma (preservation of pedicles) occur.
- Rarely, sclerotic lesions occur (1 < 3%); occasionally, an ivory vertebra.

Solitary Plasmacytoma
- Localized form of plasma cell proliferation.
- The most common bones affected are mandible, ilium, vertebrae, ribs, proximal femur, and scapula.
- 70% of solitary plasmacytoma lesions develop into diffuse multiple myeloma.
- The typical lesion has a geographic, soap bubbled, highly expansile radiographic appearance.

Treatment and Prognosis
- 90% die within 3 years.
- Treatment is usually radiotherapy, chemotherapy, and, on occasion, local excision.

CENTRAL OSTEOSARCOMA

General Considerations

Osteosarcoma (osteogenic sarcoma) is a primary malignant tumor of bone; it is derived from undifferentiated connective tissue and forms neoplastic osteoid. Osteosarcoma can be divided into five distinct clinical types: central osteosarcoma, multicentric osteosarcoma, parosteal osteosarcoma (juxtacortical osteosarcoma), secondary osteosarcoma, and extraosseous osteosarcoma. (1) The following discussion concerns central osteosarcoma.

Incidence

Central osteosarcoma is the second most common primary malignant bone tumor (multiple myeloma is the most common). Osteosarcoma is approximately twice as common as chondrosarcoma and three times more frequent than Ewing's sarcoma. (2) It is calculated that approximately 1500 cases of osteosarcoma exist at any one time in the United States. (2) Osteosarcoma represents 20% of all primary malignant bone tumors. (3)

Clinical Features

Age and Sex Distribution

Osteosarcoma is encountered most commonly in the age group from 10 to 25 years (75% of cases); few cases occur before age 5 or after age 30. (4,5) The median age for males and females is 18 and 17 years, respectively. (2) The Mayo Clinic has reported the occurrence of an osteosarcoma in a 35-month-old girl. (6) The diagnosis of primary osteogenic sarcoma in older patients should be accepted only after careful examination excludes association with other pre-existent bone disease (Paget's disease, fibrous dysplasia, irradiated bone, osteochondroma). (2)

There is a 2:1 male predominance, which does not vary in any decade of life. The average age of onset is slightly earlier in the female. It is interesting to note that patients affected by osteosarcoma have been found to be taller than their peers in the corresponding age group. (7,8) No rational explanation for this has been offered. (7,8)

Signs and Symptoms

Painful swelling at the site of the lesion is the presenting complaint in approximately 85% of patients. (9) As in most primary malignant bone tumors, a history of antecedent trauma is frequently obtained; its true relationship to the development of osteosarcoma is questionable. The cause of osteosarcoma is unknown, but it has been stated that trauma reveals more malignant growths than it produces, which is known as *traumatic determinism*. (10) Systemic manifestations, such as loss of weight, fever, cachexia, are unusual features. The pain initially is insidious and transitory; however, it eventually becomes severe and persistent. The interval between the onset of symptoms and recognition of the tumor may be 6 months or longer. Minor restriction of joint mobility may occur, creating a limp if a weight-bearing bone is involved. Rarely, the acute onset of deep venous throm-

bosis in children with osteosarcoma can occur. (11,12) The mechanism for the development of such is external compression or tumor thrombus from a grossly palpable tumor.

Location

The long bones of the extremities are the target sites for osteosarcoma. (2,4) (Fig. 11-91) The knee and shoulder are the most commonly affected joints. Huvos (2) stated that 41.5% affect the femur (most of which are in the distal portion), 16% affect the tibia and fibula (most in the proximal portion), and 15% affect the humerus (usually proximal); therefore, 58% of all osteosarcomas occur around the knee. The metaphysis abutting the physis is the classic location in 75% of cases; however, diaphyseal, as well as epiphyseal, lesions have been reported (25%). (13)

Other bones that may be involved are the calvaria, sacrum, pelvis, mandible, maxilla, scapula, clavicle, ribs, hand, calcaneus, and spine. (14–16) (Figs. 11-92 to 11-96) Primary osteosarcoma of the spine is rare, making up < 2% of all osteosarcomas. (17) The distribution is fairly equal between the lumbar and the thoracic segments, but cervical involvement is less common. (17) The vertebral body is most commonly affected, which often leads to pathologic compression fracture. Osteosarcoma also occurs in vertebrae affected by Paget's disease. (18,19)

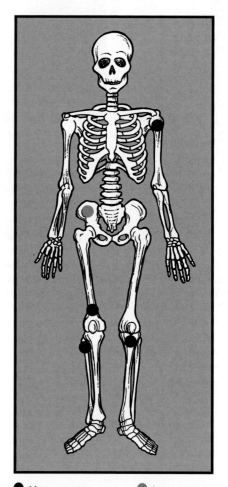

● More common   ● Less common

Figure 11-91 SKELETAL DISTRIBUTION OF OSTEOSARCOMA.

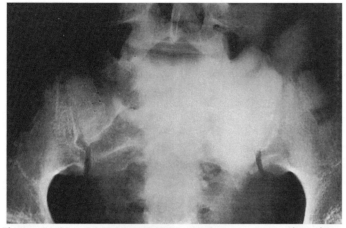

Figure 11-92   **OSTEOSARCOMA. AP Sacrum.** Note that this 15-year-old female demonstrates an ivory osteosarcoma of the sacrum. *COMMENT:* Osteosarcoma of the spine is rare; however, when present, it is most commonly found within the sacrum. (Courtesy of Terry D. Sandman, DC, DACBR, Chicago, Illinois.)

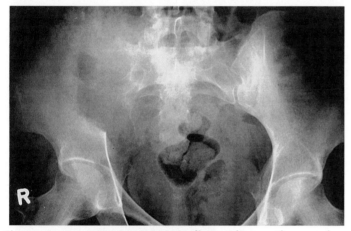

Figure 11-93   **OSTEOSARCOMA. Ilium.** Observe the grossly destructive lytic lesion on the posterior surface of the ilium, adjacent to the sacroiliac joint. This represents a lytic presentation of osteosarcoma in a 37-year-old female. (Courtesy of Friedrich H. W. Heuck, MD, Stuttgart, Germany.)

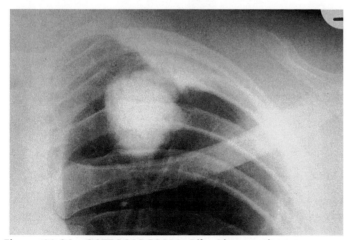

Figure 11-94   **OSTEOSARCOMA. Rib.** Observe the radiopaque osteosarcoma affecting the anterior surface of the rib. This is a rare location for osteosarcoma.

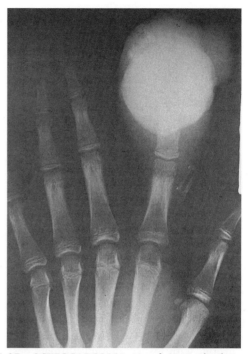

Figure 11-95   **OSTEOSARCOMA. Hand.** Note the large ivory osteosarcoma present in the distal phalanx of the index finger. There is a large soft tissue mass associated with this lesion. (Courtesy of Bryan Hartley, MD, Melbourne, Australia.)

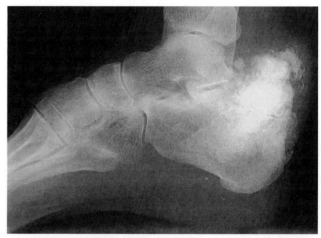

Figure 11-96   **OSTEOSARCOMA. Calcaneus.** Observe the dense, radiopaque osteosarcoma of the posterior portion of the calcaneus. The large soft tissue mass associated with this osteosarcoma shows bone production within its matrix.

Although the incidence of spinal involvement in Paget's disease is high (44%), a major study found that only 3.5% of secondary osteosarcomas arising in pagetoid bone were located in the spine. [20]

Laboratory Findings

The only pertinent and consistent laboratory finding is elevation of the alkaline phosphatase enzyme. These levels are highest with the sclerotic type of presentation and return to normal with tumor removal or treatment.

Pathologic Features

The cause of osteosarcoma is still widely unknown; however, several propagating factors leading to its development have been suggested in the recent literature. Included in this list are agents such as beryllium, viruses, radiation exposure, Paget's disease, electrical burns, and trauma. (21) The gross and microscopic pictures of osteosarcoma depend entirely on the predominant type of tumor tissue. Grossly, with little ossification, the tumor tends to be firm, but not hard, to the touch, consonant with the presence of sarcomatous stromal tissue. Yellowish dots and streaks reflect islands of new bone. When the tumor is heavily ossified, it is generally hard and densely compact. The adjacent cortex is often penetrated grossly by the tumor, with significant extension into the soft tissues. Considerable irregular periosteal reaction is the rule, with elevation of the periosteum by tumor tissue often apparent.

The histologic appearance shows spindle-shaped stromal cells, but in highly anaplastic lesions, spheroid cells with multiple hyperchromatic nuclei are present. Intercellular collagenous material is frequently observed, with the sarcomatous stromal cells enmeshed in this material. The normal osseous tissue is destroyed by the sarcomatous stromal cells or by the other tumor tissue present in the lesion, with resorption and ultimate destruction of bone trabeculae.

Osteosarcoma tends to grow in three basic patterns. Approximately half the tumors form a great deal of osseous neoplastic tissue, presenting as a sclerotic lesion (50%); the remainder are composed of sarcomatous connective tissue stroma creating a

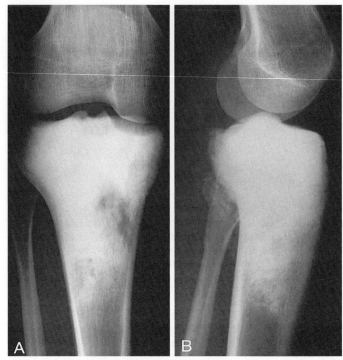

Figure 11-97   OSTEOSARCOMA: TIBIA. A. AP Knee. B. Lateral Knee. Observe the diffuse ivory osteosarcoma in the proximal tibia. *COMMENT:* Approximately 50% of the osteosarcomas present as a sclerotic lesion, rendering an ivory or sclerotic appearance.

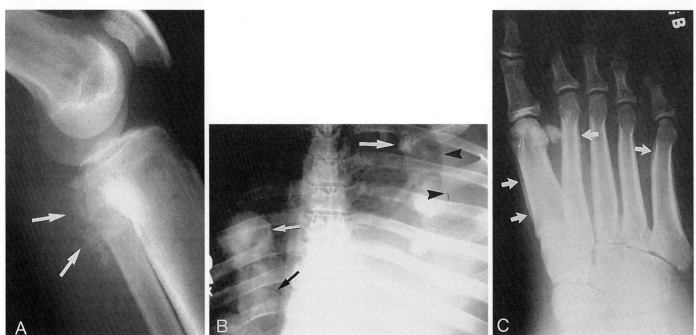

Figure 11-98   HYPERTROPHIC OSTEOARTHROPATHY DEVELOPING FROM OSTEOSARCOMA OF THE TIBIA. A. Lateral Knee. Note the destruction of the posterior surface of the tibia, with a soft tissue mass (*arrows*). This lesion represents osteosarcoma of the tibia. **B. Chest.** Observe multiple cannonball metastases in the right and left lungs (*arrows*). Massive pleural effusion is noted on the left side (*arrowheads*). **C. Foot.** Observe the solid periosteal new bone formation (*arrows*) in the diaphyseal area of all five metatarsal bones. *COMMENT:* This patient demonstrates an interesting aspect of the pathologic manifestations of osteosarcoma of bone. Metastatic lesions in the lung created hypertrophic osteoarthropathy in the foot. This is somewhat unusual in osteosarcoma because most patients die before osteoarthropathy can develop.

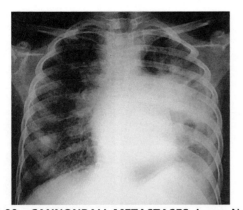

Figure 11-99 CANNONBALL METASTASES. Lung. Note the multiple radiopacities scattered throughout both lungs, representing cannonball metastases from osteosarcoma of the distal femur. These radiopacities actually represent sarcomatous growth of bone within the lung parenchyma.

lytic presentation (25%) or, if moderate osteoid matrix is present, a mixed pattern results (25%). (Fig. 11-97)

Metastases

Metastases to the lungs by the hematogenous route are common and can lead to the development of hypertrophic osteoarthropathy. (Fig. 11-98) Multiple lesions are the usual presentation, and these actually represent sarcomatous bone growths within the lungs (*cannonball metastases*). (Fig. 11-99) Spontaneous pneumothorax is relatively common because subpleural nodules that have undergone excavation lead to rupture into the pleural space. Lung resection has often proved beneficial in these patients. (22) Skeletal metastases (*skip lesions*) are also found but do not occur with the same frequency as in Ewing's sarcoma and are poor prognostic signs. (23) At autopsy, the most frequent metastatic sites are the lungs (95%), bones (50%), and kidneys (12%). (24)

Radiologic Features

Because of the relative frequency of osteosarcoma, the radiographic features are well established. (25) Osteosarcomas usually arise in the metaphyses (75%) of long bones, most frequently at the distal end of the femur, the proximal end of the tibia, and the proximal end of the humerus. Rarely, they may affect the diaphysis or epiphysis (25%) and may involve any bone, including the patella. (26,27) The epiphyseal plate functions as a barrier to tumor migration in some cases. (27) (Fig. 11-100)

The classic presentation is that of a focal lesion in the metaphysis, creating either a mottled, permeative lesion with a poorly defined zone of transition or a dense ivory or sclerotic region filling the medullary space. (Fig. 11-101) Cortical disruption is common. Periosteal new bone formation occurs and is highly irregular. This periosteal reaction often takes place within an extracortical, dense soft tissue mass that displays transverse spicules or radiating striations. (Figs. 11-102 to 11-104) This characteristic pattern of periosteal response has been referred to as sunburst, or *sunray*, and is the appearance for which osteosarcoma is best known. (28)

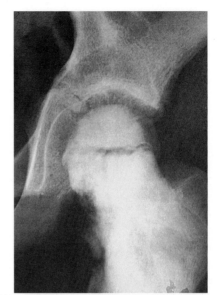

Figure 11-100 OSTEOSARCOMA. Proximal Femur. Note the numerous radiopacities scattered throughout the metaphysis of the proximal femur. This neoplastic process has extended to the femoral capital epiphysis. This is a characteristic appearance for the sclerotic presentation of osteosarcoma. *COMMENT:* It is rare for osteosarcoma to cross the epiphyseal plate, which usually functions as an effective barrier to tumor extension. (Courtesy of David P. Thomas, MD, Melbourne, Australia.)

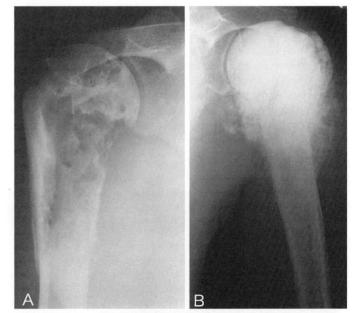

Figure 11-101 THE RADIOGRAPHIC APPEARANCE OF LYTIC VERSUS SCLEROTIC OSTEOSARCOMA. A. Lytic Presentation: Proximal Humerus. Note the focal lesion in the metaphysis of the proximal humerus, demonstrating mottled, permeative destruction. This appearance is characteristic of a lytic presentation in osteosarcoma. **B. Sclerotic Presentation: Proximal Humerus.** Note the dense radiopaque appearance to the humeral head and its metaphysis. A large soft tissue mass and spiculated periosteal response are associated with this sclerotic or ivory type of osteosarcoma. *COMMENT:* Approximately 50% of osteosarcomas present as sclerotic lesions; the remainder are lytic in presentation. Of the lytic cases, 25% have a mixed pattern if moderate osteoid matrix is present.

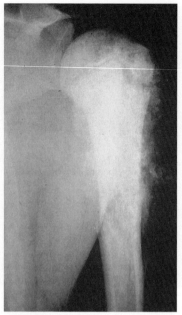

Figure 11-102 OSTEOSARCOMA. Proximal Humerus. Note the ill-defined, destructive lesion assuming the mixed pattern of presentation in the metaphysis and proximal diaphysis of the humerus. Malignant spiculated periosteal response is observed on both sides of the humeral cortex, with extension of the osteosarcoma into the soft tissue structures.

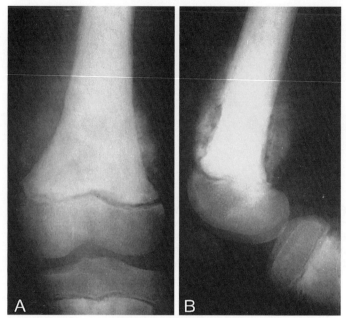

Figure 11-103 SCLEROTIC OSTEOSARCOMA: MALIGNANT PERIOSTEAL RESPONSE IN THE DISTAL FEMUR A. AP Knee. B. Lateral Knee. Observe the increase in bone density in the metaphysis and distal diaphysis of the femur. There is a sunburst or malignant spiculated periosteal response present surrounding the entire distal metaphysis of the femur. This is a classic radiographic presentation for osteosarcoma.

(Fig. 11-105) Occasionally, the periosteum is found to be elevated by tumor tissue on the upper and lower margins of the lesion, creating Codman's reactive triangles. (Fig. 11-106) This is a reactive response to the lifting of the periosteum and is not pathognomonic for osteosarcoma because it may also be found in benign conditions such as traumatic periostitis, osteomyelitis, eosinophilic granuloma, and thyroid acropathy.

As the lesions continue to grow, bone expansion may occur. Occasionally, pathologic fracture may follow some form of trivial trauma. Radiographically, 50% of these lesions are radiopaque or sclerotic and may develop a roughened lobulated margin, referred to as the *cumulus cloud* appearance. (2) (Fig. 11-107) The remaining 50% are split between a purely osteolytic lesion (25%) and a mixed lesion (25%). Soft tissue mass

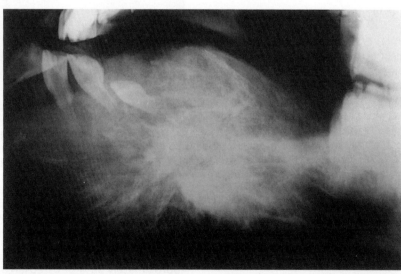

Figure 11-104 OSTEOSARCOMA OF THE MANDIBLE IN A HORSE. Observe the spiculated periosteal new bone formation with sclerotic destruction of the mandible in this thoroughbred horse. The length of the lesion (> 6 cm) suggests a primary neoplasm. The reactive skeletal changes in animals is no different than in *Homo sapiens*.

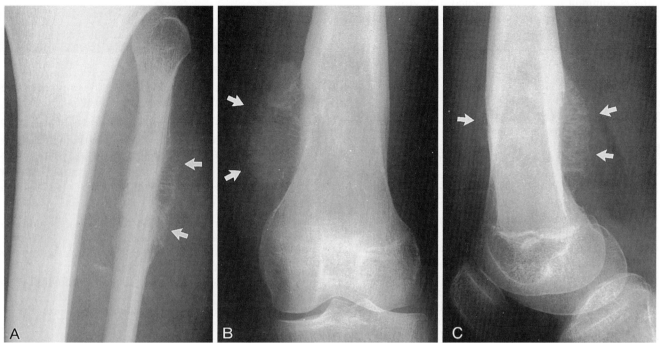

Figure 11-105 **PERIOSTEAL RESPONSE IN OSTEOSARCOMA.**
A. Fibula. Observe the spiculated periosteal response on the lateral surface of the proximal fibula (*arrows*). **B. AP Distal Femur. C. Lateral Distal Femur.** Observe the classic sunburst or spiculated periosteal response seen in the distal meta-diaphyseal area of the femur (*arrows*). This sunburst appearance, the soft tissue mass, and the destructive lesion of the medullary portion of the femur are the cardinal radiographic features of osteosarcoma.

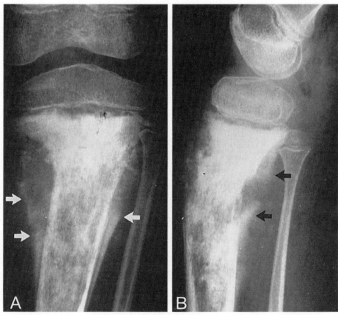

Figure 11-106 **CODMAN'S REACTIVE TRIANGLE AND OSTEOSARCOMA OF THE PROXIMAL TIBIA. A. AP Tibia. B. Lateral Tibia.** Note the mixed pattern of osteosarcoma in the proximal metaphysis of the tibia. There are large Codman's reactive triangles present surrounding the cortex of the proximal tibia (*arrows*). *COMMENT:* Codman's reactive triangle is frequently found in osteosarcoma of bone; however, it is not pathognomonic of osteosarcoma and can be found in infectious lesions, traumatic periostitis, and peculiar callus formations.

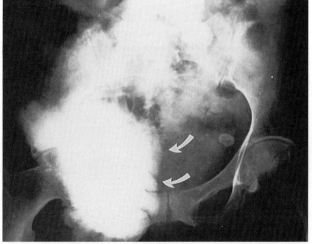

Figure 11-107 **THE CUMULUS CLOUD APPEARANCE OF OSTEOSARCOMA. Pelvis.** Observe the diffuse, sclerotic osteosarcoma affecting the ilium near the acetabulum. With closer inspection, note the lobulated margins of the medial surface of this osteosarcoma (*arrows*). This lobulated margin of osteosarcoma has been called the cumulus cloud appearance. (Courtesy of Friedrich H. W. Heuck, MD, Stuttgart, West Germany.)

formation is common in osteosarcoma and may grow to large dimensions. Ossification within this tumor mass is a frequent occurrence.

CT and MRI allow demonstration of marrow infiltration, soft tissue mass, and response to therapy, though they have not been able to offer a reliable prognosis. (29)

Treatment and Prognosis

Amputation offers the best possibility of control when the lesion is accessible and metastasis has not occurred. Radiotherapy may be given for local control and pain. (Fig. 11-108) Prognosis is poor because of the tendency for early metastasis, which occurs in up to 62% of patients. (30) Pulmonary metastases are often present before the primary lesion is discovered. Recognition of distant pulmonary metastases is important in the treatment and prognosis of osteosarcoma; the average time between recognition of pulmonary disease and death is 6 months. (31) When a solitary pulmonary metastasis is present, its removal is justifiable because of sporadic case reports of 5-year survival afterward. Generally, the sclerotic variety runs a slower, less aggressive clinical course, whereas the lytic presentation behaves in a rapidly fatal manner. (32) The best 5-year survival rate has been 20%; however, one study using intensive chemotherapy offered an 80% 5-year survival rate. (33,34) Age at diagnosis (> 19), metastasis, large tumor size, and pathologic fracture are all documented factors that decrease the prognostic outcome. (30) On the other hand, tumors of the jaw and those affecting the surface of the bone are more often associated with a good prognosis. (35) Additional studies in this area of treatment are necessary for the future generations of patients who will require treatment.

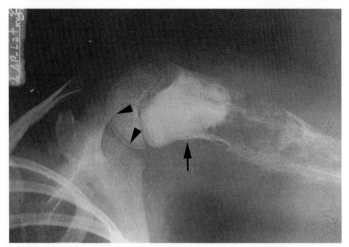

Figure 11-108 **OSTEOSARCOMA: POSTRADIATION CHANGES. AP Shoulder.** Observe the osteolytic bone destruction in the proximal diaphysis of the humerus. The dense sclerotic metaphyseal region (*arrow*) represents tumor that has responded to the radiotherapy as evidenced by the dense sclerosis. An early crescent sign (*arrowheads*) in the subarticular zone of the humeral head signifies complicating early avascular necrosis secondary to radiation.

CAPSULE SUMMARY
Central Osteosarcoma

General Considerations

- A primary malignant tumor of undifferentiated connective tissue, which forms neoplastic osteoid.

Incidence

- The second most common primary malignant bone tumor, representing 20% of all primary malignant bone tumors.
- It is twice as common as chondrosarcoma, three times more frequent than Ewing's sarcoma.

Clinical Features

- 75% of cases occur in the 10- to 25-year age range, with a 2:1 male predominance.
- Painful swelling of the involved limb is a common presenting symptom.
- The metaphyses of the distal femur, proximal tibia, and proximal humerus are the most common sites.
- Only 3.5–7% of cases occur within the spine.
- Elevation of serum alkaline phosphatase is the only consistent laboratory finding.

Pathologic Features

- Three basic patterns exist: 50% of cases are sclerotic, 25% are purely lytic, and 25% are mixed lesions.
- Metastases to the lungs by the hematogenous route are common; the multiple lesions are called cannonball metastases. Spontaneous pneumothorax is a common initial clinical presentation.
- Skeletal metastases occur, but not as frequently as in Ewing's sarcoma.

Radiologic Features

- The classic lesion presents as a permeative or ivory medullary lesion in the metaphysis of a long tubular bone.
- A sunburst or sunray periosteal response is characteristic.
- Often, Codman's reactive triangle is found associated with the destructive lesion.
- Cortical disruption with soft tissue mass formation, often growing to large dimensions, occurs. The peripheral edge of an eccentric lobulated mass whose margins are roughened and irregular may be referred to as the cumulus cloud appearance.

Treatment and Prognosis

- A 20% 5-year survival rate has been traditional; studies using intensive chemotherapy report an 80% survival rate.
- Amputation has offered the best treatment when the lesion is surgically accessible.

MULTICENTRIC OSTEOSARCOMA

General Considerations

Multicentric osteosarcoma (sclerosing osteogenic sarcomatosis, osteosarcomatosis, childhood multifocal osteosarcoma) is a rare form of osteosarcoma in which multiple independent lesions occur

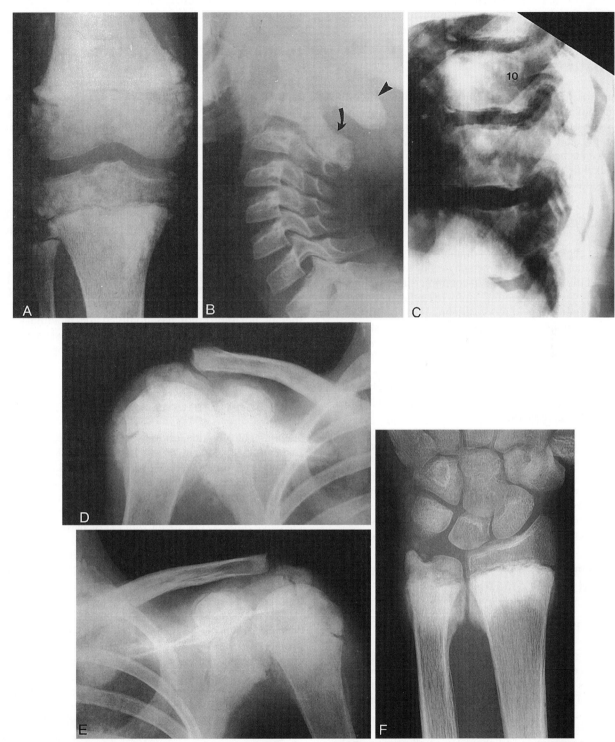

Figure 11-109   **MULTICENTRIC OSTEOSARCOMA. A. AP Knee.** Observe the radiopacities scattered throughout the entire distal metaphysis of the femur, its distal epiphysis, and the proximal epiphyses of the tibia and fibula. **B. Lateral Cervical Spine.** Note the sclerotic density of the vertebral body and neural arch of C2 (*arrow*) and the expansion and sclerotic density of the posterior arch and tubercle of C1 (*arrowhead*). **C. T10 Vertebral Body.** Note the malignant ivory vertebra at the T10 vertebral body. **D. Right Shoulder. E. Left Shoulder.** Observe the bilateral lesions of multicentric osteosarcoma in both humeral heads and the glenoid fossae and coracoid process of both scapulae. **F. Distal Radius and Ulna.** Observe the sclerotic lesions of multicentric osteosarcoma in the metaphyses of the distal radius and ulna, with associated periosteal response. *COMMENT:* Multicentric osteosarcoma (osteosarcomatosis) is a rare form of osteosarcoma, in which multiple independent lesions occur simultaneously. These multiple lesions clearly do not represent metastatic foci; therefore, multicentric osteosarcoma is a distinct and separate entity. (Courtesy of Steven P. Brownstein, MD, Springfield, New Jersey, and William E. Litterer, DC, DACBR, Fellow, ACCR, Elizabeth, New Jersey.)

simultaneously. It is not clear whether these multiple lesions represent metastatic foci or simultaneous osteosarcomas, though classically it remains a distinct and separate entity. (1,2)

Clinical Features

There are approximately 20 known cases of multicentric osteosarcoma that have been reported. (3,4) Most patients were between the ages of 5 and 10 years. The clinical course of the disease is rapid and fatal. Pulmonary metastases occur early. Pain starts as an ache and then becomes more severe and multifocal. The alkaline phosphatase enzyme is elevated because the multifocal lesions are invariably blastic in nature. (5)

Radiologic Features

The radiologic appearance is quite dramatic and easy to recognize. These lesions occur in the metaphyses of the long tubular bones; no specific bones are most common sites. Spinal involvement may occur, presenting as an irregular, nodular, radiopaque mass or creating an ivory vertebra. (Fig. 11-109, A–C) Occasionally, flat bones, such as the pelvis, sternum, skull, and ribs, may be involved. The clearly radiopaque lesions are often bilateral and symmetric in distribution. (6) (Fig. 11-109, D–F) In the early stages these lesions may resemble benign bone islands; however, as the disease progresses they fill the entire medullary canal at the metaphysis. (Fig. 11-109A) Rarely, these tumors involve the epiphyses.

The differential diagnosis may include heavy-metal poisoning (lead); however, the metaphyseal increase in density is oval or round in multifocal osteosarcoma and transverse, bandlike in metal poisoning. Other congenital disorders—such as Engelmann's disease (diaphyseal sclerosis), melorheostosis (flowing hyperostosis), osteopetrosis, or osteopoikilosis (multiple metaphyseal lesions)—can produce an increase in density; however, none assumes the classic round or large oval appearance of multifocal osteosarcoma.

PAROSTEAL SARCOMA

General Considerations

Parosteal sarcoma (juxtacortical osteosarcoma, parosteal osteosarcoma, surface osteosarcoma) is a tumor situated on the surface of a bone and is biologically different from its intramedullary counterpart. (1) This tumor is designated as a well-differentiated osteosarcoma that arises in a juxtacortical location within the periosteum. It is a relatively uncommon lesion representing 3–4% of all osteosarcomas and about 1% of all primary malignant bone tumors. (2) This tumor grows slowly in contrast to central osteosarcoma. The presenting symptoms are swelling or mass formation, with a dull, aching pain. Occasionally, the mass may interfere with joint function. Most patients have had symptoms for at least 1 year at the time of detection.

Incidence

The typical age range is from 30 to 50 years; cases have been reported in the Mayo Clinic series with a range from 12 to 58 years.

(3) There is no predilection for either sex, and no significant laboratory abnormalities are noted.

Location

The majority of cases involve the posterior surface of the distal femoral metaphysis (50% of cases). (2) Other common sites are the proximal tibia and humerus (25% of cases). Unusual sites are the ulna, radius, clavicle, metacarpal bones, phalanges, and mandible. (4–6)

Pathologic Features

Most of these tumors are quite large, varying in size from 3 to 25 cm, with an average size of 10 cm. (2) Pathologically, the tumor presents as a lobulated, sessile, bony, hard mass, having an intimate, broad-based attachment to the underlying bone. Occasionally, a periosteal fibrous tissue layer separates the tumor mass from the cortical surface, creating a cleavage plane. (7) (Fig. 11-110) It is important pathologically to determine whether or not the tumor has involved the medullary canal, because this finding affects the overall prognosis negatively. The radiologist plays a key role here because biopsies are often not deep enough to tell.

Radiologic Features

Radiographically, this lesion is a dense (radiopaque) homogenous juxtacortical mass. The classic lesion affects the popliteal surface of the distal femur. (8) (Figs. 11-111 and 11-112) A peculiar radiolucent cleft separates the majority of the ossified mass from the cortex of the femur. (8) This cleft (1 to 3 mm in width) stops abruptly at the stalk of the tumor and has been referred to as the *cleavage plane* (7) or *string sign* (2) of parosteal sarcoma. (Fig. 11-110A) This sign is present in only 30% of cases. (2) The periphery of the tumor is usually lobular in outline, and no periosteal (spiculated or laminated) new bone formation can be recognized. (8) CT cannot identify satellite lesions or distinguish between high- and low-grade tumors. (9)

The radiographic differential diagnosis is primarily with posttraumatic myositis ossificans. (10) This should not pose a real problem because most lesions of myositis are clearly separated from the bone. If, however, separation cannot be seen, the actual roentgen appearance usually provides the essential clues. The inner portions of sarcomas are uniformly dense, with a less dense peripheral margin. Myositis ossificans is less dense centrally and often has a halo-like rim of peripheral cortical bone. (11) Also, as demonstrated on serial films, myositis ossificans becomes smaller in size, whereas parosteal osteosarcoma becomes larger. These are general guidelines for radiographic differentiation; exceptions do occur.

The treatment will vary, depending on the histologic aggressiveness of the tumor. En bloc resection for the less aggressive lesions seems helpful; however, a high rate of recurrence exists (> 50%). (2) Therefore, wider margins of the tumor should be resected. Amputation should be performed only in large lesions that are determined to be highly aggressive. The 5-year survival rate is estimated to be as high as 70% following surgical excision. (12)

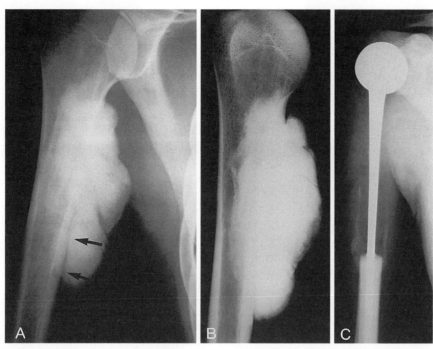

Figure 11-110   **PAROSTEAL SARCOMA. A. AP Humerus.** Observe the large homogeneous radiopaque juxtacortical mass present in the proximal metadiaphyseal area of the humerus. At the caudal end of this mass a clearly defined cleavage plane is visualized (*arrows*). **B. Specimen Radiograph. C. Prosthesis.** Observe the metal prosthesis used in the treatment of this patient's parosteal sarcoma of the proximal humerus. *COMMENT:* The cleavage plane referred to previously actually represents a periosteal fibrous tissue layer separating the tumor from the cortical surface. This has also been referred to as the string sign of parosteal sarcoma and is present in only 30% of cases. (Courtesy of Friedrich H. W. Heuck, MD, Stuttgart, West Germany.)

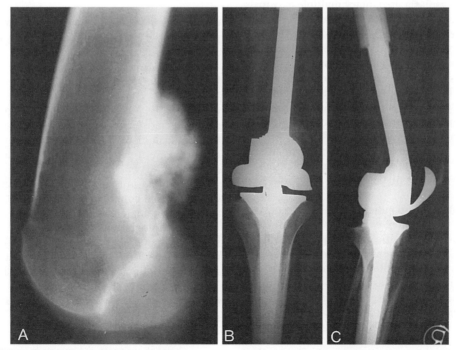

Figure 11-111   **PAROSTEAL SARCOMA: DISTAL FEMUR. A. Tomogram, Lateral Knee.** Observe the juxtacortical radiopaque mass on the posterior surface of the distal femur. **B. AP Knee. C. Lateral Knee.** Note that the postoperative radiographs demonstrate a prosthesis that has worked well for this 21-year-old patient. (Courtesy of Cynthia K. Peterson, DC, DACBR, Toronto, Canada.)

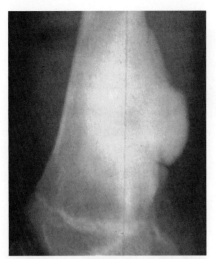

Figure 11-112 PAROSTEAL SARCOMA. Distal Femur. Observe the nodular ivory radiopaque mass on the posterior surface of the distal femur. This is the classic location for parosteal sarcoma.

SECONDARY OSTEOSARCOMA

General Considerations

Malignant degeneration of benign disorders, such as Paget's disease, polyostotic fibrous dysplasia, hereditary multiple exostosis (osteochondromas), and enchondromatosis (Ollier's disease), to osteosarcoma are documented. (1) (Fig. 11-113)

Ionizing radiation may lead to the development of bone sarcoma. These changes may result from either internal (2) or external (3) radiation sources. Martland et al. (4) documented the watch-dial painters who had inadvertently ingested radium and mesothorium during their work by wetting their paint brushes with their tongues. These people developed bone sarcomas (usually osteosarcoma) 10–15 years later.

Patients may develop postradiation sarcoma after treatment for breast cancer, Wilms' tumor, and other primary carcinomas. The latent period varies from 5 to 40 years, with 15 years being average. (2,3)

Bone sarcomas may develop in patients who have received injections of thorotrast, a radioactive contrast medium containing a 25% colloidal thorium dioxide suspension (an α emitter). (5) This contrast medium was used for arteriography and other examinations in the 1950s. Osteosarcomas have been reported with the injection of as little as 50–75 mL of thorotrast. (6) Most of the reported cases occurred 15–25 years after injection. (6) Liver and spleen toxicity with tumor formation have been documented. (6) This contrast agent is no longer in current usage.

The radiographic features of permeative, moth-eaten bone destruction with periosteal reaction and soft tissue mass is largely indistinguishable from those osteosarcomas arising de novo. (7)

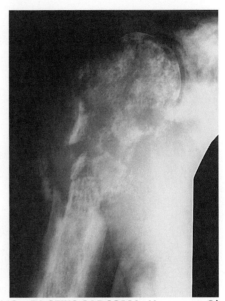

Figure 11-113 PAGET'S SARCOMA. Humerus. Observe the pathologic fracture and extensive destruction of the proximal humerus. There is extensive cortical thickening of the visualized diaphysis of the humerus. These radiographic signs are consistent with malignant degeneration of Paget's disease to osteosarcoma, as was the histologic diagnosis in this case. *COMMENT:* Malignant degeneration of Paget's disease is a rare complication, occurring in 0.9–2% of patients. The humerus, femur, tibia, pelvis, and sacrum are favorite sites. (Reprinted with permission from **Yochum TR:** *Paget's sarcoma of bone.* Radiologe 24:428, 1984.)

EXTRAOSSEOUS OSTEOSARCOMA

General Considerations

Occasionally, osteosarcomas may originate in an extraosseous site. The most common site is the soft tissues of the thigh, but they can also be found in the pleura, heart valves, dura of the brain, retroperitoneum, buttock, axilla, breast, and renal capsule. (1–3)

The prognosis is similar to osteosarcoma, with metastases to the lung being common. Most occur between 30 and 50 years of age. The histologic features are identical to osseous osteosarcoma.

The radiologic features are those of a large soft tissue mass, which is often not adjacent to a bone. The general appearance is non-specific. Occasionally, bone formation is present within the mass; this facilitates the proper diagnosis.

CHONDROSARCOMA

General Considerations

Chondrosarcoma is a malignant tumor of chondrogenic origin that remains essentially cartilaginous throughout its evolution. It arises from chondroblasts and collagenoblasts, thus producing only cartilage and collagen. Chondrosarcomas of bone are usually classified as primary, arising de novo within a given bone, or secondary, arising in a pre-existing cartilaginous lesion (e.g., osteochondroma, enchondroma). In addition, chondrosarcomas may be either central (medullary or intraosseous) or peripheral (arising on the surface of the bone). Rarely, chondrosarcoma may arise in an extraosseous site.

Incidence

Chondrosarcoma is the third most common primary malignant bone tumor, following multiple myeloma and osteosarcoma. (1) The central type is five times more common than the peripheral presentation. (2) Chondrosarcomas make up about 10% of all primary malignant bone tumors. (3)

Clinical Features

Age and Sex Distribution

Most chondrosarcomas occur after the age of 40, the usual range being 40–60 years of age. Men are affected more than women in the ratio of 2:1.

Signs and Symptoms

The initial symptom that calls attention to the presence of the tumor may be either pain or swelling, or a combination of both. Neither is diagnostic; in fact, many patients present with pain so late in the progression of the disease that it is not considered reliable in the workup of a patient suspected of chondrosarcoma. Rib lesions render pain, initially, in only one third of the cases. Peripheral chondrosarcoma is especially asymptomatic and usually presents with only minor discomfort and palpable swelling. (3) Pelvic tumors, however large, may remain hidden for a long time within the pelvic cavity. Once the mass reaches a large enough size, it will eventually compress on vital structures (bladder, bowel, lymphatic channels, blood vessels, or nerves), creating objective signs and symptoms that guide the clinician to the site of the lesion. Severe pain and disability may accompany osseous lesions when a pathologic fracture occurs, often spontaneously.

Persistent and unrelenting pain in a previously diagnosed enchondroma should raise significant suspicion about malignant degeneration. Occasionally, a rapidly expanding, high-grade, central chondrosarcoma may cause early severe pain, which is commensurate with the degree of cortical destruction and size of the soft tissue mass. (4) The duration of symptoms, as reported by patients, varies considerably; it is < 2 years for 75% of the patients and < 5 years for the rest. (5)

Location

Chondrosarcoma may arise in any bone preformed in cartilage. (Fig. 11-114) The most common sites are the pelvis and proximal femur (50%); other sites include proximal humerus (10%), ribs (15%), scapula (6%), distal femur and proximal tibia (7%), and craniofacial bones and sternum (5%). (Figs. 11-115 and

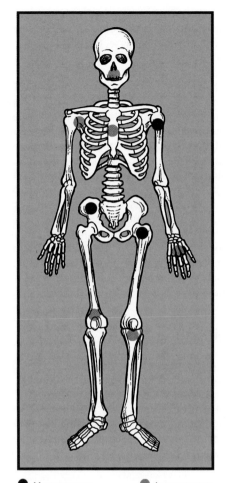

● More common   ● Less common

Figure 11-114 **SKELETAL DISTRIBUTION OF CHONDROSARCOMA.**

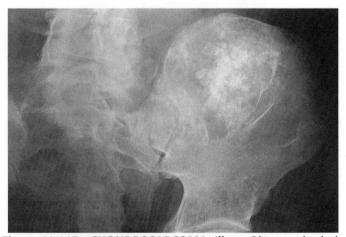

Figure 11-115 **CHONDROSARCOMA. Ilium.** Observe the lytic destructive lesion in the posterior surface of the ilium. There is mottled calcification within the central portion of the matrix of this cartilaginous tumor.

11-116) The remainder occur in the hand, foot, and spine. (6–9) When present in the foot, the lesions should be suspected as malignancies until proven otherwise. (10) Less than 2% involve the epiphysis and are usually of the clear cell variety. (11)

Chondrosarcoma is the most common primary malignant bone tumor of the hand, although representing only 4% of the total malignant tumors of the hand. (12) (Fig. 11-117) Most lesions in the hand occur in the metacarpals or phalanges; rarely, the carpal bones may be involved. Two cases in the trapezoid have been demonstrated; one case affecting the trapezium has been recorded. (6,13,14) Although the number of cases of chondrosarcoma of the vertebral column is quite small, in those reported the lesions are fairly evenly distributed throughout the spinal column. (8,9) In the spine, extramedullary defect and compression fracture may be seen, resulting in subsequent neurological deficit. (8,9) Chondrosarcoma is also the most common primary malignant bone tumor of the chest wall, including the sternum and scapula. (15–17) (Fig. 11-118) It represents the third most common primary malignancy of the pelvis, following Ewing's sarcoma and osteosarcoma. (18)

Pathologic Features

Chondrosarcomas are typically composed of faceted lobules of grayish white or bluish cartilaginous tissue and may be gritty to the touch because of the calcium contained within. These lobulated growths produce extrinsic pressure on the endosteum, creating a scalloped margin. The adjacent outer cortex is frequently broken in aggressive lesions, producing a large soft tissue mass. Cystic degeneration in a bulky tumor may be demonstrated grossly, on occasion.

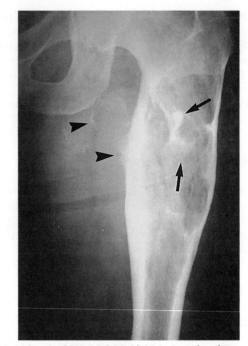

Figure 11-116 **CHONDROSARCOMA. Proximal Femur.** Note the grossly expansile lytic destructive lesion in the proximal diaphysis of the femur. Observe the central calcification present within the lesion (*arrows*). There is obvious cortical disruption, as well as a soft tissue mass, present within the inner thigh (*arrowheads*).

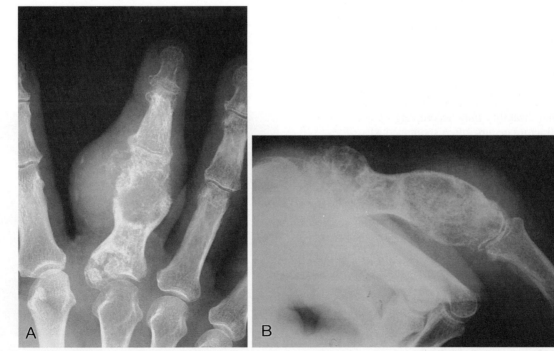

Figure 11-117 **CHONDROSARCOMA: HAND. A. PA Finger. B. Lateral Finger.** Observe the grossly destructive lesion of the proximal phalanx of the third digit. There is calcification present within the matrix of this lesion. A rather large soft tissue mass is found associated with this patient's chondrosarcoma, and calcification is also noted in the soft tissue mass.

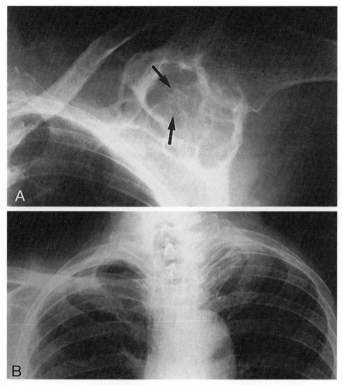

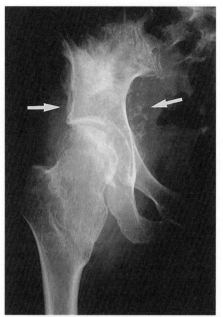

Figure 11-118 **CHONDROSARCOMA. Scapula. A. Pre-treatment.** Note the large, lytic, expansile lesion in the scapula. Observe the faint calcification in the matrix of the lesion (*arrows*). **B. Post-Treatment.** Note that the patient was treated with a radical disarticulation of his left arm and scapula, with excision of the lateral half of his clavicle. *COMMENT:* Chondrosarcoma is the most common primary malignant bone tumor of the scapula.

Figure 11-119 **CHONDROSARCOMA OF THE ILIUM SECONDARY TO MALIGNANT DEGENERATION OF A BENIGN OSTEOCHONDROMA.** Observe the broad, wide metaphysis of the proximal femur, which is characteristic of hereditary multiple exostosis (HME). There is calcification (*arrows*) within the soft tissue extensions associated with malignant degeneration of a previously benign osteochondroma of the ilium. *COMMENT:* The incidence of malignant degeneration of chondrosarcoma in HME is 20%; in a solitary osteochondroma the incidence is 1%.

Histologic sections of a typical chondrosarcoma demonstrate plump, cartilaginous cells, which contain multiple nuclei that are irregular in size. Hyperchromatism is marked, and mitotic figures may be present but generally are not numerous. Calcium is usually found on histologic section and is radiographically demonstrable in two thirds of the patients. (1) It is generally recognized that there is a relationship between the density of calcification in a chondrosarcoma and its degree of malignancy. (19) Myxoid tissue rarely calcifies, and because the degree of myxomatous histologic change is closely related to the grade of malignancy, it is not surprising that high-grade tumors are frequently associated with large areas of non-calcified tumor. (20) Approximately one third of the chondrosarcomas are purely lytic and show no matrix calcification. (1)

Secondary chondrosarcoma arises in a pre-existing cartilaginous lesion. The most common disorder to exhibit this malignant degeneration is enchondromatosis, or Ollier's disease, and hereditary multiple exostosis (HME) or multiple osteochondromas. The incidence is highest in Ollier's disease, being approximately 50% of patients; a much smaller percentage of solitary enchondromas undergo malignant change. (2,21) The incidence of malignant degeneration to chondrosarcoma in HME is 20%; in solitary osteochondroma, 1%. (2,21) (Fig. 11-119)

In general, benign cartilaginous tumors (usually enchondromas) that are close to or involve the axial skeleton have a much higher rate of malignant degeneration than those that are in the distant appendicular skeleton. Other conditions in which chondro-

sarcoma may occur secondarily include Paget's disease (22,23), fibrous dysplasia, (24) and radiation-induced sarcoma. (25)

Radiologic Features

Central Chondrosarcoma

Radiographs usually reveal a large, radiolucent, round or oval lesion with poorly defined margins. The contours of the bone are enlarged or expanded. Most lesions are in the metaphysis or diaphysis if a long bone is affected. (Fig. 11-120) Scalloping of the inner cortex (endosteum) is caused by the lobular outlines of the tumor. The cortex may be extensively eroded; this finding usually indicates an advanced stage. The slow progression of the tumor leads to fusiform expansion of the shaft and cortical thickening as a result of tumor invasion of the haversian systems. Purely epiphyseal lesions are rare; they occur in < 2% of chondrosarcomas, are usually of the *clear cell* variety, and most commonly involve the proximal femur and humerus. (11)

The matrix of the lesion may have circular radiolucencies that represent large lobules of cartilage, imparting a bubbly appearance. Less commonly, a mottled permeating destructive pattern may be seen. (Fig. 11-121) Foci of irregularly scattered calcification in the tumor matrix occur in two thirds of the cases (one third of cases are purely lytic). (Fig. 11-122) These calcifications have been called *popcorn, fluffy, stippled, cotton wool, rings, and broken rings.* Periosteal new bone formation occurs occasionally, creating a laminated or spiculated pattern.

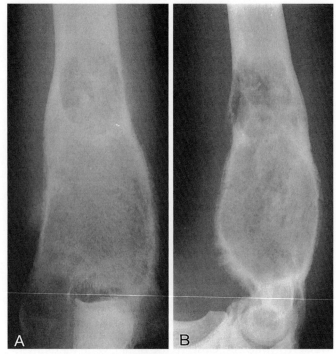

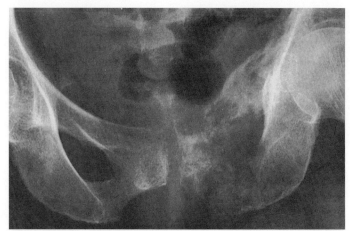

Figure 11-121 **CHONDROSARCOMA. AP Pelvis.** Note the ill-defined permeative destructive pattern present in the superior pubic ramus, inferior pubic ramus, and ischial tuberosity. Its radiographic appearance is aggressive, with a poor zone of transition surrounding the lesion. This represents a mixed infiltrating pattern of chondrosarcoma.

Figure 11-120 **CHONDROSARCOMA: DISTAL HUMERUS.**
A. AP Humerus. B. Lateral Humerus. Observe the expansile lytic lesion in the distal diaphysis and metaphysis of the humerus. A mixed pattern of bone destruction, along with periosteal new bone formation, is seen around the peripheral cortices.

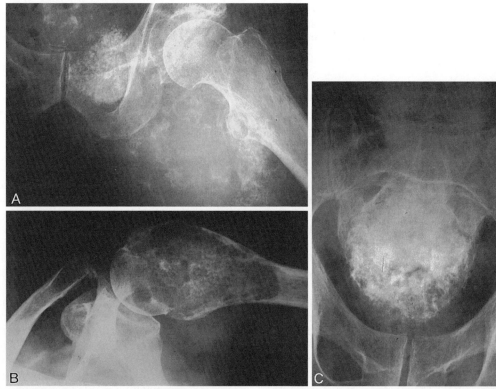

Figure 11-122 **CHONDROSARCOMA WITH MATRIX CALCIFICATION. A. Pelvis.** Observe the large soft tissue mass with matrix calcification surrounding the chondrosarcoma of the pelvis. **B. Proximal Humerus.** Note the expansile permeative lesion of the metaphysis of the proximal humerus. Stippled matrix calcification is present in the central portion of this chondrosarcoma. **C. Sacrum.** Observe the dense, homogeneous matrix calcification in the middle to lower portion of the sacrum. This lesion is characteristic of chondrosarcoma. *COMMENT:* Foci of irregularly scattered calcification in the tumor matrix of chondrosarcoma occur in two thirds of cases, with one third of cases being purely lytic. These calcifications have been called popcorn, fluffy, and stippled.

Eventually, a large soft tissue mass develops, with amorphous calcifications scattered throughout. (Fig. 11-123) In a juxtacortical or extraosseous tumor, the soft tissue mass may be the initial presenting radiologic sign when a destructive lesion in the adjacent bone may be hard to identify. An example of this is an early acetabular chondrosarcoma with a soft tissue mass extending into the pelvic cavity. (Fig. 11-124)

Peripheral Chondrosarcoma

This lesion demonstrates primarily a spiculated periosteal response and Codman's reactive triangle in the soft tissue area adjacent to the lesion. Cortical destruction may be present, but no medullary involvement occurs. The majority of the secondary chondrosarcomas present as peripheral lesions seeded from the osteocartilaginous cap of an osteochondroma. (26)

Treatment and Prognosis

Primary chondrosarcoma typically shows a slow clinical progression because spread is by direct extension rather than hematogenous routes. Irradiation and chemotherapy probably have no or little role in the curative treatment of this malignant tumor. (27,28) Radical removal of the lesion by local excision, segmented resection, or amputation is the treatment of choice. However, recent studies have suggested that total resection may increase the chance of prolonged recovery compared with partial resection. (27) In general, lesions farthest from the trunk offer the greatest possibility for initial surgical treatment by techniques other than amputation. In lesions near the trunk, radical removal at the time of initial observation is preferred because any recurrence is practically incurable. Curettage is only palliative but has been used and repeated to control some indolent lesions that are not amenable to complete removal.

The 5-year survival figures after early and adequate surgery approach 90%. (29,30) In general, more cures are attained with chondrosarcomas than with most of the other primary malignant

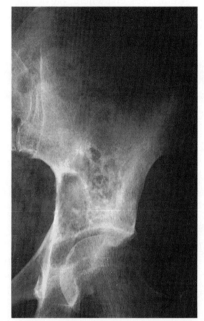

Figure 11-124   **CHONDROSARCOMA. Ilium.** Note the eccentrically placed lytic chondrosarcoma in the supra-acetabular area. Some small stippled calcifications are present within the matrix of the tumor.

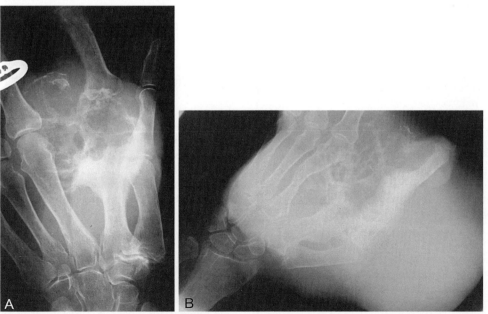

Figure 11-123   **CHONDROSARCOMA OF THE HAND, WITH A LARGE SOFT TISSUE MASS. A. Initial Radiograph.** Observe the destruction of the second metacarpal head, with a large soft tissue mass. There are scattered calcifications present throughout the destructive lesion. **B. 2-Year Follow-Up.** Note the massive progression of the destructive lesion of the second metacarpal bone, with a large soft tissue mass noted about the hand. This soft tissue mass is so large it has caused some pressure erosion on the medial cortex of the mid-diaphysis of the third metacarpal bone. *COMMENT:* At the time of the initial diagnosis, surgery was recommended but refused by the patient. This allowed the drastic progression of the tumor, creating such a large soft tissue mass. (Courtesy of Bryan Hartley, MD, Melbourne, Australia.)

bone tumors. (29,30) The location of the tumor and duration of symptoms appears not to influence the outcome, with histological grading remaining the primary marker of prognostic value. (31–33) When metastatic spread occurs, it is generally owing to invasion by the tumor of regional venous channels with access to the cardiopulmonary circulation by intravascular growth and extension. (29,30) Parenchymal metastases, usually pulmonary, are not uncommon. Metastases elsewhere, particularly to the skeleton, are infrequently encountered; similarly, extension of tumor to the regional lymph nodes is rarely reported. (2)

CAPSULE SUMMARY   Chondrosarcoma

General Considerations

- Primary chondrosarcoma arises de novo.
- Secondary chondrosarcoma arises in a pre-existing cartilaginous lesion (enchondroma, osteochondroma).
- Central chondrosarcoma arises intramedullary.
- Peripheral chondrosarcoma arises on the surface of the bone.

Incidence

- Represents the third most common primary malignant bone tumor, following myeloma and osteosarcoma.
- It makes up 10% of all primary malignant bone tumors.

Clinical Features

- Age of presentation is 40–60 years, with 2:1 male predominance.
- Pain usually presents late in the disease process, often after large soft tissue masses develop.
- Severe pain follows pathologic fracture.
- The most common sites are the pelvis, proximal femur and humerus, ribs, scapula, sternum, craniofacial bones, distal femur, and proximal tibia.

Pathologic Features

- Lobules of grayish white or bluish cartilaginous tissue.
- Malignant degeneration of Ollier's disease (enchondromatosis) is approximately 50%; HME is 20%; 1% in solitary osteochondroma.
- The closer the lesion is to the axial skeleton, the higher the potential for malignant degeneration.

Radiologic Features

- Round or oval radiolucencies with ill-defined margins evident.
- Lesions are metaphyseal or diaphyseal; < 2% are epiphyseal (clear cell variety).
- Endosteal scalloping occurs secondary to pressure erosion from the enlarging lobular mass.
- Popcorn matrix calcification in the lesion occurs in two thirds of cases; one third of the lesions are purely radiolucent.
- Laminated or spiculated periosteal response occurs.
- Metastatic disease is usually to lung; rare to bone.

Treatment and Prognosis

- Treatment consists of local excisions, segmental resection, or amputation.
- Prognosis is good, with 90% survival after early surgery.

EWING'S SARCOMA

General Considerations

Ewing's sarcoma is a primitive primary malignant tumor of bone; it is composed of tumor cells derived from the connective tissue framework of bone marrow. This highly malignant tumor was originally described in its classic form by James Ewing (1) in 1921. He described a rather specific radiographic appearance in a group of malignant pediatric bone tumors, which he called *diffuse endothelioma of bone, or endothelial myeloma.* (1) He wrote:

> The radiographs give characteristic features on which a diagnosis may be based with considerable certainty. A large portion of the whole shaft is involved, but the ends are generally spared, contrary to the rule with osteogenic sarcoma. The shaft is slightly widened, but the main alteration is a diffuse fading of the bone structure. Bone production has been entirely absent. Some of the bones appear honeycombed. Perforation of the shaft and sharp limitation of the process are wanting. The central excavation with widened bony capsule, as seen in benign giant cell tumors, is missing. The radiograph is therefore rather specific. (1)

Since Ewing's initial description, the diversity of radiographic manifestations of Ewing's sarcoma has become widely appreciated. The variety of histologic patterns that this tumor presents has caused some confusion; however, distinctive histopathologic criteria are now recognized. Oberling (2) suggested that Ewing's sarcoma originated from the marrow stem cell, which is derived from the primary reticulum; therefore, Ewing's sarcoma has been grouped with myeloma and non-Hodgkin's lymphoma (reticulum cell sarcoma) as a *round cell* tumor. These round cell tumors have a striking predilection for the marrow-rich diaphysis. Their appearance is radiographically similar, but they differ greatly in age incidence.

Incidence

Ewing's sarcoma represents approximately 7% of all primary malignant bone tumors and is the fourth most common primary malignant bone tumor, with myeloma, osteosarcoma, and chondrosarcoma occurring more frequently (in decreasing order of incidence). Ewing's sarcoma demonstrates a racial predilection affecting both American and African blacks with a significantly lower incidence than the general population. (3)

Clinical Features

Age and Sex Distribution

Ewing's sarcoma is found most commonly in the 10- to 25-year age range, with a peak at 15 years. It is rare before the age of 5 and after the age of 30; 50% of cases occur < 20 years of age. The youngest patient reported was 5 months old (4), and the oldest was age 83 years. (5) Patients in the younger age range (5–20 years) usually have lesions in the peripheral skeleton, whereas older patients (20–35 years) present with axial lesions. There is a 2:1 male to female ratio.

Signs and Symptoms

Localized pain with swelling at the site of the lesion is a consistent presenting complaint. (6) A soft tissue mass is palpable in more than one third of the cases. (6) The pain initially is dull in nature; however, it usually becomes severe and persistent a few months before diagnosis. Systemic symptoms of slight to moderate fever, secondary anemia, leukocytosis, and increased ESR are common in Ewing's sarcoma. (7) Ewing's tumor seems to be the only primary malignant bone tumor with symptoms simulating an infection. (7) Local temperature elevation with dilated veins and associated tenderness accompanies the lesion, thereby suggesting an inflammatory condition. The inflammatory-like symptoms of Ewing's sarcoma may be explained by the fact that the tumor characteristically outgrows its blood supply, resulting in extensive degeneration and necrosis. (8) With such a clinical presentation, biopsy may be the only means of diagnosis.

Location

Ewing's sarcoma is seen most frequently in the long tubular bones (50%) and in the flat bones (40%). (9) (Fig. 11-125) The lower extremity encompasses the largest portion of the tubular

involvement. The femur is most commonly involved (23%), with the tibia, fibula, and humerus following (9%). (9) The diaphysis is the classic location for these tumors; however, more cases are being seen affecting the metaphysis and metadiaphyseal region.

Of the flat bones the most frequently affected site is the pelvis (21%) (10,11), with the innominate being the most common portion involved. (Fig. 11-126) It is the most common malignant lesion of childhood to affect the ischium and pubis; 10% of all malignant rib lesions are Ewing's sarcoma. (12,13) The vast majority of the malignant costal tumors in children consist of Ewing's sarcoma. (14) Involvement of the scapula occurs in approximately 5% of cases. (9) Spinal involvement is uncommon, occurring in only 3.5–7% of all lesions in two large series. (15–17) The sacrum and lumbar spine are the most common sites. (15,17) (Fig. 11-127) Isolated cases have been reported in the feet and the mandible (horizontal ramus preferred). (18–21)

Pathologic Features

Recent research in the field of genetics has identified a genetic alteration that has been linked to the expression of a chimeric protein and possible initiation of tumors within the family of Ewing's sarcoma. (22) Upon gross inspection of Ewing's sarcoma, the lesion principally occupies the medullary cavity and is usually soft, friable, and often hemorrhagic. Cystic areas of necrosis occur. Extraosseous tumor tissue is often identified because the cortex is frequently penetrated. The overlying skin may be red, with local venous dilation; ulceration may occur.

Histologically, Ewing's sarcomas are extremely undifferentiated and consist of sheets of small, round, or oval cells in

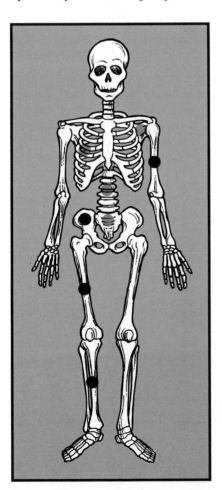

● More common ● Less common

Figure 11-125 SKELETAL DISTRIBUTION OF EWING'S SARCOMA.

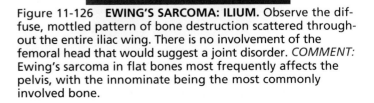

Figure 11-126 EWING'S SARCOMA: ILIUM. Observe the diffuse, mottled pattern of bone destruction scattered throughout the entire iliac wing. There is no involvement of the femoral head that would suggest a joint disorder. *COMMENT:* Ewing's sarcoma in flat bones most frequently affects the pelvis, with the innominate being the most commonly involved bone.

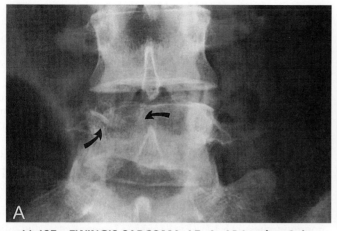

Figure 11-127   **EWING'S SARCOMA: L5. A. AP Lumbar Spine. B. Tomogram, L5.** Observe the lytic destruction of the pedicle of L5 and a portion of the vertebral body (*arrows*) in this 15-year-old patient. *COMMENT:* Ewing's sarcoma of the spine is uncommon, occurring in 3.5–7% of lesions. When present, the sacrum and lumbar spine are the most common sites.

which the nuclei are prominent and the cytoplasm is poorly visualized. The nuclei tend to be quite uniform in size and shape, and mitotic figures are numerous, while tumor giant cells and pleomorphism are conspicuously absent. This histologic pattern may be modified by large areas of ischemic necrosis (the rapidly growing tumor tends to outgrow its blood supply), so that in many tumors the preservable viable cells are found in cords or masses surrounding blood vessels with necrosis of the more remote areas.

It may be impossible to differentiate a biopsy specimen from non-Hodgkin's lymphoma, neuroblastoma, leukemia, or eosinophilic granuloma. (9) It is important to correlate the patient's age, clinical features, and radiographic presentation before a histologic diagnosis is firmly established. A special laboratory staining procedure may be helpful in the differentiation of Ewing's sarcoma and non-Hodgkin's lymphoma. The demonstration of glycogen granules upon appropriate staining of the cells is common in Ewing's sarcoma and not found in non-Hodgkin's lymphoma. (23) Fine-needle aspiration cytology in conjunction with immunocytochemistry is currently an effective, non-traumatic method for a rapid and accurate diagnosis. (24)

Radiologic Features

The classic presentation is that of a diaphyseal lesion (usually in the lower extremity), permeative in its appearance, with a wide zone of transition. (Fig. 11-128) A delicate, laminated, onion

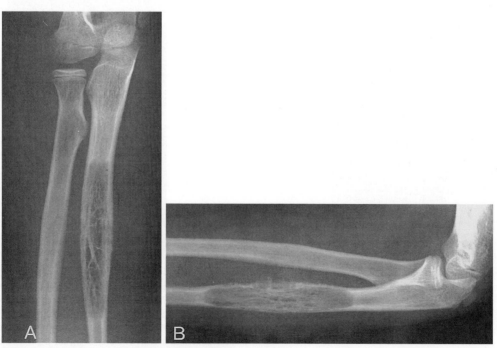

Figure 11-128   **EWING'S SARCOMA: DIAPHYSEAL INVOLVEMENT. A. AP Ulna. B. Lateral Ulna.** Observe the lytic destructive lesion in the diaphysis of the ulna. There is moderate expansion of the ulna noted. No characteristic periosteal response is present.

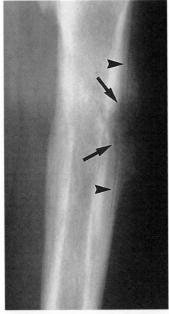

Figure 11-129   **EWING'S SARCOMA: CORTICAL SAUCERIZATION AND ONION SKIN PERIOSTEAL RESPONSE. Femur.** Observe the permeative destruction within the medullary portion of the mid-diaphysis of the femur. Disruption in the cortex, creating a saucerization appearance, is characteristic of Ewing's sarcoma (*arrows*). An additional radiographic sign of aggressive disease is the onion skin or laminated periosteal response seen adjacent to the cortical saucerization (*arrowheads*).

Table 11-16	Features of Ewing's Sarcoma

Age
   10–25 years
   Males 2:1
   Symptoms may simulate infection
Location
   Femur
   Tibia, fibula
   Humerus
   Pelvis
   Scapula
Radiologic features
   Diaphyseal
   Permeative
   Laminated or onion skin periosteal response
   Cortical saucerization

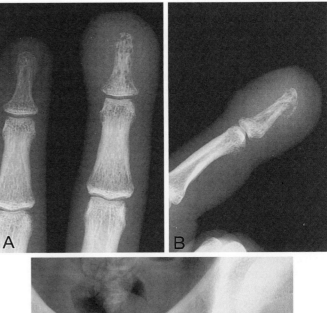

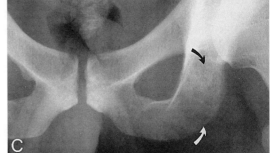

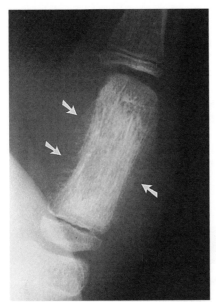

Figure 11-130   **EWING'S SARCOMA: GROOMED OR TRIMMED WHISKERS EFFECT. First Metacarpal.** Note the mottled radiolucent and radiopaque destructive pattern scattered throughout the entire first metacarpal. A fine and delicate periosteal pattern of new bone formation is present around the metaphysis and diaphysis of the first metacarpal bone, causing the groomed or trimmed whiskers appearance (*arrows*).

Figure 11-131   **EWING'S SARCOMA: METASTASIS TO BONE. A. AP Distal Phalanx. B. Lateral Distal Phalanx.** Note the aggressive permeative pattern of bone destruction present throughout the distal phalanx of the index finger. A large soft tissue mass is seen associated with this destruction. **C. Ischial Tuberosity.** Observe the ill-defined pattern of radiolucency throughout the ischial tuberosity in this 21-year-old patient whose initial complaint was that of digital pain. This ischial lesion (*arrows*) represents a secondary site of metastasis from the primary Ewing's sarcoma of the distal phalanx of his index finger. *COMMENT:* Ewing's sarcoma is the most common primary malignant bone tumor to metastasize to bone; osteosarcoma may also. (Courtesy of Bryan Hartley, MD, Melbourne, Australia.)

skin, or onion peel periosteal response is noted in only 25–50% of cases. (9) Cortical *saucerization* is an early and characteristic sign. (Fig. 11-129) This irregular defect effaces the outside of the bone occasionally, exhibiting a marginal scalloping effect. It occurs when the tumor grows through the haversian system and presents subperiosteally. Purely lytic lesions are uncommon, with a mixed lytic and sclerotic pattern predominating in the tubular bones. Approximately one third of the cases affecting flat bones demonstrate diffuse sclerosis. (25) This diffuse sclerosis represents normal bone formed as a reaction to the tumor cells rather than actual tumor bone. (25) Pathologic fracture is noted in approximately 5% of cases. (26)

Periosteal Bone Formation

The delicate parallel, laminated, onion skin, or onion peel radiographic presentation is quite striking in its appearance when present. (Fig. 11-129) This appearance is caused by the splitting and thickening of the cortex by the tumor cells. The layering is continuous, with reactive ossification in the form of Codman's triangles occurring frequently. Osteomyelitis, traumatic periostitis, osteosarcoma, and malignant lymphoma may also show a Codman's reactive triangle; therefore, it is not pathognomonic.

The sunray pattern of periosteal new bone formation may also occur in Ewing's sarcoma. These radiating spicules have been referred to as the *groomed or trimmed whiskers effect*. (27) (Fig. 11-130) It has been suggested that these perpendicular bone spicules are thinner and more hair-like than those in osteosarcoma. (28) This appearance is also found in metastatic neuroblastoma, in renal carcinoma, and, commonly, in osteosarcoma. (Table 11-16)

Metastases

Skeletal metastases occur frequently and early, leading to extensive bone destruction. Ewing's sarcoma is the most common primary malignant bone tumor to metastasize to bone. (29) (Fig. 11-131) The spine is a common site for metastasis. (17) Multiple lesions in the one bone occur and are described as *skip lesions,* a phenomenon also seen in osteosarcoma. (30) Secondary spread to the lungs is also a common occurrence, with the lung parenchyma and pleura being the favored locations. (29) (Fig. 11-132)

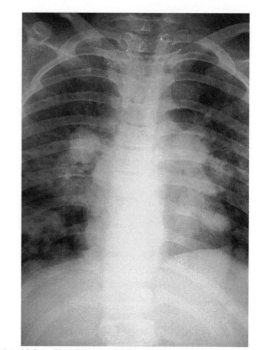

Figure 11-132 CHEST CANNONBALL METASTASES. Observe the multiple circular nodular metastatic lesions scattered throughout the central lung fields. These represent cannonball metastases, with sarcomatous growth within the lung parenchyma from Ewing's sarcoma of the femur.

Treatment and Prognosis

The 5-year survival rate has been approximately 5% for Ewing's sarcoma. Radiation therapy rendered in conjunction with effective chemotherapy in lesions detected early is increasing the survival rate. (31) Amputation may still be used in lesions around the knee. One study reported a 35% 5-year survival rate in 107 patients. (32) Early detection, adequate surgical resection, tumor size, metastasis, and age remain the key prognostic indicators for determining the outcome of the disease process. (31–34) In the event of relapse, regardless of the treatment used, the prognosis is usually fatal. (35)

CAPSULE SUMMARY Ewing's Sarcoma

General Considerations

- Originally described in 1921 by James Ewing as endothelioma of bone, or endothelial myeloma.

Incidence

- Represents 7% of all primary malignant bone tumors.
- Fourth most common primary malignant bone tumor (myeloma, osteosarcoma, and chondrosarcoma occur more frequently, in decreasing order of incidence).
- Incidence is lower among blacks in the United States and Africa.

Clinical Features

- Most cases occur in the 10- to 25-year age range; rare < 5 years and > 30 years.
- Male to female ratio is 2:1.
- Localized pain with swelling at the site of the lesion is a common symptom.
- May mimic infection; systemic signs of slight fever, secondary anemia, leukocytosis, and increased ESR are common.
- Thought to be the only primary malignant bone tumor with symptoms simulating an infection.

(continued)

CAPSULE SUMMARY   Ewing's Sarcoma (*continued*)

- The long tubular bones of the lower extremities (femur, tibia, and fibula) are the most likely sites; the innominate bone is the most common flat bone affected.

Pathologic Features

- Histologically, undifferentiated sheets of small, round, or oval cells.
- Classified as a round cell tumor, along with multiple myeloma and non-Hodgkin's lymphoma of bone.

Radiologic Features

- Classic presentation is a diaphyseal permeative lesion with a delicate onion skin or peel periosteal response.

- Cortical saucerization is a characteristic sign.
- Pathologic fracture is noted in 5% of cases.
- One third of cases affecting flat bones present with diffuse sclerosis.
- Occasionally, the sunray periosteal pattern occurs and has been called groomed, or trimmed, whiskers effect.
- The most common primary malignant bone tumor to metastasize to bone.

Treatment and Prognosis

- Amputation is still used in lesions around the knee.
- Radiation therapy along with chemotherapy in early lesions offers a 35% 5-year survival rate.

FIBROSARCOMA

General Considerations

Fibrosarcoma of bone is a primary malignant bone tumor that produces varying amounts of collagen and has no tendency to form tumor bone, osteoid, or cartilage, either in its primary site or in its metastases. (1) It presents as two types: medullary (or central) and periosteal fibrosarcoma. It is usually encountered during adult life in major long bones, especially those of the lower extremity. The majority of the medullary tumors arise de novo, but in many instances fibrosarcoma develops as a complication of a preexisting benign condition. (2)

Incidence

Fibrosarcoma of bone is relatively rare, representing only 2% of all primary malignant bone tumors. (1,2)

Clinical Features

Age and Sex Distribution

The age distribution has a wide range, from 4 to 83 years; however, they are most often found in the 30- to 50-year age range. (1,2) The median age is 38 years. A definite sex predilection has not been observed.

Signs and Symptoms

The chief complaints are local pain and swelling, which may refer to and limit the motion of the joint. (3) The average duration of symptoms at presentation is 2 years in medullary lesions and 20 months in periosteal lesions. (1) Approximately one third of the tumors present initially with a pathologic fracture. (4)

Location

The tubular bones are more frequently involved in younger patients, the flat bones in older patients. (5) The most common sites are the long bones and innominate bones, but almost 50% of cases occur around the knee. (6) (Fig. 11-133) The femur, tibia, and humerus represent sites for approximately two thirds of the tumors. (1,2) The classic locations within these bones are the condyles of the femur or the epicondyles of the humerus. (1) Other frequent sites include the innomi-nate bones, skull, and facial bones; rarely, the ribs, clavicles, scapulae, spine (Fig. 11-134), and small tubular bones may be involved. (7) It is extremely rare for multiple lesions to be present; however, in the cases reported multiple fibrosarcomas may mimic the radiologic appearance of multiple myeloma. (8)

Most fibrosarcomas are medullary lesions with a ratio of 2:1, medullary to periosteal. (1) The classic location is the metaphysis, with the typical lesion being eccentrically placed. Extension into the epiphysis and even isolated mid-diaphyseal involvement occurs. (7)

Pathologic Features

Inspection of the gross specimen reveals a fibrous mass that is fleshy, firm, and grayish white in color. (2) These tumors may grow to enormous size, creating large, hemorrhagic, necrotic central areas. (9)

Microscopically, the cellular pattern varies greatly from poorly differentiated to more mature forms. Spindle-shaped fibroblasts are commonly found in the less malignant forms, with interlaced bundles of collagen fibers. (10) In the more highly malignant (undifferentiated) lesions, considerable irregularity and marked anaplasia of the fibroblasts are commonplace, with multiple nuclei and hyperchromatism. (10) These lesions are commonly referred to as *malignant fibrous histiocytoma* (MFH). (11) Necrosis, hemorrhage, and, on occasion, secondary calcification may be observed. Bony sequestration may be found histologically and radiographically. (12) Fibrosarcoma is the only primary malignant bone tumor in which sequestration can frequently be found. (12)

Many fibrous tumors present histologically between a low grade and a high grade of cellular activity, posing a problem for

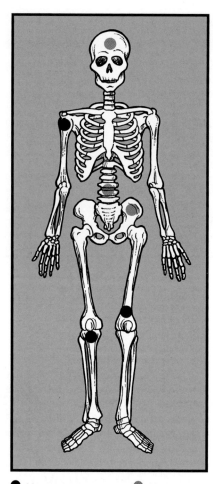

More common ● Less common ●

Figure 11-133 **SKELETAL DISTRIBUTION OF FIBROSARCOMA.**

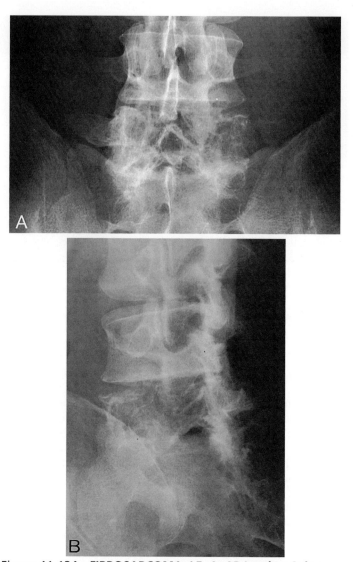

Figure 11-134 **FIBROSARCOMA: L5. A. AP Lumbar Spine. B. Oblique Lumbar Spine.** Observe the destructive osteolytic lesion of the L5 vertebral body. Destruction of the pedicle of the L5 vertebra is also noted. The destructive pattern has given a coarsened appearance to the remaining trabeculae. This is a rare site for fibrosarcoma.

the pathologist in making definitive conclusions microscopically. This is often the case in evaluating patients with fibrosarcoma. Correlation of the clinical data with the radiographic signs is heavily relied on by most pathologists. Lichtenstein (13) provided a helpful rule of thumb: "If a lesion suggests a primary malignant bone tumor but not any one in particular, then think of fibrosarcoma as a possibility, especially if the lesion is in the femur or tibia of an adult."

Radiologic Features

The radiologic findings in fibrosarcoma are generally those of a highly destructive, expanding lesion, which is usually medullary in its site of origin. The typical presentation is an eccentric, lytic lesion causing cortical thinning and endosteal erosion of a long bone. (Fig. 11-135) Most lesions at the time of detection measure > 5 cm. (2) The lytic lesion usually demonstrates no matrix calcification and appears purely radiolucent. The non-invasive (low-grade anaplastic) type of lesion may appear benign initially, but as the tumor grows, breaking the cortex and producing a well-defined soft tissue mass, its malignant nature is revealed. Fibrosarcoma is one of the most

common primary malignant bone tumors to produce a "huge" soft tissue mass, usually larger than any other neoplasm. (14) (Fig. 11-136) A permeating, destructive pattern showing poorly defined, fuzzy margins at the boundary of the tumor may be encountered. Seldom is there any significant periosteal reaction or a Codman's triangle. (Table 11-17)

Secondary Fibrosarcoma

Secondary fibrosarcoma develops in the interior of a bone at the site of a pre-existing benign bone disorder. (2) Some of the pre-existing osseous conditions in which this may occur are fibrous dysplasia, Paget's disease, postradiation, chronic osteomyelitis, and bone infarct. (15–18) A variant fibrous neoplasm has been known to complicate bone infarcts, creating a destructive lytic lesion adjacent to the infarction. It is termed *malignant fibrous histiocytoma of bone* (MFH). (19,20) Approximately 30% of the fibrosarcomas in a Mayo Clinic series were secondary to other pre-existent bone lesions or followed prior radiation. (6)

Metastases

Fibrosarcoma characteristically metastasizes late, except in the highly malignant aggressive lesions. Metastatic deposits to the lung and liver are common. This is one of the few primary bone tumors that may selectively metastasize to the lymphatic system. (12)

Treatment and Prognosis

The treatment of choice for fibrosarcoma is amputation, which usually requires some form of joint disarticulation. (1) Even after surgical interventions the probability of metastases is usually > 70%. (3) The overall 5-year survival rate is approximately 30% (7,14); age > 40 years (21) and a medullary location of the tumor signify a poorer outcome. (6) Patients with medullary lesions had a uniformly poorer prognosis (17–27% 5-year survival) compared with those with periosteal lesions (40–58% 5-year survival). (7)

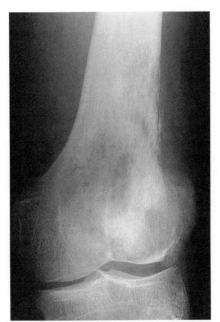

Figure 11-135 **FIBROSARCOMA. Distal Femur.** Observe the eccentric permeative lesions in the distal diaphysis, metaphysis, and subarticular portion of the distal femur. Cortical disruption suggests malignant disease.

Table 11-17	Features of Fibrosarcoma
Age	
30–50 years	
Location	
Femur, tibia (50%)	
Humerus	
Radiologic features	
Metaphyseal	
Eccentric	
Moth-eaten or permeative destruction	
Cortical disruption	
Wide zone of transition	
Large soft tissue mass	

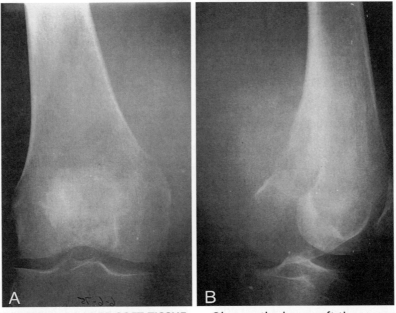

Figure 11-136 **FIBROSARCOMA WITH A LARGE SOFT TISSUE MASS. A. AP Femur. B. Lateral Femur.** Note the radiolucent destructive lesion in the medial condyle of the distal femur.

Observe the large soft tissue mass in the medial portion of the thigh and knee. This large soft tissue mass extends posteriorly, completely filling and distorting the popliteal fossa.

CAPSULE SUMMARY   Fibrosarcoma

General Considerations

- Lesion presents as two types: medullary (or central) and periosteal.
- Most arise de novo; some may complicate previous benign osseous disorders (Paget's, fibrous dysplasia, etc.).

Incidence

- Represents 2% of all primary malignant bone tumors.

Clinical Features

- Most commonly found in the 30- to 50-year age range.
- Chief complaints are localized pain and swelling, with a long duration of symptoms.
- One third of the tumors present initially with pathologic fracture.
- 50% of cases occur about the knee, with the femur, tibia, and humerus being the most common bones involved.
- The metaphysis is the classic location for this tumor.

Pathologic Features

- The only primary malignant bone tumor in which sequestration is found.

- *Lichtenstein's rule:* When any primary malignant-looking lesion in the tibia or femur is not definitively identified, fibrosarcoma should be given prime consideration.
- One of the few primary malignant bone tumors that selectively spreads to the lymphatic system.

Radiologic Features

- Highly destructive medullary lesion, lytic, and eccentrically placed within a long bone.
- Produces the largest soft-tissue mass of all the primary malignant tumors.
- Seldom is there periosteal response or Codman's triangle.

Secondary Fibrosarcoma

- Develops in the interior of the bone at the site of a pre-existing benign bone disorder.
- The most common conditions to undergo change to secondary fibrosarcoma are Paget's disease, fibrous dysplasia, osteomyelitis, postradiation, and bone infarct.
- Malignant degeneration of bone infarction to malignant fibrous histiocytoma (MFH).

Treatment and Prognosis

- Treatment of choice is amputation with joint disarticulation.
- 5-year survival rate is approximately 30%.

CHORDOMA

General Considerations

Chordoma is a rare primary malignant bone tumor that arises from the vestigial remnants of the notochord, which have persisted within the nucleus pulposus of the intervertebral disc, or from aberrant cell rests of notochordal tissue within the vertebral bodies. (1) It is a locally aggressive tumor that grows slowly, invades the surrounding soft tissue by direct extension, and seldom metastasizes. Chordomas have a distinct predilection for the ends of the axial skeleton (sacrococcygeal and spheno-occipital locations represent 85% of cases). (2,3) Unfortunately, this tumor is usually not diagnosed until it is fairly far advanced and has grown to large proportions. Until recently, almost all patients with this disease eventually died of it.

Incidence

Chordomas are relatively infrequent tumors; approximately 1000 cases have been reported, with an estimated overall incidence of 1% of all primary malignant bone tumors. (2) Some specialized major medical referral centers have reported an unusually high incidence of 4%. (2) It makes up at least 40% of sacral tumors. (4)

Clinical Features

Age and Sex Distribution

The greatest incidence of chordoma occurs between the ages of 40 and 70 years. (3) No age group is exempt, and cases have been reported in neonates. (3) Chordoma affects males more commonly than females in a ratio of approximately 2:1. (5)

Signs and Symptoms

Sacrococcygeal Chordoma. Sacrococcygeal chordoma is a slow-growing lesion that may enlarge quite silently over the course of months or even years. Symptoms are caused by the mass effect of a slowly expanding tumor. Initial symptoms are often mild, such as perineal pain and numbness, and the patient may not seek medical care until the tumor is large. Symptoms eventually result from pressure by the tumor on such adjacent extravertebral structures as the intestinal and urinary tracts and emerging nerve roots. (6) Constipation is a common complaint because of local intrapelvic pressure of the tumor mass, while rectal bleeding is rare. (6) Urinary symptoms, such as frequency, urgency, and hesitancy, may be mild at first but later in the disease may become prominent, along with the development of urinary incontinence. As the lesion infiltrates the emerging pelvic nerves (sacral, pudendal, coccygeal), sciatic nerve motor and sensory disturbances may be observed.

Patients with sacrococcygeal chordomas invariably have a presacral tumor mass that can be found on rectal examination. The mass is firm, fixed to the sacrum, and extrarectal. (5) Severe bladder dysfunction occurs late in the course of the disease as a result of either direct pressure from the mass or a neurogenic cord bladder.

Spheno-Occipital Chordoma. The symptoms of spheno-occipital chordoma result from a slowly expanding midline tumor at the base of the brain that produces increased intracranial pressure and encroachment on adjacent structures. This pressure produces early pontine or bulbar symptoms. The most consistent symptom is headache, often present for years. (2) Huvos (2) noted that > 80% of cases will present with headaches. Ocular disturbances are frequent, with complaints of blurred vision or diplopia. In most cases the tumor grows upward to produce cerebral involvement (hemiparesis), cerebellar involvement (ataxia), and cerebellar pontine angle involvement (deafness, dizziness, and tinnitus). (1) If the chordoma extends downward from the sphenoid area, it produces nasal discharge, local pain, and breathing difficulties because of nasal obstruction.

Vertebral Chordoma. Vertebral chordomas are slow-growing lesions that result in extrinsic pressure on nerve roots, the spinal cord, or adjacent extravertebral structures. In the cervical region the tumor often extends anteriorly and produces dysphagia, difficulty in breathing, and, occasionally, a palpable mass. (7) The sensory complaints include numbness in an arm or leg, usually followed by pain. Motor weakness develops in a significant number of patients, but paraplegia or quadriplegia occurs only as a late complication.

Location

Chordomas may arise anywhere in the vertebral column from the region of the spheno-occipital synchondrosis to the tip of the coccyx. (2) An extensive analysis of the reported cases in the literature reveals a predilection toward the extremes of the vertebral column with approximately 50% arising in the sacrococcygeal area (S3–S5), 35% in the clivus of Blumenbach, and only 15% in the true vertebrae. (4,7–9) (Fig. 11-137) The most common vertebral body involved by chordoma is C2 (10); the least involved area is within the thoracic spine. (11) Vertebral involvement is usually anterior, sparing the posterior elements. Intradural lesions are rare. (12)

Pathologic Features

Chordomas originate from remnants of the fetal notochord and on gross inspection range from firm to semiliquid tumors, but they are usually soft, grayish, and semitransparent. (13,14) They are lobulated and well encapsulated in the soft tissues. Discoloration owing to old or recent hemorrhage may be noted. Occasionally, a chordoma contains focal calcification or ossification. Lesions at the base of the skull are small compared with sacral ones, presumably because lesions in the head lead to death before they can become large. (8,10)

In the vertebral column usually more than one vertebral body is involved, either by spread along the posterior longitudinal ligament or by direct extension and destruction of the intervertebral disc. (10) Chordoma is the only primary malignant bone tumor that is known to cross the intervertebral disc and involve adjacent segments. (3,5,10)

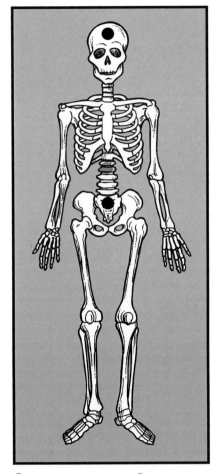

● More common   ● Less common

Figure 11-137   **SKELETAL DISTRIBUTION OF CHORDOMA.**

Microscopically, the lesions may appear highly malignant, with cellular tissue elements composed of small, round, compact cells that show very little vacuolation of the cytoplasm. In other instances grossly distended vacuolated cells are characteristic and are called physaliphorous cells. These cells contain considerable intercellular mucin, indicating a more mature type of tumor. Because of these cellular variations, a chordoma may be incorrectly diagnosed as a fibrosarcoma or chondrosarcoma, particularly because cartilage tissue and calcification can be observed in the histologic section.

Radiologic Features

The radiographic findings in almost all patients, regardless of location of the chordoma, are based on the pattern of bone involvement and the presence of a soft tissue mass. (1,10)

Sacrococcygeal Chordoma

To detect an early lesion it is essential to obtain optimum quality radiographs. These are best taken in the AP position, with a central ray angled 30° cephalad. Lateral radiographs are also helpful in detecting the presence of an anterior soft tissue mass. Tomograms may also be useful when gas and fecal material obscure the sacrum and coccyx.

Some authors (1,2) state that the sacral lesions are usually midline; however, other studies reveal that many sacral chordomas may be eccentrically placed. (15) Irregular lytic areas of bone destruction are seen in up to 80% of cases on plain film examination and at least 90% on CT. (4) The lytic defect grows slowly, assuming an oval or circular shape with scalloped margins. (Fig. 11-138) As the tumor grows it causes cortical expansion and widening of the sacrum in the AP diameter. (Fig. 11-139)

Centrally, the tumor usually contains incomplete septa and calcification. Amorphous calcification of the tumor mass may be noted on plain films in approximately 50% of the cases. (4,5,10) (Fig. 11-140) A higher percentage (approaching 85%) will show matrix calcification with the use of CT. (16) A soft tissue mass is noted on plain film in 78% of the chordoma lesions, and CT scans reveal a soft tissue mass in 93% of the patients. (16)

The differential diagnosis of sacral chordoma lesions must include osteolytic metastatic carcinoma, chondrosarcoma, giant cell tumor, aneurysmal bone cyst, and plasmacytoma. These lesions seldom have a soft tissue mass associated with bone destruction. The most difficult lesion to differentiate is chondrosarcoma because it also produces a large soft tissue mass and frequently calcifies. Biopsy may be the only means of final differentiation.

Spheno-Occipital Chordoma

The radiographic manifestations of cranial chordomas are numerous and varied and may simulate other, more common brain tumors. Most lesions occur in the midline region of the clivus of Blumenbach or adjacent to the sella turcica. Extensive bone destruction of these areas eventually occurs, often showing flocculent calcification in a large soft tissue mass. (Fig. 11-141)

Vertebral Chordoma

Roentgen signs include loss of vertebral bone density, partial or complete pathologic fracture, and often an associated large soft tissue mass. (Fig. 11-142) These radiographic signs are not unique to chordoma because myeloma and metastatic disease quite often present in a similar fashion (10); however, when contiguous vertebral bodies are involved, with destruction of the intervertebral disc, chordoma is the most likely diagnosis, providing that infection has been ruled out. Chordoma is the only primary malignant bone tumor that crosses the joint space. (10)

A radiopaque vertebral body or an ivory vertebra resulting from chordoma may occur anywhere in the spine. The C2 ver-

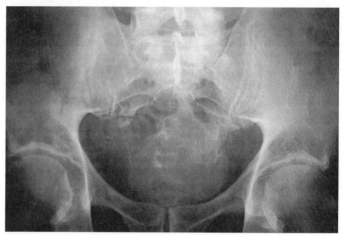

Figure 11-139   SACRAL CHORDOMA. AP Pelvis. Observe the destructive lesion in the distal surface of the sacrum.

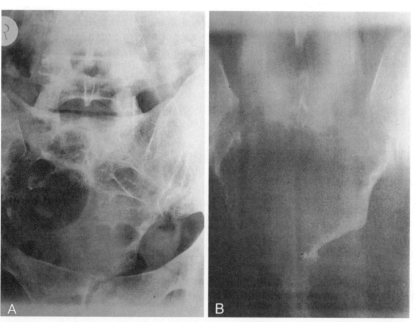

Figure 11-138   CHORDOMA. A. AP Sacrum. Observe the ill-defined loss of bone density in the middle to lower portion of the sacrum. The trabecular patterns appear to be washed out. **B. Tomogram, AP Sacrum.** Note that the tomographic evaluation of the sacral lesion reveals a large expansile chordoma of the sacrum much larger than can be appreciated on the initial plain film. (Courtesy of David P. Thomas, MD, Melbourne, Australia.)

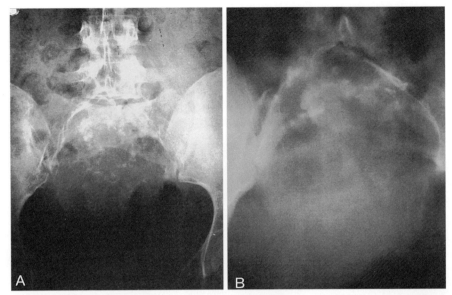

Figure 11-140   SACRAL CHORDOMA. A. AP Sacrum. B. Tomogram, AP Sacrum. Observe the grossly destructive lesion in the midportion of the sacrum. Flocculent calcification is scattered throughout the tumor matrix. *COMMENT:* Amorphous calcification of the tumor mass may be noted on plain films in approximately 50% of chordomas. (Reprinted with permission from **Yochum TR:** *Chordoma.* ACA J Chiro March, 1983.)

tebral body is the most common vertebral body site to be involved, with either lytic or blastic lesions. (Fig. 11-143) Owing to the lack of pathognomonic findings on any imaging modality, diagnosis usually is not made before biopsy. (17) (Table 11-18)

Treatment and Prognosis

The treatment for chordomas varies according to location, with surgical resection being the only hope for permanent cure. (5) Overall, irrespective of location, the median survival rate after diagnosis is approximately 6.3 years. (18) The sacrococcygeal lesions are most amenable to resection; however, historically, resection above the S2 segment has been avoided for fear of denervation of the anorectal and urogenital structures. Because of this surgical rule, many lesions were inadequately removed, and re-currence rates were extremely high. Reoccurrence will usually occur within the first 2 years of resection. (19) Studies have reported on consequences of extensive surgical sacral resections, including sacral nerve roots, and have indicated that the extensive resections are tolerated reasonably well months and years later by the patients. (20,21) Gunterberg et al. (20) reported that if just the upper half of the body of the S1 vertebra remains bilaterally, the pelvic girdle retains sufficient strength to permit standing and will not lead to collapse of the bones of the pelvis.

The treatment of intracranial chordomas is quite discouraging because the operative mortality rate is high and complete resection is rarely attainable. (2) The same is also true for the vertebral body lesions. Irradiation has been the most commonly employed treatment for clivus and vertebral body lesions; however, recently proton beam irradiation has shown to improve the prognostic outcome of any lesion that has undergone incomplete resection. (22,23)

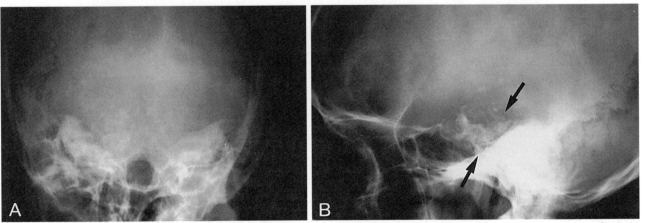

Figure 11-141   SPHENO-OCCIPITAL CHORDOMA. A. AP Towne's Projection. B. Lateral Skull. Observe the extensive destruction in the area of the clivus. Considerable flocculent calcification is present within the destructive soft tissue mass (*arrows*).

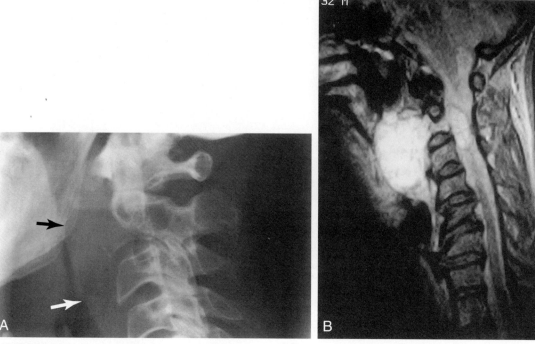

Figure 11-142 **CHORDOMA: C2. A. Lateral Upper Cervical Spine.** Observe the subtle osteolytic destruction of the vertebral body and proximal lamina of C2. The retropharyngeal interspace has been dramatically increased with the presence of a soft tissue mass (*arrows*). **B. T2-Weighted MRI, Sagittal Cervical Spine.** Observe the destruction of the C2 vertebral body with a large extension of the tumor mass to the anterior soft tissue planes at the C2–C4 levels. *COMMENT:* Approximately 50% of chordomas occur in the sacrococcygeal area, 35% in the clivus, and 15% in the spine. The most common vertebral body involved by chordoma is C2. (Reprinted with permission from **JNMS**, Vol. 5, No. 3, Fall 1997. Courtesy of Stephen F. Brown, DC, Dunmore, Pennsylvania.)

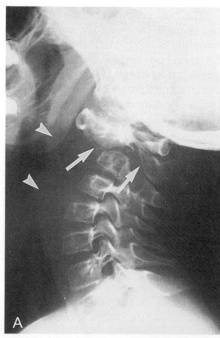

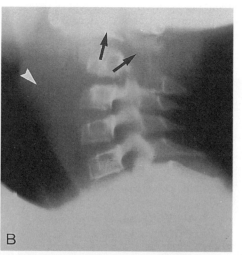

Figure 11-143 **CERVICAL CHORDOMA. A. Lateral Cervical Spine. B. Tomogram, Lateral Cervical Spine.** Note that there is nearly complete collapse of the C2 vertebral body, the neural arch, and the spinous process (*arrows*). Extension of this neoplastic process has created a large soft tissue mass, increasing the retropharyngeal interspace anterior to C2 and C3 (*arrowheads*). *COMMENT:* Vertebral chordomas represent 15% of all chordomas, with the vertebral body of C2 being the most common site. Approximately 50% of chordomas arise in the sacrococcygeal area, and 35% in the clivus of Blumenbach.

The main malignant potentials of chordoma lie in its critical locations adjacent to vital structures, its locally aggressive nature, and its extremely high recurrence rate. The prognosis for cranial chordomas is poor; they are usually fatal within 3 years of the initial diagnosis. The cranial chordomas with considerable cartilaginous calcified elements have a much better prognosis than other chordomas. Vertebral chordomas also carry a poor prognosis, with most patients succumbing to the disease within 3 years. The prognosis for sacrococcygeal chordomas is somewhat better, with 8.7% of patients surviving 5 years later. (1,10) It has been suggested that sacral chordomas affecting children are more aggressive than those affecting adults, resulting in an increased rate of morbidity in children. (24)

Table 11-18	Features of Chordoma	
Age		Expansion
50 years old		Septated
Location		Scalloped margins
Sacrococcygeal (50%)		Soft tissue mass
Clivus (35%)		Matrix calcification (50%)
Vertebrae (15%)		Ivory vertebra (rarely)
Features		
Majority central		
Lytic destruction		

CAPSULE SUMMARY   Chordoma

General Considerations

- A rare primary malignant bone tumor arising from the vestigial remnants of the notochord.
- Locally aggressive, with a slow growth rate.
- A distinct predilection for the ends of the axial skeleton, specifically, the sacrococcygeal and spheno-occipital regions.

Incidence

- A rare primary malignant bone tumor with an overall incidence of 1%.

Clinical Features

- *Sacrococcygeal chordoma:* Early on, the lesion may be clinically silent; later, as the tumor expands, localized pain with pressure symptoms from the bladder and rectum are common.
- *Spheno-occipital chordoma*
  The most consistent symptom is headaches, often present for years.
  Pressure from the enlarging midline mass may create ocular disturbances, increased intracranial pressure, ataxia, deafness, and tinnitus.
- Vertebral chordoma
  In the cervical spine, dysphagia is a common presenting symptom.
  Sensory complaints include numbness in an arm or leg, usually followed by pain.
  Motor weakness may occur, with vertebral body collapse, creating paraplegia or quadriplegia as a late complication.
- *Location:* 50% arise in the sacrococcygeal area; 35% in the clivus of Blumenbach; 15% in the true vertebrae, with the C2 body being the most common site.

Pathologic Features

- A lobulated, well-encapsulated mass is found on gross inspection.
- Most sacral lesions are not midline.
- In the spine, usually more than one vertebral body is involved.
- The only primary malignant bone tumor that is known to cross the intervertebral disc, involving adjacent spinal segments.
- Microscopically, grossly distended vacuolated cells are characteristic and are called physaliphorous cells.

Radiologic Features

- Lytic destruction, along with a soft tissue mass, is the most common roentgen sign. This destruction occurs in the sacral or base of skull area.
- 50% of the tumors show amorphous calcification on plain films, 70% with CT scans.
- Rarely, a spinal lesion can present as a solitary ivory vertebra.

Treatment and Prognosis

- Treatment varies according to location.
- Sacrococcygeal lesions are most amenable to resection.
- Treatment for intracranial chordomas is discouraging because operative mortality is high.
- Radiation therapy is the most commonly employed treatment for clival and vertebral body lesions.
- The prognosis for intracranial and vertebral lesions is poor, with most patients dying within 3 years of the initial diagnosis.
- The 5-year survival for sacrococcygeal chordomas is 8.7%.

NON-HODGKIN'S LYMPHOMA OF BONE (RETICULUM CELL SARCOMA)

General Considerations

Reticulum cell sarcoma is currently referred to as non-Hodgkin's lymphoma of bone. Older terms for the same entity are reticulosarcoma, lymphosarcoma, and round cell sarcoma. Reticulum cell sarcoma, or non-Hodgkin's lymphoma, is a rare, extranodal lymphoma histologically identical with others arising in lymphoid or soft tissues but presenting initially as a localized solitary bone lesion. (1) In 1939, Parker and Jackson (2) presented the first group of 17 cases of primary reticulum cell bone sarcoma, establishing it as a distinct clinical entity separate from the generalized form of this disease.

Incidence

Within the perspective of malignancy arising from lymphoid tissue, non-Hodgkin's lymphoma is the most common type; however, overall this tumor is rare. (3) It constitutes only 3–4% of all primary malignant bone tumors and 2.5% of all bone tumors. (4,5) The skeletal system may be secondarily involved in about 30% of malignant lymphomas. (6)

Clinical Features

Age and Sex Distribution

The majority of patients are between 20 and 40 years of age; however, a significant number of cases are recorded from 40 to 50 years of age. (4) At least 50% of the cases occur before the age of 40. (4) Most authorities show a 2:1 male preponderance.

Signs and Symptoms

Localized pain of an intermittent nature is present in almost all patients. (7) The nature of the pain is dull and aching and it is not relieved by rest. (8) One of the most striking clinical features of non-Hodgkin's lymphoma of bone is the general well-being of the patient. (2) In no other bone sarcoma is the contrast between the comparative well-being of the patient and the size of the lesion so marked. (2) More than 50% of the patients report having minor symptoms related to the lesion for > 1 year. (1) A palpable mass or soft tissue swelling is also found in many cases. (7)

Location

The femur, tibia, and humerus are the most frequently affected bones. Approximately 40% of the tumors occur around the knee. Other involved sites are pelvic bones, ribs, scapulae, and vertebrae. Most lesions are diaphyseal in location or affect the metaphysis adjacent to the diaphysis.

Pathologic Features

Upon gross examination, the tumor is generally firm but often friable tissue that is grayish white or white. Necrosis and hemorrhage are frequently present. Histologically, the tumor tissue is composed of cells that contain a fairly large ovoid or spherical single nucleus (round cell) with nucleoli often present. The cytoplasm may be sparse, and mitotic figures are commonly observed. The intercellular stroma is present in varying amounts, but in a typical lesion delicate strands of reticulum may be seen around tumor cells by using special stains. Definitive histologic differentiation of non-Hodgkin's lymphoma of bone from other lymphomas is difficult. (9)

Radiologic Features

Classically, the lesion begins in the medullary bone (bone marrow) as a permeative lytic process. (Fig. 11-144) As the tumor enlarges, patchy areas of bone destruction spread to affect the adjacent cortical bone. Periosteal response is minimal and, if present, assumes a *laminated pattern*. Midshaft lesions usually break the cortex at a later stage than do metaphyseal tumors. By the time the cortex is disrupted, the medullary lesion becomes quite large and is easily observed. (Fig. 11-145) In the later stages of the destructive process, a soft tissue mass can be demonstrated, a

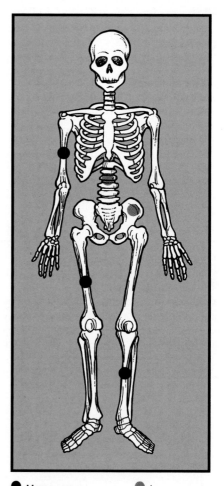

● More common　● Less common

Figure 11-144　**SKELETAL DISTRIBUTION OF NON-HODGKIN'S LYMPHOMA OF BONE (RETICULUM CELL SARCOMA).**

sequel of direct extension of tumor through cortex and periosteum. (10,11) This lytic presentation may be confused with another round cell tumor, Ewing's sarcoma; however, the periosteal reactions are much less prominent, and the patients tend to be older in non-Hodgkin's lymphoma of bone. (Fig. 11-146)

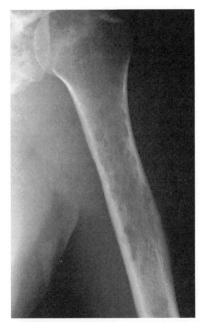

Figure 11-145 **NON-HODGKIN'S LYMPHOMA. Humerus.** Observe the multiple permeative lesions in the medullary portion of the diaphysis of the humerus. *COMMENT:* These lesions simulate the destructive appearance in multiple myeloma. Reticulum cell sarcoma, multiple myeloma, and Ewing's sarcoma are round cell tumors, and their patterns of destruction are often similar.

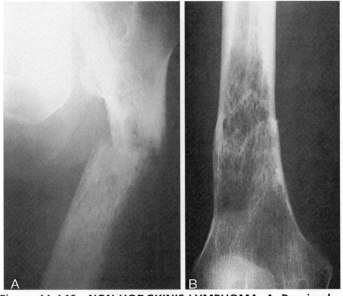

Figure 11-146 **NON-HODGKIN'S LYMPHOMA. A. Proximal Femur.** Note the extensive permeative destruction around the proximal diaphysis of the femur. Destruction of the cortices and pathologic fracture are noted. **B. Distal Femur.** Observe the permeative lesions affecting the distal diaphysis and metaphysis of the femur.

Pathologic fracture is common and may be the initial complaint. (Fig. 11-147) It occurs more frequently in this disease than with any other primary malignant bone tumor because the symptoms are so mild and the lesions are of such long duration. (12) Occasionally, the lesions may be sclerotic in presentation, mimicking an osteoblastic metastatic process. (13) Spinal involvement, including the sacrum, may cause vertebral collapse and destruction indistinguishable from metastatic disease or solitary plasmacytoma. (4,13) (Table 11-19) CT scanning will similarly reveal the osteosclerotic, osteolytic or mixed patterns during examination. (14)

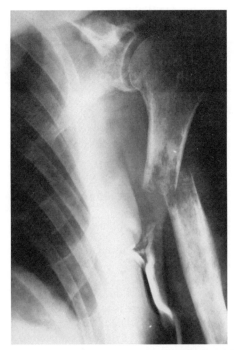

Figure 11-147 **NON-HODGKIN'S LYMPHOMA: PATHOLOGIC FRACTURE. Humerus.** Observe the pathologic fracture through the lytic destructive lesions of reticulum cell sarcoma in the proximal humerus of this 34-year-old female patient.

Table 11-19	Features of Non-Hodgkin's Lymphoma of Bone (Reticulum Cell Sarcoma)
Age	
20–40 years	
Males 2:1	
Remarkably asymptomatic	
Location	
Long bones	
Pelvis	
Ribs	
Features	
Metaphyseal, diaphyseal	
Minimal periosteal response	
Moth-eaten destruction	
Cortical disruption	
Pathologic fracture	
Soft tissue mass	

Treatment and Prognosis

The treatment of choice for primary non-Hodgkin's lymphoma of bone is radiation therapy and adjuvant chemotherapy; however, there is no substantial evidence that this combined therapy is more beneficial than isolated therapies of radiation and/or chemotherapy alone. (1,7) The prognosis for this tumor is better than that for the majority of the primary malignant bone tumors. The 5-year survival rate is approximately 48%, whereas the 10-year survival rate is 33%. (13) It is currently believed that these prognostic values are gradually increasing owing to new drug interventions in the treatment of this disease. (3) It is important to note that CT follow-up examinations will often not become negative for a period of > 1 year after treatment. (14,15)

CAPSULE SUMMARY
Non-Hodgkin's Lymphoma

General Considerations

- Also known as reticulum cell sarcoma of bone.
- A rare extranodal lymphoma presenting initially as a localized solitary bone lesion.

Incidence

- Represents only 3–4% of all primary malignant bone tumors.

Clinical Features

- 20–40 years of age is the usual range; at least 50% of the cases occur before age 40.
- Male preponderance is 2:1.
- There is localized pain of an intermittent nature.
- A striking clinical feature is the contrast between the apparent well-being of the patient and the size of the lesion.
- > 50% of patients report symptoms related to the lesion for > 1 year.
- The femur, tibia, and humerus are the most frequently affected bones.

Pathologic Features

- Histologically, the tumor tissue is composed of cells that contain a fairly large, ovoid or spheroid single nucleus (round cell).
- One of the round cell tumors, along with Ewing's sarcoma and multiple myeloma.

Radiologic Features

- A permeative medullary destruction within the diaphysis or metaphysis of a long tubular bone represents the classic location.
- Minimal laminated periosteal response may occur.
- Development of a well-defined soft tissue mass.
- Differential diagnosis includes Ewing's sarcoma, which may be done by age and the degree of periosteal response, which is greater in Ewing's sarcoma.
- Pathologic fracture is found more frequently in this disease than with any other primary malignant bone tumor.

Treatment and Prognosis

- Radiation therapy, with adjuvant chemotherapy, is the treatment of choice.
- 5-year survival rate is approximately 48%.

HODGKIN'S LYMPHOMA OF BONE

General Considerations

Hodgkin's lymphoma of bone may occur as a secondary manifestation of systemic Hodgkin's lymphoma (chest, liver, spleen, and nodes) or, rarely, as a primary bone lesion in the absence of nodal involvement. (1,2) Pain is the most common initial symptom; however, some clinically silent lesions exist and the majority of patients have other non-osseous lesions. (3) The lytic lesions are usually more symptomatic than the sclerotic ones. (4) Neurological signs may accompany spinal lesions, usually resulting from vertebral collapse and spinal cord compression. (5) Many patients report initial pain and intensification of existent pain after alcohol consumption. (6,7) Diagnosis is often difficult; however, immunohistochemical staining techniques of the involved lesions have been shown to aid in the diagnosis. (3) The prognosis of this condition has been good within the last 10 years with appropriate chemotherapeutic agents. (3,8)

Location

The primary site of skeletal involvement in Hodgkin's lymphoma is the vertebral body. The lower thoracic and upper lumbar spine is the target region. (5,9) Other bones may be involved, such as

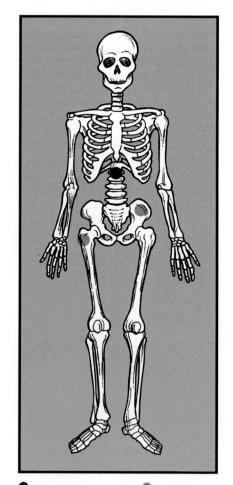

● More common   ● Less common

Figure 11-148 **SKELETAL DISTRIBUTION OF HODGKIN'S LYMPHOMA OF BONE.**

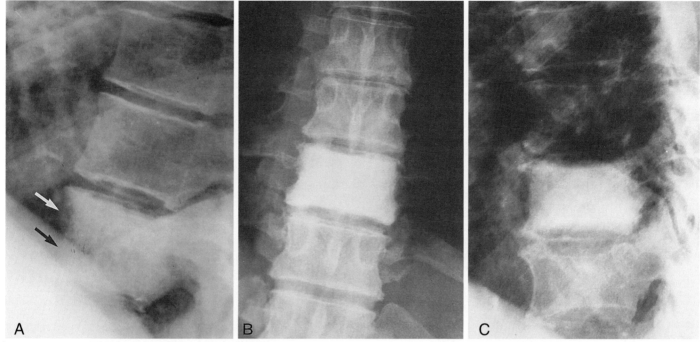

Figure 11-149 HODGKIN'S LYMPHOMA OF BONE: IVORY VERTEBRA. A. Lateral Thoracic Spine. Observe the ivory vertebra at the T12 level in this 34-year-old female who presented with an 11-year history of Hodgkin's lymphoma. There is scalloping of the anterior vertebral body (*arrows*). **B. AP Thoracic Spine. C. Lateral Thoracic Spine.** Observe the diffuse radiopacity throughout the entire vertebral body of T9 (ivory vertebra). No anterior vertebral scalloping is present in this case. *COMMENT:* The anterior and lateral scalloping of the vertebral body is characteristic in Hodgkin's lymphoma of the spine. When this radiographic sign is present in an ivory vertebra, it inevitably eliminates Paget's disease and osteoblastic metastatic disease from the differential diagnosis. (Pane A courtesy of Paul E. Siebert, MD, Denver, Colorado. Panels B and C courtesy of Steven P. Brownstein, MD, Springfield, New Jersey.)

the innominate, scapula, sternum, ribs, and femur. (Fig. 11-148) Between 10% and 20% of patients with Hodgkin's lymphoma develop skeletal disease.

Radiologic Features

Radiographically, most lesions are osteolytic (75%); sclerotic lesions also occur (15%), and mixed destruction with a periosteal response occurs in 10% of patients. (10) Polyostotic lesions are the case in two thirds of the patients. (11) With spinal involvement, scalloping of the anterior or lateral aspects of the vertebral body occurs. (11) Occasionally, a pronounced sclerotic reaction creates an ivory vertebra. (9,12) (Fig. 11-149) In the tubular bones, lytic destruction predominates, with both medullary and cortical destruction. An exuberant periosteal response may occur as the cortex is compromised.

The treatment and prognosis of Hodgkin's lymphoma is directly related to the stage of the disease at discovery. Radiation coupled with chemotherapy offers the most effective form of therapy. Previous 5-year survival rates have generally been 10%; however, with early effective treatment the current 5-year survival rate approaches 80%. (13)

SYNOVIAL SARCOMA

General Considerations

Synovial sarcoma (synovioma) is a mesenchymal sarcoma with a histologic pattern that in varying degrees mimics synovial tissue.

Synovioma is a relatively uncommon neoplasm that is predominantly observed in the 30- to 50-year age range. No sex predilection exists. Clinically, pain and a soft tissue mass at the site of the tumor are the most common complaints. A clinical impression of monoarticular arthritis may be gained. The lower limbs are more often involved, with the knee, hip, and ankle being the most common sites. (1) (Fig. 11-150) Other areas, such as the wrist, elbow, and feet, have been documented. (Fig. 11-151) The lesion is invariably solitary. Synovial sarcoma is the only primary malignant tumor that is in direct anatomic relationship with the joint surface, bursae, or tendon sheaths. Rarely, synovial sarcoma can occur in the midshaft area of a long bone as a result of dissection of synovial tissue down the tendon sheaths. (2)

Radiologic Features

Synovioma appears as a nodular soft tissue mass near a joint, averaging 7 cm in diameter. (Fig. 11-152) Calcification occurs in approximately one third of the patients, appearing as fine, granular specks within the rounded soft tissue mass. (3) (Figs. 11-153 and 11-154) Secondary bone destruction is uncommon, occurring in only 10% of cases. (3) Bony destruction takes the form of erosive changes primarily from extrinsic pressure. When actual bone invasion occurs, the margins of the lesion are ragged and ill-defined, usually having a wide zone of transition with no surrounding sclerosis or thickening. (3) MRI shows differing results, depending on size. Lesions < 5 cm often demonstrate a non-aggressive nature with homogenous signal intensity and circumscribed margins, whereas larger lesions show an inhomo-

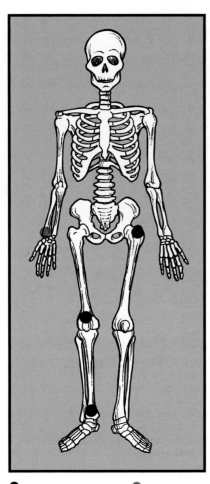

● More common   ● Less common

Figure 11-150 **SKELETAL DISTRIBUTION OF SYNOVIAL SARCOMA.**

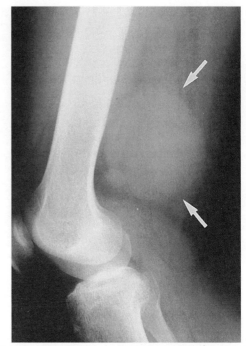

Figure 11-152 **SYNOVIAL SARCOMA. Lateral Knee.** Note the well-defined spherical soft tissue mass (*arrows*) posterior to the distal femur. This represents a synovial sarcoma in one of its more common locations. (Courtesy of C. H. Quay, MD, Melbourne, Australia.)

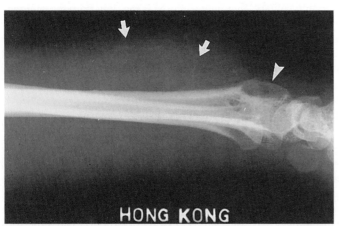

Figure 11-151 **SYNOVIAL SARCOMA. Wrist.** Note the rather large soft tissue mass on the dorsal surface of the forearm. Scattered throughout the soft tissue mass are faint linear calcifications (*arrows*). There is a lytic destructive lesion associated with this synovial sarcoma in the distal surface of the radius (*arrowhead*). (Courtesy of C. H. Quay, MD, Melbourne, Australia.)

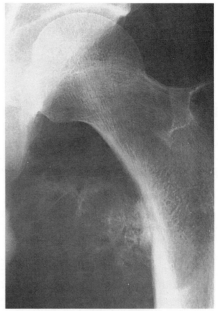

Figure 11-153 **SYNOVIAL SARCOMA. Proximal Femur.** Note the extensive destruction of the lesser trochanter. A soft tissue mass with scattered flocculent calcification is seen adjacent to the lesser trochanter. *COMMENT:* This case is somewhat interesting in that there is secondary bone destruction of the lesser trochanter and cortex of the femoral neck. Secondary bone destruction is uncommon in synovial sarcoma, occurring in only 10% of cases. The secondary destruction occurs as a result of erosion of bone from extrinsic pressure.

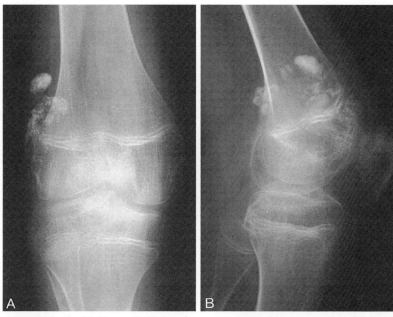

Figure 11-154 **SYNOVIAL SARCOMA. A. AP Knee. B. Lateral Knee.** Observe the nodular calcifications in the lateral portion of the soft tissues of the knee. There is no evidence of associated bone erosion in this patient. *COMMENT:* One third of patients with synovial sarcoma demonstrate fine, granular specks of calcification within the soft tissue mass.

geneous septated mass with infiltrative margins close to a joint, tendon, or bursae. (4,5)

The treatment of choice is usually surgical excision, followed by a course of irradiation (5000 R). (2) The 5-year survival rate for lower extremity lesions is 43%, and for upper extremity synoviomas, 31%. (6,7) It has been proposed that larger lesions at the time of diagnosis predispose the patient to a worse prognosis. (8) Metastasis of the lesions will occur in approximately 33% of patients. (8) The lungs, lymph nodes, and bone are the common sites of metastasis. (9)

ADAMANTINOMA

General Considerations

Adamantinoma is a rare primary malignant bone tumor with a poorly understood histogenesis. (1) It has also been referred to as malignant angioblastoma, dermal inclusion tumor, ameloblastoma, primary epidermoid carcinoma of bone, and carcinoma sarcomatodes. (2) The pathogenesis is controversial regarding whether this tumor is epithelial or mesodermal in origin. A likely explanation is that the neoplasms develop from misplaced embryonal epithelium of the enamel germ cells of the teeth, which may be present as epithelial cell rests. (3) It is impossible to definitively determine the tumor's true origin histologically at this time because there is an overlap of the epithelial and the mesodermal hypotheses. (4)

Incidence

Approximately 165 cases have been reported in the literature, with all but 18 located in the tibia. (5) (Fig. 11-155) Other bones

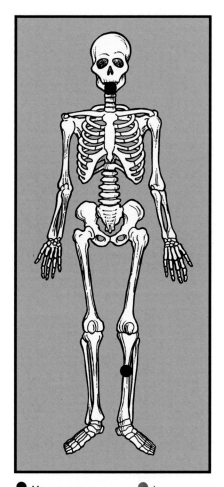

● More common ● Less common

Figure 11-155 **SKELETAL DISTRIBUTION OF ADAMANTINOMA.**

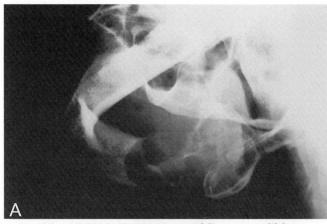

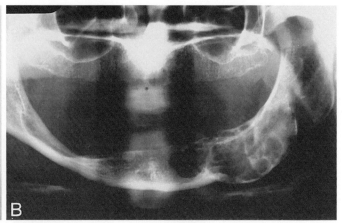

Figure 11-156 ADAMANTINOMA. A. Oblique Mandible. B. Panorex Tomogram, Mandible. Observe the osteolytic, grossly expansile lesion of the mandible. A multichambered or bubbly lesion is present. (Courtesy of Leonard B. Welsh, DC, Tamworth, New South Wales, Australia.)

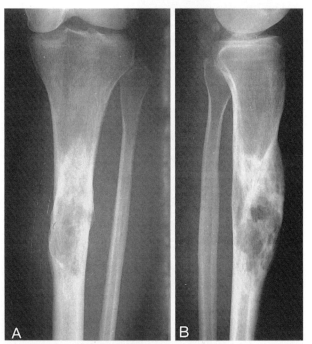

Figure 11-157 ADAMANTINOMA. A. AP Tibia. B. Lateral Tibia. Note the highly destructive lesion in the mid-diaphysis of the tibia. Observe the expansion of bone, with lytic and scalloped margins of the cortical surfaces. (Courtesy of Peter Johnston, MD, Melbourne, Australia.)

affected are the jaw, ulna, humerus, femur, and fibula. (Fig. 11-156) The mid-diaphysis of the long bones is the location in 75% of cases. (5) (Fig. 11-157) The lesions are extremely rare in the spine. (6) Most patients are between 10 and 40 years of age. (7) Pain with swelling around the growing lesion is the most common presenting symptom.

Radiologic Features

Radiographically, adamantinomas may be difficult to differentiate from other lesions because they can be situated in either the cortex or the medullary space. (1) Cortical lesions may assume a *lytic bone blister appearance*, may appear as *sawtooth loss of cortical bone* with ragged margins, or may present as a *multichambered, bubbly lesion.* (Fig. 11-156) The typical intramedullary lesion is usually one large, circumscribed area of radiolucency with a mottled increase in density scattered throughout the length of the lesion. Less commonly, a reticulated, *honeycombed type of presentation* occurs. Long-standing tumors produce marked cortical thickening and spool-shaped bulges of the outer cortex in an *eggshell fashion.* (8) (Fig. 11-157) Gradual expansion of bone with eventual cortical disruption and the development of a soft tissue mass occurs. Periosteal response is minimal and, if present, is usually of the laminated variety.

The most difficult and almost indistinguishable differential diagnosis is fibrous dysplasia, though the presence of periosteal response, moth-eaten destruction, no bowing or ground glass appearance, and younger age should allow correct diagnosis. (9,10) Special imaging procedures such as MRI are becoming more useful in differentiation and diagnosis of adamantinomas. (1,11)

The treatment of choice is amputation which has a cure rate of > 90%; however, en bloc resections have been recently shown to salvage the limb in up to 84% of cases with survival rates as high as 87% over 10 years. (12) Unfortunately, complications related to limb reconstruction is high in most of these cases. (12)

PRIMARY QUASI-MALIGNANT BONE TUMOR

GIANT CELL TUMOR

General Considerations

Giant cell tumor is a neoplasm that originates from non-bone-forming supportive connective tissue of the marrow. This highly vascular lesion is composed of spindle-shaped stromal cells interspersed among multinucleated giant cells. In 1818 Sir Astley Cooper (1) was the first to coin the term *giant cell tumor.* Since his original description, a host of bone lesions have fallen under the umbrella of giant cell tumor. Around 1940 Jaffe et al. (2) started the in-depth naming of the giant cell tumor variants. The first to be identified was pigmented villonodular synovitis, followed by benign chondroblastoma, non-osteogenic fibroma, chondromyxoid fibroma, and aneurysmal bone cyst. (3–7) All of these lesions were considered giant cell tumor variants.

Jaffe (8) classifies this tumor as being quasi-malignant because approximately 20% of the lesions are malignant, and 80% are benign. Stewart (9) in 1922 introduced the term *osteoclastoma* into the British orthopedic literature, where it has received wide and continued use.

Incidence

Giant cell tumor of bone is a relatively common primary neoplasm accounting for 5–8% of all primary malignant bone tumors (10) and 15% of all primary benign bone tumors. (11)

Clinical Features

Age and Sex Distribution

The incidence of all types of giant cell tumors is approximately the same in men and women; however, benign tumors predominate in female patients in a proportion of 3:2, the malignant tumors show a predilection for male patients in a ratio of 3:1. (12) The usual age range is 20–40 years; occurrence at other ages is exceptional. Recent research has noted an association with the formation of giant cell tumor in patients with Paget's disease occurring under the age of 50. (13,14) This association has been supported in 37 cases. (13)

Signs and Symptoms

The chief complaint is pain of an intermittent, aching nature, with localized swelling and tenderness. Often, there is restricted movement of the involved adjacent joint. No physical signs or symptoms are characteristic of this tumor, which occasionally can grow to enormous size and remain clinically silent. Pathologic fracture often may be the precipitating factor to symptom production.

Location

The most common sites are the distal femur, proximal tibia, distal radius, and proximal humerus, in decreasing order of incidence. (15) (Fig. 11-158) Involvement of the distal radius carries a more serious prognosis because most of these lesions are malignant. (Fig. 11-159) The sacrum is the most common spinal site, representing 8% of cases. (12) Giant cell tumor is the most common benign tumor of the sacrum. (15) (Figs. 11-160 and 11-161) Spinal sites above the sacrum are rare. Other infrequent sites are the calcaneus, innominate, rib, carpal bones, and patella. (16–20) (Fig. 11-162)

Patellar neoplastic disease is uncommon; however, most patellar tumors are benign (73%) and are cartilaginous in origin (chondroblastomas or enchondromas) or giant cell tumors. (21) Giant cell tumor is the most common neoplasm of the patella. (22)

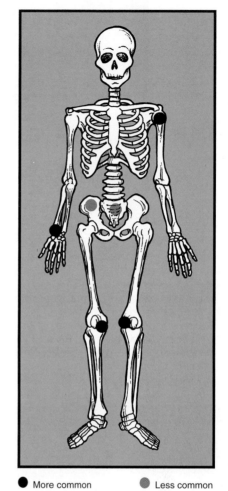

● More common   ● Less common

Figure 11-158   **SKELETAL DISTRIBUTION OF GIANT CELL TUMOR.**

Rarely, metastatic disease from any origin may affect the patella; this is the most common cause for malignancy in the patella. Multifocal giant cell tumors have been reported but are rare. (23) It is always important to rule out multiple brown tumors of hyperparathyroidism when polyostotic lesions are encountered.

This tumor usually begins in the metaphyseal end of a long bone in or adjacent to the ossified epiphyseal line. It usually extends to the end of a long bone, abutting its joint surface, leaving the lesion subarticular. (Fig. 11-163). The lesion is limited to the metaphysis in only 1% of cases. (24)

Pathologic Features

Pathologically, a typical lesion consists of varying amounts of connective tissue stromal cells and giant cells. The stromal cells vary in appearance, being either plump, spindle shaped, or ovoid, generally with large nuclei. The giant cells are multinucleated, with a tendency for the nuclei to be in the center of the cell. The proportion of stromal cells to giant cells determines whether the lesion has a benign or malignant propensity. Many giant cells are found in the most benign lesions, and few or no giant cells in truly malignant lesions. The spindle cell stroma of the giant cell tumors requires the most meticulous attention, for it is on the

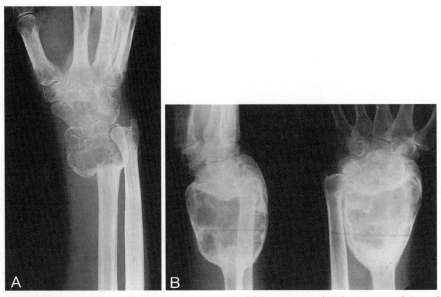

Figure 11-159   GIANT CELL TUMOR: DISTAL RADIUS.
A. Oblique Wrist. Observe the subarticular radiolucent expansile lesion of the entire distal surface of the radius, with a pathologic fracture. Of incidental notation is spotty disuse osteoporosis scattered throughout the carpal bones and the bases of the visualized metacarpals. **B. PA and Lateral Wrist.** Observe the grossly expansile, heavily trabeculated or soap bubble geographic lesion involving the subarticular surface of the distal radius. Owing to the extensive bone expansion, there is posterior and lateral displacement of the ulna. *COMMENT:* Giant cell tumor involving the distal radius carries a sinister prognosis because most of these lesions are malignant.

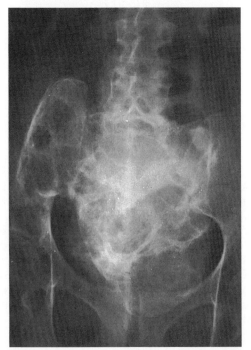

Figure 11-160   **GIANT CELL TUMOR. AP Sacrum.** Observe the grossly expansile, geographic lesion involving the entire sacrum. This giant cell tumor was found in an 18-year-old male. Note that the peripheral margins of the majority of this lesion are well defined; however, this is a malignant giant cell tumor. *COMMENT:* Approximately 80% of giant cell tumors are benign and 20% are malignant. It is impossible to predict the histologic nature of giant cell tumors from a radiograph, even when they appear to fill the criteria for benign lesions. The only means for appropriate diagnosis is biopsy. (Courtesy of William E. Litterer, DC, DACBR, Fellow, ACCR, Elizabeth, New Jersey.)

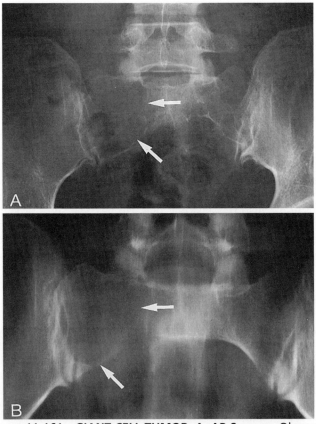

Figure 11-161   **GIANT CELL TUMOR. A. AP Sacrum.** Observe the eccentric geographic lesion present within the sacral ala (*arrows*) without matrix calcification. **B. Tomogram, AP Sacrum.** Note that tomographic evaluation of the sacrum demonstrates a large geographic area of destruction limited to the sacral ala and not affecting the sacroiliac joint (*arrows*). (Courtesy of Allan J. Warrener, DC, Melbourne, Australia.)

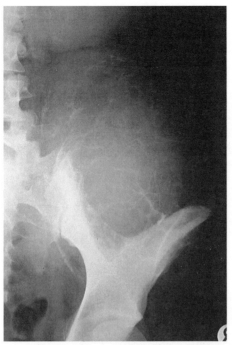

Figure 11-162 **GIANT CELL TUMOR. Ilium.** Observe the grossly expansile lytic lesion of the middle and posterior surfaces of the ilium. Note also the soap bubble matrix in this large malignant giant cell tumor of the ilium.

regularity or anaplasia in these cells that the clinical behavior of the tumor hinges.

Giant cells are ubiquitous; they may be present in any lesion of bone, benign, malignant, or reactive. Their presence must be gauged in the context of other associated findings. The mere presence of occasional or even numerous giant cells does not permit tumor identification or classification.

Radiologic Features

The radiographic appearance of giant cell tumor is characteristic. It is an eccentric, metaphyseal, multilobed radiolucent lesion of a long bone. (25) In an adult, it is located adjacent to the articular surface of the bone (subarticular). (Fig. 11-164) It is also subarticular in flat bones, occurring near the sacroiliac joint and acetabulum in the innominate. The cortex is thinned and expanded, and the endosteal margins show a wide zone of transition, suggesting a malignant lesion. (25) (Fig. 11-165) The lesion may traverse the entire shaft in a relatively thin bone, such as the fibula or ulna. (Fig. 11-166) A delicate periosteal reaction may develop, independent of infractions of the cortex.

This sharply circumscribed lesion often expands bone, with a rather characteristic soap bubble pattern. (24) (Fig. 11-167) Most cases are purely lytic (60%), and the soap bubble pattern is present in 40% of cases. (24) These bubbles and delineating lines are really reactive trabeculae of bone formed by appositional bone growth and do not actually chamber the lesion because of their peripheral location. Thus the giant cell tumor, removing numerous trabeculae by its neoplastic growth, prompts reinforcement of the remaining trabeculae, resulting in the soap bubble pattern. (Fig. 11-168) If the tumor is very aggressive, a purely

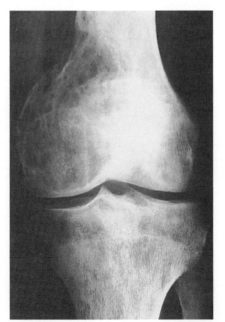

Figure 11-163 **GIANT CELL TUMOR. Distal Femur.** Observe the eccentric lytic destruction of the medial condyle and metaphysis of the distal femur. There is a moderate soap bubble matrix alteration present within the central portion of the lesion. The location of this giant cell tumor is classic, in that it presents eccentrically and at the subarticular surface of the distal femur.

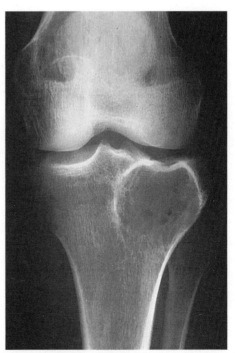

Figure 11-164 **GIANT CELL TUMOR. Proximal Tibia.** Observe the well-defined geographic lesion within the lateral portion of the proximal tibia. This lesion is in its classic subarticular location and is eccentrically placed, typical for a giant cell tumor.

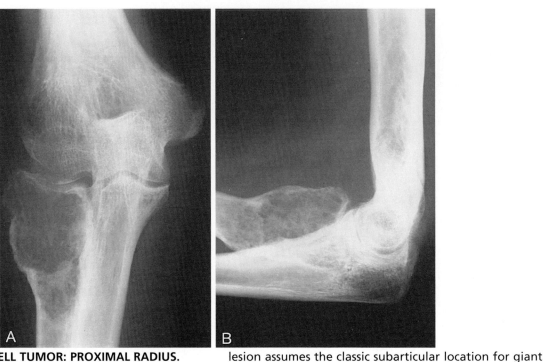

Figure 11-165 **GIANT CELL TUMOR: PROXIMAL RADIUS.**
A. AP Elbow. B. Lateral Elbow. Observe the expansile, geographic lesion within the radial head and metaphysis. This lesion assumes the classic subarticular location for giant cell tumor.

lytic radiolucent lesion will be seen with cortical breakthrough and the development of a soft tissue mass. (Fig. 11-169)

Involvement of flat bones, such as the ilium, rib, and sacrum, demonstrate the same roentgen appearance of an expanding, radiolucent, soap bubble lesion. Spinal involvement above the sacrum with expansion and lytic destruction of a vertebral body or neural arch is usually called an osteoblastoma or ABC radiographically, before biopsy. The cervical and lumbar spine are the most common sites. (Fig. 11-170) The radiologist alone cannot predict with any accuracy whether the giant cell tumor is benign or malignant. (Fig. 11-171) The approach to definitive diagnosis must be correlated by three means: radiologic, clinical, and histologic. Some of the most benign-appearing lesions have metastasized to distant sites, proving fatal for the patient. (Table 11-20)

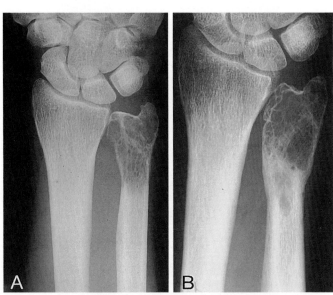

Figure 11-166 **GIANT CELL TUMOR: DISTAL ULNA. A. PA Wrist.** Observe the lytic destructive lesion at the distal subarticular surface of the ulna. The soap bubble appearance is present in the matrix of this lesion. **B. 6-Month Follow-Up, PA Wrist.** Note the extensive expansion of the previously recognized giant cell tumor of the distal ulna. A heavier trabeculation or soap bubble appearance is present within the distal ulna.

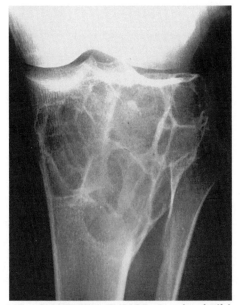

Figure 11-167 **GIANT CELL TUMOR. Proximal Tibia.** Note the grossly expansile, heavily trabeculated, geographic lesion involving the entire subarticular surface of the proximal tibia. (Courtesy of Joseph W. Howe, DC, DACBR, Fellow, ACCR, Los Angeles, California.)

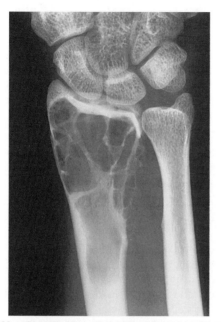

Figure 11-168   GIANT CELL TUMOR, SOAP BUBBLE PATTERN. Distal Radius. Observe the subarticular, expansile, geographic lesion in the distal portion of the radius. This tumor has removed numerous trabeculae by its neo-plastic growth, prompting reinforcement of the remaining trabeculae and rendering a classic soap bubble pattern. *COMMENT:* Giant cell tumors in the distal radius carry a higher incidence of malignancy than giant cell tumors at any other skeletal site.

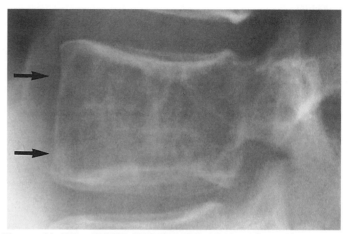

Figure 11-170   GIANT CELL TUMOR. L3 Vertebra. Observe the lytic expansile lesion of the vertebral body and a portion of the pedicle of the L3 vertebra. Note the loss of the anterior concavity of the vertebral body secondary to bony expansion (*arrows*) and the slightly chambered appearance. (Courtesy of Kelvin E. Brinsmead, DC, Kiama, New South Wales, Australia.)

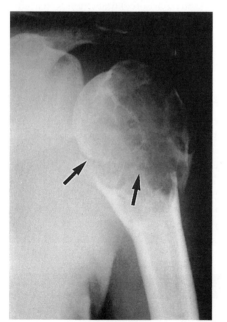

Figure 11-169   PATHOLOGIC FRACTURE IN GIANT CELL TUMOR. Proximal Humerus. Observe the subarticular, expansile giant cell tumor of the proximal humerus. Heavy trabeculation or soap bubble trabecular changes are scattered throughout the lesion. Note the pathologic fracture and cortical offset through the metaphysis (*arrows*).

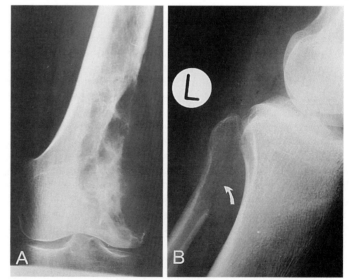

Figure 11-171   MALIGNANT GIANT CELL TUMOR. A. Distal Femur. Observe the gross cortical destruction of the distal femur and the medial condyle. There is an eccentric lytic lesion, with scalloping of the endosteum. This radiographic presentation strongly suggests a malignant giant cell tumor, which was confirmed at biopsy. **B. Proximal Fibula.** Observe the lytic destruction of the subarticular surface of the proximal fibula. There is a permeative pattern of bone destruction scattered throughout the matrix of the tumor, along with a break in the proximal cortex (*arrow*).

Table 11-20	Features of Giant Cell Tumor

Age
 20–40 years
Location
 Distal femur, proximal tibia
 Distal radius
 Proximal humerus
 Sacrum, ilium
Features
 Eccentric
 Metaphyseal–epiphyseal
 Subarticular
 Expansion
 Thin cortex
 Geographic
 Internal septation (soap bubble)

Treatment and Prognosis

It is important to ensure that the giant cell tumor is completely removed the first time surgical intervention is performed. (25) The surgeon must plan an excision to minimize the likelihood of recurrence, while trying to preserve function of the involved limb. It has been suggested that incomplete excision is the primary risk factor for determining the risk of recurrence (26) owing to the contents of the tumor "spilling over" and contaminating nearby tissues. (27) In cases of incomplete excision, follow-up radiation therapy is recommended by some (28,29), whereas others have advocated that radiotherapy is associated with an increased risk of malignant degeneration and thus should be avoided when possible. (30,31) The surgeon contemplating curettage should remember that giant cell tumors tend to invade adjacent structures slowly. The trabeculae that are permeated by the osteoclasts of the tumor will persist for some time after involvement; the tumor, therefore, extends beyond the inner ridge of trabeculae.

Recurrence rates of 12–50% have been reported after curettage combined with liquid nitrogen freezing, bone packing, or grafting. (32) Curettage removes only the contents of the cavity. There is no removal of the contents of the area beyond the cavity that is formed by the reactive remnants of bone, unless a conscious effort is made to curette the ridge of trabeculae forming the outer shell of the cavity. Failure to do so accounts for the high recurrence rate. Sterilization of the cavity by means of phenol or liquid nitrogen is quite effective. (33) The cavity is usually reconstructed with an acrylic cement, which has also shown good results. (34) Complete resection is required occasionally, especially around the knee. Spinal lesions are usually inoperable, leaving radiation therapy as the only option for obtaining a cure. (33)

The prognosis is excellent for the benign giant cell tumor; however, its malignant counterpart carries a poor prognosis with < 10% of cases having a 5-year survival rate (33) resulting from recurrence or metastasis. Although distant metastasis is relatively rare, it has been suggested that the expression of the p53 gene may predispose the patient to this unfortunate event. (35,36) Metastasis has been documented in only 50 cases, primarily affects the lung, and usually occurs within 3 years of surgical resection. (35) More recent studies have suggested that chemotherapy in combination with surgical excision may be of benefit in increasing the survival rates for patients with malignant variants of the tumor. (37)

CAPSULE SUMMARY Giant Cell Tumor

General Considerations

- Sir Astley Cooper in 1818 was the first to use the term giant cell tumor.
- Quasi-malignant tumor: 80% benign and 20% malignant.
- Osteoclastoma is a British term that has been used for giant cell tumor.

Incidence

- Represents 5–8% of all primary malignant bone tumors and 15% of all primary benign bone tumors.

Clinical Features

- Benign tumors predominate in female patients in a proportion of 3:2; the malignant tumors affect males in a ratio of 3:1.
- 20–40 years is the usual age range.
- Localized pain of an aching nature, which often restricts movement of the involved adjacent joint.
- Most common sites of involvement are distal femur, proximal tibia, distal radius, and proximal humerus, in decreasing order of incidence.
- The sacrum is the most common spinal site, representing 8% of cases.
- The most common benign tumor of the sacrum.

Radiologic Features

- Most lesions begin in the metaphysis and subsequently extend to the subarticular location, once the epiphyseal line has closed.
- Characteristic lesion in a long bone is a radiolucent, eccentric metaphyseal defect that extends to a subarticular location.
- Significant bone expansion with the production of a soap bubble appearance is noted.
- Radiologic differentiation of benign versus malignant lesions is not feasible.

Treatment and Prognosis

- Treatment of choice is surgical curettage combined with liquid nitrogen freezing, bone packing, or grafting. Recurrence rates of 12–50% are reported, with recurrence being merely an expression of inadequate removal.
- Spinal lesions are usually inoperable, requiring radiation therapy for cure.
- Prognosis for benign lesions is excellent; only 10% survive 5 years with malignant lesions.

PRIMARY BENIGN BONE TUMORS

SOLITARY OSTEOCHONDROMA

General Considerations

Osteochondroma is a bony exostosis projecting from the external surface of a bone; it usually has a hyaline-lined cartilaginous cap. The first person to describe and clearly illustrate osteochondroma was Sir Astley Cooper, surgeon and anatomist at St. Thomas' and Guy's Hospitals, London, in 1818. (1) When the lesion is seen in a single bone, it is called solitary osteochondroma; if two or three bones are involved, with no familial history, the condition is called multiple osteochondromas; when the tumors are widespread throughout the skeleton, there is usually a familial history and the condition is called hereditary multiple exostosis. The cause is not known, but it is thought that the solitary lesions arise from displaced cartilage from the physis and that hereditary multiple exostoses (HME) represents a congenital dysplasia leading to a tumor-like growth abnormality at the metaphysis.

Incidence

Osteochondroma represents the most common benign skeletal growth or tumor. (2) Including all forms of osteochondroma and HME, it represents 50% of all benign bone neoplasms and 10–15% of all primary bone tumors. (3) These figures could be higher because many lesions go unreported because of their silent nature.

Clinical Features

Age and Sex Distribution

Most osteochondromas are encountered in childhood and adolescence, with 75% of cases occurring before the age of 20. (4) Often, the lesions are not detected until later in life, when the patient is radiographed for other reasons. A 2:1 male predominance has been noted. (4)

Signs and Symptoms

Most osteochondromas are asymptomatic unless they disturb surrounding blood vessels or nerves or are large enough to impair adjacent joint function. The most frequent complaint is a hard, painless mass near a joint. Occasionally, a fracture through the stalk of an osteochondroma causes a patient to present with severe pain and swelling. Some patients will present for surgical removal of an osteochondroma for cosmetic purposes, particularly if the mass is large and in a tightly compartmentalized space (hand, foot, forearm). Large spinal osteochondromas have been reported to produce bizarre neurological symptoms from cord compression, sciatica, and scoliosis. (5–7) Rarely, a traumatic popliteal artery pseudo-aneurysm may result from perforation or penetration of a sharply pointed osteochondroma arising from the posterior surface of the femur. (8) A rare case of death has occurred, complicating an odontoid osteochondroma. (9) Huge osteochondromas of the pelvis can produce symptoms of obstructive uropathy. (10)

Pain and rapid growth may indicate malignant degeneration, requiring immediate removal. Complications include fracture (7%), deformity with subsequent loss of motion (23%), vascular injury (7%), neurological compromise (10%), adventitious bursae formation (27%), and mechanical irritation. (11,12)

Location

Osteochondroma can occur in any bone preformed in cartilage. It usually affects the long tubular bones: the femur (34%), humerus (18%), tibia (15%). Other locations include the pelvis (8%), scapula (5%), and ribs (3%). (13) Sporadic cases have been reported in the metacarpal bones, condylar process of the mandible, base of the skull, astragalus (talus), calcaneus, and the spine. (14–18) (Fig. 11-172) Spinal lesions usually are located near the

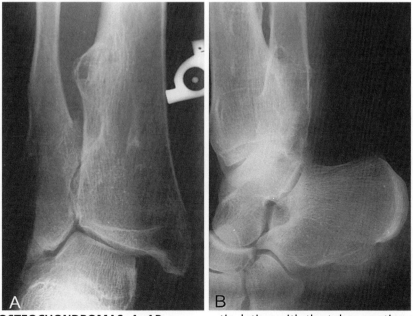

Figure 11-172 **MULTIPLE OSTEOCHONDROMAS. A. AP Ankle.** Observe the metaphyseal broad-based (sessile) osteochondromas affecting the distal tibia and fibula. There is a significant alteration of the angulation of the tibia in its articulation with the talus, creating a tibial–talar slant. **B. Lateral Ankle.** Note the broad-based (sessile) osteochondroma on the plantar surface of the calcaneus.

secondary centers of ossification at the tips of the transverse processes, spinous processes, laminae, and costovertebral joints. (19) Scapular lesions are not uncommon and arise from the inferior angle, superior angle (Luschka's tubercle), and coracoid process. (20) (Fig. 11-173) A rare case of osteochondroma has been documented at the distal clavicle, resulting in shoulder impingement syndrome of the rotator cuff. (21)

Pathologic Features

Grossly, osteochondroma's most common form of presentation is as an exostosis arising from the metaphyseal region of a long bone. There are two types: *sessile* and *pedunculated*. Sessile osteochondroma is characterized by its flat plateau-like stalk producing a broad-based protuberance. Of the two types, this is the least common variety but seen most often in the proximal humerus and scapula. Conversely, pedunculated osteochondroma exhibits a base that has an elongated bony stalk merging continuously with the host bone. The cap of the exostosis is cartilaginous (hyaline) and is often lobulated in its appearance. The knee, hip, and ankle are the most common sites for the pedunculated osteochondroma.

Osteochondromas can vary in size, with some reaching 10 cm. Histologically, the appearance of an actively growing osteochondroma shows foci of actively proliferating cartilage cells that closely resemble the normal epiphyseal growth plate. Consequently, an osteochondroma ceases to grow after closure of the normal epiphyseal growth plates.

Malignant degeneration of a solitary osteochondroma occurs in approximately 1% of cases, in contrast to the 20% rate in the familial form of HME. (22) Most lesions, when they degenerate, transform to chondrosarcoma, but osteosarcoma and fibrosarcoma also occur. The pathologic distinction between an osteochondroma and an exostotic chondrosarcoma is often difficult because most of the chondrosarcomas are low grade, with only subtle malignant histologic features. (23) Patients with malignant degeneration of an osteochondroma average around 30 years of age, whereas the average age of those with chondrosarcoma is about 45. Plain radiographic distinction between these benign and malignant lesions is difficult. The thickness of the cartilaginous cap at the periphery of the tumor may provide a clue to malignancy because chondrosarcomas tend to have thicker cartilage, generally 3 cm or more. (24) The most com-

mon regions to be involved are the pelvis and shoulder girdle. (3,24) A cortical break or a growing soft tissue mass suggests malignancy. (Table 11-21)

Osteochondromas can develop as sequelae of radiation therapy for an unrelated malignant disorder. Most reported cases are included in evaluations of spinal changes after irradiation in childhood, usually for either Wilms' tumor or neuroblastoma, which are two tumors that are more commonly irradiated.

Radiologic Features

The knee (tibia and femur) is the location most commonly involved, with the metaphysis being the common place of origin.

Table 11-21	Features of Osteochondroma Suggesting Malignant Transformation
Clinical	
30 years of age	
Pelvis, shoulder	
< 1% of solitary osteochondromas; 20% in HME	
Increasing pain and mass at site of known osteochondroma	
Chondrosarcoma most common	
Radiologic	
Thick, irregular calcified cap	
Bone destruction	
Soft tissue mass	
Altered appearance on sequential studies	

HME, hereditary multiple exostosis.

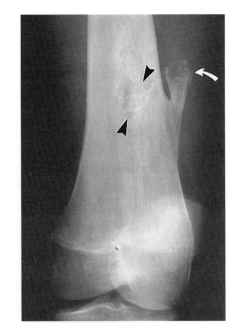

Figure 11-174 **OSTEOCHONDROMA AND NON-OSSIFYING FIBROMA. Distal Femur.** Observe the solitary pedunculated osteochondroma of the metaphysis of the distal femur (*arrow*). In addition, there is a geographic lesion with endosteal scalloping noted in the medullary portion of the distal femur, which represents a non-ossifying fibroma (*arrowheads*). This is a coincidental occurrence of these two benign bone tumors.

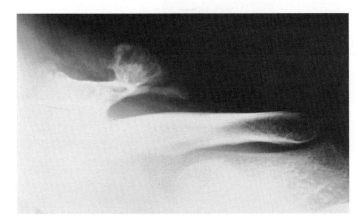

Figure 11-173 **SOLITARY OSTEOCHONDROMA, LUSCHKA'S TUBERCLE. Scapula.** Note the solitary osteochondroma arising from the superior angle of the scapula (Luschka's tubercle). Observe the calcified osteocartilaginous cap.

The pedunculated type has an osteocartilaginous domed cap on a long, slender stalk. (Figs. 11-174 and 11-175) The cartilaginous cap usually shows irregularity and amorphous, spotty calcification, leaving the calcified areas dense and radiopaque. (Figs. 11-176 and 11-177) These exostoses invariably project away from the joint, owing to muscle pull; thus Greenfield (25) used the term *coat hanger exostosis.* (Fig. 11-178) En face visualization of an osteochondroma reveals a dense ring of cortex surrounding the base as it is seen superimposed upon the cartilage cap. (25) (Fig. 11-179)

Malignant transformation should be suspected when a cartilage cap is visualized that is > 2 cm in adults and > 3 cm in children. (12) It is also important to note that the cortex and spongiosa of the osteochondroma blend imperceptibly with the cortex and spongiosa of the host bone. (13) This feature differentiates an osteochondroma from parosteal sarcoma and periosteal chondrosarcoma, which show a *cleavage plane* between the normal bone and the neoplasm. Occasionally, the stalk of a pedunculated osteochondroma may fracture. (Fig. 11-180)

The sessile osteochondroma creates a broad-based exostosis lacking an elongated projection and creating a long, asymmetric widening of the bone. (Fig. 11-181) Amorphous, spotty calcification is lacking. These lesions are found in the metaphyseal–diaphyseal portion of the bone. The proximal humerus, scapula, and proximal femur are the most common sites. Osteochondromas are not found in the epiphyseal end of the bone, but an epiphyseal growth similar to osteochondroma does occur (Trevor's disease). (See Chapter 8.) In the pelvis most osteochondromas occur near the anterosuperior iliac spine or the ischiopubic synchondrosis, creating an amorphous localized area of spotty calcification. Similar lesions are seen affecting the anterior surface of the ribs. If large enough, these lesions have been designated *cauliflower exostoses.* Large osteochondromas affecting the neural arch of the vertebrae may create an appearance called the *cauliflower spine.* (Fig. 11-182; Table 11-22)

MRI is useful in determining the presence of malignant transformation. Thin cartilage caps down to 1 mm can be identified, as well as the overlying perichondrium. (26) In malignancy the cap thickens to > 3 cm, and the perichondrium will be breached.

Treatment and Prognosis

Most solitary osteochondromas are asymptomatic and never require treatment. Large lesions that create symptoms should be widely surgically excised, with care taken to include the periosteal surface, helping ensure an effective cure.

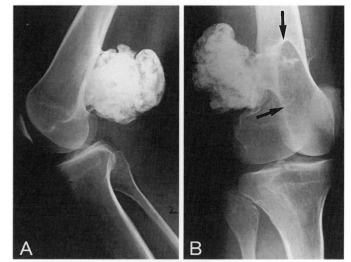

Figure 11-176 **OSTEOCHONDROMA WITH A LARGE OSTEOCARTILAGINOUS CAP. A. Lateral Knee.** Observe the dense calcification within the cartilaginous cap of this large osteochondroma arising from the posterior cortical surface of the distal femur. **B. Oblique Knee.** Note the distinct stalk arising from the femoral metaphysis. The triangular radiolucency (*arrows*) represents the region of origin of the osteochondroma. (Courtesy of Paul E. Siebert, MD, Denver, Colorado.)

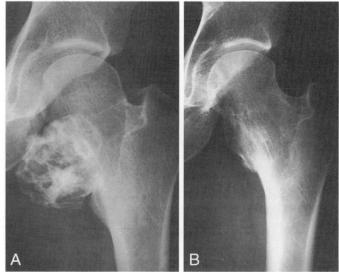

Figure 11-177 **CAULIFLOWER OSTEOCHONDROMA. A. Lesser Trochanter of the Femur.** Observe the cauliflower exostosis arising from the lesser trochanter of the proximal femur. There are areas of increased density scattered throughout the osteochondroma, representing calcified islands of cartilage. **B. Postsurgery.** Because this solitary osteochondroma created some mechanical pressure on vital structures in the area of the groin, it was surgically removed.

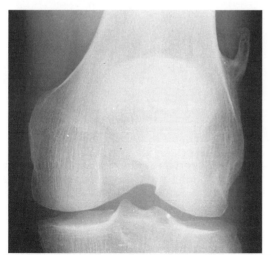

Figure 11-175 **SOLITARY OSTEOCHONDROMA. Distal Femur.** Note the pedunculated solitary osteochondroma, arising from the distal metaphysis of the femur.

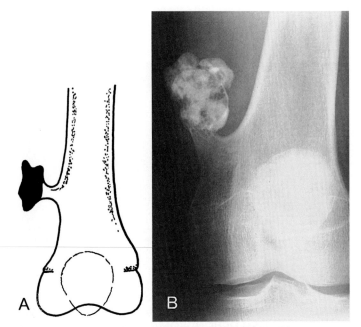

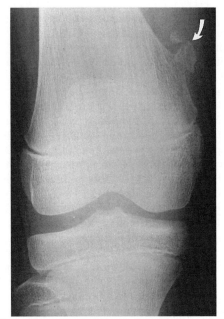

Figure 11-178 **COAT HANGER EXOSTOSIS. A. Diagram. B. Distal Femur.** Observe the solitary osteochondroma arising from the metaphyseal cortex of the distal femur. These exostoses project away from the joint because of muscle pull and have been referred to as coat hanger exostoses. Note also the dense flocculent calcification of the cartilaginous cap. (Courtesy of Keith H. Charlton, DC, Brisbane, Queensland, Australia.)

Figure 11-180 **FRACTURE OF AN OSTEOCHONDROMA. AP Femur.** Observe the small osteochondroma on the medial metaphysis of the distal femur, with a fracture of its distal surface (*arrow*).

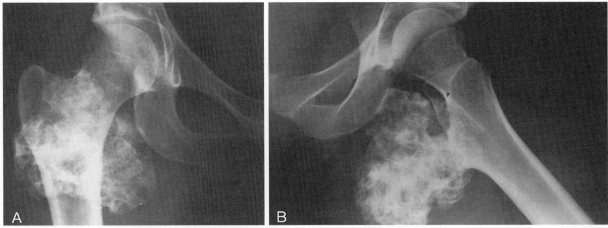

Figure 11-179 **CAULIFLOWER OSTEOCHONDROMA. A. AP Femur.** Note the large, lobulated solitary osteochondroma arising from the lesser trochanter of the femur. Its true point of origin cannot be determined from this frontal radiograph. **B. Oblique (Frog-Leg Projection) Femur.** Note that the point of origin of the large osteochondroma is now clearly seen to be the lesser trochanter of the proximal femur. Observe the flocculent areas of calcification scattered throughout this large osteochondroma. (Courtesy of Terry D. Sandman, DC, DACBR, Chicago, Illinois.)

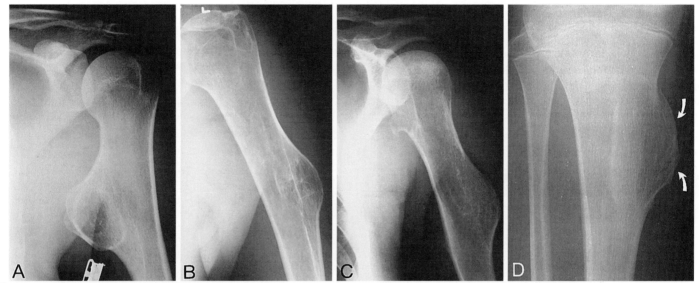

Figure 11-181 **SESSILE OSTEOCHONDROMAS. A–C. Humerus. D. Proximal Tibia.** Observe the broad-based exostoses along the cortical surfaces of the midportions of the humeri and the medial metaphysis of the proximal tibia. The radiolucent central matrix of all four lesions represents uncalcified cartilage (*arrows*). (Courtesy of Thomas G. Asbel, DC, Lakeville, Minnesota.)

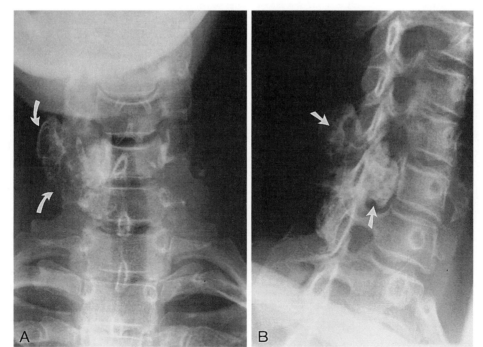

Figure 11-182 **CAULIFLOWER SPINE. A. AP Lower Cervical Spine.** Observe the eccentric lobulated exostosis occurring off the articular pillar of C6 (*arrows*). **B. Oblique Cervical Spine.** Note the large, cauliflower exostosis arising from the articular pillar of C6 (*arrows*). *COMMENT:* Osteochondromas affecting the neural arch of the vertebrae are referred to as the cauliflower spine.

Subungual Exostosis

A specific type of solitary osteochondroma that arises from the distal portion of the terminal phalanx of the toes, especially the great toe, is termed a subungual exostosis. (27) (Fig. 11-183) Its site of origin differs from the classic osteochondroma because it stems from the tip of the terminal phalanx, extending beneath or adjacent to the nail bed (28) and not in the metaphyseal portion of the bone. Its cap is fibrocartilaginous, in contrast to the hyaline cap of the typical osteochondroma. (29) These lesions may be painful and often require surgical removal. They typically occur in the 2nd–3rd decade of life and have a 2:1 female predominance. (27)

Table 11-22	Radiologic Features of Osteochondroma

Knee, shoulder, hip
Pedunculated type
   Thin, elongated stalk
   Metaphyseal
   Blends with cortex and spongiosa
   Projects away from joint (coat hanger)
   Lucent when en face
   Calcified cartilage cap (cauliflower, spotty)
Sessile type
   Broad based
   Metaphyseal
   Wide, broad metaphysis
   Lucent when en face
   Calcified cartilage cap (uncommon)

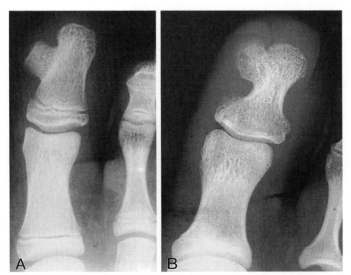

Figure 11-183 SUBUNGUAL EXOSTOSIS. A. Great Toe. Observe the broad-based subungual exostosis occurring off the medial cortical surface of the distal phalanx. **B. Great Toe.** Note the bilobed subungual exostosis present involving the distal phalanx of the great toe. Notice the shadow of a separate nail covering the distal exostosis. (Courtesy of David M. Walker, DPM, Melbourne, Australia.)

CAPSULE SUMMARY
Solitary Osteochondroma

General Considerations

- First described and illustrated by Sir Astley Cooper, surgeon and anatomist.
- Represents a bony exostosis on the external surface of a bone and usually has a hyaline-lined cartilaginous cap.

Incidence

- The most common benign skeletal growth or tumor; represents 50% of all benign bone tumors and 10–15% of all primary bone tumors.

Clinical Features

- 75% occur before age 20.
- Male predominance is 2:1.
- Most are asymptomatic, unless they disturb surrounding blood vessels or nerves.
- The most frequent complaint is a painless hard mass near a joint.
- Occasionally, a fractured stalk creates pain and swelling.
- Cord compression from a spinal osteochondroma occasionally occurs.
- Large pelvic osteochondromas may produce symptoms of obstructive uropathy.
- Pain and rapid growth may herald the appearance of malignant degeneration.
- The most common sites of involvement are the femur, humerus, tibia, pelvis, ribs, and scapula. Scapular involvement of the superior angle has been called Luschka's tubercle.

Pathologic Features

- Two types exist:
  Sessile: a broad, flat base and no stalk; common in the humerus and scapula.
  Pedunculated: a long stalk attaching it to the host bone. Its cap is of hyaline cartilage and frequently calcifies. Common in the knee, hip, and ankle.
- Vary in size, with some reaching 10 cm.
- Histologically resembles the normal epiphyseal growth plate.
- Malignant degeneration occurs in 1% of cases, appears around 30 years of age, and most commonly affects the bones of the pelvis and shoulder girdle.

Radiologic Features

- Coat hanger exostoses represent pedunculated lesions growing away from the joints on the metaphysis of the involved bones.
- En face visualization reveals a dense ring of cortex surrounding the base.
- The cortex and spongiosa of both the lesion and host bone blend imperceptibly, representing a key radiologic feature.
- Sessile form appears as an asymmetric bump lacking a stalk and having a broad-based attachment.

(continued)

CAPSULE SUMMARY
Solitary Osteochondroma (*continued*)

- Pedunculated lesions appear as a lobulated cauliflower mass with a dense, amorphous calcified cap.
- Large, dense spinal lesions may be called the cauliflower spine.

Treatment and Prognosis

- No treatment is necessary in most cases because the lesions are clinically silent.
- Symptomatic, large lesions are effectively treated by surgical excision.

HEREDITARY MULTIPLE EXOSTOSIS

General Considerations

Hereditary multiple exostosis (HME) is an inherited autosomal dominant metaphyseal overgrowth that is characterized by multiple osteochondromas. (1) (Fig. 11-184) It was described originally in 1814 by Boyer. (2) It has also been called multiple osteochondromatosis, external chondromatosis and, by Keith and the British, diaphyseal aclasis— *aclasis* referring to an alteration of the modeling process. (3,4) It is most frequently discovered between the ages of 2 and 10 years. Both sexes are equally affected; however, the condition appears to be somewhat less severe in female patients. (5) Genetic investigations have identified the responsible genes and further studies have revealed an association of growth disturbances among affected individuals. (6) The number of osteochondromas varies from a few to hundreds, with an average of 10. The metaphyseal portions of the long bones of the knee, ankle, shoulder, and wrist are most commonly affected; however, flat bone involvement has been reported. (7,8) (Fig. 11-185) The distribution is usually bilateral and may be symmetric. The elbows are usually spared. (Fig. 11-186) The hands are often involved in advanced cases. (Fig. 11-187)

Radiologic Features

The chief clinical complaint is painless, lumpy joints. This clinical presentation is the same as solitary osteochondroma (discussed earlier in this chapter). A characteristic *bayonet hand deformity* occurs about the wrist as a result of retardation of bone growth; the deformity is characterized by shortening of the ulna, outward bowing of the radius, and a subluxation of the radioulnar joint. (Fig. 11-188) This deformity occurs in about 30% of patients. (4) Large osteochondromas in the distal tibia or fibula often cause pressure erosions of the adjacent bone, leaving a scalloped margin to the outer cortex. (Fig. 11-189)

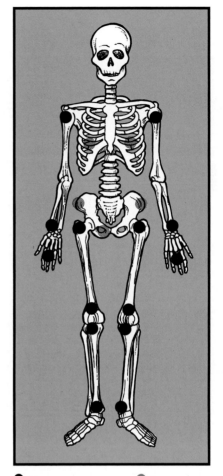

● More common   ◐ Less common

Figure 11-184 **SKELETAL DISTRIBUTION OF HEREDITARY MULTIPLE EXOSTOSIS.**

Pelvic lesions can become cauliflower-like and appear dense and large. (Fig. 11-190) At times differentiation from chondrosarcoma may be difficult radiographically. The ribs are most frequently involved at the costochondral junctions. (Fig. 11-191) Spinal cord compression can occur with a large vertebral lesion. (9) (Table 11-23)

Malignant degeneration occurs in 5–25% of cases. (10) Dahlin (11) believed this figure to be closer to 20%. Most lesions develop into chondrosarcoma; however, fibrosarcoma and osteosarcoma have been reported. The pelvis and shoulder girdle are the most common sites. (12) (Fig. 11-192) The clinician must be suspicious of malignant degeneration when a known HME patient complains of pain or renewed growth of an osteochondroma.

The treatment is surgical and is usually for cosmetic rather than symptomatic reasons. Recurrence of the tumor after adequate excision is highly suggestive of an aggressive lesion. Malignant degeneration, or the suspicion of such, is cause for surgical removal.

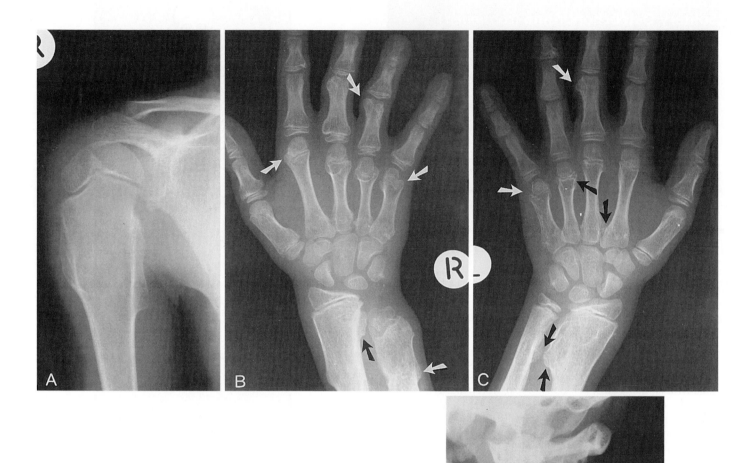

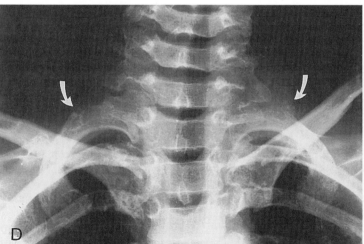

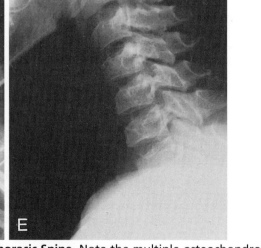

Figure 11-185 **HEREDITARY MULTIPLE EXOSTOSIS.**
A. AP Shoulder. Note the several sessile osteochondromas involving the cortical margins of the proximal metaphysis of the humerus. **B and C. Bilateral Hands.** Observe multiple small osteochondromas (*arrows*) throughout the metacarpals, phalanges, distal radius, and ulna bilaterally. **D. AP** **Cervicothoracic Spine.** Note the multiple osteochondromas (*arrows*) involving the posterior surfaces of the first rib bilaterally. **E. Lateral Cervical Spine.** Observe the sessile osteochondroma arising from the posterior arch of the atlas (*arrow*). (Courtesy of David P. Thomas, MD, Melbourne, Australia.)

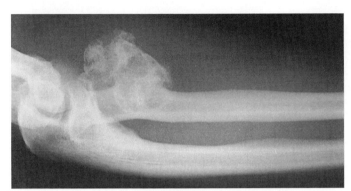

Figure 11-186 **OSTEOCHONDROMA. Lateral Elbow.** Note the large, cauliflower exostosis arising from the radial tuberosity. Observe the flocculent calcification scattered throughout this cauliflower exostosis.

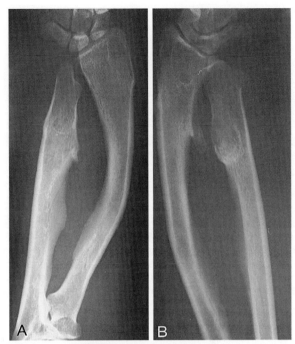

Figure 11-188 **BAYONET HAND DEFORMITY. A. Left Forearm. B. Right Forearm.** Observe the small osteochondromas, affecting the radius and ulna bilaterally. *COMMENT:* The bayonet hand deformity is found in approximately 30% of patients with hereditary multiple exostosis affecting the wrist. This deformity occurs as a result of retardation of bone growth and is characterized by shortening of the ulna, outward bowing of the radius, and subluxation of the radioulnar joint.

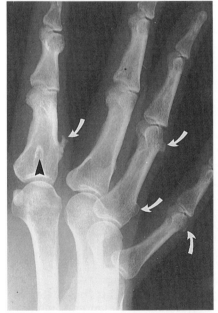

Figure 11-187 **MULTIPLE OSTEOCHONDROMAS. Hand.** Observe the small osteochondromas scattered throughout the proximal phalanges (*arrows*). A clearly outlined osteochondroma seen en face is present in the proximal phalanx of the second digit (*arrowhead*).

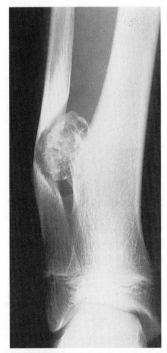

Figure 11-189 **PRESSURE EROSION FROM OSTEO-CHONDROMA.** Note the large cauliflower exostosis occurring off the cortex of the distal tibia, which has produced a significant pressure erosion of the adjacent fibula.

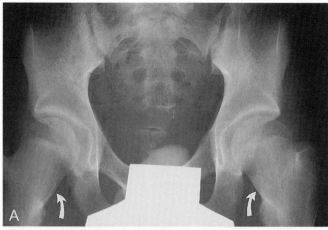

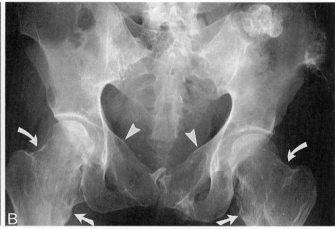

Figure 11-190 **HEREDITARY MULTIPLE EXOSTOSIS (HME): SESSILE TYPE. A. AP Pelvis.** Observe the broad thickening of the metaphysis of both femora (*arrows*). This is a characteristic appearance for HME involving the proximal femur. **B. AP Pelvis.** Observe the multiple cauliflower exostoses along the anterior margins of the pelvis. Note the broad femoral necks, a characteristic sign of HME (*arrows*). In addition, there are sessile osteochondromas affecting the pubic rami bilaterally, creating a deformed and expanded appearance (*arrowheads*).

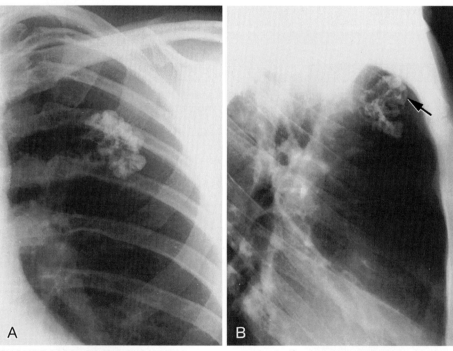

Figure 11-191 **OSTEOCHONDROMA: COSTOCHONDRAL JUNCTION. A. PA Chest.** Note the large, lobulated, and calcified osteochondroma present at the anterior surface of the second rib. Matrix calcification is present throughout the osteocartilaginous cap. **B. Lateral Chest.** Note that the calcified lesion is projected into the anterior mediastinum (*arrow*).

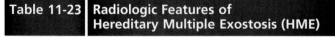

Table 11-23	Radiologic Features of Hereditary Multiple Exostosis (HME)

Multiple, painless lumps and bumps around joints
Bayonet deformity of the wrist
Broad metaphyses
Calcified cauliflower cartilaginous caps

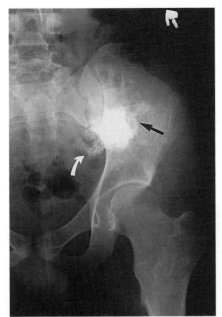

Figure 11-192 **HEREDITARY MULTIPLE EXOSTOSIS: MALIGNANT DEGENERATION. Pelvis.** Observe the sessile osteochondromas affecting the proximal metaphysis of the right femur. There is a radiopaque density extending from the anterior midportion of the right ilium. This density represents malignant degeneration of an osteochondroma, with an associated soft tissue mass extending into the pelvic basin (*arrows*).

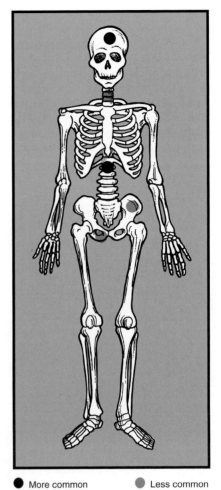

● More common   ● Less common

Figure 11-193 **SKELETAL DISTRIBUTION OF HEMANGIOMA.**

HEMANGIOMA

General Considerations

Hemangioma, a primary benign neoplasm, is a slowly growing lesion of bone composed of newly formed capillary, cavernous, or venous blood vessels. Most lesions are clinically silent.

Incidence

Hemangiomas represent about 1% of all primary bone tumors and 2–3% of all radiographically perceptible spinal tumors. Schmorl and Junghans (1) found asymptomatic vertebral hemangiomas in 11% of 3829 consecutive, serially sectioned vertebral columns removed at autopsy. Many of these lesions are not demonstrated on radiographs but are frequently seen on MRI. Hemangioma is the most common benign bone tumor of the spine. (2,3)

Clinical Features

Age and Sex Distribution

Most spinal hemangiomas develop after puberty, and the majority of the lesions are seen in adults > 40 years. There is a slightly higher incidence in female patients. (3)

Signs and Symptoms

Most hemangiomas at any site are clinically silent. Symptomatic vertebral hemangiomas usually present with localized pain and surrounding muscle spasm. Neurological compromise may be noted with symptoms of hypesthesia, hyperesthesia, radiculitis, and localized pain owing to spinal stenosis. Those spinal lesions that become symptomatic do so as a result of cord compression, which may occur in any of four ways: (*a*) hypertrophy and ballooning of the vertebral body owing to angiomatous invasion, (*b*) extension of the hemangioma into the epidural space, (*c*) compression fracture of the involved vertebra, and (*d*) hemorrhage. (3) Most of the symptomatic spinal lesions are in the midthoracic region because the larger size of the cord relative to the size of the spinal canal in this region is a predisposing factor. Fracture of the involved vertebra causing spinal cord compression is a rare finding; a few sporadic cases have been reported. (4,5)

Hemangiomas of the maxilla and mandible must be noted, particularly by dentists, because tooth extraction in the area of a hemangioma could prove fatal because of exsanguination. (6,7)

Lesions of the long bones are rare but present, with dull, vague pains that gradually attract clinical attention.

Location

The most common sites for hemangioma are the spine and skull, representing 75% of lesions. (8) (Fig. 11-193) Spinal lesions are most common in the lower thoracic and upper lumbar area. Most lesions affect a portion or all of the vertebral body. Extension into the neural arch occurs in 10–15% of the cases, usually following initial vertebral body involvement. (9) Most lesions in the skull affect the frontal bone. Sporadic cases have been reported in the cervical spine, long tubular bones, mandible and maxilla, patella, the metacarpals, ribs, scapula, and the soft tissues. (5,8–12) (Fig. 11-194)

Pathologic Features

Pathologically, two types of hemangiomas of bone are recognized: *capillary* and *cavernous*. The capillary type consists of fine capillary loops tending to spread outward in a *sunburst* fashion; this type, when present, is usually encountered in flat bones

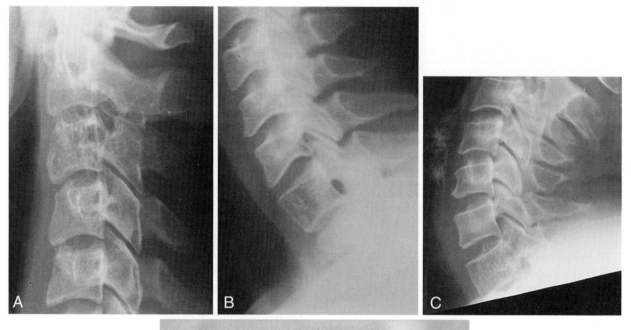

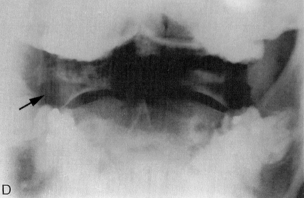

Figure 11-194 **CERVICAL SPINE HEMANGIOMA. A. C3 Vertebral Body.** Note the characteristic coarsening of the trabecular patterns found within the C3 vertebral body, articular pillar, and lamina. This appearance is consistent with hemangioma. **B. C7 Vertebral Body.** Note the coarsening of the trabecular patterns, with bone expansion noted, and loss of bone density throughout the C7 vertebral body. The patient presented with no symptoms in this area, and the appearance is characteristic of hemangioma of bone. **C. C7 Vertebral Body.** Note the vertical striations scattered throughout the vertebral body, assuming a corduroy cloth appearance. There is no thickening of the endplate; however, expansion of the vertebral body is noted. There is minimal extension of the hemangiomatous process into the pedicle and superior articular pillar. This 42-year-old female presented with suboccipital headaches and an asymptomatic C7 cervical hemangioma. **D. Atlas.** Note the unilateral involvement of the lateral mass, evidenced by the coarse trabecular patterns and slight expansion (*arrow*). (Panel A courtesy of R. A. Fladland, DC, Milwaukee, Wisconsin. Special thanks to Gary A. Longmuir, DC, DACBR, Phoenix, Arizona, for his assistance in obtaining this case. Panel B courtesy of Appa L. Anderson, DC, DACBR, Fellow, ACCR, Portland, Oregon. Panel C reprinted with permission from **Yochum TR:** *Spinal hemangioma.* ACA J Chiro April, 1983. Courtesy of Karsten Hviid, DC, Arhus, Denmark. Panel D courtesy of Appa L. Anderson, DC, DACBR, Fellow, ACCR, Portland, Oregon.)

(ribs, innominate) and in the metaphyseal ends of long bones. Capillary hemangiomas are relatively uncommon. The cavernous type consists of large, thin-walled blood vessels and sinuses, lined by a single layer of endothelial cells, surrounded by resorbed bony trabeculae. The cavernous type is the most common type of hemangioma and frequently involves the vertebrae and skull. On occasion, reactive new bone may be observed in both the capillary and the cavernous types of hemangioma.

Radiologic Features

Hemangiomas in bone usually present a characteristic appearance; however, this varies with the anatomic site. (Table 11-24)

Spine

Most spinal hemangiomas are solitary; however, double or triple lesions have been reported. (13) (Fig. 11-195) The radiologic appearance of vertebral hemangioma includes coarse vertical striations in the vertebral body, separated by more lucent zones. There is a slight, overall loss of bone density to the affected ver-

tebra, which occurs as a result of replacement of the normal architecture by the angiomatous vessels. The vertical striations create what has been called the *corduroy cloth appearance*, which is best appreciated in the lateral view. (13) (Fig. 11-196) This appearance has also been called the *striated vertebra*. (14) Most spinal lesions affect primarily the vertebral bodies, with but a few cases extending into the neural arch. Vertebral body

Table 11-24	Radiologic Features of Hemangioma
Spine	
Thoracolumbar region	
Vertebral body	
Coarse vertical striations (corduroy cloth or striated vertebra)	
Paravertebral swelling	
Differential diagnosis: Paget's disease, osteoporosis	
Skull	
Frontal bone	
Round, oval	
Geographic lesion radiating spicules (sunray or spoked wheel)	
Long bones	
Expansile	
Coarsened trabeculae (honeycomb)	

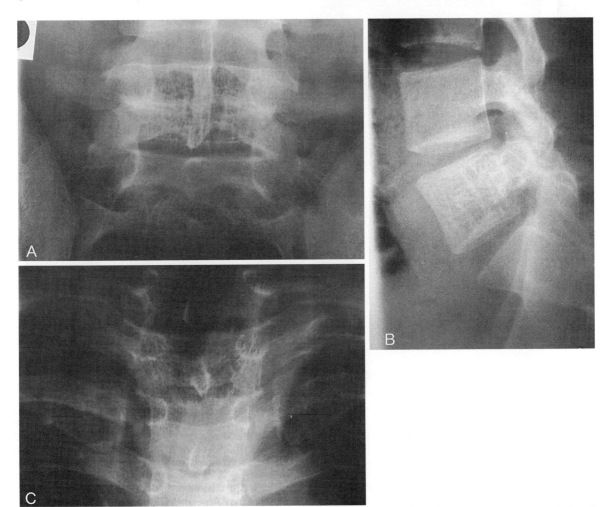

Figure 11-195 **DOUBLE HEMANGIOMAS. A. AP L5. B. Lateral L5.** Observe the coarsened trabecular pattern, creating the corduroy cloth appearance of the L5 vertebral body. This has also been called the striated vertebra. **C. AP Thoracic Spine.** Note that in the same patient there is coars-ening of the trabecular patterns characteristic of spinal hemangioma involving the T2 vertebral body. (Reprinted with permission from **Yochum TR:** *Spinal hemangioma.* ACA J Chiro April, 1983.)

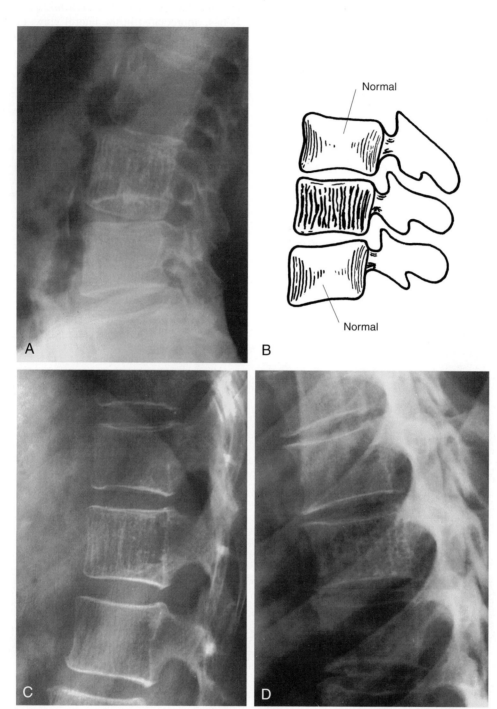

Figure 11-196 **SPINAL HEMANGIOMA: CORDUROY CLOTH APPEARANCE. A. Lateral Lumbar Spine.** Observe the coarsened trabecular patterns throughout the L3 vertebral body. **B. Diagram. C. Lateral Thoracolumbar Spine.** Note the accentuation of the vertical trabecular patterns throughout the vertebral body of the L1 vertebra. This appearance is characteristic of spinal hemangioma and has been referred to as the striated vertebra. **D. T9 Vertebra.** Observe the coarsening of the trabecular patterns throughout the vertebral body of T9, consistent with an intraosseous spinal hemangioma. *COMMENT:* The most common sites for hemangioma are the spine and skull, making up 75% of all such lesions. Spinal hemangiomas are most common in the lower thoracic and upper lumbar areas. Most lesions affect a portion or all of the vertebral body, with 10–15% of the cases extending into the neural arch after initial vertebral body involvement. (Panel A courtesy of Stephen F. Kesler, DC, Salt Lake City, Utah.)

expansion is a rare occurrence in hemangioma but, when present, often leads to symptoms secondary to spinal stenosis. (15)

The roentgen pattern of hemangioma may be simulated by other conditions. One of the major disease processes that can mimic the coarsened trabecular patterns of spinal hemangioma is Paget's disease. Because hemangiomas rarely expand bone and vertebral Paget's disease often does, the differential diagnosis is usually made on the basis of bone expansion. (9) An additional sign supportive of Paget's disease is the thickening of the cortical endplates, which has been called the *picture frame appearance.* (Fig. 11-197) Cortical thickening is not a feature of hemangioma, leaving the vertebral endplates crisp and unaffected. (9) Patients with senile or postmenopausal osteoporosis may demonstrate prominent vertical trabeculae within the vertebral bodies. This occurs as a result of the preferential resorption of the transverse trabeculae and accentuation of the remaining vertical trabeculae. This process creates a *pseudo-hemangiomatous* appearance of multiple vertebrae in patients with diffuse osteoporosis. (9) One should hesitate to conclude that a geriatric patient has more than one vertebral hemangioma (on plain films) because it is more likely the patient has simple osteoporosis.

An unusual roentgen sign that has been rarely seen is the presence of a paravertebral mass with spinal hemangioma. Only a few case studies have been reported. (16,17) The paravertebral mass may be large or only a localized bulge of the thoracic paraspinal line, usually on the left side. It may occur because of the extension of the tumor through the cortex of the vertebral body into the adjacent soft tissues. (16) On CT and MRI predominantly fatty stroma types are less likely to be associated with spinal cord compression. (18) Another possible cause is a compression fracture of the involved vertebra, which can lead to an increase in the transverse diameter of the vertebral body and a hematoma in the paravertebral space, causing a segmental bulge. (17)

Skull

Although hemangioma may occur anywhere in the skull, it is most commonly found in the frontal bone. (19) (Fig. 11-198) The lesion varies from 1 to 7 cm in diameter and is a round or oval radiolucency when viewed en face. The lytic defect often has dense, fine spicula radiating from its centrum, creating a *sunburst* or *spoked-wheel appearance.* (9,19) (Fig. 11-199) The intense nature of the radiating spicules of bone can mimic osteosarcoma, particularly in tangential or profile views. Ordinarily, the hemangioma extends outward, well beyond the normal contour of the bone. Often accompanying this external bulging is an erosion or disappearance of the outer table of the skull, while the integrity of the inner table is usually preserved. The profile view frequently discloses vertical striations, which produce the characteristic sunray effect. (20)

Other Bones

Involvement of bones other than the skull and spine is uncommon; however, the radiographic appearance is that of an expansile, lytic,

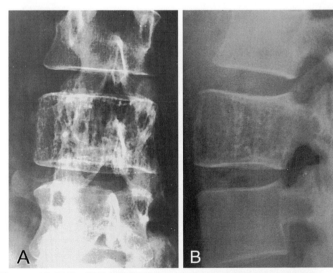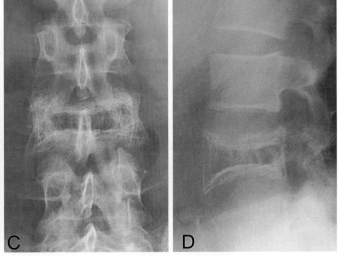

Figure 11-197 **HEMANGIOMA VERSUS PAGET'S DISEASE: DIFFERENTIAL DIAGNOSIS. A. Hemangioma: AP Lumbar Spine. B. Lateral Lumbar Spine.** Observe the loss of bone density and accentuation of the vertical trabecular patterns throughout the L3 vertebral body. There is a loss of the anterior concavity of the vertebral body, caused by bony expansion. There is no thickening of the vertebral endplates. This appearance is characteristic of an expanding spinal hemangioma. **C. Paget's Disease: AP Lumbar Spine. D. Lateral Lumbar Spine.** Observe the thickening of the trabecular patterns throughout the vertebral body and neural arch of L3. This trabecular thickening is reminiscent of the changes characteristically found in the corduroy cloth appearance of spinal hemangioma. There is bone expansion noted, with significant thickening of the vertebral endplates, creating a *pic-*

ture frame appearance. There is central depression of the vertebral body, suggesting a pathologic fracture. These radiographic signs secure the diagnosis of Paget's disease. *COMMENT:* Because occasionally Paget's disease may mimic the appearance of a hemangioma in the vertebral body, differential diagnosis is essential. Cortical thickening at the vertebral endplates reminiscent of the *picture frame* appearance is characteristically seen in Paget's disease, but is not found in hemangioma. The vertebral endplates are crisp and unaffected in spinal hemangioma. The radiographic sign of bony expansion, which usually suggests Paget's disease, does occur in a small percentage of patients with hemangioma. The differential radiographic sign, therefore, is thickening of the vertebral endplates in Paget's disease, a sign not present with hemangioma.

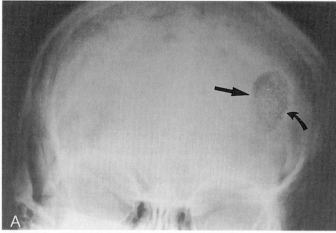

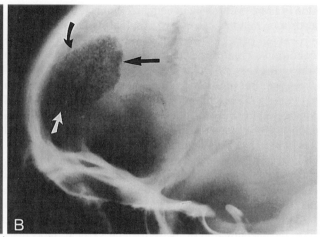

Figure 11-198 **HEMANGIOMA: FRONTAL BONE. A. PA Skull. B. Lateral Skull.** Observe the oval radiolucent defect in the frontal bone (*arrows*). The central portion of this radiolucency demonstrates a *sunburst* or *spoked-wheel* appearance, which is characteristic of hemangioma. *COMMENT:* Although hemangioma may occur anywhere in the skull, it is most commonly found in the frontal bone; this represents the second most common site of intraosseous hemangioma. The lesion varies from 1 to 7 cm in diameter and is a round or oval radiolucency when viewed en face.

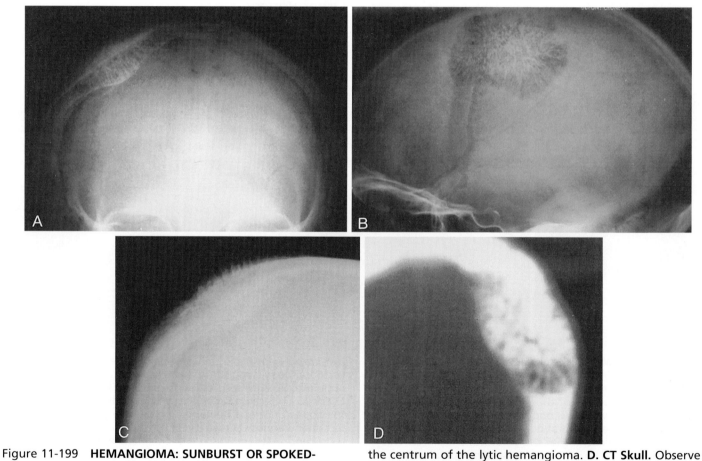

Figure 11-199 **HEMANGIOMA: SUNBURST OR SPOKED-WHEEL APPEARANCE. A. PA Skull. B. Lateral Skull.** Note the circular radiolucent defect present primarily within the temporal bone, with minimal extension into the frontal bone. There is an intense, radiating spiculation of bone from the central portion of the lytic defect, creating the *sunburst* or *spoked-wheel* appearance of an intraosseous hemangioma. **C. Tangential Skull.** Observe the fine spicula radiating from the centrum of the lytic hemangioma. **D. CT Skull.** Observe the large, radiating hemangioma present within the table of the skull. *COMMENT:* Hemangiomas affecting the calvaria often present with dense, fine spicula radiating from the centrum, creating a *sunburst* or *spoked-wheel* appearance. The intense nature of the radiating spicules of bone can mimic osteosarcoma, particularly in tangential or profile views.

fine, lacy network or honeycombing lesion. The radiating coarse linear strands diverging from the center also occur, leaving a sun-ray appearance. (Fig. 11-200)

Soft Tissue Hemangioma

Soft tissue hemangioma is the cause of a palpable soft tissue mass usually found in the forearm, lower leg, or paravertebral area. (Figs. 11-201 and 11-202) Spherical calcifications occur within the mass, representing phleboliths, and characterizing the vascular nature of the mass.

Treatment and Prognosis

Most hemangiomas are clinically silent, requiring no treatment. Symptomatic spinal lesions are either fractured or expanding bone, creating spinal stenosis and impending paraplegia. Surgical de-

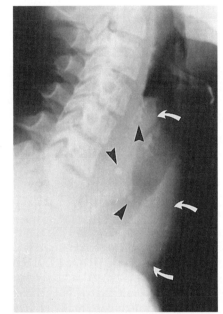

Figure 11-202 SOFT TISSUE HEMANGIOMA. Lateral Cervical Spine. Observe the large hemangioma present in the soft tissue structures of the lower neck (*arrows*). There are small circular calcifications scattered throughout the soft tissue hemangioma that represent phleboliths (*arrowheads*).

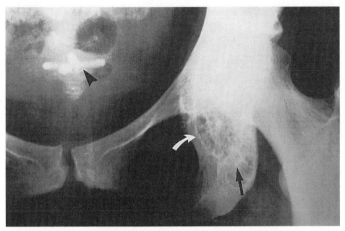

Figure 11-200 HEMANGIOMA. AP Pelvis. Observe the radiating trabecular patterns scattered throughout an oval hemangioma involving the ischium (*arrows*). Of incidental notation is an intrauterine device present in the pelvic basin (*arrowhead*). (Courtesy of Richard T. Coade, MIR, DC, Kempsey, New South Wales, Australia.)

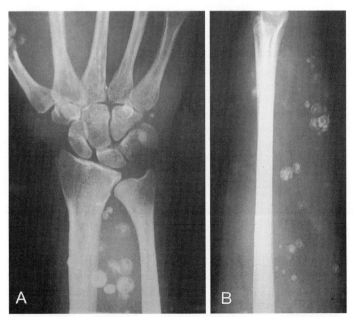

Figure 11-201 SOFT TISSUE HEMANGIOMA. A. PA Forearm. B. Lateral Forearm. Observe the multiple laminated soft tissue densities lying within the soft tissues, consistent with phleboliths. *COMMENT:* These are a characteristic finding of soft tissue hemangioma.

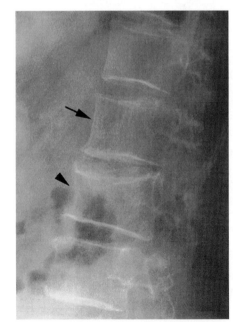

Figure 11-203 HEMANGIOMA WITH ADJACENT COMPRESSION FRACTURE. Observe the L1 hemangioma (*arrow*) and the subadjacent compression fracture at L2 (*arrowhead*). *COMMENT:* This attests to the inherent strength of the hemangioma. (Courtesy of Kevin J. La Londe, DC, Duxbury, Massachusetts.)

compression is to be performed only on those lesions that are creating cord compression.

A question arises concerning the integrity of the spinal hemangioma and as to the incidence of compression fracture. Review of the literature finds < 15 cases of hemangiomatous vertebral collapse. (5,21,22) Holta (5) stated that a hemangiomatous vertebra is reinforced by thick, sclerotic vertical trabeculae, secondary to appositional new bone formation and is, therefore, stronger than the adjacent normal vertebrae. (Fig. 11-203) Because so few of

these lesions fracture, one wonders how valid it is to severely curb a patient's activities because of the mere presence of a vertebral body hemangioma.

Occasionally, radiation therapy may be given to a symptomatic, inoperable vertebral hemangioma. Symptomatic hemangiomas of the skull are treated quite effectively by en bloc excision, with a low recurrence rate and favorable prognosis. (23) Such is also the case with hemangiomas in other sites. If the lesion is in a bone that can be spared (rib, nasal bone), local resection is indicated. (23)

CAPSULE SUMMARY Hemangioma

General Considerations

- A vascular solitary neoplasm that is slow growing and composed of newly formed capillary, cavernous, or venous blood vessels.
- A benign neoplasm with no malignant potential.

Incidence

- Represents 1% of all radiographically demonstrable primary bone tumors, 2–3% of all spinal tumors.
- Schmorl and Junghans found 11% of 3829 sectioned autopsy specimens to have asymptomatic vertebral lesions; many of these lesions are not demonstrable on radiographs.
- The most common benign bone tumor of the spine.

Clinical Features

- Most lesions are seen in patients > 40 years of age; however, lesions often develop after puberty and go undetected until later in life.
- Slightly higher incidence in females exists.
- Most lesions at any site are asymptomatic.
- Most symptomatic spinal lesions are the result of expansion leading to the development of spinal stenosis. These patients may present with signs of impending paraplegia.
- 75% of lesions occur in the spine and skull, the lower thoracic and upper lumbars are the target areas with the frontal bone being the most common bone affected in the skull.
- Most spinal lesions are in the vertebral body, with 10–15% extending into the neural arch.

Pathologic Features

- Two types exist.
  Capillary: consists of fine capillary loops that spread outward in a sunburst fashion, usually affecting flat bones. This type is uncommon.

Cavernous: consists of large, thin-walled blood vessels and sinuses lined by endothelial cells. This is the most common type, frequently affecting the vertebrae and skull.

Radiologic Features

- The classic spinal lesion is one with coarse vertical striations within the vertebral body and has been called the *corduroy cloth* appearance or the *striated* vertebra.
- Rarely, a paravertebral mass may be found associated with vertebral hemangioma.
- A *pseudo-hemangiomatous* appearance occurs throughout the spine in patients with senile or postmenopausal osteoporosis. Because most lesions are solitary, the clinician should hesitate to conclude that a patient has multiple hemangiomas because it is usually as a result of the vertical trabecular accentuation of osteoporosis.
- Vertebral expansion may rarely occur, creating a similar appearance to Paget's disease of the spine. Differentiation is made by the lack of the cortical endplate thickening in hemangioma, which is so characteristic of Paget's disease (*picture frame appearance*).
- Most skull lesions are in the frontal bone, creating a round or oval radiolucency, a radiating *sunburst* or *spoked-wheel* appearance that extends from the center of the lytic defect.

Treatment and Prognosis

- Most lesions are clinically silent and require no treatment.
- Symptomatic spinal lesions are either fractured or are expanding bone creating spinal stenosis; surgical decompression may be necessary under these circumstances.
- Radiation treatment may be used occasionally in inoperable vertebral hemangioma.
- Skull lesions are easily treated by en bloc excision and have a favorable prognosis.

OSTEOMA

General Considerations

Osteomas are benign bone tumors that arise in membranous bones. Because most osteomas are asymptomatic, their true incidence is not known. (1) Several studies of patients from oto-

laryngology clinics reveal a < 1% incidence; however, osteomas represent the most common benign tumor of the nose and paranasal sinuses. (1–3) Most lesions are clinically silent and occur in the frontal and ethmoid sinuses or affect the outer or inner tables of the skull. (4) (Fig. 11-204) If symptoms develop it is usually not until the 2nd–5th decades of life (3) and shows neither signs of progression nor malignant change. If the lesions interfere with the drainage of the involved sinus, they can lead to chronic sinusitis with retro-orbital pressure, headaches, muco-

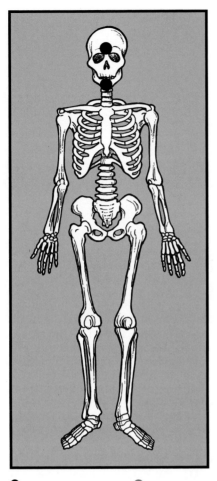

Figure 11-204 **SKELETAL DISTRIBUTION OF OSTEOMA.**

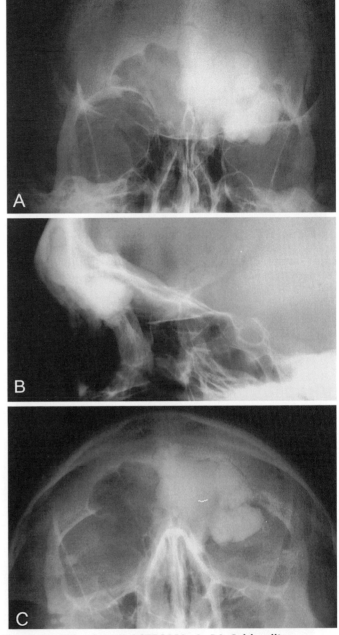

Figure 11-205 **GIANT OSTEOMA. A. PA Caldwell's Projection Sinus. B. Lateral Sinus. C. AP Waters' Projection Sinus.** Observe the giant, ivory osteoma present in the frontal sinus. *COMMENT:* Patients with lesions of this magnitude often experience proptosis, a variety of ocular disturbances, and exophthalmos. (Courtesy of David P. Thomas, MD, Melbourne, Australia.)

celes, and, rarely, brain abscess. (5,6) Although infrequent, osteomas of the frontal sinus have been associated with posterior protrusion into the cranial cavity, resulting in life-threatening situations. (7)

Most osteomas never reach a size > 2 cm, and they are most often found by coincidence. Occasionally, these lesions can become large, nearly filling the entire sinus cavity (*giant osteomas*). (Fig. 11-205) These patients may experience a variety of ocular disturbances, including proptosis, headaches, and recurrent sinusitis. (8) Mandibular osteomas create mechanical and cosmetic problems (Fig. 11-206) and, rarely, may cause bizarre defects in vision and balance by virtue of their close proximity to the carotid sinus and internal carotid artery. (8) A 3:1 female to male ratio has been noted. (9) It is believed that these lesions develop in response to embryologic tissue growth defects, infection, or trauma. (4) Histologically, there are two types: the *ivory* or *compact* osteoma and the *trabecular* or *spongy* osteoma. They are differentiated by their point of origin within the bone.

Radiologic Features

The radiographic appearance of osteoma is that of a round or oval, well-circumscribed, radiopaque structure. (6) (Figs. 11-207 and 11-208) Rarely does one attain a size > 2 cm. (Fig. 11-209)

If a sinus osteoma is large (*giant osteoma*), it occasionally causes expansion of the sinus walls. (Table 11-25) Rarely, osteoma may occur off of the outer skull table and can become quite large. (Figs. 11-210 to 11-212)

The symptomatic osteomas are best treated by surgical excision. (10) Recurrence after excision seldom occurs. (10) Most osteomas require no treatment because they are asymptomatic lesions. (10,11)

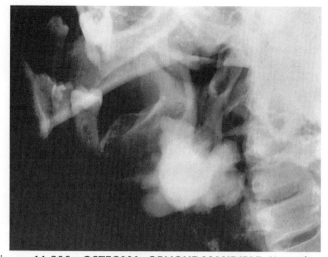

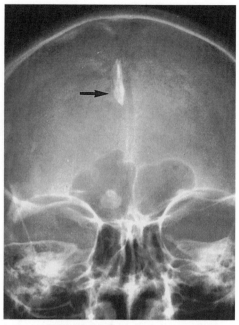

Figure 11-206 **OSTEOMA: OBLIQUE MANDIBLE.** Note the large, lobulated, ivory osteoma projecting off the angle of the mandible. (Courtesy of Bryan Hartley, MD, Melbourne, Australia.)

Figure 11-207 **OSTEOMA: FRONTAL SINUS.** Observe the well-circumscribed radiopaque osteoma present within the frontal sinus. Of incidental notation is a plaque-like area of calcification present within the falx cerebri (*arrow*), a normal variant. (Courtesy of Thomas F. Bergmann, DC, Minneapolis, Minnesota.)

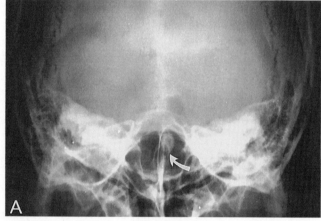

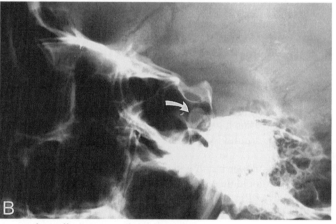

Figure 11-208 **OSTEOMA: SPHENOID SINUS. A. AP Towne's Projection, Skull. B. Lateral Projection, Sinuses.** Observe the oval, well-circumscribed osteoma on the posterior surface of the sphenoid sinus (*arrows*).

Table 11-25	Radiologic Features of Osteoma
Arise in membranous bones	
Sinuses—frontal, ethmoids	
Mandible	
Skull bones	
Homogeneously opaque	

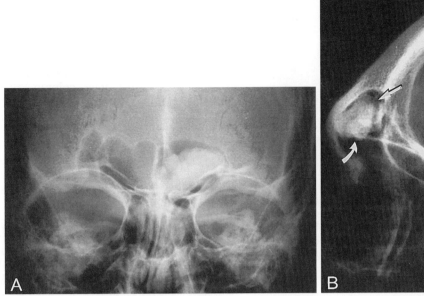

Figure 11-209 GIANT OSTEOMA: FRONTAL SINUS. A. PA Caldwell's Projection: Frontal Sinuses. B. Lateral Close-Up of **Frontal Sinus.** Observe the giant osteoma of the frontal sinus, with a lobulated peripheral margin (*arrows*).

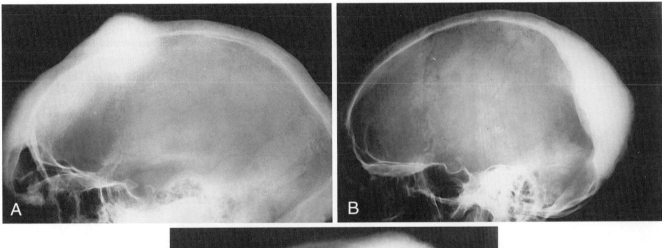

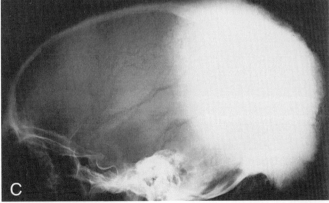

Figure 11-210 GIANT OSTEOMA: CALVARIA. A. Lateral Skull. Note the homogeneous, ill-defined, radiopaque osteoma involving the frontal bone. This alters the shape and contour of the skull table. **B. Lateral Skull.** Observe the large, dense osteoma affecting the posterior portion of the parietal bone and extending into the occiput. Significant ex- pansion of the outer table is noted. **C. Lateral Skull.** Note the gigantic ivory osteoma projecting from the posterior sur- face of the skull. Owing to the significant bony expansion and cosmetic deformity, this was surgically removed. (Courtesy of Bryan Hartley, MD, Melbourne, Australia.)

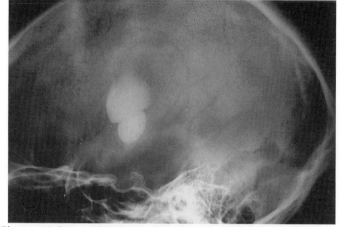

Figure 11-211 **OSTEOMA: TEMPORAL BONE.** Observe the well-circumscribed radiopaque osteoma affecting the temporal bone. This is a somewhat unusual location for an osteoma. (Courtesy of Klaus W. Weber, MD, Fort Wayne, Indiana.)

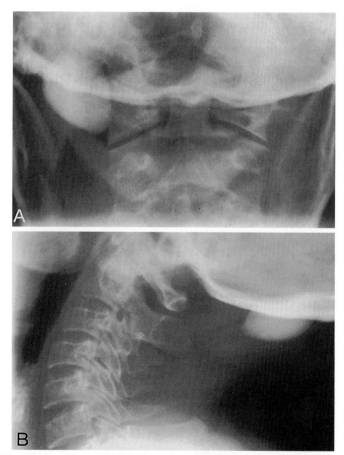

Figure 11-212 **OSTEOMA: OCCIPUT. A. AP Open Mouth. B. Lateral Cervical Spine.** Note the large, oval, radiopaque osteoma protruding from the outer table of the occiput. (Courtesy of Margaret A. Seron, DC, DABCO, DACBR, Denver, Colorado.)

GARDNER'S SYNDROME

General Considerations

Gardner's syndrome may be defined as a triad of abnormal growths: multiple osteomas, colonic polyposis, and soft tissue fibromas. (1) This syndrome is transmitted as an autosomal Mendelian dominant. Variable reports occur in the literature regarding the incidence of osseous manifestations. Approximately 45% of patients with Gardner's display all of the classic lesions and symptoms. (2) In a survey of 280 patients with this syndrome, 40 (14%) showed bone lesions. (2) The osteomas appear as protuberant, oval, dense, occasionally lobulated masses, which are usually attached to the cortex. (Fig. 11-213) These lesions are polyostotic and quite distinctive in appearance. The most common bones involved are the frontal, mandible (near the mandibular angle), maxilla, sphenoid, ethmoid, zygoma, and the small tubular bones of the hands and feet. It should be emphasized that, when present, the bone lesions usually precede the polyps and skin lesions. (Fig. 11-214)

The polyposis of the colon should be considered premalignant, and any patient who has multiple osteomas should have the colon examined. (3) Other members of the family should be examined as well because of the inheritability of the condition. Prophylactic resection of the bowel is the treatment of choice.

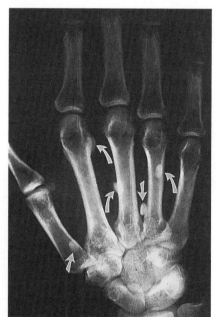

Figure 11-213 **GARDNER'S SYNDROME. PA Hand.** Observe the small, well-defined osteomas projecting from the metacarpal bones (*arrows*). *COMMENT:* Gardner's syndrome may be defined as a triad of abnormal growths: multiple osteomas, colonic polyps, and soft tissue fibromas. The bones most commonly involved are the frontal, mandible, maxilla, and small tubular bones of the hands and feet. It should be emphasized that in Gardner's syndrome the bone lesions usually precede the colonic polyps and skin lesions. The polyps of the colon are considered premalignant, and any patient who has multiple osteomas should have a colon examination. Owing to the familial nature of this syndrome, all family members need to be evaluated.

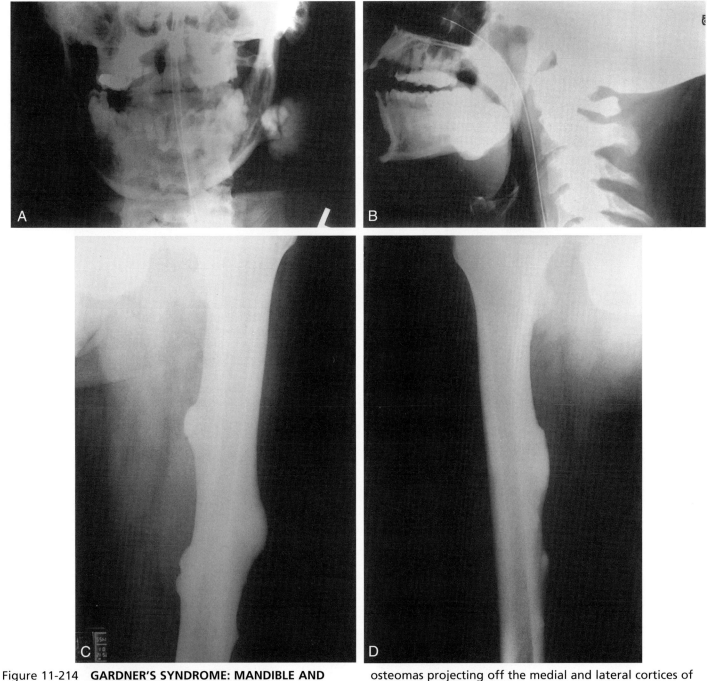

Figure 11-214   **GARDNER'S SYNDROME: MANDIBLE AND FEMORA. A. AP Mandible. B. Lateral Mandible.** Observe the giant ivory-like osteoma projecting off the left mandible near its angle. **C. and D. Bilateral Femora.** Observe the large osteomas projecting off the medial and lateral cortices of the mid-diaphysis of both femora. (Courtesy of Mathew Pardy, MD, Department of Radiology, University Hospital, Denver, Colorado.)

BONE ISLAND

General Considerations

A solitary discrete area of sclerosis in the skeleton, usually called a bone island (endosteoma), is an entity well known to the practitioner and radiologist. (Fig. 11-215) It is usually asymptomatic and in most cases an incidental finding. These bone islands are particularly common in the ischium, ilium, sacrum, and proximal femur but may be found in the humerus, vertebra, talus, scaphoid, and ribs. (Fig. 11-216 to 11-219) The only location in which bone islands do not occur is the skull. (1)

Clinical Features

Bone islands may be found at any age but are far more common in adults than in children. They are asymptomatic and clinically insignificant lesions. They are usually unchanged in size over many years but occasionally may grow. (2) (Fig. 11-220) Bone islands

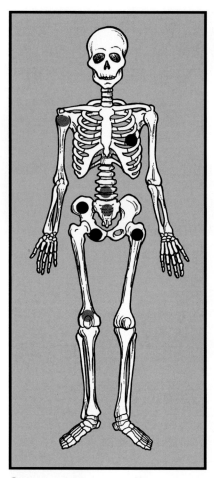

● More common ● Less common

Figure 11-215 **SKELETAL DISTRIBUTION OF BONE ISLAND.**

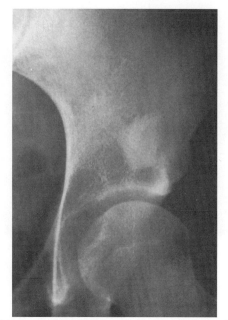

Figure 11-217 **BONE ISLAND. AP Ilium.** Observe the large radiopaque bone island in the supra-acetabular area. (Courtesy of James R. Brandt, DC, DABCO, Coon Rapids, Minnesota.)

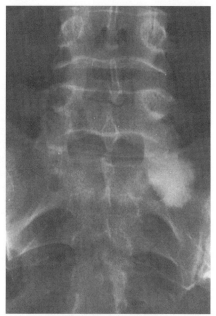

Figure 11-218 **BONE ISLAND. AP Sacrum.** Observe the large, lobulated bone island within the sacral ala. *COMMENT:* Bone islands, which are found in the ilium, sacrum, and lumbar spine, may mimic the appearance of early osteoblastic metastasis. To differentiate these two entities appropriately, serial radiographs may be helpful; however, the definitive evaluation to rule out osteoblastic metastatic disease is the bone scan. The majority of bone islands will not be active on bone scan, whereas metastatic osteoblastic lesions will appear as hot spots. (Courtesy of Kenneth E. Yochum, DC, St. Louis, Missouri.)

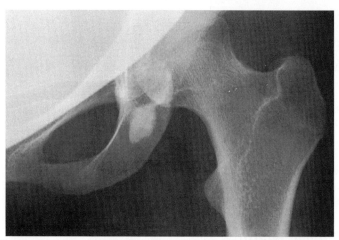

Figure 11-216 **BONE ISLAND. AP Ischium.** Note the oval radiopacity within the ischium, which represents a large bone island. Of incidental notation is a radiopaque ovarian shield seen obscuring the pelvic basin and a portion of the pelvic brim. (Courtesy of Gary M. Guebert, DC, DACBR, St. Louis, Missouri.)

are not generally thought to be active lesions, although a change in their size with prolonged observation has been well documented. (3) Onitsuka (4) reported a 31.9% incidence of change in size in 138 bone islands for which sequential roentgenograms over intervals ranging from 1 to 23 years were available. Most of his patients showed an increase in size of the bone islands, although a few is-

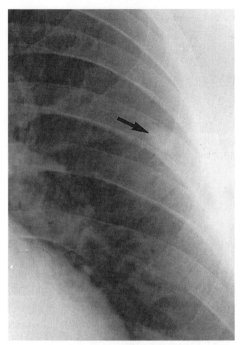

Figure 11-219 **BONE ISLAND. Rib.** Note the oval bone island within the posterolateral surface of the rib (*arrow*).

lands decreased in size. Included in his study were examples of bone islands enlarging in proportion to adolescent growth. In general, approximately 30% enlarge over a period of years. Although most bone islands appear stable, changes in them may be so slow that observation over many years is necessary. Hoffman and Campbell (5) reported a case of a bone island that disappeared with the development of hyperparathyroidism, as a result of resorption of bone, and reappeared after treatment by removal of a benign parathyroid adenoma. This finding further emphasizes the fact that bone islands are not inert areas of sclerosis; rather, they are areas of dynamic compact bone and subject to the same metabolic influences that affect the skeletal system in general. (6)

A routine blood profile shows no significant changes. The slow growth of bone islands results in normal levels of serum alkaline phosphatase. (7)

The development of a bone island has little significance except for its recognition and differential diagnosis. (8) The cause of these lesions remains obscure and relatively unknown. (8,9)

Pathologic Features

A bone island represents a focus of compact lamellar bone located within normal spongiosa. The histologic appearance of a bone island is in fact the same as that seen in osteopoikilosis. The radiologic features of the two conditions are also similar, except that the former is usually solitary, whereas the latter consists of multiple areas of sclerosis. It has been observed that the sclerotic areas in osteopoikilosis can become more radiopaque with age but show no significant change in size over an extended number of years. (3) They produce sclerotic, well-defined intramedullary densities on radiographs. (Fig. 11-221)

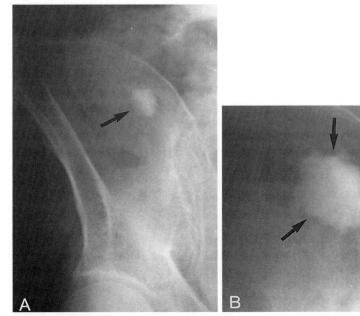

Figure 11-220 **GROWING BONE ISLAND. A. Ilium.** Note the small, oval bone island in the posterior portion of the ilium in an adult male patient (*arrow*). **B. 6-Year Follow-Up.** Observe the enlargement of the previously noted bone island. Observe the thorn-like radiating spicules of bone sur-

rounding the peripheral border of the bone island (*arrows*). This thorn-like appearance strongly suggests a bone island rather than an osteoblastic metastatic focus. This lesion was asymptomatic. (Courtesy of Wolfgang Lediner, DC, Mountain Home, Arkansas.)

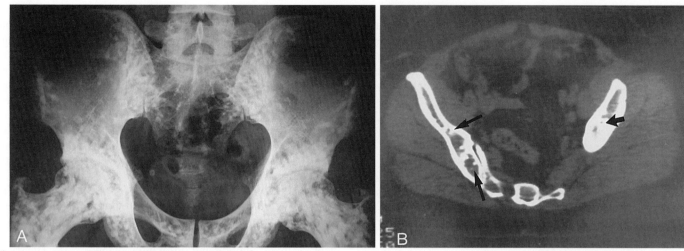

Figure 11-221 OSTEOPOIKILOSIS. A. AP Pelvis. Observe the multiple, well-defined bone islands scattered throughout the pelvis, sacrum, and proximal femora. This appearance is characteristic of osteopoikilosis. **B. CT Pelvis.** Observe the small, spherical bone islands within the medullary portion of the ilium, representing osteopoikilosis (*arrows*). (Courtesy of Bryan Hartley, MD, Melbourne, Australia.)

Radiologic Features

The radiologic findings in bone islands are usually intramedullary ovoid, round, or oblong radiopaque densities that are aligned with the long axis of the trabecular architecture. (6,8) (Fig. 11-222) The margins are sharply demarcated and in many cases have thorn-like radiating spicules of bone (*brush border*) intermingled with the trabeculae of the spongiosa. (Fig. 11-220*B*) No protrusion from the cortical surface of the involved bones can be identified. The majority of small bone islands are seen in the femoral neck and the intertrochanteric space of the proximal femur. (Fig. 11-223) Distinctively, they are located either in the epiphysis or metaphysis but never in the diaphysis. Bone islands are notably rare in the spine. (8) When present, it is usually the lumbar vertebral body that is involved, though neural arch sites have been recorded. (9) (Figs. 11-224 and 11-225) Bone islands, especially in the pelvis, can be > 1 cm and are referred to as *giant bone islands*. (8,10) (Fig. 11-217)

Bone Scan

The increased localization of bone-scanning agents in a variety of sclerotic bone lesions is well known, but uptake in a bone island has not been described with any great frequency in the literature. (2) (Fig. 11-225) Radionuclide bone scanning has been suggested as a means of differentiating bone islands from osteoblastic metastases and other lesions with focally increased bone density because this distinction cannot always be made by radiographs. The skeletal uptake of technetium-tagged phosphorus compounds is thought to be owing primarily to increased regional blood flow. Thus the usual absence of focal bone scan abnormality in bone islands has been attributed to normal regional blood flow resulting from presumed metabolic inactivity; however, instances of positive bone scans have been described in patients with growing and biopsyproven bone islands. (3,6) It would seem that increased new bone production should occur as a bone island is being formed, presumably accompanied by increased regional blood flow; how-

ever, this is usually slight because growth is slow. Relatively rapid growth periods have been reported in some bone islands, occasionally doubling or tripling in size in 5–7 years, rendering a positive, or hot, bone scan at the time of growth potential. (Table 11-26)

Differential Diagnosis

Anatomic location is an important factor in deciding whether or not a radionuclide study of a suspected bone island is necessary. The characteristic solitary lesion in the proximal third of the femur is classically of no clinical concern. However, regions of radiopacity in the sacrum, ilium, and lumbar vertebral bodies may be foci of osteoblastic metastasis. For that reason, a definitive diagnosis of benign bone island of the sacrum, ilium, or lumbar spine can be made only with the report of a negative bone scan.

Although most bone islands are usually stable in size, some may exhibit growth, as noted earlier; therefore, the major importance in recognizing bone islands is the need to distinguish them from other, significant pathologic processes, such as the following.
Osteoblastic Metastasis. An osteoblastic metastasis is usually well defined and not as dense as a bone island. When a bone island shows *thorn-like* radiations, or a *brush border,* there is little problem in differentiation because these features are not commonly found in metastasis. Osteoblastic metastasis is often polyostotic, whereas the incidence of multiple bone islands is far less common. (1,10)
Osteoid Osteoma. Osteoid osteoma is not usually a diagnostic problem because patients with this disease complain of quite severe nocturnal pain. Commonly, a central nidus with or without calcification may be seen within an area of exuberant reactive sclerosis of bone. (1)
Osteoma. Osteomas protrude from the surface of the bone, whereas bone islands are within the spongiosa. The majority of osteomas are in the head and neck area, particularly within the frontal sinuses, but bone islands are distinctly unusual in the skull. In patients with the rare Gardner's syndrome, osteomas may be found in any part of the skeleton. (1)

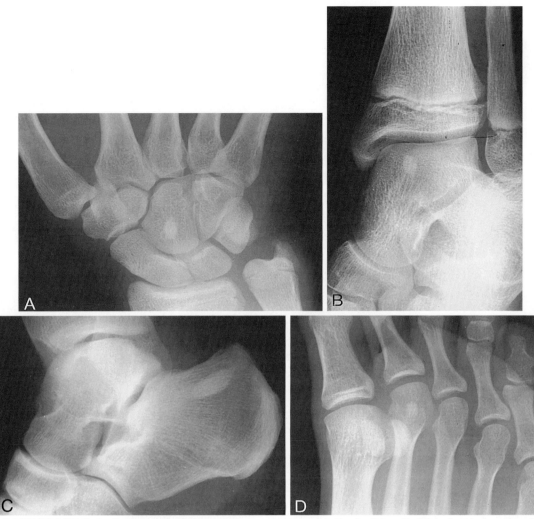

Figure 11-222 **BONE ISLANDS. A. Capitate. B. Talus. C. Calcaneus. D. Second Metatarsal Head.** (Panel C courtesy of Peter M. Davis, BAppSc (Chiro), Warnambool, Victoria, Australia.)

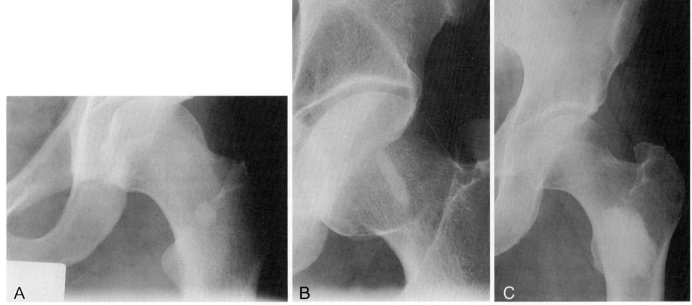

Figure 11-223 **BONE ISLAND. A. AP Femur.** Note the oval bone island in the intertrochanteric space of the proximal femur. This is the most common location for a bone island. **B. AP Femur.** Observe the oblong radiopacity representing a somewhat unusual radiographic presentation for a bone island. **C. AP Femur.** Observe the thorn-like border at the periphery of this lesion, suggesting the possibility of a bone island. Osteoblastic metastatic disease could mimic this appearance, and further clinical follow-up may be indicated in patients who present with lesions such as this and who have localized symptoms. (Panel A courtesy of Richard T. Coade, MIR, DC, Kempsey, New South Wales, Australia.)

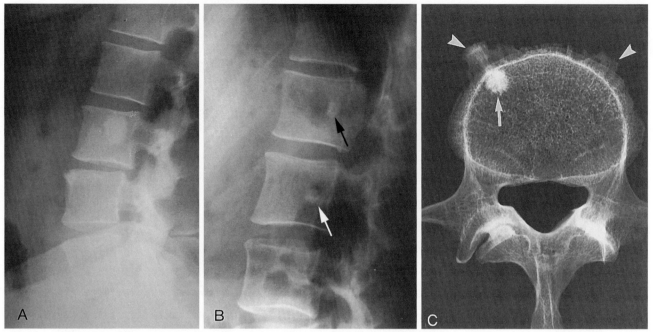

Figure 11-224 **BONE ISLAND. A. Lateral Lumbar Spine.** Note the large, circular bone island within the L3 vertebral body. **B. Lateral Lumbar Spine.** Note that two focal bone islands are seen in the L2 and L3 vertebral bodies, respectively (*arrows*). **C. Specimen Radiograph.** This specimen demonstrates clearly the discrete bone island present within the lumbar vertebral body (*arrow*). Spondylophyte formation is noted around the anterior surface of this vertebral body (*arrowheads*).

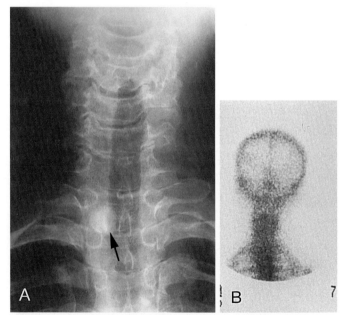

Figure 11-225 **BONE ISLAND: THORACIC SPINE. A. Plain Film.** Note the oval bone island in the T1 vertebral body (*arrow*). **B. Bone Scan.** Note the even distribution of tracer uptake with no focal accumulation at T1. *COMMENT:* Bone islands in the cervical and thoracic spine are rare. A failure for bone islands to exhibit uptake is typical of these lesions, though, on occasion, especially with large lesions, some activity can be seen. (Courtesy of Lawrence T. Sellers, DC, DACBR, Portland, Oregon.)

Table 11-26	Radiologic Features of Bone Islands
Epiphyseal, metaphyseal	
Medullary	
Round-oval: long axis oriented along lines of stress	
Smooth or radiating border	
Homogeneously opaque	
Normal adjacent cortex	
May change size	
Occasionally positive on isotopic scanning	

A large or growing bone island should be included in the differential diagnosis of any sclerotic bone lesion that is positive on bone scan. The absence of a primary tumor, the slow rate of growth of the sclerotic focus over years, the absence of pain at the site involved, and the presence of a clearly demarcated margin of the dense radiographic shadow favor the diagnosis of a growing bone island. If these criteria are applied, it should be possible to differentially diagnose a bone island from a primary or secondary bone tumor. In patients with a complicated history, as in those who present with a previous malignancy, the definitive diagnosis becomes more difficult. In some cases, the only definitive mechanism for final diagnosis may be biopsy.

OSTEOID OSTEOMA

General Considerations

Osteoid osteoma was first described by Henry Jaffe (1) in 1925; however, for several decades the orthopedic community rejected his findings and considered osteoid osteoma to be a variant of osteomyelitis. (2,3) Osteoid osteoma has since been accepted as a distinct benign bone disorder, most likely a neoplasm. Well-documented radiographic findings of osteoid osteoma and a typical clinical presentation have been described in the literature (4,5); however, the typical radiographic and clinical patterns do not always occur, and often a confusing picture of a young patient with bone pain emerges, which presents a diagnostic dilemma to both the radiologist and the clinician.

Incidence

Osteoid osteoma makes up approximately 2.6% of all excised bone tumors and approximately 11% of all benign bone tumors. (6)

Clinical Features

Age and Sex Distribution

This lesion occurs predominantly in young patients between the ages of 10 and 25 years. The youngest patient reported was an 8-month-old child with a lesion in the tibia. (7) Approximately 12% of cases occur before the age of 10, and 13% after the age of 30. (8) The ratio of male to female is 2:1. (5,8)

Signs and Symptoms

Pain is characteristic of this lesion and may be accompanied by vasomotor disturbances, primarily, profuse sweating and increased skin temperature in the affected region. The classic description is of a gradual onset of increasingly severe, deep, aching pain, which however, only 65% of patients have the classic presentation of night pain relieved by aspirin. (9) Because of localized bone pain, many patients are seen initially by a rheumatologist for evaluation. The diagnosis usually is not readily apparent, and the clinical manifestations of osteoid osteoma resemble inflammatory arthritis, degenerative arthritis, and septic arthritis. In 30% of patients the pain is referred to a nearby joint so that the roentgen examination may be misdirected. It is important to note that the clinical evidence of pain may be present many months before roentgen evidence of the lesion.

Localized swelling and point tenderness are frequent findings. Limitation of motion, painful limp, stiffness, and weakness of nearby joints may be noted; muscle atrophy and limp occur as a result of joint involvement.

Painful, rigid scoliosis resulting from a lesion located on the concave side of the curve is the classic clinical presentation of a lumbar or thoracic osteoid osteoma. When a cervical vertebra is involved, torticollis and secondary contracture of the sternocleidomastoid muscle may be noted. Lesions in the spinous processes do not produce torticollis or scoliosis, but rather localized pain and spinal stiffness. (10) A lesion of the proximal femur or lumbar vertebrae may simulate a herniated disc; however, on physical examination true sciatica is not demonstrated. (11)

Location

Osteoid osteoma can occur in nearly any bone; however, 50% of cases occur in the femur and tibia. (12) (Figs. 11-226 and 11-227)

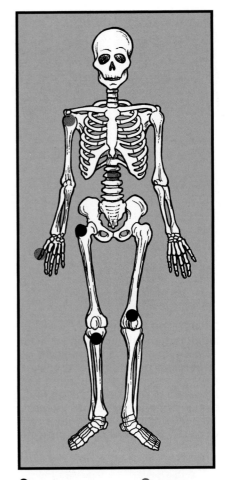

● More common   ● Less common

Figure 11-226 **SKELETAL DISTRIBUTION OF OSTEOID OSTEOMA.**

There is a predilection for the upper end of the femur, particularly the neck and trochanters. Approximately 10% of cases occur within the spine, most of these affecting the neural arch. The lamina, pedicle, facet, and spinous process are involved in descending order of frequency. Other sites include the ribs, clavicle, humerus, fibula, mandible, skull, carpals, and thumb. (13–16) (Fig. 11-228)

Pathologic Features

The actual lesion of osteoid osteoma is a nidus that grossly appears as a soft, reddish brown, vascularized tumor that is usually ≤ 1 cm in diameter. The nidus appears radiolucent on the radiograph, and the second component of the osteoid osteoma is a significant reactive sclerosis with cortical thickening and a solid periosteal response encompassing the nidus. (Fig. 11-229) The nidus is initially uncalcified but, upon maturity, may develop a fleck of target calcification within the center of the nidus.

The microscopic appearance of the nidus demonstrates small, spherical nodules of highly vascularized fibrous connective tissue, with benign giant cells within an interlacing network of osteoid trabeculae, which are usually thin and contain a variable amount of mineralization.

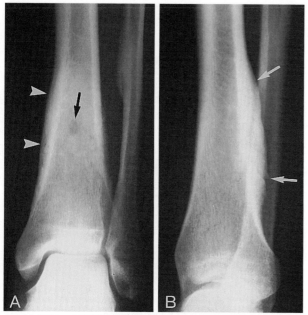

Figure 11-227 **OSTEOID OSTEOMA. A. AP Tibia.** Observe the radiolucent tumor nidus within the central medullary portion of the distal tibia (*arrow*). There is significant reactive sclerosis of bone surrounding the radiolucent nidus, some of which is periosteal new bone formation, assuming a solid pattern (*arrowheads*). **B. Lateral Tibia.** Note the significant cortical and periosteal new bone formation on the posterior surface of the distal tibia (*arrows*). The tumor nidus of the osteoid osteoma is not clearly visualized on this projection.

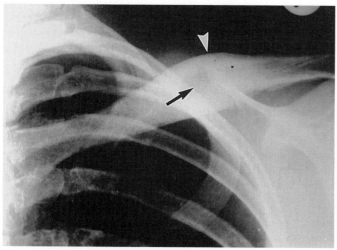

Figure 11-228 **OSTEOID OSTEOMA. Clavicle.** Note the large, radiolucent tumor nidus in the mid-diaphysis of the clavicle (*arrow*). There is exuberant reactive sclerosis around the tumor nidus, creating bone expansion and enlargement of the clavicle (*arrowhead*). This is a rare location for osteoid osteoma. (Courtesy of David P. Thomas, MD, Melbourne, Australia.)

There are three specific anatomic locations for osteoid osteoma: cortical (most common), cancellous (intramedullary), and subperiosteal. Their histologic and radiographic appearances vary significantly, depending on the specific location.

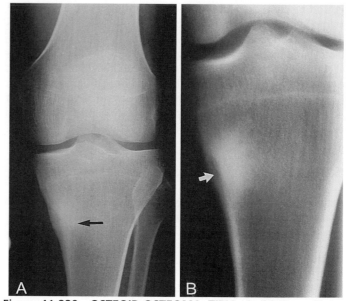

Figure 11-229 **OSTEOID OSTEOMA: TIBIA. A. AP Knee.** Note the ill-defined area of increased cortical new bone in the medial metaphysis of the proximal tibia (*arrow*). **B. Tomogram, AP Tibia.** Observe that the previously noted reactive sclerosis in the medial cortical surface of the tibia is visualized. A small radiolucent tumor nidus is also seen (*arrow*). *COMMENT:* This patient presented with pain that was worse at night and that was dramatically relieved by the use of aspirin. This is the characteristic history of patients with both osteoid osteoma and Brodie's abscess.

Radiologic Features

The radiographic appearance of a well-developed lesion is as a characteristic lucent nidus with surrounding florid perifocal reactive sclerosis. (17) (Fig. 11-230) This is the typical appearance of a cortically placed osteoid osteoma. The initial lesion is a small area of increased bony density that surrounds an oval or round lucent nidus usually ≤ 1 cm in diameter. (18) (Fig. 11-231) The osteoid osteoma can cause so much surrounding sclerosis that the nidus is obscured on a single roentgenographic view. (Fig. 11-232) Occasionally, a central fleck of calcification can be seen on plain films within the radiolucent nidus. (Fig. 11-233) When plain films are negative, CT or radioisotope bone scans are often necessary to identify the lesion.

Intramedullary lesions that are intracapsular (such as those in the femoral neck) provoke much less reactive sclerosis because of the low rate of bone production from the intracapsular periosteum. Lesions in this location are much more difficult to detect because the lucent nidus is often the only abnormality visualized. (Fig. 11-234)

Spinal osteoid osteomas are elusive lesions. (19,20) Patients often undergo numerous radiographic studies before the correct diagnosis is reached. Lumbosacral strain, psychogenic back pain, cervical strain, herniated nucleus pulposus, and biomechanical back pain are frequent prior diagnoses. As in other areas of the skeleton, osteoid osteomas may produce pain before radiographic changes, and in the spine the changes are difficult to detect on plain films. The neural arch is the classic location, and early lesions may be found only with the use of CT and bone scanning; CT through an area of increased radionuclide uptake may demonstrate the lucent nidus. The most common site for spinal osteoid

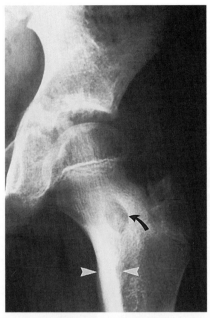

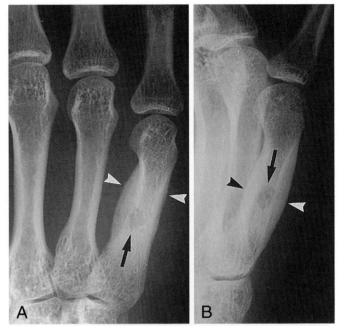

Figure 11-230 **OSTEOID OSTEOMA. Femoral Neck.** Note the well-defined radiolucent tumor nidus within the neck of the proximal femur (*arrow*). A significant degree of reactive sclerosis of bone is seen adjacent to the tumor nidus (*arrowheads*), with the greatest changes seen caudal to the radiolucent nidus. This is a characteristic presentation for osteoid osteoma at this site. (Reprinted with permission from the **Center for Devices and Radiological Health, FDA, and the American College of Radiology:** *Learning File, Skeletal Section, SK-935.*)

Figure 11-231 **OSTEOID OSTEOMA: HAND. A. and B. Fifth Metacarpal.** Observe the well-defined radiolucent tumor nidus within the medullary component of the diaphysis of the fifth metacarpal (*arrows*). Reactive sclerosis and appositional periosteal new bone surround the tumor nidus (*arrowheads*). (Courtesy of Bryan Hartley, MD, Melbourne, Australia.)

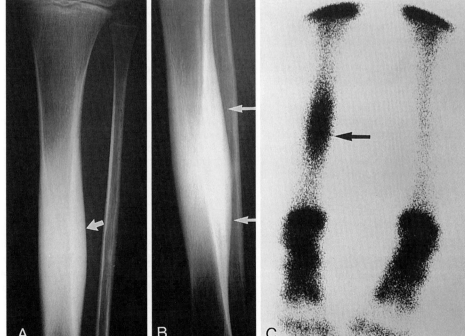

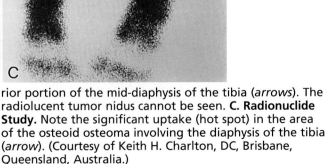

Figure 11-232 **OSTEOID OSTEOMA. A. AP Tibia.** Note the significant reactive sclerosis of bone in the mid-diaphysis of the tibia. Periosteal new bone formation thickens the cortex and obscures the observer's ability to differentiate the medullary and cortical portions of the bone (*arrow*). **B. Lateral Tibia.** Observe the significant periosteal new bone formation, along with thickening of the cortex, in the poste- rior portion of the mid-diaphysis of the tibia (*arrows*). The radiolucent tumor nidus cannot be seen. **C. Radionuclide Study.** Note the significant uptake (hot spot) in the area of the osteoid osteoma involving the diaphysis of the tibia (*arrow*). (Courtesy of Keith H. Charlton, DC, Brisbane, Queensland, Australia.)

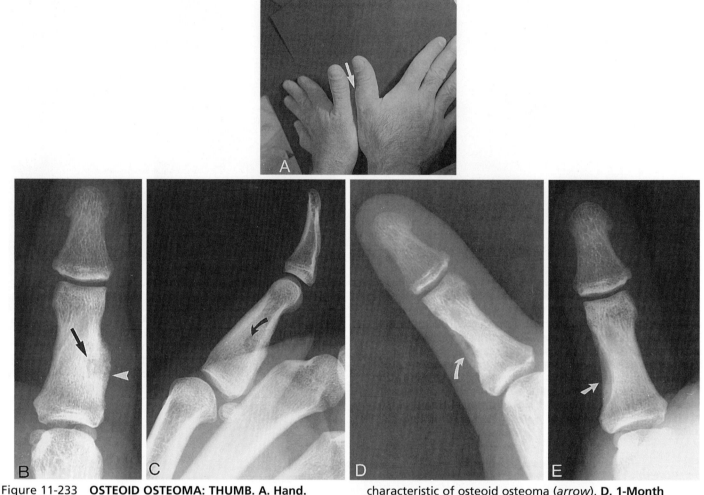

Figure 11-233 OSTEOID OSTEOMA: THUMB. A. Hand. Observe the soft tissue swelling present around the base of the thumb (*arrow*). This patient was complaining of pain, which was worse at night, aggravated by activity, and alleviated with the use of aspirin. **B. PA Thumb.** Note the small, radiolucent nidus within the medullary portion of the proximal phalanx (*arrow*). A florid reaction of periosteal new bone formation is present, creating enlargement of the phalanx (*arrowhead*). **C. Oblique Thumb.** Observe the radiolucent tumor nidus present in the central portion of the proximal phalanx. Close observation reveals a central fleck of calcification seen within the radiolucent tumor nidus, which is characteristic of osteoid osteoma (*arrow*). **D. 1-Month Postsurgery.** Note that the tumor nidus has been removed surgically. There is a moderate degree of periosteal new bone formation present in the area where the tumor nidus was located (*arrow*). The patient received dramatic relief of his pain following surgery. **E. 2-Year Follow-Up.** Note the area from which the tumor was removed still shows a moderate degree of cortical new bone (*arrow*). (Reprinted with permission from **Yochum TR:** *Osteoid osteoma of the thumb.* ACA Council Roent November, 1979. Courtesy of Mark Baum, DC, Miami, Florida.)

osteoma is the lumbar spine (60%), with lesions less common in the cervical, thoracic, and sacral vertebrae (27%, 12%, and 2%, respectively). (21) Vertebral body lesions are uncommon (7%); most lesions are in the neural arch. (21) The initial radiographic sign is a lucent nidus, which often goes undetected. The more mature lesion incites reactive sclerosis, leaving a dense or ivory pedicle or lamina. (Figs. 11-235 and 11-236) Often, the lesion will be on the concave side of a painful scoliosis. (Fig. 11-237) This appearance must be differentiated from the stress response opposite a unilateral spondylolysis, congenital agenesis of the contralateral pedicle, osteoblastoma, and, rarely, osteoblastic metastatic carcinoma. (22–24) Vertebral body lesions may produce an ivory vertebra or focal sclerosis, usually close to the endplate. (Fig. 11-238)

Angiography can be helpful in selected cases of osteoid osteoma for definitive diagnosis. (25) The area of the lesion is highly vascularized, with an intensely homogenous vascular blush appearing in the arterial phase and persisting late into the venous phase. This is the definitive means of distinguishing osteoid osteoma from a Brodie's abscess, which shows no such vascular blush within its necrotic cavity.

In most cases of osteoid osteoma, plain roentgenograms are sufficient to demonstrate the lesion, providing the diagnosis in > 75% of cases. (8) CT may be helpful for localizing the nidus, especially where plain roentgenograms are equivocal. If the roentgenogram is negative but the clinical history suggests a lesion, then a bone scan or MRI should be performed. (26) Bone scans will show a regional increase in uptake with an intense

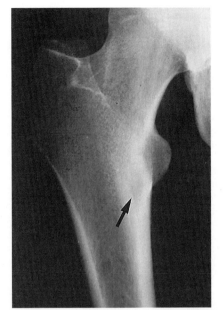

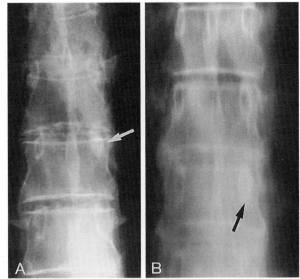

Figure 11-236   **OSTEOID OSTEOMA: THORACIC SPINE. A. AP Thoracic.** Observe the dense radiopacity affecting the pedicle of the T9 vertebra (*arrow*). **B. Tomogram, AP T9.** Tomographic evaluation clearly defines the sclerotic pedicle at T9 (*arrow*). *COMMENT:* Approximately 10% of the cases of osteoid osteoma occur within the spine, with most of these affecting the neural arch. The lamina, pedicle, facet, and spinous process are involved, in descending order of frequency. The most common site for spinal osteoid osteoma is the lumbar region (60%), with lesions less commonly found in the cervical, thoracic, and sacral vertebrae (27%, 12%, and 2%, respectively).

Figure 11-234   **OSTEOID OSTEOMA IN A HARD-TO-SEE AREA. Proximal Femur.** Observe the subtle radiolucent tumor nidus just inferior to the lesser trochanter (*arrow*). The minimal reactive sclerosis that surrounds this lesion is hard to perceive because of the confluence of the cortex at this anatomic site. *COMMENT:* Osteoid osteomas that occur adjacent to the lesser trochanter are often difficult to visualize. This is a relatively common location for osteoid osteoma.

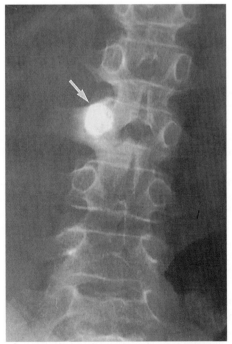

Figure 11-235   **OSTEOID OSTEOMA. AP Lumbar Spine.** Observe the densely radiopaque pedicle of the L3 vertebra (*arrow*). This 12-year-old patient presented with pain that was worse at night and was dramatically alleviated by aspirin. (Courtesy of John E. MacRae, DC, DACBR, Toronto, Ontario, Canada.)

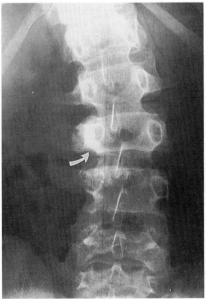

Figure 11-237   **OSTEOID OSTEOMA. AP Lumbar Spine.** Observe the reactive sclerosis in the area of the lamina and pedicle of L3 (*arrow*). *COMMENT:* This patient presented with a painful scoliosis, and an osteoid osteoma involving the neural arch was found. The osteoid osteoma is on the concave side of the scoliosis, which is the classic presentation. (Courtesy of Jack Edeiken, MD, Houston, Texas.)

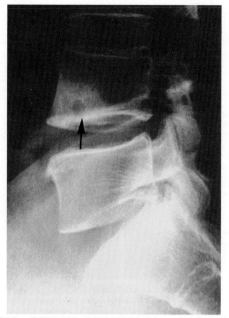

Figure 11-238 OSTEOID OSTEOMA. Vertebral Body. Observe the radiolucent nidus in the sub-endplate region (*arrow*). Reactive sclerosis extends into the vertebral body. (Courtesy of Merritt L. Armstrong, DC, Freeport, Maine.)

Table 11-27	Radiologic Features of Osteoid Osteoma

Spine
    Antalgic scoliosis, lesion on concave side
    Dense pedicle, facet, transverse process, lamina
Long bones
    Metaphyseal, diaphyseal
    Geographic lesion (nidus)
        Eccentric
        < 1 cm in size
        Central calcific fleck
        Surrounding rim of sclerosis
        Adjacent solid periosteal response
Additional studies
    Angiogram: arterial blush, venous retention
    Bone scan: localized increased uptake
    CT: clear demonstration of the nidus
Differential diagnosis
    Brodie's abscess: lacks angiographic changes, nidus usually
        > 2 cm
    Stress fracture: linear fracture line demonstration, time sequence
        changes

focal zone of uptake superimposed (*double-density sign*). (9,27) This is particularly true with spinal lesions. If the bone scan is positive, then CT is helpful in defining the nature of the lesion. If these studies are equivocal, angiography may be necessary to finally locate and provide the correct diagnosis. (Table 11-27) MRI usually exhibits surrounding marrow edema, which in turn may improve the conspicuity of the nidus. (28,29) In general, MRI is a reliable modality in the demonstration of the nidus. (29)

Differential Diagnosis

Garré's Chronic Sclerosing Osteomyelitis. In the current literature Garré's osteomyelitis has been disregarded as a singular and distinct disease process. (See Chapter 12.) Although described by Garré as chronic sclerosing osteomyelitis, it is considered probable that many of the lesions formerly regarded as being inflammatory in origin were in fact osteoid osteomas.

Brodie's Abscess. The clinical and radiologic presentation of Brodie's abscess may resemble osteoid osteoma. Pain that is worse at night and alleviated by aspirin is a characteristic shared by both osteoid osteoma and Brodie's abscess. The radiolucent nidus of Brodie's abscess is normally much larger (> 1 cm and often closer to 2 cm in diameter) than that of osteoid osteoma. (16) The *halo rim* of sclerosis surrounding the radiolucent nidus of an abscess is frequently thicker and more irregular than that found associated with osteoid osteoma. The *vascular blush* on angiographic studies is found in osteoid osteoma and not Brodie's abscess. There are, of course, exceptions to these differential points, and Brodie's abscess must be considered in a differential diagnosis when the radiologic appearance seems to be that of osteoid osteoma and the clinical presentation is equally similar. (16)

Stress Fracture. A stress fracture frequently produces focal changes that may mimic osteoid osteoma clinically and radiologically. Sequential studies over time and images usually demonstrate healing of the fracture.

Treatment and Prognosis

In general, most osteoid osteomas require no treatment because their natural history is self-limiting; however, in patients who will not comply or who are unwilling to sustain a regime of non-steroidal anti-inflammatory drugs (NSAIDs) until the pain resolves, more invasive measures are available. (30) Radiotherapy and thermocoagulation have recently gained interest because they require less invasion of the tissues than does surgery. (31–33) Thermocoagulation has shown success rates of approximately 92% in recent studies. (33) With respect to surgery, the treatment of choice, is wide en bloc excision with removal of a small portion of the surrounding sclerotic bone. (Fig. 11-239) Most patients have dramatic relief of symptoms after surgery, and recurrence is rare, provided complete excision of the nidus is accomplished. (34,35) Surgical procedures are becoming more effective with CT guidance to ensure removal of the nidus. (36,37) Some surgeons may delay surgery until the nidus is of adequate size to be clearly demonstrated by CT, to ensure effective surgical treatment. It is not necessary to remove the reactive sclerosis, even though this may form the major part of the radiologic presentation.

Spontaneous regressions have been reported; however, an extended time span is necessary for this to occur, and most patients cannot tolerate the pain for this period of time (> 10 years). (38) Spinal lesions are treated by excision, unless they occur in the vertebral body, in which case they are then treated with irradiation.

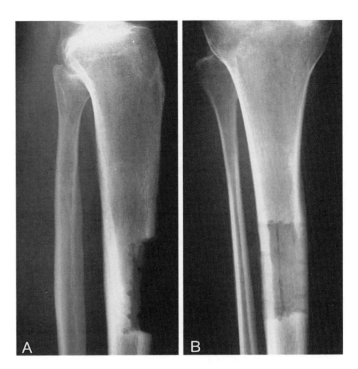

Figure 11-239 **OSTEOID OSTEOMA: EN BLOC EXCISION.**
A. Lateral Tibia. B. AP Tibia. Note the large, postsurgical de-
fect on the anterior cortex of the mid-diaphysis of the tibia.
This represents an en bloc excision for a previously diag-
nosed osteoid osteoma. (Courtesy of Jack Edeiken, MD,
Houston, Texas.)

CAPSULE SUMMARY   Osteoid Osteoma

General Considerations

- First described by Henry Jaffe in 1925.
- Radiographic and clinical findings are characteristic.

Incidence

- Makes up 2.6% of all excised bone tumors and approximately 11% of all benign bone tumors.

Clinical Features

- There is a 2:1 male predominance; 10- to 25-year age range
  is most common.
- Severe pain, worse at night, that is dramatically alleviated
  by the use of aspirin occurs in 65% of cases.
- Muscle atrophy and limp occur in long-standing lesions of
  the lower extremities.
- Painful and rigid scoliosis, with the lesion on the concave
  side of the curve, usually occurs in the lumbar spine.
- 50% occur in the femur and tibia; 10% occur within the
  spine, usually in the neural arch.

Pathologic Features

- The tumor consists of a nidus, that is usually ≤ 1 cm in
  diameter.
- Target calcification may occur in the center of the radiolucent nidus.
- The most common location within the bone is in the cortex,
  with intramedullary and subperiosteal lesions also occurring.

Radiologic Features

- The characteristic appearance of a cortical lesion is as a
  radiolucent nidus surrounded by florid perifocal reactive
  sclerosis.
- Often, CT and bone scans are necessary to demonstrate the
  nidus, especially in the spine.
- Intramedullary lesions that are intracapsular (such as the
  femoral neck) provoke much less reactive sclerosis.
- 60% of the spinal lesions are in the lumbar spine, usually
  creating an ivory pedicle or neural arch.

Differential Diagnosis

- Brodie's abscess is the prime clinical and radiographic disease entity to mimic osteoid osteoma. This differentiation
  cannot be made clinically because patients with either present with a similar history. Radiographic differentiation is
  suggested by observing the nidus, usually > 2 cm in Brodie's
  abscess.

Treatment and Prognosis

- In surgically accessible lesions a wide en bloc excision is
  the treatment of choice.
- It is not necessary to remove the reactive sclerosis, even
  though this may form the major part of the radiologic
  presentation.
- Vertebral body lesions are often treated with irradiation.
- Prognosis is good, with little chance of recurrence when
  complete surgical excision of the nidus is accomplished.

OSTEOBLASTOMA

General Considerations

Osteoblastoma is a rare primary benign bone tumor that usually presents within the spine. In 1954 Dahlin and Johnson (1) described a large, benign neoplastic lesion, which on histology was similar to osteoid osteoma and which they defined as *giant osteoid osteoma*. A benign osteoblastic neoplasm with many similar morphologic features was designated a *benign osteoblastoma* by Jaffe (2) in 1956. For a long time these two entities (osteoblastoma and osteoid osteoma) have been considered separately. In fact, the two lesions differ in size, location, and roentgen appearance, but they share a common age range and similar microscopic appearance.

Incidence

Osteoblastoma is an uncommon tumor that accounts for about 1% of all primary bone tumors, with approximately 400 cases reported in the literature. (3)

Clinical Features

Age and Sex Distribution

The age range is from 3 to 78 years. (4) Approximately 70% of the cases occur before the age of 20, with the peak range being 10–20 years of age. (4) There is a predilection for males in a ratio of 2:1.

Signs and Symptoms

The chief complaint is pain that is less severe than that of osteoid osteoma. It is also not nocturnal and is not particularly relieved by aspirin. The duration of pain varies from a few months to as long as 2 years. Extremity lesions produce local tenderness and a palpable mass of increasing size. Spinal lesions in the thoracic and lumbar area present with a *painful scoliosis* in > 50% of cases. (5) Benign osteoblastoma and osteoid osteoma are the most common neoplastic causes of scoliosis provoked by pain. (4,6) Local muscle spasm and rigidity may be noted. Other symptoms of referred pain, paresthesias, weakness, or even paraplegia as a sequela of spinal stenosis may occur. (7)

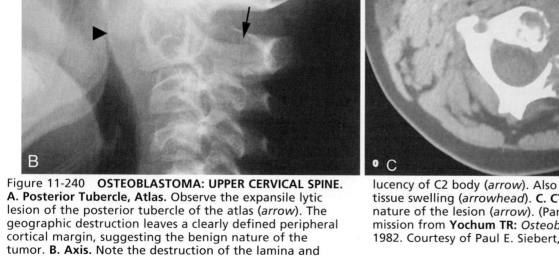
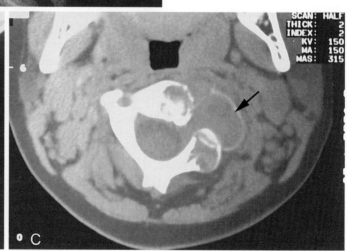

**Figure 11-240   OSTEOBLASTOMA: UPPER CERVICAL SPINE.
A. Posterior Tubercle, Atlas.** Observe the expansile lytic lesion of the posterior tubercle of the atlas (*arrow*). The geographic destruction leaves a clearly defined peripheral cortical margin, suggesting the benign nature of the tumor. **B. Axis.** Note the destruction of the lamina and lucency of C2 body (*arrow*). Also note the prevertebral soft tissue swelling (*arrowhead*). **C. CT, Axis.** Note the expansile nature of the lesion (*arrow*). (Panel A reprinted with permission from **Yochum TR:** *Osteoblastoma.* ACA J Chiro May, 1982. Courtesy of Paul E. Siebert, MD, Denver, Colorado.)

Osteoblastomas of the cervical spine most frequently present with non-specific, dull, aching pain and slight to moderate cervical tenderness of several months duration. Neurological signs are not common in cervical spine osteoblastomas because most of the lesions arise in the spinous process rather than in the neural arch, whereas the thoracic and lumbar lesions causing neurological symptoms arise from the laminae and pedicles. (8) In addition, the intervertebral canal is largest in the cervical region; and, despite the cervical cord enlargement, there is greatest room for expansion in this area before neural tissue is compressed. (7)

Location

The most common location for osteoblastoma is the spine, femur, and foot and ankle, in order of frequency. (9) Within the spine, the neural arch is primarily affected, chiefly the spinous process, transverse process, and laminae. (7) The vertebral body is only rarely involved primarily but can be a site of secondary extension from a neural arch lesion. (10) A rare site in the cervical spine is the atlas. (11) (Fig. 11-240) The cervical segments most commonly involved are the C4, C5, and C6 vertebrae. The lower thoracic and upper lumbar areas are the target sites for

osteoblastoma to occur (10) with only rare incidences at L5. (8) The long bones of the appendicular skeleton, usually the lower extremity, are involved in 30% of cases. The metaphysis and diaphysis are the most common locations within the bone. There is a predilection for the dorsal surface of the talus when present in the foot. (12) Other sites include the small bones of the hands, the skull, maxilla, mandible, and ribs. (12–16) (Figs. 11-241 and 11-242) Rarely, multicentric osteoblastomas have been reported. (17)

Pathologic Features

The gross appearance is as a violet red hemorrhagic, gritty, friable mass. The nidus is usually > 2 cm and is softer than that of osteoid osteoma. The overall size of the lesion is usually from 2 to 10 cm. Microscopically, it may be nearly impossible to differentiate osteoblastoma from osteoid osteoma. The osteoblasts appear prominent and plump, surrounding woven bone, highly vascular tissue, and there is a more orderly pattern of broader and longer osteoid trabeculae than is found in osteoid osteoma. Most osteoblastomas produce thick trabeculae of osteoid and woven bone with irregular serrated borders. Cartilage has not been reported in association with the osteoblastoma, and unequivocal anaplasia is lacking. The lack of cellular anaplasia helps differentiate this lesion from a malignant osteosarcoma, which, on occasion, an inexperienced pathologist has mistakenly diagnosed.

Radiologic Features

In contrast to osteoid osteoma, plain roentgenograms are usually sufficient to confirm the diagnosis of osteoblastoma, but CT and, occasionally, a nuclear bone scan can also be helpful. The radiologic appearance of osteoblastoma varies, depending on the anatomic location of the lesion. (Table 11-28)

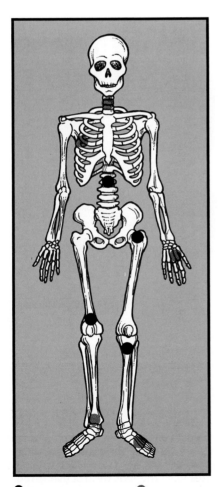

● More common   ● Less common

Figure 11-241 **SKELETAL DISTRIBUTION OF OSTEOBLASTOMA.**

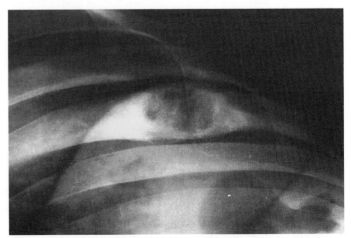

Figure 11-242 **OSTEOBLASTOMA. Rib.** Observe the large lytic defect within the midshaft of the sixth rib. A minimal degree of reactive sclerosis surrounds this lesion. This is an unusual site for osteoblastoma. (Reprinted with permission from **Yochum TR:** *Osteoblastoma.* ACA J Chiro May, 1982. Courtesy of Paul E. Siebert, MD, Denver, Colorado.)

Spine

The characteristic appearance is that of an expansile lesion, usually affecting the neural arch, with a clearly defined, eggshell-thin cortical rim at the periphery of the lesion. (Fig. 11-243) Most spinal lesions are purely radiolucent; however, a mixture of mottled blastic and lytic changes, as well as radiopaque lesions, may occur. (Figs. 11-244 to 11-246) Most spinal lesions are 4–6 cm in size; occasionally, they can appear larger. CT imaging will better delineate the nature of the lesion, and MRI is useful for assessing the involvement of adjacent structures from the bony expansion. (Fig. 11-247) The lesion that can mimic the lytic form of osteo-

Table 11-28	Radiologic Features of Osteoblastoma

Spine
  Neural arch
  Expansile
  Thin peripheral cortical rim
  Matrix usually lytic; occasionally mixed or purely sclerotic
Long bones
  Metaphyseal, diaphyseal
  Expansile, lytic
  Thin peripheral cortical rim
  > 2 cm

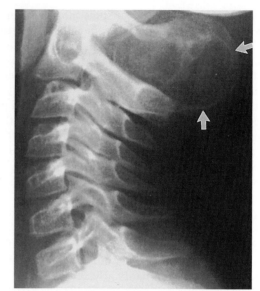

Figure 11-243 OSTEOBLASTOMA. Lateral Cervical Spine. Note the grossly expansile lytic lesion of the posterior tubercle of the atlas. The peripheral cortex of this huge osteoblastoma is clearly defined and eggshell thin (*arrows*). There is a slight osteoid matrix scattered throughout this radiolucent osteoblastoma. (Courtesy of Bryan Hartley, MD, Melbourne, Australia.)

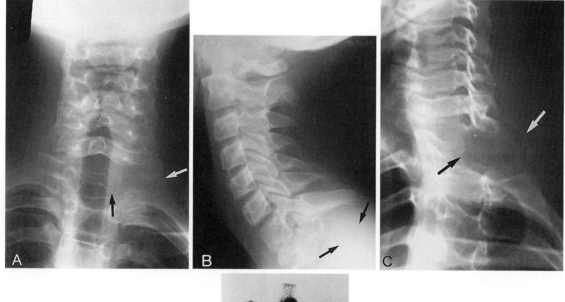

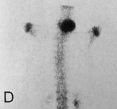

Figure 11-244 OSTEOBLASTOMA: THORACIC SPINE. A. AP Cervicothoracic Spine. Note the lytic destruction of the pedicle, lamina, transverse process, and spinous process of the T1 vertebra (*arrows*). **B. Lateral Cervical Spine.** Observe the gross lytic destruction of the spinous process and lamina of the T1 vertebra (*arrows*). **C. Oblique Cervical Spine.** Note the gross lytic destruction of the neural arch and spinous process of the T1 vertebra (*arrows*). **D. Bone Scan.** Note the diffuse area of increased uptake of radionuclide substance (hot spot), which correlates with the lytic destructive osteoblastoma of the neural arch of T1. (Courtesy of David P. Thomas, MD, Melbourne, Australia.)

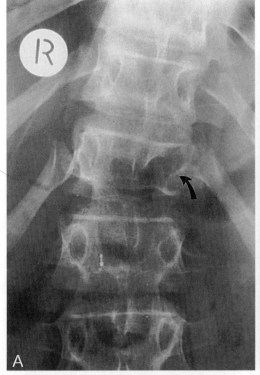

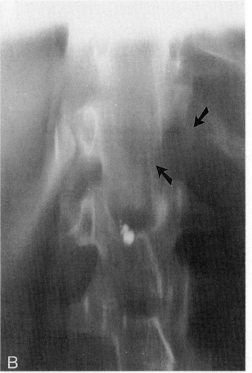

Figure 11-245 **OSTEOBLASTOMA: THORACIC SPINE. A. AP T12.** Note the lytic destruction of the pedicle, lamina, and vertebral body of T12 (*arrow*). **B. AP Tomogram, T12.** Observe the extensive osteolytic destruction of the pedicle, lamina, spinous process, and vertebral body of T12 (*arrows*).

COMMENT: The majority of patients with osteoblastomas in the spine present with purely radiolucent lesions; however, a mixture of mottled blastic and lytic changes, as well as radiopaque lesions, may occur.

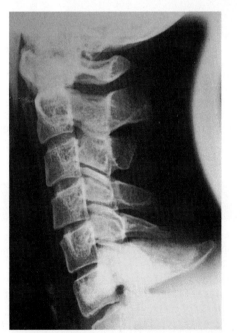

Figure 11-246 **OSTEOBLASTOMA: CERVICAL SPINE.** Note the grossly expansile, radiopaque osteoblastoma involving the spinous process, lamina, and articular pillar, with extension into the vertebral body of the C6 vertebra. *COMMENT:* This is one of the few cases of osteoblastoma that present in a truly sclerotic form. (Reprinted with permission from **Yochum TR:** *Osteoblastoma.* ACA J Chiro May, 1982. Courtesy of Trevor G. Williams, DC, Broken Hill, New South Wales, Australia.)

blastoma in the spine is aneurysmal bone cyst (ABC). Both lesions favor involvement of the neural arch of the spine, with ABC having a greater tendency to create huge expansion with a soap bubble appearance. The sclerotic osteoblastomas are not a differential problem because ABC does not present in a sclerotic fashion. (18,19) (Fig. 11-246)

Extremities

Involvement of the tubular bones generally affects the metaphysis or diaphysis in a lytic and expansile fashion. (18,19) The epiphysis is usually spared. Often, the cortex is thin, as the lesion expands the bone, leaving a radiolucent nidus, which is usually > 2 cm. (18,19) (Fig. 11-242) There is no surrounding dense halo of new bone adjacent to the nidus as is the case in osteoid osteoma. (15,16) Most lesions occur around the knee and hip.

Treatment and Prognosis

With small lesions, simple excision or surgical curettage will suffice. Recurrence rates are low, averaging about 5%. Spinal lesions that are large may require bone grafting. Radiation therapy may be used as a last resort if the spinal lesion is inoperably placed, making complete removal impossible.

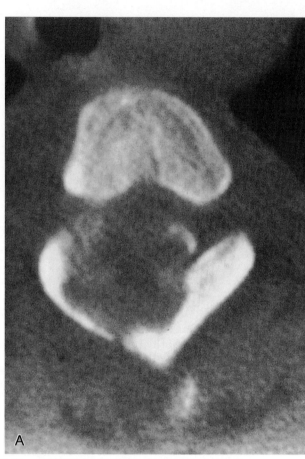

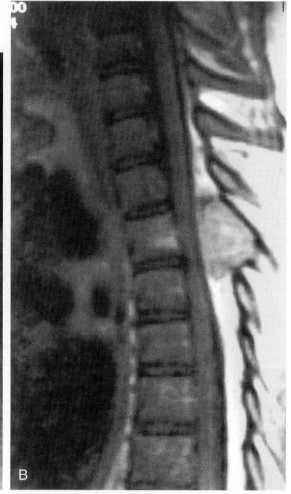

**Figure 11-247   OSTEOBLASTOMA: THORACIC SPINE.
A. CT, Axial T9.** Note the expansile osteolytic lesion affecting the lamina of the T9 vertebra. Observe the bony matrix within the destructive lesion. **B. T1-Weighted MRI, Sagittal Thoracic Spine.** Observe the large expansile lesion in the T9 lamina. This has produced posterior compression on the subarachnoid space and spinal cord. A slight degree of marrow change is seen in the posteroinferior vertebral body of T9, suggesting tumor extension to this level. *COMMENT:* This 16-year-old patient complained of lower thoracic pain. Plain film radiographs detected an expansile lesion of the T9 lamina and spinous process, and more sophisticated imaging was then performed. Note the bony matrix within the lesion. (Courtesy of Matthew Evitts, DO, Department of Radiology, University Hospital, Denver, Colorado.)

CAPSULE SUMMARY   Osteoblastoma

General Considerations

- Dahlin and Johnson described this lesion originally as a giant osteoid osteoma.
- Jaffe coined the term osteoblastoma in 1956.

Incidence

- A rare primary benign bone tumor, representing 1% of all primary bone tumors.

Clinical Features

- 70% occur before the age of 20; peak range is 10–20.
- There is a 2:1 male predilection.
- Localized pain, which is not nocturnal and is of less severity than osteoid osteoma.

- Painful scoliosis in > 50% of cases.
- Neurological deficit may occur with expansile spinal lesions creating spinal stenosis.
- The neural arch of the spine is the most common location, with spinous process, transverse process, and laminae involved in 40% of cases.
- 30% of cases affect the long bones of the appendicular skeleton.

Pathologic Features

- Microscopically, it may be nearly impossible to differentiate osteoblastoma from osteoid osteoma.
- Produces thick trabeculae of osteoid and woven bone with irregular serrated borders.

(continued)

CAPSULE SUMMARY   Osteoblastoma (*continued*)

Radiologic Features

- Spinal lesions are usually radiolucent and expansile, affecting the neural arch.
- Tubular bone involvement creates a metaphyseal or diaphyseal lytic lesion with a nidus > 2 cm. There is no reactive sclerosis surrounding the radiolucent nidus.

Treatment and Prognosis

- Small lesions are treated effectively by curettage or simple excision.
- 5% recurrence rate exists.
- Spinal lesions are often inoperable and require radiation therapy.

SOLITARY ENCHONDROMA

General Considerations

Solitary enchondroma is a common benign bone tumor arising in residual islands of cartilage left in the metaphysis as the physis grows away. It appears as a single lesion within the interior of the bone with a great predilection for the bones of the hand and foot, although it may occur in any bone preformed in cartilage. It is often found by the coincidence of trauma because most lesions of the hand are asymptomatic, unless pathologic fracture occurs secondary to structural weakening. It is also called a central chondroma.

Incidence

Solitary enchondroma represents the most common benign bone tumor of the hand. (1) It makes up 10% of all benign bone tumors. (2) The second most common tumor of the hand that secondarily affects bone is pigmented villonodular synovitis. (3)

Clinical Features

Age and Sex Distribution

The tumor arises during the growth period, and most tumors are seen between the ages of 10 and 30 years; peak incidence is usually in the 3rd decade. Males and females are equally affected.

Signs and Symptoms

The most frequent mode of presentation is that of a painless tumor, which is found in the hands and feet. Because the lesion has been present for an extended period of time before it creates any symptoms, the duration of symptoms is short. A pathologic fracture following some trivial trauma usually precipitates localized pain and swelling. (4) (Fig. 11-248) Many patients live a normal life span with an enchondroma in the hand or foot and never develop any symptoms or even take notice of its presence.

Lesions affecting the long tubular bones (femur and humerus) may also be asymptomatic, but enchondromas in these locations tend to be more symptomatic than those of the small tubular bones of the hands and feet. Sudden onset of pain without any history of trauma may indicate active growth and herald the onset of malig-

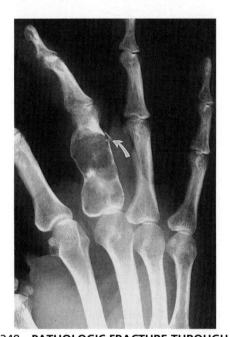

Figure 11-248   PATHOLOGIC FRACTURE THROUGH AN ENCHONDROMA. Oblique Hand. Observe the expansile, geographic lesion present in the proximal phalanx of the third finger. This enchondroma has weakened the bone and allowed a pathologic fracture to occur following trivial trauma (*arrow*).

nant degeneration, an event that occurs much more frequently in long bone enchondromas than in the short tubular bones of the hands and feet. (5)

Location

Approximately 50% of all enchondromas occur in the small tubular bones of the hand, with the phalanges accounting for 40% and the metacarpals 10%. (6) (Fig. 11-249) Only rarely is the thumb affected. (1) Enchondromas occur more commonly on the ulnar than on the radial side of the hand. (7,3) With respect to the phalanges, distal phalanges involvement is rare (8), and the tumor is usually near the proximal end. (9) In the metacarpals the lesion is toward the distal end. (9) The proximal phalanges, distal metacarpals, and middle and distal phalanges are the involved areas, in decreasing order of incidence. Occasionally, the foot will be involved. (Fig. 11-250) Other sites include the femur (14%), humerus (13%), and ribs (13%). (6) The malignant potential of enchondroma increases dramatically the closer the lesion is to the

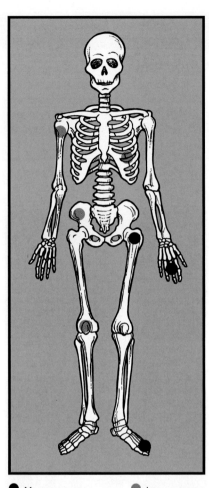

● More common   ● Less common

Figure 11-249 SKELETAL DISTRIBUTION OF SOLITARY ENCHONDROMA.

axial skeleton. (5,10) Enchondromas have been documented within the patella. (11) Tumors of the patella are uncommon; however, when present they are usually benign and of cartilaginous origin. Other obscure sites documented are the mandible, skull base, and vertebrae. (12–14) Flat bones, such as the pelvis and sternum, are only rarely involved and carry a high potential for malignant degeneration. (6)

Pathologic Features

The gross characteristics are rarely evident in surgical specimens because the standard form of treatment is curettage of the lesion, and all that is received are small granules or *rice-like fragments* of cartilaginous material, sometimes embedded in spicules of bone, where the tumor abuts on the surrounding normal tissue. Histologically, the tumor is composed of small masses or nodules of hyaline cartilage, separated by a scant, sometimes richly vascularized fibrous stroma. Foci of calcification are sometimes encountered in the cartilage; this occurs in approximately 50% of cases and can be seen on radiographs. All tumors of cartilage matrix have a great predilection for calcification, including other cartilaginous tumors, such as osteochondroma and chondroblastoma. It is often difficult to differentiate enchondromas from malignant cartilage tumors histologically. Correlation with the clinical and radiographic data, including CT, MRI, and bone scans, is absolutely necessary to avoid an incorrect diagnosis and needless surgery. (15)

Radiologic Features

Enchondroma presents as a geographic area of radiolucency that expands and may deform bone. (Fig. 11-251) The margins are well defined. The cortex remains intact, although it may be con-

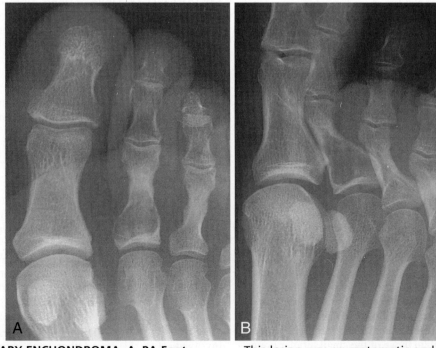

Figure 11-250 SOLITARY ENCHONDROMA. A. PA Foot. B. Oblique Foot. Note the geographic, expansile lesion of the base of the proximal phalanx of the second toe. No pathologic fracture or stippled calcification is demonstrated.

This lesion was asymptomatic and found upon radiographic examination to rule out fracture. (Courtesy of David M. Walker, DPM, Melbourne, Australia.)

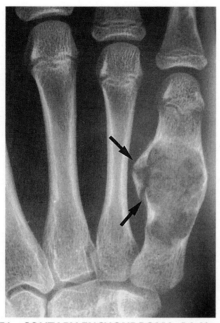

Figure 11-251 SOLITARY ENCHONDROMA. PA Hand. Observe the large geographic area of radiolucency within the mid-diaphysis of the fifth metacarpal. Significant expansion, endosteal scalloping, bone deformity, and pathologic fracture are noted (*arrows*). Matrix calcification is evident.

siderably thinned because of endosteal scalloping and expansion. Most singular lesions are centrally placed, within the metaphysis; however, the occasional eccentric lesion is noted, which may create quite a large mass. (Fig. 11-252) Stippled or punctate matrix calcification is found scattered randomly throughout the lucent defect in 50% of cases. (Fig. 11-253)

Without such calcification enchondroma must be differentiated from fibrous dysplasia, simple bone cyst, chondroblastoma, giant cell tumor, and osteoblastoma. If the lesion is placed in the distal phalanx, an epidermoid inclusion cyst or glomus tumor is the prime differential consideration. (Fig. 11-254) Epidermoid inclusion cyst represents post-traumatic implantation of epidermoid tissue within the bone. This cyst is found most often in patients who do a lot of sewing and who are likely to have needles penetrate the skin. The lack of calcification and the history of trauma are helpful points to clarify the diagnosis; both lesions are often asymptomatic. The glomus tumor is a painful, lucent defect affecting the distal phalanx by means of pressure erosion. An abnormal dilatation of blood vessels in a tightly compartmentalized area like the distal phalanx creates the characteristic pressure destructive lesions. Bone scan evaluations may reveal increased radiotracer uptake in the areas of enchondromas. (16)

In long bones it is important to be able to differentiate enchondroma with heavy calcification (*calcifying enchondroma*) (14) from a medullary bone infarct. The pattern of calcification is often helpful with the enchondroma providing so-called *rings* or *broken*

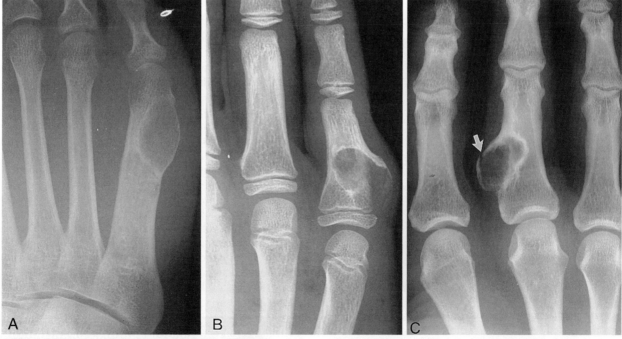

Figure 11-252 SOLITARY ENCHONDROMA: ECCENTRIC EXPANSILE LESION. A. Foot. Observe the eccentric, geographic, expansile lesion present in the metaphysis of the distal surface of the fifth metatarsal. **B. Hand.** Note the grossly expansile, radiolucent lesion involving the base of the proximal phalanx of the fifth digit. This lesion has broken the cortex and produced a rather large soft tissue mass.

C. Hand. Observe the eccentric expansile lesion of the proximal phalanx of the third digit. Significant bony expansion has produced a large soft tissue mass and cosmetic deformity. The cortex is thin, and a small pathologic fracture is noted (*arrow*). (Panel A courtesy of Robin F. Birchall, DC, Lilydale, Victoria, Australia.)

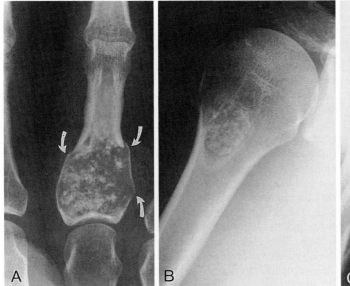

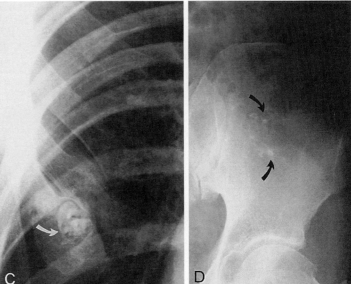

Figure 11-253 SOLITARY ENCHONDROMA: STIPPLED CALCIFICATION. A. Hand. Observe the large, geographic, expansile lesion at the base of the proximal phalanx of the fourth digit. There is classic, heavy, stippled calcification scattered throughout the entire matrix of this enchondroma. There is also an associated pathologic fracture (*arrows*). **B. Humerus.** Observe the geographic radiolucency within the metaphysis of the proximal humerus. There is characteristic stippled calcification throughout this solitary enchondroma. **C. Rib.** Note the expansile solitary enchondroma, with heavy matrix calcification, in the anterior surface of the seventh rib (*arrow*). **D. Ilium.** Note the large, geographic radiolucency within the midportion of the iliac fossa. Note the moderate stippled calcification associated with this solitary enchondroma (*arrows*). (Panel A courtesy of Gerald A. Fitzgerald, MD, Sydney, Australia. Panel D courtesy of Bryan Hartley, MD, Melbourne, Australia.)

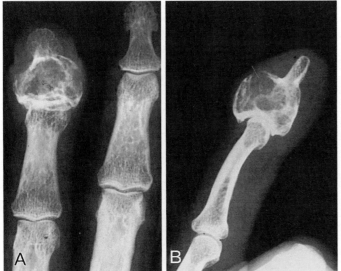

Figure 11-254 ENCHONDROMA. A. PA Hand. B. Lateral Hand. Note the grossly expansile, radiolucent solitary enchondroma involving the base of the distal phalanx of the ring finger. Endosteal scalloping, with a slight interruption in the cortex, is noted. *COMMENT:* When solitary enchondromas are found in the distal phalanx, an epidermoid inclusion cyst or glomus tumor must be considered in the differential diagnosis. Epidermoid inclusion cysts represent post-traumatic implantation of epidermoid tissue in the bone. A glomus tumor is a painful lucent defect of the distal phalanx that is caused by pressure erosion from abnormal dilatation of blood vessels in this tightly compartmentalized space.

rings—small, rounded calcification surrounded by a lucent matrix. In contrast, a bone infarct creates a streaky, roughened calcification with peripheral borders that have been called *serpiginous* in appearance. In addition, the infarct is often surrounded by a characteristic fibro-osseous margin, which may assume a well-defined straight line on one side of the lesion, a feature seldom observed in an enchondroma. The roentgen sign of bone expansion favors enchondroma because a medullary bone infarct does not expand bone. (Fig. 11-255; Table 11-29)

Malignant transformation of a solitary enchondroma to a chondrosarcoma is rare. It appears to occur in the bones closest to the axial skeleton. Malignant changes are more frequent in the long tubular bones than in the small bones of the hand or feet. (17) Patients develop unrelenting pain in a lesion that was previously asymptomatic. The radiologic features that suggest malignant transformation are cortical disruption, focal malignant periosteal reaction, a poor zone of transition, and a large, soft tissue mass. (Figs. 11-256 and 11-257)

Table 11-29	Radiologic Features of Enchondroma
Hands, feet	
Geographic lesion	
Central	
Endosteal scalloping	
Thinned cortex	
Expansion	
Stippled calcification (50%)	
Pathologic fracture	
Occasional malignant transformation	

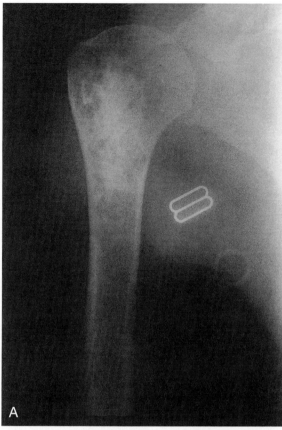

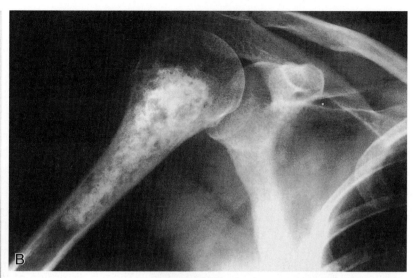

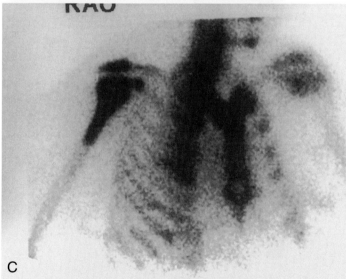

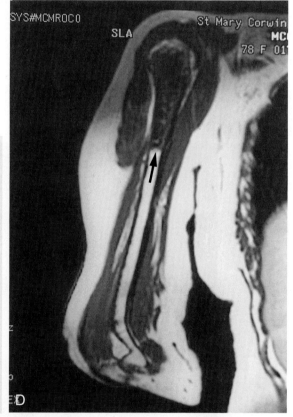

Figure 11-255 **BENIGN ENCHONDROMA VERSUS CHONDRO-SARCOMA OR BONE INFARCT. A. AP Humerus in 1984.**
B. Baby-Arm Humerus in 1997. Observe the focal serpiginous calcification within the matrix of the proximal diaphysis and metaphysis of the left humeral head. Over the 13-year time frame the lesion has minimally enlarged. No obvious evidence of cortical breakthrough or soft tissue mass is identified. **C. Planar Bone Scan, 1997.** Note the intense focal uptake of radionuclide affecting the area of involvement in the humerus seen on the plain film. No other areas of uptake are identified. **D. T1-Weighted MRI, Semisagittal Left Humerus, 1997.** Observe the low signal intensity in the proximal humerus with marrow replacement (*arrow*). Part of the low signal intensity is related to the dense matrix calcification. There is no cortical breakthrough or soft tissue mass.

COMMENT: Clinicians are often presented with areas of irregular calcification within the marrow of the distal femur, proximal tibia, or proximal humerus, which have the appearance of a bone infarct. The possibility of a slow-growing enchondroma or low-grade chondrosarcoma must be ruled out. The first examination of choice should be a bone scan. Because it is metabolically inactive, the diagnosis of bone infarct is easily made. If the bone scan is positive, an MRI study should be the next examination of choice to rule out soft tissue extension and cortical breakthrough. Biopsy of these lesions is often challenging for the pathologist because low-grade chondrosarcoma and enchondroma may be similar histologically. This patient's biopsy diagnosis was a benign enchondroma; at the 2003 follow-up examination, the patient's shoulder was asymptomatic.

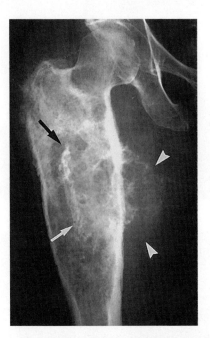

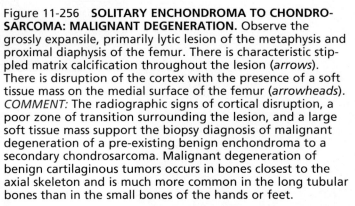

Figure 11-256 **SOLITARY ENCHONDROMA TO CHONDRO-SARCOMA: MALIGNANT DEGENERATION.** Observe the grossly expansile, primarily lytic lesion of the metaphysis and proximal diaphysis of the femur. There is characteristic stippled matrix calcification throughout the lesion (*arrows*). There is disruption of the cortex with the presence of a soft tissue mass on the medial surface of the femur (*arrowheads*). *COMMENT:* The radiographic signs of cortical disruption, a poor zone of transition surrounding the lesion, and a large soft tissue mass support the biopsy diagnosis of malignant degeneration of a pre-existing benign enchondroma to a secondary chondrosarcoma. Malignant degeneration of benign cartilaginous tumors occurs in bones closest to the axial skeleton and is much more common in the long tubular bones than in the small bones of the hands or feet.

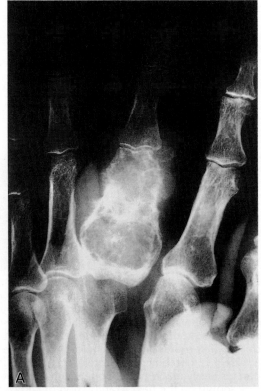

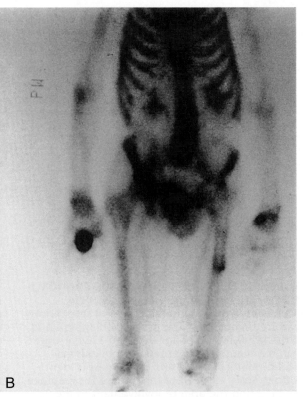

Figure 11-257 **ENCHONDROMA TO CHONDROSARCOMA: MALIGNANT DEGENERATION. A. PA Hand.** Observe the expansile, lytic, highly destructive lesion of the proximal phalanx of the third digit of the hand. There is cortical destruction and the presence of a soft tissue mass. There is stippled calcification in the matrix of the lesion. **B. Planar**

Bone Scan. Observe the intense uptake of the radionuclide within the area of the third digit. An additional area of uptake is seen at the base of the thumb, consistent with erosive osteoarthritis. A third area of small focal uptake is noted within the area of the elbow, consistent with the injection site. No other abnormalities are identified. (*continued*)

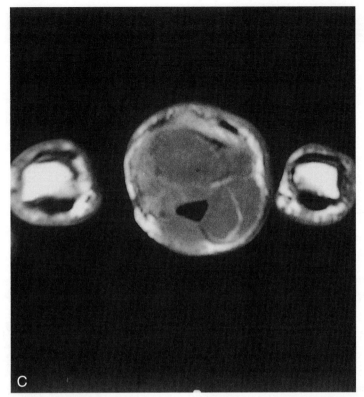

Figure 11-257 (*continued*)   **C. CT, Axial Midshaft of Proximal Phalanges of the Hand.** Observe the highly expansile destructive process affecting the proximal phalanx of the third digit along with considerable extension into the surrounding soft tissues. *COMMENT:* Malignant degeneration of a previously benign enchondroma is most commonly found in the axial skeleton and less frequently in the peripheral skeleton. The incidence of malignant degeneration of a solitary enchondroma is ≤ 1%, whereas that of multiple enchondromatosis (Ollier's disease) has been reported as high as 50%, but may more realistically be 10%. (Courtesy of Sean Bryant, MD, Department of Radiology, University Hospital, Denver, Colorado.)

Treatment and Prognosis

Most lesions in the hands or feet that create no cosmetic deformity require no treatment at all; however, if pathologic fracture occurs, casting and curettage are usually recommended. (18,19) Enchondromas in the long tubular bones or that create significant expansion in the small tubular bones require careful curettage followed by cryosurgery with bone chips) or cement packing. (20,21) The closer the enchondroma is to the axial skeleton, the higher the potential for malignant degeneration; therefore, some surgeons will remove these lesions prophylactically when they are in this location. Irradiation of benign cartilaginous lesions is absolutely contraindicated.

CAPSULE SUMMARY   Enchondroma

General Considerations
- May form in any bone preformed in cartilage.
- It is also called central chondroma.

Incidence
- Most common benign bone tumor of the hand, making up 10% of all benign bone tumors.

Clinical Features
- This tumor arises in the 10–30 age range.
- No sex predilection exists.
- This lesion is usually asymptomatic in the hands and feet until trauma draws attention to it.

- Lesions of the long bones are usually more symptomatic.
- 50% of all enchondromas occur in the hands and feet: phalanges, 40%; metacarpals, 10%. Other sites include femur, 14%; humerus, 13%; ribs, 13%.

Pathologic Features
- Histologically, composed of small masses of hyaline cartilage, separated by scant, sometimes richly vascularized fibrous stroma.
- 50% of cases show matrix calcification via radiographs.

(*continued*)

CAPSULE SUMMARY   Enchondroma (*continued*)

Radiologic Features

- Patients present with a geographic, expansile lytic lesion usually of a phalanx of the hand.
- The lesion usually occurs within the metaphysis of the bone, centrally placed.
- Stippled or punctate matrix calcification is seen within the lesion.
- Malignant degeneration to a chondrosarcoma appears to occur more often when the enchondromas are multiple and when they are closer to the axial skeleton; cortical disrup-

tion, malignant periosteal response, and a soft tissue mass are radiographic signs of malignant change.

Treatment and Prognosis

- Most lesions require no treatment because they are usually asymptomatic.
- Symptomatic lesions, usually in the long tubular bones, require careful curettage, followed by cryosurgery and bone chips.
- Irradiation of benign cartilaginous lesions is contraindicated.

MULTIPLE ENCHONDROMATOSIS (OLLIER'S DISEASE)

General Considerations

The presence of central chondromas or enchondromas in multiple sites is referred to as enchondromatosis. The initial description of this condition was by a French physician who denoted a unilateral form of the disease that now bears his name, Ollier's disease. (1) Today, however, enchondromatosis occurs most often bilaterally, and Ollier's disease has also been used in association with bilateral lesions. Jaffe (2) preferred the term *multiple enchondromatosis* over Ollier's disease. Enchondromatosis is a cartilage dysplasia of bone representing an inborn anomaly of enchondral bone formation. (3) This anomalous malformation leaves unossified cartilage remnants in the diaphyses and metaphyses.

Clinical Features

Pain is rarely found associated with multiple enchondromas, unless there is superimposed trauma and pathologic fracture. If the lesions are large, deformity and loss of limb function may occur. The most frequent location is in the small bones of the hands and feet. (4) The femur and tibia are frequently affected, and the iliac crest is the most commonly involved flat bone. (3) (Fig. 11-258)

Radiologic Features

Radiographically, these lesions are similar to solitary enchondromas, with a round or oval radiolucency that creates a symmetric widening of the bone. (Fig. 11-259) Central matrix calcification is common. (Figs. 11-260 to 11-262) Occasionally, these lesions can be eccentrically placed, causing a larger expansion of bone. Often, with central metaphyseal lesions, *streak-like or vertical bands of radiolucencies* can be seen projecting toward the diaphysis of the bone. (5) (Figs. 11-263 and 11-264)

Malignant degeneration of enchondromas in patients with enchondromatosis has been reported. (6) Jaffe (2) stated a rate of

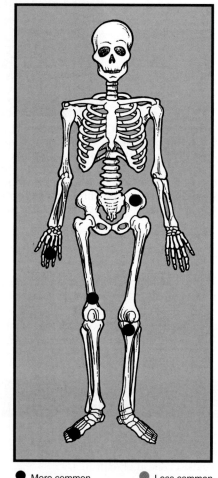

● More common   ● Less common

Figure 11-258   SKELETAL DISTRIBUTION OF MULTIPLE ENCHONDROMATOSIS (OLLIER'S DISEASE).

50%, which may be high; 10% may be more realistic. (7) Malignant changes can occur in any bone; however, the pelvic bones and the shoulder girdle are the most common sites (Fig. 11-265). (3) MRI is useful in detecting any malignant transformation. (8)

The treatment for deforming or symptomatic lesions is surgical curettage or en bloc excision. (9)

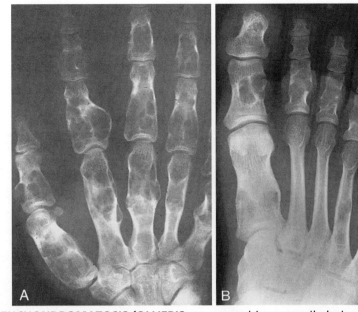

Figure 11-259 **MULTIPLE ENCHONDROMATOSIS (OLLIER'S DISEASE). A. Hand.** Observe the geographic, expansile, soap bubble lesions affecting nearly every bone visualized within the hand. Slight matrix calcification is noted in the metacarpal bones. **B. Foot.** Observe the multiple, geographic, expansile lesions scattered throughout the proximal phalanges of the foot. The first metatarsal and the diaphysis of the fourth metatarsal also contain expansile enchondromas. The expansion of bone has widened the diaphysis of most of the affected bones.

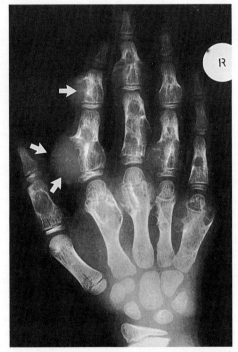

Figure 11-260 **MULTIPLE ENCHONDROMATOSIS (OLLIER'S DISEASE). Hand.** Note the multiple, geographic, expansile lesions scattered throughout nearly all of the tubular bones of the hand. There is gross eccentric expansion of the medial cortex of the middle and proximal phalanges of the second digit, creating a rather large soft tissue mass and cosmetic deformity (*arrows*). Similar expansion, but to a lesser extent, is seen throughout the metacarpal bones and proximal phalanges. Scattered matrix calcification is seen within several of the enchondromas. (Courtesy of David P. Thomas, MD, Melbourne, Australia.)

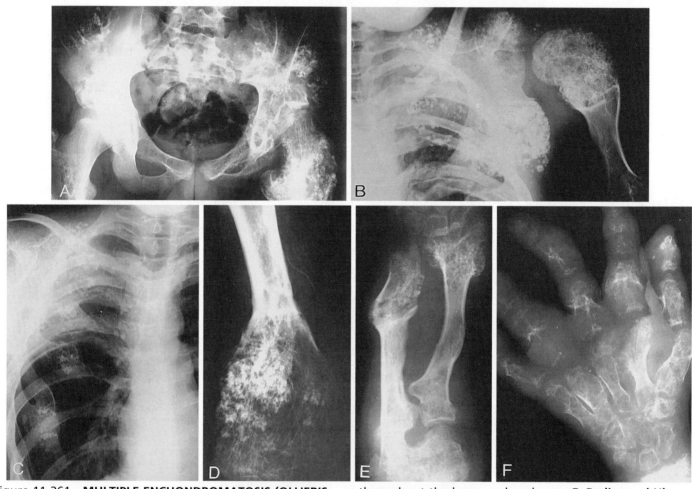

Figure 11-261 **MULTIPLE ENCHONDROMATOSIS (OLLIER'S DISEASE): DIFFUSE SKELETAL INVOLVEMENT. A. Pelvis.** Observe the multiple enchondromas scattered throughout the pelvis and proximal femora. There is a heavy matrix of stippled calcification throughout these lesions. **B. Left Shoulder.** Note the extensive enchondromatosis involving the scapula, ribs, and proximal humerus. Dense, stippled calcification is seen associated with the multiple enchondromas. **C. Right Shoulder and Ribs.** Note the multiple enchondromas at the anterior surfaces of several ribs as well as in the scapula; these demonstrate classic punctate or stippled calcification. **D. Distal Femur.** Observe the gross expansion of the distal femur, with stippled calcification throughout the large enchondroma. **E. Radius and Ulna.** Observe the expansion of the distal radius and ulna, with stippled calcification within the radiolucent lesions. Additional enchondromas are seen in the distal humerus and in the radial head and tuberosity. **F. Hand.** Note the multiple enchondromas involving all of the tubular bones of the hand. Because of the gross expansile nature of these lesions, the peripheral cortex is poorly visualized throughout, giving the appearance of a malignant disorder. Advanced cases of multiple enchondromatosis, with gross expansion, may often present this pattern of bone destruction. (Courtesy of Bryan Hartley, MD, Melbourne, Australia.)

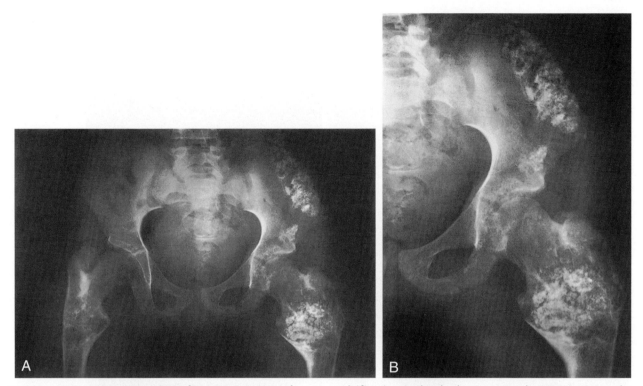

Figure 11-262 **ENCHONDROMATOSIS (OLLIER'S DISEASE): ILIUM AND PROXIMAL FEMUR. A. AP Pelvis. B. AP Hip.** Observe the multiple enchondromas affecting the proximal femora and ilium. The characteristic punctate or stippled calcification is clearly demonstrated. *COMMENT:* Enchondroma of the ilium are somewhat unusual, although the proximal femur is a common site. (Courtesy of Michael T. Buehler, DC, DACBR, Durango, Colorado.)

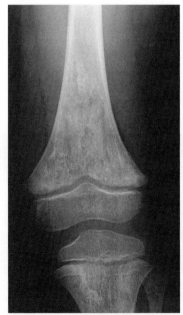

Figure 11-263 **MULTIPLE ENCHONDROMATOSIS (OLLIER'S DISEASE): STREAK-LIKE METAPHYSEAL VERTICAL RADIO-LUCENCIES. AP Knee.** Observe the streak-like radiolucencies throughout the metaphysis of the distal femur and proximal tibia. This appearance is typical of the cartilaginous lesions affecting the metaphyses of long tubular bones in multiple enchondromatosis.

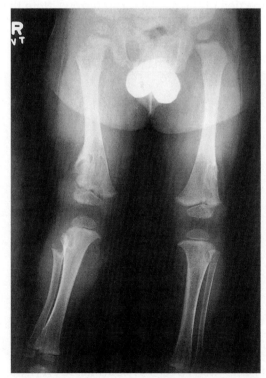

Figure 11-264 **MULTIPLE ENCHONDROMATOSIS (OLLIER'S DISEASE). AP Bilateral Lower Legs.** Observe the radiolucent streak-like appearance within the metaphysis of the proximal and distal femur, tibia, and fibula. *COMMENT:* The streak-like metaphyseal vertical radiolucencies seen in this case are characteristic of the early metaphyseal changes of Ollier's disease in pediatric patients, usually < 3 years of age. (Courtesy of Douglas Elliott, MD, Department of Radiology, University Hospital, Denver, Colorado.).

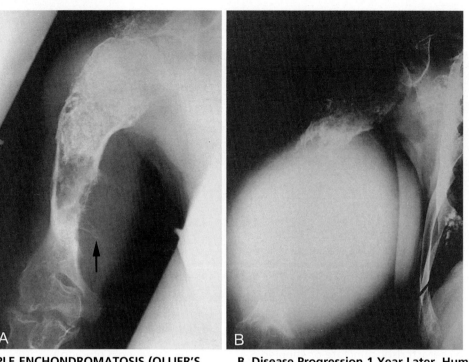

Figure 11-265 **MULTIPLE ENCHONDROMATOSIS (OLLIER'S DISEASE): MALIGNANT DEGENERATION. A. Humerus.** Note the destruction of the medial cortex (*arrow*). Note the multiple enchondromas of the proximal humerus and acromion.

B. Disease Progression 1 Year Later, Humerus. Note that the lesion has progressed, with gross bone destruction and a large soft tissue mass. (Courtesy of Lawrence A. Cooperstein, MD, Pittsburgh, Pennsylvania.)

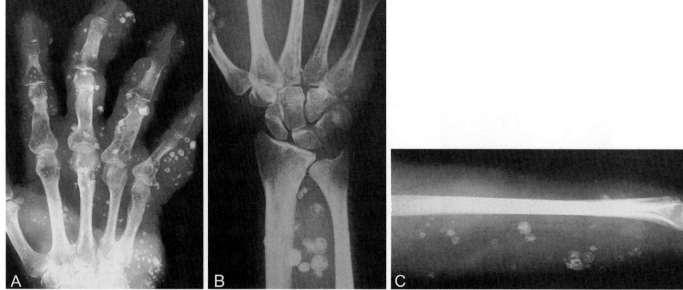

Figure 11-266 **MAFFUCCI'S SYNDROME. A. PA Hand.** Observe the large soft tissue cavernous hemangiomas throughout the hand, with associated phlebolith calcification within the masses. These phleboliths appear as circular radiopacities within the soft tissue masses. **B. PA Wrist. C. Lateral Forearm.** Note the large, circular calcifications throughout the soft tissues of the wrist and forearm. These calcifications represent phleboliths within adjacent soft tissue cavernous hemangiomas. Note the relatively radiolucent center present within the calcifications, which is a characteristic presentation of phleboliths. *COMMENT:* Maffucci's syndrome is defined as multiple enchondromatosis with soft tissue cavernous hemangiomas. (Panel A courtesy of Jack Edeiken, MD, Houston, Texas.)

MAFFUCCI'S SYNDROME

General Considerations

In 1881 Maffucci (1) described a syndrome of enchondromatosis of bone and soft tissue cavernous hemangiomas. This syndrome is quite rare and not of a hereditary nature. (2) Symptoms of the disease are not present at birth but will usually present before puberty. (3) There has been only 90 cases reported in the world literature. Most cases are seen in the hand, with multiple phalangeal enchondromas and an adjacent soft tissue cavernous hemangioma. The hemangiomas present as soft tissue masses containing phleboliths, which appear radiographically as radiopaque concretions around a relatively lucent center. (4) (Fig. 11-266) There is a greater tendency (as high as 25%) toward malignant degeneration of the enchondromas in Maffucci's syndrome than there is in Ollier's disease (enchondromatosis without hemangiomas). (4,5) Except for the soft tissue hemangiomas, the radiographic features of Maffucci's syndrome are identical to those of Ollier's disease, which substantiates the necessity to search carefully for hemangiomas in any patient diagnosed with Ollier's disease. (4,6) One recent study recommends the use of full body MRI to avoid misdiagnosis and erroneous expectations of the prognosis. (6) The outcome of Maffucci's syndrome is widespread, ranging from minor lifestyle alterations to total incapacitation. (7)

PERIOSTEAL CHONDROMA

General Considerations

Periosteal chondroma is a slowly growing, benign cartilaginous tumor of limited size that develops within and beneath the periosteum on the surface of cortical bone. The first description of periosteal chondroma as a distinctive entity was by Lichtenstein and Hall in 1952. (1) Jaffe (2) in 1956 described additional cases and coined the term *juxtacortical chondroma*, which is synonymous with periosteal chondroma. Approximately 80 cases have been reported, with no sex predilection. Most patients present with a painless mass; however, a significant number may complain of mild pain, often of long duration. A bony lump may be palpable.

Incidence

The most common location for periosteal chondroma is in the small bones of the hands and feet. (3) The humerus is also a common site, but other sites, such as the femur, tibia, radius, ulna, and fibula, have been reported. (4) These lesions occur most often in young adults and may reach 3–4 cm in diameter.

Radiologic Features

The radiographic features of periosteal chondroma are somewhat characteristic. (3,5) The typical tumor presents as a metaphyseal lesion in a tubular bone that appears as an area of cortical indentation, resulting in a *scalloped, or saucerized depression* of the outer cortex, with a well-defined inner margin. The superior and inferior edges may be overhanging. (Fig. 11-267) Within this area of saucerization some recognizable cartilage matrix is often present; this is seen more frequently in the smaller lesions. A demonstrable soft tissue mass is present in approximately one third of patients. (6) A ledge or buttress of periosteal bone may extend from the adjacent cortex around a portion of the chondroma, especially at its proximal end, and a dense rind of lamellar bone usually separates the tumor from the medullary cavity. The lesions most likely to cause a problem in differential diagnosis are fibrous cortical defect, periosteal desmoid, periosteal chondrosarcoma, and aneurysmal bone cyst. (3,6,7)

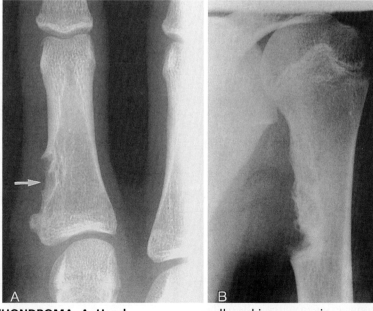

Figure 11-267   **PERIOSTEAL CHONDROMA. A. Hand.** Observe the juxtacortical radiolucency present within the metaphysis of the proximal phalanx (*arrow*). There is a cortical indentation, with scalloping or a saucerized depression of the outer cortex and a well-defined inner margin. **B. Humerus.** Note the rather large cortical indentation with scalloped inner margins present on the medial aspect of the metaphysis of the proximal humerus. The classic cortical saucerized depression at the outer cortex, with a well-defined inner margin, is visualized at the caudal aspect of this lesion. This is a characteristic appearance for a periosteal chondroma (juxtacortical chondroma).

Knowledge of and familiarity with the radiographic features of periosteal chondroma are important, because in many cases, the final diagnosis must be made by combining the pathologic and radiographic features. (8) MRI can aid in the diagnosis because 100% of the lesions are bordered by a hypointense rim and will reveal a soft tissue mass of hypointensity on T1-weighted sequences and hyperintensity on T2-weighted images. (9,10) Pressure erosions of the adjacent cortex will be well visualized. (9)

Many periosteal chondromas are treated by en bloc excision, and wide excision is recommended for all tumors > 3 cm owing to the difficulty in differentiating benign and malignant tumors. (8) Recurrence is rare; thus it is important that a radiographic diagnosis be available before biopsy to avoid unnecessary procedures. Although the three classic features of periosteal chondroma are not always seen in combination, the majority of cases present with sufficient scalloping of the outer cortex, a slight overhanging of bony edges, and an evident calcified cartilaginous matrix, allowing a proper diagnosis to be made. (7)

CHONDROBLASTOMA

General Considerations

Benign chondroblastoma is a rare primary benign bone tumor of cartilaginous origin. (1) It is usually seen before epiphyseal closure and primarily affects the long tubular bones of the lower extremity. Ewing (2) in 1928 was the first to focus on this tumor and called it a calcifying giant cell tumor. It has also been referred to as cartilage-containing giant cell tumor by Kolodny (3); and in 1931, when Codman (4) described the tumor in some detail, he too felt this lesion to be a giant cell variant and referred to it as an epiphyseal chondromatous giant cell tumor. It was not until 1942, through the work of Jaffe and Lichtenstein (5), that benign chondroblastoma became established as a separate and distinct entity. The basic concepts that they set forth at that time have since been firmly established. Chondroblastoma is often called Codman's tumor, a term that is still in use today.

Incidence

Chondroblastoma is rare, representing < 1% of all primary bone tumors. More than 550 cases are reported in the world literature. (6)

Clinical Features

Age and Sex Distribution

Although the age range of patients is wide, most lesions occur in patients who are between 10 and 25 years old. (7) This lesion almost always develops and manifests itself in the 2nd decade of life. (8) That the chondroblastoma arises from the cells of the enchondral plate after the osseous nucleus is well developed is doubtless the reason it occurs so consistently in the 2nd decade of life. This lesion appears approximately twice as frequently in males. (9)

Signs and Symptoms

Most patients present with the chief complaint of pain, which is often referred to the adjacent joint. (10) Local tenderness and swelling may also be encountered. Muscle atrophy and weakness may affect the involved limb because symptomatology of months' or even years' duration is often the case. The pain is usually mild and dull.

Location

Classically, chondroblastomas present within the epiphyseal region of a long tubular bone, with occasional extension into the metaphyseal region. Diaphyseal lesions do not occur. The lesions vary in size, with 3–6 cm being average; 90% of the lesions are found in the medullary cavity, and 10% affect the cortex. (11) When the lesion affects both the metaphysis and the epiphysis, it is usually eccentric.

The most common locations are proximal femur, including trochanters (23%), distal femur (20%), proximal tibia (17%), proximal humerus (17%), tarsal bones (9%), and innominates (5%). (12) (Fig. 11-268) Pelvic chondroblastoma has a marked predilection for the triradiate cartilage of the innominate bone. (11) Codman originally described this lesion to be almost exclusive to the humerus, which has since been shown to be incorrect. (4) He was the first, however, to appreciate the great predilection for the tuberosities of the humerus over the humeral head epiph-

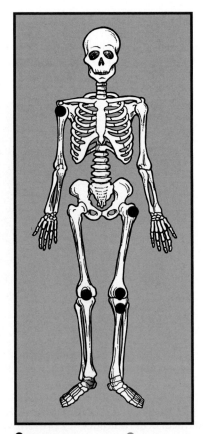

● More common   ● Less common

Figure 11-268 **SKELETAL DISTRIBUTION OF CHONDRO-BLASTOMA.**

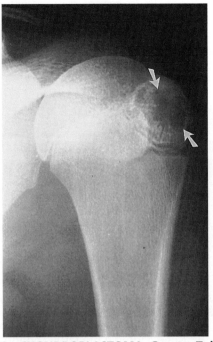

Figure 11-269 **CHONDROBLASTOMA. Greater Tuberosity of the Humerus.** Observe the oval, geographic lesion within the greater tuberosity apophysis (*arrows*). This is a characteristic location for chondroblastoma.

ysis. (Figs. 11-269 and 11-270) This anatomic preference still holds true today. A similar situation exists with lesions in the upper end of the femur, where the lesion arises more often in the trochanters than adjacent to the articular surface of the femoral head. (Fig. 11-271)

Sporadic cases have been reported in such unusual locations as the skull, mandibular condyle, mastoid, manubrium, vertebral column, metacarpals, finger, rib, and patella. (13–17) Generally, tumors of the patella are benign (73%) and of cartilaginous origin. (18) Giant cell tumor is the most common benign bone tumor of the patella, followed by chondroblastoma. (19,18)

Pathologic Features

Microscopic examination of the tissue reveals the lesion to consist of uniform, small polyhedral cells with sharp cytoplasmic margins. The lesion also includes giant cells, and small amounts of chondroid material presenting a *chicken wire calcification*, which is the hallmark of this lesion. (20) This calcification is associated with matrix secretion that stains positively with Alcian blue, helping differentiate it from the typical giant cell tumor. (20) The multinucleated giant cells seen histologically are secondary to the occurrence of hemorrhage and necrosis and may occasionally cloud the issue, allowing an erroneous diagnosis of giant cell tumor to be made. (20)

Some cases of malignant chondroblastomas have been reported in patients without prior irradiation (21,22) with subsequent metastasis to the lung. (1) Perhaps those cases actually represented low-grade chondrosarcoma rather than benign chondroblastoma of bone. The issue of malignant chondroblastomas has not been resolved within the literature at this time.

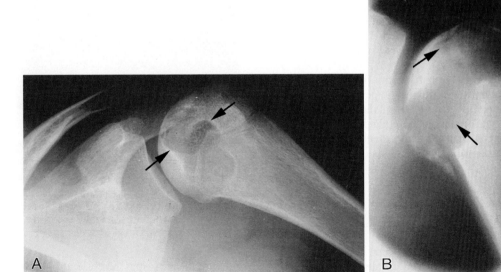

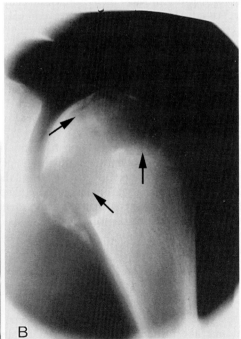

Figure 11-270 **CHONDROBLASTOMA. Head of Humerus. A. Plain Film.** Note the geographic lesion within the epiphysis of this skeletally immature patient (*arrows*). No matrix calcification is visible. **B. Tomogram.** Observe the epiphyseal nature of the lesion (*arrows*). (Courtesy of Michael J. Silverstein, MD, St. Louis, Missouri.)

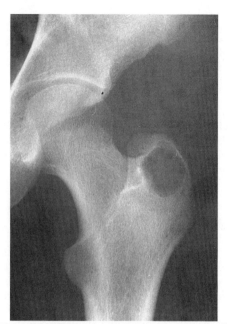

Figure 11-271 CHONDROBLASTOMA. Greater Trochanter of the Femur. Note the oval, geographic lesion within the greater trochanter of the proximal femur. This appearance and location are characteristic for chondroblastoma.

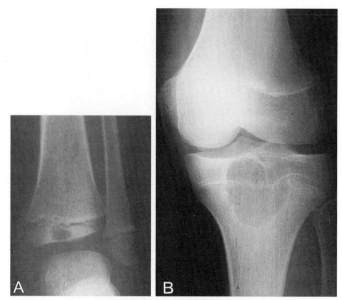

Figure 11-272 CHONDROBLASTOMA: EPIPHYSEAL AND METAPHYSEAL EXTENSION. A. AP Ankle. Note the oval, radiolucent lesion within the central portion of the tibial epiphysis. **B. AP Knee.** Observe the large chondroblastoma affecting the tibial epiphysis, with extension into the metaphysis. Observe the sharp zone of transition and clearly defined margins of this lesion. *COMMENT:* Chondroblastoma and giant cell tumor are the two most common neoplasms to affect the epiphysis.

Radiologic Features

Radiologically, chondroblastoma characteristically consists of a medullary oval or round lytic lesion involving the epiphysis or neighboring metaphysis in a long bone of an adolescent patient. (23) (Fig. 11-272) Most lesions are eccentric, but a few can be centrally located. (Fig. 11-273) The zone of transition is quite sharp, along with a slight marginal rim of sclerosis, denoting the benign nature of the lesion. Most chondroblastomas are radiolucent lesions that are geographic in appearance and that lack any soap bubble compartmentalization of the interior, whereas up to 17% may take a cystic appearance. (24) (Fig. 11-274) Like most cartilaginous tumors, matrix calcification occurs, leaving the lesion with a *punctate or stippled interior* or an appearance of *fluffy cotton wool.* (25) Edeiken (26) stated that approximately 50% of chondroblastomas demonstrate calcification. MRI correlates these findings with a low signal intensity rim with low signal intensity foci stippled throughout the interior. (27)

Periosteal bone apposition occurs in almost two thirds of patients. (28,29) Most epiphyseal lesions will show solid periosteal new bone formation on the metaphyseal portions of the bone, leaving a characteristic buttress type of response. (28) Pathologic fracture rarely occurs. As the lesions mature with growth, bone expansion and deformity are noted, coupled with peripheral sclerosis and fluffy matrix calcifications. (Table 11-30) Up to 15% of cases are associated with an aneurysmal bone cyst. (30)

Differential Diagnosis

The key lesions to be differentiated are Brodie's abscess, eosinophilic granuloma, and ischemic necrosis of the epiphysis. In Brodie's abscess, the associated periosteal response is usually adjacent to the lesion, not in the adjacent metaphysis. Eosinophilic granuloma rarely affects the epiphysis; when it does, the lesions are usually more centrally placed. Eosinophilic granu-

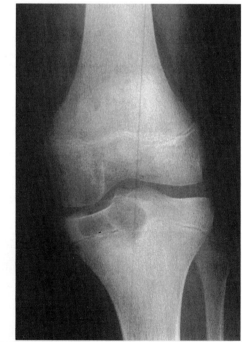

Figure 11-273 CHONDROBLASTOMA. Knee. Note the multiloculated, geographic lesion within the medial tibial epiphysis. This lesion is somewhat eccentrically located and represents a chondroblastoma.

loma and ischemic necrosis may not be radiographically separable, and biopsy may prove to be the definitive means of distinction. The early crescent sign and sharp step-off defects found in the lytic stage of ischemic necrosis provide adequate roentgen signs to allow differentiation because the lesions of chondro-

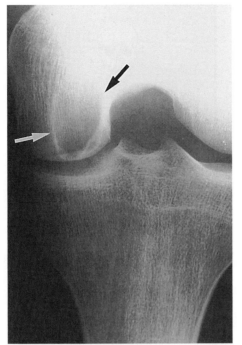

Figure 11-274 CHONDROBLASTOMA. Knee. Note the geographic subarticular lesion involving the lateral surface of the medial condyle of the distal femur (*arrows*).

Table 11-30	Radiologic Features of Chondroblastoma
	Epiphyseal
	Geographic lesion
	Eccentric
	Round, oval
	Sclerotic rim
	Central calcification (50%)
	Metaphyseal periostitis

blastoma are quite smooth and well margined. Giant cell tumor is another epiphyseal lesion that usually presents as a geographic lucency, but it usually develops after closure of the epiphysis, whereas chondroblastoma develops while the growth plate is open.

Treatment and Prognosis

Surgical treatment of these tumors is effective, showing success in up to 90% of cases. (31,32) Thorough curettage is performed, accompanied by packing of the cavity with cancellous bone chips. Resection is the best form of treatment in expendable bones, such as ribs, patella, or a digit. (31) Local recurrence is seen in 20% of uncomplicated lesions in 3-year follow-up studies. (10) A higher rate of recurrence exists when lesions are inadequately resected in the area of the hip (femur, greater trochanter, and pelvis) (33) and in lesions complicated by secondary development of an aneurysmal bone cyst. Recently, percutaneous radiofrequency heat ablation techniques have been studied and have shown promising results as an alternative to invasive surgical interventions. (34)

CAPSULE SUMMARY   Chondroblastoma

General Considerations

• Jaffe and Lichtenstein established benign chondroblastoma as a distinct clinicoradiologic entity.
• An often used synonym is Codman's tumor.

Incidence

• A rare primary benign bone tumor representing < 1% of all primary bone tumors.

Clinical Features

• 10- to 25-year age range is customary, with a 2:1 male predominance.
• Chief complaint is pain referred to the adjacent joint.
• Symptoms may be present for months or even years.
• The classic location is the epiphysis, with occasional extension into the metaphysis.
• Most lesions are 3–6 cm.
• 90% are medullary; 10% are cortical.
• 77% of the lesions occur about the knee, hip, and shoulder.
• Codman stressed the great anatomic preference for the tuberosities of the humerus rather than for the epiphysis of the humeral head. A similar predilection exists for the trochanters of the proximal femur.

Pathologic Features

• Microscopically, a chicken wire type of calcification of the chondroid matrix is characteristic of chondroblastoma.

Radiologic Features

• Oval or round lytic lesion in the epiphysis of a long tubular bone is characteristic.
• Most lesions are eccentrically placed.
• 50% of the lesions demonstrate a fluffy cotton wool calcification of the matrix.
• Periosteal bone apposition occurs in the adjacent metaphysis in one third of patients.
• Mature lesions will show bone expansion and marginal sclerosis.

Differential Diagnosis

• Brodie's abscess, eosinophilic granuloma, and ischemic necrosis of the epiphysis are the key lesions in differential diagnosis. Giant cell tumor, while radiologically similar, usually affects an older age group.

Treatment and Prognosis

• Curettage, accompanied by packing with cancellous bone chips, is recommended.
• Resection is the form of treatment in expendable bones.
• Local recurrence rate is 20% in a 3-year follow-up period, recurrence being a reflection of inadequate initial treatment.

CHONDROMYXOID FIBROMA

General Considerations

Chondromyxoid fibroma is a rare, benign primary neoplasm of bone composed of chondroid, fibrous, and myxoid tissues in varying proportions. The tumor was first described by Jaffe and Lichtenstein (1) in 1948; they reported eight cases and distinguished the neoplasm from chondrosarcoma, giving it the name it bears today. Despite its name, the neoplasm is generally classified as a tumor of cartilage origin, and the suggested alternative name of fibromyxoid chondroma is not generally accepted. (2)

Incidence

Chondromyxoid fibroma is a rare bone tumor; in total, it accounts for < 1% of all bone neoplasms, both benign and malignant. (3) The lesion is usually found within two distinct age ranges, with 60% of the lesions occurring between the ages of 10 and 30. (4) Another peak in incidence generally occurs between 50 and 70 years of age. (5) No sex predilection exists.

Clinical Features

The chief complaint is localized pain with occasional swelling. These symptoms are slow in evolving, sometimes taking months or years to become fully established. (6) Rarely, a patient may be totally asymptomatic, the lesion being discovered on routine radiographs taken for other reasons. Pathologic fracture is rare.

The most common location is the tibia, usually the proximal third; Greenfield (7) stated that 50% of the tumors occur in the tibia. At least 50% of lesions occur at the knee. (8) Other common sites are the femur, humerus, fibula, ribs, innominate, and the small bones of the hands and feet. (9) (Fig. 11-275) Rarely, the vertebrae are affected, with only seven reported cases in the cervical spine. (10) In the tubular bones the origin of the lesion is primarily metaphyseal. (11) Extension into the epiphysis rarely occurs, whereas isolated diaphyseal involvement has been noted. (12)

Pathologic Features

Histologically, the lesion consists of a varied mixture of elements, including a fibrous component, chondroid ground substance, and giant cells. The extreme variability of the chondroid, myxoid, and fibrous patterns associated with these lesions is characteristic, and giant cells may abound. The histologic features, although varied, are clearly benign and demonstrate minimal pleomorphism. (2)

Radiologic Features

The radiographic features are that of a lucent lesion from 1 to 10 cm in diameter, with an average of 3 cm. (3) The typical presentation reveals an eccentric oval or round geographic lesion, usually metaphyseal in location. (13) (Fig. 11-276) Most lesions

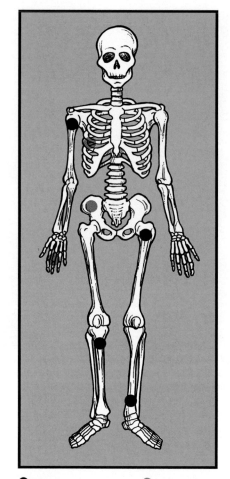

● More common　　● Less common

Figure 11-275　**SKELETAL DISTRIBUTION OF CHONDRO-MYXOID FIBROMA.**

are in the tibia (proximal third). (Fig. 11-277) This ovoid lesion has its long axis parallel to the bone. (14) Many have a scalloped, sclerotic margin, which may be thinner on the cortical side, while remaining well defined and sclerotic on the medullary side. (13,14) Because the lesion grows in a lobular fashion, pressure erosion on the endosteum, creating a scalloped margin, is to be expected. (8,15) (Figs. 11-277 and 11-278) Tumors of a fibrous or cartilaginous nature have a great predilection for creating endosteal scalloping. (14,15) Often, the lesion will be trabeculated (chambered or soap bubbled) in appearance. These trabeculations do not exemplify the formation of true bony septa because they are incomplete, the result of ridges and grooves with scalloping at the periphery of the lesion. (4,8) They have been referred to as pseudo-trabeculations. (3) Calcification within the lesion that can be demonstrated on radiographs is rare but is seen in 25% of cases microscopically. (6,14) (Table 11-31) MRI reveals low signal intensity on T1-weighted images and heterogeneous high signal intensity on T2-weighted images. (16)

Treatment by curettage or excision is usually successful, but occasionally the tumor recurs (10% of cases). (4) Recurrence seems to be more likely in young patients, < 15 years of age, and with tumors that contain much myxoid material and large, atypical nuclei. (15) Recurrent tumors are adequately treated by recurettage, coupled with cauterization or cryosurgery. (15)

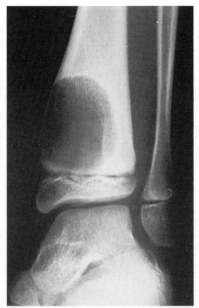

Figure 11-276 **CHONDROMYXOID FIBROMA. Distal Tibia.** Observe the large, radiolucent lesion in the distal metaphysis of the tibia. There is minimal cortical expansion, with a sharp zone of transition. *COMMENT:* One lesion that should be considered in the differential diagnosis of such a radiographic presentation in the tibia is a simple bone cyst.

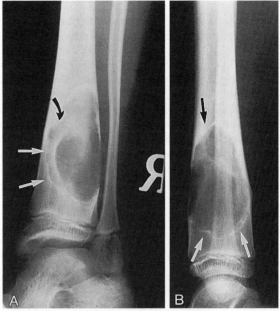

Figure 11-278 **CHONDROMYXOID FIBROMA: DISTAL TIBIA. A. Medial Oblique Ankle.** Note the large, oval, radiolucent lesion filling the entire medullary surface of the distal tibia. There is minimal expansion of bone on its lateral surface. Endosteal scalloping is present throughout, denoting a cartilage or fibrous lesion (*arrows*). **B. Lateral Ankle.** Observe the sharp zone of transition around the large chondromyxoid fibroma of the distal tibia (*arrows*). The sharp zone of transition and sclerotic border denote a benign lesion.

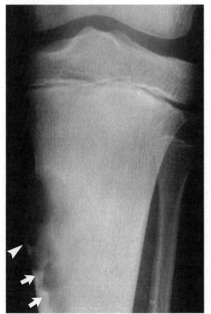

Figure 11-277 **CHONDROMYXOID FIBROMA. Proximal Tibia.** Note the eccentric, metaphyseal, geographic lesion in the proximal third of the tibia. Endosteal scalloping (*arrows*), along with bone expansion, is noted (*arrowhead*). *COMMENT:* The most common location for chondromyxoid fibroma is the proximal third of the tibia, as seen in this case. About 50% of chondromyxoid fibromas occur in the tibia, with other common sites being the femur, humerus, fibula, ribs, and small bones of the hands and feet.

Table 11-31	Radiologic Features of Chondromyxoid Fibroma
Tibia (50% occur here) Metaphyseal Geographic lesion Eccentric Oval, round Endosteal scalloping Expansion Soap bubble appearance Rarely, calcification in matrix	

Radiation therapy has shown to be of benefit when resection is not feasible; however, therapy of this nature increases the risk of future malignancies. (5)

FIBROUS XANTHOMA OF BONE: NON-OSSIFYING FIBROMA

General Considerations

Fibrous xanthoma of bone is a term that encompasses several lesions known under two major names: non-ossifying fibroma (NOF) and fibrous cortical defect (FCD). Most researchers believe that these two entities are the identical lesion seen in different age ranges and stages of growth. Indeed, the only differentiating factor is the patient's age, with fibrous cortical defect appearing in 4- to 8-year-olds and non-ossifying fibroma being seen in 8- to 20-year-olds. NOF has a number of synonyms: non-osteogenic fibroma, metaphyseal fibrous defect, solitary xanthoma, xanthogranuloma of bone, and fibrous medullary defect. (1,2) Jaffe (3) was the first to use the term non-ossifying fibroma, distinctly separating this lesion from the giant cell tumor variants. Dahlin (4), Aegerter and Kirkpatrick (5), and others noted that this lesion is entirely non-neoplastic and emphasized that the spontaneous resolution, which so often occurs, is supportive evidence that this lesion represents faulty ossification, rather than a true neoplasm.

Incidence

The true incidence is difficult to determine because the majority of the lesions are asymptomatic and never discovered. (6) Between 30% and 40% of normal children have FCD, with NOF being somewhat less common. (7)

Clinical Features

Age and Sex Distribution

The usual age range is 8–20 years, with the average age being 14. (8) Males predominate in a 2:1 ratio.

Signs and Symptoms

Most lesions are asymptomatic and found by coincidence when the patient is being radiographed for some other reason, usually following trauma. Large lesions, > 8 cm, often cause persistent pain and may significantly weaken the bone, allowing pathologic fracture to occur, especially in active adolescents. (9)

Location

This lesion commonly affects the bones of the lower extremity, with the distal tibia being the most frequent site. (10) Other sites include the proximal tibia, distal femur, fibula, and proximal humerus. (Fig. 11-279) Isolated cases are seen in the ribs and ilium. Most lesions are diametaphyseal and eccentric in position. The eccentric location on one side of the bone is characteristic but is not always identifiable in some of the thinner bones, particularly the fibula or ribs.

Pathologic Features

The histologic picture of an NOF and that of a FCD are identical. This consists of a whorled bundle of spindle-shaped, stromal connective tissue cells with varying amounts of intercellular, collagenous material interspersed. Foam cells containing lipid and giant cells are frequently present.

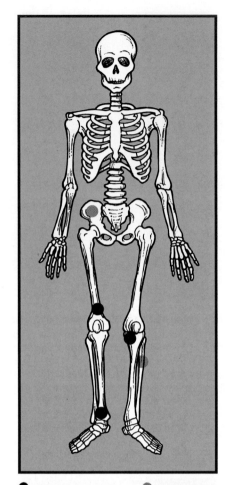

● More common　　● Less common

Figure 11-279 **SKELETAL DISTRIBUTION OF NON-OSSIFYING FIBROMA.**

Radiologic Features

The radiographic appearance of NOF is so characteristic that biopsy is seldom necessary. The typical lesion is solitary, radiolucent, eccentric, and generally ovoid; it often thins and may expand the cortex. (Fig. 11-280) The margins are scalloped, and there is often a multilocular, bubbly appearance. (Fig. 11-281) The osteolytic area may vary from 2 to 7 cm in diameter and has a narrow zone of transition. The medullary portion of the lesion has a dense sclerotic border, leaving the cortical margin thin (Fig. 11-282). Larger lesions may actually involve the entire width of a long bone (e.g., the fibula). Periosteal response occurs only with pathologic fracture. (Fig. 11-283) Epiphyseal lesions are rare, and on occasion the metaphyseal lesion is carried by growth into the diaphysis of the long bone. Malignant transformation does not occur.

Multiple NOFs do occur in association with neurofibromatosis. (11) Their appearance is that of rather large lesions that are somewhat bilateral and symmetrically involve the metaphyses of the lower extremity. (Table 11-32) In the absence of neurofibromatosis, NOFs may be multiple in 10% of cases. (12) Healing of the lesion does occur and is characterized by sclerotic filling in of the matrix. (Fig. 11-284)

NOF and FCD show minimal to mild uptake on bone scan examination. (13) The uptake is low compared with malignant

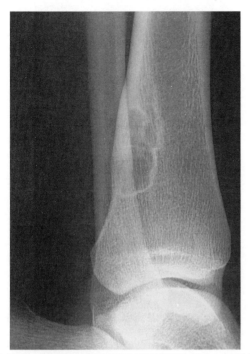

Figure 11-280 **NON-OSSIFYING FIBROMA. Distal Tibia.** Note the eccentric, solitary, radiolucent lesion on the posterior surface of the distal tibia. This lesion demonstrates a bubbly appearance and an encapsulated sclerotic margin.

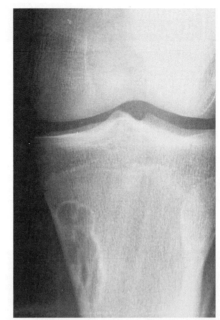

Figure 11-282 **NON-OSSIFYING FIBROMA. Proximal Tibia.** Note the eccentric, geographic lesion in the medial metaphysis of the proximal tibia. Observe the sclerotic margin and endosteal scalloping, creating a bubbly matrix.

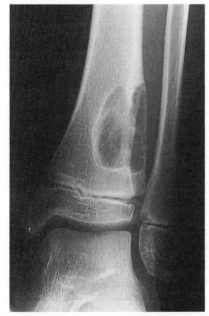

Figure 11-281 **NON-OSSIFYING FIBROMA. Distal Tibia.** Note the eccentric, geographic radiolucency in the distal metaphysis of the tibia. Observe the well-delineated sclerotic margin, the endosteal scalloping, and the bubbly appearance in the matrix of the lesion. This location and radiographic presentation are typical for non-ossifying fibroma. *COMMENT:* These lesions are usually asymptomatic and found when patients are radiographed after trauma to rule out fracture. Most lesions spontaneously regress, filling in with new bone in a period of 4–5 years.

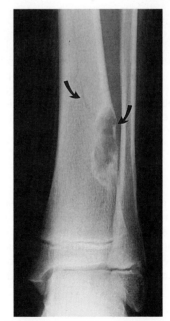

Figure 11-283 **NON-OSSIFYING FIBROMA: PATHOLOGIC FRACTURE. Ankle.** Observe the eccentric non-ossifying fibroma in the distal metaphysis of the tibia. This patient experienced an inversion injury to the ankle and developed a pathologic fracture through a pre-existing, asymptomatic nonossifying fibroma (*arrows*).

Table 11-32	Radiologic Features of Nonossifying Fibroma

Lower extremity; distal femur, proximal and distal tibia
Metaphyseal
Geographic lesion
   Eccentric
   Tapered distally and elongated (flame-shaped)
   Oval
   Expansion
   Thinned cortex
   Scalloped, sclerotic margin
Pathologic fracture
Multiple in neurofibromatosis

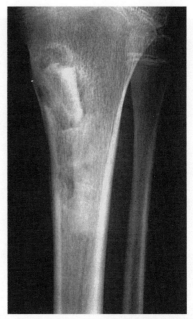

Figure 11-285 NON-OSSIFYING FIBROMA: BONE CHIP THERAPY. AP Knee. Observe the areas of increased bone density surrounding the previous non-ossifying fibroma. This patient's non-ossifying fibroma was surgically curetted, and bone chips were placed within the lesion. *COMMENT:* It is somewhat unusual for a non-ossifying fibroma to require surgery and bone chip therapy; however, if the lesion is persistently symptomatic or causes a great deal of bone expansion, this treatment is often used.

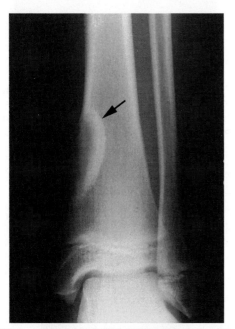

Figure 11-284 NON-OSSIFYING FIBROMA: HEALED FORM. AP Ankle. Note the characteristic eccentric, elongated nature of the lesion well demarcated with a sclerotic border (*arrow*). Evidence of healing is inferred from the overall increase in density of the lesion matrix.

nign bone tumors known to consistently regress without treatment. As regression occurs, initially the lytic defect fills in with solid bone, leaving a dense sclerotic focus. Over a period of 4–5 years, this radiopaque area loses its density until it eventually blends in with the surrounding cortex.

Large, symptomatic lesions are usually treated by curettage or block excision. (9) (Fig. 11-285) Those lesions with superimposed pathologic fracture may be treated conservatively by means of casting immobilization; most fractures will heal, leaving the lesion still present. (15) Occasionally, the lesion may get larger after trauma, and surgical intervention is then the treatment of choice. (15)

FIBROUS XANTHOMA OF BONE: FIBROUS CORTICAL DEFECTS

General Considerations

FCD is sometimes referred to as subperiosteal cortical defect or Caffey's defect. (1) This lesion was originally described by Sontag and Pyle (2) when they evaluated 200 children by serial radiographs, finding a high incidence of metaphyseal lytic lesions in the lower extremities. Caffey (1) performed a more extensive clinical and radiologic study of 1000 healthy children and found 41.8% of the boys and 31% of the girls to have FCD.

lesions and other benign tumors, such as osteoblastoma, osteoid osteoma, and aneurysmal bone cyst. The only distinguishing finding on MRI is a hypointense signal and septation on T2-weighted images. (14) Generally, the intensity of the signals found on MRI depend on the amount of fibrous tissue, hemosiderin, hemorrhage, collagen, histiocytes and bone trabeculae found within the lesion. (14)

Treatment and Prognosis

Because most lesions are asymptomatic, no treatment or surgery is indicated. Spontaneous regression is the usual clinical outcome, taking from 2 to 5 years. NOFs, along with FCDs, are the only be-

Incidence

Between 30% and 40% of children in the 4- to 8-year range have one or more FCDs.

Clinical Features

Age and Sex Distribution

The most common age range is 4–8 years, and the lesions are rarely found in children < 2 years of age. (3) The duration of the lesions is longer in males (4 years) than in females (2 years). The lesion is seen more frequently in males in the ratio of 2:1.

Signs and Symptoms

These lesions are invariably asymptomatic and are usually discovered as an accidental finding because of a roentgen survey done for unrelated reasons.

Location

The bones of the lower extremity are most commonly affected. (Fig. 11-286) The most common site is the posterior-medial surface of the distal femur. (Fig. 11-287) Other common sites include the tibia, fibula, proximal femur, proximal humerus, ribs, and ilium.

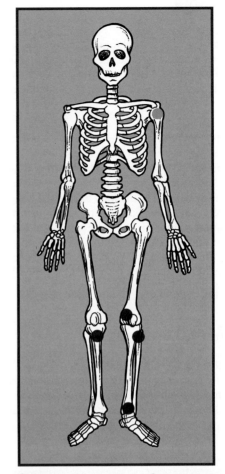

● More common   ● Less common

Figure 11-286 SKELETAL DISTRIBUTION OF FIBROUS CORTICAL DEFECT.

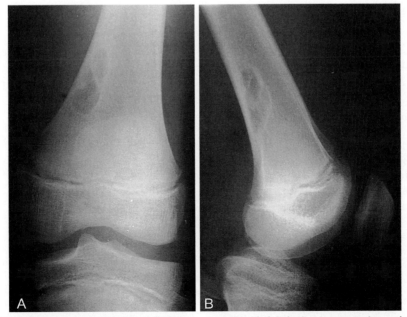

Figure 11-287 FIBROUS CORTICAL DEFECT: DISTAL FEMUR. A. AP Knee. B. Lateral Knee. Note the eccentric, radiolucent lesion within the distal medial metaphysis of the femur. Observe the sclerotic margin and sharp zone of transition around this lesion, suggesting a benign response. This fibrous cortical defect was asymptomatic and found coincidentally on radiographic examination to rule out a fracture.

Pathologic Features

The cortical defects represent fibrous cell rests or originate from the underlying periosteum. More recently it has been proposed that the lesion is precipitated by avulsion fracture at a muscle attachment. (4) FCD and NOF are histologically identical.

Radiologic Features

FCDs are eccentric, lytic, geographic lesions that are located within the metaphysis of long tubular bones. Most lesions appear round and extend parallel to the long axis of the bone. Smaller lesions are purely lytic, whereas larger lesions may present with a bubbly appearance. (Fig. 11-288) The peripheral rim of the lesion usually is sclerotic, providing a sharp zone of transition, confirming its benign nature. The FCDs are often multiple in presentation, which is somewhat rare for NOFs, except when found in association with neurofibromatosis. (5)

Treatment and Prognosis

Because most lesions regress totally within 2 years, no treatment is necessary. (6) These lesions are rarely symptomatic and seldom require any medical care. FCDs and NOFs are the only benign bone tumors that heal spontaneously within 2–5 years. (3,4)

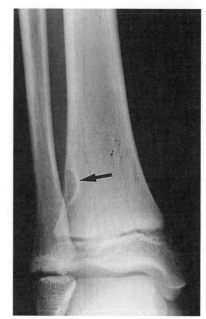

Figure 11-288 FIBROUS CORTICAL DEFECT. Distal Tibia. Observe the small, eccentric, geographic lesion surrounded by a heavy halo of sclerosis in the distal metaphysis of the tibia (*arrow*). This lesion is typical of fibrous cortical defect.

CAPSULE SUMMARY   Non-ossifying Fibroma and Fibrous Cortical Defect (Fibrous Xanthomas)

General Considerations
• Thought to be faulty ossification and do not represent true neoplasms.

Incidence
• 30–40% of normal children have FCD; NOF is slightly less common.

Clinical Features
• 8–20 years is the age range for NOF, 4–8 years is the range for FCD.
• There is a 2:1 male predominance.
• Most lesions are asymptomatic and found by coincidence when a patient is radiographed.
• Large lesions, > 8 cm, may be symptomatic and often lead to pathologic fracture, especially in active adolescents.
• Distal tibia is the most common site for NOF, with distal femur, proximal tibia, humerus, and fibula also being affected.
• Posterior medial surface of the distal femur is the most common site for FCD.

Pathologic Features
• The histologic findings of NOF and FCD are identical, consisting of whorled bundles of spindle-shaped stromal connective tissue cells with intercellular collagenous material.

Radiologic Features
• The radiographic appearance is such that biopsy is seldom necessary.
• The lesion is solitary, eccentric, radiolucent ovoid, bubbly, usually located in the metaphysis.
• Cortical expansion and thinning occurs.
• Most lesions are 2–7 cm in diameter.
• Periosteal response occurs only secondary to pathologic fracture.
• Malignant transformation does not occur.
• The presence of bilateral symmetric NOF may occur in association with neurofibromatosis.
• It shows mild uptake on bone scan.

Treatment and Prognosis
• Most lesions are asymptomatic and never require any form of treatment.
• The only benign bone tumors that consistently regress without treatment (2–5 years).

SIMPLE BONE CYST

General Considerations

Simple bone cyst (SBC), sometimes referred to as a unicameral bone cyst (UBC), solitary bone cyst, or juvenile bone cyst, is not a true neoplasm of bone but rather a fluid-filled cyst that is lined with a thin layer of fibrous tissue. Nonetheless, it is frequently classified under the heading of primary bone tumors. Jaffe and Lichtenstein (1), who described the first cases in 1942, clearly delineated this cyst as a distinct disease entity, naming it unicameral bone cyst. The term *unicameral,* meaning "one house," has actually created some confusion because many lesions present with a bubbly or chambered appearance; it is not single chambered at all. All of the cases that Jaffe and Lichtenstein originally reported were of the single-chamber cystic variety, which led them to use the term unicameral initially. However, many multichambered lesions have been reported since, which are better termed simple bone cysts rather than unicameral. In fact, histologically they are the same lesion.

Incidence

SBCs represent slightly more than 3% of biopsied primary bone tumors. (2)

Clinical Features

Age and Sex Distribution

An SBC most commonly occurs between the ages of 3 and 14 years (80% of cases). (3) They have been reported in a 2-month-old infant (4) and in patients > 50 years. (4) Males predominate 2:1.

Signs and Symptoms

Most lesions are totally asymptomatic until a pathologic fracture occurs, not uncommonly in athletic activities. (5,6) Approximately two thirds of the SBCs eventually undergo pathologic fracture. (7)

Location

Most lesions occur in the proximal humerus and proximal femur (75% of cases). (8) (Fig. 11-289) Humeral lesions are twice as common as those found in the femur. Of the patients who are < 17 years of age, with open growth plates and who have SBCs, 81% of the lesions occur in the humerus or femur; after 17 years of age with closure of the growth plate, 52% occur in the pelvis and calcaneus. Sporadic cases are noted in the ribs (9), fibula, tibia, sacrum, clavicle, and the small bones of the hand. There is a predilection for involvement of the anterior portion of the calcaneus. (10)

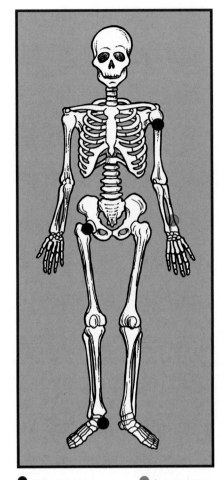

● More common   ● Less common

Figure 11-289   **SKELETAL DISTRIBUTION OF SIMPLE BONE CYST.**

The origin of the lesion is in the metaphysis, immediately adjacent to the epiphyseal cartilage plate. Most lesions are central, with the long axis parallel to the long axis of the host bone. SBCs in this location were called *active* by Jaffe and Lichtenstein (1), and they maintain their growth potential. Those cysts that are displaced from the growth plate by the normal process of enchondral bone growth are termed *latent* cysts. (1) The latent cysts are more mature and may occasionally reach the mid-diaphysis of the humerus or femur. (Fig. 11-290) It has been stated that the latent cysts carry no significant growth potential, compared with the active cysts within the metaphysis. (1,9) However, many latent cysts do retain their growth activity, even if they are a good distance from the growth plate, leaving a significant degree of normal bone interspersed. Perhaps the term latent cyst is inappropriate at this time.

Pathologic Features

SBC is a fluid-filled cavity located in the metaphyseal portion of the growing long bone. The lining of the cyst consists of fibrous connective tissue with a mesothelial surface and a layer of reactive

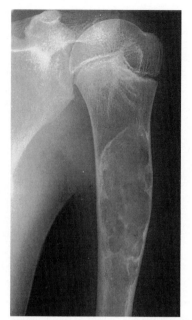

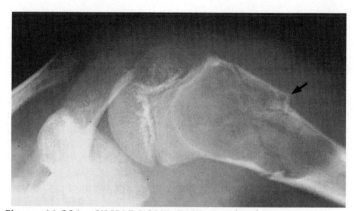

Figure 11-291 **SIMPLE BONE CYST. Proximal Humerus.** Note the large, geographic, expansile lesion affecting the metaphysis and proximal diaphysis of the humerus. This cystic radiolucency deforms the medial metaphysis of the humerus and has weakened the bone to the extent that a pathologic fracture has occurred along with a *hinged fragment sign* (arrow).

Figure 11-290 **SIMPLE BONE CYST: LATENT CYST. Humerus.** Note the large, expansile, geographic lesion within the diaphysis of the humerus. A multiloculated appearance is present throughout the matrix of the lesion. *COMMENT:* This represents a latent cyst because it has been displaced from the growth plate by the normal process of enchondral bone growth. Latent cysts are more mature and may occasionally reach into the mid-diaphysis of the humerus or femur.

A characteristic radiologic sign may be seen when a pathologic fracture complicates this lesion. This is the *fallen fragment sign* (12,13) and represents a small, detached, floating bone fragment, which will change position within the lytic defect from the recumbent to the upright position. This sign is seen in 10% of the SBCs that fracture. (14) (Fig. 11-294) If the fragment remains attached, it may swing into the cavity and may even move (*hinged fragment sign*). (6) (Fig. 11-295)

It is interesting to note that SBC of the calcaneus has a characteristic radiographic appearance and location: a geographic

bone reinforcing the cavity margin. Multiple smaller spaces are often noted at the periphery of the larger central cyst. These are embedded in the adjacent connective tissue; are similarly lined by single-layered, flattened mesothelium; and are the source of the recurrent cysts if not removed at time of excision. The fibrous lining of the cyst is capable of metaplasia into osseous structures (*cementum-like product*), a change that suggests fibrous dysplasia. Myxoid tissue, giant cells, and cholesterol clefts may be present, and tissue from the cyst lining may occasionally become malignant. (11) The fluid within the cyst may be clear, straw yellow, or sanguinous, and there may be clots within the cavity.

Radiologic Features

The classic appearance is that of a geographic or cystic radiolucency that is broad at the metaphyseal end and narrower at the diaphyseal end. (Fig. 11-291) The long axis is greater than the diameter, leaving the formation of a truncated cone appearance. The lesion is radiolucent, except for the thin septa, which creates a bubbly or loculated appearance. The loculation is incomplete or pseudo because no complete septation occurs. Endosteal scalloping occurs, rather than true bony bridging, which aids in the production of the pseudo-loculation.

Bone expansion frequently occurs but seldom extends beyond the diametric confines of the epiphyseal plate. (Fig. 11-292) Cortical disruption and soft tissue mass formation does not occur. No periosteal changes occur, except after a fracture. (Fig. 11-293) Matrix calcification is rare.

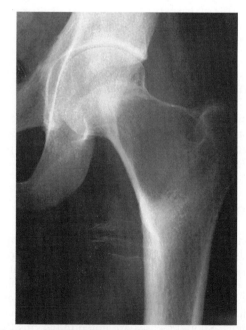

Figure 11-292 **SIMPLE BONE CYST. Proximal Femur.** Note the large, oval, geographic lesion expanding the femoral neck and metaphysis of the proximal femur. The zone of transition is clear and distinct, and there is no evidence of pathologic fracture.

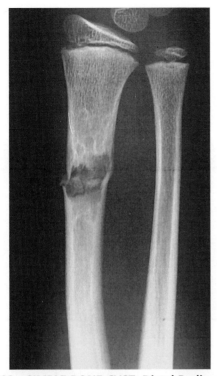

Figure 11-293   **SIMPLE BONE CYST. Distal Radius.** Note the radiolucent defect filling the entire medullary portion of the distal diaphysis of the radius. The central matrix of this lesion is somewhat bubbly, and the peripheral cortical margins demonstrate a pathologic fracture.

lesion placed at the base of the calcaneal neck just inferior to the anterior portion of the posterior facet. (2) (Fig. 11-296) The anterior margin of the cyst is usually straight and vertical, whereas the posterior border is typically curvilinear. The cyst is purely lytic, being completely void of bone structure. Most of these lesions are asymptomatic and seldom fracture or need treatment. On the axial projection, the cysts are noted to be consistently lateral to the midline and only rarely are medial or central. (2) This location may be helpful in the differential diagnosis of other lytic lesions in this region, such as chondroblastoma and giant cell tumor, which tend to be central lesions, as seen on the axial projection. (2) (Table 11-33) A common variant in the calcaneus is a triangular lucency with the apex directed superiorly, which often is a demonstration of a central vascular nutrient foramen. (15)

Treatment and Prognosis

The traditional treatment of choice has been surgical curettage with cauterization of the cyst. Newer techniques allow curettage to be performed by endoscopic procedures reducing the incisional area and invasion of the skin. (16) Packing of the hollow cavity with bone chips following surgery is necessary. (Fig. 11-297) As with the curettage techniques, percutaneous injection of demineralized bone matrix can be accomplished to reduce invasiveness. (17,18) However, recurrence rates with this technique have been high, 30–40%. (19) More recently, the injection of steroids has significantly reduced the recurrence rates, thus providing effective treatment for the cyst. (6,20–22)

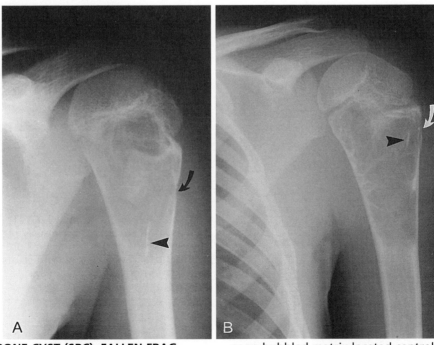

Figure 11-294   **SIMPLE BONE CYST (SBC): FALLEN FRAGMENT SIGN. A. AP Humerus.** Observe the large metaphyseal SBC with a cortical fracture (*arrow*). The fractured fragment is demonstrated in the most caudal portion of the radiolucent defect, representing a fallen fragment sign (*arrowhead*). **B. AP Humerus.** Observe the radiolucent SBC with soap-bubbled matrix located centrally within the proximal metaphysis of the humerus. There is a small cortical fracture (*arrow*) with a fallen fragment sign within the cystic radiolucencies (*arrowhead*). *COMMENT:* About 10% of patients with SBC present with a fallen fragment sign.

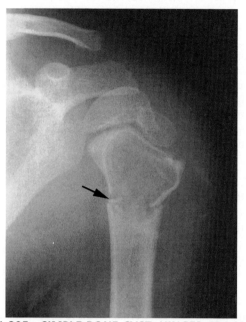

Figure 11-295 SIMPLE BONE CYST: HINGED FRAGMENT SIGN. Humerus. Note the characteristic lesion within the proximal metaphysis. Observe the pathologic fracture extending through the lesion and the displaced cortical bone flake remaining attached to the adjacent cortex, referred to as the *hinged fragment sign* (*arrow*). (Courtesy of Lawrence A. Cooperstein, MD, Pittsburgh, Pennsylvania.)

Table 11-33	Radiologic Features of Simple Bone Cyst

Proximal humerus, proximal femur, calcaneus
Metaphyseal, diaphyseal (latent)
Geographic lesion
   Central
   Elongated lesion
   Expansion (truncated)
   Endosteal scalloping
   No periosteal reaction
Pathologic fracture
   Fallen fragment sign (10% of cases)

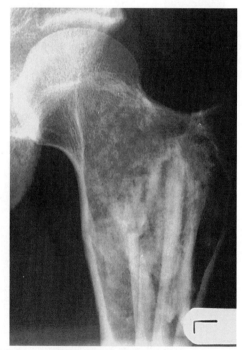

Figure 11-297 SIMPLE BONE CYST: BONE CHIP THERAPY. AP Femur. Note that a previously recognized cyst of the proximal third of the femur was present. The lesion was drained of its serous fluid, and struts of bone were placed within the hollow cavity.

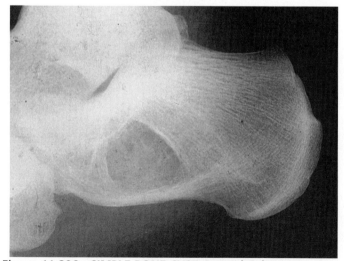

Figure 11-296 SIMPLE BONE CYST. Lateral Calcaneus. Note the oval, geographic radiolucency in the subtalar region of the anterior calcaneus. This radiographic appearance, along with its location, is characteristic of simple bone cyst.

CAPSULE SUMMARY   Simple Bone Cyst

General Considerations
- Synonyms are unicameral bone cyst, solitary bone cyst, and juvenile bone cyst.
- Not a true neoplasm.
- Jaffe and Lichtenstein in 1942 described and named this lesion unicameral bone cyst.

Incidence
- Represents slightly > 3% of primary bone tumors.

Clinical Features
- 80% occur in the 3- to 14-year age range, with a 2:1 male predominance.
- Most lesions are clinically silent until pathologic fracture occurs, which occurs in two thirds of cases.
- 75% of lesions occur in the humerus and proximal femur, humeral lesions being twice as common as those found in the femur.
- Active cysts are metaphyseal in origin and are centrally located, immediately adjacent to the epiphyseal plate, maintaining their growth potential.
- Latent cysts represent those that are displaced from the growth plate and may reach the mid-diaphysis. Their growth potential is somewhat less than the active cysts.

Pathologic Features
- The cystic lesion is lined with fibrous connective tissue of a mesothelial nature.
- The lesion is filled with fluid, which may be clear, straw yellow, or sanguinous.

Radiologic Features
- The classic lesion is an expansile, geographic defect that is pseudo-loculated.
- The metaphyseal end of the lesion is larger than the diaphyseal end, creating a truncated cone appearance.
- Bony expansion frequently occurs but seldom extends beyond the diametric confines of the epiphyseal plate.
- Matrix calcification is rare.
- 10% of cases show a *fallen fragment sign* after pathologic fracture, representing a cortical fragment of bone that falls to the dependent portion of the lesion.
- An incomplete cortical fracture may show a *hinged fragment sign.*

Treatment and Prognosis
- Surgical curettage and bone chip replacement has been the usual mode.
- Recurrence rate for curettage is 30–40%.
- Steroid injection appears to be the most effective recent treatment, with a much lower recurrence rate.

ANEURYSMAL BONE CYST

General Considerations

ABC is a non-neoplastic solitary lesion of bone consisting of a cystic cavity filled with blood. (1) Before 1942, ABC was regarded as a variant of giant cell tumor of bone. (2) In 1942, while reporting cases of SBC, Jaffe and Lichtenstein (3) used the term *aneurysmal bone cyst* to describe two cases. In the 1950s, the term became popular. ABC is the only bone lesion that derives its name from its roentgen appearance rather than from its histology. (4) The lesion is neither an aneurysm nor a true cyst but is made of channels containing flowing blood. The cut surface has a sponge-like appearance without elastic properties. The true pathogenesis of aneurysmal bone cyst is still unknown. (5)

Incidence

ABCs represent approximately 1% of biopsied primary bone tumors. (5)

Clinical Features

Age and Sex Distribution

ABC occurs in patients between 5 and 20 years of age in 75% of the cases. (6) Approximately 60% occur in females. (5,6)

Signs and Symptoms

The chief complaint of patients with ABC is acute onset of pain at the affected site with a rapid increase in severity over a short period of time. (7) Pathologic fractures are frequent, particularly with markedly destructive and expanding lesions. (7) Spinal ABCs may produce neurological deficits and even complete paraplegia. (8,9) This occurs because of the lesion's marked predilection for the neural arch, resulting in spinal stenosis and an extradural defect or complete block on myelographic investigation. (10) Systemic signs and symptoms, such as anorexia, fever, and an increased ESR, are generally absent. An antecedent history of trauma is not infrequently obtained in a young patient presenting with an ABC.

Location

In 80% of cases the cysts are in the long tubular bones and spine. (11) (Fig. 11-298) The remainder affect the flat bones and short tubular bones. The femur and tibia are the most common long tubular bones affected. (6) The thoracic and lumbar spine are the most common spinal areas, with a great predilection for the neural arch (spinous process, transverse process, and lamina). (12) Vertebral body involvement is not frequent; however, when present, it is usually associated with an already existing neural arch lesion.

Most lesions in the long tubular bones are primarily eccentric lesions affecting the metaphysis, but also appearing in the diaphysis. Lesions of the short tubular bones are usually central and

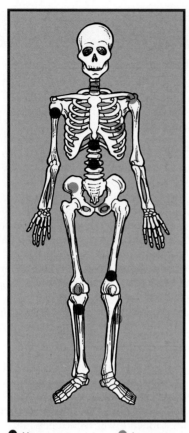

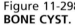

● More common   ● Less common

Figure 11-298 **SKELETAL DISTRIBUTION OF ANEURYSMAL BONE CYST.**

diaphyseal in location. (13) Aneurysmal bone cyst is the most common benign bone tumor of the clavicle. (6,14) Other sporadic sites of occurrence are the fibula, patella, calvaria (most common bone is the occiput), orbit, and ribs. (14–18)

Pathologic Features

ABC represents a proliferation of the vascular component of the marrow, with bone erosion and cyst formation secondary to pressure on the adjacent osseous structures. The gross pathologic findings consist of a bulging shell of bone containing large, blood-filled, cystic cavities. Distended thin-walled blood spaces are identified, without blood clot.

ABC has been designated as *primary* and *secondary,* the latter term being used when the histology indicates a co-existing lesion, either benign or malignant. A primary ABC is defined histologically as anastomosing fibrous-walled channels or lacunae that are blood filled. Some authors have suggested a hereditary component to the formation of primary ABC's. (19) The blood-filled channels may have either a complete or an incomplete lining of endothelial cells; but unlike true blood vessels, they contain no elastic lamina or muscle layer. Typically, the fibrous walls contain red blood cells, granules of hemosiderin, foreign-body giant cells, and spicules of reactive bone. A secondary ABC has the same microscopic characteristics but with additional histologic findings indicating another entity. It is not known whether the second entity develops before, after, or simultaneously with the ABC. The relationship of the two is unknown. The bone lesions occurring in conjunction with a secondary ABC are, in the order of decreasing frequency, giant cell tumor, osteosarcoma, simple (unicameral) bone cyst, NOF, and fibrous dysplasia. (14)

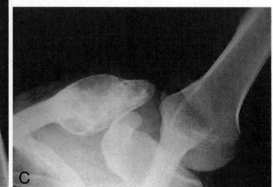

Figure 11-299 **ANEURYSMAL BONE CYST (ABC): TYPICAL LOCATIONS. A. Proximal Fibula.** Note the large, geographic expansion of the metaphysis of the proximal fibula, creating a lytic lesion with a thin cortical margin. This lesion demonstrates the characteristic radiographic sign of a blown-out appearance of bone. **B. Proximal Humerus.** Observe the eccentric, cortical expansion of the medial metaphysis of the proximal humerus. **C. Distal Clavicle.** Note the significant expansion of the distal third of the clavicle associated with a multiloculated radiolucent ABC. ABC is the most common benign bone tumor of the clavicle. (Panel A reprinted with permission from **Yochum TR:** *Aneurysmal bone cyst—A case study.* ACA J Chiro January, 1982. Panel C reprinted with permission from **Center for Devices and Radiological Health, FDA, and the American College of Radiology:** *The Learning File, Skeletal Section, SK-215.*)

Radiologic Features

The radiologic features may vary, but the basic pattern usually consists of an expanding, rapidly growing, saccular lytic lesion in the involved bone, sharply demarcated by a thin subperiosteal shell. (Fig. 11-299) In long bones the lesion tends to be eccentric, creating a saccular protrusion with multiple fine septae internally and sharply demarcated, bulging, scalloped borders. (Fig. 11-300) Most lesions are metaphyseal; however, they extend to the epiphyseal end of the bone after the growth plate has closed. Rarely, ABC crosses the growth plate to involve the epiphysis secondarily. ABC is the only benign bone tumor known to do this. (14)

Many lesions may reach 8–10 cm in size. The characteristic cortical change is a marked ballooning of a thinned cortex. This cortical bulge has been described as having a *blown-out appearance* or as the *finger-in-the-balloon sign.* (20) (Fig. 11-301) Most lesions are purely osteolytic; however, on occasion a soap bubble pattern within the lesion, caused by residual or newly formed ridges of cortex, may be observed. Periosteal new bone formation near the margins of the lesion, creating a buttressing effect, is characteristic of ABC, thus helping differentiate an SBC. (Fig. 11-302) The peripheral edges of this lesion are outlined by a paper thin, or *eggshell,* rim of new bone formation. (20) Gross distension of the cortex to the point of it almost becoming invisible may occur with rapidly growing lesions. Therefore, because of its markedly expansive and destructive quality, ABC may simulate a malignant neoplasm.

On CT and MRI several fluid levels (*fluid–fluid*) can be seen within this multicystic lesion. (21,22) These are probably owing to settling of degraded blood products and can also be seen in osteosarcoma, giant cell tumor, and chondroblastoma. On these modal-

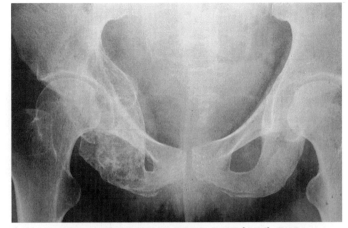

Figure 11-301 ANEURYSMAL BONE CYST (ABC): THE BLOWN-OUT APPEARANCE. Note the grossly expansile, radiolucent lesion affecting the pelvic brim, medial acetabulum, and ischium. The peripheral cortical margin of this lesion is intact. This is a typical radiographic appearance of an ABC involving the pelvis. (Courtesy of Richard T. Coade, MIR, DC, Kempsey, New South Wales, Australia.)

ities individual chambers are separated by septae surrounded by a thin peripheral rim of low signal intensity on T1- and T2-weighted images. (22)

A spinal ABC creates a grossly expansile lytic lesion, usually of the neural arch (spinous process, transverse process, or lamina), which usually lacks any septation. (Fig. 11-303) This appearance may be called the *inflated spine.* (Fig. 11-304) The thoracic and lumbar spine are predisposed. The other major entity in the differential diagnosis of neural arch spinal expansile lesions is

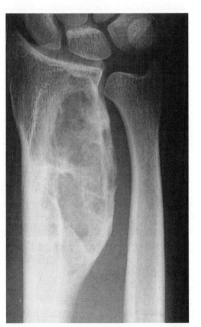

Figure 11-300 ANEURYSMAL BONE CYST (ABC): THE ECCENTRIC LESION. Distal Radius. Observe the long, eccentric radiolucency present within the distal metaphysis of the radius. Significant expansion of bone with a bubbly appearance of the central matrix is noted. This is a typical radiographic appearance of ABC.

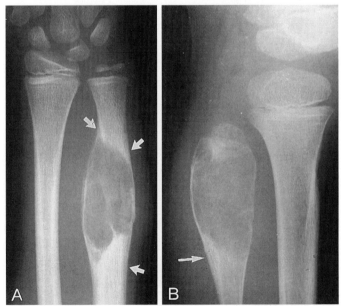

Figure 11-302 ANEURYSMAL BONE CYST (ABC): THE PERIOSTEAL BUTTRESS. A. Distal Ulna. Note the large, expansile ABC affecting the distal portion of the ulna. Periosteal new bone formation near the peripheral margins of the lesion creates a buttressing effect, which is characteristic of ABC (*arrows*). **B. Proximal Fibula.** Observe the large, geographic, expansile ABC of the proximal fibula. The typical periosteal buttressing effect is present at the proximal surface of the lytic lesion (*arrow*).

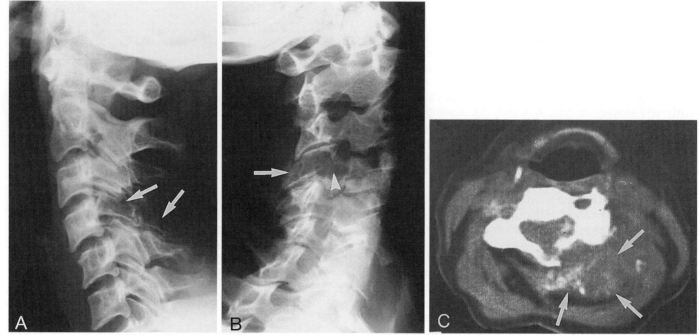

Figure 11-303 ANEURYSMAL BONE CYST (ABC): C4 VERTEBRA. A. Lateral Cervical. Note the grossly destructive, expansile lytic lesion in the articular pillar, lamina, and spinous process of the C4 vertebra (*arrows*). **B. Oblique Cervical.** Note the extensive lytic destruction of the articular pillar (*arrow*) and pedicle (*arrowhead*) of the C4 vertebra. **C. Axial CT: C4.** Observe the large, expansile ABC affecting the lamina and spinous process of the C4 vertebra (*arrows*). Osseous debris is scattered throughout the radiolucent lesion.

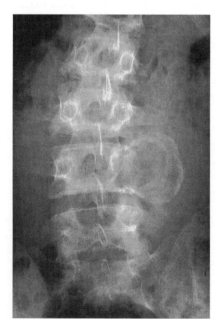

Figure 11-304 ANEURYSMAL BONE CYST (ABC): THE INFLATED SPINE. AP Lumbar. Note the grossly expansile, geographic lesion affecting the pedicle and transverse process of the L4 vertebra. The gross expansion of a neural arch by an ABC may be referred to as the *inflated* spine. COMMENT: ABCs, when affecting the spine, have a great predilection to destroy the neural arch, as do osteoblastomas. (Reprinted with permission from **Yochum TR:** *Aneurysmal bone cyst—A case study.* ACA J Chiro January, 1982. Courtesy of Robin Canterbury, DC, DACBR, Davenport, Iowa.)

Table 11-34	Radiologic Features of Aneurysmal Bone Cyst

Long bones: metaphysis, diaphysis
Spine: neural arch, inflated spine
Geographic
   Eccentric
   Expansile
   Very thin peripheral cortex
   Light septations
Marginal periosteal buttress
Fluid–fluid levels on MRI

osteoblastoma. The age range i have greater expansile properties. An osteoblastoma may present as a radiopaque lesion occasionally, facilitating the differential diagnosis. Most osteoblastomas in the spine, however, are lytic lesions, and a biopsy may be the only means of final differentiation. (Table 11-34)

Treatment and Prognosis

Surgical curettage with bone chip replacement is currently the usual mode of therapy; however recent research is identifying less invasive measures for treatment. (23,24) Studies have suggested that intralesional injection with Ethibloc (25) or calcitonin and methylprednisolone (26) are promising treatments without surgical intervention. Furthermore, with more invasive surgical measures, recurrence rates are high, often approaching 50%. (27)

Radiation therapy creates sclerosis of the vessels, helping reduce recurrence rates. Most spinal lesions are treated with a 2000- to 3000-rad tumor dose because they are often inoperable. Radiation therapy must be used cautiously because it carries with it a potential for postradiation sarcoma as a sequela many years later. Therefore, surgical curettage remains the treatment of choice. Most patients have a favorable prognosis for complete restoration of normal function.

CAPSULE SUMMARY   Aneurysmal Bone Cyst

General Considerations

- Jaffe and Lichtenstein offered the term aneurysmal bone cyst in describing two cases.
- The only bone lesion that derives its name from its roentgen appearance rather than from its histology.
- The true pathogenesis is unknown.

Incidence

- Represents 1% of biopsied primary bone tumors.

Clinical Features

- 75% of cases present between the ages of 5 and 20 years.
- 60% occur in females.
- Pain at the site, which is of a relatively acute onset, occurs.
- An antecedent history of trauma is common.
- Spinal lesions may produce neurological deficits or paraplegia as a result of the grossly expansile tumor in the neural arch causing spinal stenosis and cord compression.
- 80% of the lesions are in the long tubular bones (femur and tibia) and spine.
- Spinal lesions affect the neural arch, spinous process, transverse process, and lamina. The thoracic and lumbar spine are the most common regions involved.

Pathologic Features

- Represents a proliferation of the vascular component of the marrow, with removal of bone and cyst formation.

- Two types exist: primary and secondary (ABC plus a superimposed benign or malignant tumor).
- Gross findings are a bulging shell of bone lined by periosteum and new bone, containing large, blood-filled, cystic cavities.

Radiologic Features

- In long bones the lesion is an eccentric, metaphyseal, saccular protrusion of the bone.
- The only benign bone tumor known to cross the epiphyseal plate.
- Some lesions may reach 8–10 cm and are purely lytic.
- The cortical ballooning has been termed the *blown-out appearance* or the *finger-in-the-balloon sign*.
- Periosteal buttressing at the edge of the lesion is characteristic.
- Spinal lesions in the neural arch must be differentiated from osteoblastoma. ABC is usually more expansile and will not present as a radiopaque lesion, which osteoblastoma may occasionally do.
- MRI demonstrates a classic *fluid–fluid* level.

Treatment and Prognosis

- Surgical curettage, along with replacement bone chip therapy, is still the mode of therapy.
- Recurrence rates are as high as 50% following curettage.
- Occasionally, radiation therapy is used with inoperable lesions, usually in the spine.

INTRAOSSEOUS LIPOMA

General Considerations

Primary intraosseous lipoma is a rare cause of a lytic lesion, actually representing the rarest primary benign bone tumor. (1) Approximately 200 cases have been reported in the world literature. (2) DeLee (3) reported the first case in 1901. Soft tissue and subperiosteal lipomas are more common than the intraosseous lesions and can secondarily involve the skeleton by extrinsic pressure on the cortex. (4) (Fig. 11-305)

Incidence

A wide age range exists, between 5 and 70 years of age. The peak decade is the 4th. (4) No sex predilection exists. Most lesions are asymptomatic and are discovered accidentally when radiographs are taken for other reasons. Occasionally, the patient presents with pain, the duration of symptoms being variable. (5) The most common anatomic sites are the metaphyses of long bones, particularly the tibia and fibula, calcaneus and metatarsals. (6,7) (Fig. 11-306) They are rare in the spine. (8)

Pathologic Features

Pathologically, the gross specimens show lesions of variable size (2–13 cm), bright yellow in color, which are well demarcated from the rest of the bone. (9) The composition of the fatty tissue is identical to the frequently occurring soft tissue lipomas. (3,5)

Radiologic Features

Radiologically, the intraosseous lipoma produces an osteolytic lesion with a well-defined and/or sclerotic border. (10) A narrow zone of transition indicates the slow growth pattern of this nonaggressive neoplasm. A metaphyseal predilection exists, and in half of the reported cases the lesion expands the bone at the expense of the inner margin of the cortex. A characteristic appearance in long bones is an ovoid, elongated appearance with a wedge-shaped end on its diaphyseal surface.

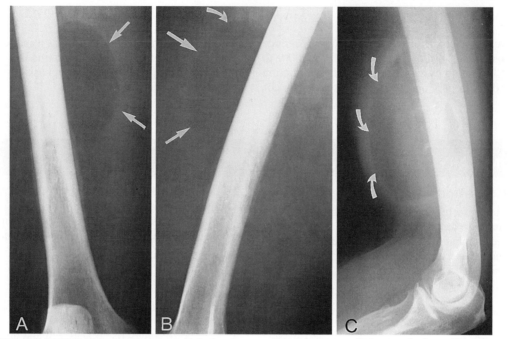

Figure 11-305 **SOFT TISSUE LIPOMAS. A. AP Femur. B. Lateral Femur.** Note the large, radiolucent soft tissue lipoma within the anterior soft tissues of the thigh (*arrows*). **C. Lateral Humerus.** Observe the well-defined, radiolucent, soft tissue lipoma anterior to the distal diaphysis of the humerus (*arrows*). *COMMENT:* Soft tissue lipomas appear radiographi-cally as large, radiolucent lesions since fat appears as a radiolucent or black density on the final radiograph. The radiopaque densities surrounding the above lipomas represent the normal soft tissue density of water in the adjacent musculature.

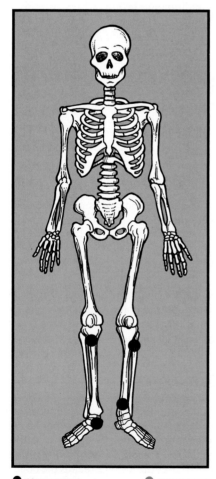

● More common   ● Less common

Figure 11-306 **SKELETAL DISTRIBUTION OF INTRAOSSEOUS LIPOMA.**

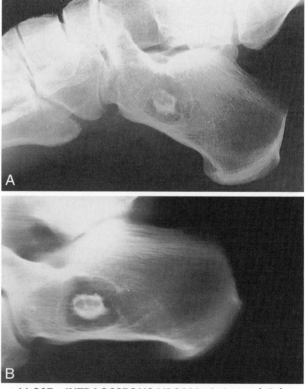

Figure 11-307 **INTRAOSSEOUS LIPOMA. A. Lateral Calcaneus. B. Tomogram, Lateral Calcaneus.** Note the well-defined, geographic lesion in the subtalar anterior surface of the calcaneus. A characteristic target or doughnut-shaped sequestrum calcification is present within the central portion of the intraosseous lipoma. (Courtesy of Steven P. Brownstein, MD, Springfield, New Jersey.)

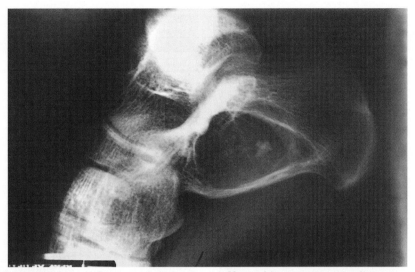

Figure 11-308 INTRAOSSEOUS LIPOMA. Calcaneus. Note the well-defined geographic lytic expansile lesion in the subtalar region of the calcaneus. Note the convex expansion of the floor of the calcaneus. Observe the small area of central target or doughnut-shaped sequestrum calcification within the lesion. *COMMENT:* The most common bones affected by interosseous lipoma are the tibia and fibula, as well as the calcaneus. The main differential diagnosis for a calcaneal lytic expansile lesions is simple bone cyst; however, they do not have a target central calcification. (Courtesy of John Duda, MD, Department of Radiology, University Hospital, Denver, Colorado.)

The shape of the calcaneal lesion is also unusual in that it is trapezoidal, with a broad base and a narrow, truncated superior surface. (11) They usually appear in the base of the calcaneal neck (12) and an additional radiologic sign of intraosseous lipoma is the *target* or *doughnut-shaped sequestrum,* which represents a radiopacity of central necrosis. (Figs. 11-307 and 11-308) This central, round density of the lipoma differs from the calcification of the cartilage tumors, which are characterized by small multiple rings or broken rings, and also differs from the calcification of infarcts, which is peripheral rather than central in location. Thus a well-defined, ovoid, lobulated, expanding intramedullary lesion, particularly with a central density, should suggest the possibility of an intraosseous lipoma. (Fig. 11-309) Occasionally, the lipoma may not show a target calcific nidus. (13)

CT offers a definitive means of diagnosis by measuring the attenuation numbers of the lesion, which fall within the range of fatty tissue. (14) Those lipomas that do not have central calcification are often called SBCs from plain films. (14) A CT or MRI

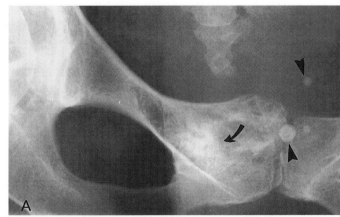

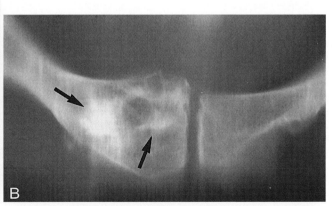

Figure 11-309 INTRAOSSEOUS LIPOMA. A. AP Pubic Bone. Note the lytic lesion expanding and deforming the pubic bone, with a heavy area of intraosseous calcification (*arrow*). Of incidental notation are the circular phleboliths present near the pubic rami (*arrowheads*). These are a frequent finding and are of no clinical significance to the patient. **B. Tomogram, Pubic Bone.** Note that the tomographic projection of the pubic articulation clearly defines the lytic expansile lesion, with a target calcified nidus (*arrows*). *COMMENT:* This young female patient presented with back pain, and the asymptomatic expansile lesion within the pubic bone was found coincidentally on initial radiographs. This lesion was initially thought to represent an enchondroma or perhaps a low-grade chondrosarcoma, and biopsy surprised all concerned when an intraosseous lipoma was confirmed. This is a rare location for intraosseous lipoma. (Courtesy of Steven B. Klayman, DC, Austin, Texas.)

Table 11-35	Preferential Site of Origin of Various Bone Tumors

Epiphysis
 Chondroblastoma
 Giant cell tumor after fusion of growth plate
Metaphysis
 Osteosarcoma
 Parosteal sarcoma
 Chondrosarcoma
 Enchondroma
 Chondromyxoid fibroma
 Fibrosarcoma
 Non-ossifying fibroma
 Giant cell tumor before fusion of growth plate
 Simple bone cyst
 Aneurysmal bone cyst
 Osteoblastoma
 Osteochondroma
 Bone island (long bone)
Diaphysis
 Myeloma
 Ewing's tumor
 Non-Hodgkin's lymphoma
 Adamantinoma

Adapted from **Greenfield GB:** *Radiology of Bone Diseases,* ed 3. Philadelphia, JB Lippincott, 1980.

Table 11-36	Preferential Time of Occurrence of Various Bone Tumors

Tumor	Age of Maximum Incidence (decades)
Osteosarcoma	2, 3 (smaller peak at 7)
Parosteal sarcoma	4, 5
Chondrosarcoma	4, 5, 6
Fibrosarcoma	4
Giant cell tumor	3, 4
Ewing's tumor	2
Non-Hodgkin's lymphoma	3, 4
Multiple myeloma	5, 6, 7
Chondroblastoma	2
Chondromyxoid fibroma	2, 3
Non-ossifying fibroma	2
Osteoid osteoma	2, 3
Osteoblastoma	2, 3
Simple bone cyst	1, 2
Aneurysmal bone cyst	2, 3

Adapted from **Greenfield GB:** *Radiology of Bone Diseases,* ed 3. Philadelphia, JB Lippincott, 1980.

Table 11-37	Most Common Locations of Bone Tumors

Type	Tumor	Skeletal Sites
Malignant	Chondrosarcoma	Pelvis, scapula, sternum, femur, humerus
	Chordoma	Sacrococcygeal, skull base, C2
	Ewing's sarcoma	Pelvis, femur, humerus
	Fibrosarcoma	Femur, tibia
	Multiple myeloma	Pelvis, spine, sternum, femur, humerus, skull
	Osteosarcoma	Femur, tibia, humerus
	Parosteal sarcoma	Femur
	Non-Hodgkin's lymphoma	Femur, humerus, pelvis, spine
Quasi-malignant	Giant cell tumor	Femur, tibia, radius
Benign	Aneurysmal bone cyst	Femur, tibia, humerus, spine (neural arch)
	Bone island	Pelvis, femur
	Chondroblastoma	Humerus, femur
	Chondromyxoid fibroma	Tibia, rib, ulna
	Enchondroma	Metacarpals, phalanges, metatarsals, femur
	Fibrous cortical defect	Femur, tibia
	Hemangioma	Spine, skull
	Non-ossifying fibroma	Femur, tibia
	Osteoblastoma	Femur, humerus, spine (neural arch)
	Osteochondroma	Femur, tibia, humerus
	Osteoid osteoma	Femur, tibia, spine

TUMOR-LIKE PROCESSES

PAGET'S DISEASE

General Considerations

Paget's disease, named osteitis deformans by Sir James Paget (1) in 1877, is a bone disease of unknown origin characterized by osteolysis followed by extensive attempts at repair. It should be remembered that Sir James identified and described this disease without the use of radiographs, and his initial discussions were with five patients. (1) He called this slowly progressive entity *osteitis deformans,* thinking a chronic inflammatory process led to the deformity. It is most commonly found in the axial skeleton, but it has been found in nearly every bone of the human skeleton. Because of its unique ability throughout the various stages of the disease process to mimic many other diseases, Paget's disease, together with fibrous dysplasia, has been referred to as the "great imitators of bone disease."

examination should give the correct diagnosis in these cases, with MRI revealing high signal intensities on both T1- and T2-weighted images. (14,15)

Symptomatic lesions require curettage and bone packing into the defect. (12) Asymptomatic lesions are best left alone. (16)

Tables 11-35 through 11-37 briefly outline the sites of origin and preferential time of occurrence of primary bone tumors.

Historic Note: Sir James Paget

James Paget was born in Yarmouth, England, in 1814, the son of a wealthy merchant banker. At the age of 15 he was apprenticed to a local general practitioner with whom he pursued studies both in medicine and in botany. When he was 21, he became an anatomy demonstrator at St. Bartholomew's Hospital in London, teaching medical students anatomy and physiology while pursuing his own interests of pathology and surgery. At the early age of 30, he was among the first people to be elected a Fellow of the Royal College of Surgeons and at the age of 33 was appointed Professor of Anatomy and Pathology at the Royal College of Surgeons in London. He became a Fellow of the Royal Society at 37 years of age and was knighted 6 years later, at which time he commenced his observations on the first patient with the bone disease that was later to bear his name. At the age of 47 he was appointed Senior Assistant Surgeon at St. Bartholomew's Hospital and 6 years later became Surgeon to Queen Victoria and the Prince of Wales. At the time he presented his first patient with osteitis deformans in London he considered the bone lesion to be inflammatory. He died on December 30, 1899, by which time he had recorded 23 patients with osteitis deformans, 5 of whom had died from malignant degeneration.

Incidence

The true prevalence of Paget's disease is difficult to determine because it is most often asymptomatic and is usually detected when roentgenograms are obtained for other reasons. The most effective and reliable data in the literature on the incidence of Paget's disease can be found in the work of Schmorl (2) of Germany. Schmorl found 138 cases of Paget's disease out of 4614 necroscopies of an unselected population > 40 years of age, representing an incidence of 3%. (1) Up to 12% will have a first-degree relative with Paget's disease, a percentage that is seven times greater than the normal population. (3)

The incidence of Paget's disease is low in some countries, such as Asia, Africa, and Scandinavia, whereas in the United Kingdom, Australia, and New Zealand it is high. (4) Although the incidence of Paget's disease varies throughout certain regions of the United Kingdom, the mean incidence is 5%, the highest in the world. (5) The prevalence in Australia and New Zealand may be explained by the original colonization of these countries with immigrants from the United Kingdom. This hypothesis is supported by evidence that the prevalence of Paget's disease is slightly higher among recent immigrants to Australia than in offspring born in Australia. (5) The disease has been found only once in an Australian Aborigine. (6) Variable prevalence within the United States is present, with the northern states having a higher incidence than the southern states (New York, 3.8%; Atlanta, Georgia, 1.1%). (5) In both centers the prevalence among blacks and whites is approximately equal. This contrasts sharply to the apparent rarity of the bone disease in African blacks, whereas Paget's disease is clearly recognized in white immigrants into Southern Africa. The incidence in the Scandinavian countries is 0.4%. (5)

These geographic variations suggest that an environmental factor may be operating. Because there is good radiologic evidence from Anglo-Saxon skeletons that the disease has been present in the United Kingdom for at least 1000 years, it seems highly unlikely that there could be an environmental agent associated with modern industries unless these are producing naturally occurring

end products. In support of this are pagetic changes noted in the skull of a Neanderthal man (7) and in a skeleton in an ancient Egyptian tomb. (8) An analysis of Beethoven's skeletal remains has suggested that Paget's disease may have contributed to the composer's loss of hearing. (9)

Cause

There have been many hypotheses as to the cause of Paget's disease; however, none has been properly substantiated. Thus the origin of this disease remains unknown. (10) (Table 11-38) Theories proposed are that of an inflammatory disorder, endocrine disorder, autoimmune disorder, inborn error of connective tissue metabolism, vascular disorder, and neoplasm. (1,11–15) Some investigators have classified Paget's disease as a metabolic disorder; however, it is not generalized, and normal bone can always be identified. (16) The fact that Paget's disease is localized to some, but not all, bones is offered as strong evidence against its being a metabolic or endocrine disorder. (16)

More recent studies using the electron microscope have shown that characteristic fibrillar intranuclear inclusions are present in the osteoclasts of patients with Paget's disease. (17) These inclusions resemble the measles virus nucleocapsids, suggesting that a slow virus infection is the causal agent. The paramyxovirus family has been strongly implicated. (18) These inclusions have also been reported in patients with giant cell tumor, which on occasion occurs with Paget's disease. (19) The long incubation period of some viruses may explain the geographic variation in migrant populations and the late onset and slow progression of the disease. (17,19) Further research and studies may prove Sir James Paget correct in his suggestion of nearly a century ago that the cause of this disease is inflammatory in nature. Paget's disease is included in this text as a tumor-like process of bone, which should not be misinterpreted as suggesting its definitive cause.

Clinical Features

Age and Sex Distribution

Paget's disease is a common skeletal disorder, particularly in the middle-aged and geriatric patient. It is rare before the age of 40, and affects 3–4% of the population > 40 years of age. (20) Most patients are > 55 years of age at the time of diagnosis. (21) There is a 2:1 male prevalence in Paget's disease. (21)

Table 11-38	Causal Theories for Paget's Disease of Bone
Inflammatory disorder	
Endocrine disorder	
Autoimmune disorder	
Inborn error of connective tissue metabolism	
Vascular disorder	
Metabolic disorder	
Neoplasm	
Chronic viral infection: measleslike virus[a]	

[a] The most current theory.

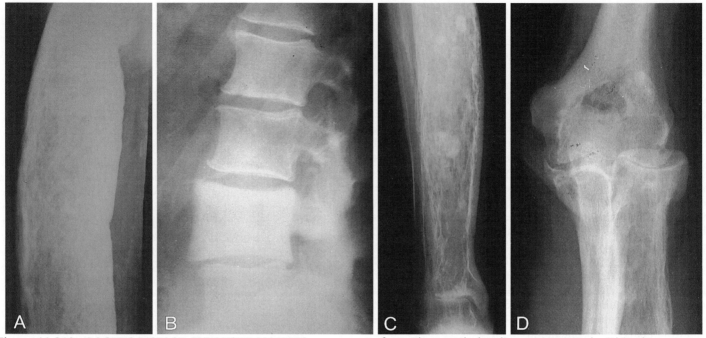

Figure 11-310 **PAGET'S DISEASE: EXPANSILE MANIFES-TATIONS. A. AP Femur.** Observe the thickening of the cortex, affecting the diaphysis of the femur. **B. L4 Vertebral Body.** Note the significant expansion of the L4 vertebral body, along with the typical changes of an ivory vertebra. **C. AP Tibia and Fibula.** Observe the gross expansion and cortical thickening of the tibia, with subarticular involvement of its distal surface. The mottled radiopacities noted within the medullary portion of the tibia represent the characteristic cotton wool appearance. **D. AP Elbow.** Observe the expansion of the proximal radius, affecting its subarticular surface. (Panel B courtesy of Joseph W. Howe, DC, DACBR, Fellow, ACCR, Los Angeles, California.)

Signs and Symptoms

The onset of Paget's disease is insidious, and up to 90% of patients are asymptomatic. (22,23) The most common symptom is pain of a dull nature, which ensues from several factors, including stress owing to mechanical disruption of bone, joint destruction, increased blood flow through the bone, and multiple microscopic fractures. (24) This pain is of low intensity, boring in nature, present both at rest and at night, and not aggravated by exertion. The diagnosis is frequently made on routine radiographs obtained for other purposes.

Because of hypervascularity, temperature differences of up to 5°C may be found between a normal and an affected side of the body. (25) Enlargement of bone is a common feature of Paget's disease. (Fig. 11-310) Patients with Paget's disease of the skull may complain of a continuously enlarging hat size. (26) Similarly, in the foot, enlargement of the heel may prevent a patient from fitting into normal-size shoes. (Fig. 11-311)

Complications

See Table 11-39 for a compilation of the complications of Paget's disease.

Deformity. A common problem for which patients with Paget's disease seek care is deformity. (Fig. 11-312) This usually occurs in weight-bearing bones, with bowing of the femur or tibia a common finding. The femoral neck usually yields under pressure, creating a coxa vara and the *shepherd's crook deformity.* Anterior bowing of the tibia occurs and has been called *sabre shin deformity.* (Fig. 11-313) Occasionally, lateral bowing of the femur and tibia create a genu varum deformity (*bowleg*). Other deformities include basilar invagination, protrusio acetabuli, and leontiasis ossea (lion-like facies), which is a result of facial bone involvement and increased frontal and parietal bossing. (27) (Fig. 11-314)

Basilar Invagination. The weight of the enlarged, softened calvaria and brain leads to molding of the skull base upon the upper cervical segments, creating basilar invagination. This complication occurs in approximately one third of patients and is more common

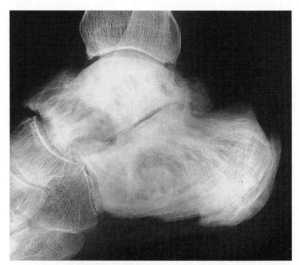

Figure 11-311 **PAGET'S DISEASE: TALUS AND CALCANEUS.** Note the classic Paget's disease affecting the talus and calcaneus, creating significant expansion of the anterior surface of the talus near its articulation with the tarsal navicular.

Table 11-39	Complications of Paget's Disease
Common	**Uncommon**
Deformities	Anemia
Shepherd's crook[a]	High-output cardiac failure
Saber shin	
Otto's pelvis	Ureteric colic
Leontiasis ossea	Pseudo-fractures
Basilar invagination	Spinal stenosis
Genu varum	Joint degeneration
Pathologic fracture	Malignant degeneration (0.9–2%)
(banana-like in type)	

[a] The most common complication that usually affects the proximal femur.

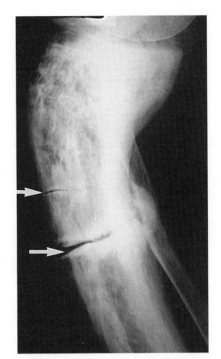

Figure 11-313 **PAGET'S DISEASE: SABER SHIN DEFORMITY.**
Observe the significant anterior bowing of the tibia, along with cortical thickening and expansion of bone, creating the characteristic saber shin deformity from Paget's disease. Pseudo-fractures affecting the anterior surface of the tibia are also noted (*arrows*).

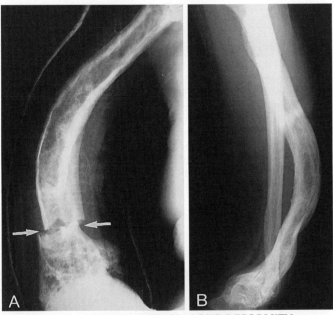

Figure 11-312 **PAGET'S DISEASE: BONE DEFORMITY.**
A. AP Humerus. Observe the significant lateral bowing of the entire surface of the humerus. Note the cortical thickening and accentuated trabecular patterns consistent with Paget's disease. There is a transverse pathologic fracture noted in the distal surface of the humerus (*arrows*).
B. Lateral Forearm. Note the significant dorsal bowing deformity of the entire radius, as a result of underlying Paget's disease.

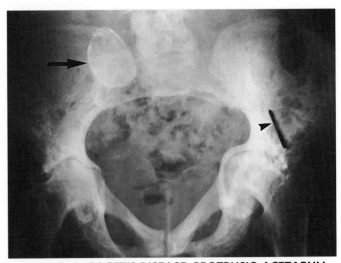

Figure 11-314 **PAGET'S DISEASE: PROTRUSIO ACETABULI.**
Note the extensive Paget's disease affecting the bones of the pelvis. Bilateral medial progression of the femoral heads through the deformed acetabuli, secondary to Paget's disease, is noted. This deformity is referred to as protrusio acetabuli. A porcelain gallbladder is incidentally noted in the right lower portion of the abdomen (*arrow*). An artifact is present above the hip joint (*arrowhead*).

in skulls with the mixed form of Paget's disease. The degree of involvement at the base does not necessarily parallel the involvement of the vault. Basilar invagination may lead to brainstem compression, syringomyelia, or obstructive hydrocephalus. (26,28)

Symptoms from these changes tend to be gradual in development and progressive in character. Cranial nerve palsies involving the third, sixth, and seventh nerves may occur. Nerve deafness may be complicated by severe auditory canal stenosis from bone expansion. In doubtful cases, where symptoms might be a result of basilar invagination, use of the spinographic measurement of Chamberlain's line may be helpful. Generally, the tip of the odontoid should not lie > 3 mm above this line, which takes as its points of origin the posterior surface of the hard palate and the inner margin of the foramen magnum. (Fig. 11-315) The main cause of an osseous-induced basilar artery syndrome in the adult is extensive

Paget's disease of the skull. This may cause various neurological symptoms, such as headaches, giddiness, or vertigo, including signs of ischemia of the spinal cord.

Pathologic Fracture. This represents the most common complication of Paget's disease. (29) The fractures are usually trans-

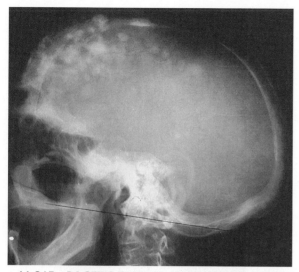

Figure 11-315 PAGET'S DISEASE: BASILAR INVAGINATION. Lateral Skull. Observe the typical, cotton wool pagetoid changes affecting primarily the frontal and parietal portion of the calvaria. Involvement of the skull base has allowed basilar invagination to occur. This is demonstrated by the odontoid process migrating significantly above Chamberlain's line.

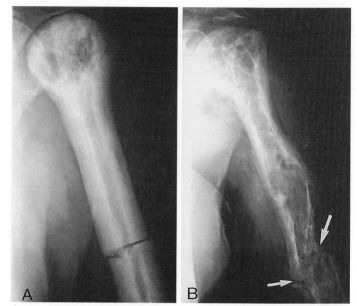

Figure 11-316 PAGET'S DISEASE: PATHOLOGIC FRACTURE. A. AP Humerus. Note the transverse fracture of the mid-diaphysis of the humerus. This fracture occurs through pagetoid bone and has been referred to as *banana-like* in patients with fractures complicating Paget's disease. **B. AP Humerus.** Note the extensive Paget's disease affecting the entire surface of the humerus, which has allowed the pathologic fracture to occur in its distal surface (*arrows*). (Courtesy of Alf Turner, MIR, BAppSc (Chiro), DACBR, Bournemouth, England.)

verse in their orientation and, when the tubular bones are involved, have been referred to as *banana-like* in type. (30) (Figs. 11-316 and 11-317) The most common sites are those areas that are under the greatest weight-bearing stress. The most frequently affected site is the proximal third of the femur, in particular, the femoral neck and subtrochanteric region. (5) (Fig. 11-318) Fractures of the lumbar vertebral bodies and tibia are also common sites. (30) Most of the fractures occur during the mixed (biphasic) or sclerotic phase of the disease and not in the lytic (destructive) phase. (5)

Pseudo-Fractures. Pseudo-fractures (Looser's lines, increment fractures, Milkman's syndrome, umbau zonen) are local areas of demineralization within the bone, which are replaced by fibrous tissue. They may represent healing reactions to infractions and are often asymptomatic. Occasionally, they may predispose the patient to complete transverse fractures (*banana-like*). (Fig. 11-312) The most common sites involved are the femoral neck, subtrochanteric region of the femur, scapula, pubic and ischial rami, and proximal ulna and tibia. (30) Frequently, they present as bilateral and symmetric radiolucent bands. Those affecting the subtrochanteric region of the femur do so on the convex surface of the outer cortex. (Fig. 11-319) Pseudo-fractures are also present in the following diseases: osteomalacia, florid rickets, fibrous dysplasia, and hyperphosphatasia, as well as in diseases in which osteomalacia is a secondary feature (e.g., Wilson's disease).

Spinal Stenosis. Because of the expansile capacity of Paget's disease, vertebral body and neural arch involvement can lead to compressive neuropathy. It is estimated that about one third of all patients with spinal involvement will have stenosis. (31) Spinal cord and nerve root compression may result from the pressure of distorted soft bones or pathologic fractures. In the former instance symptoms are slow in appearance; in the latter they are rapid. It is most frequent in the upper thoracic spine; however, cases in the cervical spine, at the axis, and in the lumbar spine, causing cauda equina syndrome, are also recorded. (32–35) (Figs. 11-320 to 11-322) The upper thoracic spine predilection

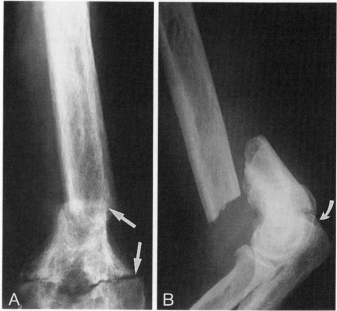

Figure 11-317 PAGET'S DISEASE: COMPLICATING PATHOLOGIC FRACTURE. A. AP Elbow. B. Lateral Elbow. Note the two pathologic fractures through the pagetoid bone affecting the distal humerus (*arrows*). Significant malalignment associated with the transverse pathologic fracture is present, affecting the distal portion of the humerus.

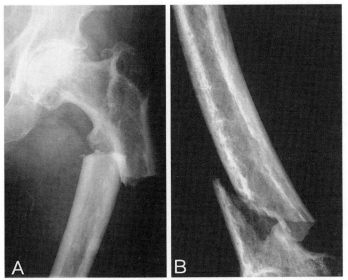

Figure 11-318 **PAGET'S DISEASE: PATHOLOGIC FRACTURE.**
A. Proximal Femur. Note the transverse, *banana-like* pathologic fracture affecting the intratrochanteric area of the proximal femur. This is the most frequent site for pathologic fracture in Paget's disease. **B. Distal Femur.** Observe the spiral pathologic fracture of the distal metadiaphyseal surface of the femur.

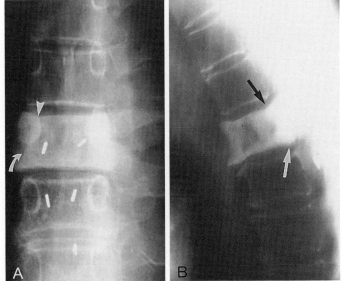

Figure 11-320 **PAGET'S DISEASE: SPINAL STENOSIS.**
A. AP Thoracic Spine. Observe the ivory vertebra affecting the midthoracic spine (*arrow*). There is significant expansion and involvement of the pedicle (*arrowhead*) of the affected vertebra. Of incidental notation are metallic surgical clips following decompressive laminectomy. **B. Lateral Thoracic Spine.** Note the expansion of the involved thoracic ivory vertebra (*arrows*). This bone expansion, along with neural arch involvement, created spinal stenosis in this patient, requiring surgical decompression.

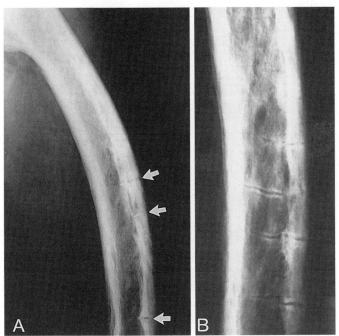

Figure 11-319 **PAGET'S DISEASE: PSEUDO-FRACTURES.**
A. AP Femur. Note the extensive Paget's disease of the entire visualized surface of the femur. Observe the radiolucent defects affecting the cortex of the lateral convex surface of the femur, which is characteristic of pseudo-fractures (*arrows*). **B. AP Femur.** Observe the large areas of pseudo-fracture formation through the pagetoid bone.

is owing to the fact that the cord is largest at this level and the spinal canal is the smallest.

Most patients are between 40 and 60 years of age. The specific neurological symptoms are varied and may manifest as weakness of the legs, urinary incontinence, or sensory disturbance. (32) Rarely, ossification of extradural fat has caused the cauda equina syndrome in patients with Paget's disease. These changes in the size of the spinal canal are best demonstrated by CT scans. (36,37)

Anemia. Patients with long-standing Paget's disease may develop anemia because of bone marrow replacement by fibrous tissue. This complication is not common, though, because of the abundance of hematopoietic reserves. (38)

Joint Degeneration. Paget's disease may also give rise to an arthritis that is particularly common about the hip (Paget's coxopathy). The arthritis is thought to be secondary to accelerated enchondral ossification and replacement of cartilage by pagetic bone. (39,40) The joint space narrowing is usually concentric or symmetric, affecting both the femur and acetabulum. A further feature is protrusio acetabuli, which predisposes the patient to premature secondary degenerative joint disease. (Fig. 11-323) Other causes for the joint space narrowing are cartilage necrosis over the diseased bone and secondary to accelerated subchondral ossification owing to increased vascularity of the underlying bone. In addition to the hip, the knee may demonstrate joint changes resulting from Paget's disease. Intradiscal invasion and fusion in the spine can produce intersegmental ankylosis. (41)

Ureteric Colic. Paget's disease predisposes to urinary calculus formation. This is associated with the hypercalcemia and hypercalciuria that may occur in Paget's disease, particularly at times

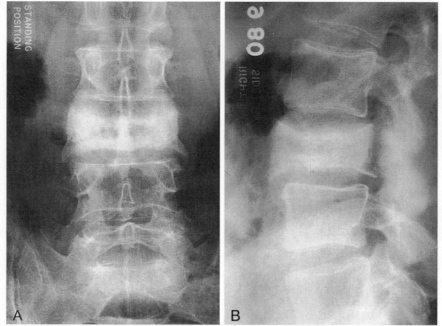

Figure 11-321 **PAGET'S DISEASE: SPINAL STENOSIS. A. AP Lumbar Spine. B. Lateral Lumbar Spine.** Observe the significant expansion of the L3 vertebral body, with an ivory appearance. There is central depression of the vertebral endplates, suggestive of fracture. Observe the ivory density of the pedicle and lamina of L3, indicating pagetoid involvement.

COMMENT: This patient presented with signs and symptoms suggestive of a large central disc herniation, mimicking cauda equina syndrome. A laminectomy was performed. (Courtesy of Gary G. Coleman, MIR, BAppSc (Chiro), Traralgon, Victoria, Australia)

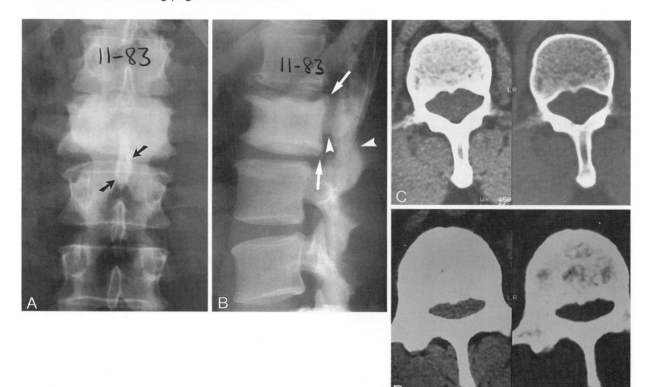

Figure 11-322 **PAGETIC SPINAL STENOSIS MIMICKING CAUDA EQUINA SYNDROME. A. AP Lumbar Spine.** Observe the ivory vertebra affecting L2, with expansion of the spinous process (*arrows*). **B. Lateral Lumbar Spine.** Observe the characteristic changes of Paget's disease, creating an ivory vertebra at L2. Cortical thickening with expansion of the posterior vertebral endplates is noted (*arrows*). Observe the increase in density in the pedicle and lamina area suggestive of pagetoid extension to the neural arch (*arrowheads*). **C. Normal Axial CT, L1.** Note the normal circumference of the spinal canal at L1. **D. Axial**

CT, L2 Ivory Vertebra. Observe the significant reduction of the dimensions of the spinal canal secondary to the extensive expansion of the vertebral body and neural arch from pagetoid involvement. *COMMENT:* This 42-year-old patient presented with symptoms of an L2–L3 disc mimicking cauda equina syndrome. Patients with spinal stenosis, as demonstrated in this case, usually require emergency decompression laminectomy. (Courtesy of Lawrence A. Cooperstein, MD, Pittsburgh, Pennsylvania.)

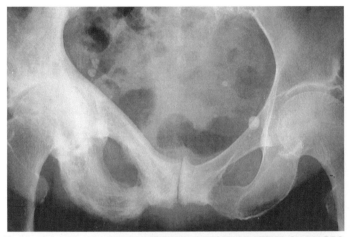

Figure 11-323 PAGET'S DISEASE: DEGENERATIVE CHANGES. Note the extensive pagetoid involvement of the hemipelvis, with classic cortical thickening and bone expansion. There is uniform narrowing of the hip joint as a result of premature degenerative joint disease, which is a frequent complication of Paget's disease. Of incidental notation is degenerative arthrosis of the pubic articulation.

of immobilization. It is suggested that the incidence of urinary calculus formation is 10 times the expected incidence in Paget's disease, compared with an otherwise normal population of this age range. (5)

High-Output Cardiac Failure. Pagetic bone develops a vastly increased blood supply, perhaps 20 times the normal vascularity, and the presence of microscopic multiple arteriovenous shunts has been noted. In patients with extensive involvement, this may lead to high output type of cardiac congestive failure. At least one third of the skeleton must be involved to produce congestive heart failure (5); however, lesser degrees of skeletal involvement may result in a hyperdynamic circulation. This is a rare complication of Paget's disease. (29)

Malignant Degeneration

In the original description of this basic disorder of bone, Sir James noted an association of sarcoma in 2 of the 5 original cases. (1) By 1889 he had collected a total of 23 cases, 5 of which had undergone malignant degeneration. (42)

Incidence. Because the exact incidence of uncomplicated Paget's disease is not known, it is extremely difficult to establish an accurate statistic for the percentage of malignant degeneration of this disease process. The incidence suggested in the literature ranges from 0.9% to 20%. The reason for this wide range is the biased patient population source used in the early articles written on this topic. When only patients with advanced, polyostotic, and clinically obvious or symptomatic Paget's disease have been included in a study (as has been the case throughout the early articles in the literature), the frequency of sarcomatous degeneration climbs to 7–20%. (43) However, when large numbers of patients with asymptomatic Paget's disease of minimal extent are included, the recorded frequency is considerably less, ranging from 0.9 to 2%. (44)

Age and Sex Distribution. Paget's sarcoma is rare before the age of 40 (44), most authorities agree, with a general range for

the average age being 57–66 years. (43) There is an approximate 2:1 male preponderance.

Signs and Symptoms. The most common presenting symptoms of malignant degeneration are those of severe localized pain, creating local disability, and an occasional pulsatile mass. Because Paget's disease is often asymptomatic, unless weight-bearing deformities create localized discomfort, the onset of pain in the patient known to have Paget's disease should seriously suggest the development of a sarcoma of bone. (43) The duration of symptoms varies from 1 to 8 months, with an average of 4.5 months. (45) Spontaneous or pathologic fractures as a result of trivial trauma are dramatic features in patients with Paget's disease, both in the early and late phases. Schajowicz et al. (46) have reported a 21% incidence of pathologic fractures after reviewing 62 cases of Paget's sarcoma.

Site Distribution. Sarcoma complicating Paget's disease has a distribution similar to uncomplicated Paget's disease, except for the relatively high incidence of neoplasia in the humerus and the relatively low frequency in the vertebrae. (43) The femur is the most commonly involved bone, followed, in decreasing order of frequency, by the humerus, innominate bone, skull, and tibia. (43) (Figs. 11-324 to 11-332) Unusual sites include the calcaneus, talus, rib, fibula, ulna, and radius. (43) (Figs. 11-333 and 11-334) Most lesions affect the diaphyseal medullary canal. Vertebral Paget's sarcoma is rare. (43,45) Only eight cases involving the spine have been reported, with the lumbar spine being the most common site. (43–47) (Fig. 11-335) Huang et al. (47) reported a 63-year-old male with Paget's sarcoma involving the L4 vertebral body. Records show two cases in the thoracic spine and one in the cervical spine. (43)

Pathologic Findings. The most common histologic tumor type complicating Paget's disease is osteosarcoma. (46) The second most common tumor type is fibrosarcoma, with chondrosarcoma, malignant fibrous histiocytoma, and reticulosarcoma representing a small number in the cell types of malignant degeneration of Paget's disease. The gross appearance and microscopic characteristics of Paget's sarcoma are no different from those of osteosarcoma arising in a bone unaffected by Paget's disease. (48) Giant cell tumor has also been found to complicate Paget's disease as a benign or malignant neoplasm.

Radiologic Findings. The most common radiologic presentation is a focal lytic area of destruction as a result of neoplastic proliferation of fibrous stromal tissue. The earliest radiographic feature is a small focus of subcortical destruction of bone. (Fig. 11-336) The typical lesion stands out clearly as a small or large oval area of radiolucency blanketed against a background of pagetic bone. (Fig. 11-337) Although the lytic type of presentation predominates (> 50%), both a mixed and sclerotic presentation also exist, with the sclerotic form representing approximately 25% of cases. (43) (Fig. 11-338) Periosteal response is usually absent. Pathologic fracture and soft tissue mass formation are common signs in advanced cases. (Fig. 11-339) Patients frequently develop *cannonball metastasis* to the lung, leading to early death.

Treatment and Prognosis. Standard treatment for Paget's sarcoma is surgical resection or, occasionally, radiation therapy. These approaches are often followed by chemotherapy in an attempt to limit metastatic disease. The use of radiation therapy as a primary therapeutic approach is reserved only for such tumors that are not amenable to surgery. Paget's sarcoma is the most threatening sarcoma of bone (49) with a 5-year survival rate of only 8%.

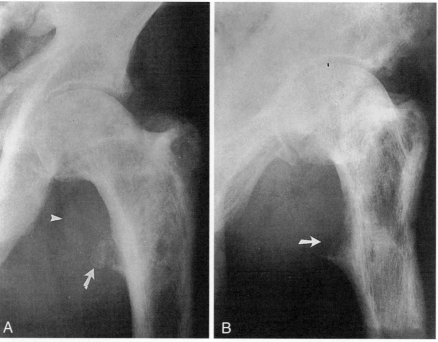

Figure 11-324 PAGET'S DISEASE: MALIGNANT DEGEN-ERATION. A. AP Hip. Observe the pagetoid changes seen throughout the proximal femur. There is cortical destruction of the lesser trochanter (*arrow*), along with a soft tissue mass (*arrowhead*), as a result of malignant degeneration of the preexisting benign Paget's disease. **B. Oblique Hip.**

Note the extensive sarcomatous destruction of the lesser trochanter is noted (*arrow*). *COMMENT:* The incidence of malignant degeneration of Paget's disease is 0.9–2.0%. (Courtesy of Gerald A. Fitzgerald, MD, Sydney, Australia.)

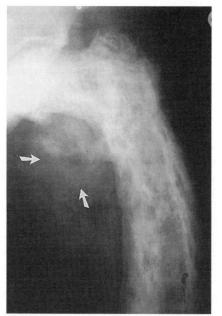

Figure 11-325 PAGET'S DISEASE: MALIGNANT DEGENER-ATION. AP Hip. Observe the extensive expansion of the proximal femur, with a lateral bowing deformity. There is cortical destruction present in the area of the femoral neck and lesser trochanter, with a large soft tissue mass (*arrows*), suggesting sarcomatous degeneration. (Reprinted with permission from **Yochum TR:** *Paget's sarcoma of bone.* Radiologe 24:428, 1984.)

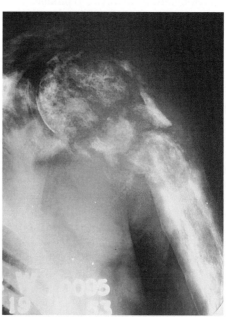

Figure 11-326 PAGET'S DISEASE: MALIGNANT DEGEN-ERATION. AP Shoulder. Note the extensive Paget's disease affecting the entire proximal humerus. Observe the pathologic fractures through the area of malignant degeneration of the preexisting benign Paget's disease. (Reprinted with permission from **Yochum TR:** *Paget's sarcoma of bone.* Radiologe 24:428, 1984.)

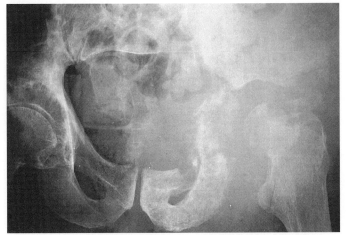

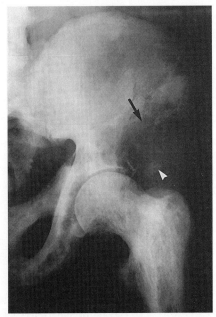

Figure 11-327 **PAGET'S DISEASE: MALIGNANT DEGEN-ERATION. AP Pelvis.** Note the extensive destruction of the acetabulum and pelvic rim as a result of malignant degeneration of Paget's disease. Observe the lack of destruction of the femoral head, which negates the possibility of septic arthritis. Note also the increase in density of the remaining superior pubic rami and ischial tuberosity characteristic of Paget's disease. Similar changes of Paget's disease affect the opposite pelvis and iliopectineal line. (Reprinted with permission from **Yochum TR:** *Paget's sarcoma of bone.* Radiologe 24:428, 1984.)

Figure 11-329 **PAGET'S DISEASE, ILIUM: MALIGNANT DEGENERATION. AP Hip.** Note the extensive Paget's disease affecting the sacrum, entire ilium, and proximal femur. There is cortical destruction affecting the ilium in the supra-acetabular area (*arrow*). Some bone debris secondary to the malignant degeneration is seen in the soft tissue mass (*arrowhead*). (Courtesy of Bryan Hartley, MD, Melbourne, Australia.)

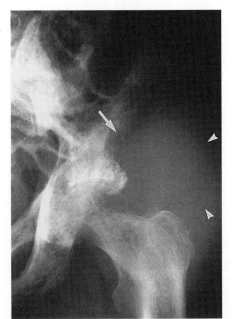

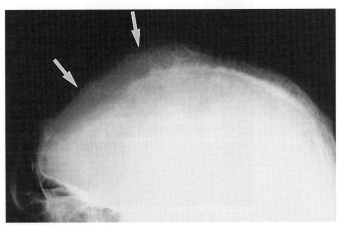

Figure 11-328 **PAGET'S DISEASE: MALIGNANT DEGEN-ERATION. AP Hip.** Observe the pagetoid changes present within the ilium, with cortical destruction of the supra-acetabular area, suggestive of malignant change (*arrow*). There is a large soft tissue extension creating a well-defined mass (*arrowheads*) associated with the malignant degeneration. (Reprinted with permission from **Yochum TR:** *Paget's sarcoma of bone.* Radiologe 24:428, 1984.)

Figure 11-330 **PAGET'S DISEASE: MALIGNANT DEGEN-ERATION. Lateral Skull.** Note the extensive Paget's disease affecting the visualized calvaria. There is cortical destruction and soft tissue mass formation of the frontal bone as a result of malignant degeneration (*arrows*).

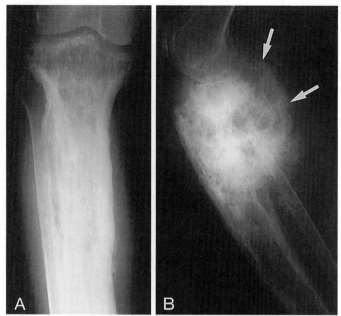

Figure 11-331 **PAGET'S DISEASE: MALIGNANT DEGEN-ERATION. A. AP Tibia. B. Lateral Tibia.** Observe the pagetoid changes affecting the tibia. There is extensive cortical de-struction and a large sarcomatous soft tissue mass present on the posterior proximal surface of the tibia (*arrows*). This soft tissue mass demonstrates a sunburst periosteal response, which is somewhat atypical in Paget's sarcoma. (Reprinted with permission from **Yochum TR:** *Paget's sarcoma of bone.* Radiologe 24:428, 1984.)

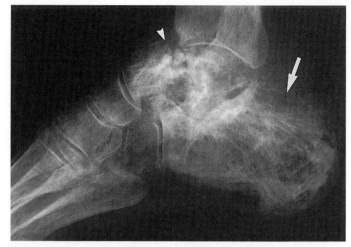

Figure 11-333 **MULTIFOCAL PAGET'S SARCOMA. Lateral Ankle.** Note the extensive Paget's disease involving the entire talus and calcaneus. Observe the cortical destruction sec-ondary to malignant degeneration affecting the superior as-pect of the calcaneus (*arrow*) and the neck of the talus (*arrowhead*). *COMMENT:* Multifocal involvement of Paget's sarcoma is extremely rare. (Reprinted with permission from **Yochum TR:** *Paget's sarcoma of bone.* Radiologe 24:428, 1984.)

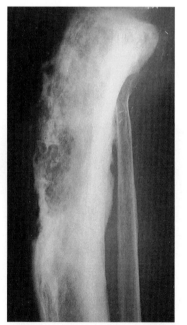

Figure 11-332 **PAGET'S DISEASE: MALIGNANT DEGEN-ERATION. Lateral Tibia.** There is extensive pagetoid involve-ment of the proximal tibia. Note the characteristic cortical thickening present on the posterior surface of the tibia, with destruction of the anterior tibial cortex as a result of malig-nant degeneration. (Reprinted with permission from **Yochum TR:** *Paget's sarcoma of bone.* Radiologe 24:428, 1984.)

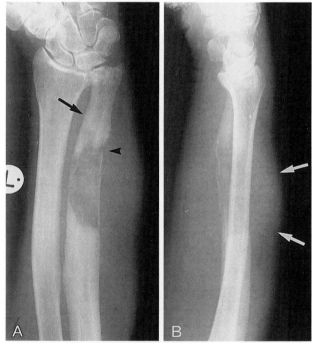

Figure 11-334 **PAGET'S DISEASE: MALIGNANT DEGEN-ERATION. A. PA Forearm.** Observe the cortical thickening of the distal shaft of the ulna, suggesting pagetoid change (*arrow*). There is a large, lytic lesion within the mid-diaphysis of the ulna, with cortical disruption (*arrowhead*). **B. Lateral Forearm.** Observe the large soft tissue mass associated with the lytic destructive lesion in the ulna (*arrows*). (Reprinted with permission from **Yochum TR:** *Paget's sarcoma of bone.* Radiologe 24:428, 1984.)

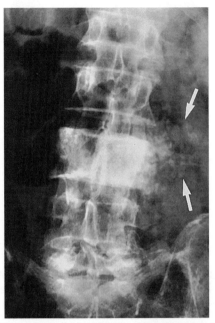

Figure 11-335 **PAGET'S DISEASE: MALIGNANT DEGEN-ERATION. L3 Vertebra.** Observe the pagetoid changes in the L3 vertebral body, creating an increase in bone density. A large soft tissue mass is associated with the malignant degeneration of the pagetoid ivory vertebra (*arrows*). *COMMENT:* Paget's sarcoma of the spine is rare, with < 10 cases reported. The majority of cases reported are in the lumbar spine. (Courtesy of Sharon A. Jaeger, DC, DACBR, Los Angeles, California.)

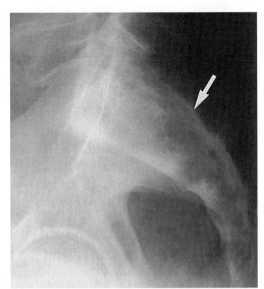

Figure 11-336 **PAGET'S DISEASE: MALIGNANT DEGEN-ERATION. Sacrum.** Observe the pagetoid changes throughout the entire sacrum. There is a lytic area of destruction within the midportion of the sacrum (*arrow*) at the site of malignant degeneration. (Courtesy of Bryan Hartley, MD, Melbourne, Australia.)

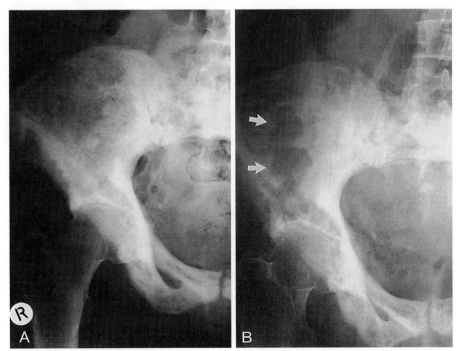

Figure 11-337 **PAGET'S DISEASE: MALIGNANT DEGEN-ERATION, A SERIAL STUDY. A. AP Pelvis.** Observe the typical changes of Paget's disease affecting the entire hemipelvis and sacrum. **B. 1-Year Follow-Up, AP Pelvis.** Note the large lytic defects present within the midportion of the hemipelvis (*arrows*). The lytic areas represent focal malignant degeneration of Paget's disease. (Reprinted with permission from **Yochum TR:** *Paget's sarcoma of bone.* Radiologe 24:428, 1984.)

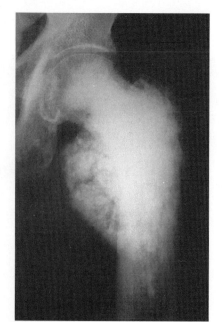

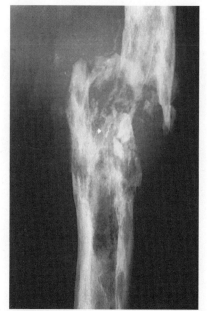

Figure 11-338 **PAGET'S DISEASE: MALIGNANT DEGEN-ERATION. Femur.** Observe the dense, radiopaque changes within the femoral neck and proximal diaphysis. A large, soft tissue mass is noted along the inner surface of the femoral neck and shaft. These changes represent the sclerotic presentation of malignant degeneration of Paget's disease to an osteosarcoma. (Reprinted with permission from **Yochum TR:** *Paget's sarcoma of bone.* Radiologe 24:428, 1984.)

Figure 11-339 **PAGET'S DISEASE: MALIGNANT DEGEN-ERATION. Pathologic Fracture of the Femur.** Observe the pagetoid changes present throughout the mid-diaphysis of the femur. A pathologic fracture has occurred through a site of malignant degeneration. (Courtesy of Bryan Hartley, MD, Melbourne, Victoria, Australia.)

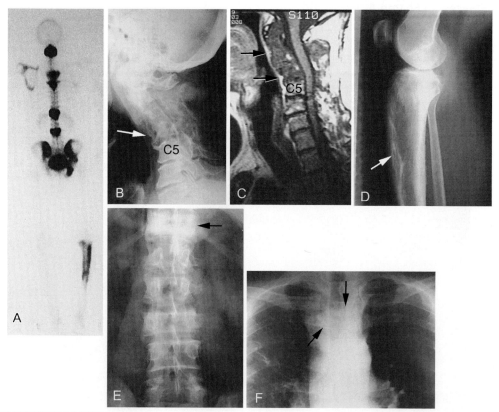

Figure 11-340 **POLYOSTOTIC PAGET'S DISEASE. A. Nuclear Bone Scan.** Observe all dark regions of the visualized skeleton corresponding to sites of Paget's disease, other than the bladder and sacroiliac joints. **B. Cervical Spine.** Note that Paget's disease involves the contiguous segments C2–C4 and has also produced intradiscal fusion (*arrow*). **C. T1-Weighted MRI, Sagittal Cervical.** Observe that the Paget's diseased seg- ments show low signal intensity (*arrows*). **D. Tibia.** Note the characteristic cortical thickening and trabecular accentuation (*arrow*). **E. Lumbar Spine.** Note that the T12 and L3 vertebrae are increased in density and expanded (*arrow*). **F. Manubrium.** Note the manubrium is sclerotic and expanded (*arrows*). (Courtesy of Gary L. Smith, DC, DACBR, Portland, Oregon.)

(50) The prognosis for Paget's sarcoma is grave and often rapidly fatal. (43)

Location

Paget's disease is often found at initial presentation to be polyostotic. (Fig. 11-340) The bones most commonly affected by Paget's disease, in diminishing order of frequency, are the pelvis (including the sacrum), femur, skull, tibia, vertebrae, clavicle, humerus, and ribs. (Figs. 11-341 to 11-345) The lesions vary in their distribution from a single bone to a widespread, almost complete skeletal involvement. The fibula is the bone least likely to be involved; involvement of all other bones, including those of the hand, foot (usually the calcaneus or talus), as well as the patella, and other sesamoid bones has been reported. Within the spine there is a definite variation in distribution, with preferential involvement of the L3 and L4 vertebrae, lower thoracic vertebrae, and the upper two cervical vertebrae. (50–54) (Figs. 11-346 to 11-352) The involvement of the lower extremity is more than twice that of the upper extremity. There is also a tendency for the right side of the skeleton to be involved more than the left. (5)

In tubular bones involvement invariably includes the subarticular end of the bone; seldom does the lesion stop at the me-taphysis. (Fig. 11-353) The extent of the lesion usually reaches the mid-diaphysis. This subarticular location is a helpful differential point when fibrous dysplasia is being considered because these lesions usually stop at the metaphysis.

Laboratory Findings

The serum alkaline phosphatase is almost invariably raised in Paget's disease. This enzyme is liberated by osteoblasts and is produced in great quantity as accelerated new bone formation attempts to compensate for the increased rate of bone resorption. In the active polyostotic state these values may be as high as 20 times that of normal values (55); however, in the monostotic involvement the levels may be slightly elevated or normal. The increased rate of osteoclastic resorption causes destruction of bone collagen and a concomitant increase in urinary excretion of hydroxyproline.

Ordinarily, the serum calcium and inorganic phosphorus values are normal in cases of Paget's disease. One would expect to find the serum calcium levels to be elevated in generalized

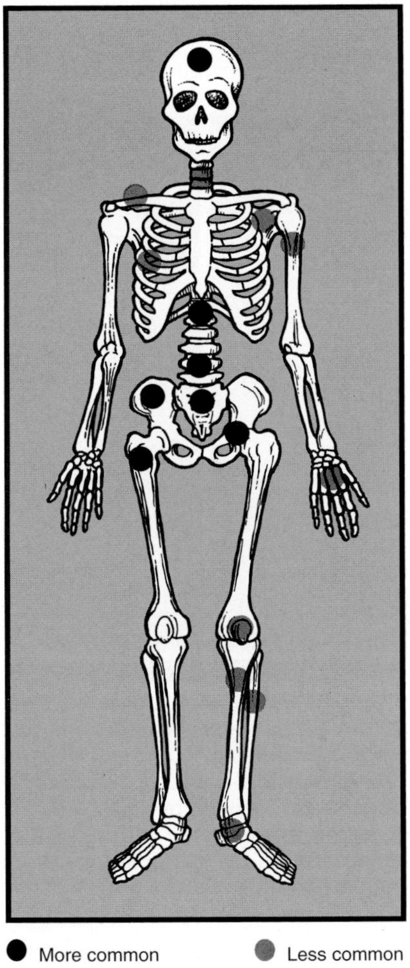

Figure 11-341 **SKELETAL DISTRIBUTION OF PAGET'S DISEASE.** ● More common ● Less common

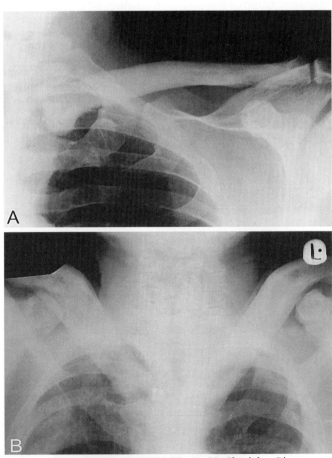

Figure 11-342 **PAGET'S DISEASE. A. AP Clavicle.** Observe the pagetoid expansion and cortical thickening of the entire clavicle. Note the subarticular involvement at both ends of the clavicle. **B. Bilateral Clavicles.** Observe the extensive cortical thickening and bone expansion at both the medial and distal portions of the clavicles. Pagetoid changes are also noted in both scapulae, with significant expansion of the coracoid processes. There are some changes in the ribs that are also suggestive of Paget's disease.

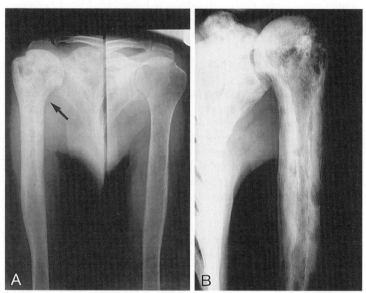

Figure 11-343 **PAGET'S DISEASE: HUMERUS. A. Bilateral AP Shoulders.** Observe the pagetoid changes of cortical thickening, radiolucent cystic changes, bone expansion, and subarticular involvement affecting the humeral head and proximal diaphysis (*arrow*). The opposite shoulder in this patient was normal. **B. AP Shoulder.** Observe the extensive cortical thickening and subarticular pagetoid changes in the visualized humerus. Similar changes of Paget's disease are present in the visualized portion of the scapula, particularly the coracoid process, which is expanded.

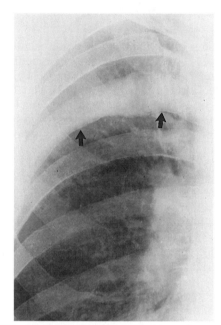

Figure 11-345 **PAGET'S DISEASE. Rib.** Note the cortical thickening and an increase in density of the posterolateral surface of the fifth rib consistent with Paget's disease (*arrows*).

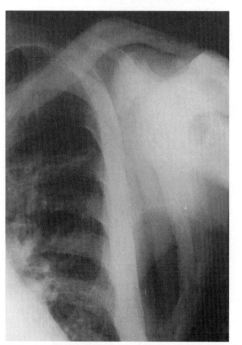

Figure 11-344 **PAGET'S DISEASE. Thorax and Shoulder.** Observe the pagetoid changes involving the clavicle, scapula, humeral head, and ribs.

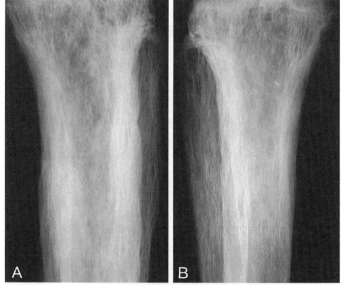

Figure 11-346 **PAGET'S DISEASE. A and B. Bilateral Tibia and Fibula.** Observe the extensive cortical thickening of the tibia and coarsening of the trabecular patterns of both the tibia and fibula. Bone expansion is also noted. *COMMENT:* The fibula is the bone least likely to be involved in Paget's disease; however, when present, the radiographic changes are consistent with all other sites. (Courtesy of Bryan Hartley, MD, Melbourne, Australia.)

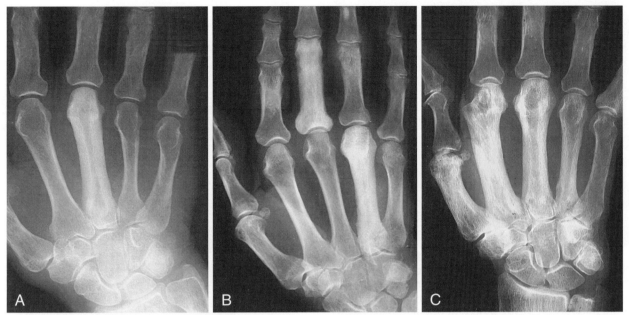

Figure 11-347   **PAGET'S DISEASE. A. PA Hand: Monostotic Involvement.** Note the extensive cortical thickening, increase in density, with subarticular extension of the pagetoid process involving the entire third metacarpal bone. Compare the thin cortices of the normal metacarpals adjacent with the thickened cortices of the pagetoid third metacarpal. **B. PA Hand: Polyostotic Involvement.** Observe the increase in bone density, bone expansion, and subarticular involvement of Paget's disease involving the fourth metacarpal and proximal phalanx of the third digit. Of incidental notation is a bone island in the distal phalanx of the fourth digit. **C. PA Hand: Polyostotic Involvement.** Observe the coarsening of the trabecular patterns, cortical thickening, and subarticular extension of the pagetoid changes affecting the first, second, third, and fourth metacarpals, as well as the proximal phalanx of the fifth digit. (Courtesy of Bryan Hartley, MD, Melbourne, Australia.)

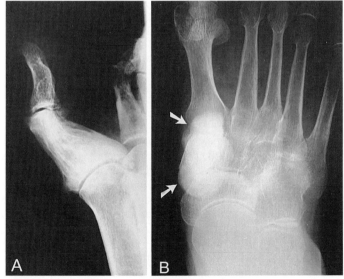

Figure 11-348   **PAGET'S DISEASE: FOOT. A. Great Toe.** Observe the pagetoid changes involving the proximal phalanx of the great toe. There is significant expansion of the base of the proximal phalanx, with coarsening of the trabecular patterns. **B. Dorsal Plantar Foot.** Observe the ivory-like density of the first cuneiform. Significant expansion of the first cuneiform, along with the sclerotic changes, supports the diagnosis of Paget's disease (*arrows*).

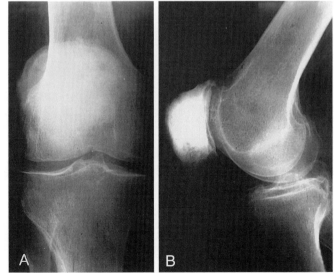

Figure 11-349   **PAGET'S DISEASE: PATELLA. A. AP Knee. B. Lateral Knee.** Note the sclerotic alteration of the trabecular patterns affecting the entire patella, creating significant expansion. (Courtesy of John W. Hawrylak, DC, DACBR, Phoenix, Arizona.)

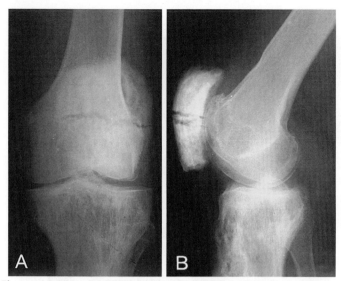

Figure 11-350 PAGET'S DISEASE: GIANT PATELLA. A. AP Knee. Observe the significant expansion and cortical thickening of the patella. Pagetoid changes are also noted in the proximal tibia. **B. Lateral Knee.** Note the pathologic fracture through the midportion of the pagetoid patella. Observe the pagetoid changes in the proximal tibia. (Courtesy of David P. Thomas, MD, Melbourne, Australia.)

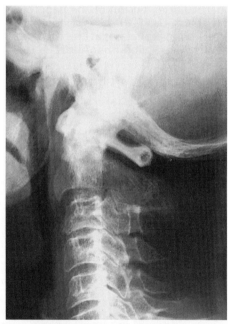

Figure 11-351 PAGET'S DISEASE: CERVICAL SPINE. Note the accentuation of the trabecular patterns affecting the vertebral body and neural arch of C2. Observe the significant expansion of the vertebral body of C2. Similar trabecular changes of Paget's disease are noted in the posterior arch and tubercle of C1, along with the occiput. (Courtesy of David P. Thomas, MD, Melbourne, Australia.)

Paget's disease during the destructive stage, yet this is usually not the case. This may be explained by the fact that in the natural course of the disease new osteoid is laid down and mineralized in the wake of the destructive process. This new bone probably uses most of the calcium that is liberated. (56)

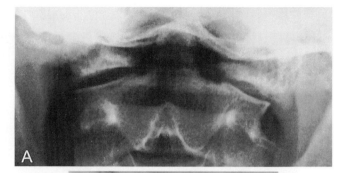

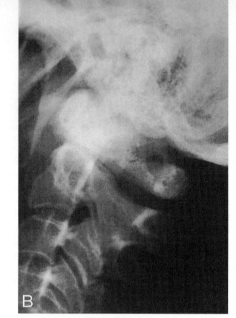

Figure 11-352 PAGET'S DISEASE: ATLAS. A. AP Open Mouth. Observe the accentuation of the trabecular patterns and bone expansion affecting the lateral masses of the atlas. **B. Lateral Cervical Spine.** Observe the cortical trabecular changes and expansion of bone affecting the posterior arch and tubercle of the atlas. These changes are consistent with Paget's disease.

Pathologic Features

The lesions of Paget's disease are characterized by marked vascularity and fibrosis. In the early osteolytic stage normal bone is replaced by fibrous tissue and osteoid, which may be completely calcified, and hemorrhage and necrosis also occur. Because destruction and repair occur repeatedly in the same areas, there is a bizarre and pattern-less arrangement of the cement lines, which has been called the *mosaic structure of Paget's disease.* In the bone- forming phase, considerable new bone formation occurs, with a predominance of cortical accretion. As the new bone grows into the spongiosa, the demarcation line between the cortex and the spongiosa is obliterated and an actual increase in the size of the affected bone takes place. The lesions are generally highly vascular, particularly the osteolytic lesions, with a high rate of bone metabolism reflected by an elevated uptake of bone-seeking radionuclides. It has been suggested that the excessive vascularity is associated with multiple, microscopic arteriovenous malformations in the affected bone. This hypervascularity may result in high-output cardiac failure in rare instances.

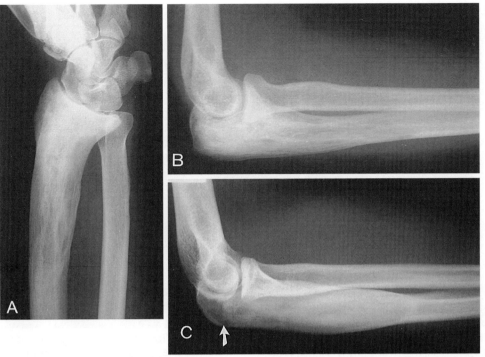

Figure 11-353 PAGET'S DISEASE: SUBARTICULAR EXTENSION. A. Distal Radius. Observe the pagetoid expansion and coarsening of the trabecular patterns involving the subarticular surface of the distal radius. **B. Lateral Elbow, Paget's Disease.** Note the pagetoid expansion of the olecranon process, with subarticular extension of the disease process. **C. Lateral Elbow, Fibrous Dysplasia.** Note the radiographic changes of fibrous dysplasia noted within the olecranon process, which are limited proximally, at the level of the metaphysis, without extending to the full distal subarticular surface of the ulna (*arrow*).

Stages of Paget's Disease

The four stages of Paget's disease are well documented and are outlined as follows (Table 11-40):

Stage One: Osteolytic, Destructive, or Monophasic Stage. In stage one of pagetic involvement, osteoclastic overactivity creates gross loss of bone density. This destructive phase is frequently associated with the radiographic sign *osteoporosis circumscripta.* (Fig. 11-354)

Stage Two: Combined, Mixed, or Biphasic Stage. Stage two is the one most frequently encountered clinically. It is a reflection of both underlying destruction and production of bone. It is characterized by cortical thickening, with an overall increased radiopacity and accentuation of trabecular patterns with lucent areas intermixed. Bone expansion is a common finding. The entire process is basically one of extensive repair, with cheap fibrous bone replacement secondary to the osteoclastic lytic destruction. (10)

Stage Three: Sclerotic or Ivory Stage. In stage three there is a uniform thickening of trabeculae with increased radiopacity simulating an ivory appearance of the bone. Bone expansion may or may not be present. This stage is most commonly seen in the innominate or the vertebrae.

Table 11-40	Four Stages of Paget's Disease
Stage one: osteolytic, destructive, or monophasic	
Stage two: combined, mixed, or biphasic	
Stage three: sclerotic or ivory	
Stage four: malignant degeneration	

Stage Four: Malignant Degeneration. Stage four is the lethal stage and is discussed thoroughly under "Complications."

Metastatic Disease and Paget's Disease

It is of interest to note the relative infrequency of metastatic disease superimposed on pre-existing uncomplicated Paget's disease. One might expect that, because of the pathologic state of hypervascularity in pagetic bone, the incidence of metastatic disease would be higher in bones affected by Paget's disease than in the normal skeleton. (43) In fact, pagetic bone is much less likely to develop metastatic lesions than normal bone. It has been suggested that as a result of the rapid osteoclastic and osteoblastic response in pagetic bone the environment or soil for the proliferation of secondary tumor cells is poor. (43) In addition, patients who develop primary carcinoma with metastasis are usually elderly. Perhaps by this time the pagetoid changes are more quiescent and the vascular supply is lessened. The definitive answer to this question remains unknown. The literature to date offers but a few case reports of metastatic disease developing in pre-existing uncomplicated Paget's disease, the largest series (12 cases) being reported by Wilner and Sherman. (57)

Radiologic Features

The radiologic features of Paget's disease strikingly mirror the pathologic changes. Plain film radiography is usually adequate; however, bone scans may be helpful in seeking the location of

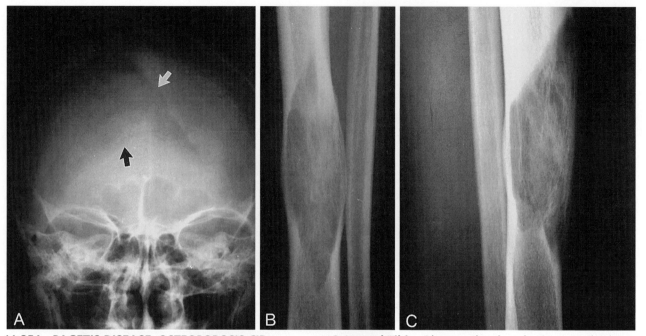

Figure 11-354 PAGET'S DISEASE: OSTEOPOROSIS CIR-CUMSCRIPTA. A. PA Skull. Observe the sharply demarcated area of radiolucency present throughout the frontal bone (*arrows*), which is characteristic of the osteolytic phase of Paget's disease (*osteoporosis circumscripta*). **B. AP Tibia.**

C. Lateral Tibia. Observe the sharply circumscribed area of loss of bone density present within the mid-diaphysis of the tibia. This radiolucency has been called the *candle flame, V-shaped,* or *blade of grass appearance.*

additional lesions once a single bony site has been observed. Because pagetic bone has an increased metabolic activity, as much as five times that of adjacent normal bone, lesions of Paget's disease will render a positive, or hot, bone scan. (58) (Fig. 11-355) It should be reemphasized that bone scans are sensitive to abnormal areas of bone metabolism but are totally non-specific. Therefore, areas that show increased radionuclide uptake on a bone scan should be followed by routine radiologic examination to confirm Paget's disease. (58)

General Features

The radiologic features of Paget's disease vary in appearance, depending on the stage of involvement and the bone affected; however, distinctive signs of Paget's disease include changes in bone density, coarsened trabeculae, cortical thickening, bone expansion, subarticular distribution, pseudo-fractures, bowing deformities, and pathologic fracture. (Table 11-41) In the initial acute osteolytic phase, a typical sharply defined lytic area with

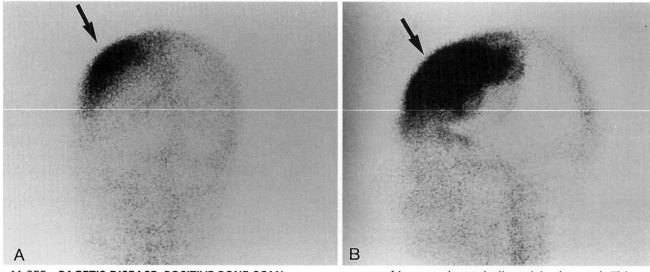

Figure 11-355 PAGET'S DISEASE: POSITIVE BONE SCAN. A. PA Skull. B. Lateral Skull. Observe the focal area of increased uptake of the radionuclide substance consistent with

an area of increased metabolic activity (*arrows*). This patient's plain films demonstrated characteristic radiographic signs of Paget's disease.

Table 11-41	General Radiographic Features of Paget's Disease
Thickened cortex Coarsened trabeculae Bone expansion Increased or decreased density Subarticular extension Long lesion Deformity	

Table 11-42	Named Radiographic Signs of Paget's Disease
Skull	Osteoporosis circumscripta Cotton wool appearance
Spine	Picture frame appearance Ivory vertebra
Pelvis	Brim or rim sign obliterating Kohler's teardrop
Femur and tibia	Blade of grass appearance, V lesion, or candle flame appearance

a narrow zone of transition is observed. Consonant with the general predilection of Paget's disease for hematopoietic areas of the skeleton, the calvaria, innominates, and long bones are most often affected. Occasionally, other areas, such as the tubular bones of the hand and foot, may be involved. In the calvaria and pelvis, the lytic area tends to be spherical, whereas in a long bone the radiolucent lesion is often elongated, ending in a V with a sharp border and giving a *flame-shaped appearance*. The lesion virtually always starts in the end of a long bone (subarticular location) and progresses shaftward, if it does not remain stationary. An osteolytic lesion may be highly expansile as it thins and balloons the cortices. Pathologic fracture through a lesion is not uncommon. A periosteal reaction may be observed in highly aggressive lesions. In this acute phase, partially calcified osteoid may also be detected.

In the spine well-defined lytic areas are unusual in the osteolytic phase. More commonly observed are one or several collapsed vertebral bodies, with the vertebral appendages frequently involved in the process. Of aid in distinguishing osteolytic Paget's disease of a vertebra from other causes (e.g., metastasis, plasmacytoma) is the early appearance of new bone in the Paget's lesion with subsequent enlargement of the vertebra.

Specific Locations

The radiographic signs of Paget's disease are best described by regional location. (Table 11-42)
Skull. The skull is commonly involved in the polyostotic form of this disease. The disease begins as a maplike or geographic

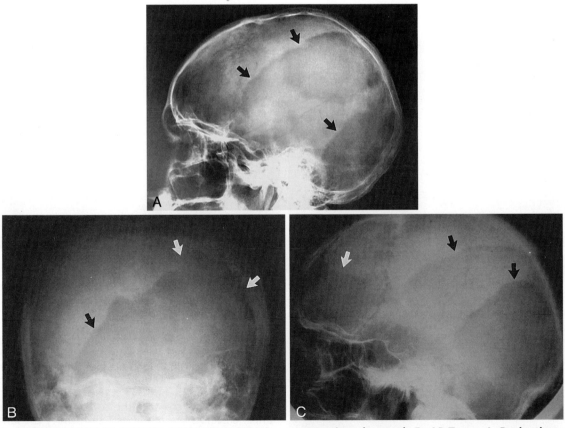

Figure 11-356 **PAGET'S DISEASE: VARIED MANIFESTATIONS OF OSTEOPOROSIS CIRCUMSCRIPTA. A. Lateral Skull.** Note the large areas of map-like radiolucencies scattered throughout the skull table, representing osteoporosis circumscripta (*arrows*). **B. AP Towne's Projection. C. Lateral Skull.** Observe the large areas of loss of bone density throughout the bony calvaria, consistent with the lytic phase of Paget's disease (*arrows*). *(continued)*

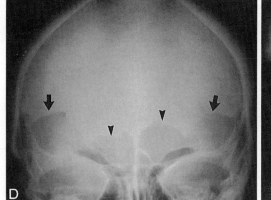

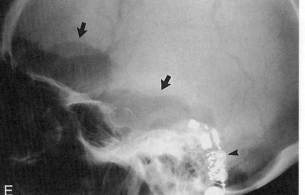

Figure 11-356 (continued) D. PA Caldwell's Projection. Note the well-demarcated area of radiolucency throughout the frontal and parietal bone, which represents osteoporosis circumscripta of Paget's disease (*arrows*). This should not be confused with the normal landmarks of the frontal sinus (*arrowheads*). **E. Lateral Skull.** Observe the lytic areas affecting the frontal and parietal bone, characteristic of osteoporosis circumscripta of Paget's disease (*arrows*). Of incidental notation is a metallic density seen superimposed over the mastoid air cells, which represents the patient's hearing aid (*arrowhead*).

resorption of bone, most commonly in the frontal and occipital areas, progressing gradually to encompass the entire calvaria. The outer table is destroyed from within, whereas the inner table is spared, and the suture lines provide no barrier to the bone destruction. This process has been referred to as *osteoporosis circumscripta* and is representative of the early, lytic stage of Paget's disease of the skull. (21) (Fig. 11-356)

In the second stage (combined phase), reparative processes begin as a sclerosis of the inner table. At this stage the disease becomes quiescent, with irregular patches of radiopacity in the thickened diploe. This pattern in the skull is characteristic and diagnostic of Paget's disease; it is termed the *cotton wool appearance* because of the fuzzy, poorly defined edges of the sclerotic areas. (21) (Fig. 11-357)

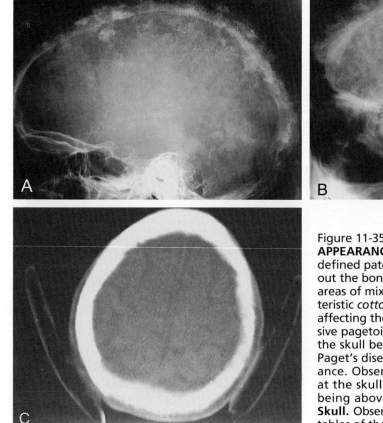

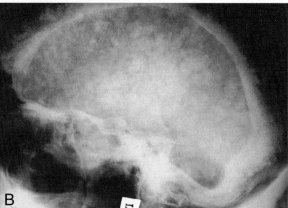

Figure 11-357 PAGET'S DISEASE: COTTON WOOL APPEARANCE. A. Lateral Skull. Observe the ill-defined patches of radiopacity scattered throughout the bony calvaria. These changes, with some areas of mixed radiolucencies, represent the characteristic *cotton wool* appearance of Paget's disease affecting the skull. **B. Lateral Skull.** Note the extensive pagetoid expansion of the bony calvaria, with the skull being involved in the mixed phase of Paget's disease, creating the *cotton wool* appearance. Observe the platybasia deformity present at the skull base, with the odontoid process being above Chamberlain's line. **C. Axial CT Skull.** Observe the extensive thickening of the tables of the skull as a result of Paget's disease.

Spine. The lumbar spine is commonly involved in the mixed stages of Paget's disease and may involve a single vertebra or affect multiple vertebrae. (Figs. 11-358 and 11-359) The vertebral body is enlarged with a rim of thickened cortex, giving the appearance of a *squared-off, picture frame vertebra.* (30) (Fig. 11-360) Accentuation of the trabecular pattern, especially in the

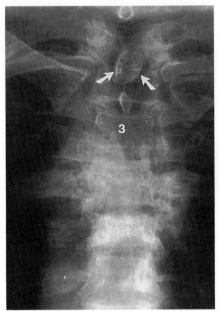

Figure 11-358 POLYOSTOTIC SPINAL PAGET'S DISEASE. Thoracic Spine. Note the pagetoid changes in the T1, T3, T4, T5, and T6 vertebral bodies. Observe the coarsening of the trabecular patterns throughout these vertebral segments and, more specifically, the significant expansion of the spinous process of T1 (*arrows*).

vertical plane, may simulate the *striated* appearance of a vertebral hemangioma.

Monostotic Paget's disease of the spine may also be seen in the sclerotic stage. (Fig. 11-361) The vertebral body and posterior elements appear extensively radiopaque, giving the characteristic *ivory vertebra* appearance. (57) Although this is a classic appearance, it must be differentiated from other diseases that can develop a dense vertebral body. The three most common causes for an *ivory vertebra* are (*a*) osteoblastic metastatic carcinoma (usually from the prostate gland), (*b*) Paget's disease (osteitis deformans), and (*c*) Hodgkin's disease (lymphoma). (Fig. 11-362, Tables 11-43 and 11-44) With a singular vertebral body involved and no other bones affected, differentiation is essential.

The radiographic differential diagnosis of a solitary *ivory vertebra* may sometimes be accomplished by inspecting the anterior aspect of the vertebra. The normal concavity of the vertebral body will be unaltered in patients with osteoblastic metastasis because bone expansion is not a common feature. Paget's disease, however, usually creates a squaring off or bulging of the anterior surface of the vertebral body as a result of the inherent cortical thickening and bone expansion. Rarely, Paget's disease may not expand the vertebral body and, if no other bony lesions are present, a biopsy may be required for final diagnosis.

The sclerotic changes of the vertebral body affected by Hodgkin's occur secondary to hematogenous metastases. In Hodgkin's lymphoma there is often anterior scalloping of the ivory vertebral body, thus accentuating the anterior vertebral concavity. The pathogenesis of this is thought to be from contiguous lymph nodal tissue pressing on the vertebral body as a result of transmitted aortic pulsations. Not all ivory vertebrae from Hodgkin's disease will demonstrate anterior scalloping; however, it is a classic sign when present and should always be searched for. Clinical information is also helpful because most Hodgkin's patients are generally much younger (20- to 40-year age range),

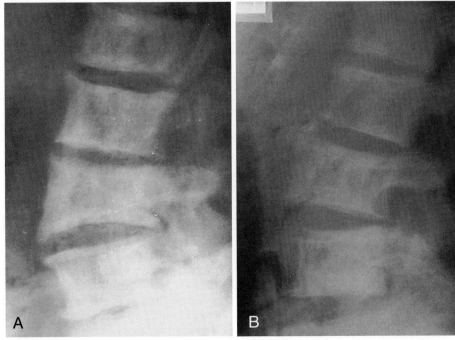

Figure 11-359 POLYOSTOTIC PAGET'S DISEASE: LUMBAR SPINE. A and B. Lateral Lumbar Spine. Note the extensive pagetoid change, creating significant vertebral body expansion, along with coarsening of the trabecular patterns throughout the entire lumbar spine of both patients.

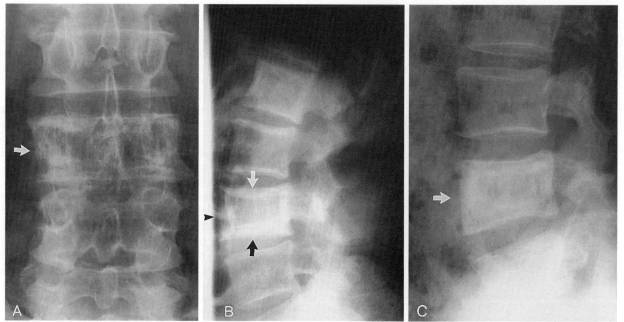

Figure 11-360 **PAGET'S DISEASE: PICTURE FRAME VERTEBRA. A. AP Lumbar Spine.** Note the accentuation of the trabecular patterns throughout the L3 vertebra, with significant bone expansion, creating the characteristic *picture frame* appearance (*arrow*). **B. Lateral Lumbar Spine.** Observe the characteristic picture frame vertebra at the L4 vertebra. Considerable thickening of the vertebral end-plates (*arrows*) and loss of the anterior concavity of the vertebral body, suggesting bone expansion (*arrowhead*), are characteristic signs of Paget's disease. **C. Lateral Lumbar Spine.** Observe the characteristic *picture frame* appearance at the L4 vertebra (*arrow*).

whereas Paget's disease and osteoblastic metastatic carcinoma both occur in the > 50-year age group. The alkaline phosphatase blood test is elevated in all three conditions, but the acid phosphatase should be elevated only when the blastic lesions are from the prostate gland as a primary source.

Pelvis. The pelvis is one of the more common sites of pagetoid change and is usually affected by the combined stages of the disease. The involvement may affect only half of the pelvis, or the whole pelvis including the sacrum. (Fig. 11-363) The characteristic findings are cortical thickening and expansion of the pubis and ischium. The roentgen appearance is one of patchy areas of sclerosis, with intermittent lucent defects and increased trabecular markings. There is usually a thickening of cortical margins along the pelvic rim and obliteration of Köhler's teardrop, which is called the *rim,* or *brim, sign.* (21,30) (Fig. 11-364) Weakening of the pelvic bones may result in protrusio acetabuli. Sacral involvement as a monostotic presentation is also quite common. (30) (Fig. 11-365)

Femur. The femur is usually involved in the mixed stage of this disease process. The disease begins as a subarticular lesion extending into the metaphysis and diaphysis of the bone. (Fig. 11-366) This subarticular location is characteristically found in pagetoid involvement of long or short tubular bones. It provides a strong differential point between fibrous dysplasia and other disease processes that do not include subarticular bone involvement. The roentgenographic appearance is one of expanded femoral cortices with coarse trabecular patterns, particularly in the vertical plane, and obliteration of the marrow cavity in advanced stages. (Fig. 11-367) Pseudo-fractures may be present in the subtrochanteric region of the femur, usually on the lateral or convex surface of the cortex. Bone softening results in a varus deformity of the hip, referred to as the *shepherd's crook deformity.*

Tibia. The tibia is the second most common site of lytic Paget's disease. (30) The radiologic appearance is one of a radiolucent defect beginning in the subarticular end of the proximal tibia and extending down the shaft in a characteristic *candle flame* or V-shaped appearance, which is often referred to as a *blade of grass appearance.* (Fig. 11-368) This flame-shaped lytic defect indicates the advancing edge of osteoclastic resorption of bone. (Fig. 11-369) With extensive involvement anterior bowing of

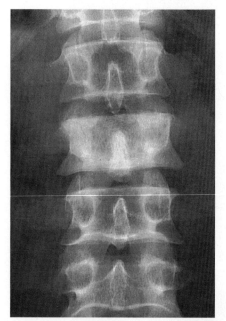

Figure 11-361 **PAGET'S DISEASE: IVORY VERTEBRA. Lumbar Spine.** Observe the diffuse radiopacity throughout the L2 vertebral body, with associated bony expansion of the spinous process.

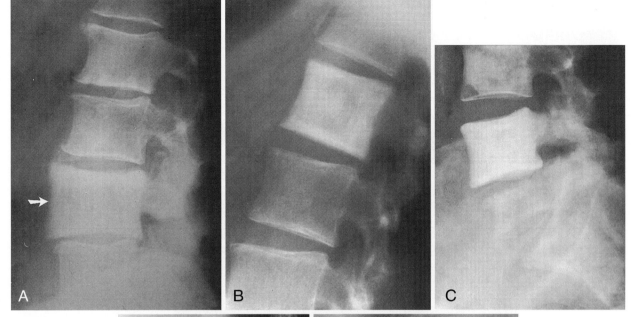

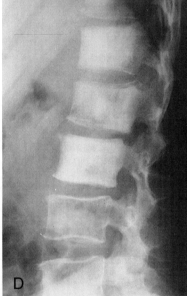

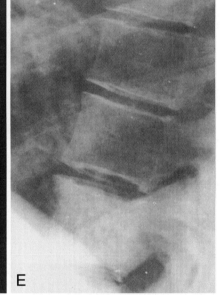

Figure 11-362 **IVORY VERTEBRA: DIFFERENTIAL DIAGNOSIS.**
A. Paget's Disease: Lateral Lumbar Spine. Note the solitary
ivory vertebra at the L4 vertebral body. Vertebral body expansion, with loss of the anterior concavity (*arrow*), suggests the
diagnosis of Paget's disease. **B–D. Osteoblastic Metastasis:
Lateral Lumbar Spine.** Observe the solitary or multiple ivory
vertebrae throughout these lumbar spines. Preservation of the
anterior concavity of the vertebral body, without evidence of
cortical thickening or vertebral body expansion, suggests the

diagnosis of a malignant ivory vertebra. **E. Hodgkin's
Lymphoma: Lower Thoracic Spine.** Observe the solitary ivory
vertebra affecting the T12 vertebral segment. There is deep
anterior scalloping of the vertebral body, which accentuates
the anterior concavity of this vertebral segment and occurs as
a result of direct extension from malignant lymphadenopathy.
(Panel A courtesy of Joseph W. Howe, DC, DACBR, Fellow,
ACCR, Los Angeles, California. Panel E courtesy of Paul E.
Siebert, MD, Denver, Colorado.)

Table 11-43	Differential Diagnosis of an Ivory Vertebra		
Factor	Blastic Metastases	Paget's Disease	Hodgkin's Disease
Age	> 45	> 50	20–40
Increased density	+++	+++	+++
Expansion	—	+++	—
Anterior scalloping	—	—	+++
Acid phosphatase	+++[a]	—	—
Alkaline phosphatase	++	+++	++

[a] Males, prostate.
—, Does not occur; +, seldom occurs; ++, often occurs; +++, very commonly occurs.

Table 11-44	Solitary Ivory Vertebra	
Common Causes		Uncommon Causes
Osteoblastic metastasis		Sarcoidosis
Hodgkin's lymphoma		Chordoma
Paget's disease		Myeloma
Degenerative sclerosis		Osteosarcoma
Osteomyelitis (fungal or chronic)		Ewing's sarcoma
		Osteoid osteoma
		Osteoblastoma
		Bone island

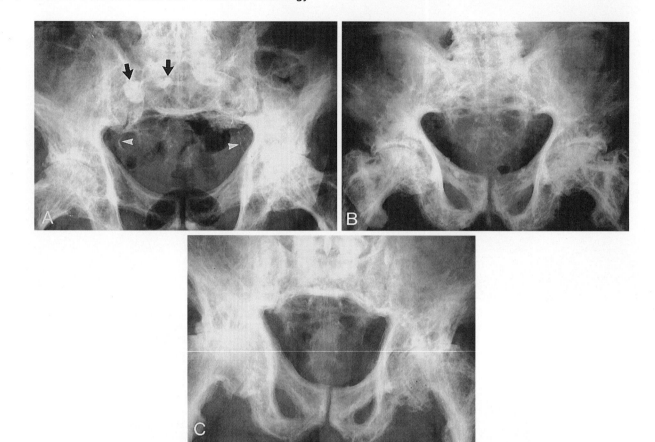

Figure 11-363 PAGET'S DISEASE: DIFFUSE INVOLVEMENT. A. AP Pelvis. Observe the coarsened, irregular trabecular patterns scattered throughout the pelvis, sacrum, and proximal femora. Of incidental notation are calcified mesenteric lymph nodes (*arrows*) and vascular calcifications (*arrowheads*) within the pelvic basin. **B. AP Pelvis.** Note this example of the diffuse coarsening of the trabecular patterns seen in extensive Paget's disease of all of the bones of the pelvis and proximal femora. **C. AP Pelvis.** Observe the Paget's disease within the pelvis, sacrum, and proximal femora. Because of the extensive alteration in weight bearing present within the hip joint articulations, there is premature degenerative joint disease.

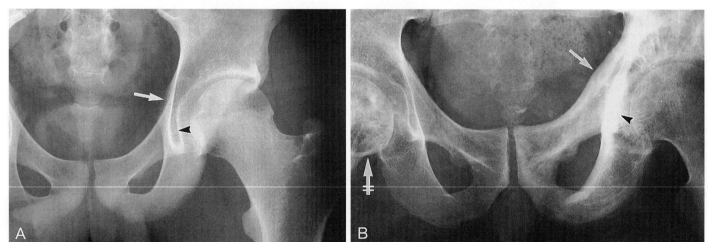

Figure 11-364 PAGET'S DISEASE: BRIM SIGN AND OBLITERATION OF KÖHLER'S TEARDROP. A. AP Hip: Normal. Observe the normal pelvic rim at the area of the iliopectineal line (*arrow*). The caudal aspect of the iliopectineal line forms the normal Köhler's teardrop (*arrowhead*). Observe also the trabecular patterns and cortical margins of the normal skeleton. **B. AP Hip.** Note the extensive pagetoid thickening of the trabecular patterns as it affects the iliopectineal line, creating the brim sign (*arrow*). Obliteration of Köhler's teardrop (*arrowhead*) as a result of pagetoid changes in the pubic rami and ischial tuberosity is noted. Compare the trabecular changes and increase in bone density of the pagetoid portion of the pelvis to the normal cortical trabecular patterns, Köhler's teardrop, pubic rami, and ischial tuberosities of the opposite side. For observers with a Sherlock Holmes eye, note the pagetoid subarticular involvement of the proximal femur in the opposite femoral head (*crossed arrow*). (Courtesy of Kenneth E. Yochum, DC, St. Louis, Missouri.)

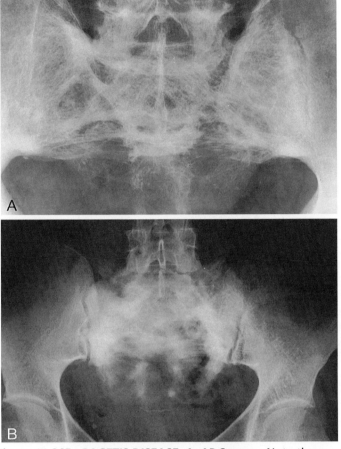

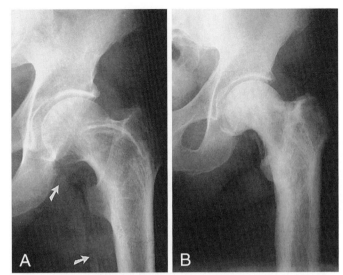

Figure 11-367 **PAGET'S DISEASE: FEMUR. A. AP Hip.** Note the coarsening of the trabecular patterns, particularly in the vertical plane, seen throughout the femoral head and neck. Of incidental notation is extensive vascular calcification in the soft tissues of the inner thigh (*arrows*). **B. AP Hip.** Observe the increase in radiopacity involving the femoral head and cortices of the diaphysis. Coarsening of the trabecular patterns, along with expansion of bone, is a sign of Paget's disease.

Figure 11-365 **PAGET'S DISEASE. A. AP Sacrum.** Note the extensive coarsening of the trabecular patterns throughout the sacrum. The expansion of the sacral ala has distorted the appearance of the sacroiliac joint, giving the appearance of ankylosis. **B. AP Sacrum.** Observe the sclerotic changes of the sacrum, along with bony expansion, consistent with Paget's disease.

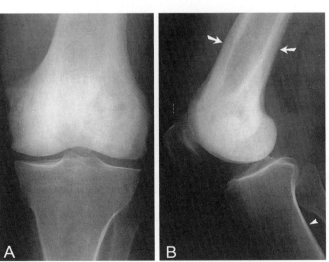

Figure 11-366 **PAGET'S DISEASE: SUBARTICULAR INVOLVEMENT. A. AP Knee. B. Lateral Knee.** Observe the sclerotic appearance of the visualized distal femur, with subarticular extension of the pagetoid process. There is extensive cortical thickening noted in the distal diaphysis of the femur (*arrows*), compared with the normal cortical width on the posterior surface of the proximal tibia (*arrowhead*).

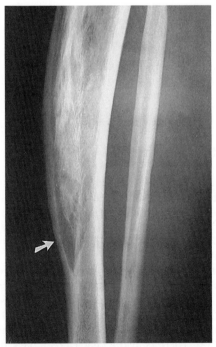

Figure 11-368 **PAGET'S DISEASE: BLADE OF GRASS APPEARANCE. Tibia.** Observe the radiolucent defect at the caudal aspect of the pagetoid tibia (*arrow*). This presentation in Paget's disease has been referred to as the *blade of grass appearance* or *candle flame* or *V-shaped* lytic defect. (Courtesy of Joseph W. Howe, DC, DACBR, Fellow, ACCR, Los Angeles, California.)

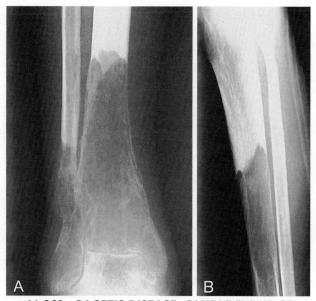

Figure 11-369 PAGET'S DISEASE: CANDLE FLAME OR V-SHAPED LYTIC DEFECT. A. AP Ankle. Note the extensive deossification of bone affecting the distal portion of the tibia and fibula. Observe the advancing flame-shaped lytic defect present in the proximal portion of the tibia and fibula, which indicates the advancing edge of osteoclastic resorption of bone (*osteoporosis circumscripta*). There is a malalignment of the distal fibula, suggesting an area of previous fracture. **B. Lateral Tibia and Fibula.** Observe the focal osteoporosis present in the middle and lower diaphysis of the tibia. The sharp border to this lytic defect assumes a *candle flame* or *V-shaped* appearance. This is typical of the early lytic phase of Paget's disease, particularly in the tibia.

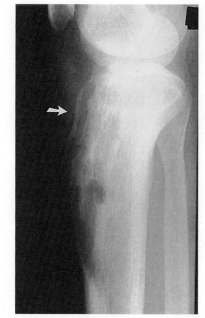

Figure 11-370 PAGET'S DISEASE: AVULSION FRACTURE. Lateral Tibia. Observe the pagetoid changes present in the proximal portion of the tibia. An avulsion of the tibial tuberosity is noted (*arrow*).

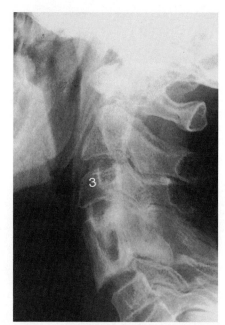

Figure 11-371 PAGET'S DISEASE OCCURRING WITHIN A BLOCK VERTEBRA. Lateral Cervical Spine. There is a congenital block vertebra present at C4 and C5 with fusion of the vertebral bodies, facets, lamina, and spinous processes. Paget's disease has developed at C4 and C5 with complete involvement of each vertebra. (Courtesy of Michael T. Buehler, DC, DACBR, Durango, Colorado.)

the tibia occurs and has been called the *saber shin deformity* (a similar deformity is found in congenital syphilis). (Fig. 11-296) Rarely, an avulsion fracture of the tibial tuberosity can occur. (Fig. 11-370)

Differential Diagnosis

Paget's disease should be included in a differential diagnosis in any osteosclerotic condition of the skeletal system in adults because the most common presentation of Paget's disease is in the mixed stage (Fig. 11-371). However, it must be remembered that radiology is only one method of diagnosis and clinical correlation is essential.

The two most common entities that may be difficult in differentiation are osteolytic or osteoblastic metastatic carcinoma and, in the spine, hemangioma of bone. The main diagnostic differential points in metastatic carcinoma are the lack of thickening of the cortex and frequent disruption of the cortex as a result of aggressive destruction. There is also a characteristic lack of significant bone expansion found with metastasis, which is usually one of the classic radiologic signs found in Paget's disease. (Fig. 11-372) In addition, a lesion in a tubular bone that is not located in the subarticular region is less likely to be Paget's disease.

Hemangioma of the vertebral bodies produces a vertically striated pattern, which may closely mimic the coarse vertical trabeculae of Paget's disease. A small percentage of the capillary type of hemangioma of the vertebral bodies may also allow expansion of bone. When this occurs, the differential diagnosis of a monostotic lesion of Paget's disease from a hemangioma may be extremely difficult. A helpful roentgen sign is the lack of corti-

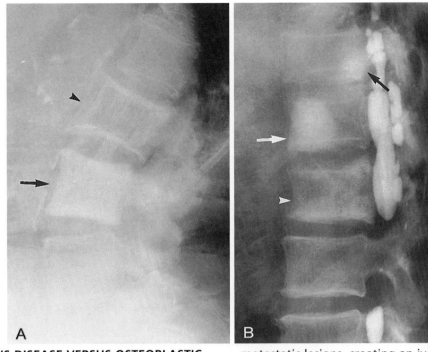

Figure 11-372 **PAGET'S DISEASE VERSUS OSTEOBLASTIC METASTATIC DISEASE. A. Lateral Lumbar Spine.** Observe the homogeneous ivory vertebra at the L3 level (*arrow*). There is preservation of the anterior concavity of the vertebral body, without bone expansion. These signs suggest a malignant, metastatic, ivory vertebra. Observe the cortical thickening of the vertebral endplates, coarsening of the trabecular patterns, and loss of the anterior concavity of the L2 vertebra (*arrowhead*). These radiographic signs confirm Paget's disease. Of incidental notation is diffuse atherosclerotic plaquing in the abdominal aorta. **B. Lateral Thoracolumbar Spine.** Observe the nodular, radiopaque, metastatic lesions, creating an ivory appearance within the T11 and T12 vertebral bodies (*arrows*), representing osteoblastic metastatic disease. There is cortical thickening, with posterior vertebral endplate expansion at the L1 vertebral body, consistent with the radiographic signs of Paget's disease (*arrowhead*). The radiopaque densities in the spinal canal represent residual contrast media from a previous myelographic examination. *COMMENT:* The cardinal radiographic features differentiating osteoblastic metastatic disease from Paget's disease are cortical thickening and bone expansion in Paget's disease, signs seldom found in osteoblastic metastasis.

cal thickening of the vertebral endplate in hemangioma, the presence of which is often the hallmark of spinal Paget's disease. (Fig. 11-373) Most solitary hemangiomas are of the cavernous type and show no significant expansion of bone, providing a useful differential point. (54)

Treatment and Prognosis

The main thrust in the medical treatment of Paget's disease has been to inhibit bone resorption with the use of salmon and human calcitonin. (59) Paget's disease arises when some unknown stimulus causes a considerable increase in the number and activity of osteoclasts. The ability of calcitonin to inhibit osteoclastic bone resorption by decreasing the activity and proliferation of osteoclasts led to the proposal that it be used in the treatment of Paget's disease, and experience over the last 10 years has in fact confirmed its therapeutic effect. (59)

Calcitonin has proved effective in giving pain relief, beginning usually between 2 and 8 weeks after the initiation of treatment. If pain relief has not been achieved within 3 months of starting treatment with calcitonin, it is almost certainly not going to be accomplished. For that reason, when using therapeutic trials of calcitonin for pain, a period of 3 months has been chosen as the optimum time. There seems no point in providing calcitonin treatment for any shorter period in Paget's disease. (59)

Generally, most drug therapy (calcitonin and diphosphonate) is used to suppress osteoclastic activity with the hope that osteoblastic activity will normalize soon after. Preradiographic and postradiographic changes showing improvement in patients with Paget's disease on medication have been demonstrated by numerous authors. There are, however, a number of patients who do not respond; the explanation for this is not presently available. (59)

Supportive braces to prevent extensive bone deformity in the weight-bearing bones is an adjunctive aid to the clinician in managing patients with extensive Paget's disease.

The natural progress of Paget's disease is extremely slow and poorly documented. It is exceedingly difficult to predict the behavior of Paget's, as it is quite certain that many of the monostotic lesions of this disease may be asymptomatic throughout life. The radiologic appearance may remain static for a decade or more. The normal course for the disease seems to be one of slow progression over many years, with increasing sclerosis, bony enlargement, and deformity. Until the true cause of this disease is ascertained, treatment will remain limited and prognosis uncertain. Further research is necessary to establish the specific origin of this peculiar and relatively common disease.

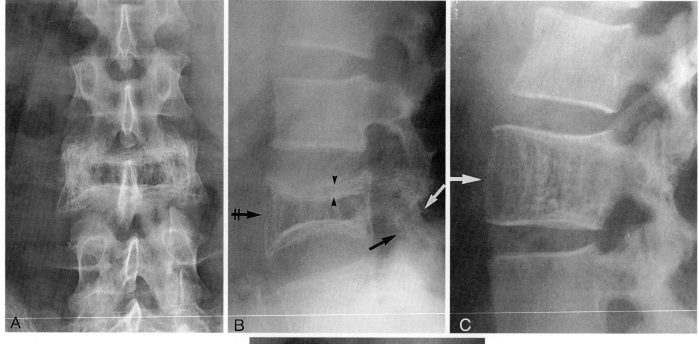

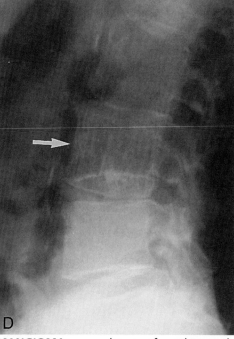

Figure 11-373 **PAGET'S DISEASE VERSUS HEMANGIOMA: DIFFERENTIAL DIAGNOSIS. A. AP Lumbar Spine: Paget's Disease.** Note the extensive coarsening of the trabecular patterns in the vertical distribution throughout the vertebral body. **B. Lateral Lumbar Spine: Paget's Disease.** Note the vertical accentuation of the trabecular patterns, accompanied by thickening of the vertebral endplates (*arrowheads*) and an overall expansion of the vertebral body and visualized neural arch (*arrows*). There is distinct loss of the anterior concavity of the vertebral body associated with bone expansion (crossed *arrow*). **C. Lateral Lumbar Spine: Hemangioma.** Note the accentuation of the vertical trabecular patterns throughout the vertebral body of L2. There is also loss of the concavity of the anterior surface of the vertebral body as a result of bony expansion (*arrow*). Observe the normal width of the vertebral endplates of the affected L2 vertebral body. This appearance within the vertebra has

been referred to as the *corduroy cloth* appearance of hemangioma. **D. Lateral Lumbar Spine: Hemangioma.** Observe the characteristic *corduroy cloth* appearance of a vertebral body hemangioma affecting the L3 segment (*arrow*). The normal anterior concavity of the vertebral body is preserved, with no bony expansion noted. Of incidental notation is scattered atherosclerotic plaquing throughout the abdominal aorta. *COMMENT:* The cardinal roentgen signs for the differential diagnosis of hemangioma versus Paget's disease in its combined phase of presentation in the spine are (*a*) a lack of cortical thickening of the vertebral endplate in hemangioma is contrasted to extensive endplate thickening in Paget's disease and (*b*) the radiographic sign of vertebral body expansion may be found in both Paget's disease and hemangioma; however, it is more commonly found in Paget's disease. (Panel D courtesy of Stephen F. Kesler, DC, Salt Lake City, Utah.)

CAPSULE SUMMARY   Paget's Disease

General Considerations

- Sir James Paget in 1877 described a disorder of bone that today bears his name.
- Also known as osteitis deformans, it is a great imitator of bone diseases, along with fibrous dysplasia.

Incidence

- 3% of the adult population > 40 years old have the disease.
- Highest incidence is in United Kingdom (5% of the population); high in Australia and New Zealand; rare in Asia, Africa, and Scandinavia.
- In the United States it is more common in the northern states and is somewhat uncommon in the southern states.

Cause

- Many theories have been offered, but none substantiated: inflammatory disorder, endocrine disorder, autoimmune disorder, inborn error of connective tissue metabolism, vascular disorder, metabolic disorder, neoplasm, and chronic viral infection—a measles-like virus, which is the most current theory.

Clinical Features

- 2:1 male predominance.
- Rare before age 40, most common after 55.
- 90% of patients are asymptomatic.
- Pain, when present, is of low intensity and may be associated with bowing deformities or fractures.
- An increasing hat size is common because of enlargement of the calvaria.
- The most common bones affected in uncomplicated disease are the pelvis, vertebrae, clavicle, humerus, and ribs; the fibula is the bone least likely to be involved.
- Subarticular location is characteristic, which usually extends into the diaphysis.

Complications

- Deformity of bone is a common complication, including shepherd's crook deformity of the proximal femur (coxa vara), saber shin deformity (anterior tibial bowing), protrusio acetabuli, leontiasis ossea, frontal and parietal bossing, and basilar invagination.
- Pathologic fracture of the vertebral body and transverse banana-like fracture of long bones is common.
- Pseudo-fractures are noted representing local areas of demineralization within the bone, which are replaced by fibrous tissue.
- Spinal stenosis may occur as a result of bony expansion of a vertebra, leading to compressive neuropathy.
- Anemia may rarely occur as a result of fibrous tissue replacing the bone marrow.
- Paget's coxopathy represents articular cartilage destruction with secondary degenerative changes.
- Ureteric colic occurs secondary to hypercalcemia and hypercalcuria, creating urinary calculus formation, which seems to occur more readily in patients who have been immobilized.

- High-output cardiac failure is a rare complication, occurring when at least one third of the skeleton is involved.
- *Malignant degeneration:* incidence is 0.9 to 2%; rare under age 40, average age, 57–66. Symptoms of localized pain in a patient with known Paget's disease may herald the development of malignant degeneration; most common bones are the femur, humerus, innominate, skull, and tibia; only nine cases are reported in the vertebrae. Osteosarcoma is the most common tumor to complicate Paget's disease (50% of cases); radiologically, 50% of lesions are lytic, 25% sclerotic, and 25% mixed; treatment is radiation therapy or surgical resection; 5-year survival rate is poor (8%).

Laboratory Findings

- Owing to osteoclastic resorption there is an enhanced destruction of bone collagen, leading to an increase in urinary excretion of hydroxyproline.
- A significant increase in alkaline phosphatase occurs, occasionally 20 times the normal values.
- Hypercalcemia may occur.

Pathologic Features

- The pattern-less replacement of normal bone by pagetic, vascular, and fibrotic bone has been called the mosaic structure of Paget's disease.
- *Four stages:* stage one—osteolytic, destructive, monophasic; stage two—combined, mixed, biphasic; stage three—sclerotic or ivory; stage four—malignant degeneration.

Radiologic Features

- *Bone scan:* pagetic lesions will be hot on bone scan.
- *Skull:* early skull lesions demonstrate the lytic stage of osteoporosis circumscripta, whereas more advanced changes of the combined stage create the cotton wool appearance.
- *Spine:* vertebral involvement causes a thickened and enlarged vertebral endplate, creating the squared-off, picture frame vertebra; these changes occur in the biphasic stage.
- Homogenous increase in radiopacity of a vertebral body creates the ivory vertebra. The three most common causes for an ivory vertebra are osteoblastic metastatic carcinoma, Paget's disease, and Hodgkin's lymphoma.
- *Pelvis:* the fundamental roentgen signs of Paget's disease are cortical thickening and bone expansion. These changes are classically manifested in the pelvis with thickening of the iliopectineal line, obliterating Köhler's teardrop, which has been called the rim or brim sign.
- *Long bones:* the tibia is the second most common site of lytic Paget's disease (the skull being the most common). The changes of a radiolucent defect usually begin in the subarticular end of the proximal tibia, extending down the shaft in a characteristic candle flame or V-shaped appearance, often referred to as a blade of grass appearance.

Treatment and Prognosis

- Medical treatment has consisted of salmon and human calcitonin, an osteoclast inhibitor.
- Supportive braces to prevent extensive bone deformity are helpful.

FIBROUS DYSPLASIA

General Considerations

Fibrous dysplasia of bone is a disorder of unknown cause in which skeletal aberrations constitute the cardinal feature. Certain endocrinopathies and abnormal pigmentations of the skin may form a part of the total disease process. Because of this, three basic forms of the disease are currently recognized: the monostotic form (affecting one bone), the polyostotic form (affecting many bones), and the polyostotic form with associated endocrine abnormalities.

Fibrous dysplasia of bone is a fairly common, well-recognized, locally circumscribed, slowly progressing, benign disorder of fibro-osseous tissue. Fibrous dysplasia was not recognized as a distinct clinical entity until Lichtenstein (1) in 1938 reported eight cases with detailed studies of bone lesions. He proposed the term fibrous dysplasia, or polyostotic fibrous dysplasia in the presence of multiple bone lesions. Although recognized clinically as a distinct entity only in recent decades, fibrous dysplasia has affected the human skeleton for centuries. Several reports of the disease have appeared in literature of paleontopathology. In the years before 1938 many patients who actually had fibrous dysplasia of bone were diagnosed as having osteitis fibrosa cystica (von Recklinghausen). Because both diseases produce significant deossification of the skeleton with multiple cyst-like accumulations in bone, it is easy to understand how these two diseases could have been originally poorly differentiated. Similarly, cases of hyperparathyroidism producing multiple osseous brown tumors were also mistakenly diagnosed as fibrous dysplasia before a full understanding of these diseases was gained. (2) The present and outdated terms for fibrous dysplasia, hyperparathyroidism, and neurofibromatosis are outlined in Table 11-45. Because of their varied radiographic manifestations and ability to mimic other disease processes, fibrous dysplasia and Paget's disease have been referred to as the *"great imitators* of bone disease."

Incidence

The fact that the number of reported cases exceeded 1500 by 1971 confirms that fibrous dysplasia is a common disease. (3) Available data seem to indicate that the monostotic form accounts for about 70%, the polyostotic form without endocrine disturbances about 27%, and the polyostotic form with endo-

crine disturbances (McCune-Albright syndrome) about 3%. (4) The actual incidence of each form, however, cannot be assessed precisely because the monostotic form may remain asymptomatic, only to be detected accidentally, and thus can often escape clinical detection. Even the polyostotic form may occasionally exist unnoticed for decades and present as an incidental finding.

Clinical Features

Age and Sex Distribution

Fibrous dysplasia generally makes its appearance in late childhood; some severe forms, however, may manifest themselves in infancy. Each form of the disease has a different average age of onset. The monostotic form manifests itself initially around the age of 14, the polyostotic form without endocrine disorders, around the age of 11, and the polyostotic form associated with endocrine disturbances, around the age of 8. (5) Although it is not uncommon for certain lesions to be detected during later decades of life, there is good evidence that the majority, if not all, bone lesions develop during the period of skeletal growth. (6)

According to Uehlinger (7), monostotic and polyostotic fibrous dysplasia not accompanied by endocrine disorders reveals an even sex distribution. By contrast, polyostotic fibrous dysplasia with endocrine disorders displays an obvious predilection for females.

Signs and Symptoms

The symptoms of fibrous dysplasia depend on the location of the lesion and often its size. Many lesions are completely asymptomatic and are found accidentally after a radiologic examination is initiated for some other reason. Lesions in the upper end of the femur often present with a limp and complaints of intermittent pain. Persistent pain with long bone involvement often occurs as a result of pathologic fracture.

Polyostotic disease usually presents with a more pronounced deformity and bowing of the bones and a greater tendency toward pathologic fracture. Harris et al. (8) found leg length discrepancy to be the most common physical deformity, this being the result of an extreme coxa vara and bowing deformity of the femur. This appearance has been referred to as the *shepherd's crook deformity.* (5)

Asymmetric enlargement and deformity of the cranial and facial bones may lead to unilateral cranial hyperostosis. Asymmetric enlargement and deformity of the cranial and facial bones may lend the face a *leonine* appearance. *Leontiasis ossea,* however, occurs in a number of other skeletal disorders and is, therefore, not a specific feature of this disease. Rib involvement may produce a localized bony prominence in the thoracic cage. In rare instances a lesion can reach enormous proportions, to the extent that enlargement of a single rib can obliterate a large portion of the thoracic cavity. (9) Occasionally, involvement of the ethmoid and sphenoid bone can cause obstruction of the entire nasal cavity.

Cutaneous Abnormalities

Café au Lait Spots. Abnormal cutaneous pigmentation is the most common of the extraskeletal expressions of fibrous dysplasia. These pigmented skin macules are referred to as *café au lait*

Table 11-45	Terms Used to Describe Fibrous Dysplasia	
Present	**Past**
Monostotic fibrous dysplasia	Osteitis fibrosa cystica localisata
Polyostotic fibrous dysplasia and Albright's syndrome	Osteitis fibrosa cystica disseminata
Hyperparathyroidism	Osteitis fibrosa cystica generalisata or von Recklinghausen's disease of bone
Neurofibromatosis of von Recklinghausen	Fibrocystic disease (multiple)

Adapted from **Wilner D:** *Radiology of Bone Tumors and Related Disorders.* Philadelphia, WB Saunders, 1982.

spots and may occasionally be confused with those found in neurofibromatosis. The pigmented areas are caused by an increased amount of melanin in the basal cells of the epidermis. The color varies from dark brown to chestnut or yellowish. They are not raised above the adjacent skin, and they are generally distributed about the midline. The most common locations for the lesions are the lower lumbar region, buttocks, back of the neck, shoulders, chest, and oral mucosa. (4) Their margins are irregular and they are few in number. Their size, however, may vary considerably and, generally, their location coincides with the side of skeletal involvement. Similarly, when the bone lesions are distributed bilaterally, so are the skin pigmentations. (4) The irregular margins have been referred to as the *coast of Maine appearance,* which is in contrast to the smooth, well-defined margins found in the café au lait spots of neurofibromatosis, representing the *coast of California appearance.* (Fig. 11-374) The lesions found in fibrous dysplasia tend to be somewhat darker than the café au lait spots of neurofibromatosis. In order for the clinician to feel confident that the skin pigmentations of neurofibromatosis actually represent café au lait spots, there must be a minimum of six lesions, each being 1.5 cm or larger in size. Therefore, the irregularity of the margins of the café au lait spots and, histologically, the absence of the giant pigment granules in the malpighian cells or melanocytes differentiates café au lait spots in fibrous dysplasia from the similar pigmented skin areas encountered in neurofibromatosis. (4)

The café au lait spots are usually present at birth, but may develop later and precede the skeletal and endocrinologic manifestations. Although quite unusual, café au lait spots may be found in the monostotic form. (8) In the polyostotic form without endocrine disturbances, they are present in > 30% of patients. In the polyostotic form with endocrine disturbances, they are found in nearly all patients. (4)

Location and Distribution

Fibrous dysplasia may present as a solitary lesion (monostotic form) or as multiple lesions in several bones (polyostotic form). (Fig. 11-375) Polyostotic fibrous dysplasia may be limited to a

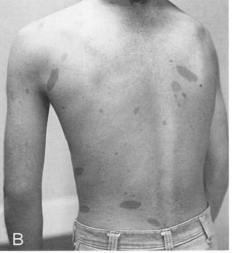

● More common   ● Less common

Figure 11-375   SKELETAL DISTRIBUTION OF FIBROUS DYSPLASIA (POLYOSTOTIC).

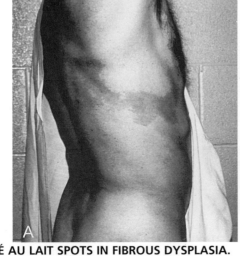

Figure 11-374   CAFÉ AU LAIT SPOTS IN FIBROUS DYSPLASIA.
A. Fibrous Dysplasia. Observe the large café au lait spot surrounding the thorax of this patient with fibrous dysplasia. Note the irregular margins, which have been referred to as the *coast of Maine appearance* in fibrous dysplasia.
B. Neurofibromatosis. Observe the multiple café au lait spots on this patient's back. The margins to these skin lesions are smooth, representing the *coast of California appearance* of café au lait spots in neurofibromatosis. *COMMENT:* Note those spots in fibrous dysplasia tend to be larger than neurofibromatosis.

single limb (monomelic distribution) or may involve both sides of the skeleton (bilateral distribution).

Monostotic Fibrous Dysplasia. The monostotic form is neither a forme fruste nor a precursor of the polyostotic form. So far, there has been no report of a transition from a monostotic to a polyostotic manifestation of fibrous dysplasia. In spite of an identical histologic appearance, the two forms are different clinically; the monostotic form is much less likely to develop fractures and deformities. It would, therefore, appear appropriate to regard the two forms as relatively independent clinical entities.

Of patients with monostotic fibrous dysplasia 75% present with lesions in the ribs, femur (proximal), tibia, or skull. An additional 10% of lesions are found within the pelvis and humerus. With monostotic involvement of the jaws the maxilla is usually twice as frequently affected (64%) as the mandible (36%). A rare, cortical form of fibrous dysplasia exists, which is in direct contrast to the usual diametaphyseal medullary location. This cortical fibrous dysplasia occurs in the anterior proximal surface of the tibia. (Fig. 11-376) Fibrous dysplasia of the rib is the most common benign rib lesion and usually measures > 4 cm in length. (Fig. 11-377) Isolated cases in the clavicle, scapula, tarsal and carpal bones, other long bones, and the spine (10,11) have been reported. (Fig. 11-378)

Polyostotic Fibrous Dysplasia. The polyostotic form most commonly affects the femur, skull, tibia, humerus, ribs, fibula, radius, and ulna, in decreasing order of incidence. This form distinguishes itself from the monostotic form by the following features: (*a*) in the extension of the skeletal involvement to the shoulder and pelvic girdle and in the more frequent involvement of the craniofacial skeleton and vertebral column; (*b*) in the tendency to affect entire limbs; (*c*) in the severity of deformities, which may lead to extensive crippling (e.g., shepherd's crook deformity of the prox-

imal femur); and (*d*) in the higher incidence of spontaneous and often recurrent fractures. (7)

Spinal changes in polyostotic fibrous dysplasia are somewhat uncommon; when present, however, they usually affect more than one spinal segment, and then they affect the vertebral body.

The number of bones involved in polyostotic fibrous dysplasia varies; it may be high. Hopf (12) described a 43-year-old female with 79 separate lesions involving 75 bones, who was followed radiographically for > 20 years. This represents about a 39% in-

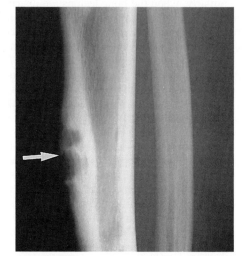

Figure 11-376 CORTICAL FIBROUS DYSPLASIA. Tibia. Observe the geographic, radiolucent lesions in the anterior tibial cortex (*arrow*). *COMMENT:* The anterior proximal surface of the tibia is the most common site for cortical fibrous dysplasia, which is rare.

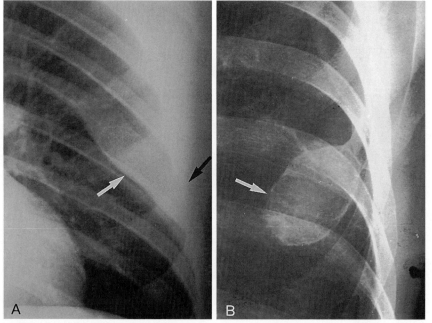

Figure 11-377 FIBROUS DYSPLASIA: RIB INVOLVEMENT. A. PA Ribs. Observe the radiolucent, expansile lesion present within the midportion of the left eighth rib (*arrows*). Observe the *ground glass appearance* of the matrix of this lesion. **B. PA Rib.** Observe the geographic, expansile lesion in the anterior surface of the right fourth rib (*arrow*). The central matrix of the lesion is *ground glass* in appearance.

The peripheral cortical border of this lesion is thin; however, no disruption in the cortex is noted. *COMMENT:* Fibrous dysplasia of the rib is the most common benign rib lesion; it usually measures > 4 cm in length. The most common sites for monostotic fibrous dysplasia are the proximal femur and the rib structures.

volvement of the entire skeleton. In some instances of monomelic distribution, every bone of the entire extremity may be involved. The incidence of craniofacial involvement is about 10% in monostotic disease and about 50% in polyostotic disease with moderate skeletal involvement, but reaches 100% in polyostotic disease with extensive skeletal involvement. (13,14) The majority of the cranial lesions display an asymmetric distribution and include the mandible in approximately 20% of cases. (13)

Endocrine Abnormalities

McCune-Albright syndrome is defined as polyostotic fibrous dysplasia associated with skin pigmentation and precocious sexual development. There is a tendency for the bone lesions in this syndrome to be unilateral in distribution. The area of skin pigmentation may be large and affects primarily the neck, chest, back, shoulder, and pelvic girdle. McCune-Albright syndrome is encountered almost exclusively in females. Precocious sexual development manifests itself in females by premature occurrence of irregular menstrual bleedings at the age of 5–6 years, and occasionally much earlier. The development of secondary sexual characteristics follows the precocious menarche. There is good evidence to support the fact that the precocious sexual development represents true precocious puberty. Benedict (15) collected five cases of McCune-Albright syndrome in males, which is quite unusual. The prognosis for patients with McCune-Albright syndrome is generally poor. (16)

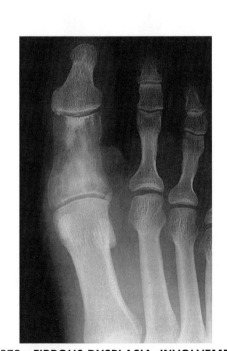

Figure 11-378 **FIBROUS DYSPLASIA: INVOLVEMENT OF THE GREAT TOE. PA Foot.** Note the expansion and alteration of the trabecular patterns of the proximal phalanx of the great toe. A mottled area of radiopacity throughout this radiolucent lesion is noted, as a result of the characteristic *ground glass appearance. COMMENT:* Most tubular bone involvement in fibrous dysplasia does not extend to the subarticular surface of the bone; however, when a small tubular bone is involved, the subarticular extension point of differentiation from Paget's disease is no longer applicable.

Laboratory Findings

Laboratory studies are usually within normal values, except for the occasional elevation of serum alkaline phosphatase and osteocalcin. (17) This slight elevation usually occurs during periods of exacerbation of the disease process or consolidation of a spontaneous fracture. The serum calcium and phosphorus levels are normal.

Cherubism

Cherubism is a familial fibrous dysplasia of the jaws (18) characterized by swelling of the lower face. It is inherited as an autosomal dominant trait, with an 80% penetrance. It is usually recognized between the ages of 18 months and 2 years, and then becomes stationary and regresses spontaneously during puberty. (18) It affects primarily the mandible but occasionally the maxilla. Multilocular cystic lesions with asymmetric distribution in the mandible and maxilla are responsible for the characteristic changes in facial configuration. (19) (Fig. 11-379) Swelling of the cheeks stretches the skin and retracts the lower eyelids, which in turn produces a slight upward turning of the eyes, so that the lower half of the sclera is exposed abnormally. The eyes then appear to assume an *eyes-raised-to-heaven attitude.* (20) Histologically, cherubism is indistinguishable from giant cell reparative granuloma. (21)

Pathologic Features

Fibrous dysplasia is an abnormality in which normal bone undergoing physiologic resorption is replaced by an abnormal proliferation of an isomorphous fibrous tissue of spindle cells and poorly formed bony trabeculae of woven bone. (22) Recent studies have suggested the cause of the disease stems from mutagenic change in the *GNAS1* gene of a somatic cell. (23) The trabeculae have an irregular size, form, or distribution; they display no orientation or apparent relation to the function of the affected cylindrical or flat bone. The disease has been considered as an arrest of bone matu-

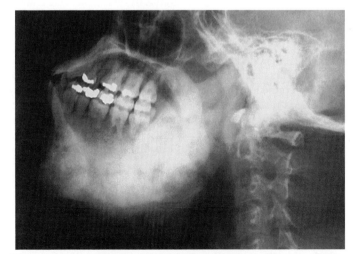

Figure 11-379 **FIBROUS DYSPLASIA: CHERUBISM. Mandible.** Observe the diffuse sclerosis and expansion of the mandible secondary to extensive fibrous dysplasia. (Courtesy of Norman W. Kettner, DC, DACBR, St. Louis, Missouri.)

ration at the immature stage of woven bone, as a disturbance of postnatal cancellous bone maintenance, or as a misdifferentiation of the bone-forming mesenchyme. (6,24,25) This proliferation process may sooner or later extend beyond normal boundaries and give rise to expansion, distortion, and structural weakness. It involves primarily the cancellous and seldom the cortical bone formation. Lesions replace normal cortex by erosion from within, creating endosteal scalloping, but in most instances are covered with a shell, however thin, of normal cortical bone.

The macroscopic appearance of bones affected by fibrous dysplasia is that of a fusiform or spherical enlargement, with a surface of thin, intact, cortical bone. The enlargement may measure up to several centimeters in diameter. On a longitudinal section the cancellous bone has been replaced by a yellowish white, resilient tissue, which occasionally includes small cysts filled with an amber fluid. The transition to normal bone is usually quite abrupt. A cross section of a tubular bone with a fibrous dysplastic lesion generally reveals a widening of the shaft and a thinning of the cortex, with significant endosteal scalloping. Endosteal scalloping of bone is a characteristic pathologic and radiologic sign of fibrous or cartilaginous lesions of bone. Replacement of the medulla by connective tissue eccentrically expands the bone and leaves a firm and rubbery substance irregularly scattered throughout. Disseminated throughout the fibrous lesion are various spicules of bone, creating a radiopaque appearance to some lesions of fibrous dysplasia. Radiographically, this results in the *ground glass appearance*. As a rule, the fibrous tissue may be readily cut with a knife. The poorly ossified bone spicules lend it a certain elastic, gritty consistency comparable to *sand embedded in putty*. A cut surface of a dysplastic lesion in general reveals a grayish or whitish color and considerable variation in vascularity.

Lesions in the base of the skull or maxilla generally possess a firmer consistency than those in the ribs or long bones because they include a greater amount of bone spicules. Skull lesions, therefore, commonly display a much greater radiopacity than lesions seen in the tubular bones or flat bones of the pelvis. Aside from the bones of the skull, the olecranon process is the only other site where fibrous dysplasia consistently appears significantly more radiopaque than in other bony structures. (Figs. 11-380 and 11-381)

The histologic appearance of fibrous dysplasia presents a fairly characteristic picture of irregular trabeculae of woven bone varying in size, shape, and distribution, without apparent functional orientation. These trabeculae are embedded in a loosely or densely textured, cellular, and vascular connective tissue stroma. This histologic appearance is the end result of a probable metaplasia proliferating connective tissue. The matrix surrounding the bony trabeculae is made up of cellular fibrovascular connective tissue. The morphologic pattern of the stroma varies with the age of the lesion. In a younger lesion, the stroma displays a looser arrangement, and there is less collagen formation. In an older lesion, the stroma is usually quite dense.

Sarcomatous Transformation

In rare instances fibrous dysplasia may be associated with malignant change. (26) This phenomenon was first described by Coley and Stewart. (27) The true incidence of sarcomatous transformation in fibrous dysplasia is 0.5%. (28) This percentage might be somewhat high, considering that there are presently no accurate

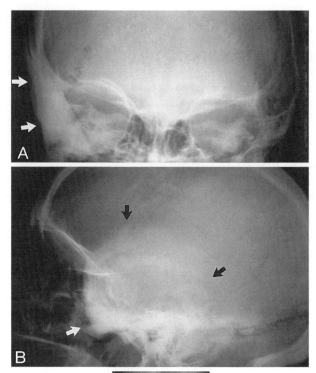

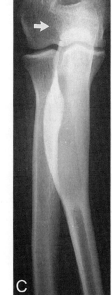

Figure 11-380 **SCLEROTIC FIBROUS DYSPLASIA. A. PA Skull.** Observe the sclerotic changes associated with fibrous dysplasia of the temporoparietal area of the skull (*arrows*). **B. Lateral Skull.** Note a significant area of increased radiopacity as a result of fibrous dysplasia affecting the temporal area of the skull (*arrows*). **C. AP Elbow.** Observe the expansion of the medullary portion of the proximal ulna as a result of extensive fibrous dysplasia. The lesion in the ulna demonstrates a characteristic *ground glass appearance,* with a heavier osteoid matrix, creating a sclerotic presentation. Note the lack of subarticular extension of fibrous dysplasia in the proximal portion of the olecranon process (*arrow*). This is a helpful point in differentiating fibrous dysplasia from Paget's disease in tubular bones. Paget's disease usually extends to the subarticular surface of the bone.

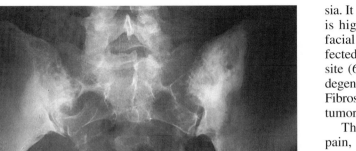

Figure 11-381 **SCLEROTIC FIBROUS DYSPLASIA MIMICKING OSTEOBLASTIC METASTASIS.** Observe the diffuse areas of increased radiopacity, with mottled radiolucencies affecting the posterior surfaces of the ilium bilaterally. There is no involvement of the sacrum or sacroiliac joints. These lesions were initially thought to represent metastatic tumors, with symptoms in the local area. This was a biopsy-confirmed sclerotic fibrous dysplasia. (Courtesy of Lynton G. F. Giles, DC, PhD, Townsville, Queensland, Australia.)

figures available on incidence of clinically manifested, asymptomatic forms of the disease. The age range at which sarcomatous transformation has been recognized varies from 8 to 61 years, with a mean of 32 years. The latency period between the diagnosis of fibrous dysplasia and subsequent sarcomatous degeneration varies between 2 and 30 years. The sarcoma, on the average, develops within 14 years after the initial diagnosis of fibrous dyspla-

sia. It is somewhat more prevalent among males, and the incidence is higher in the polyostotic form. In the monostotic form the facial bones and bones of the cranial vault are most frequently affected (50%). In the polyostotic form, the femur is the common site (62%). (Figs. 11-382 and 11-383) Other sites for malignant degeneration include the tibia, humerus, scapula, pelvis, and fibula. Fibrosarcoma and osteosarcoma are the most common malignant tumors to complicate fibrous dysplasia.

The clinical features of malignant transformation include pain, local swelling, and radiologically demonstrable bone destruction with cortical disruption. (5,7) The cause of malignant transformation is still unknown. In a few instances radiation therapy may be a precipitating factor. In the majority of instances, however, the same unidentified factor that induces the proliferation of the fibro-osseous tissue might also produce a sarcomatous transformation. (28)

Radiologic Features

The skeletal lesions of fibrous dysplasia are not usually present at birth; they are present, however, several years before puberty and often progress throughout the entire life of the patient. Because of the progressive turnover of bone, patients with fibrous dysplasia will have a positive bone scan. (29) All of the bones of the body may be involved; however, there is a particular site predilection for monostotic and polyostotic involvement. (Table 11-46)

Monostotic Fibrous Dysplasia

The most common location for monostotic fibrous dysplasia is in the proximal third of the femur and the ribs. (30) Most lesions

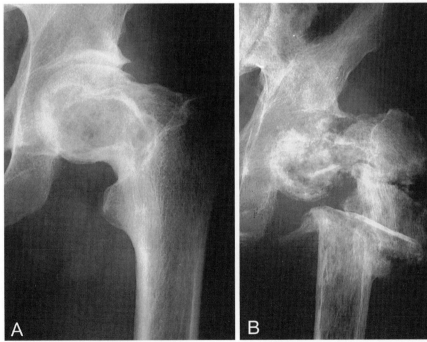

Figure 11-382 **FIBROUS DYSPLASIA: MALIGNANT DEGENERATION. A. AP Hip.** Observe the large, geographic lesion, with a heavy rind or rim of sclerosis encapsulating it, which is characteristic of benign fibrous dysplasia. **B. 11-Year Follow-Up: AP Hip.** Note the pathologic fracture and exten-

sive destruction of bone affecting the femoral head, neck, and proximal diaphysis. The radiographic presentation suggests malignant degeneration. This was a biopsy-confirmed malignant degeneration of fibrous dysplasia to fibrosarcoma.

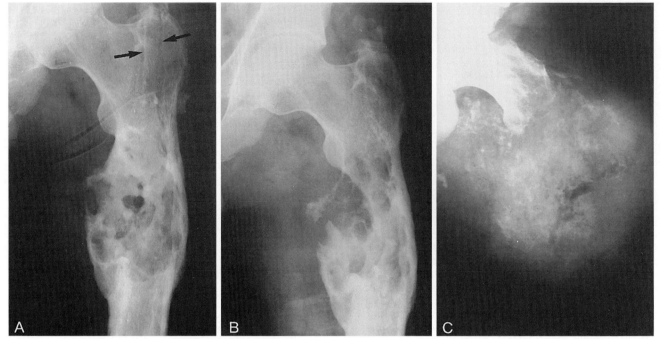

Figure 11-383 FIBROSARCOMA COMPLICATING FIBROUS DYSPLASIA. A. AP Femur. Note the large, expansile lesion of fibrous dysplasia within the proximal diaphysis of the femur. This patient experienced a pathologic fracture before these radiographs were taken, and an intermedullary pin had been placed to immobilize the lesion. Observe the remnant electroplating of the bone from the previously placed intramedullary pin *(arrows)*. **B. 3-Year Follow-Up: AP Femur.** Observe the cortical destruction as a result of underly-ing malignant degeneration. The patient presented with local-ized pain in the area of the inner thigh. **C. AP Femur.** Observe that as a result of malignant degeneration to fibrosarcoma, this patient received an amputation of the lesion. Unfortu-nately, postsurgical infection and tumor recurrence in the soft tissue areas complicated the surgical procedure. (Courtesy of Bryan Hartley, MD, Melbourne, Australia.)

Table 11-46	Radiologic Features of Fibrous Dysplasia

Monostotic
  Proximal femur, ribs
  Diametaphyseal
  Geographic
    Lucent, smoky (ground glass)
    Thick sclerotic margin (rind)
    Occasionally septated (soap bubble)
  Expansion
  Cortical thinning and scalloping
  Elongated lesion
  Pathologic fracture
Polyostotic
  Multiple lesions; may be unilateral
  Pseudo-fractures
  Deformities
    Femur: coxa vara, shepherd's crook
    Rib: extrapleural sign
    Pelvis: protrusio acetabulae
  Spine rarely involved
Complications
  Malignancy (0.5%)
  Fractures
  Deformities

affecting the long bones are placed in the diametaphysis and spare the subarticular surface of the bone. This anatomic predilection is helpful in the differential diagnosis of Paget's disease. Paget's dis-ease on occasion may mimic fibrous dysplasia; however, involve-ment of the tubular bones in Paget's disease invariably extends to include subarticular bone. (Fig. 11-384)

The lesions of monostotic fibrous dysplasia are usually radio-lucent, often having a loculated or trabeculated appearance. (Fig. 11-385) Scattered throughout the fibrous lesion, there is an ap-pearance of radiopacity. (Fig. 11-386) This represents the classic *ground glass* or *smoky appearance* of bone. As described earlier, this represents a base matrix of fibrous tissue with scattered os-teoid, which Murrary and Jacobson (31) so appropriately called the *wipe out of the trabecular patterns appearance*. Many students of radiology have struggled with the phrase *ground glass appear-ance of bone*. After hearing numerous explanations, the most plau-sible one offered suggests the appearance of glass after a grinder is used on its surface to disturb its glistening sheen. This renders a homogenous, ill-defined density across the surface of the glass, which is characteristic of the appearance within the medullary canal of the bones involved in fibrous dysplasia.

These geographic cystic lesions are often well demarcated and, in the monostotic form, usually have a thick, sclerotic bor-der, referred to by Murray and Jacobson (31) as the *rind of scle-rosis*. (Fig. 11-387) There is a widening of the medullary canal, and the endosteum is often thinned and scalloped. Expansion of bone is a common finding. Deformity of bone, particularly in weight-bearing bones, is often found and occasionally is associ-ated with pathologic fracture. There is no evidence of periosteal response, except in those cases following pathologic fracture or malignant change. Most of these lesions render a typical and characteristic appearance, allowing the radiologist to establish the correct diagnosis in a high percentage of cases. In question-

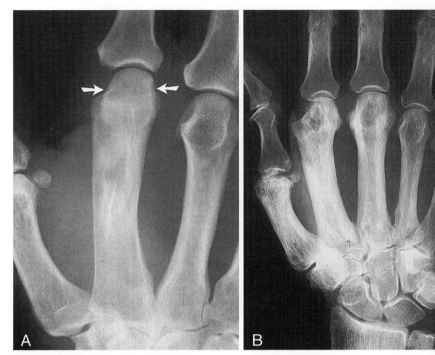

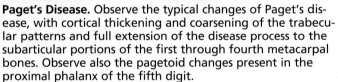

Figure 11-384 **ANATOMIC DISTRIBUTION OF FIBROUS DYSPLASIA VERSUS PAGET'S DISEASE. A. PA Hand: Fibrous Dysplasia.** Observe expansion of the second metacarpal bone, with the characteristic *ground glass* or *smoky appearance.* Note the lack of subarticular extension of the disease process, since it stops at the distal metaphysis (*arrows*). **B. PA Hand:**

Paget's Disease. Observe the typical changes of Paget's disease, with cortical thickening and coarsening of the trabecular patterns and full extension of the disease process to the subarticular portions of the first through fourth metacarpal bones. Observe also the pagetoid changes present in the proximal phalanx of the fifth digit.

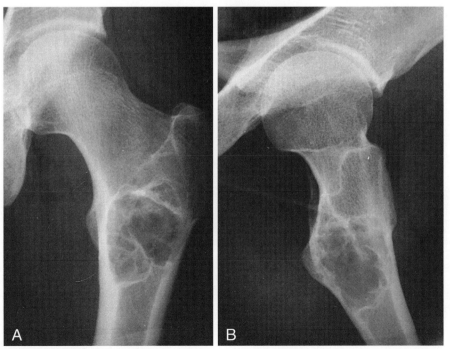

Figure 11-385 **MONOSTOTIC FIBROUS DYSPLASIA. A. AP Femur. B. Oblique Femur.** Observe the large, geographic, multiloculated lesion present in the intertrochanteric region of the femur. This lesion is asymptomatic and is characteristic of monostotic fibrous dysplasia.

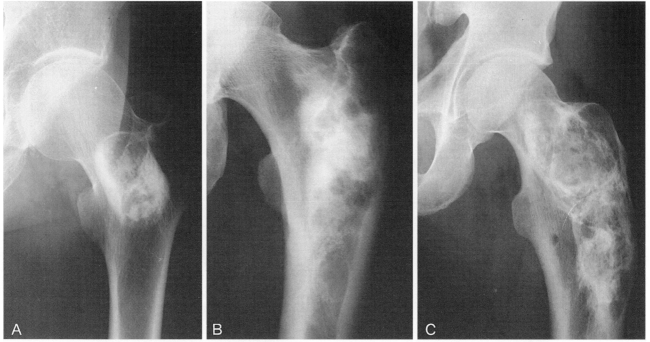

Figure 11-386 MONOSTOTIC FIBROUS DYSPLASIA: VARIED MANIFESTATIONS. A–C. AP Hip. Observe the varied manifestations of mixed sclerosis and radiolucency in these three patients.

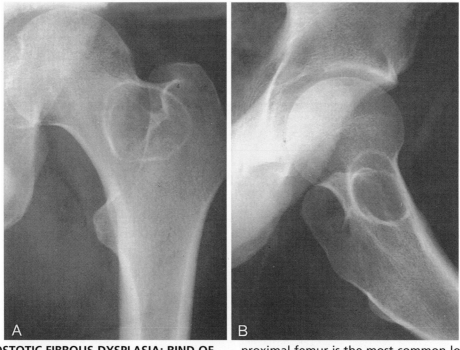

Figure 11-387 MONOSTOTIC FIBROUS DYSPLASIA: RIND OF SCLEROSIS. A. AP Hip. B. Oblique Hip. Observe the large, geographic radiolucency within the intertrochanteric space of the femur. There is a dense encapsulated *rind* or rim of sclerosis. *COMMENT:* The intertrochanteric space of the proximal femur is the most common location for monostotic fibrous dysplasia. The ribs are the second most common site. The *rind* of sclerosis around the fibrous dysplastic lesion is characteristic. These lesions usually are asymptomatic.

able circumstances, bone scintigraphy may aid in the confirmation of fibrous dysplasia. Bone scanning will generally reveal an area of marked uptake. (17) When only slight or no radiotracer uptake is present fibrous dysplasia should be ruled out of the differential. (32)

Polyostotic Fibrous Dysplasia

Lesions of polyostotic fibrous dysplasia are more often symptomatic than those of the monostotic form. This is the result of bowing deformities and pathologic fracture. (Fig. 11-388) Most

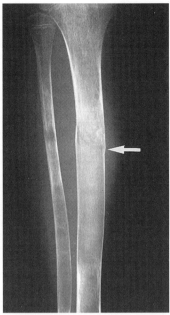

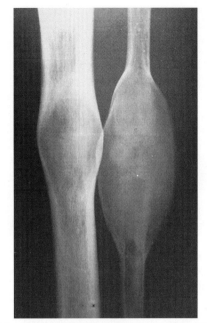

**Figure 11-388 PATHOLOGIC FRACTURE IN FIBROUS DYSPLA-
SIA. AP Tibia and Fibula.** Observe the extensive diaphyseal
involvement of both the tibia and the fibula, with the characteristic *ground glass appearance.* There is a pathologic fracture
present through the proximal diaphysis of the tibia (*arrow*).

**Figure 11-390 POLYOSTOTIC FIBROUS DYSPLASIA: TYPICAL
GROUND GLASS APPEARANCE.** Observe the significant expansion of the mid-diaphysis of the tibia and fibula, with
the characteristic *ground glass appearance* to the matrix of
the fibrous dysplastic lesions.

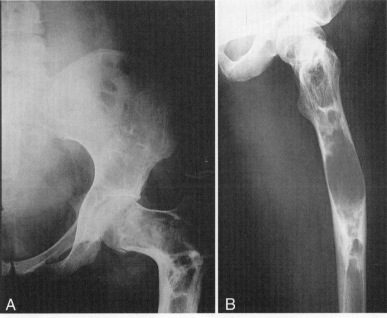

**Figure 11-389 FIBROUS DYSPLASIA: SHEPHERD'S CROOK
DEFORMITY. A. AP Hip. B. Oblique (Frog-Leg) Hip.** Observe
the polyostotic lesions, consistent with fibrous dysplasia,
present within the ilium, proximal femur, and diaphysis of
the femur. There is a coxa vara deformity present, creating
the characteristic *shepherd's crook deformity.* A typical
ground glass appearance of the mid-diaphyseal area of the
femur is noted.

bowing deformities occur in weight-bearing bones, particularly the proximal femur, where the classic *shepherd's crook
deformity* occurs. This *shepherd's crook deformity* represents a
reduction in the femoral angle of incidence to near 90°, creating
a coxa vara deformity. (Fig. 11-389) The lesions of polyostotic fibrous dysplasia most often involve the entire diaphysis of the
long tubular bone, creating widening of the medullary canal with

thinning and scalloping of the endosteum. These lesions more often
demonstrate the *ground glass appearance* rather than the characteristic, completely radiolucent lesion that is seen so often in the
monostotic form. (Fig. 11-390) Incomplete septa or ridges create
loculation throughout the lesion.

In the polyostotic form of fibrous dysplasia, pseudo-fractures
(increment fractures) occur affecting the weight-bearing bones

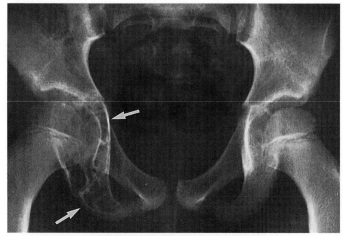

Figure 11-391 **FIBROUS DYSPLASIA. AP Pelvis.** Observe the geographic, multiloculated lesion affecting the medial portion of the acetabulum and ischial tuberosity (*arrows*). This lesion is characteristic of fibrous dysplasia.

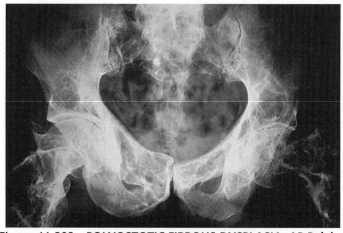

Figure 11-392 **POLYOSTOTIC FIBROUS DYSPLASIA. AP Pelvis.** Observe the polyostotic, multiloculated, geographic lesions scattered throughout the pelvis, pubic rami, and proximal femora. These lesions are typical of fibrous dysplasia.

usually on the convex surface of the deformed cortex. The phrase *increment fractures* refers to the regular intervals at which these pseudo-fractures occur along the length of the bone. Similar pseudo-fractures are found in Paget's disease, osteomalacia, and rickets.

The bones more frequently involved in polyostotic fibrous dysplasia are those of the pelvis, lower extremity, upper extremity, ribs, and skull. In the pelvis, as elsewhere in the skeleton, the disease tends toward a unilateral distribution, and often one side is much more severely involved. (Fig. 11-391) If the pelvis is in-

volved on one side, invariably, the proximal femur will be as well. (Fig. 11-392) Rib lesions produce the characteristic *extrapleural sign;* gross expansion with loculation of bone is often the presentation. (Fig. 11-393) The involvement may be unilateral or bilateral in distribution, but is often asymmetric. In general, most rib lesions remain asymptomatic, only to be detected incidentally during routine chest films. Spontaneous fracture may also bring the lesion to attention. Fibrous dysplasia is said to be the most common cause of a benign long lesion of a rib (> 4 cm). (30,31) (Fig. 11-394) Bone scans are of use to identify the

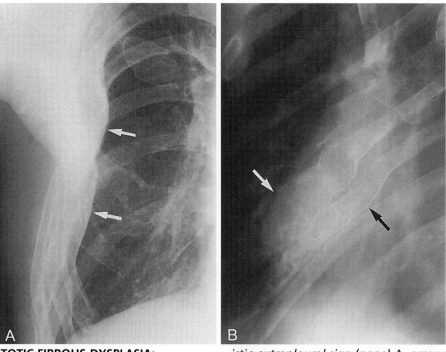

Figure 11-393 **POLYOSTOTIC FIBROUS DYSPLASIA: CREATING THE EXTRAPLEURAL SIGN. A. PA Ribs. B. Oblique Ribs.** Observe the polyostotic changes of fibrous dysplasia within the lateral margins of the ribs, creating the character-

istic *extrapleural sign* (panel A, *arrows*). There is significant fibrous replacement of bone, creating the *ground glass* or *smoky appearance* to the matrix of these rib lesions (panel B, *arrows*).

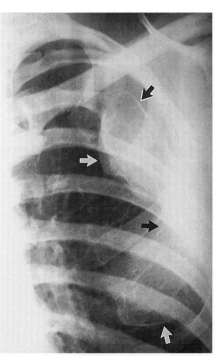

Figure 11-394 **FIBROUS DYSPLASIA. Rib.** Observe the considerable expansion of nearly the entire left fourth rib from extensive fibrous dysplasia (*arrows*). This lesion is > 4 cm and is characteristic for the long lesion presentation of fibrous dysplasia. *COMMENT:* Lesions of fibrous dysplasia within the rib structures can be aggressive in appearance and, at times, may mimic malignant neoplasms. This was the case in this patient because the peripheral cortical margins are poorly demonstrated. The presence of other skeletal lesions of fibrous dysplasia often helps in the definitive diagnosis of fibrous dysplasia.

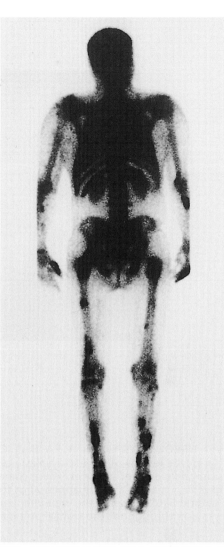

Figure 11-395 **FIBROUS DYSPLASIA: POSITIVE BONE SCAN.** Note that this adult with polyostotic fibrous dysplasia shows intense uptake in multiple lesions throughout the entire skeleton. Active lesions in polyostotic fibrous dysplasia will show intense uptake on nuclear medicine scans. (Courtesy of Reza Sazgari, MD, Department of Radiology, University Hospital, Denver, Colorado.)

location of the lesions in the polyostotic form of the disease. (Fig. 11-395)

Pseudo-arthrosis has been documented in fibrous dysplasia, usually affecting the bones of the lower extremity as a complication of pathologic fracture that has not healed. Neurofibromatosis and fibrous dysplasia are the two most common disorders of bone to produce pseudo-arthrosis.

Involvement of the skull by polyostotic fibrous dysplasia occasionally may mimic the combined biphasic form of Paget's disease. Lesions of the lytic variety, leading to loculations and expansion of bone, most commonly occurring in the skull vertex, create no differential diagnostic problem with Paget's disease (31); however, fibrous dysplasia involving the skull base often is bone forming and sclerotic, as are the changes of Paget's disease. (Figs. 11-396 and 11-397) Often, the bones of the maxilla and mandible are involved, which provides some aid in differential diagnosis because these bones are much less commonly involved in Paget's disease. The broadened calvaria often displays localized, diffuse areas of radiolucency and increased radiopacity side by side. This co-existence of bone resorption and sclerosis strongly resembles Paget's disease. It is the thinning of the external table in fibrous dysplasia versus cortical thickening in Paget's disease that aids in the definitive differential diagnosis. (33)

The vertebral column is infrequently involved in fibrous dysplasia. If present, it is invariably found associated with the polyostotic form of the disease. Most lesions affect the vertebral body but may occasionally extend into the neural arch. (Fig. 11-398) Vertebral collapse is most commonly found in the lumbar spine, as are the majority of the lesions. The vertebral lesions appear homogeneously radiolucent, lacking the classic *ground glass appearance.* Murray and Jacobson (31) stated that narrowing of the disc spaces is common with spinal involvement in polyostotic fibrous dysplasia. No explanation as to the pathogenesis of this radiographic sign is offered. Although we have seen this sign associated with polyostotic fibrous dysplasia, there are many cases with spinal involvement that lack disc space narrowing.

It should be emphasized that there are no radiographic findings that rule out the presence of one or more specific endocrine disorders known to occur in association with fibrous dysplasia.

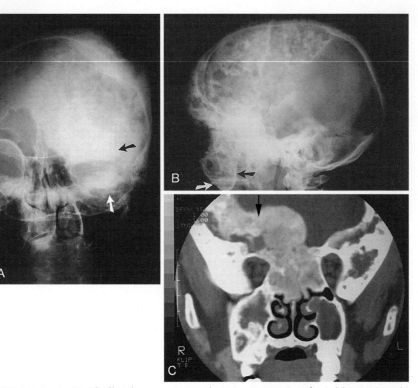

Figure 11-396 **FIBROUS DYSPLASIA. A. PA Skull.** Observe the sclerotic and lytic lesions of fibrous dysplasia affecting half of the skull table and facial bones. These changes have distorted the orbit, creating a dense appearance to its floor (*arrows*). **B. Lateral Skull.** Observe the well-delineated lesions of fibrous dysplasia throughout the frontal and parietal bones. Extensive facial bone involvement has produced bony expansion, with a well-defined cortical margin (*arrows*). **C. Coronal CT Scan.** Note the dense ground glass appearance to the matrix of the lesion extending along the petrous ridge of the temporal bone (*arrow*) into the ethmoid sinuses. (Courtesy of Joan Sutcliffe, MD, Denver, Colorado.)

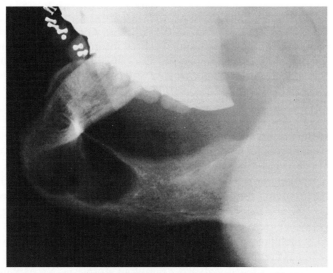

Figure 11-397 **FIBROUS DYSPLASIA: MANDIBLE.** Observe the large, geographic, expansile lesion of the mandible, representing fibrous dysplasia.

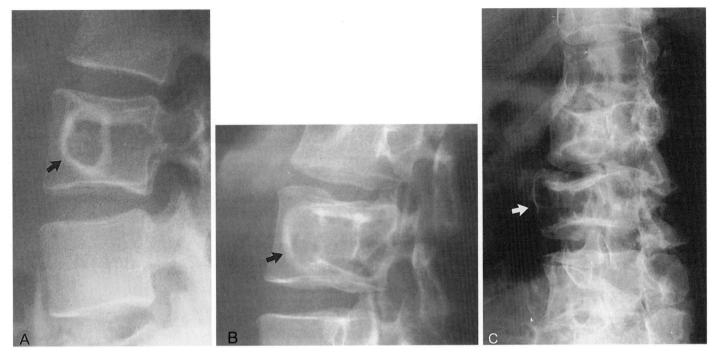

Figure 11-398 **FIBROUS DYSPLASIA: VERTEBRAL INVOLVE-MENT. A. Lateral Lumbar Spine. B. Oblique Lumbar Spine.** Observe the large, geographic lesion within the vertebral body of L3. There is a characteristic thick, encapsulated rim of sclerosis associated with this vertebral body lesion, creating the *rind of sclerosis* appearance (*arrows*). **C. Oblique Lumbar Spine.** Observe the polyostotic lesions of fibrous dysplasia affecting the vertebral body and neural arch of the lower thoracic segments and lumbar spine. There is significant expansion of the vertebral body of L2 (*arrow*), along with vertebral arch involvement. *COMMENT:* Fibrous dysplasia of the vertebrae is uncommon.

CAPSULE SUMMARY   Fibrous Dysplasia

General Considerations

- Lichtenstein in 1938 was the first to recognize and name the disease entity.
- Originally, this disease was confused with hyperparathyroidism.
- It has been called a *great imitator* of bone disease along with Paget's disease.

Incidence

- Not an uncommon disorder; however, the actual incidence is difficult to ascertain, since most lesions are asymptomatic.

Clinical Features

- Age of presentation varies from 8 to 14 years.
- An even sex distribution, except for the associated McCune-Albright syndrome, which is almost exclusively found in females.
- Most lesions are asymptomatic. Bowing deformities and pathologic fracture are the most common causes of symptoms (i.e., shepherd's crook deformity).
- *Café au lait spots:* chestnut-pigmented, non-elevated macules, present in 30% of patients with polyostotic fibrous dysplasia. The serrated irregular margins have been referred to as the coast of Maine appearance. Also found in neurofibromatosis, but these margins are smooth and are referred to as the coast of California appearance.

- Monostotic fibrous dysplasia (solitary lesion) is most commonly found in the ribs, femur (proximal), tibia (anterior cortex), and skull (75% of cases).
- Polyostotic fibrous dysplasia (multiple bones) is most commonly found in the femur, skull, tibia, humerus, ribs, fibula, radius, and ulna.
- Vertebral involvement is rare; when present, it affects the vertebral body rather than the arch and is found usually in the polyostotic form of the disease.
- McCune-Albright syndrome represents polyostotic fibrous dysplasia associated with skin pigmentation and precocious sexual development.
- Cherubism represents a familial fibrous dysplasia of the jaws.

Pathologic Features

- Represents an abnormality in which normal bone undergoes physiologic resorption and replacement with abnormal proliferation of fibrous tissue.
- The fibrous lesion often creates widening of the medullary canal, thinning of the cortex, and endosteal scalloping; scalloping of the endosteum is a sign seen in lesions of fibrous and cartilaginous matrix.
- The fundamental lesion of fibrous dysplasia is that of a fibrous-based matrix with scattered bony spicules intermixed. This renders an increase in radiopacity to the existing

(continued)

CAPSULE SUMMARY Fibrous Dysplasia (*continued*)

radiolucent lesion and has been called the ground glass appearance.
- Sarcomatous transformation is rare (0.5%). The femur and skull are the target sites, with fibrosarcoma and osteosarcoma being the most common complicating tumor types.

Radiologic Features
- Skeletal lesions are not present at birth; they occur several years before puberty.
- Most lesions are radiolucent, loculated, or trabeculated in appearance.
- Ground glass or smoky appearance of the radiolucent lesion is classic. Murray and Jacobson called this the wipe out of the trabecular patterns.

- Most lesions demonstrate an encapsulated sclerotic border around the geographic lesion, which has been called the rind of sclerosis.
- Bone expansion with widening of the medullary canal, endosteal thinning, and scalloping occurs.
- Shepherd's crook deformity of the femur is common.
- Expansile rib lesions often create the extrapleural sign.
- Pseudo-arthrosis occurs as a complication of pathologic fracture and non-union. The lower extremity is most often affected. Neurofibromatosis and fibrous dysplasia are the two most common disorders of bone to produce pseudo-arthrosis.

NEUROFIBROMATOSIS

General Considerations

Neurofibromatosis (NF) is an inherited disorder, transmitted as an autosomal dominant, with variable gene expression. (1) Although original reports of Tiresius (2) in 1773 and Smith (3) in 1849 antedated that of von Recklinghausen (4) in 1882, he was given credit for drawing the association of neural and cutaneous fibrous elements to this disease.

Neurofibromatosis is classified into two clinical forms: neurofibromatosis 1 (von Recklinghausen's: café au lait spots, neurofibromas, bone changes) and neurofibromatosis 2 (acoustic nerve tumors). Neurofibromatosis 1 is a neuroectodermal and mesodermal dysplasia. It is characterized by a triad of pigmented cutaneous lesions (café au lait spots), multiple soft, elevated, cutaneous tumors (fibroma molluscum), and various osseous alterations of the axial and appendicular skeleton. The extent of involvement ranges from minimal to an extensive generalized deforming disease process. The condition affects primarily the peripheral nerves; however, the central nervous system may rarely be involved, occasionally leaving the patient mentally retarded.

Incidence

The incidence of neurofibromatosis is estimated as 1/3000 births, and a family history of neurofibromatosis can be found in approximately 60% of patients, inherited as an autosomal dominant trait. (5)

Clinical Features

Age and Sex Distribution

Neurofibromatosis occurs with equal incidence in both male and female, as well as white and black, patients. Patients with neurofibromatosis are born with this disorder; however, some may not manifest signs at birth, only developing the classic signs in early childhood. Diagnosis is made based on clinical criteria. (1)

Cutaneous Abnormalities

Café au Lait Spots. The cutaneous macules are non-elevated chestnut, melaniferous pigmentations most commonly found on the back, chest, and abdomen and represent the second most common skin manifestation of this disorder. Most patients have smoothly marginated café au lait spots (*coast of California appearance,* which is geographically smooth), in contrast to the jagged margins of the café au lait spots found in fibrous dysplasia (*coast of Maine appearance,* which is geographically jagged). (6) (Fig. 11-399) Café au lait spots develop in 50% of patients with neurofibromatosis; however, 15% of the normal population will have one or two café au lait spots as a normal variant, and 1% of the normal population will have more than two. Strict criteria are necessary to establish the diagnosis of neurofibromatosis. (6,7) Six or more café au lait spots measuring 1.5 cm or more in diameter provide an essential factor in establishing the diagnosis of neurofibromatosis. (5) It should be noted that café au lait spots are age related because they are not always present at birth; they tend to increase in number, size, and pigmentation up to the 3rd decade. Occasionally, they may fade in intensity with age. Café au lait spots are also found in patients with fibrous dysplasia (33% of cases) and less commonly in tuberous sclerosis. (7)

Fibroma Molluscum. Fibroma molluscum are multiple, asymptomatic cutaneous nodules, which are usually elevated above the skin surface. They are soft, nipplelike, pedunculated, or sessile skin tabs that vary in size from tiny pinhead dots to masses of 5 cm or more. They may be few and widely dispersed or virtually may cover the entire body. (Fig. 11-400) Fibroma molluscum represents the most frequent and best diagnostic cutaneous feature of neurofibromatosis. (8)

Elephantiasis Neuromatosa. The term applied to the large soft tissue masses that create skin folds is elephantiasis neuromatosa. These masses actually represent diffuse plexiform neurofibromas. Plexiform neurofibromas are currently included in the

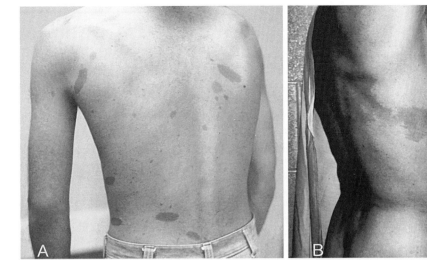

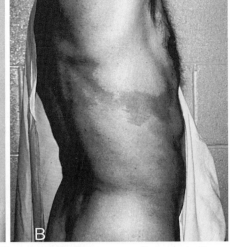

Figure 11-399 CAFÉ AU LAIT SPOTS. A. Neurofibromatosis. Observe the multiple café au lait spots on this patient's back, which are smoothly marginated and assume the characteristic *coast of California appearance.* **B. Fibrous Dysplasia.** Observe the large, geographically jagged café au lait spot present on this patient's thorax, creating the characteristic *coast of Maine appearance. COMMENT:* Café au lait spots are the second most common skin manifestation of neuro- fibromatosis; fibroma molluscum is the most common. Of patients with neurofibromatosis, 50% develop café au lait spots; 30% of patients with the polyostotic form of fibrous dysplasia develop these spots. Six or more café au lait spots measuring 1.5 cm or more in diameter present an essential fact in establishing the diagnosis of neurofibromatosis. Of the normal population, 15% will have one or two café au lait spots, as a normal variant.

diagnostic criteria for neurofibromatosis (9) and may lead to massive enlargement of the skin, soft tissues, and underlying bony structures (focal giantism). Other than creating a disfiguring appearance plexiform neurofibromas are associated with functional impairment and substantial morbidity. (10) Transformation into malignant peripheral nerve sheath tumors is a complication and surgical resection is the treatment of choice. (10)

Signs and Symptoms

The signs and symptoms of neurofibromatosis are widely varied. The specific symptoms will depend on the location of the abnormality.

Skull. Neurofibroma of the optic nerve may produce blurred vision, scotoma, and transient blindness. A defect in the posterior

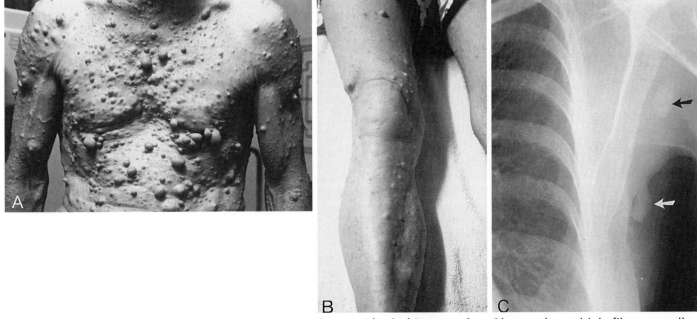

Figure 11-400 NEUROFIBROMATOSIS: FIBROMA MOLLUS- CUM. A. Thorax: Physical Presentation. Observe the multiple, asymptomatic nodules that are characteristic of fibroma molluscum in patients with neurofibromatosis. **B. Lower Leg:** **Physical Presentation.** Observe the multiple fibroma molluscum affecting the anterior thigh and lower leg. **C. PA Axilla.** Observe the large fibroma molluscum in the axilla area of this patient with neurofibromatosis (*arrows*).

superior orbital wall may allow drooping of the upper eyelid, dislocation of the eyeball, or even pulsating exophthalmos. Pulsating exophthalmos occurs as a result of direct contact with the meninges, cerebrospinal fluid pulsations, and the orbital contents. The absence of the bony separation allows for transmission of intracranial vascular pulsation to the globe. (11) There is no suggestion within the literature that pulsating exophthalmos associated with neurofibromatosis is progressive or that there is any long-term threat to vision. Ocular pulsation may also be found with intra-orbital aneurysms and vascular anomalies, and these conditions should be considered in the differential diagnosis of pulsating exophthalmos. (11) Facial asymmetry is often present, representing more of a cosmetic problem than a functional one.

Spine. Neurofibromas affecting the spinal nerves often render localized pain and various motor symptoms, including, in advanced cases, paraplegia. Severe kyphoscoliosis, so frequently found in neurofibromatosis, may be asymptomatic or be complicated by cord compression and paraplegia. (12) Rarely, laxity of the ligaments supporting the atlantoaxial joints occurs in neurofibromatosis, leading to atlantoaxial subluxation. (13,14) This creates symptoms of suboccipital headache and motor weakness to the upper extremities.

Pathologic Features

The typical neurofibroma is indistinguishable from a schwannoma (neurinoma) or neuroma and grossly appears as a grayish brown or gray, firm, rubbery mass. Histologically, interlacing strands of elongated foam cells and pigment are arranged in a characteristic palisading pattern. The rate of malignant degeneration in neurofibromatosis is reported to be approximately 5% (15); most transform to a neurofibrosarcoma, and clinical suspicion of malignant degeneration should be raised if there is progressive enlargement and pain related to a mass lesion. (16) This transformation occurs more often in internal tissues than in superficial cutaneous lesions. (16) It has been suggested that repeated biopsies of these lesions predisposes to malignant degeneration.

Radiologic Features

The most frequently involved areas are the spine and skull, and characteristic radiographic changes often allow the clinician to establish the diagnosis of neurofibromatosis. (Fig. 11-401) Approximately 50% of the patients with neurofibromatosis develop skeletal lesions. (8) (Table 11-47)

Spine

The most common radiographic feature of neurofibromatosis is the development of a scoliosis, occurring in approximately 50% of patients. (8,17,18) Classically, the scoliosis involves a short segment (5–7 vertebrae) and is acutely angular in presentation. Kyphoscoliosis is the most common form and usually affects the lower thoracic spine. (12,18) The cause of the scoliosis is unknown, and paraplegia may accompany advanced cases.

Cervical kyphosis is a common feature of neurofibromatosis, creating an acutely angular reversal of the normal lordosis. (7,18) Posterior vertebral body scalloping is usually seen, along with deformity of the vertebral bodies, as a result of the underlying

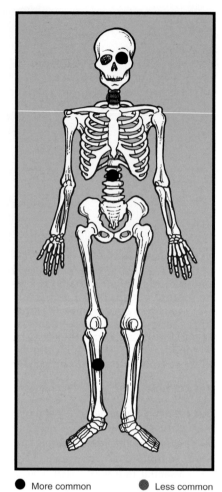

● More common   ● Less common

Figure 11-401 SKELETAL DISTRIBUTION OF NEUROFIBROMATOSIS.

Table 11-47	Radiologic Features of Neurofibromatosis

Spine
　　Scoliosis: short, angular, kyphosis
　　Vertebral scalloping
　　　　Posterocentral
　　　　Eccentric unilateral
　　Intrathoracic meningocele
Skull
　　Orbital defects
　　　　Sphenoid wing agenesis (bare orbit)
　　　　Optic canal expansion
　　Lambdoidal defect or asterion defect
　　Macrocranium
Ribs
　　Scalloped, irregular (twisted ribbons)
Long bones
　　Pseudo-arthrosis (tibia)
　　Non-ossifying fibromas
　　Focal giantism
Extraskeletal
　　Multisystem involvement

mesodermal dysplasia. (Fig. 11-402) This appearance could be confused with spinal tuberculosis; however, lack of disc space narrowing and the presence of posterior vertebral body scalloping strongly suggest the diagnosis of neurofibromatosis.

Vertebral Scalloping. Scalloping of the posterior surface of the vertebral body commonly occurs in neurofibromatosis. (12,19) Two forms of erosive defects exist: posterocentral and eccentric, unilateral scalloping. Posterocentral scalloping, usually affecting more than one vertebral level, is secondary to dural ectasia, which is a recognized manifestation of neurofibromatosis. (Fig. 11-403) Eccentric unilateral scalloping may also occur. This pattern is suggestive of a localized, dumbbell neurofibroma arising from a spinal nerve root and protruding through the adjacent intervertebral foramina (IVF). (20) (Fig. 11-404) This usually affects an isolated level, and the cervical, lower thoracic, and upper lumbar areas are most often involved. (Fig. 11-405) Erosion of the posterior body and adjacent pedicle results in an enlarged IVF. (Fig. 11-406) Similar extrinsic erosions can occur from neurofibromas affecting the extremities. (Fig. 11-407) A paraspinal mass is seen on the AP thoracic or PA chest radiograph as a result of either a large, dumbbell neurofibroma or, more frequently, an intrathoracic meningocele. (Fig. 11-408)

Intrathoracic Meningocele. Intrathoracic meningocele is a protrusion of the dura and arachnoid through a thoracic intervertebral foramen and posterior aspect of the rib cage into the extrapleural thoracic cavity. (8) These lesions occur in approximately 66% of cases and vary in size from 1 to 6 cm. (21) Most lesions are first seen as an asymptomatic posterior mediastinal mass and are erroneously interpreted as a neurofibroma. Most meningoceles occur laterally, on the right side. (8) Myelography reveals filling with contrast material of the meningocele; this does not occur in a neurofibroma, which is a solid tumor. (Fig. 11-409) Because saccular dilatation of the meninges extends into the chest through the intervertebral foramen in the same manner as a dumbbell neurofibroma, it is capable of producing enlargement of the intervertebral foramen, erosion of the posterior surface of the vertebral body, and pressure defects on the pedicles and posterior ribs at the level of the meningocele. (8) (Fig. 11-410)

Skull

Orbital Defects. Agenesis or hypoplasia of the posterior wall of the orbit, wings of the sphenoid, and the orbital plate of the frontal bone is a common finding in neurofibromatosis. This creates what has been referred to as the *bare orbit.* (8) (Fig. 11-411) This abnormality allows direct contact of the temporal lobe of the brain and its meninges with the orbital soft tissues. This anatomic relationship often creates pulsating exophthalmos. These changes are usually unilateral.

Neurofibroma affecting the optic nerve may lead to enlargement of the optic foramen. Detailed radiographs of the orbit, often including CT, are necessary to visualize these changes. Approximately 20% of patients with an optic glioma have neurofibromatosis.

Lambdoidal Defect. A radiolucent defect is sometimes seen in the calvaria adjacent to the lambdoidal suture, just posterior to the parietal–mastoid and occipital–mastoid sutures, and is virtually diagnostic of neurofibromatosis. (Fig. 11-412) This defect is more common on the left side. Because neurofibromatous tissue is characteristically lacking within the calvarial defect, this

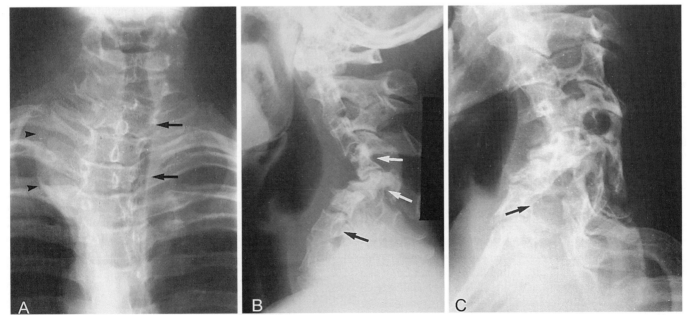

Figure 11-402 **NEUROFIBROMATOSIS: CERVICAL SPINE.**
A. AP Cervicothoracic. Observe the deviation of the trachea (*arrows*) as the result of a large intrathoracic meningocele in the right upper lung apex (*arrowheads*). **B. Lateral Cervical.** Observe the acute angular reversal of the normal cervical lordosis, associated with dysplastic changes of the vertebral bodies of C4, C5, and C6 as a result of underlying neurofibromatosis. There is posterior vertebral body scalloping (*arrows*).

C. Oblique Cervical. Observe the extensive vertebral body scalloping and the pedicle destruction at the first thoracic segment (*arrow*). The pedicle destruction at the T1 vertebra creates a large intervertebral foramina at this level. (Reprinted with permission from **Yochum TR:** *Neurofibromatosis or von Recklinghausen's disease—A case study.* ACA J Chiro June, 1980. Courtesy of Clayton F. Thomsen, DC, Sydney, Australia.)

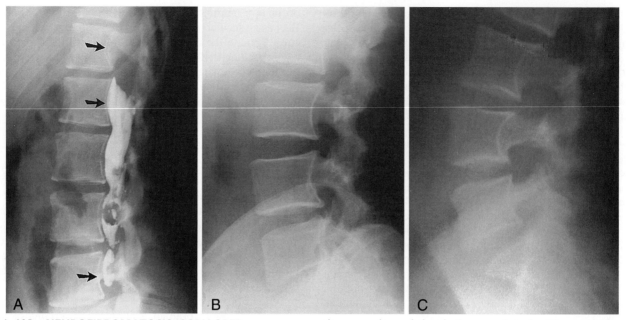

Figure 11-403 NEUROFIBROMATOSIS: SCALLOPED VERTEBRAE. A. Myelogram, Lateral Lumbar Spine. Observe the fine sclerotic margins, representing scalloping of the posterior vertebral body margins in neurofibromatosis (*arrows*). **B. Lateral Lumbar Spine.** Note the extensive posterior vertebral body scalloping secondary to neurofibromatosis. **C. Lateral Lumbar Spine.** Observe the deep, posterior vertebral body indentations secondary to scalloping from the mesodermal dysplasia, associated with neurofibromatosis. *COMMENT:* Posterocentral vertebral body scalloping in neurofibromatosis that affects more than one vertebral level is secondary to the pathologic changes of dural ectasia. (Panel B reprinted with permission: **Yochum TR:** *A radiographic anthology of vertebral names.* J Manipulative Physiol Ther 8:87, 1985. Panel C courtesy of Reed B. Phillips, DC, DACBR, PhD, Los Angeles, California.)

actually represents an area of hypoplasia or agenesis of bone. Radiographically, it appears as a geographic loss of bone density, which may vary in size, occasionally reaching 10 cm. Hypoplasia of the ipsilateral mastoid process has been associated. (22) This lambdoidal calvarial lesion has been referred to as the *asterion defect.* (23)

Macrocranium. A poorly recognized but frequently present radiographic sign of neurofibromatosis is macrocranium and macroencephaly. Actually, this sign was one of the more prominent features in one of the earliest documented cases of neurofibromatosis, the so-called elephant man reported by Treves. (24)

Ribs

An additional expression of neurofibromatosis is the thin, irregular, scalloped, attenuated appearance of the ribs. This deformity of the ribs has been called the *twisted ribbon appearance.* (12,17) Intercostal neurofibromas may produce erosions on the inferior surface of the ribs, occasionally mimicking coarctation of the aorta. Mesodermal dysplasia and hypoplasia may also play a part in the rib deformities because often no neurofibromas can be isolated in the neighboring structures. A similar twisted appearance can occur in the small tubular bones of the extremities. (Fig. 11-413)

Pseudo-Arthrosis of a Long Bone

Pseudo-arthrosis is an entity characterized by pathologic fracture and inability to form normal callus in healing; deossification and bending of weight-bearing bones may also occur. (Fig. 11-414) Of patients with pseudo-arthrosis, 50% manifest some stigmata of neurofibromatosis. The tibia in its lower two thirds is the most commonly affected bone. There is no evidence of neurofibromatous tissue in or near the site of the deformed pseudo-arthrosis. (Fig. 11-415) Rarely, fibrous dysplasia patients may develop similar pseudo-arthrosis lesions in bone.

Association of Multiple Non-Ossifying Fibromas

Neurofibromatosis may occasionally present with cystic central or intramedullary lesions in the metaphysis of the long tubular bones. (Fig. 11-416) Histologically, most of these lesions prove to be non-ossifying fibromas and are often multiple, bilateral, and much larger than the typical lesion. (25) The bones of the lower extremities are the most frequently affected.

Focal Giantism

Localized skeletal enlargement or focal giantism is perhaps the most bizarre and fascinating aspect of neurofibromatosis. The hypertrophy may involve a single bone or the entire extremity. (Fig. 11-417) The bones are usually normal in shape, and the associated muscles and joints are proportionately enlarged, along with the surface soft tissues. The pathogenesis is the result of chronic hyperemia owing to hemangiomas and lymphangiomatous lesions associated with neurofibromatosis.

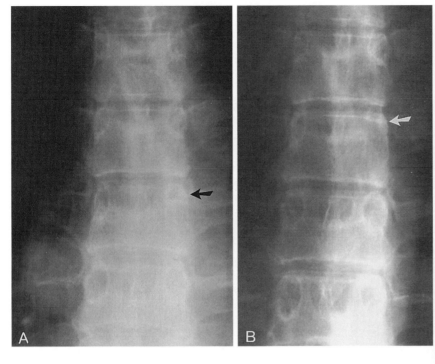

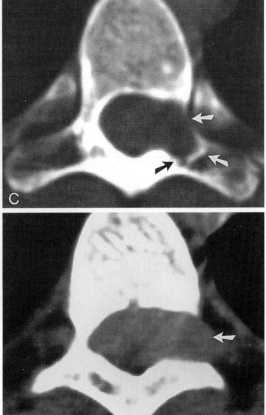

Figure 11-404 **THE DUMBBELL NEUROFIBROMA. A. AP Thoracic Spine.** Observe the destruction of the caudal aspect of the T10 pedicle (*arrow*). **B. 3-Year Follow-Up: AP Thoracic Spine.** Note the nearly complete destruction of the pedicle at the T10 vertebra (*arrow*). **C. Axial CT, T10.** Observe the extensive pressure erosions affecting the pedicle, lamina, and transverse process of the involved vertebra (*arrows*). **D. Axial CT, T10.** Observe the significant enlargement of the neuroforamina (*arrow*) as a result of complete destruction of the pedicle of T10 on the involved side. (Courtesy of Margaret A. Seron, DC, FACO, DACBR, Denver, Colorado.)

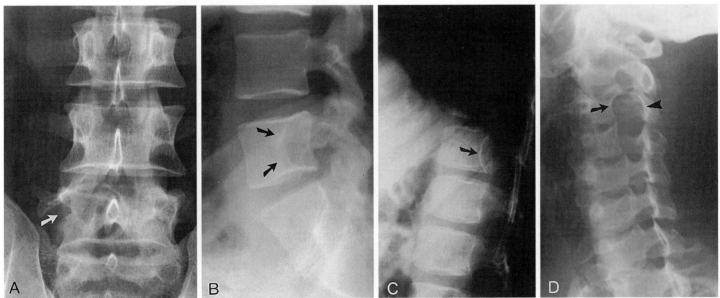

Figure 11-405 **VERTEBRAL EROSION ASSOCIATED WITH A DUMBBELL NEUROFIBROMA. A. AP Lumbar Spine.** Observe the unilateral destruction of the pedicle of the L5 vertebra (*arrow*) secondary to a localized neurofibroma. **B. Lateral Lumbar Spine.** Observe the posterior vertebral body scalloping of L5, with an anterior sclerotic margin (*arrows*). **C. Lateral Thoracolumbar Spine.** Observe the deep posterior vertebral body scalloping affecting the T12 vertebra (*arrow*). **D. Oblique Cervical Spine.** Note the significant enlargement of the intervertebral foramina between C3 and C4. There is destruction of the pedicle unilaterally at C3 and scalloping of the posterior margin of the body of C3 (*arrow*). Observe the sclerotic margin around the enlarged intervertebral foramina (*arrowhead*). (Panel B courtesy of Lawrence A. Cooperstein, MD, Pittsburgh, Pennsylvania.)

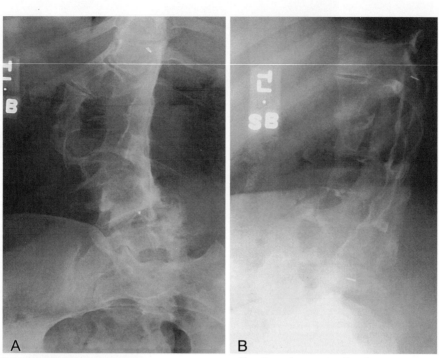

Figure 11-406 **NEUROFIBROMATOSIS: EXTENSIVE VERTEBRAL INVOLVEMENT. A. AP Lumbar Spine. B. Lateral Lumbar Spine.** Observe the extensive posterior vertebral body erosion and expansion of the intervertebral foramina affecting the entire lumbar spine and lower thoracic vertebrae. (Courtesy of Lawrence A. Cooperstein, MD, Pittsburgh, Pennsylvania.)

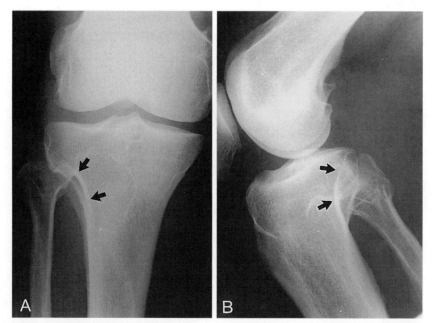

Figure 11-407 **EXTRINSIC SKELETAL EROSIONS FROM NEUROFIBROMA. A. AP Knee. B. Lateral Knee.** Observe the extrinsic pressure erosions on the posterolateral aspect of the tibia (*arrows*). These have occurred secondary to a slowly growing neurofibroma.

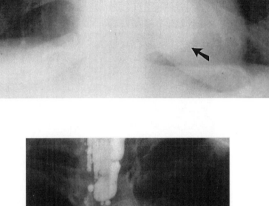

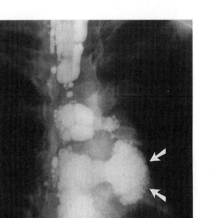

Figure 11-408 **NEUROFIBROMA PRESENTING AS A POSTE-RIOR MEDIASTINAL MASS. PA Chest.** Observe the dense radiopaque nodular lesion seen through the left ventricle of the heart (*arrows*). This lesion is in the posterior mediastinum and represents a neurofibroma.

Figure 11-409 **NEUROFIBROMATOSIS: INTRATHORACIC MENINGOCELE. AP Thoracic Myelogram.** Note the protrusion of the dura and arachnoid through a midthoracic intervertebral foramen into the posterior aspect of the rib cage (*arrows*). This represents an intrathoracic meningocele associated with neurofibromatosis.

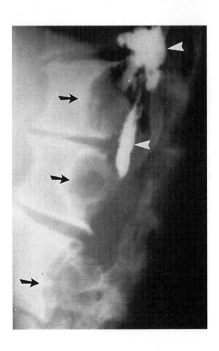

Figure 11-410 **NEUROFIBROMATOSIS: VERTEBRAL EROSION SECONDARY TO MENINGOCELES.** Note the large, posterior vertebral body scalloped erosions present affecting the T12, L1, and L2 vertebral bodies (*arrows*). The radiopaque density present in the spinal canal represents residual contrast material from the previous myelographic investigation (*arrowheads*). (Courtesy of Antonio Baciocco, MD, and Peter Christensson, DC, Rome, Italy.)

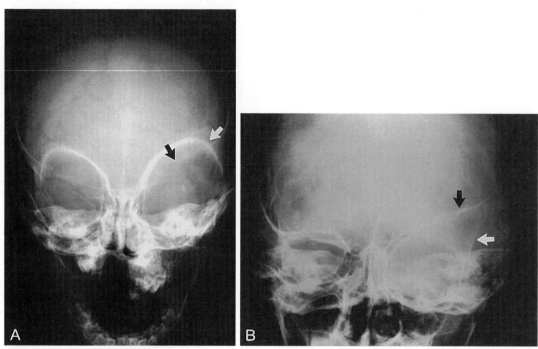

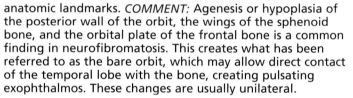

Figure 11-411 NEUROFIBROMATOSIS: BARE ORBIT. A. PA Skull. Note the hypoplasia of the posterior wall of the orbit as a result of underdevelopment of the sphenoid bone (*arrows*). **B. PA Skull.** Observe the distortion of the greater and lesser wing of the sphenoid (*arrows*) as a result of hypoplasia. Close observation of the central portion of the involved orbit reveals distortion of the normal landmarks, giving the appearance of the orbit being bare of its normal anatomic landmarks. *COMMENT:* Agenesis or hypoplasia of the posterior wall of the orbit, the wings of the sphenoid bone, and the orbital plate of the frontal bone is a common finding in neurofibromatosis. This creates what has been referred to as the bare orbit, which may allow direct contact of the temporal lobe with the bone, creating pulsating exophthalmos. These changes are usually unilateral.

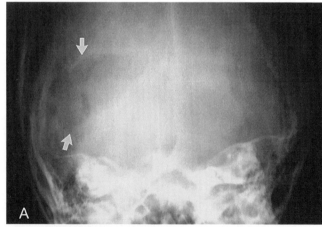

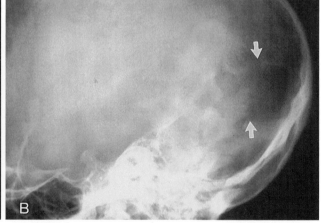

Figure 11-412 NEUROFIBROMATOSIS: LAMBDOIDAL DEFECT OR ASTERION DEFECT. A. AP Towne's Projection, Skull. Observe the rather sharply demarcated area of radiolucency present near the lambdoidal suture (*arrows*). **B. Lateral Skull.** Note the focal area of radiolucency associated with the lambdoid suture (*arrows*). This represents the lambdoidal defect of neurofibromatosis and has been referred to as the *asterion defect*. *COMMENT:* This radiolucent defect is seen adjacent to the lambdoidal suture, just posterior to the parietal mastoid and occipital mastoid sutures and is virtually diagnostic of neurofibromatosis. The defect actually represents an area of hypoplasia or agenesis because no neurofibromatous tissue is seen within the calvarial defect. Hypoplasia of the ipsilateral mastoid process has been associated, a radiographic finding that was not present in this case.

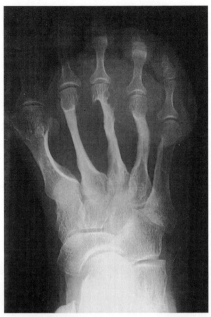

Figure 11-413 NEUROFIBROMATOSIS: FOOT. Observe the thin, irregular, scalloped appearance of the metatarsal bones. This deformity in the metatarsal bones is likened to the twisted ribbon appearance seen affecting the ribs in neurofibromatosis. Mesodermal dysplasia is the underlying pathologic process allowing this radiographic appearance to occur in neurofibromatosis.

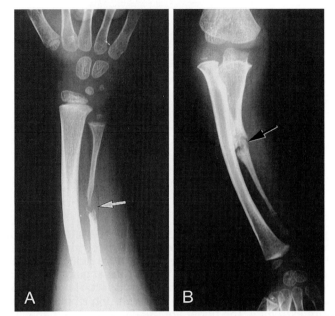

Figure 11-415 NEUROFIBROMATOSIS: PSEUDO-ARTHROSIS. A and B. Ulna. Observe the pseudo-arthrosis in the mid-diaphysis of the ulna (*arrows*). *COMMENT:* Of patients with pseudo-arthrosis, 50% manifest some stigmata of neurofibromatosis. The tibia in its lower two thirds is the most commonly affected bone. There is no evidence of neurofibromatous tissue in or near the site of the deformed pseudo-arthrosis. Rarely, fibrous dysplasia patients may develop similar pseudo-arthrosis lesions in bone.

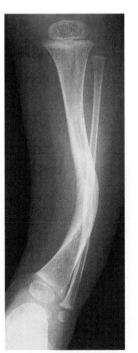

Figure 11-414 NEUROFIBROMATOSIS: DEFORMITY. Observe the bowing deformity of the tibia, with alteration of the bony texture as a result of the underlying changes of neurofibromatosis. (Courtesy of C. H. Quay, MD, Melbourne, Australia.)

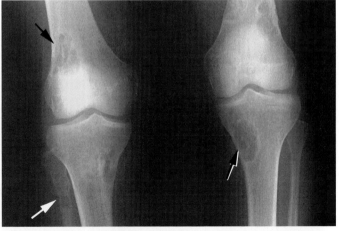

Figure 11-416 NEUROFIBROMATOSIS: MULTIPLE NON-OSSIFYING FIBROMAS. Note the distinctive, multiple, eccentrically elongated lesions in the lower extremity bilaterally (*arrows*).

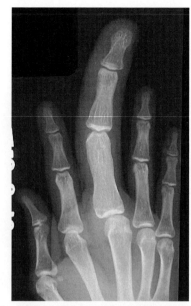

Figure 11-417 FOCAL GIANTISM IN NEUROFIBROMATOSIS.
Observe the localized skeletal enlargement or focal giantism, affecting the skeletal structures of the third digit. Soft tissue hypertrophy is also noted. *COMMENT:* Focal giantism is perhaps the most bizarre and fascinating aspect of neurofibromatosis. The hypertrophy may involve a single bone or the entire extremity. The bones are usually normal in shape, and the associated muscles and joints are proportionately enlarged, along with the surface soft tissues. The pathogenesis is the result of chronic hyperemia owing to hemangiomas and lymphangiomatous lesions associated with neurofibromatosis. (Courtesy of David P. Thomas, MD, Melbourne, Australia.)

Table 11-48	Propensity of Malignant Degeneration in Benign Skeletal Tumors and Tumor-Like Processes	
		Reference[a]
Solitary osteochondroma	1.0%	Dahlin (17)
HME	20%	Dahlin (7)
Solitary enchondroma	Rare (< 1.0%)	Hamlin (12)
Multiple enchondromatosis (Ollier's disease)	50%	Jaffe (2)
Maffucci's syndrome	> 50%	Howard (2)
Paget's disease	0.9–2.0%	McKenna (35)
Fibrous dysplasia	Rare (0.5%)	Huvos (19)
Neurofibromatosis	5%	Patel (11)

[a]Numbers refer to the section in which the particular disease entity is discussed. HME, hereditary multiple exostosis.

Table 11-49	Differential Diagnosis of Polyostotic Benign Tumor or Tumor-Like Conditions of Bone (TRY 7)
	Paget's disease
	Fibrous dysplasia
	Histiocytosis X
	Neurofibromatosis
	Hereditary multiple exostoses
	Ollier's disease
	Brown's tumors (hyperparathyroidism)

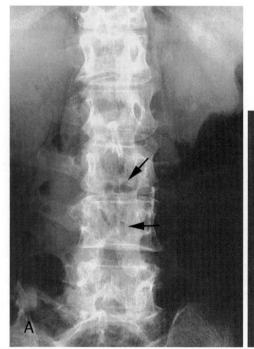

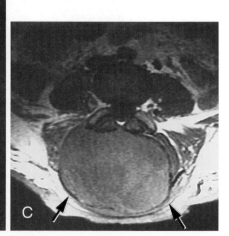

Figure 11-418 NEUROFIBROMATOSIS: MALIGNANT DEGENERATION, NEUROFIBROSARCOMA. A. AP Lumbar Spine. Note the destruction of the L3 and L4 spinous processes (*arrows*). **B. T2-Weighted MRI, Sagittal Lumbar Spine with Contrast.** Observe the soft tissue mass in the paraspinal musculature (*arrows*). **C. T1-Weighted MRI, Axial Lumbar Spine.** Note the soft tissue mass in the midline (*arrows*). (Courtesy of Joan Sutcliffe, MD, Denver, Colorado.)

Extraskeletal Manifestations

Extraskeletal manifestations of neurofibromatosis are varied and relatively common, as a result of the widespread mesodermal nature of this disease. They include intracranial neurofibromas and intramural gastrointestinal lesions, as well as lesions in the lung, mediastinum, and soft tissues throughout the body. Renal artery stenosis occurs, which predisposes these patients to the development of renal hypertension. (26) In addition, there is a strong association between the presence of adrenal pheochromocytoma and neurofibromatosis; 20% of patients with this neoplasm also have neurofibromatosis. However, only 1% of patients with neurofibro-

matosis develop pheochromocytoma. Malignant degeneration to neurofibrosarcoma does occur. (Fig. 11-418) Therefore, a hypertensive adult patient with neurofibromatosis should be carefully investigated for renal artery stenosis and pheochromocytoma as an organic cause for their hypertension. (26) Osteomalacia, presumably owing to renal tubular dysfunction, is rarely found in patients with long-standing neurofibromatosis. The radiographic signs of osteomalacia in an adult or rickets in a child do not provide a means for determining the presence or absence of neurofibromatosis. (Table 11-48) Neurofibromatosis is one of seven bone disorders to be considered in the differential diagnosis of benign polyostotic tumor-like lesions. (Table 11-49)

CAPSULE SUMMARY   Neurofibromatosis

General Considerations

- An inherited disorder, transmitted as an autosomal dominant.
- In 1882 von Recklinghausen drew the first association of neural and cutaneous fibrous elements in a disease called neurofibromatosis.
- A triad of findings is characteristic: café au lait spots, fibroma molluscum, and osseous deformities and lesions.

Incidence

- 1/3000 births is the approximate incidence of neurofibromatosis.
- 60% of patients have a familial history.

Clinical Features

- Equal male to female ratio.
- 50% of patients with neurofibromatosis develop café au lait spots.
- Café au lait spots are non-elevated, chestnut skin pigmentations, which are smoothly marginated (coast of California).
- The presence of six or more café au lait spots measuring 1.5 cm or more is considered diagnostic of neurofibromatosis.
- 15% of the normal population has one or two café au lait spots.
- 1% of the normal population may have more than two café au lait spots.
- Fibroma molluscum is a multiple asymptomatic cutaneous nodule, which is elevated above the skin's surface; this is the most common cutaneous manifestation of neurofibromatosis.
- Elephantiasis neuromatosa represents thick large soft tissue folds in neurofibromatosis.
- Pulsating exophthalmos may be a presenting sign occurring as a result of a temporal lobe herniation through the deficient posterior surface of the orbit.
- Spinal involvement may include paraplegia, kyphoscoliosis, and atlantoaxial subluxation.

Pathologic Features

- Grossly, the lesions of neurofibroma appear as a grayish brown, firm, rubbery mass.
- Histologically, interlacing strands of elongated cells are arranged in a palisading pattern, containing foam cells and pigment.
- Malignant degeneration to neurofibrosarcoma occurs in 5% of cases; a higher incidence of sarcomatous degeneration occurs with those lesions that have been repeatedly biopsied.

Radiologic Features

- 50% of cases develop skeletal lesions.
- Kyphoscoliosis is the most common spinal roentgen sign, occurring in 50% of patients. The kyphoscoliosis is classically acutely angular and is short segmented (5 to 7 vertebrae), usually affecting the lower thoracic spine.
- Scalloping of the posterior surface of the vertebral bodies is characteristic. Two types of scalloping exist: posterocentral scalloping at multiple levels that is secondary to dural ectasia, and eccentric unilateral scalloping usually at a single level occurs as a result of a dumbbell neurofibroma, creating enlargement of the IVF.
- An eccentric paraspinal mass is often seen on the AP thoracic or PA chest radiograph.
- Intrathoracic meningoceles represent a common cause for the presence of a posterior mediastinal mass in a patient with neurofibromatosis. Most meningoceles occur laterally and on the right side.
- Unilateral agenesis or hypoplasia affecting the sphenoid portion of the posterior wall of the orbit, creating a bare orbit, is characteristic. It is this bony abnormality that allows pulsating exophthalmos to occur.
- A radiolucent defect in the lambdoidal suture represents underlying hypoplasia of bone and not neurofibromatous erosion. This lesion is most common on the left side and may have hypoplasia of the ipsilateral mastoid process associated. This associated lambdoidal lesion has been called the asterion defect.
- Scalloping irregularities of the ribs create the twisted ribbon appearance.
- Pseudo-arthrosis of the tibia occurs in 50% of cases.
- Multiple large bilateral non-ossifying fibromas have been documented to occur in association.
- Focal giantism (local overgrowth or hypertrophy of both the skeletal and soft tissue structures), usually of the lower extremities, is perhaps the most bizarre and fascinating roentgen sign.
- Renal artery stenosis occurs in association, creating hypertension.
- 1% of patients with neurofibromatosis have a pheochromocytoma; 20% of patients with pheochromocytoma have neurofibromatosis.
- Osteomalacia may rarely occur in association, owing to renal tubular dysfunction.

Medicolegal Implications

SKELETAL TUMORS

- Recognition of bone tumors requires the clinical decision to obtain a radiograph. Key points in the history must be sought, including past history of malignancy, loss of appetite, weight loss, and night pain. Unresponsiveness to care and worsening of symptoms are clinical indicators that necessitate further consideration. Failure to recognize these important red flags results in a delay in appropriate patient management.
- Even though plain films are relatively insensitive, requiring between 30% and 50% loss of bone mass before it becomes radiographically visible, they remain, for the most part, the best initial study for these lesions.
- Knowledge of the locations, age frequencies, and appearance of individual bone tumors is essential for appropriate recognition and clinical decision making.

- Radiographs need to be of the highest quality, with adequate views. Failure to fulfill these criteria is a medicolegal risk.
- The interpreter should be able to accurately describe the lesion and make some conclusions on the behavior of the lesion. The necessity for second opinion review depends on the individual circumstances, but it is to be encouraged wherever there is doubt on the patient's status or if a tumor is suspected.
- Advanced imaging (e.g., bone scan, CT, MRI) should be given consideration when the radiographs are normal and the clinical findings don't resolve or progressively worsen with conservative management.
- Sophisticated imaging modalities don't render a histologic diagnosis but rather provide further characterization of the lesion, as well as the extent of tumor infiltration. This aids in surgical planning and helps monitor the patient's response to the chosen therapy.

■ *References*

METASTATIC BONE TUMORS

1. **Jaffe HJ:** *Tumors and Tumorous Conditions of the Bones and Joints.* Philadelphia, Lea & Febiger, 1958.
2. **Abrams HL, Spiro R, Goldstein N:** *Metastases in carcinoma: Analysis of 1000 autopsied cases.* Cancer 3:74, 1950.
3. **Johnson AD:** *Pathology of metastatic tumors in bone.* Clin Orthop 73:8, 1970.
4. **Radford M, Gibbons CL:** *Management of skeletal metastases.* Hosp Med 63(12):772, 2002.
5. **Willis RA:** *The Spread of Tumors in the Human Body.* London, Butterworths, 1973.
6. **Napoli LD, Hansen HH, Muggia FM:** *The incidence of osseous involvement in lung cancer, with special reference to the development of osteoblastic changes.* Radiology 108:17, 1973.
7. **Kanis JA, McCloskey EV, Powles T, et al.:** *A high incidence of vertebral fracture in women with breast cancer.* Br J Cancer 79(7–8):1179, 1999.
8. **Kriteman L, Sanders WH:** *Normal alkaline phosphatase levels in patients with bone metastases due to renal cell carcinoma.* Urology 51(3):397, 1998.
9. **Ataus S, Citci A, Alici B, et al.:** *The value of serum prostate specific antigen and other parameters in detecting bone metastases in prostate cancer.* Int Urol Nephrol 31(4):481, 1999.
10. **Wymenga LF, Boomsma JH, Groenier K, et al.:** *Routine bone scans in patients with prostate cancer related to serum prostate-specific antigen and alkaline phosphatase.* Br J Urol Int 88(3):226, 2001.
11. **Lin K, Szabo Z, Chin BB, Civelek AC:** *The value of baseline bone scan in patients with newly diagnosed prostate cancer.* Clin Nucl Med 24(8):579, 1999.
12. **Batson OV:** *The function of the vertebral veins and their role in the spread of metastases.* Ann Surg 112:138, 1940.
13. **Deutsch A, Resnick D:** *Eccentric cortical metastases to the skeleton from bronchogenic carcinoma.* Radiology 137:49, 1980.
14. **Hendrix RW, Rogers LF, Davis TM Jr:** *Cortical bone metastasis.* Radiology 181:409, 1991.
15. **Milch RA, Changus GW:** *Response to tumor invasion.* Cancer 9:340, 1956.
16. **McDougall IR:** *Skeletal scintigraphy.* West J Med 130:503, 1979.
17. **Galasko CSB:** *The pathological basis for skeletal scintigraphy.* J Bone Joint Surg 57A:353, 1975.
18. **Litterer WE:** *Nuclear bone scanning—Skeletal imaging.* J Clin Chiro 3(2):7, 1980.
19. **Wu PS, Chiu NT, Lee BF, et al.:** *Clinical significance of solitary rib hot spots on bone scans in patients with extraskeletal cancer: Correlation with other clinical manifestations.* Clin Nucl Med 27(8):567, 2002.
20. **Han LJ, Au-Yong TK, Tong WC, et al.:** *Comparison of bone single-photon emission tomography and planar imaging in the detection of vertebral metastases in patients with back pain.* Eur J Nucl Med 25(6):635, 1998.
21. **Citrin DL, Hougen C, Zweibel W:** *Use of serial bone scans in assessing response of bone metastases to systemic treatment.* Cancer 47:680, 1981.
22. **Lee YTN:** *Bone scanning in patients with early breast carcinoma: Should it be a routine staging procedure?* Cancer 47:486, 1981.
23. **Charkes ND, Malmud LS, Caswell T:** *Preoperative bone scans: Use in women with early breast cancer.* JAMA 233:516, 1975.
24. **DeSantos LA, Libshitz HI:** *Adult bone.* In: HI Libshitz HI, ed, *Diagnostic Roentgenology of Radiotherapy Change.* Baltimore, Williams & Wilkins, 1979.
25. **Bachman AS, Sproul EE:** *Correlation of radiographic and autopsy findings in suspected metastases in the spine.* Bull NY Acad Med 44:169, 1940.
26. **Sedonja I, Budihna NV:** *The benefit of SPECT when added to planar scintigraphy in patients with bone metastases in the spine.* Clin Nucl Med 24(6):407, 1999.
27. **Krishnamurthy GT, et al.:** *Distribution pattern of metastatic bone disease. A need for total body skeletal image.* JAMA 237:2504, 1977.
28. **Steinborn MM, Heuck AF, Tiling R, et al.:** *Whole-body bone marrow MRI in patients with metastatic disease to the skeletal system.* J Comput Assist Tomogr 23(1):123, 1999.
29. **Mysorekar VV, Dandekar CP, Rao SG:** *Metastatic bone tumors.* J Indian Med Assoc 96(3):74, 1998.
30. **Yuh WTC, Zachar CK, Barloon TJ, et al.:** *Vertebral compression fractures: Distinction between benign and malignant causes with MR imaging.* Radiology 172:215, 1989.
31. **Shih TT, Huang KM, Li YW:** *Solitary vertebral collapse: Distinction between benign and malignant causes using MR patterns.* J Magn Reson Imaging 9(5):635, 1999.

32. **Fourney DR, Schomer DF, Nader R, et al.:** *Percutaneous verte-broplasty and kyphoplasty for painful vertebral body fractures in cancer patients.* J Neurosurg 98(1 Suppl):21, 2003.
33. **Resnick D, Niwayama G:** *Diagnosis of Bone and Joint Disorders,* ed 2. Philadelphia, WB Saunders, 1988.
34. **Abdelwahab IF, Miller TT, Herman G, et al.:** *Transarticular inva-sion of joints by bone tumors: Hypothesis.* Skeletal Radiol 20:279, 1991.
35. **Silberstein M, Hennessy O, Lau L:** *Neoplastic involvement of the sacroiliac joint: MR and CT features.* Australas Radiol 36:334, 1992.
36. **Algra PR, Heimans JJ, Valk J, et al.:** *Do metastases in vertebrae begin in the body or the pedicles? Imaging study in 45 patients.* AJR 158:1275, 1992.
37. **Greenfield GB:** *Radiology of Bone Diseases,* ed 3. Philadelphia, JB Lippincott, 1980.
38. **Macnab I:** *Backache.* Baltimore, Williams & Wilkins, 1977.
39. **Wackenheim A:** *Radiodiagnosis of the Vertebra in Adults.* Chicago, Yearbook, 1983.
40. **Albers VL:** *Congenital absence of a lumbar pedicle with sclerosis and hypertrophy of the contralateral pedicle.* ACA J Chiro, 1984.
41. **Yochum TR:** *Case of the missing pedicle.* ACA Council Roentgenol, 1981.
42. **Genant HK, Wilson JS, Bovill EG, et al.:** *Computed tomography of the musculoskeletal system.* J Bone Joint Surg 61A:1088, 1980.
43. **LaBan MM, Newman JM:** *Occult sternal metastasis identified by laminography in patients with chest pain.* Arch Phys Med Rehabil 65:203, 1984.
44. **Phillips CD, Pope TL, Jones JE, et al.:** *Nontraumatic avulsion of the lesser trochanter: A pathognomonic sign of metastatic disease?* Skeletal Radiol 17:106, 1988.
45. **Wu KK, Guise ER:** *Metastatic tumors of the foot.* South Med J 71:807, 1978.
46. **Moeller FA:** *Pulmonary adenocarcinoma: Metastasis to a lesser toe.* J Am Pod Assoc 61:297, 1971.
47. **Strang R:** *Phalangeal metastases as a first clinical sign of broncho-genic carcinoma.* Br J Surg 39:372, 1952.
48. **Mulvey RB:** *Peripheral bone metastasis.* AJR 91:155, 1964.
49. **Johnson LC:** *A general theory of bone tumors.* Bull NY Acad Med 29:164, 1953.
50. **Galmarini CM, Kertesz A, Oliva R, et al.:** *Metastasis of broncho-genic carcinoma to the thumb.* Med Oncol 4:282, 1998.
51. **Lehrer HZ, Maxfield WS, Nice CM:** *The periosteal "sunburst" pattern in metastatic bone tumors.* AJR 108:154, 1970.
52. **Hove B, Gyldensted C:** *Spiculated vertebral metastases from pros-tate carcinoma. Report of first two cases.* Neuroradiology 32:337, 1990.
53. **Clain A:** *Secondary malignant disease of bone.* Br J Cancer 19:15, 1965.
54. **Fidler M:** *Incidence of fracture through metastases in long bones.* Acta Orthop Scand 52:623, 1981.
55. **Berquist TH, Ehman RL, King BF, et al.:** *Value of MR imaging in differentiating benign from malignant soft tissue masses: Study of 95 lesions.* AJR 155:1251, 1990.
56. **Coombes RC, Dady P, Parsons C, et al.:** *Assessment of response of bone metastases to systemic treatment in patients with breast cancer.* Cancer 52:610, 1983.
57. **Perez EA:** *Metastatic bone disease in breast cancer: the patient's perspective.* Semin Oncol 28(Suppl 11):60, 2001.
58. **Finley RS:** *Bisphophonates in the treatment of bone metastases.* Semin Oncol 29(Suppl 4):132, 2002.
59. **Ciray I, Astrom G, Andreasson I, et al.:** *Evaluation of new scle-rotic bone metastases in breast cancer patients during treatment.* Acta Radiol 41(2):178, 2000.
60. **Rossleigh MA, Lovegrove FTA, Reynolds PM, et al.:** *The assess-ment of response to therapy of bone metastases in breast cancer.* Aust NZ J Med 14:19, 1984.
61. **Janjan NA, Payne R, Gillis T, et al.:** *Presenting symptoms in patients referred to a multidisciplinary clinic for bone metastases.* J Pain Symptoms Manage 16(3):171, 1998.

NEUROBLASTOMA
1. **Groncy P, Finkelstein JZ:** *Neuroblastoma.* Pediatr Ann 7:548, 1978.
2. **Eklof O, Gooding CA:** *Intrathoracic neuroblastoma.* AJR 100:202, 1967.
3. **Bond JV:** *Clinical features of neuroblastoma.* Br J Hosp Med 145:43, 1975.
4. **Eklof O, Gooding CA:** *Paravertebral widening in cases of neuro-blastoma.* Br J Radiol 40:358, 1967.
5. **Johnson LC:** *A general theory of bone tumors.* Bull NY Acad Med 29:164, 1953.

PRIMARY MALIGNANT BONE TUMORS
MULTIPLE MYELOMA
1. **Clamp JR:** *Some aspects of the first recorded case of multiple mye-loma.* Lancet 2:1354, 1967.
2. **Bence Jones H:** *On a new substance occurring in the urine of a patient with mollities ossium.* Philos Trans R Soc Lond (Biol) 1:55, 1848.
3. **von Rustizky J:** *Multiples myeloma.* Dtsch Z Chir 3:162, 1873.
4. **Kahler O:** *Zur Symptomatologie des multiplen Myeloms.* Wien Med Presse 30:209, 1889.
5. **Longsworth LG, Shedlovsky T, MacInnes DA:** *Electrophoretic patterns of normal and pathological human blood serum and plasma.* J Exp Med 70:399, 1939.
6. **Grabar P, Williams CA:** *Methode permettant l'etude coniugu;aaee des proprietes electrophoretiques et immunochimiques d'un m;aae-lange de proteines: Application au serum sanguin.* Biochem Biophys Acta 10:193, 1953.
7. **Mirra JM:** *Bone Tumors—Diagnosis and Treatment.* Philadelphia, JB Lippincott, 1980.
8. **Kyle RA:** *Multiple myeloma—Review of 869 cases.* Mayo Clin Proc 50:29, 1975.
9. **Hewell GM, Alexanian R:** *Multiple myeloma in young persons.* Ann Intern Med 84:441, 1976.
10. **Wilner D:** *Radiology of Bone Tumors and Allied Disorders.* Philadelphia, WB Saunders, 1982.
11. **Huvos AG:** *Bone Tumors—Diagnosis, Treatment and Prognosis.* Philadelphia, WB Saunders, 1979.
12. **Kyle RA:** *Clinical aspects of multiple myeloma and related disorders including amyloidosis.* Pathol Biol (Paris) 47(2):148, 1999.
13. **Zaidi AA, Vesole DH:** *Multiple myeloma: an old disease with new hope for the future.* CA Cancer J Clin 51(5):273, 2001.
14. **Irish AB, Winearls CG, Littlewood T:** *Presentation and survival of patients with severe renal failure and myeloma.* Q J Med 90(12):773, 1997.
15. **Gordon DA, Pruzanski T, Waldemar F, et al.:** *Amyloid arthritis simulating rheumatoid disease in five patients with multiple myeloma.* Am J Med 55:142, 1973.
16. **Wiernik PH:** *Amyloid joint disease.* Medicine 51:465, 1972.
17. **Mulder JD, van Rijssel THG:** *Amyloid tumor of the sternum as part of a solitary plasmacytoma* [Case Report 233]. Skeletal Radiol 10:53, 1983.
18. **Ludwig H, Kumpan W, Sinzinger H:** *Radiography and bone scin-tigraphy in multiple myeloma: A comparative analysis.* Br J Radiol 55:173, 1982.
19. **Leonard RCF, Owen JP, Proctor SJ, et al.:** *Multiple myeloma: Radiology or bone scanning?* Clin Radiol 32:291, 1981.
20. **Heiser S, Schartzman JJ:** *Variations in roentgen appearance of skeletal system in myeloma.* Radiology 58:178, 1952.
21. **Murray RO, Jacobson HG:** *The Radiology of Skeletal Disorders,* ed 2. New York, Churchill Livingstone, 1977.
22. **Jacobson HG, Poppel MH, Shapiro JH, et al.:** *The vertebral pedi-cle sign. A roentgen finding to differentiate metastatic carcinoma from multiple myeloma.* AJR 80:817, 1958.
23. **Cohen DM, Svien HJ, Dahlin DC:** *Long-term survival of patients with myeloma of the vertebral column.* JAMA 187:914, 1964.
24. **Brown TS, Paterson CR:** *Osteosclerosis in myeloma.* J Bone Joint Surg 55B:621, 1973.

25. **Clarisse PDT, Staple TW:** *Diffuse bone sclerosis in multiple myeloma.* Radiology 99:327, 1971.

26. **Schreiman JS, McLeod RA, Kyle RA, et al.:** *Multiple myeloma: Evaluation by CT.* Radiology 154:483, 1985.

27. **Libshitz HI, Malthouse SR, Cunningham D, et al.:** *Multiple myeloma: Appearance at MR imaging.* Radiology 182:833, 1992.

28. **Yochum TR, Molyneux TP:** *Multiple myeloma.* ACA J Chiro, 1983.

29. **Kyle RA, Gertz MA, Witzig TE, et al.:** *Review of 1027 patients with newly diagnosed multiple myeloma.* Mayo Clin Proc 78(1):21, 2003.

30. **Corso A, Klersy C, Lazzarino M, Bernasconi C:** *Multiple myeloma in younger patients: The role of age as a prognostic factor.* Ann Hematol 76(2):67, 1998.

31. **Weber DM:** *Newly diagnosed multiple myeloma.* Curr Treat Options Oncol 3(3):235, 2002.

32. **Berenson JR:** *Myeloma—The therapeutic challenge.* Med Klin 95(Suppl 2):19, 2000.

SOLITARY PLASMACYTOMA

1. **Mirra JM:** *Bone Tumors—Diagnosis and Treatment.* Philadelphia, JB Lippincott, 1980.

2. **Lane SL:** *Plasmacytoma of the mandible.* Oral Surg 5:434, 1952.

3. **Ganesh M, Sankar NS, Jagannathan R:** *Extramedullary plasmacytoma presenting as upper back pain.* J R Soc Health 120(4):262, 2000.

4. **Roberts M, Rinaudo PA, Vilinskas J, et al.:** *Solitary sclerosing plasma-cell myeloma of the spine.* J Neurosurg 40:125, 1974.

5. **Tanaka M, Shibui S, Nomura K, Nakanishi Y:** *Solitary plasmacytoma of the skull: A case report.* Jpn J Clin Oncol 28(10):626, 1998.

6. **Baba H, Maezawa Y, Furusawa N, et al.:** *Solitary plasmacytoma of the spine associated with neurological complications.* Spinal Cord 36(7):470, 1998.

7. **Miller FR, Lavertu P, Wanamaker JR, et al.:** *Plasmacytomas of the head and neck.* Otolaryngol Head Neck Surg 119(6):614, 1998.

8. **Liebross RH, Ha CS, Cox JD, et al.:** *Clinical course of solitary extramedullary plasmacytoma.* Radiother Oncol 52(3):245, 1999.

9. **Alexiou C, Kau RJ, Dietzfelbinger H, et al.:** *Extramedullary plasmacytoma: tumor occurrence and therapeutic concepts.* Cancer 85(11):2305, 1999.

CENTRAL OSTEOSARCOMA

1. **Edeiken J:** *Roentgen Diagnosis of Diseases of Bone,* ed 3. Baltimore, Williams & Wilkins, 1981.

2. **Huvos AG:** *Bone Tumors—Diagnosis, Treatment and Prognosis.* Philadelphia, WB Saunders, 1979.

3. **Dahlin DC, Coventry MB:** *Osteogenic sarcoma—A study of 600 cases.* J Bone Joint Surg 49A:101, 1967.

4. **Chindia ML:** *Osteosarcoma of the jaw bones.* Oral Oncol 37(7):545, 2001.

5. **Cade S:** *Osteogenic sarcoma.* JR Coll Surg Edinb 1:79, 1955.

6. **Siegal GP, Dahlin DC, Sim FH:** *Osteoblastic osteogenic sarcoma in a 35-month-old girl. Report of a case.* Am J Clin Pathol 63:886, 1975.

7. **Scranton PE Jr, DeCicco FA, Totten RS, et al.:** *Prognostic factors in osteosarcoma. A review of 20 years' experience at the University of Pittsburgh Health Center Hospitals.* Cancer 36:2179, 1975.

8. **Fraumeni JF Jr:** *Stature and malignant tumors of bone in childhood and adolescence.* Cancer 20:967, 1967.

9. **Widhe B, Widhe T:** *Initial symptoms and clinical features in osteosarcoma and Ewing sarcoma.* J Bone Joint Surg 82A:667, 2000.

10. **Ewing J:** *Bulkley lecture: Modern attitude toward traumatic cancer.* Arch Pathol 19:690, 1935.

11. **McKenna RJ, Schwinn CP, Soong KY, et al.:** *Sarcomata of the osteogenic series—An analysis of 552 cases.* J Bone Joint Surg 48A:1, 1966.

12. **Levine AM, Chretien P:** *Deep venous occlusion as the initial presentation of osteogenic sarcoma of the sacrum.* J Bone Joint Surg 61A:775, 1979.

13. **Gold RH, Mirra JH:** *Highly anaplastic epiphyseal osteosarcoma.* Skeletal Radiol 3:69, 1978.

14. **Findelstein JB:** *Osteosarcoma of the jaw bones.* Radiol Clin North Am 8:425, 1970.

15. **Salmon M:** *Osteosarcome de l'omoplate chez une enfant. Radiotherapie—Scapulectomie.* Chirurgie 99:887, 1973.

16. **Carrol RE:** *Osteogenic sarcoma in the hand.* J Bone Joint Surg 39A:325, 1957.

17. **Marsh HO, Choi CB:** *Primary osteogenic sarcoma of the cervical spine originally mistaken for benign osteoblastoma—A case report.* J Bone Joint Surg 52A:1467, 1970.

18. **Espinosa GA, Platt H:** *Two cases of osteosarcoma of the spine arising from Pagetic bone.* App Radiol 12:59, 1983.

19. **Yochum TR:** *Paget's sarcoma of bone.* Radiologe 24:428, 1984.

20. **McKenna RF, Schwinn CP, Soong KY, et al.:** *Osteogenic sarcoma arising in Paget's disease.* Cancer 17:42, 1964.

21. **Fuchs B, Pritchard DJ:** *Etiology of osteosarcoma.* Clin Orthop 397:40–52, 2002.

22. **St. James AT:** *Resection of multiple metastatic pulmonary lesions of osteogenic sarcoma.* JAMA 169:943, 1959.

23. **Wuisman P, Enneking WF:** *Prognosis for patients who have osteosarcoma with skip metastasis.* J Bone Joint Surg 72A:60, 1990.

24. **Price CHG, Jeffree GM:** *Metastatic spread of osteosarcoma.* Br J Cancer 28:515, 1973.

25. **Kumar R, David R, Madewell JE, et al.:** *Radiographic spectrum of osteogenic sarcoma.* AJR 148:767, 1987.

26. **Goodwin MA:** *Primary osteosarcoma of the patella.* J Bone Joint Surg 43B:338, 1961.

27. **Norton KI, Hermann G, Abdelwahab IF, et al.:** *Epiphyseal involvement in osteosarcoma.* Radiology 180:813, 1991.

28. **Hingorani CB, Sharma OP:** *Osteosarcoma—A roentgenographic study.* Indian J Cancer 10:285, 1973.

29. **Holscher HC, Bloem JL, Vanel D, et al.:** *Osteosarcoma: Chemotherapy-induced changes at MR imaging.* Radiology 182:839, 1992.

30. **Carsi B, Rock MG:** *Primary osteosarcoma in adults older than 40 years.* Clin Orthop 397:53, 2002.

31. **Sweetnam R, Knowelden J, Jedden H:** *Bone sarcoma; treatment by irradiation, amputation, or a combination of the two.* Br Med J 2:363, 1971.

32. **Copeland MM:** *Primary malignant tumors of bone—Evaluation of current diagnosis and treatment.* Cancer 20:738, 1967.

33. **Price CHG:** *The prognosis of osteosarcoma—An analytical study.* Br J Radiol 39:181, 1966.

34. **Smith J, Huvos AG, et al.:** *Radiographic changes in primary osteogenic sarcoma following intensive chemotherapy.* Radiology 143:355, 1982.

35. **Unni KK:** *Osteosarcoma of bone.* J Orthop Sci 3:287, 1998.

MULTICENTRIC OSTEOSARCOMA

1. **Amstutz HC:** *Multiple osteogenic sarcomata—Metastatic or multicentric? Report of two cases and review of the literature.* Cancer 24:923, 1969.

2. **Hopper KD, Moser RP, Haseman DB, et al.:** *Osteosarcomatosis.* Radiology 175:233, 1990.

3. **Owen LB, Eskey CW, Kashatus WC, et al.:** *Multiosseous osteosarcoma: Report of one case and review of the literature.* Radiol Clin Biol 35:43, 1966.

4. **Price CHG, Truscott DE:** *Multifocal osteogenic sarcoma. Report of a case.* J Bone Joint Surg 39B:524, 1957.

5. **Silverman G:** *Multiple osteogenic sarcoma.* Arch Pathol 21:88, 1936.

6. **Lowbeer L:** *Multifocal osteosarcomatosis—A rare entity.* Bull Pathol 9:52, 1968.

PAROSTEAL SARCOMA

1. **Lichtenstein L:** *Tumors of periosteal origin.* Cancer 8:1060, 1955.

2. **Huvos AG:** *Bone Tumors—Diagnosis, Treatment and Prognosis.* Philadelphia, WB Saunders, 1979.

3. **Unni KK, Dahlin DC, Beabout JW, et al.:** *Parosteal osteogenic sarcoma.* Cancer 37:2466, 1976.
4. **Sanchis Olmos V, Ferrer Torelles M, Fernandez Criado M:** *Osteoma parostal de clavicula.* Acta Orthop Traumatol Iber 4:471, 1956.
5. **Stark HH, Jones FE, Jernstrom P:** *Parosteal osteogenic sarcoma of a metacarpal bone. A case report.* J Bone Joint Surg 53A:147, 1971.
6. **Som M, Peimer R:** *Juxtacortical osteogenic sarcoma of the mandible.* Arch Otolaryngol 74:532, 1961.
7. **Lodwick GS:** *The Bones and Joints.* Chicago, Year Book Medical, 1973.
8. **Edeiken J, et al.:** *Parosteal sarcoma.* AJR 3:579, 1971.
9. **Hudson TM, Springfield DS, Benjamin M, et al.:** *Computed tomography of parosteal osteosarcoma.* AJR 144:961, 1985.
10. **Kenan S, Abdelwahab IF, Klein MJ, et al.:** *Parosteal osteosarcoma involving the left radius. Case report 835.* Skeletal Radiol 23:229, 1994.
11. **Yochum TR:** *Post traumatic myositis ossificans.* ACA J Chiro, 1982.
12. **Unni KK, Beabout JW, et al.:** *High-grade surface osteosarcomas.* Am J Surg Pathol 8:81, 1984.

SECONDARY OSTEOSARCOMA

1. **Yochum TR:** *Paget's sarcoma of bone.* Radiologe 24:428, 1984.
2. **Castle WB, Drinker KR, Drinker CK:** *Necrosis of the jaw in workers employed in applying a luminous paint containing radium.* J Indust Hyg 7:371, 1925.
3. **Yoneyama T, Greenlaw RH:** *Osteogenic sarcoma following radiotherapy for retinoblastoma.* Radiology 93:1185, 1969.
4. **Martland HS, et al.:** *The late effects of internally deposited radioactive materials in man.* Medicine 31:221, 1952.
5. **Huvos AG:** *Bone Tumors—Diagnosis, Treatment and Prognosis.* Philadelphia, WB Saunders, 1979.
6. **Tsuya A, Tanaka T, Mori T, et al.:** *Four cases of Thorotrast injury and estimation of absorbed tissue dose in critical organs.* J Radiat Res 4:126, 1963.
7. **Lorigan JG, Libshitz HI, Peuchot M:** *Radiation-induced sarcoma of bone: CT findings in 19 cases.* AJR 153:791, 1989.

EXTRAOSSEOUS OSTEOSARCOMA

1. **Das Guptz TK, Hajdu SI, Foote FW Jr:** *Extraosseous osteogenic sarcoma.* Ann Surg 168:1011, 1968.
2. **Lowry K Jr, Haynes CD:** *Osteogenic sarcoma of extraskeletal soft tissues: A case report.* Am Surg 30:97, 1964.
3. **Salm R:** *A case of primary osteogenic sarcoma of extraskeletal soft tissue.* Br J Cancer 13:614, 1959.

CHONDROSARCOMA

1. **Greenfield GB:** *Radiology of Bone Diseases,* ed 3. Philadelphia, JB Lippincott, 1980.
2. **Jaffe HJ:** *Tumors and Tumorous Conditions of the Bones and Joints.* Philadelphia, Lea & Febiger, 1969.
3. **Lichtenstein L, Jaffe HL:** *Chondrosarcoma of bone.* Am J Pathol 19:553, 1943.
4. **O'Neal LW, Ackerman LV:** *Chondrosarcoma of bone.* Cancer 5:551, 1952.
5. **Marcove RC, Mike V, Hutter RVP, et al.:** *Chondrosarcoma of the pelvis and upper end of the femur. An analysis of factors influencing survival time in 113 cases.* J Bone Joint Surg 54A:561, 1972.
6. **Dahlin DC, Salvador AH:** *Chondrosarcomas of the bones of the hands and feet—A study of 30 cases.* Cancer 34:755, 1974.
7. **Roberts PH, Price CHG:** *Chondrosarcoma of the bones of the hand.* J Bone Joint Surg 59B:213, 1977.
8. **Blaylock RL, Kempe LG:** *Chondrosarcoma of the cervical spine [Case Report 44].* J Neurosurg 4:500, 1976.
9. **Camins MB, Duncan AW, Smith J, et al.:** *Chondrosarcoma of the spine.* Spine 3(3):202, 1978.
10. **Lo EP, Pollak R, Harvey CK:** *Chondrosarcoma of the foot.* J Am Podiatr Med Assoc 90(4):203, 2000.

11. **Present D, Bacchini P, Pignatti G, et al.:** *Clear cell chondrosarcoma of bone. A report of 8 cases.* Skeletal Radiol 20:187, 1991.
12. **Palmieri TJ:** *Chondrosarcoma of the hand.* J Hand Surg 9:332, 1984.
13. **Scott WW, Fishman EK, Lubbe WJ:** *Chondrosarcoma of the right trapezoid bone [Case Report 259].* Skeletal Radiol 11:137, 1984.
14. **Granberry WM, Bryan W:** *Chondrosarcoma of the trapezium [Case Report 3].* J Hand Surg 3(3):277, 1978.
15. **Somers J, Faber LP:** *Chondroma and chondrosarcoma.* Semin Thorac Cardiovasc Surg 11(3):270, 1999.
16. **Smith J, McLachlan DL, Huvos AG, et al.:** *Primary tumors of the clavicle and scapula.* Am J Roentgenol Radium Ther Nucl Med 124:113, 1975.
17. **Martini N, Huvos AG, Smith J, et al.:** *Primary malignant tumors of the sternum.* Surg Gynecol Obstet 138:391, 1974.
18. **Somville J, Van Bouwel S:** *Surgery for primary bone sarcomas of the pelvis.* Acta Orthop Belg 67(5):442, 2001.
19. **Feldman F:** *Cartilaginous tumors and cartilage forming tumor-like conditions of the bones and soft tissues.* In: K Ranniger, ed, *Encyclopedia of Medical Radiology.* Vol 5, part 6. Berlin: Springer, 1977.
20. **Sweet DE, Madewell JE, Ragsdale BD:** *Radiologic and pathologic analysis of solitary bone lesions. Part III: Matrix patterns.* Radiol Clin North Am 19:785, 1981.
21. **Lichtenstein L:** *Bone Tumors,* ed 4. St. Louis, CV Mosby, 1972.
22. **Schajowicz F, Aravjo ES, Berenstein A:** *Sarcoma complicating Paget's disease of bone.* J Bone Joint Surg 65B:299, 1983.
23. **Yochum TR:** *Paget's sarcoma of bone.* Radiologe 24:428, 1984.
24. **Huvos AG, Higinbotham NL, Miller TR:** *Bone sarcomas arising in fibrous dysplasia.* J Bone Joint Surg 54A:1047, 1972.
25. **Fitzwater JE, Cabaud HE, Farr GH:** *Irradiation induced chondrosarcoma.* J Bone Joint Surg 58A:1037, 1976.
26. **Norman A, Sissons HA:** *Radiographic hallmarks of peripheral chondrosarcoma.* Radiology 151:589, 1984.
27. **York JE, Berk RH, Fuller GN, et al.:** *Chondrosarcoma of the spine: 1954 to 1997.* J Neurosurg 90(1 Suppl):73, 1999.
28. **Rizzo M, Ghert MA, Harrelson JM, Scully SP:** *Chondrosarcoma of bone: Analysis of 108 cases and evaluation for predictors of outcome.* Clin Orthop (391):224, 2001.
29. **Eriksson AI, Schiller A, Mankin HJ:** *The management of chondrosarcoma of bone.* Clin Orthop 153:44, 1980.
30. **Sanerkin NG, Gallagher P:** *A review of the behavior of chondrosarcoma of bone.* J Bone Joint Surg 61B:395, 1979.
31. **Bruns J, Elbracht M, Niggemeyer O:** *Chondrosarcoma of bone: An oncological and functional follow-up study.* Ann Oncol 12(6):859, 2001
32. **Fiorenza F, Abudu A, Grimer RJ, et al.:** *Risk factors for survival and local control in chondrosarcoma of bone.* J Bone Joint Surg 84B:93, 2002.
33. **Rozeman LB, Hogendoorn PC, Bovee JV:** *Diagnosis and prognosis of chondrosarcoma of bone.* Expert Rev Mol Diagn 2(5):461, 2002.

EWING'S SARCOMA

1. **Ewing J:** *Diffuse endothelioma of bone.* Proc Pathol Soc 21(n.s.):17, 1921.
2. **Oberling C:** *Les reticulo sarcomes et les reticulo endotheliosarcomes de la moelle osseuse (sarcomes d'Ewing).* Bull Assoc Fr Etude Cancer 17:259, 1928.
3. **Fraumenti JF Jr, Glass AG:** *Rarity of Ewing's sarcoma among U.S. Negro children [Letter].* Lancet 1:366, 1970.
4. **Coley BL, Higinbotham NL, Bowden L:** *Endothelioma of bone (Ewing's sarcoma).* Ann Surg 128:533, 1948.
5. **Bhansali SK, Desai PB:** *Ewing's sarcoma. Observations on 107 cases.* J Bone Joint Surg 45A:541, 1955.
6. **Widhe B, Widhe T:** *Initial symptoms and clinical features in osteosarcoma and Ewing sarcoma.* J Bone Joint Surg 82A:667, 2000.
7. **Lichtenstein L, Jaffe HL:** *Ewing's sarcoma of bone.* Am J Pathol 23:43, 1947.
8. **Aegerter E, Kirkpatrick JA Jr:** *Orthopedic Diseases,* ed 4. Philadelphia, WB Saunders, 1975.

9. **Wilner D:** *Radiology of Bone Tumors and Allied Disorders.* Philadelphia, WB Saunders, 1982.
10. **Rosen G, Caparros B, Huvos AG, et al.:** *Ewing's sarcoma. Ten years' experience with adjuvant chemotherapy.* Cancer 47:2204, 1981.
11. **Li WK, Lane JM, Rosen G, et al.:** *Pelvic Ewing's sarcoma.* J Bone Joint Surg 65A:738, 1983.
12. **Kozlowski K, Campbell J, Beluffi G, et al.:** *Primary bone tumors of the pelvis in childhood—Ewing's sarcoma of the ilium, pubis and ischium. (Report of 30 cases). Part 1.* Australas Radiol 33:354, 1989.
13. **Levine E, Levine C:** *Ewing tumor of rib: Radiologic findings and computed tomography contribution.* Skeletal Radiol 9:227, 1983.
14. **Staalman CR:** *Ewing's sarcoma in rib.* J Belgisch Radiol 65:329, 1982.
15. **Dahlin DC:** *Ewing's tumor. Bone Tumors,* ed 3. Springfield, Charles C. Thomas, 1978.
16. **Whitehouse GH, Griffiths GJ:** *Roentgenologic aspects of spinal involvement by primary and metastatic Ewing's tumor.* J Can Assoc Radiol 27:290, 1976.
17. **Grubb MR, Currier BL, Pritchard DJ, et al.:** *Primary Ewing's sarcoma of the spine.* Spine 19:309, 1994.
18. **Bonanone V, Cardani R:** *An unusual case of Ewing's tumor on the foot.* Minerva Ortop 24:441, 1973.
19. **Dunn EJ, Yuska KH, Judge DM, et al.:** *Ewing's sarcoma of the great toe. A case report.* Clin Orthop 16:203, 1976.
20. **Potdar GG:** *Ewing's tumor of the jaws.* J Oral Surg 29:505, 1970.
21. **Blakemore JR, Stein M:** *Primary Ewing's sarcoma of the mandible: Report of a case.* J Oral Surg 33:376, 1975.
22. **West DC:** *Ewing sarcoma family of tumors.* Curr Opin Oncol 12(4): 323, 2000.
23. **Schajowicz F:** *Ewing's sarcoma and reticulum cell sarcoma of bone. With special reference to the histochemical demonstration of glycogen as an aid to differential diagnosis.* J Bone Joint Surg 41A:349, 1959.
24. **Frostad B, Tani E, Brosjo O, et al.:** *Fine needle aspiration cytology in the diagnosis and management of children and adolescents with Ewing sarcoma and peripheral primitive neuroectodermal tumor.* Med Pediatr Oncol 38:33, 2002.
25. **Shirley SK, Gilula LA, Siegal GP, et al.:** *Roentgenographic-pathologic correlation of diffuse sclerosis in Ewing sarcoma of bone.* Skeletal Radiol 12:69, 1984.
26. **Aufranc OE, Jones WN, Turner RH:** *Pathologic fracture of the proximal femur.* JAMA 199:107, 1967.
27. **Garber CZ:** *Reactive bone formation in Ewing's sarcoma.* Cancer 4:839, 1951.
28. **Geschickter CF, Maseritz IH:** *Ewing's sarcoma.* J Bone Joint Surg 21A:26, 1939.
29. **Telles NC, Rabson AS, Pomeroy TC:** *Ewing's sarcoma: An autopsy study.* Cancer 41:2321, 1978.
30. **Sundaram M, Merenda G, McGuire MM:** *A skip lesion in association with Ewing sarcoma.* J Bone Joint Surg 71A:764, 1989.
31. **Hoffmann C, Ahrens S, Dunst J, et al.:** *Pelvic Ewing sarcoma: A retrospective analysis of 241 cases.* Cancer 85(4):869, 1999.
32. **Dwyer AJ, Glaubiger DL, Ecker JG, et al.:** *The radiographic follow-up of patients with Ewing sarcoma: A demonstration of a general method.* Radiology 145:327, 1982.
33. **Jenkin RD, Al-Fawaz I, Al-Shabanah MO, et al.:** *Metastatic Ewing sarcoma/PNET of bone at diagnosis: prognostic factors—A report from Saudi Arabia.* Med Pediatr Oncol 37(4):383, 2001.
34. **Cotterill SJ, Ahrens S, Paulussen M, et al.:** *Prognostic factors in Ewing's tumor of bone: Analysis of 975 patients from the European Intergroup cooperative Ewing's Sarcoma Study Group.* J Clin Oncol 18:3108, 2000.
35. **Shankar AG, Ashley S, Craft AW, Pinkerton CR:** *Outcome after relapse in an unselected cohort of children and adolescents with Ewing sarcoma.* Med Pediatr Oncol 40(3):141, 2003.

FIBROSARCOMA

1. **Huvos AG:** *Bone Tumors—Diagnosis, Treatment and Prognosis.* Philadelphia, WB Saunders, 1979.

2. **Wilner D:** *Radiology of Bone Tumors and Allied Disorders.* Philadelphia, WB Saunders, 1982.
3. **Papagelopoulos PJ, Galanis EC, Trantafyllidis P, et al.:** *Clinicopathologic features, diagnosis, and treatment of fibrosarcoma of bone.* Am J Orthop 31(5):253, 2002.
4. **Larsson SE, Lorentzon R, Boquist L:** *Fibrosarcoma of bone.* J Bone Joint Surg 58B:412, 1976.
5. **Jaffe HL:** *Tumors and Tumorous Conditions of the Bones and Joints.* Philadelphia, Lea & Febiger, 1958.
6. **Dahlin DC:** *Fibrosarcoma of bone. A study of 114 cases.* Cancer 23:35, 1969.
7. **Cunningham MP, Arlen M:** *Medullary fibrosarcoma of bone.* Cancer 21:31, 1968.
8. **Kabukcuoglu Y, Kabukcuoglu F, Carter S, et al.:** *Multiple diffuse fibrosarcoma of bone.* Am J Orthop 28(12):715, 1999.
9. **Tarasov BP:** *Diagnosis of fibrosarcoma of the bone.* Arkh Patol 32:23, 1969.
10. **Antonescu CR, Erlandson RA, Huvos AG:** *Primary fibrosarcoma and malignant fibrous histiocytoma of bone—A comparative ultrastructural study: Evidence of a spectrum of fibroblastic differentiation.* Ultrastruct Pathol 24(2):83, 2000.
11. **Smith SE, Kransdorf MJ:** *Primary musculoskeletal tumors of fibrous origin.* Semin Musculoskelet Radiol 4(1):73, 2000.
12. **Greenfield GB:** *Radiology of Bone Diseases,* ed 3. Philadelphia, JB Lippincott, 1980.
13. **Lichtenstein L:** *Bone Tumors,* ed 4. St. Louis, CV Mosby, 1972.
14. **Eyre-Brook AL, Price CHG:** *Fibrosarcoma of bone.* J Bone Joint Surg 51B:20, 1969.
15. **Huvos AG, Higinbotham NL, Miller TR:** *Bone sarcomas arising in fibrous dysplasia.* J Bone Joint Surg 54A:1047, 1972.
16. **Yochum TR:** *Paget's sarcoma of bone.* Radiologie 24:428, 1984.
17. **Akbarnia BA, Wirth CR, Colman N:** *Fibrosarcoma arising from chronic osteomyelitis.* J Bone Joint Surg 58A:123, 1976.
18. **Dorfman HD, Norman A, Wolf H:** *Fibrosarcoma complicating bone infarction in a caisson worker. A case report.* J Bone Joint Surg 48A:528, 1966.
19. **Heselson NG, Med M, Price SK:** *Two malignant fibrous histiocytomas in bone infarcts—Case report.* J Bone Joint Surg 65A:166, 1983.
20. **Ros PR, Viamonte M Jr, Rywlin AM:** *Malignant fibrous histiocytoma: Mesenchymal tumor of ubiquitous origin.* AJR 142:753, 1984.
21. **Papagelopoulos PJ, Galanis E, Frassica FJ, et al.** *Primary fibrosarcoma of bone. Outcome after primary surgical treatment.* Clin Orthop 373:88, 2000.

CHORDOMA

1. **Wilner D:** *Radiology of Bone Tumors and Allied Disorders.* Philadelphia, WB Saunders, 1982.
2. **Huvos AG:** *Bone Tumors—Diagnosis, Treatment and Prognosis.* Philadelphia, WB Saunders, 1979.
3. **Higinbotham NL, Phillips RF, Farr HW, et al.:** *Chordoma: Thirty-five-year study at Memorial Hospital.* Cancer 20:1841, 1967.
4. **Smith J, Ludwig RL, Marcove RC:** *Sacrococcygeal chordoma. A clinicoradiolical study of 60 patients.* Skeletal Radiol 16:37, 1987.
5. **Dahlin DC, MacCarty CS:** *Chordoma: A study of fifty-nine cases.* Cancer 5:1170, 1952.
6. **Utne JR, Pugh DG:** *The roentgenologic aspects of chordoma.* AJR 74:593, 1955.
7. **Kamrin RP, Potanos JN, Pool JL:** *An evaluation of the diagnosis and treatment of chordoma.* J Neurol Neurosurg Psychiatry 27:157, 1964.
8. **Mabrey RE:** *Chordoma: A study of 150 cases.* Am J Cancer 25: 501, 1935.
9. **Seaton RW, Weaver EN:** *The chordoma.* VA Med Mon 89:34, 1962.
10. **Yochum TR:** *Chordoma of the sacrum.* ACA J Chiro, 1983.

11. **Topsakal C, Bulut S, Erol FS, et al.:** *Chordoma of the thoracic spine—Case report.* Neurol Med Chiro (Tokyo) 42(4):175, 2002.
12. **Tashiro T, Fukuda T, Inoue Y, et al.:** *Intradural chordoma: Case report and review of the literature.* Neuroradiology 36:313, 1994.
13. **Crapanzano JP, Ali SZ, Ginsberg MS, Zakowski MF:** *Chordoma: A cytologic study with histologic and radiologic correlation.* Cancer 93:40, 2001.
14. **Warakaulle DR, Anslow P:** *A unique presentation of retroclival chordoma.* J Postgrad Med 48(4):285, 2002.
15. **Mindell ER:** *Chordoma—Current concepts review.* J Bone Joint Surg 63A:501, 1981.
16. **Meyer JE, Lepke RA, Lindfors KK, et al.:** *Chordomas: Their CT appearance in the cervical, thoracic, and lumbar spine.* Radiology 153:693, 1984.
17. **Manzone P, Fiore N, Forlino D, et al.:** *Chordoma of the lumbar L2 vertebra: Case report and review of the literature.* Eur Spine J 7(3):252, 1998.
18. **McMaster ML, Goldstein AM, Bromley CM,, et al.:** *Chordoma: incidence and survival patterns in the United States: 1973–1995.* Cancer Causes Control 12(1):1, 2001.
19. **York JE, Kaczaraj A, Abi-Said D,, et al.:** *Sacral chordoma: 40-year experience at a major cancer center.* Neurosurgery 44:74, 1999. [Discussion 44:79, 1999.]
20. **Gunterberg B, Romanus B, Stener B:** *Pelvic strength after major amputation of the sacrum.* Acta Orthop 47:635, 1976.
21. **Stener B, Gunterberg B:** *High amputation of the sacrum for extirpation of tumors.* Spine 3:351, 1978.
22. **Cheng EY, Ozerdemoglu RA, Transfeldt EE, Thompson RC Jr:** *Lumbosacral chordoma. Prognostic factors and treatment.* Spine Aug 24:1639, 1999.
23. **Colli B, Al-Mefty O:** *Chordomas of the craniocervical junction: follow-up review and prognostic factors.* J Neurosurg 95:933, 2001.
24. **Iwasa Y, Nakashima Y, Okajima H, Morishita S:** *Sacral chordoma in early childhook: Clinicopathological and immunohistochemical study.* Pediatr Dev Pathol 1:420, 1998.

NON-HODGKIN'S LYMPHOMA OF BONE (RETICULUM CELL SARCOMA)

1. **Huvos AG:** *Bone Tumors—Diagnosis, Treatment and Prognosis.* Philadelphia, WB Saunders, 1979.
2. **Parker F Jr, Jackson H Jr:** *Primary reticulum cell sarcoma of bone.* Surg Gynecol Obstet 68:45, 1939.
3. **Dranitsaris G:** *Treatment of non-Hodgkin's lymphoma.* Anticancer Drugs 9(10):879, 1998.
4. **Murray RO, Jacobson HG:** *The Radiology of Skeletal Disorders,* ed 2. New York, Churchill Livingstone, 1977.
5. **Ivins JC, Dahlin DC:** *Malignant lymphoma (reticulum cell sarcoma).* Proc Mayo Clin 38:375, 1963.
6. **Coles WC, Schultz MD:** *Bone involvement in malignant lymphoma.* Radiology 50:458, 1948.
7. **Baar J, Burkes RL, Gospodarowicz M:** *Primary non-Hodgkin's lymphoma of bone.* Semin Oncol 26(3):270, 1999.
8. **Wang CC, Fleischli DJ:** *Primary reticulum cell sarcoma of bone: With emphasis on radiation therapy.* Cancer 22:994, 1968.
9. **Jones D, Kraus MD, Dorfman DM:** *Lymphoma presenting as a solitary bone lesion.* Am J Clin Pathol 111(2):171, 1999.
10. **Sherman RS, Snyder RE:** *The roentgen appearance of primary reticulum cell sarcoma of bone.* AJR 58:291, 1947.
11. **Wilson TW, Pugh DG:** *Primary reticulum cell sarcoma of bone, with emphasis on roentgen aspects.* Radiology 65:343, 1955.
12. **Edeiken J:** *Roentgen Diagnosis of Diseases of Bone,* ed 3. Baltimore, Williams & Wilkins, 1981.
13. **Ackerman L, Drunen MV, Reyes CV:** *Malignant large cell lymphoma of sacrum* [Case report 836]. Skeletal Radiol 23:232, 1994.
14. **Israel O, Mekel M, Bar-Shalom R, et al.:** *Bone lymphoma: 67 Ga scintigraphy and CT for prediction of outcome after treatment.* J Nucl Med 43(10):1295, 2002.
15. **Francis KC, Higinbotham NL, Coley BL:** *Primary reticulum cell sarcoma of bone. Report of 44 cases.* Surg Gynecol Obstet 92(2):142, 1954.

HODGKIN'S LYMPHOMA OF BONE

1. **Fucilla IS, Hamann A:** *Hodgkin's disease in bone.* Radiology 77:53, 1961.
2. **Dyttert V:** *Primary osseous lymphogranuloma. A contribution.* Neoplasma 13:105, 1966.
3. **Donaldson SS:** *Pediatric Hodgkin's disease—Up, up, and beyond.* Int J Radiat Oncol Biol Phys 54(1)1, 2002.
4. **Stuhlbarg J, Ellis FW:** *Hodgkin's disease of bone. Favorable prognostic significance?* AJR 93:568, 1965.
5. **Clark A, Stanish WD:** *An unusual cause of back pain in a young athlete. A case report.* Am J Sports Med 13:51, 1985.
6. **Conn HO:** *Alcohol-induced pain as a manifestation of Hodgkin's disease.* Arch Intern Med 100:241, 1957.
7. **Callahan BC, Coe R, Place HM:** *Hodgkin's disease of the spine presenting as alcohol-related pain.* J Bone Joint Surg 76A:119, 1994.
8. **Chandi L, Kumar L, Kochupillai V, et al.:** *Hodgkin's disease: A retrospective analysis of 15 years experience at a large referral center.* Natl Med J India 11(5):212, 1998.
9. **Rowe LJ:** *Hodgkin's lymphoma of the thoracic spine.* J Can Chiro Assoc 28:212, 1984.
10. **Granger W, Whitaker R:** *Hodgkin's disease in bone, with special reference to periosteal reaction.* Br J Radiol 40:939, 1967.
11. **Pear BL:** *Skeletal manifestations of the lymphomas and leukemias.* Semin Roentgenol 9:229, 1974.
12. **Hulten O:** *Ein Fall von "Elfenbeinwirbel" bei Lymphogranulomatose.* Acta Radiol 8:245, 1927.
13. **Newcomer LN, Silverstein MB, Cadman EC, et al.:** *Bone involvement in Hodgkin's disease.* Cancer 49:338, 1982.

SYNOVIAL SARCOMA

1. **Mackenzie DH:** *Synovial sarcoma, a review of 58 cases.* Cancer 19:169, 1966.
2. **Lazarus JA, Marks MS:** *Synovial sarcoma.* Surgery 13:290, 1943.
3. **Lewis RW:** *Roentgen recognition of synovioma.* AJR 44:170, 1940.
4. **Blacksin MF, Siegel JR, Benevenia J, Aisner SC:** *Synovial sarcoma: frequency of nonaggressive MR characteristics.* J Comput Assist Tomogr 21(5):785, 1997.
5. **Morton MJ, Berquist TH, McLeod RA, et al.:** *MR imaging of synovial sarcoma.* AJR 156:337, 1991.
6. **Raben M, Calabrese A, Higinbotham NL, et al.:** *Malignant synovioma.* AJR 93:145, 1965.
7. **Wright PH, Sim FH, Soule EH, et al.:** *Synovial sarcoma.* J Bone Joint Surg 64A:112, 1982.
8. **Skytting BT, Bauer HC, Perfekt R, et al.:** *Clinical course in synovial sarcoma: a Scandinavian sarcoma group study of 104 patients.* Acta Orthop Scand 70(6):536, 1999.
9. **Valenzuela RF, Kim EE, Seo JG, et al.:** *A revisit of MRI analysis for synovial sarcoma.* Clin Imaging 24(4):231, 2000.

ADAMANTINOMA

1. **Judmaier W, Peer S, Drejzi T, et al.:** *MR findings in tibial adamantinoma. A case report.* Acta Radiol 39(3):276, 1998.
2. **Lichtenstein L:** *Bone Tumors,* ed 5. St. Louis, CV Mosby, 1977.
3. **Fischer B:** *Über ein primäres adamantinoma der tibia.* Frankfurter Zeitschr Pathol 12:422, 1913.
4. **Unni KK, Dahlin DC, Beabout JW, et al.:** *Adamantinomas of long bones.* Cancer 34:1796, 1974.
5. **Wilner D:** *Radiology of Bone Tumors and Allied Disorders.* Philadelphia, WB Saunders, 1982.
6. **Nerubay J, Chechick A, Horoszowski H, et al.:** *Adamantinoma of the spine.* J Bone Joint Surg 70A:467, 1988.
7. **Sarisozen B, Durak K, Ozturk C:** *Adamantinoma of the tibia in a nine-year-old child.* Acta Orthop Belg 68(4):412, 2002.
8. **Huvos AG, Marcove RC:** *Adamantinoma of long bones.* J Bone Joint Surg 57A:148, 1975.
9. **Kuruvilla G, Steiner GC:** *Osteofibrous dysplasia-like adamantinoma of bone: a report of five cases with immunohistochemical and ultrastructural studies.* Hum Pathol 29:809, 1998.

10. **Bloem JL, van der Heul RO, Schuttevaer HM, et al.:** *Fibrous dysplasia vs adamantinoma of the tibia: Differentiation based on discriminant analysis of clinical and plain film findings.* AJR 156:1017, 1991.

11. **Torriani M, Derkigil SS, Etchebehere M, Amstalden EM:** *Magnetic resonance imaging of tibial classic adamantinoma at 2 tesla.* J Comput Assist Tomogr 26:844, 2002.

12. **Qureshi AA, Shott S, Mallin BA, Gitelis S:** *Current trends in the management of adamantinoma of long bones. An international study.* J Bone Joint Surg 82A:1122, 2000.

PRIMARY QUASI-MALIGNANT BONE TUMOR

GIANT CELL TUMOR

1. **Cooper A, Travers B:** *Surgical Essays,* ed 3. London, Cox & Son, 1818.

2. **Jaffe HL, Lichtenstein L, Portis RB:** *Giant cell tumor of bone; its pathologic appearance, grading, supposed variants, and treatment.* Arch Pathol 30:993, 1940.

3. **Jaffe HL, Lichtenstein L, Sutro CJ:** *Pigmented villonodular synovitis, bursitis, and tenosynovitis.* Arch Pathol 31:731, 1941.

4. **Jaffe HL, Lichtenstein L:** *Benign chondroblastoma of bone.* Am J Pathol 18:969, 1942.

5. **Jaffe HL, Lichtenstein L:** *Non-osteogenic fibroma of bone.* Am J Pathol 18:205, 1942.

6. **Jaffe HL, Lichtenstein L:** *Chondromyxoid fibroma of bone.* Arch Pathol 45:541, 1948.

7. **Lichtenstein L:** *Aneurysmal bone cyst, a pathological entity commonly mistaken for giant cell tumor and occasionally for hemangioma and osteogenic sarcoma.* Cancer 3:279, 1950.

8. **Jaffe HL:** *Tumors and Tumorous Conditions of the Bones and Joints.* Philadelphia, Lea & Febiger, 1958.

9. **Stewart MJ:** *The histogenesis of myeloid sarcoma.* Lancet 2:1106, 1922.

10. **Schajowicz F:** *Tumors and Tumor-Like Lesions of Bone and Joints.* New York, Springer-Verlag, 1981.

11. **Dahlin DC:** *Giant cell tumor. Bone Tumors,* ed 2. Springfield, Charles C Thomas, 1967.

12. **Hutter RVP, Worcester JN Jr, Francis KC, et al.:** *Benign and malignant giant cell tumors of bone. A clinicopathological analysis of the natural history of the disease.* Cancer 15:653, 1962.

13. **Gebhart M, Vandeweyer E, Nemec E:** *Patet's disease of bone complicated by giant cell tumor.* Clin Orthop 352:187, 1998.

14. **Magitsky S, Lipton JF, Reidy J, et al.:** *Ultrastructural features of giant cell tumors in Patet's disease.* Clin Orthop 401:213, 2002.

15. **Huvos AG:** *Bone Tumors—Diagnosis, Treatment and Prognosis.* Philadelphia, WB Saunders, 1979.

16. **Sheth RD, Shah SN:** *Osteoclastoma of the os calcis.* Int Surg 57:748, 1972.

17. **Locher GW, Kaiser G:** *Giant-cell tumors and aneurysmal bone cysts of ribs in childhood.* J Pediatr Surg 10:103, 1975.

18. **Fitzpatrick DJ, Bullough PG:** *Giant cell tumor of the lunate bone: A case report.* J Hand Surg 2:269, 1977.

19. **Srivastava TP, Tuli SM, Varma BP, et al.:** *Giant cell tumor of metacarpals.* Indian J Cancer 12:164, 1975.

20. **Kelikian H, Clayton I:** *Giant-cell tumor of the patella.* J Bone Joint Surg 39A:414, 1957.

21. **Mercuri M, Casadei R:** *Patellar tumors.* Clin Orthop 389:35, 2001.

22. **Faris WF, Rubin BD, Fielding JW:** *Aneurysmal bone cyst of the patella.* J Bone Joint Surg 60A:711, 1978.

23. **Singson R, Feldman F:** *Multicentric giant cell tumors of bone* [Case report 229]. Skeletal Radiol 9:276, 1983.

24. **Wilner D:** *Radiology of Bone Tumors and Allied Disorders.* Philadelphia, WB Saunders, 1982.

25. **Roux S:** *Giant cell tumors of bone.* Rev Rhum Engl Educ 65:139, 1998.

26. **Chakravarti A, Spiro IJ, Hug EB, et al.:** *Megavoltage radiation therapy for axial and inoperable giant-cell tumor of bone.* J Bone Joint Surg 81A:1566, 1999.

27. **Fidler NW:** *Surgical treatment of giant cell tumours of the thoracic and lumbar spine: Report of nine patients.* Eur Spine J 10:69, 2001.

28. **Verhagen WI, Bartels RH, Schaafsma HE, Rob de Jong TH:** *A giant cell tumor of the sacrum or a soft tissue giant cell tumor. A case report.* Spine 23(14):1609, 1998.

29. **Miszczyk L. Wydmanski J, Spindel J:** *Efficacy of radiotherapy for giant cell tumor of bone: Given either postoperatively or as sole treatment.* Int J Radiat Oncol Biol Phys 49(5):1239 2001.

30. **Briccoli A, Malaguti C, Iannetti C, et al.:** *Giant cell tumor of the rib.* Skeletal Radiol 32(2):107, 2003.

31. **Garcia-Bravo A, Sanchez-Enriquez J, Mendez-Suarez JL, et al.:** *Secondary tetraplegia due to giant-cell tumors of the cervical spine.* Neurochirurgie 48(6):527, 2002.

32. **Goldenberg RR, Campell CJ, Bonfiglio M:** *Giant cell tumor of bone.* J Bone Joint Surg 52A:619, 1970.

33. **Hudson TM, Schiebler M, Springfield DS, et al.:** *Radiology of giant cell tumors of bone: Computed tomography, arthro-tomography, and scintigraphy.* Skeletal Radiol 11:85, 1984.

34. **Wada T, Kaya M, Nagoya S, et al.:** *Complications associated with bone cementing for the treatment of giant cell tumors of bone.* J Orthop Sci 7(2):194, 2002.

35. **Kitano K, Shiraishi T, Okabayashi K, et al.:** *A lung metastasis from giant cell tumor of bone at eight years after primary resection.* Jpn J Thorac Cardiovasc Surg 47(12):617, 1999.

36. **Masui F, Ushigome S, Fujii K:** *Giant cell tumor of bone: A clinicopathologic study of prognostic factors.* Pathol Int 48(9):723, 1998.

37. **Anract P, De Pinieux G, Cottias P, et al.:** *Malignant giant-cell tumours of bone. Clinico-pathological types and prognosis: a review of 29 cases.* Int Orthop 22(1):19, 1998.

PRIMARY BENIGN BONE TUMORS

SOLITARY OSTEOCHONDROMA

1. **Cooper A:** *Exostosis.* In: A Cooper, B Travers, eds, *Surgical Essays,* ed 3. London, Cox & Son, 1818.

2. **Cannon JF:** *Hereditary multiple exostosis.* Am J Hum Genet 6:419, 1954.

3. **Huvos AG:** *Bone Tumors—Diagnosis, Treatment and Prognosis.* Philadelphia, WB Saunders, 1979.

4. **Harsha WN:** *The natural history of osteocartilaginous exostoses (osteochondroma).* Am Surg 20:65, 1954.

5. **Gokay H, Bucy PC:** *Osteochondroma of lumbar spine. Report of a case.* J Neurosurg 12:72, 1955.

6. **Fiumara E, Scarabino T, Guglielmi G, et al.:** *Osteochondroma of the L-5 vertebra: A rare cause of sciatic pain. Case report.* J Neurosurg 91(2 Suppl):219, 1999.

7. **Jose Alcaraz Mexia M, Izquierdo Nunez E, Santonja Garriga C, Maria Salgodo Salinas R:** *Osteochondroma of the thoracic spine and scoliosis.* Spine 26:1082, 2001.

8. **Wilner D:** *Radiology of Bone Tumors and Allied Disorders.* Philadelphia, WB Saunders, 1982.

9. **Rose EF, Fekete A:** *Odontoid osteochondroma causing sudden death. Report of a case and review of the literature.* Am J Clin Pathol 42:606, 1964.

10. **Lee FA:** *Solitary cartilaginous exostosis of the ilium presenting as an abdominal mass.* Am J Dis Child 114:195, 1967.

11. **Mehta M, White LM, Knapp T, et al.:** *MR imaging of symptomatic osteochondromas with pathological correlation.* Skeletal Radiol 27(8):427, 1998.

12. **Woertler K, Lindner N, Gosheger G, et al.:** *Osteochondroma: MR imaging of tumor-related complications.* Eur Radiol 10(5):832, 2000.

13. **Mirra JM:** *Bone Tumors—Diagnosis and Treatment.* Philadelphia, JB Lippincott, 1980.

14. **Mangini U:** *Tumors of the skeleton of the hand.* Bull Hosp Joint Dis 28:61, 1967.

15. **Eller DJ, Blakemore JR, Stein M, et al.:** *Transoral resection of a condylar osteochondroma: Report of a case.* J Oral Surg 35:409, 1977.

16. **List CF:** *Osteochondromas arising from base of skull.* Surg Gynecol Obstet 76:480, 1943.
17. **Milch RA:** *Osteochondroma of the astragalus.* Am J Surg 87:145, 1954.
18. **Ilgenfritz HC:** *Vertebral osteochondroma.* Am Surg 17:917, 1951.
19. **Inglis AE, Rubin RM, Lewis RJ, et al.:** *Osteochondroma of the cervical spine. Case report.* Clin Orthop 126:127, 1977.
20. **Wouters HW, Szepesi K, Kullmann L:** *Solitary osteochondroma of the scapula. A report on six cases.* Arch Chir Neerl 26:63, 1974.
21. **Reichmister J, Reeder JD, Gold DL:** *Osteochondroma of the distal clavicle: An unusual cause of rotator cuff impingement.* Am J Orthop 29(10):807, 2000.
22. **Dahlin DC:** *Bone Tumors: General Aspects and Data on 6,221 Cases,* ed 3. Springfield, Charles C Thomas, 1978.
23. **Coley BI, Higinbotham NL:** *Secondary chondrosarcoma.* Ann Surg 139:547, 1954.
24. **Hudson TM, Springfield DS, Spanier SS, et al.:** *Benign exostoses and exostotic chondrosarcomas: Evaluation of cartilage thickness by CT.* Radiology 152:595, 1984.
25. **Greenfield GB:** *Radiology of Bone Diseases,* ed 3. Philadelphia, JB Lippincott, 1980.
26. **Lee JK, Yao L, Wirth CR:** *MR imaging of solitary osteochondromas: Report of eight cases.* AJR 149:557, 1987.
27. **Lokiec F, Ezra E, Krasin E, et al.:** *A simple and efficient surgical technique for subungual exostosis.* J Pediatr Orthop 21:76, 2001.
28. **Letts M, Davidson D, Nizalik E:** *Subungual exostosis: Diagnosis and treatment in children.* J Trauma 44(2):346, 1998.
29. **Evison G, Price CH:** *Subungual exostosis.* Br J Radiol 39:451, 1966.

HEREDITARY MULTIPLE EXOSTOSIS

1. **Kivioja A, Ervasti H, Kinnunen J, et al.:** *Chondrosarcoma in a family with multiple hereditary exostoses.* J Bone Joint Surg 82B(2):261, 2000.
2. **Boyer A:** *Traite des Maladies Chirurgicales.* Vol 3. Paris, VeMigneret, 1814.
3. **Keith A:** *Studies on the anatomical changes which accompany certain growth disorders of the human body. The nature of the structural alterations in the disorder known as multiple exostoses.* J Anat 54:101, 1920.
4. **Ellis UH, Taylor JG:** *Diaphyseal aclasis.* J Bone Joint Surg 33B:100, 1951.
5. **Harsha WN:** *The natural history of osteocartilaginous exostoses (osteochondroma).* Am Surg 20:65, 1954.
6. **Porter DE, Emerton ME, Villanueva-Lopez F, Simpson AH:** *Clinical and radiographic analysis of osteochondromas and growth disturbance in hereditary multiple exostoses.* J Pediatr Orthop 20(2):246, 2000.
7. **Felix NA, Mazur JM, Loveless EA:** *Acetabular dysplasia associated with hereditary multiple exostoses. A case report.* J Bone Joint Surg 82B:555, 2000.
8. **Paik NJ, Han TR, Lim SJ:** *Multiple peripheral nerve compressions related to malignantly transformed hereditary multiple exostoses.* Muscle Nerve 23(8):1290, 2000.
9. **Madigan R, Worral T, McClain EJ:** *Cervical cord compression in hereditary multiple exostosis.* J Bone Joint Surg 56A:401, 1974.
10. **Flatt AE:** *Chondrosarcoma supervening on diaphyseal aclasis.* Br J Surg 43:85, 1955.
11. **Dahlin DC:** *Bone Tumors: General Aspects and Data on 6,221 Cases,* ed 3. Springfield, Charles C Thomas, 1978.
12. **Garrison RC, Dahlin DC, Unni KK, et al.:** *Chondrosarcoma arising in osteochondroma.* Cancer 49:1890, 1982.

HEMANGIOMA

1. **Schmorl G, Junghans H:** *The Human Spine in Health and Disease,* ed 2. New York, Grune & Stratton, 1971.
2. **Bailey P, Bucy PC:** *Cavernous hemangioma of the vertebrae.* JAMA 92:1748, 1929.
3. **Mohan V, Gupta SK, Tuli SM, et al.:** *Symptomatic vertebral hemangiomas.* Clin Radiol 31:575, 1980.
4. **Manning HJ:** *Symptomatic hemangioma of the spine.* Radiology 56:58, 1951.
5. **Holta O:** *Hemangioma of the cervical vertebra with fracture and compression myelomalacia.* Acta Radiol 23:423, 1942.
6. **Broderick RA, Round H:** *Cavernous angioma of the maxilla. Fatal hemorrhage after teeth extraction.* Lancet 2:13, 1933.
7. **Macansh JD, Owen MD:** *Central cavernous hemangioma of the mandible.* J Oral Surg 30:293, 1972.
8. **Ogose A, Hotta T, Morita T, et al.:** *Solitary osseous hemangioma outside the spinal and craniofacial bones.* Arch Orthop Trauma Surg 120:262, 2000.
9. **Yochum TR:** *Spinal hemangiomas.* ACA J Chiro, 1983.
10. **Lund BA, Dahlin DC:** *Hemangiomas of the mandible and maxilla.* J Oral Surg 22:234, 1964.
11. **Bansal VP, Singh PC, Grewal DS, et al.:** *Hemangioma of the patella. A report of two cases.* J Bone Joint Surg 56B:139, 1974.
12. **Tunon BJ, Gonzalez PF:** *Angiomatosis of the metacarpal skeleton.* Hand 9:88, 1977.
13. **Sherman RS, Wilner D:** *The roentgen diagnosis of hemangioma of bone.* AJR 86:1146, 1961.
14. **Wackenheim A:** *Radiodiagnosis of the Vertebra in Adults.* New York, Springer-Verlag, 1983.
15. **McAllister VL, Kendall BE, Bull JWD:** *Symptomatic vertebral hemangiomas.* Brain 98:71, 1975.
16. **Bery K, Chawla S:** *Hemangioma of the spine with compression of the cord.* Indian J Radiol 21:117, 1967.
17. **Mohan V:** Roentgen evaluation of thoracic paraspinal line in health and disease [Thesis]. Banaras Hindu University, 1975.
18. **Laredo JD, Assouline E, Gelbert F, et al.:** *Vertebral hemangiomas: Fat content as a sign of aggressiveness.* Radiology 177:467, 1990.
19. **Kelemen G, Holmes EM:** *Cavernous hemangioma of the frontal bone.* J Laryngol Otol 72:557, 1948.
20. **Wilner D:** *Radiology of Bone Tumors and Allied Disorders.* Philadelphia, WB Saunders, 1982.
21. **Bell RL:** *Hemangioma of a dorsal vertebra with collapse and compression myelopathy.* J Neurosurg 12:570, 1955.
22. **Bergstrand A, Hook O, Lidvall H:** *Vertebral hemangiomas compressing the spinal cord.* Acta Neurol Scand 39:59, 1963.
23. **Cushing H:** *Surgical end results in general with case of cavernous hemangioma of skull in particular.* Surg Gynecol Obstet 36:303, 1923.

OSTEOMA

1. **Childrey JH:** *Osteomas of the sinuses, of the frontal and sphenoid bone.* Arch Otolaryngol 30:63, 1939.
2. **Schertel L:** *Die H;auohlenosteome.* Radiologie 15:62, 1975.
3. **Kim AW, Foster JA, Papay FA, Wright KW:** *Orbital extension of a frontal sinus osteoma in a thirteen-year-old girl.* JAAPOS 4(2):122, 2000.
4. **Namdar I, Edelstein DR, Huo J, et al.:** *Management of osteomas of the paranasal sinuses.* Am J Rhinol 12(6):393, 1998.
5. **Shady JA, Bland LI, Kazee AM, et al.:** *Osteoma of the frontoethmoid sinus with secondary brain abscess and intracranial mucocele: Case report.* Neurosurgery 34:920, 1994.
6. **Greenspan A:** *Benign bone-forming lesions: Osteoma, osteoid osteoma, and osteoblastoma.* Skeletal Radiol 22:485, 1993.
7. **Johnson D, Tan L:** *Intraparenchymal tension pneumatocele complicating frontal sinus osteoma: case report.* Neurosurgery 50:878, 2002. [Discussion 50;880, 2002.]
8. **Bullough PG:** *Ivory exostosis of the skull.* Postgrad Med J 41:277, 1965.
9. **Maclennan WD, Brown RD:** *Osteoma of the mandible.* Br J Oral Surg 12:219, 1974.
10. **Montgomery WW:** *Osteoma of the frontal sinus.* Ann Otol Rhinol Laryngol 69:245, 1960.
11. **Lautenbach E:** *Klinische und histologische Studien an Osteomen.* Dtsch Zahn Mund Kieferheilkd 43:434, 1964.

GARDNER'S SYNDROME

1. **Gardner EJ:** *Discovery of the Gardner syndrome.* Birth Defects 13:48, 1972.

2. **Watne AL, Core SK, Carrier JM:** *Gardner's syndrome.* Surg Gynecol Obstet 141:53, 1975.
3. **McNab AA:** *Orbital osteoma in Gardner's syndrome.* Aust N Z J Ophthalmol 26(2):169, 1998.

Bone Island

1. **Smith J:** *Giant bone islands.* Radiology 107:35, 1973.
2. **Trombetti A, Noel E:** *Giant bone islands: a case with 31 years of follow-up.* Joint Bone Spine 69(1):81, 2002.
3. **Blank N, Lieber A:** *The significance of growing bone islands.* Radiology 85:508, 1965.
4. **Onitsuka H:** *Roentgenologic aspects of bone islands.* Radiology 123:607, 1977.
5. **Hoffman RR Jr, Campbell RE:** *Roentgenologic bone island instability in hyperparathyroidism.* Radiology 103:307, 1972.
6. **Sickle EA, Genant HK, Hoffer PB:** *Increased localization of 99M TE-Pyrophosphate in a bone island: Case report.* J Nucl Med 17:113, 1976.
7. **Davies JA, Hall FM, Goldberg RP, et al.:** *Positive bone scans in bone islands.* J Bone Joint Surg 61a:6, 1979.
8. **Greenspan A, Steiner G, Knutzon R:** *Bone island (enostosis): Clinical significance and radiologic and pathologic correlations.* Skeletal Radiol 20:85, 1991.
9. **Gower DJ, Tytle T, Brumback R:** *Enlarging endostoma (bone island) of the spinous process.* Neurosurgery 30:608, 1992.
10. **Yochum TR:** *Giant bone island of the right innominate with osteolytic metastatic carcinoma of the right innominate from a previous malignant breast neoplasm.* ACA J Chiro, 1981.

Osteoid Osteoma

1. **Jaffe HL:** *Osteoid osteoma—A benign osteoblastic tumor composed of osteoid and atypical bone.* Arch Surg 31:709, 1935.
2. **Freiberger RH, Loitman BS, Helpern M:** *Osteoid osteoma: A report on 80 cases.* AJR 82:194, 1959.
3. **Byers PD:** *Solitary benign osteoblastic lesions of bone: Osteoid osteoma and benign osteoblastoma.* Cancer 22:43, 1968.
4. **Sim FH, Dahlin DC, Beabout JW:** *Osteoid osteoma: Diagnostic problems.* J Bone Joint Surg 57A:154, 1975.
5. **Schajowicz F, Lemos C:** *Osteoid osteoma and osteoblastoma.* Acta Orthop Scand 41:272, 1970.
6. **Dahlin DC:** *Bone Tumors,* ed 3. Springfield, Charles C Thomas, 1978.
7. **Habermann ET, Stern RE:** *Osteoid osteoma of the tibia in an eight-month-old boy. A case report.* J Bone Joint Surg 56A:633, 1974.
8. **Cohen MD, Harrington TM, Ginsburg WW:** *Osteoid osteoma: 95 cases and a review of the literature.* Semin Arthritis Rheumatol 12(3):265, 1983.
9. **Helms CA, Hattner RS, Vogler JB III:** *Osteoid osteoma: Radionuclide diagnosis.* Radiology 151:779, 1984.
10. **Paus BC, Kim TK:** *Osteoid osteoma of the spine.* Acta Orthop Scand 33:24, 1963.
11. **Flaherty RA, Pugh DG, Dockerty MB:** *Osteoid osteoma.* AJR 76:1041, 1956.
12. **Sabannos AO, Bickel WH, Moe JH:** *Natural history of osteoid osteoma.* Am J Surg 91:880, 1956.
13. **Foss EL, Dockerty MB, Good CA:** *Osteoid osteoma of the mandible.* Cancer 8:592, 1955.
14. **Reinhardt K:** *Osteoid osteom im os parietale.* Fortschr Geb Roentgenstr Nuklearmed 116:563, 1972.
15. **Arazi M, Memik R, Yel M, Ogun TC:** *Osteoid osteoma of the carpal bones.* Arch Orthop Trauma Surg 121:119, 2001.
16. **Yochum TR:** *Osteoid osteoma of the thumb* [Roentgen Brief]. ACA Council, Nov 1979.
17. **Greenspan A:** *Benign bone-forming lesions: osteoma, osteoid osteoma, and osteoblastoma.* Skeletal Radiol 22:485, 1993.
18. **Jaffe HL:** *Osteoid osteoma of bone.* Radiology 45:319, 1945.
19. **Macleelan DI, Wilson FC Jr:** *Osteoid osteoma of the spine.* J Bone Joint Surg 49A:111, 1967.

20. **Caldicott WJH:** *Diagnosis of spinal osteoid osteoma.* Radiology 92:1192, 1969.
21. **Gamba JL, Martinez S, Apple J, et al.:** *Computed tomography of axial skeletal osteoid osteomas.* AJR 142:769, 1984.
22. **Yochum TR:** *Reactive sclerosis of a pedicle due to unilateral spondylolysis—A case study.* ACA J Chiro, 1980.
23. **Albers VL:** *Congenital absence of a lumbar pedicle with sclerosis and hypertrophy of the contralateral pedicle.* ACA J Chiro, 1984.
24. **Yochum TR:** *Case of the missing pedicle* [Roentgen Brief]. ACA Council Roentgenol, Feb 1981.
25. **Lindbom A, Lindvall W, Soderberg G, et al.:** *Angiography in osteoid osteoma.* Acta Radiol 54:327, 1960.
26. **Georgoulis AD, Papageorgiou CD, Moebius UG, et al.:** *The diagnostic dilemma created by osteoid osteoma that presents as knee pain.* Arthroscopy 18(1):32, 2002.
27. **Swee RG, McLeod RA, Beabout JW:** *Osteoid osteoma: Detection, diagnosis, localization.* Radiology 130:117, 1979.
28. **Azouz EM:** *Bone marrow edema in osteoid osteoma* [Letter]. Skeletal Radiol 23:53, 1994.
29. **Spouge AR, Thain LM:** *Osteoid osteoma: MR imaging revisited.* Clin Imaging 24(1):19, 2000.
30. **Ilyas I, Younge DA:** *Medical management of osteoid osteoma.* Can J Surg 45(6):435, 2002.
31. **Torriani M, Rosenthal DI:** *Percutaneous radiofrequency treatment of osteoid osteoma.* Pediatr Radiol 32(8):615, 2002.
32. **Osti OL, Sebben R:** *High-frequency radio-wave ablation of osteoid osteoma in the lumbar spine.* Eur Spine J 7(5):422, 1998.
33. **Vanderschueren GM, Taminiau AH, Obermann WR, Bloem JL:** *Osteiod osteoma: Clinical results with thermocoagulation.* Radiology 224:82, 2002.
34. **Sluga M, Windhager R, Pfeiffer M, et al.:** *Peripheral osteoid osteoma. Is there still place for traditional surgery?* J Bone Joint Surg 84B:249, 2002.
35. **Buhler M, Binkert C, Exner GU:** *Osteoid osteoma: Technique of computed tomography-controlled percutaneous resection using standard equipment available in most orthopaedic operating rooms.* Arch Orthop Trauma Surg 121(8):458, 2001.
36. **Katz K, Kornreich L, David R, et al.:** *Osteoid osteoma: Resection with CT guidance.* Isr Med Assoc J 2(2):151, 2000.
37. **Parlier-Cuau C, Champsaur P, Nizard R, et al.:** *Percutaneous removal of osteoid osteoma.* Radiol Clin North Am 36(3):559, 1998.
38. **Vickers CW, Pugh DC, Ivins JC:** *Osteoid osteoma. A 15-year follow-up of an untreated patient.* J Bone Joint Surg 41A:357, 1959.

Osteoblastoma

1. **Dahlin DC, Johnson EW Jr:** *Giant osteoid osteoma.* J Bone Joint Surg 36A:559, 1954.
2. **Jaffe HL:** *Benign osteoblastoma.* Bull Hosp Joint Dis 17:141, 1956.
3. **Lichtenstein L, Sawyer WR:** *Benign osteoblastoma. Further observations and report of twenty additional cases.* J Bone Joint Surg 46A:755, 1964.
4. **McLeod RA, Dahlin DC, Beabout JW:** *The spectrum of osteoblastoma.* AJR 126:321, 1976.
5. **Mehdian H, Faraj AA, Weatherley C:** *Painful scoliosis secondary to osteoblastoma of the vertebral body.* Eur Spine J 7(3):246, 1998.
6. **Mehta MH, Murray RO:** *Scoliosis provoked by painful vertebral lesions.* Skeletal Radiol 1:223, 1977.
7. **MacClellan DI, Wilson FC Jr:** *Osteoid osteoma of the spine.* J Bone Joint Surg 49A:111, 1967.
8. **Sonel B, Yagmuriu B, Tuncer S, et al.:** *Osteoblastoma of the lumbar spine as a cause of chronic low back pain.* Rheumatol Int 21(6): 253, 2002.
9. **Temple HT, Mizel MS, Murphey MD, Sweet DE:** *Osteoblastoma of the foot and ankle.* Foot Ankle Int 19(10):698, 1998.
10. **Yochum TR:** *Osteoblastoma.* ACA J Chiro, 1982.
11. **Gelberman RH, Olson CO:** *Benign osteoblastoma of the atlas.* J Bone Joint Surg 56A:808, 1974.

12. **Maar D, Dornetzhuber V:** *Benign osteoblastoma ossis tali resembling ostiitis tuberculosa.* Acta Chir Orthop Traumatol Cech 41:362, 1974.
13. **Ronis ML, Obando M, Bucko MI, et al.:** *Benign osteoblastoma of the temporal bone.* Laryngoscope 84:857, 1974.
14. **Borello ED, Sedano HO:** *Giant osteoid osteoma of the maxilla.* Oral Surg 23:563, 1967.
15. **Brady CL, Browne RM:** *Benign osteoblastoma of the mandible.* Cancer 30:329, 1972.
16. **Rosensweig J, Mikail M, Mayman A:** *Benign osteoblastoma: Report of an unusual rib tumor and review of the literature.* Can Med Assoc J 89:1189, 1963.
17. **Schajowicz F, Lemos C:** *Osteoid osteoma and osteoblastoma. Closely related entities of osteoblastic derivation.* Acta Orthop Scand 41:272, 1970.
18. **Marsh BW, Bonfiglio M, Brady LP, et al.:** *Benign osteoblastoma: Range of manifestations.* J Bone Joint Surg 57A:1, 1975.
19. **Pochaczevsky R, Yen YM, Sherman RS:** *The roentgen appearance of benign osteoblastoma.* Radiology 75:429, 1960.

SOLITARY ENCHONDROMA

1. **Takigawa K:** *Chondroma of the bones of the hand—A review of 110 cases.* J Bone Joint Surg 53A:1591, 1971.
2. **Dahlin DC:** *Bone Tumors,* ed 2. Springfield, Charles C Thomas, 1967.
3. **Poznanski AK:** *The Hand in Radiologic Diagnosis.* Philadelphia, WB Saunders, 1974.
4. **Ablove RH, Moy OJ, Peimer CA, Wheeler DR:** *Early verses delayed treatment of enchondroma.* Am J Orthop 29(10):771, 2000.
5. **Levy WM, Aegerter EE, Kirkpatrick JA Jr:** *The nature of cartilaginous tumors.* Radiol Clin North Am 2:327, 1964.
6. **Wilner D:** *Radiology of Bone Tumors and Allied Disorders.* Philadelphia, WB Saunders, 1982.
7. **Montero LM, Ikuta Y, Ishida O, et al.:** *Enchondroma in the hand retrospective study—Recurrence cases.* Hand Surg 7:7, 2002.
8. **Chandy J, Wade PJ, Chen K:** *Malignant transformation of a solitary enchondroma.* Hosp Med 62(3):180, 2001.
9. **Edeiken J:** *Roentgen Diagnosis of Diseases of Bone,* ed 3. Baltimore, Williams & Wilkins, 1981.
10. **Braddock GTF, Hadlow VD:** *Osteosarcoma in enchondromatosis (Ollier's disease). Report of a case.* J Bone Joint Surg 48B:145, 1966.
11. **Lammot TR:** *Enchondroma of the patella. A case report.* J Bone Joint Surg 14A:1230, 1968.
12. **Potdar GG, Srikhande SS:** *Chondrogenic tumors of the jaws.* Oral Surg 30:649, 1970.
13. **Bell MS:** *Benign cartilaginous tumors of the spine.* Br J Surg 58:707, 1971.
14. **Laurence W, Franklin EL:** *Calcifying enchondroma of long bones.* J Bone Joint Surg 35B:224, 1953.
15. **Flemming DJ, Murphey MD:** *Enchondroma and chondrosarcoma.* Semin Musculoskelet Radiol 4(1):59, 2000.
16. **Dobert N, Menzel C, Ludwig R, et al.:** *Enchondroma: A benign osseous lesion with high F-18 FDG uptake.* Clin Nucl Med 27(10):695, 2002.
17. **Hamlin JA, Adler L, Greenbaum EI:** *Central enchondroma—A precursor to chondrosarcoma?* J Can Assoc Radiol 22:206, 1971.
18. **Marco RA, Gitelis S, Brebach GT, Healey JH:** *Cartilage tumors: Evaluation and treatment.* J Am Acad Orthop Surg 8(5):292, 2000.
19. **McVey MJ, Kettner NW:** *Pathologic fracture of metacarpal enchondroma: Case study and differential diagnosis.* J Manipulative Physiol Ther 25(5):340, 2002.
20. **Jewusiak EM, Spence KF, Sell KW:** *Solitary benign enchondroma of the long bones of the hand. Results of curettage and packing with freeze-dried cancellous bone allograft.* J Bone Joint Surg 53A:1587, 1971.
21. **Bickets J, Wittig JC, Kollender Y, et al.:** *Enchondromas of the hand: treatment with curettage and cemented internal fixation.* J Hand Surg 27A:870, 2002.

MULTIPLE ENCHONDROMATOSIS (OLLIER'S DISEASE)

1. **Ollier M:** *Dyschondroplasie.* Lyon Med 93:23, 1900.
2. **Jaffe HL:** *Tumors and Tumorous Conditions of the Bones and Joints.* Philadelphia, Lea & Febiger, 1958.
3. **Huvos AG:** *Bone Tumors—Diagnosis, Treatment and Prognosis.* Philadelphia, WB Saunders, 1979.
4. **Mosher JF:** *Multiple enchondromatosis of the hand. A case report.* J Bone Joint Surg 58A:717, 1976.
5. **Mainzer F, Minagi H, Steinbach HL:** *The variable manifestations of multiple enchondromatosis.* Radiology 99:377, 1971.
6. **Cowan WK:** *Malignant change and multiple metastases in Ollier's disease.* J Clin Pathol 18:650, 1965.
7. **Schwartz HS, Zimmerman MA:** *The malignant potential of enchondromatosis.* J Bone Joint Surg 69A:269, 1987.
8. **Unger EC, Kessler HB, Kowalyshyn MJ, et al.:** *MR imaging of Maffucci syndrome.* AJR 150:351, 1988.
9. **Giannikas AC:** *Treatment of metacarpal enchondromata. Report of three cases.* J Bone Joint Surg 48B:333, 1966.

MAFFUCCI'S SYNDROME

1. **Maffucci A:** *Di un caso di encondroma ed angioma multiplo. Contributione alla genesi embrionale dei tumori.* Mov Med Chir 13:399, 1881.
2. **McDermott AL, Dutt SN, Chavda SV, Morgan DW:** *Maffucci's syndrome: Clinical and radiological features of a rare condition.* J Laryngol Otol 114(10):845, 2001.
3. **Nakamura K, Matsushita T, Haga N, et al.:** *Swelling of the dorsum of the hand and/or foot can be a first sign of Maffacci syndrome.* Arch Orthop Trauma Surg 119:470, 1999.
4. **Howard FM, Lee RE Jr:** *The hand in Maffucci's syndrome.* Arch Surg 103:752, 1971.
5. **Unger EC, Kessler HB, Kowalyshyn MJ, et al.:** *MR imaging of Maffucci syndrome.* AJR 150:351, 1988.
6. **Ahmed SK, Lee WC, Irving RM, Walsh AR:** *Is Ollier's disease an understaging of Maffucci's syndrome?* J Laryngol Otol 113(9):861, 1999.
7. **Kuwahara RT, Skinner RB Jr:** *Maffucci syndrome: a case report.* Cutis 69(1):21, 2002.

PERIOSTEAL CHONDROMA

1. **Lichtenstein L, Hall JE:** *Periosteal chondroma. A distinctive benign cartilage tumor.* J Bone Joint Surg 34a:691, 1952.
2. **Jaffe HL:** *Juxtacortical chondroma.* Bull Hosp Joint Dis 17:20, 1956.
3. **deSantos LA, Spjut HJ:** *Periosteal chondroma: A radiographic spectrum.* Skeletal Radiol 6:15, 1981.
4. **Meyer R:** *Juxtacortical chondroma.* Br J Radiol 31:106, 1958.
5. **Bauer TW, Dorfman HD, Latham JT Jr:** *Periosteal chondroma.* Am J Surg Pathol 6:631, 1982.
6. **Rockwell MA, Saiter ET, Enneking WF:** *Periosteal chondroma.* J Bone Joint Surg 54A:102, 1972.
7. **Boriani S, Bacchini P, Bertoni F, et al.:** *Periosteal chondroma.* J Bone Joint Surg 65A:205, 1983.
8. **Robinson P, White LM, Sundaram M, et al.:** *Periosteal chondroid tumors: radiologic evaluation with pathologic correlation.* AJR Am J Roentgenol 177(5):1183, 2001.
9. **Woertler K, Blasius S, Brinkschmidt C, et al.:** *Periosteal chondroma: MR characteristics.* J Comput Assist Tomogr 25:425, 2001.
10. **Yamamoto T, Nagira K, Kurosaka M:** *Periosteal chondroma presenting as a subcutaneous mass in the thumb.* Clin Imaging 25:432, 2001.

CHONDROBLASTOMA

1. **Masui F, Ushigome S, Kamitani K, et al.:** *Chondroblastoma: A study of 11 cases.* Eur J Surg Oncol 28(8):869, 2002.
2. **Ewing J:** *Neoplastic Diseases. A Treatise on Tumors,* ed 3. Philadelphia, WB Saunders, 1928.
3. **Kolodny A:** *Bone sarcoma.* Surg Gynecol Obstet 44:1, 1927.

4. **Codman EA:** *Epiphyseal chondromatous giant cell tumors of the upper end of the humerus.* Surg Gynecol Obstet 52:543, 1931.

5. **Jaffe HL, Lichtenstein L:** *Benign chondroblastoma of bone. A reinterpretation of the so-called calcifying or chondromatous giant cell tumor.* Am J Pathol 18:969, 1942.

6. **Huvos AG:** *Bone Tumors—Diagnosis, Treatment and Prognosis.* Philadelphia, WB Saunders, 1979.

7. **Kunkel MG, Dahlin DC, Young HH:** *Benign chondroblastoma.* J Bone Joint Surg 38A:817, 1956.

8. **Trebse R, Rotter A, Pisot V:** *Chondroblastoma of the patella associated with and aneurysmal bone cyst.* Acta Orthop Belg 67(3):290, 2001.

9. **Treasure ER:** *Benign chondroblastoma of bone.* J Bone Joint Surg 37B:462, 1955.

10. **McBryde A Jr, Goldner JL:** *Chondroblastoma of bone.* Am Surg 36:94, 1970.

11. **McLeod RA, Beabout JW:** *The roentgenographic features of chondroblastoma.* AJR 118:464, 1973.

12. **Wilner D:** *Radiology of Bone Tumors and Allied Disorders.* Philadelphia, WB Saunders, 1982.

13. **Ilaslan H, Sundaram M, Unni KK:** *Vertebral chondroblastoma.* Skeletal Radiol 32(2):66, 2003.

14. **Kudo T, Okada K, Hirano Y, Sageshima M:** *Chondroblastoma of a metacarpal bone mimicking an aneurysmal bone cyst: A case report and a review of the literature.* Tohoku J Exp Med 194(4):251, 2001.

15. **Neviaser RJ, Wilson JN:** *Benign chondroblastoma of the finger.* J Bone Joint Surg 54A:389, 1972.

16. **Assor D:** *Chondroblastoma of the rib. Report of a case.* J Bone Joint Surg 55A:208, 1973.

17. **Cohen J, Cahen I:** *Benign chondroblastoma of the patella; a case report.* J Bone Joint Surg 45A:824, 1963.

18. **Mercuri M, Casadei R:** *Patellar tumors.* Clin Orthop 389:35, 2001.

19. **Kelikian H, Clayton I:** *Giant cell tumor of the patella.* J Bone Joint Surg 39A:414, 1957.

20. **Mirra J:** *Bone Tumors, Diagnosis and Treatment.* Philadelphia, JB Lippincott, 1980.

21. **Kahn LB, Wood FM, Ackerman LV:** *Malignant chondroblastoma. Report of two cases and review of the literature.* Arch Pathol 88:371, 1969.

22. **Sirsat MV, Doctor VM:** *Benign chondroblastoma of bone: Report of a case of malignant transformation.* J Bone Joint Surg 52B:741, 1970.

23. **Rischke B, Engels C, Pietsch E, et al.:** *[Chondroblastoma of the patella with pathological fracture]* Unfallchirurg 103:898, 2000.

24. **Otsuka T, Kobayashi M, Yonezawa M, et al.:** *Treatment of chondroblastoma of the calcaneus with a secondary aneurysmal bone cyst using endoscopic curettage without bone grafting.* Arthroscopy 18(4):430, 2002.

25. **Greenfield GB:** *Radiology of Bone Diseases,* ed 3. Philadelphia, JB Lippincott, 1980.

26. **Edeiken J:** *Roentgen Diagnosis of Diseases of Bone,* ed 3. Baltimore, Williams & Wilkins, 1981.

27. **Oxtoby JW, Davies AM:** *MRI characteristics of chondroblastoma.* Clin Radiol 51(1):22, 1996.

28. **Braunstein E, Martel W, Weatherbee L:** *Periosteal bone apposition in chondroblastoma.* Skeletal Radiol 4:34, 1979.

29. **Brower AC, Moser RP, Kransdorf MJ:** *The frequency and diagnostic significance of periostitis in chondroblastoma.* AJR 154:309, 1990.

30. **Crim JR, Gold RH, Mirra JM, Eckardt J:** *Case report 748: Chondroblastoma of the femur with an aneurysmal bone cyst.* Skeletal Radiol 21(6):403, 1992.

31. **Varma BP, Gupta IM:** *Atypical chondroblastoma of tibia. Report of recurrent lesion.* Clin Orthop 89:241, 1972.

32. **Blitch E, Mendicino RW:** *Chondroblastoma of the calcaneus: literature review and case presentation.* J Foot Ankle Surg 35(3):250, 1996

33. **Ramappa AJ, Lee FY, Tang P, et al.:** *Chondroblastoma of bone.* J Bone Joint Surg 82A(8):1140, 2000.

34. **Erickson JK, Rosenthal DI, Zaleske DJ, et al.:** *Primary treatment of chondroblastoma with percutaneous radio-frequency heat ablation: Report of three cases.* Radiology 221(2):463, 2001.

CHONDROMYXOID FIBROMA

1. **Jaffe HL, Lichtenstein L:** *Chondromyxoid fibroma of bone. A distinctive benign tumor likely to be mistaken especially for chondrosarcoma.* Arch Pathol 45:541, 1948.

2. **Schajowicz F, Gallardo H:** *Chondromyxoid fibroma (fibromyxoid chondroma) of bone.* J Bone Joint Surg 53B:198, 1971.

3. **Feldman F, Hecht HL, Johnston AD:** *Chondromyxoid fibroma of bone.* Radiology 94:249, 1970.

4. **Huvos AG:** *Bone Tumors—Diagnosis, Treatment and Prognosis.* Philadelphia, WB Saunders, 1979.

5. **Durr HR, Lienemann A, Nerlich A, et al.:** *Chondromyxoid fibroma of bone.* Arch Orthop Trauma Surg 120:42, 2000.

6. **Rahimi A, Beabout JW, Ivins JC, et al.:** *Chondromyxoid fibroma: A clinicopathologic study of 76 cases.* Cancer 30:726, 1972.

7. **Greenfield GB:** *Radiology of Bone Diseases,* ed 3. Philadelphia, JB Lippincott, 1980.

8. **Wilson AJ, Kyriakos M, Ackerman LV:** *Chondromyxoid fibroma: Radiographic appearance in 38 cases and in a review of the literature.* Radiology 179:513, 1991.

9. **Hau MA, Fox EJ, Rosenberg AE, Mankin HJ:** *Chondromyxoid fibroma of the metacarpal.* Skeletal Radiol 30:719, 2001.

10. **Lopez-Ben R, Siegal GP, Hadley MN:** *Chondromyxoid fibroma of the cervical spine: Case report.* Neurosurgery 50(2):409, 2002.

11. **Feit EM, Dobbs BM:** *Chondromyxoid fibroma of the fourth metatarsal.* J Am Posdiatr Med Assoc 90(4):211, 2000.

12. **Ralph LL:** *Chondromyxoid fibroma of bone.* J Bone Joint Surg 44B:7, 1962.

13. **Turcotte B, Pugh DG, Dahlin DC:** *The roentgenologic aspects of chondromyxoid fibroma of bone.* AJR 87:1085, 1962.

14. **Murphy NB, Price CHG:** *The radiological aspects of chondromyxoid fibroma of bone.* Clin Radiol 22:261, 1971.

15. **Beggs IG, Stoker DJ:** *Chondromyxoid fibroma of bone.* Clin Radiol 33:671, 1982.

16. **Park SH, Kong KY, Chung HW, et al.:** *Juxtacortical chondromyxoid fibroma arising in an apophysis.* Skeletal Radiol 29:466, 2000.

FIBROUS XANTHOMA OF BONE: NON-OSSIFYING FIBROMA

1. **Lefebvre J, Hassan M:** *Fibromes non ossifiants.* Rev Prat 19:2133, 1969.

2. **Adams JP, Goldner JL:** *Fibrous lesions of bone.* South Med J 46:529, 1953.

3. **Jaffe HL:** *Tumors and Tumorous Conditions of the Bones and Joints.* Philadelphia, Lea & Febiger, 1948.

4. **Dahlin DC:** *Bone Tumors,* ed 3. Springfield, Charles C Thomas, 1978.

5. **Aegerter E, Kirkpatrick JA Jr:** *Orthopedic Diseases,* ed 4. Philadelphia, WB Saunders, 1975.

6. **Compere CL, Coleman SS:** *Nonosteogenic fibroma of bone.* Surg Gynecol Obstet 105:588, 1957.

7. **Caffey J:** *On fibrous defects in cortical walls of growing tubular bones.* Adv Pediatr 7:13, 1955.

8. **Maudsley RH, Stansfeld AG:** *Nonosteogenic fibroma of bone.* J Bone Joint Surg 38B:714, 1956.

9. **Drennan DB, Maylahn DJ, Fahey JJ:** *Fractures through large nonossifying fibromas.* Clin Orthop 103:82, 1974.

10. **Young JWR, Levine AM, Dorfman HD:** *Nonossifying fibroma of the tibia [Case Report 293].* Skeletal Radiol 12:294, 1984.

11. **Goodnough CP, Kuhlmann RP, Stark E:** *Von Recklinghausen's neurofibromatosis—With nonosteogenic fibroma.* NY State J Med 75:2407, 1975.

12. **Kumar R, Swischuk LE, Madewell JE:** *Benign cortical defect: Site for an avulsion fracture.* Skeletal Radiol 15:553, 1986.

13. **Brenner RJ, Hattner RS, Lilien D:** *Scintigraphic features of nonosteogenic fibroma.* Radiology 131:727, 1979.
14. **Jee WH, Choe BY, Kang HS, et al.:** *Nonossifying fibroma: Characteristics at MR imaging with pathologic correlation.* Radiology 209:197, 1998.
15. **Arata MA, Peterson HA, Dahlin DC:** *Pathological fractures through nonossifying fibromas.* J Bone Joint Surg 63A:980, 1981.

FIBROUS XANTHOMA OF BONE: FIBROUS CORTICAL DEFECTS
1. **Caffey J:** *On fibrous defects in cortical walls of growing tubular bones.* Adv Pediatr 7:13, 1955.
2. **Sontag LW, Pyle SI:** *The appearance and nature of cystlike areas in the distal femoral metaphysis of children.* AJR 46:185, 1941.
3. **Marek FM:** *Fibrous cortical defect.* Bull Hosp Joint Dis 16:77, 1955.
4. **Moser RP, Sweet DE, Haseman DB, et al.:** *Multiple skeletal fibroxanthomas: Radiologic-pathologic correlation of 72 cases.* Skeletal Radiol 16:353, 1987.
5. **Goodnough CP, Kuhlmann RP, Stark E:** *Von Recklinghausen's neurofibromatosis—With nonosteogenic fibroma.* NY State J Med 75:2407, 1975.
6. **Bullough PG, Walley J:** *Fibrous cortical defect and nonossifying fibroma.* Postgrad Med J 41:672, 1965.

SIMPLE BONE CYST
1. **Jaffe HL, Lichtenstein L:** *Solitary unicameral bone cyst, with emphasis on the roentgen picture, the pathologic appearance and the pathogenesis.* Arch Surg 44:1, 1942.
2. **Mirra JM:** *Bone Tumors—Diagnosis and Treatment.* Philadelphia, JB Lippincott, 1980.
3. **Margau R, Babyn P, Cole W, et al.:** *MR imaging of simple bone cysts in children: Not so simple.* Pediatr Radiol 30(8):551, 2000.
4. **Jaffe HL:** *Tumors and Tumorous Conditions of the Bones and Joints.* Philadelphia, Lea & Febiger, 1958.
5. **Garceau GJ, Gregory CF:** *Solitary unicameral bone cyst.* J Bone Joint Surg 36A:267, 1954.
6. **Rowe LJ, Brandt JR:** *Simple bone cysts in athletes.* Chiro Sports Med 2:33, 1988.
7. **Wilner D:** *Radiology of Bone Tumors and Allied Disorders.* Philadelphia, WB Saunders, 1982.
8. **Hagberg S:** *The solitary bone cyst.* Acta Chir Scand 138:25, 1967.
9. **Shulman HS, Wilson SR, Cruickshank KB, et al.:** *Unicameral bone cyst in a rib of a child.* AJR 128:1058, 1977.
10. **Abdelwahab IF, Lewis MM, Klein MJ, et al.:** *Simple (solitary) bone cyst of the calcaneus. Case report 515.* Skeletal Radiol 17: 607, 1989.
11. **Jaffe HL, Lichtenstein L:** *Solitary unicameral bone cyst.* J Bone Joint Surg 36A:267, 1954.
12. **Johnson LC, Vetter H, Putschar WGJ:** *Sarcomas arising in bone cysts.* Virchows Arch Pathol Anat 335:428, 1962.
13. **McGlynn FJ, Mickelson MR, El-Khoury GY:** *The fallen fragment sign in unicameral bone cyst.* Clin Orthop 156:157, 1981.
14. **Reynolds J:** *The "fallen fragment sign" in the diagnosis of unicameral bone cysts.* Radiology 92:949, 1969.
15. **Keats TE, Harrison RB:** *The calcaneal nutrient foramen: A useful sign in the differentiation of true from simulated cysts.* Skeletal Radiol 3:239, 1979.
16. **Bonnel F, Canovas F, Faure P:** *Treatment of a simple bone cyst of the calcaneus by endoscopic curettage with cancellous bone injection.* Acta Orthop Belg 65(4):528, 1999.
17. **Killian JT, Wilkinson L, White S, Brassard M:** *Treatment of unicameral bone cyst with demineralized bone matrix.* J Pediatr Orthop 18(5):621, 1998.
18. **Rougraff BT, Kling TJ:** *Treatment of active unicameral bone cysts with percutaneous injection of demineralized bone matrix and autogenous bone marrow.* J Bone Joint Surg 84A(6):921, 2002.
19. **Smith RW, Smith CF:** *Solitary unicameral bone cyst of the calcaneus.* J Bone Joint Surg 56A:49, 1974.
20. **Capanna R, Albisinni U, Campanacci M, et al.:** *Contrast examination as a prognostic factor in the treatment of solitary bone cyst by cortisone injection.* Skeletal Radiol 12:97, 1984.
21. **Capanna R, DalMonte A, Campanacci M:** *The natural history of unicameral bone cyst after steroid injection.* Clin Orthop 166:204, 1982.
22. **Scaglietti O, Marchetti PG, Bartolozzi P:** *Final results obtained in the treatment of bone cysts with methylprednisolone acetate (depomedral) and a discussion of results achieved in other bone lesions.* Clin Orthop 165:33, 1982.

ANEURYSMAL BONE CYST
1. **Papagelopoulos PJ, Choudhury SN, Frassica FJ, et al.:** *Treatment of aneurysmal bone cysts of the pelvis and sacrum.* J Bone Joint Surg 83A:1674, 2001.
2. **Ewing J:** *Neoplastic Diseases: A Treatise on Tumors,* ed 4. Philadelphia, WB Saunders, 1940.
3. **Jaffe HL, Lichtenstein L:** *Solitary unicameral bone cyst, with emphasis on the roentgen picture, the pathologic appearance, and the pathogenesis.* Arch Surg 44:1, 1942.
4. **Carson DH, Wilkinson RH, Bhakkaviziam A:** *Aneurysmal bone cysts in children.* AJR 116:644, 1972.
5. **Donaldson WF:** *Aneurysmal bone cyst.* J Bone Joint Surg 44A:25, 1962.
6. **Tillman BP, Dahlin DC, Lipscomb PR, et al.:** *Aneurysmal bone cyst: An analysis of ninety-five cases.* Mayo Clin Proc 43:478, 1968.
7. **Bollini G, Jouve JL, Cottalorda J, et al.:** *Aneurysmal bone cyst in children: analysis of twenty-seven patients.* J Pediatr Orthop B 7:274, 1998.
8. **Chen SH, Huang TJ, Hsueh S, et al.:** *Unusual bleeding of aneurysmal bone cyst in the upper thoracic spine.* Chang Gung Med J 25(3): 183, 2002.
9. **Chan MS, Wong YC, Yuen MK, Lam D:** *Spinal aneurysmal bone cyst causing acute cord compression without vertebral collapse: CT and MRI findings.* Pediatr Radiol 32(8):601, 2002.
10. **Besse BE Jr, Dahlin DC, Pugh DG, et al.:** *Aneurysmal bone cysts: Additional considerations.* Clin Orthop 7:93, 1956.
11. **Wilner D:** *Radiology of Bone Tumors and Allied Disorders.* Philadelphia, WB Saunders, 1982.
12. **Hay MC, Paterson D, Taylor TKF:** *Aneurysmal bone cysts of the spine.* J Bone Joint Surg 60B:406, 1978.
13. **Burkhalter WC, Schroeder FC, Eversmann WW Jr:** *Aneurysmal bone cysts occurring in the metacarpals.* J Hand Surg 3:579, 1978.
14. **Yochum TR:** *The aneurysmal bone cyst (fibula).* ACA J Chiro, 1982.
15. **Faris WF, Rubin BD, Fielding JW:** *Aneurysmal bone cyst of the patella.* J Bone Joint Surg 60A:711, 1978.
16. **Burns-Cox CJ, Higgins AT:** *Aneurysmal bone cyst of the frontal bone.* J Bone Joint Surg 51B:344, 1969.
17. **Hino N, Ohtsuka K, Hashimoto M, Sakata M:** *Radiographic features of an aneurysmal bone cyst of the orbit.* Ophthalmologica 212(3):198, 1998.
18. **Bossart PA, Fitzpatrick HF:** *Aneurysmal bone cyst of rib.* Arch Surg 88:229, 1964.
19. **DiCaprio MR, Murphy MJ, Camp RL:** *Aneurysmal bone cyst of the spine with familial incidence.* Spine 25(12):1589, 2000.
20. **Mirra JM:** *Bone Tumors—Diagnosis and Treatment.* Philadelphia, JB Lippincott, 1980.
21. **Vilanova JC, Dolz JL, Maestro de Leon JL, et al.:** *MR imaging of a malignant schwannoma and an osteoblastoma with fluid-fluid levels. Report of two new cases.* Eur Radiol 8(8):1359, 1998.
22. **Munk PL, Helms CA, Holt RG, et al.:** *MR imaging of aneurysmal bone cysts.* AJR 153:99, 1989.
23. **Otsuka T, Kobayashi M, Sekiya I, et al.:** *A new treatment of aneurysmal bone cyst by endoscopic curettage without bone grafting.* Arthroscopy 17(7):E28, 2001.
24. **Ramirez N, Perez C, Rivera YC:** *Distal third fibular aneurysmal bone cyst: en bloc resection and proximal third fibular reconstruction.* Am J Orthop 30(3):237, 2001.

25. **Garg NK, Carty H, Walsh HP, et al.:** *Percutaneous Ethibloc injection in aneurysmal bone cysts.* Skeletal Radiol 29(4):211, 2000.
26. **Gladden ML Jr, Gillingham BL, Hennrikus W, Vaughan LM:** *Aneurysmal bone cyst of the first cervical vertebrae in a child treated with percutaneous intralesional injection of calcitonin and methylprednisolone. A case report.* Spine 25:527, 2000. [Discussion 25:531, 2000.]
27. **Murray RO, Jacobson HG:** *The Radiology of Skeletal Disorders,* ed 2. London, Churchill Livingston, 1977.

INTRAOSSEOUS LIPOMA

1. **Yamamoto T, Akisue T, Marui T, et al.:** *Intraosseous lipoma of the humeral head: MR appearance.* Clin Imaging 25:428, 2001.
2. **Yildiz HY, Altinok D, Saglik Y:** *Bilateral calcaneal intraosseous lipoma: A case report.* Foot Ankle Int 23(1):60, 2002.
3. **DeLee JC:** *Intraosseous lipoma of the proximal part of the femur.* J Bone Joint Surg 61A:601, 1973.
4. **Hart JAL.:** *Intraosseous lipoma.* J Bone Joint Surg 55B:624, 1973.
5. **Smith WE, Feinberg R:** *Intraosseous lipoma of bone.* Cancer 10:1151, 1957.
6. **Onguru O, Pabuccu Y, Celasun B:** *Intraosseous lipoma of the fibula.* Clin Imaging 26(1):55, 2002.
7. **Weinfeld GD, Yu GV, Good JJ:** *Intraosseous lipoma of the calcaneus: a review and report of four cases.* J Foot Ankle Surg 41(6): 398, 2002.
8. **Milgram JW:** *Intraosseous lipomas: Radiologic and pathologic manifestations.* Radiology 167:155, 1988.
9. **Matsubayashi T, Nakajima M, Tskada M:** *Intraosseous lipoma* [Case Report 118]. Skeletal Radiol 5:131, 1980.
10. **Milgram JW:** *Involuted intraosseous lipoma of the sacrum.* Spine 16:243, 1991.
11. **Poussa M, Holmstrom T:** *Intraosseous lipoma of the calcaneus.* Acta Orthop Scand 47:570, 1976.
12. **Bertram C, Popken F, Rutt J:** *Intraosseous lipoma of the calcaneus.* Langenbecks Arch Surg 386(5):313, 2001.
13. **Appenzeller J, Weitzner S:** *Intraosseous lipoma of the os calcis.* Clin Orthop 101:171, 1974.
14. **Ketyer S, Brownstein S, Cholankeril J:** *CT diagnosis of intraosseous lipoma of the calcaneus.* J Comput Assist Tomogr 7(3):546, 1983.
15. **Hatori M, Hosaka M, Ehara S, Kokubun S:** *Imaging features of intraosseous lipomas of the calcaneus.* Arch Orthop Trauma Surg 121(8):429, 2001.
16. **Goldman AB, Marcove RC, Huvos AG, et al.:** *Intraosseous lipoma of the tibia* [Case Report 280]. Skeletal Radiol 12:209, 1984.

TUMOR-LIKE PROCESSES

PAGET'S DISEASE

1. **Paget J:** *On a form of chronic inflammation of bones (osteitis deformans).* Med Chir Trans 60:37, 1877. [Rpt Clin Orthop 49:12, 1966.]
2. **Schmorl G:** *über ostitis deformans Paget.* Virchows Arch Pathol Anat Physiol 283:694, 1932.
3. **Siris E:** *Epidemiological aspects of Paget's disease: Family history and relationship to other medical conditions.* Semin Arthritis Rheum 23:222, 1994.
4. **Rosenbaum HD, Hanson DJ:** *Geographical variation in the prevalence of Paget's disease of bone.* Radiology 92:959, 1969.
5. **Guyer PB:** *Research into Paget's disease—Clues to the etiology and clinical significance.* Radiography 48:185, 1982.
6. **Barry HC:** *Paget's Disease of Bone.* London, Churchill Livingstone, 1969.
7. **Butlin T:** *Pathological Society of London—Osteitis deformans.* Lancet 1:519, 1885.
8. **Hutchinson J:** *On osteitis deformans.* Illus Med News 2:169, 1889.
9. **Naiken VS:** *Did Beethoven have Paget's disease?* Ann Intern Med 74:995, 1971.
10. **Edeiken J:** *Roentgen Diagnosis of Disease of Bone,* ed 3. Baltimore, Williams & Wilkins, 1981.

11. **Berman L:** *The endocrine treatment of Paget's disease.* Endocrinology 16:109, 1932.
12. **Luxton RW:** *Paget's disease of bone associated with Hashimoto's stroma lymphomatosa. A clue to the pathogenesis of Paget's disease.* Lancet 1:441, 1957.
13. **Francis MJO, Smith R:** *Evidence of a generalized connective tissue defect in Paget's disease of bone.* Lancet 1:841, 1974.
14. **Moore S:** *Osteitis deformans. A theory of its etiology.* J Bone Joint Surg 33A:421, 1951.
15. **Rassmussen H, Bordier P:** *The Physiology and Cellular Basis of Metabolic Bone Disease.* Baltimore, Williams & Wilkins, 1974.
16. **Albright F, Reifenstein EC Jr:** *The Parathyroid Glands and Metabolic Bone Disease. Selected Studies.* Baltimore, Williams & Wilkins, 1948.
17. **Mills BG, Singer FR:** *Nuclear inclusions in Paget's disease of bone.* Science 194:201, 1976.
18. **Rima BK:** *Paramyxoviruses and their role in disease.* Semin Arthritis Rheum 23:230, 1994.
19. **Welsh RA, Meyer AT:** *Nuclear fragmentations and associated fibrils in giant cell tumor of bone.* Lab Invest 22:63, 1970.
20. **Smith SE, Murphey MD, Motamedi K, et al.:** *From the archives of the AFIP. Radiologic spectrum of Paget's disease of bone and its complications with pathologic correlation.* Radiographics 22:1191, 2002.
21. **Edeiken J, DePalma AF, Hodes PJ:** *Paget's disease: Osteitis deformans.* Clin Orthop 146:141, 1966.
22. **Schneider D, Hofmann MT, Peterson JA:** *Diagnosis and treatment of Paget's disease of bone.* Am Fam Physician 65(10):2069, 2002.
23. **Dalinka MK, Aronchik JM, Haddad JG Jr:** *Paget's disease.* Orthop Clin North Am 14:243, 1983.
24. **Steinbach HL:** *Some features of Paget's disease.* AJR 86:950, 1961.
25. **Snapper I:** *Bone Diseases in Medical Practice,* ed 3. New York, Grune & Stratton, 1957.
26. **Siris ES, Jacobs JP, Canfield RE:** *Paget's disease of bone.* Bull NY Acad Med 56:285, 1980.
27. **Jaffe HL:** *The classic Paget's disease of bone.* Clin Orthop 127:4, 1977.
28. **Pryce AP, Wiener SN:** *Syringomyelia associated with Paget's disease of the skull.* AJR 155:881, 1990.
29. **Theros EG:** *Professional Self-Evaluation and Continuing Education Program, Set 2: Bone disease syllabus, ACR.* Chicago, Waverly Press, 1972.
30. **Yochum TR:** *Paget's disease—A clinical review.* J Clin Chiro 3(2):68, 1980.
31. **Hadjipavlou AG, Gaitanis LN, Katonis PG, Lander P:** *Paget's disease of the spine and its management.* Eur Spine J 10(5):370, 2001.
32. **Clarke PR:** *Neurological manifestations of Paget's disease.* J Neurol Sci 38:171, 1978.
33. **Ramaamurthi B, Visvanathan GS:** *Paget's disease of the axis causing quadraplegia.* J Neurosurg 14:580, 1957.
34. **Klenerman L:** *Cauda equina and spinal cord compression in Paget's disease.* J Bone Joint Surg 48B:365, 1966.
35. **Alpers BJ, Mancall EL:** *Clinical Neurology,* ed 6. Philadelphia, FA Davis, 1971.
36. **Clarke PR, Williams HI:** *Ossification in extradural fat in Paget's disease of the spine.* Br J Surg 62:571, 1975.
37. **Hadjipavlou A, Shaffer N, Lander P, et al.:** *Pagetic spinal stenosis with extradural pagetoid ossification.* Spine 13:128, 1988.
38. **Aegerter E, Kirkpatrick JA:** *Orthopedic Diseases,* ed 4. Philadelphia, WB Saunders, 1975.
39. **Machtey I, Rodnan GP, Benedek TG:** *Paget's disease of the hip joint.* Am J Med Sci 251:524, 1966.
40. **Altman RD:** *Articular complications of Paget's disease of bone.* Semin Arthritis Rheum 23:248, 1994.
41. **Lander P, Hadjipavlou A:** *Intradiscal invasion of Paget's disease of the spine.* Spine 16:46, 1991.
42. **Paget J:** *Remarks on osteitis deformans.* Illus Med News 2:181, 1889.

43. **Yochum TR:** *Paget's sarcoma of bone.* Radiologe 24:428, 1984.
44. **McKenna RJ, Schwinn CP, Soong KY, et al.:** *Osteogenic sarcoma arising in Paget's disease.* Cancer 17:42, 1964.
45. **Porretta CA, Dahlin DC, Janes JM:** *Sarcoma in Paget's disease of bone.* J Bone Joint Surg 39A:1314, 1957.
46. **Schajowicz F, Aravjo ES, Berenstein A:** *Sarcoma complicating Paget's disease of bone.* J Bone Joint Surg 65B:299, 1983.
47. **Huang TL, Cohen NJ, Sahgal S, et al.:** *Osteosarcoma complicating Paget's disease.* Clin Orthop 141:50, 1979.
48. **Dehner LP, Anderson JT, Brown D:** *Orthopedic and pathologic aspects of Paget's disease.* Minn Med 60:422, 1977.
49. **Jattiot F, Goupille P, Azais I, et al.:** *Fourteen cases of sarcomatous degeneration in Paget's disease.* J Rheumatol 26(1):150, 1999.
50. **Friedman AC, Orcutt J, Madewell JE:** *Paget's disease of the hand: Radiographic spectrum.* AJR 138:691, 1982.
51. **Rubin RP, Adler JJ, Adler DP:** *Paget's disease of the calcaneus.* J Am Pod Assoc 73:263, 1983.
52. **Weinert CR, Wiss DA:** *Paget's disease of the patella.* Clin Orthop 142:139, 1979.
53. **Brown HP, LaRocca H, Wickstrom JK:** *Paget's disease of the atlas and axis.* J Bone Joint Surg 53A:1441, 1971.
54. **Yochum TR:** *Cervical Paget's disease.* ACA J Chiro 1982.
55. **Hadley LA:** *Anatomico—Roentgenographic Studies of the Spine,* ed 3. Springfield, Charles C Thomas, 1976.
56. **Krane SM:** *Paget's disease of bone.* Clin Orthop 127:24, 1977.
57. **Wilner D, Sherman RS:** *Roentgen diagnosis of Paget's disease (osteitis deformans).* Med Radiogr Photogr 42:35, 1966.
58. **Miller SW, Castronovo FP Jr, Pendergrass HP, et al.:** *Technetium 99m labeled diphosphonate bone scanning in Paget's disease.* Am J Roentgenol Radium Ther Nucl Med 121:177, 1974.
59. **Martin TJ:** *Treatment of Paget's with calcitonins.* Aust NZ J Med 9:36, 1979.

FIBROUS DYSPLASIA

1. **Lichtenstein L:** *Polyostotic fibrous dysplasia.* Arch Surg 36:874, 1938.
2. **Hunter D, Turnbull HL:** *Hyperparathyroidism: Generalized osteitis fibroma.* Br J Surg 32:203, 1931.
3. **Slow IN, Stern D, Friedman EW:** *Osteogenic sarcoma arising in pre-existing fibrous dysplasia: Report of a case.* J Oral Surg 29:126, 1971.
4. **Van Tilburg W:** *Fibrous dysplasia.* In: PJ Vinken, GW Bruyn, eds, *Handbook of Clinical Neurology.* Vol 14, Amsterdam, North Holland, 1972.
5. **Van Horn PE Jr, Dahlin DC, Bickel WH:** *Fibrous dysplasia: A clinical pathologic study of orthopedic surgical cases.* Proc Mayo Clin 38:175, 1963.
6. **Lichtenstein L, Jaffe HL:** *Fibrous dysplasia of bone.* Arch Pathol 33:777, 1942.
7. **Uehlinger E:** *Fibrose dysplasia.* In: HR Schinz, WE Baensch, W Frommhold, et al., eds, *Lehrbuch der R;auontgendiagnostik,* ed 6. Stuttgart, Georg Thieme Verlag, 1979.
8. **Harris WH, Dudley HR Jr, Barry JR:** *Natural history of fibrous dysplasia.* J Bone Joint Surg 44A:207, 1962.
9. **Fries JW:** *The roentgen features of fibrous dysplasia of the skull and facial bones: A critical analysis of thirty-nine pathologically proven cases.* AJR 77:71, 1957.
10. **Isefuku S, Hatori M, Ehara S, et al.:** *Fibrous dysplasia arising from the calcaneus.* Tohoku J Exp Med 189(3):227, 1999.
11. **Resnik CS, Lininger JR:** *Monostotic fibrous dysplasia of the cervical spine: Case report.* Radiology 151:49, 1984.
12. **Hopf M:** *Zur Kenntnis der polyostotischen fibrosen Dysplasie.* Radiol Clin (Basel) 28:129, 1949.
13. **Gurler T, Alper M, Gencosmanoglu R, et al.:** *McCune-Albright syndrome progressing with sever fibrous dysplasia.* J Craniofac Surg 9(1):79, 1998.
14. **Windolz F:** *Cranial manifestations of fibrous lesions of bone.* AJR 58:51, 1947.
15. **Benedict PH:** *Sexual precocity and polyostotic fibrous dysplasia.* Am J Dis Child 111:426, 1966.
16. **Keijser LC, Van Tienen TG, Schreuder HW, et al.:** *Fibrous dysplasia of bone: management and outcome of 20 cases.* J Surg Oncol 76:157, 2001. [Discussion 767:167, 2001.]
17. **Di Leo C, Ardemagni A, Bestetti A, et al.:** *A rare case of poly-ostotic fibrous dysplasia assessed by bone scintigraphy with Tc-99m methylene diphosphonate (MDP).* Nuklearmedizin 38(5):169, 1999.
18. **Yucel OT, Genc E, Kaya S:** *Cherubism: A radiological and clinical presentation.* Turk J Pediatr 40(3):453, 1998.
19. **Cornelius EA, McClenden JL:** *Cherubism—Hereditary fibrous dysplasia of the jaws.* AJR 104:136, 1969.
20. **Jones WA, Gerrie J, Pritchard J:** *Cherubism—A familial fibrous dysplasia of the jaws.* J Bone Joint Surg 32B:334, 1950.
21. **Yamaguchi T, Dorfman HD, Eisig S:** *Cherubism: Clinicopathologic features.* Skeletal Radiol 28:350, 1999.
22. **Sirvanci M, Karaman K, Onoat L, et al.:** *Monostatic fibrous dysplasia of the clivus: MRI and CT findings.* Neuroradiology 44(10): 847, 2002.
23. **Cohen MM Jr, Howell RE:** *Etiology of fibrous dysplasia and McCune-Albright syndrome.* Int J Oral Maxillofac Surg 28(5):366, 1999.
24. **Reed RJ:** *Fibrous dysplasia of bone.* Arch Pathol 75:480, 1963.
25. **Aegerter EE, Kirkpatrick JA Jr:** *Orthopedic Diseases,* ed 3. Philadelphia, WB Saunders, 1968.
26. **Kaushik S, Smoker WR, Frable WJ:** *Malignant transformation of fibrous dysplasia into chondroblastic osteosarcoma.* Skeletal Raiol 31:103, 2002.
27. **Coley RL, Stewart FW:** *Bone sarcoma in polyostotic fibrous dysplasia.* Ann Surg 121:872, 1945.
28. **Huvos AG, Higinbotham NL, Miller TR:** *Bone sarcomas arising in fibrous dysplasia.* J Bone Joint Surg 54A:1047, 1972.
29. **Edeiken J:** *Roentgen Diagnosis of Diseases of Bone,* ed 3. Baltimore, Williams & Wilkins, 1981.
30. **Gibson MJ, Middlemiss JH:** *Fibrous dysplasia of bone.* Br J Radiol 44:1, 1971.
31. **Murray RO, Jacobson HG:** *The Radiology of Skeletal Disorders,* ed 2. London, Churchill Livingstone, 1977.
32. **Han J, Ryu JS, Shin MJ, et al.:** *Fibrous dysplasia with barely increased uptake on bone scan: a case report.* Clin Nucl Med 25(10): 785, 2000.
33. **Tehranzadeh J, Fung Y, Donohue M, et al.:** *Computed tomography of Paget's disease of the skull versus fibrous dysplasia.* Skeletal Radiol 27:664, 1998.

NEUROFIBROMATOSIS

1. **Korf BR:** *Diagnosis and management of neurofibromatosis type 1.* Curr Neurol Neurosci Rep 1(2):162, 2001.
2. **Tiresius TWC:** *Historia Pathologica Singularius Cutis Turpitudinis.* Leipzig, SL Crusius, 1793.
3. **Smith RW:** *A Treatise on the Pathology, Diagnosis and Treatment of Neuroma.* Dublin, Hodges & Smith, 1849.
4. **von Recklinghausen K:** *Über die Multiplen Fibrome der Haut und ihre Beziehung zu den Multiplen Neuromen.* Berlin, A Hirschwald, 1882.
5. **Crowe FW, Schull WJ, Neel JV:** *A Clinical, Pathological, and Genetic Study of Multiple Neurofibromatosis.* Springfield, Charles C Thomas, 1956.
6. **Albright F, Reifenstein EC Jr:** *The Parathyroid Glands and Metabolic Bone Disease: Selected Studies.* Baltimore, Williams & Wilkins, 1948.
7. **Yochum TR:** *Neurofibromatosis or von Recklinghausen's disease.* ACA J Chiro 1980.
8. **Wilner D:** *Radiology of Bone Tumors and Allied Disorders.* Philadelphia, WB Saunders, 1982.
9. **Blitz NM, Hutchinson B, Grabowski MV:** *Pedal plixiform neurofibroma: Review of the literature and case report.* J Foot Ankle Surg 41(2):117, 2002.

10. **Korf BR:** *Plexiform neurofibromas.* Am J Med Genet 89(1):31, 1999.
11. **Wiesenfeld D, James PL:** *Pulsating exophthalamos associated with neurofibromatosis.* J Max Fac Surg 12:11, 1984.
12. **Funasaki H, Winter RB, Lonstein JB, et al.:** *Pathophysiology of spinal deformities in neurofibromatosis.* J Bone Joint Surg 76A:692, 1994.
13. **Samoto T, Watanabe Y, Suda A, et al.:** *Atlantoaxial dislocation with neurofibromatosis—A case report.* Orthop Traum Surg 24:289, 1981.
14. **Isu T, Miyasaka K, Abe H:** *Atlantoaxial dislocation associated with neurofibromatosis—Report of three cases.* J Neurosurg 58:451, 1983.
15. **Patel YD, Morehouse HT:** *Neurofibrosarcomas in neurofibromatosis: Role of CT scanning and angiography.* Clin Radiol 33:555, 1982.
16. **Hunt K, Jager RM, Garreston HD, et al.:** *Neurofibrosarcoma complicating von Recklinghausen's disease.* J Kentucky Med Assoc 74:346, 1976.
17. **Holt JF, Wright EM:** *Radiologic features of neurofibromatosis.* Radiology 51:647, 1948.
18. **Edeiken J:** *Roentgen Diagnosis of Diseases of Bone.* ed 3. Baltimore, Williams & Wilkins, 1981.
19. **Casselman ES, Mandell GA:** *Vertebral scalloping in neurofibromatosis.* Radiology 131:89, 1979.
20. **Angtuaco EJC, Binet EF, Flanigan S:** *Value of computed tomographic myelography in neurofibromatosis.* J Neurosurg 13:666, 1983.
21. **Biondetti PR, Vigo M, Fiore D, et al.:** *CT appearance of generalized von Recklinghausen neurofibromatosis.* J Comput Assist Tomogr 5:866, 1983.
22. **Klatte EC, Franken EA, Smith JA:** *The radiographic spectrum in neurofibromatosis.* Semin Roentgenol 11:17, 1976.
23. **Reeder MM, Felson B:** *Gamuts in Radiology.* Cincinnati, Audiovisual Radiology of Cincinnati, 1975.
24. **Treves F:** *Congenital deformity.* Br Med J 2:1140, 1884.
25. **Goodnough CP, Kuhlmann RP, Stark E:** *von Recklinghausen's neurofibromatosis—With nonosteogenic fibroma.* NY State J Med 75:2407, 1975.
26. **Halpern M, Currarino G:** *Vascular lesions causing hypertension in neurofibromatosis.* N Engl J Med 273:248, 1965.

Infection 12

Lindsay J. Rowe and Terry R. Yochum

SUPPURATIVE OSTEOMYELITIS

General Considerations

Skeletal sepsis has always affected humankind, and evidence of skeletal infection has been found in fossil creatures that lived 250 million years ago. (1) Evidence from ancient Egyptian mummies and from skeletons in medieval burial grounds confirms its presence in early times. (2) Nelaton (3) coined the term *osteomyelitis* in 1844. He gave experimental animals intravenous injections of *Staphylococcus* and described the hematogenous osteomyelitis that resulted. (2,3) At that time the mortality among affected children was 30%. (4) The advent of antibiotic therapy has diminished mortality rates to extremely low levels, but late diagnosis or inappropriate management still carries serious consequences. (4)

Incidence

With the advent of modern chemotherapy in the 1930s there has been a significant reduction in deformity and mortality from osteomyelitis. Recently, there has been an increased frequency of osteomyelitis in immunosuppressed patients (cortisone induced, etc.), alcoholics, newborns, and drug addicts. The worldwide incidence of osteomyelitis has been reduced with the introduction of antibiotics. In countries in which the general health standards are low and the population is high, osteomyelitis and its sequelae remain relatively common disorders.

Cause

The list of microorganisms that can invade the osseous structures is long and varied; however, specific species are more frequently found than others. *Staphylococcus aureus* is responsible for approximately 90% of all bone and joint infections. In the immunosuppressed patient (e.g., newborn infant, AIDS patient, alcohol or drug abuser, patient on corticosteroid therapy), organisms other than *Staphylococcus* are more commonly involved; these include *Haemophilus influenzae, Diplococcus pneumoniae, Mycobacterium, Pseudomonas,* fungal, and Gram-negative organisms. *Streptococcus* group B is often the invasive organism in infants when the humerus is involved. (5)

There are four major pathways by which suppurative osteomyelitis invades bone: (6)

- *Hematogenous spread of infection:* This represents a deposition into the bloodstream of organisms that may reach distant skeletal sites. This is the most common source of osteomyelitis.
- *Spread from a contiguous source of infection:* Infection can extend into the bone from an adjacent contaminated site. Cutaneous, sinus, and dental infections are common sites of origin for adjacent osteomyelitis.
- *Direct implantation of infection:* This usually occurs as a result of direct penetrating injuries or puncture wounds, such as would be caused by a nail, splinter, or glass; such infections are most common in the feet. Open fractures are an additional source of direct implantation.
- *Postoperative infection:* Contamination of surgical sites continues to be an important cause of suppurative osteomyelitis.

Clinical Features

The clinical presentation of pyogenic osteomyelitis has changed dramatically since the beginning of modern chemotherapy in the 1930s. Before then, the disease was often an acute, virulent disorder that resulted in death from septic complications before a

1373

diagnosis could be made. Current drug therapies modify the severity, duration, course, and prognosis of suppurative osteomyelitis.

The clinical features of suppurative osteomyelitis vary significantly among infants, young children, and adults. Infants and young patients present with an acute process characterized by fever, chills, pain, and swelling over the affected body part. There is frequently an extensive loss of limb function. Elevated white blood cell counts with a Schilling's shift to the left and an increase in the erythrocyte sedimentation rate (ESR) frequently occur relatively early. The signs and symptoms in an adult patient are often varied and reflect a more chronic or insidious process. The usual mode of presentation is fever, malaise, edema, erythema, and pain over the affected area. Pre-existing infection of other organ systems, most commonly the skin, respiratory tract, and genitourinary tract, is identified in 50% of cases.

Suppurative osteomyelitis occurs most often between the ages of 2 and 12 years, with a 3:1 male predominance, which is thought to be explained by the observation that boys have a greater exposure to trauma. Most commonly, the large tubular bones of the extremities are affected. The femur is the most common bone involved; the tibia, humerus, and radius are also favored sites. Clavicle involvement is rare (7), as is involvement of the pelvis. (8) When involvement of the pelvis does occur it commonly affects the ilium and is rarely preceded by trauma. (8)

A major predisposing factor to the development of suppurative osteomyelitis is intravenous drug addiction, such as heroin. The most common microbes are *Staphylococcus aureus* and *Pseudomonas* (mainliners' syndrome). (9,10) An unusual predilection for the axial skeleton has been noted. The greatest involvement is that of the *S joints:* **s**pine, **s**acroiliac, **s**ymphysis pubis, and **s**ternoclavicular. (6) In addition, diabetic, steroid-immunosuppressed, and hemodialysis patients are all particularly vulnerable (6,11–13). In diabetic patients a *sausage* appearance or deformity of a pedal digit is a reliable physical sign of osteomyelitis. (14)

Pathologic Features

Vascular Anatomy

To better understand the pathologic and radiologic features of suppurative osteomyelitis, a close inspection of the vascular anatomy is essential. The radiologic and pathologic features of osteomyelitis differ in the infant, child, and adult. These differences are inherent to the blood supply of the various vital centers of growth within the bone. (Fig. 12-1)

Infantile Pattern. In infants the fetal vascular compartment may persist in some tubular bones up to the age of 1 year. (6) As a result of this persistence, metaphyseal and diaphyseal vessels may penetrate the physis (growth plate). Trueta (15) found that the vascular barrier at the growth plate became evident at the age of 8 months and was fully formed by the 18th month. Until the age of 8 months, the physis forms no effective barrier to the spread of infection into the epiphyses and the joint. (15) This anatomic relationship explains the high incidence of septic arthritis with epiphyseal involvement in infantile osteomyelitis. (6)

Childhood Pattern. The childhood pattern occurs between 1 year and the time the open physis fuses. The blood flow through the metaphysis is slow and turbulent, creating a natural environment for the proliferation of microbes. No metaphyseal blood vessels penetrate the physis and the epiphyseal blood supply is distinct and separate; therefore, it is easy to understand why there

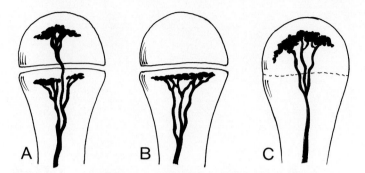

Figure 12-1 NORMAL VASCULAR SUPPLY IN TUBULAR BONES: CHILD, INFANT, AND ADULT. A. Infant. Note that a small percentage of the metaphyseal blood vessels may penetrate the cartilaginous growth plate and supply the epiphysis. **B. Child.** Observe the vascular supply in the metaphysis; it does not cross the growth plate. **C. Adult.** Note that because the growth plate is no longer present, blood supplies to the metaphysis and the distal end of the bone are continuous. (Adapted from **Resnick D, Niwayama G:** *Diagnosis of Bone and Joint Disorders.* Philadelphia, WB Saunders, 1981.)

is a unique predilection for hematogenous osteomyelitis to affect the metaphysis and spare the epiphysis or joint. (6)

Adult Pattern. In the adult, the metaphyseal vessels gradually penetrate the vanishing physis, re-establishing communication between the metaphysis and the subarticular end of the bone (previously the epiphysis). (6) With such vascular communication, organisms may gain rapid access to the subarticular bone and its adjacent joint. This explains the increased incidence of septic arthritis secondary to osteomyelitis in adult patients.

Pathophysiology

Hematogenous osteomyelitis begins in the bone with implantation of the offending organism, usually in the medullary tissues, followed by a vascular and cellular response. Initially, the localized suppurative edema creates an increased intramedullary pressure, resulting in mechanical compression of the capillaries and sinusoids in the marrow cavity. This precipitates infarction of marrow fat, hematopoietic tissue, and bone. Adjacent to the marginal area of infarction there is active hyperemia, as is the case in other soft tissue infarction. The hyperemia is accompanied by osteoclastic activity, which causes focal osteolysis and regional osteoporosis. An inflammatory exudate forms at the margin of the infarct.

Eventually, the inflammatory process penetrates the endosteum (inner cortex) and enters the Haversian and lacunar systems of the bone to reach the subperiosteal space. This process occurs readily in infants because they have few Sharpey's fibers and the periosteum is easily stripped from the bone. This produces exuberant periostitis, owing to the increased pressure in the subperiosteal space. The involvement of periosteal and subperiosteal areas causes a loss of blood supply to the cortical bone, rendering it necrotic. Cortical and medullary infarcts result in the formation of a *sequestrum,* or dead bone (Latin: "to set apart"). (Fig. 12-2) A ring sequestrum may complicate pin tract osteomyelitis. (16) The sequestered bone fragments are usually removed by osteoclasts when small; larger fragments may require surgical removal. As the pus lifts the periosteum, it causes a modest degree of new

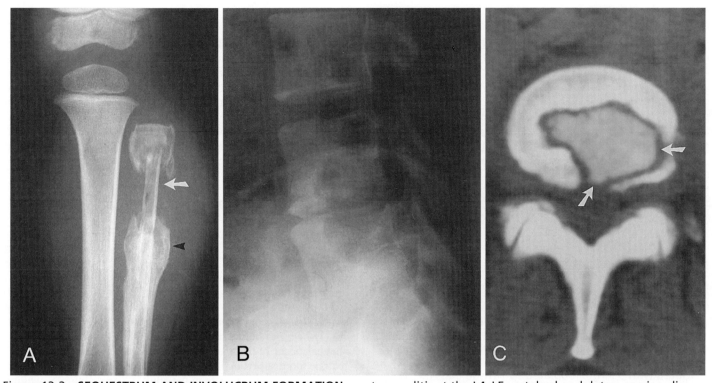

Figure 12-2 **SEQUESTRUM AND INVOLUCRUM FORMATION.**
A. AP Tibia and Fibula. Note the central necrotic bone
(sequestrum) (*arrow*), which is surrounded by an extensive
periosteal collar of new bone (involucrum) (*arrowhead*).
B. Lateral Lumbar Spine. C. Axial CT, L5. Note that the CT
scan nicely demonstrates sequestrum formation in the L5
vertebral body (*arrows*), a rare finding in the spine. This 23-
year-old AIDS patient had *Staphylococcus aureus* osteomyelitis at the L4–L5 vertebral endplates, causing disc
space narrowing and large lytic abscesses in the vertebral
bodies. (Panel A reprinted with permission from the **Center
for Devices and Radiological Health, FDA, and the American
College of Radiology:** *The Learning File, Skeletal Section, SK-
401.* Panels B and C courtesy of Steven P. Brownstein, MD,
Springfield, New Jersey.)

bone proliferation and pain. The periosteal new bone is the body's
attempt to wall off the infective process. This bony collar is
often referred to as an *involucrum* (Latin: "to wrap or cover").
(Fig. 12-2) The thick bony sleeve usually envelops the affected
segment of the shaft; and in cases of extensive lesions, almost the
entire shaft may become encased in involucrum.

The occurrence of a defect that may develop in the involucrum is referred to as a *cloaca*. The function of these defects is
to allow the continued discharge (decompression) of inflammatory products from the bone and has been referred to as *empyema
necessitatis*. (17) These cloacae are most frequently associated
with chronic osteomyelitis, which is stubborn in its response to
conventional antibiotic therapy.

One rare but significant complication of the draining sinus
(cloaca) is the development of a squamous cell carcinoma within
the channel of the cloaca. (6,18) This ulcerative channel and malignant transformation is found only with chronic osteomyelitis
and may be referred to as a *Marjolin's ulcer*. (17,19) (Fig. 12-3)
This lesion is quite deep within the involved limb; the femur and
tibia are the most common sites. A 20- to 30-year latent period
is typical from the onset of osteomyelitis to the development of
neoplasm (6), thus regular biopsies should be performed on all
chronic ulcers for early diagnosis and detection of malignant degeneration. (19) Amputation is often the most reliable treatment
for Marjolin's ulcers. (20)

In more chronic forms of osteomyelitis a thickened irregular
cortex and dense sclerotic bone may surround the focal areas of
osteolytic destruction. In addition, a heavy involucrum is formed,
and the persistent draining sinus allows the infection to seed the
soft tissues chronically. Many patients have chronic osteomyelitis
for years, even with the use of antibiotic therapy.

Radiologic Features

Extremity Involvement

It must be emphasized that there are no radiologic plain film
changes in the early phase of marrow osteomyelitis. The radiographic *latent period* for extremities is approximately 10 days. For
spinal lesions this may approach 3 weeks. The latent period represents the time that it takes for osseous destruction to be appreciated on radiographs. The most accurate means of detecting early
destructive activity is by nuclear bone scan; findings may be positive within the first few hours of the onset of clinical symptoms.
(21–23) The most common radiopharmaceuticals currently used
are technetium–methylene diphosphonate (^{99m}Tc-MDP) and
gallium-67 citrate. Basically, there will be an increased uptake of
radionuclide as a response to the increased inflammation and destruction within the bone within all three phases of the study.

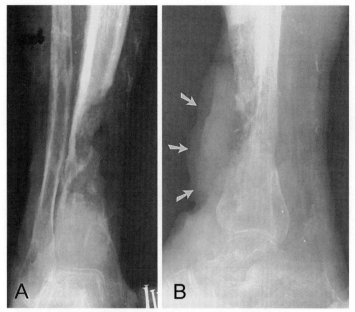

Figure 12-3 MARJOLIN'S ULCER. A. AP Tibia. Note the grossly destructive osteolytic lesion in the diametaphyseal area of the distal tibia. **B. Lateral Tibia.** Observe the lytic destructive lesion on the anterior surface of the tibia, associated with a large, lobulated soft tissue mass (*arrows*). *COMMENT:* Marjolin's ulcer represents the complication of a squamous cell carcinoma developing within the ulcerative channel of the draining sinus (cloaca). This is found only in chronic osteomyelitis and is a rare complication. A 20- to 30-year latent period is typical from the onset of osteomyelitis to the development of neoplasm.

(21,23) This increase in uptake is usually referred to as a *hot spot* on the final image. (21) (Figs. 12-4 and 12-5) Therefore, when there is even a remote clinical suspicion of infection in a patient, a bone scan should be obtained, even if initial radiographs appear normal. T1-weighted MRI studies show low signal, while T2-weighted images show high signal. (24,25) (Fig. 12-6) These MRI features, when involving the juxta-physeal medullary aspect of the bone, are virtually diagnostic of infection in children. (26) The plain film radiographic diagnosis of osteomyelitis is made on the basis of abnormalities in soft tissue and bone, as demonstrated on standard radiographs. (Table 12-1)

Soft Tissue Alterations

Often the earliest radiologic signs of infection involve the soft tissues rather than bone. These signs may be seen within 3 days of the bacterial contamination of the bone. (27) Swelling of the deep soft tissues, usually around the metaphysis in infants and children, may be the earliest radiographic sign. (6) (Fig. 12-7) Such swelling often elevates the lucent fat planes from the adjacent bone. The adjacent edema and cellulitis of the soft tissues will slowly begin to obliterate the myofascial marginal planes. These changes occur in the deep myofascial structures first and then affect the more superficial levels. (27) These soft tissue changes are more difficult to appreciate in the adult. If the soft tissue swelling is immense, it may resemble the mass-like density of a soft tissue neoplasm. The neoplasm, however, displaces and deforms the soft tissue margins without obliterating them, making differentiation possible. (28)

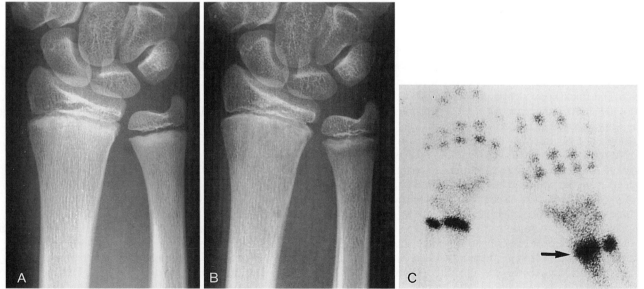

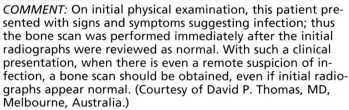

Figure 12-4 BONE SCAN: EARLY DETECTION OF OSTEO-MYELITIS. A. Initial Plain Film. Note that the initial radiographic examination shows no destructive changes in this 12-year-old patient who presented with pain in the wrist. **B. 10-Day Follow-Up.** Note the permeative pattern of bone destruction in the metaphysis of the distal radius. **C. Bone Scan, Initial Presentation.** Note that this examination, performed at the same time as panel A, reveals an area of increased uptake (a hot spot) (*arrow*) of technetium.

COMMENT: On initial physical examination, this patient presented with signs and symptoms suggesting infection; thus the bone scan was performed immediately after the initial radiographs were reviewed as normal. With such a clinical presentation, when there is even a remote suspicion of infection, a bone scan should be obtained, even if initial radiographs appear normal. (Courtesy of David P. Thomas, MD, Melbourne, Australia.)

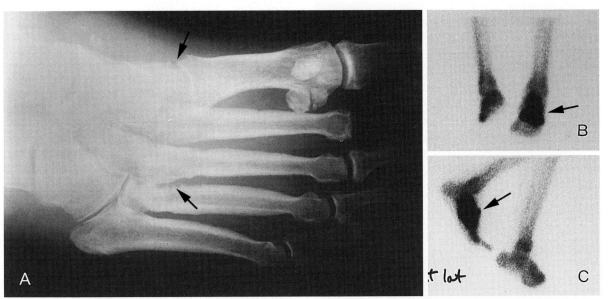

Figure 12-5 BONE SCAN: EARLY DETECTION OF OSTEO-MYELITIS. A. Plain Film. Note that diffuse soft tissue swelling is evident over the tarsometatarsal junction. A few subtle bone erosions can be appreciated (*arrows*). **B and C. Bone Scan.** Note the diffuse increase in uptake over the tarso-metatarsal region (*arrows*). *COMMENT:* In this diabetic patient, the bone scan was decisive in identifying an infection that could rapidly progress and place the limb at risk. On bone scan, a second infective site was isolated in the shoulder. (Courtesy of Michael A. Fox, MD, Memphis, Tennessee.)

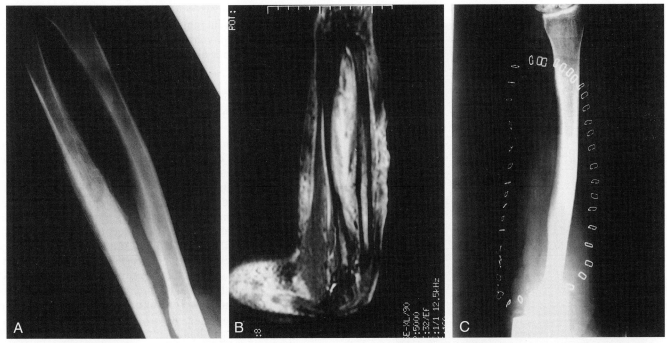

Figure 12-6 OSTEOMYELITIS: IV DRUG USER. A. PA Forearm. Observe the focal bone destruction and periosteal new bone formation within the ulna. There is some pressure erosion seen on the lateral margin of the mid-diaphysis of the radius from the associated soft tissue mass. **B. T2-Weighted Coronal MRI, Forearm.** Note that the destructive ulnar lesion can be identified. There is bright signal intensity within the soft tissues surrounding the interosseous membrane, suggesting an inflammatory response consistent with osteomyelitis with secondary extension to the adjacent soft tissues. An increase in compartmental pressure may have caused extrinsic pressure erosion of the radius. **C. PA Postsurgical Forearm.** The patient could not be treated effectively by antibiotic therapy, and a complete ulnar resection was performed. *COMMENT:* This 27-year-old female IV drug abuser presented with severe pain in the forearm and an enlarging soft tissue mass. (Courtesy of Kenneth J. McCabe, MD, and Joyce D. Schroeder, MD, Department of Radiology, University Hospital, Denver, Colorado.)

Table 12-1	Radiologic Signs of Osteomyelitis

Early signs
  Latent period
    10 days in the extremities
    21 days in the spine
  Soft tissue
    Elevation and displacement of fat planes
    Obliteration of fat planes
    Increased density
  Bone
    Moth-eaten or permeative medullary and cortical destruction
    Periosteal new bone (solid, laminated, Codman's triangle)
Late signs
  Soft tissue
    Draining sinus (secondary carcinoma of tract)
    Debris
  Bone
    Destruction of adjacent cortex
    Involucrum
    Cloaca
    Sequestrum
    Sclerosis and moth-eaten sclerosis
  Joint
    Loss of joint space
    Healing by bony ankylosis

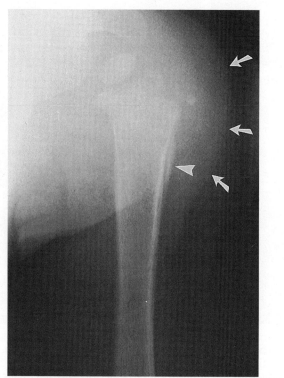

Figure 12-7 OSTEOMYELITIS: EARLY RADIOGRAPHIC SIGNS. Humerus. Note the large soft tissue swelling (*arrows*) representing an early radiographic sign of osteomyelitis in this pediatric patient. Observe also the lifting of the periosteum as a result of the infectious process, creating a *solid-type* periosteal reaction (*arrowhead*).

Osseous Alterations

The stage has now been set for the underlying pathologic process to be visible on the skeletal radiograph. Essentially, two changes will be apparent: bone destruction and periosteal response.

Bone Destruction. The early lesion is that of a *moth-eaten* or permeative destructive pattern, creating a focal loss of bone density usually affecting the metaphysis. (Figs. 12-8 and 12-9) This destructive focus, if not treated early, may disseminate to the epiphysis or diaphysis of the bone. Its extension across the growth plate depends on the patient's age. Eventually, large medullary destructive osteolytic lesions occur, which often reach the cortex. (Fig. 12-10) Bone sequestrum formation appears 3–6 weeks after the initial onset of symptoms. These necrotic fragments actually retain their original radiographic density. As a result, they appear sclerotic relative to the adjacent osteopenic bone. With cortical disruption, the purulent exudate gains access to the soft tissues through the cloaca.

Periosteal Response. With suppurative infections, periosteal new bone formation often assumes a *laminated or lamellar pattern.* (Fig. 12-11) This sign is most common in infants and children. An occasional Codman's reactive triangle may be seen, and its appearance in acute pyogenic osteomyelitis cannot be differentiated from that of a primary malignant neoplasm or even traumatic periostitis. (28) Significant lifting of the periosteum by pus not only creates a laminated response but, with continued periosteal new bone production, a large involucrum may occur. This involucrum is composed of more rapidly formed woven bone and is, therefore, less dense radiographically. As a result, there is a radiographic contrast between dense infarcted sequestrum and the less dense involucrum. Once the infection has been treated and subsides, this involucrum will be remodeled and resorbed, leaving only a minor alteration in contour near the original site of the infection.

Spinal Involvement

Incidence. Suppurative infections of the spine make up only 2–4% of all cases of osteomyelitis. (29) Spinal infections of all causes represent only 10% of skeletal lesions; the overwhelming majority of osseous infections (90%) involve the appendicular skeleton. The highest incidence of suppurative spondylitis occurs in debilitated patients in the 5th–6th decade. Males are affected more frequently than females. The most common site is the lumbar spine, followed by the thoracic spine. *Staphylococcus aureus* is the most common infectious agent, representing 90% of both adult and childhood infections. Other Gram-positive organisms that produce suppurative spondylitis include *Streptococcus* and *Pneumococcus.* Gram-negative infections resulting from *Escherichia coli, Pseudomonas, Salmonella, Klebsiella,* and *Corynebacterium* are much less common than the Gram-positive infections. (29) Brucellosis (*Brucella abortis, B. melitensis, B. suis*) causes joint infection in almost 30% of cases; of these, up to 25–50% involve the spine, and 40–70% involve the sacroiliac joint. (30,31)

Clinical Features. The signs and symptoms, as well as the course of suppurative spondylitis, depend on a balance between the virulence of the organism, the extent of the disease process, and the host resistance. (29) A history of a recent primary infection (furunculosis, urinary tract, or upper respiratory tract infection), recent surgery, or instrumentation (catheterization, cystoscopy, or

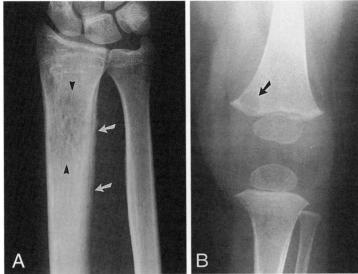
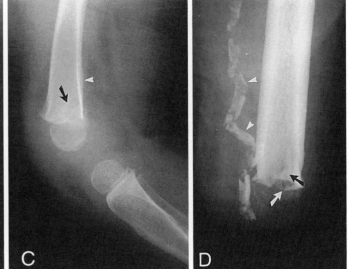

Figure 12-8 **OSTEOMYELITIS: BONE DESTRUCTION. A. Distal Radius.** Observe the moth-eaten pattern of lytic bone destruction (*arrowheads*) in the diametaphyseal area of the distal radius. There is a poor zone of transition around this destructive lesion, which is characteristic of aggressive disorders of bone such as osteomyelitis. Observe the solid periosteal response on the cortical surface of the distal radius (*arrows*), which occurs as a result of pus elevating the periosteal envelope. **B and C. Knee.** Note the large infectious destructive lesion in the medial metaphysis of the distal femur (*arrows*). An additional sign of osteomyelitis is the periosteal response on the posterior surface of the distal femur (*arrowhead*). **D. Stump Infection.** Observe the moth-eaten lesions (*arrows*) in the distal portion of the femur in this diabetic patient. Note the extensive vascular calcification (*arrowheads*) in the soft tissue structures of the remaining portion of the thigh. This patient had undergone amputation of his lower limb as a result of long-standing diabetes. Vascular calcification is a common complication of long-standing diabetes. (Courtesy of Bryan Hartley, MD, Melbourne, Australia.)

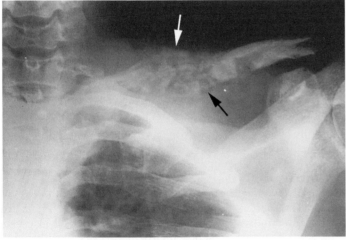

Figure 12-9 **OSTEOMYELITIS. Clavicle.** Observe the diffuse moth-eaten destruction of the clavicle shaft (*arrows*). This is an extremely uncommon site of involvement but graphically displays the cardinal signs of aggressive bone destruction simulating a neoplasm. (Courtesy of Michael J. Silberstein, MD, St. Louis, Missouri.)

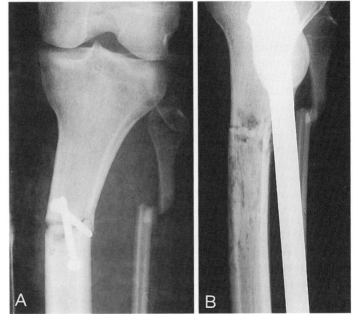

Figure 12-10 **POSTSURGICAL OSTEOMYELITIS. A. AP Tibia and Fibula.** Observe the fracture dislocation of the fibula. This young adult male suffered a severe injury in a motorcycle accident. Open reduction and surgical pinning of the complete fracture of the tibia were performed. **B. Lateral Tibia.** Just 4 weeks after the surgical intervention, the patient complained of persistent pain at the area of the fracture site. Note the typical moth-eaten destructive lesions of osteomyelitis.

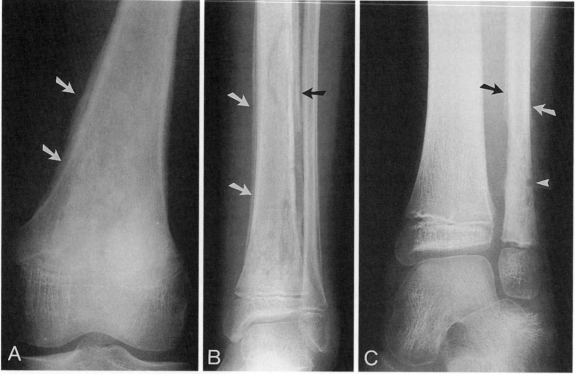

Figure 12-11   OSTEOMYELITIS: PERIOSTEAL RESPONSE.
A. Distal Femur. Observe the thick collar of periosteal new bone (*arrows*) in the distal femur. Observe also the destructive lesions in the metaphysis of the distal femur occurring as a result of osteomyelitis. **B. Distal Tibia.** Note the extensive laminated periosteal response affecting the diaphysis and metaphysis of the distal tibia (*arrows*). The scattered areas of radiolucency throughout the tibia represent infective destructive lesions. **C. Distal Fibula.** Note the laminated periosteal response (*arrows*) in the distal portion of the fibula in this pediatric patient. There are lytic destructive lesions noted in the distal portion of the fibula (*arrowhead*), representing the infectious focus.

bowel surgery) may be elicited in a significant number of cases. (29,32) A high association between suppurative spondylitis and urinary tract infection exists, with the spread of the infection occurring primarily via Batson's venous plexus. Spontaneous pyogenic vertebral osteomyelitis caused by *Staphylococcus aureus* and *Escherichia coli* may occur in older patients with several underlying illnesses. (33) Regardless of the cause, back pain is the most common complaint and is usually insidious in onset and constant. The pain may be radicular in distribution and be aggravated by motion.

Physical examination reveals local tenderness and decreased motion. Fever is infrequent in adults and occurs in only one third of affected children. (4,29) Laboratory findings reveal an elevated ESR. Often, the white blood cell count is normal or only minimally elevated in patients with spinal disease. Elevated white blood cell counts are more common when there is appendicular involvement. Owing to the absence of fever and the ability to reproduce the pain mechanically, the incidence of misdiagnosis in patients with vertebral osteomyelitis is estimated at approximately 33%. (34) Commonly these misinterpretations of symptoms are labeled as a herniated disc, spinal stenosis, metastatic carcinoma, and vertebral strain. (34)

The drug abuser presents with a higher incidence of Gram-negative infections; the offending organism is often *Aerobacter, Klebsiella,* or *Pseudomonas.* These patients often have multiple sites of infection affecting the *S joints.* (6) There is frequent involvement of the cervical spine, which is an unusual site in other types of suppurative spondylitis. (35)

Radiologic Patterns in Children and Adults. The age of the patient determines location, rate of spread, and thus the radiologic features of spondylitis. In children < 20 years of age the vascular channels to the disc still exist and provide a pathway for disc infection before vertebral disease. (4,6,29) With initial disc involvement there is a narrowing of the overall disc height. This is usually associated with paraspinal edema (abscess formation). Eventually, the vertebral endplate is destroyed, creating patchy areas of osteolysis throughout the vertebral body.

In adults the initial focus occurs at the anterior vertebral endplate. This appears as an area of radiolucency and irregularity. The vertebral endplate contains vascular channels, which allow nutrition of the intervertebral disc and also provide a site for entry of septic microemboli. Because the adult disc is avascular, organisms frequently lodge in the low-flow end-organ vascular arcades adjacent to the subchondral plates and involve the discs secondarily. (Fig. 12-12) Vertebral destruction and collapse ensues, with soft tissue paraspinal swelling. (Figs. 12-13 to 12-15)

Intradiscal gas is extremely uncommon in spinal infection, though in rare instances it may be seen on CT in clostridia, brucellosis, tuberculosis, and streptococcus. (36) Soft tissue swelling is evidenced radiographically by widening of the retropharyngeal and retrotracheal spaces in cervical spine infections, displacement of the paraspinal lines in thoracic spine infections, and paravertebral or psoas abscess in the lumbar spine. (Figs. 12-16 and 12-17) Complicating epidural abscess is best depicted on MRI with a low signal on T1-weighted images and a high signal on

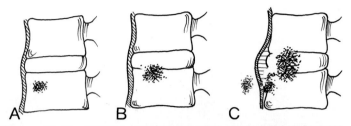

Figure 12-12 **SPINAL OSTEOMYELITIS: PATHOPHYSIOLOGY OF SEQUENTIAL DEVELOPMENT. A. Early.** An early infectious lesion occurs in the anterosuperior corner of the vertebral body. **B. Middle.** The infectious process extends through the vertebral endplate. **C. Late.** With further dissemination of the infectious process, a subligamentous pathway of spread may occur. This may allow for scalloped erosions on the anterior surface of the vertebral body or rupture of the anterior longitudinal ligament. (Adapted from **Resnick D, Niwayama G:** *Diagnosis of Bone and Joint Disorders.* Philadelphia, WB Saunders, 1981.)

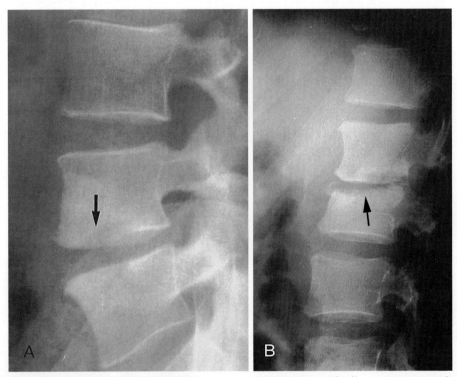

Figure 12-13 **CARDINAL PLAIN FILM FEATURES OF SPINAL INFECTION. A. L4–L5.** Observe the disc space narrowing at the L4–L5 level, with destruction of the subchondral vertebral endplate (*arrow*). **B. L2–L3.** A more advanced stage of presentation with disc space narrowing and vertebral endplate destruction (*arrow*). (Panel A courtesy of Graham J. Tripp, DC, Tweed Heads, New South Wales, Australia.)

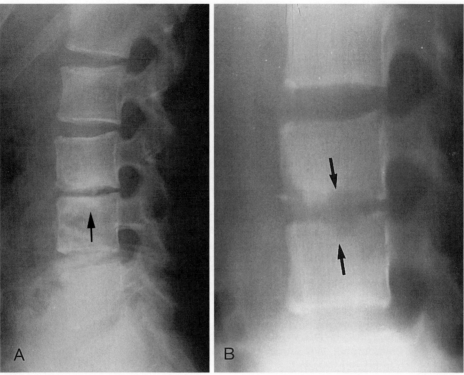

Figure 12-14 **EARLY SPINAL INFECTION: L3–L4. A. Plain Film: Lateral Lumbar.** Note the marked disc space narrowing between the L3 and the L4 vertebral segments, with no obvious evidence of vertebral endplate destruction (*arrow*). **B.**

Tomography: Lateral Lumbar. Observe that the tomographic examination reveals lytic destruction of the inferior endplate of L3 and the superior endplate of L4 (*arrows*). The extensive disc space narrowing is clearly recognizable.

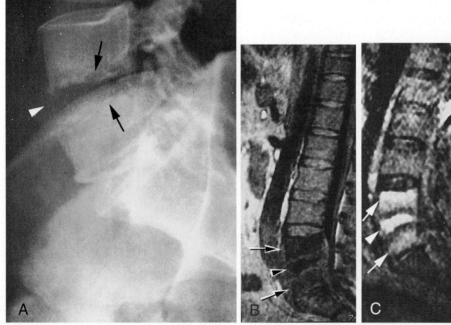

Figure 12-15 **LUMBAR SPINE INFECTION. A. Plain Film.** Note that at the L4–L5 interspace there is loss of disc space (*arrowhead*) and vertebral body endplates (*arrows*). **B. T1-Weighted MRI, Sagittal Lumbar.** Note that the signal is diffusely decreased (*blackened areas*) throughout the L4 and L5 vertebral bodies owing to marrow inflammation (*arrows*). The L4 intervertebral disc exhibits a low signal compared with adjacent discs (*arrowhead*). **C. T2-Weighted MRI,**

Sagittal Lumbar. Note that on this study the signal throughout the L4 and L5 vertebral bodies is high (*whitened areas*), consistent with edema (*arrows*). Similarly, the L4 intervertebral disc is of high signal intensity owing to edema (*arrowhead*). *COMMENT:* These MRI findings are quite specific for disc infection: low signal on T1-weighted studies and high signal on T2-weighted studies. (Courtesy of Craig P. Church, DC, DACBR, Toledo, Ohio.)

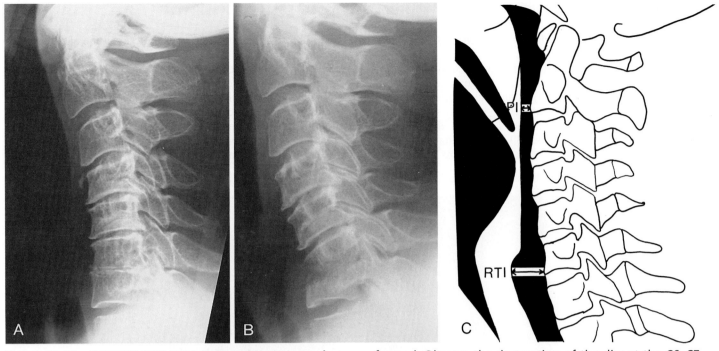

Figure 12-16 **STAPHYLOCOCCAL INFECTION. A. Lateral Cervical Spine, Initial Study.** This 55-year-old patient presented with cervical spine pain. Note that the initial radiograph was interpreted as representing extensive degenerative disc space narrowing. Observe the disc space narrowing at the C6–C7 level, without obvious additional degenerative findings such as osteophytes or endplate sclerosis. **B. 1-Month Follow-Up, Lateral Cervical Spine.** The patient remained unresponsive to conservative care and, with more persistent symptoms, a follow-up radiograph was performed. Observe the destruction of the disc at the C6–C7 level. There is extensive destruction of the vertebral endplates of C6 and C7 as well. Also note the large retrolaryngeal abscess anterior to the C6 and C7 segments. **C. Normal Prevertebral Soft Tissue Interspaces.** On the lateral radiograph the retropharyngeal interspace (RPI) should not be > 7 mm at the C2 level. The retrotracheal interspace (RTI) should not be > 20 mm at the C6 level. Observe that in panel B the retrotracheal space is approaching 30 mm, owing to a prevertebral abscess.

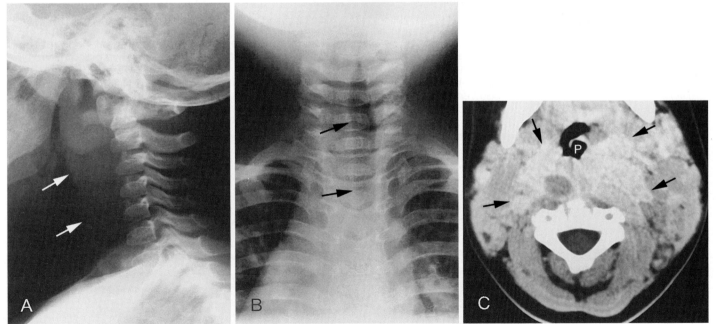

Figure 12-17 **RETROPHARYNGEAL ABSCESS. A. Lateral Cervical Spine.** Note the marked prevertebral swelling extending from the retropharyngeal to retrolaryngeal interspaces (arrows). There is no spinal involvement. **B. Frontal Cervical Spine.** Observe the lateral shift of the trachea (arrows). **C. CT, Axial Cervical Spine.** Note that the pharynx (P) is displaced well anterior. A diffuse area of high attenuation can be seen throughout the prevertebral space (arrows). *COMMENT:* This 2-year-old female presented with a history of upper respiratory tract infection and swelling of the left side of the neck with palpable tenderness. This collection of soft tissue mass represents purulent debris and edema from an infectious origin, which has arisen within the prevertebral space (quinsy) but has not infiltrated the adjacent vertebral segments. (Courtesy of David Neal, MD, Columbus, Ohio.)

T2-weighted studies. (37) Spontaneous osseous ankylosis may occur as a late sequela. (Fig. 12-18)

Brucella spondylitis exhibits these features of diminished disc height; loss of vertebral endplate; and, in approximately 15% of cases, a soft tissue abscess. (30,38) Additional manifestations are anterior discovertebral erosions simulating Schmorl's nodes with a normal disc, *ivory vertebra*, peripheral vacuum phenomenon, and frequent anterior osteophytes. (30,39) The lumbar spine is the most common site involved, particularly the low lumbar ver-

tebrae. (30,31,39) Bone scan reveals increased uptake in at least 90% of cases. (31)

Sacroiliac joint infection is less common. A higher incidence occurs in intravenous drug users and in those who may have had ileotomy as a donor site for bone grafting, sacroiliac arthrography, or therapeutic injection. (40) Between 40% and 70% of brucellosis joint infections involve the sacroiliac articulation. (31) The radiographic signs on plain film and CT consist of loss of the articular cortex, erosions of the subchondral bone, and some re-

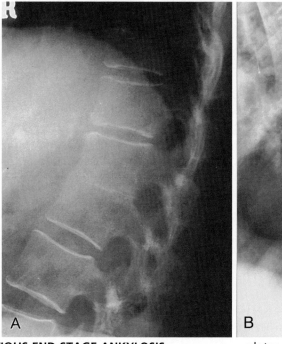

Figure 12-18 **INFECTIOUS END-STAGE ANKYLOSIS.**
A. Lateral Lumbar Spine. Observe the bony ankylosis of the L1 and L2 vertebral segments. This patient was treated with antibiotics early, before extensive destruction of the endplates occurred. **B. Lateral Thoracic Spine.** Note the extensive destruction of the intervertebral discs and vertebral end-

plates of the T9 and T10 segments. Complete ankylosis at this level has occurred as a result of the final stages of the infectious process. *COMMENT:* Suppurative osteomyelitis in its end stage creates bony ankylosis, whereas the end-stage ankylosis of tuberculosis tends to be of a more fibrous nature.

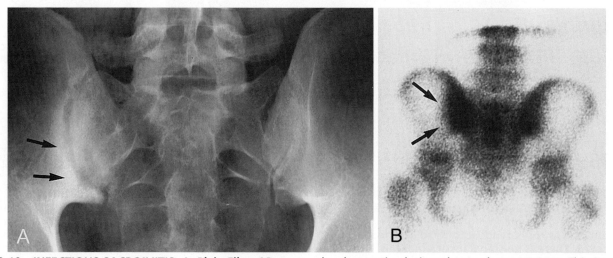

Figure 12-19 **INFECTIOUS SACROILIITIS. A. Plain Film: AP Sacrum.** Observe the destruction of the cortical bone of the sacrum and ilium. There is considerable reactive sclerosis in the inferior portion of the sacroiliac joint (*arrows*). **B. Bone Scan.** Note the increased activity (hot spot) in the area of

the destructive lesions (*arrows*). *COMMENT:* This 24-year-old patient presented with acute pain in the sacroiliac joint. Aspiration of the sacroiliac joint and culturing produced *Staphylococcus aureus* organisms. (Courtesy of Gerald A. Fitzgerald, MD, Sydney, Australia.)

active sclerosis. (Fig. 12-19) These signs may be identical to inflammatory sacroiliitis such as seen in Reiter's syndrome or psoriatic arthritis. On MRI, findings include decreased signal on T1- and increased signal on T2-weighted scans within the joint, subchondral bone, and iliopsoas muscle. (41)

Treatment and Prognosis

The key to effective treatment is early diagnosis. Once the proper diagnosis is established, antibiotic therapy may successfully abort the infection before appreciable bone necrosis occurs. If such measures fail, more extensive destruction can be anticipated, and it is frequently necessary to resort to surgical drainage and débridement of sequestered fragments. In most cases antibiotic therapy is an effective cure of the local infectious process; however, antimicrobial therapies should be prolonged because the reoccurrence rate may be as high as 14%. (42) More than 30% of patients can expect residual disability (42) in which the course of the infection may lead to pathologic fracture of the weakened bone or septic arthritis by extension. It must be remembered that in addition to the local destruction there may be distant hematogenous spread of infection. This often leads to the development of pyemic abscesses and focal cellulitis elsewhere. The overall prognosis is generally good, with a mortality rate estimated at only 11% as long as early diagnosis and effective treatment have been initiated. (42)

Medicolegal Implications

SUPPURATIVE OSTEOMYELITIS

- Early diagnosis is extremely important. The single most important factor in making the diagnosis is suspecting its presence through an adequate history and examination, obtaining basic blood parameters (white cells, ESR, C-reactive protein), and acquiring plain films. If these remain equivocal (radiographic latent period of plain films is a minimum of 10 days in the extremities, 21 days in the spine) but the clinical picture remains unclear, a nuclear bone scan is the technique of choice to detect its presence.
- Undetected osteomyelitis may lead to considerable morbidity and even mortality. Spread into a contiguous joint, especially in the young, may lead to permanent disability. In the spine, the major risk is spinal cord involvement, which can be catastrophic. Septicemia may seed the infection to distant sites such as the lungs, heart, and brain.

CAPSULE SUMMARY   Suppurative Osteomyelitis

General Considerations

- Systemic or localized infections have been recognized for many years.
- Immunosuppressed patients, alcoholics, newborns, and drug addicts are predisposed.
- Antibiotics have significantly reduced the sepsis-related mortality.

Cause

- *Staphylococcus aureus* causes 90% of all bone and joint infections.
- Pathways for the spread of infection: hematogenous, contiguous source, direct implantation, and postoperative.

Clinical Features

- Early diagnosis is important, and clinical signs and symptoms precede plain film findings by 7–10 days in the appendicular skeleton and 21 days in the spine.
- Young patients present with acute systemic symptoms.
- Adult patients present with symptoms that vary and tend to be more chronic.
- The most frequently affected age range is 2–12 years; 3:1 males.
- Affects large tubular bones, most commonly the femur.
- Drug addicts are predisposed to *Pseudomonas* infections involving the S joints.

Pathologic Features

- *Sequestrum formation:* necrotic cortical or medullary bone.
- *Involucrum:* cortical collar of new bone.

- *Cloaca:* draining sinus.
- *Empyema necessitatis:* empyema in which the pus can make a spontaneous escape.
- *Marjolin's ulcer:* malignant degeneration of squamous cell lining of cloaca.

Radiologic Features

- Bone scans are the earliest means of diagnosis.
- *Radiographic latent period (for plain films):* extremities, 10 days; spine, 21 days.
- *Soft tissue alterations:* elevated fat planes, obliterated fat planes, increased density, and paraspinal edema.
- *Bone changes:*
  Moth-eaten bone destruction, usually metaphyseal in origin.
  Periosteal new bone formation (solid, laminated, Codman's triangle).
  Sequestrum.
  Involucrum.
  Joint space destruction (osseous ankylosis).
  Epiphysis often spared if physis is open.
  Loss of disc height, with spine involvement.
  Vertebral destruction and collapse.

Treatment and Prognosis

- *Treatment:* antibiotics; surgical débridement (late).
- *Prognosis:* good, if diagnosed early.

OTHER ASSOCIATED ENTITIES

BRODIE'S ABSCESS

Clinical Features. Brodie's abscess was first described by Brodie in 1832. (1) It is defined as a localized, aborted form of suppurative osteomyelitis. The classic clinical presentation is that of localized limb pain, which is often nocturnal and dramatically alleviated by aspirin. This mimics the typical presenting symptoms of patients with osteoid osteoma. Patients often have a history of recent distant infection or have even undergone dental surgery that has *seeded* to bone. Brodie's abscess is most common in male children. The metaphyses of the tubular bones are most commonly affected, particularly the distal tibia, proximal tibia, distal femur, proximal or distal fibula, and distal radius (listed in decreasing order of incidence). (Figs. 12-20 and 12-21) Less frequently seen is Brodie's abscess affecting the diaphyses of tubular bones or flat bones. (2) (Figs. 12-22 to 12-25)

Pathologic Features. The abscess lies within a bone cavity that is incarcerated by a wall of inflammatory granulation tissue. The adjacent spongy bone becomes sclerotic. The cavity contains necrotic debris and purulent or mucoid fluid (3) from which the offending microorganism may or may not be cultured. *Staphylococcus aureus* is the most common bacterial agent to be isolated. Often, the abscess is sterile and no microorganisms can be found. Pathologically, a Brodie's abscess is often misdiagnosed as chronic recurrent multifocal osteomyelitis. (4)

Radiologic Features. The abscess is depicted as an oval, elliptical, or serpiginous radiolucency with no visible matrix surrounded by a *halo* or *doughnut rim* of heavy reactive sclerosis. (5)

The radiolucency is usually ≥ 1.0 cm, with no associated bony enlargement or cortical break through. (5) As a differential point, the radiolucent nidus of osteoid osteoma is invariably < 1.0 cm and may have a target center of calcification. The nidus of an osteoid osteoma is composed of a vascular stroma, and the presence

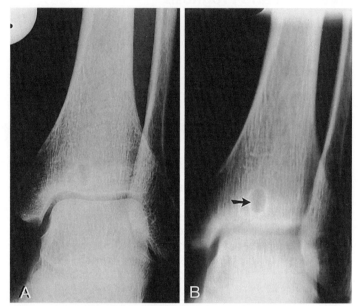

Figure 12-20 **BRODIE'S ABSCESS: VALUE OF TOMOGRAPHY.** **A. AP Ankle.** Note the small geographic lucency within the distal tibia. **B. Tomography, AP Ankle.** Observe that the lesion is better delineated and a rim of sclerosis is appreciated (*arrow*). *COMMENT:* Tomography is useful in defining if there is a tract leading into the joint and for evaluating the matrix of the lesion. CT now replaces tomography to detect early lesions.

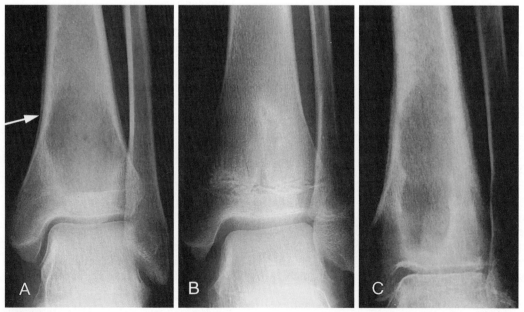

Figure 12-21 **BRODIE'S ABSCESS: SPECTRUM OF APPEARANCES. A. Tibia: Large, Sclerosis Absent.** Note that this appearance makes it difficult to conclude with a convincing diagnosis of infection. There is a single periosteal lamination of the medial cortex (*arrow*), signifying the lesion is active, excluding an indolent lesion such as simple bone

cyst from the differential diagnosis. **B. Tibia: Elongated, Linear Form.** Note that this presentation is virtually diagnostic of a Brodie's abscess, with a reactive rim of sclerosis. **C. Tibia: Loculated, Sclerosis Limited.** Note the lesion is long, lacks a dense reactive rim of sclerosis, and is associated

(continued)

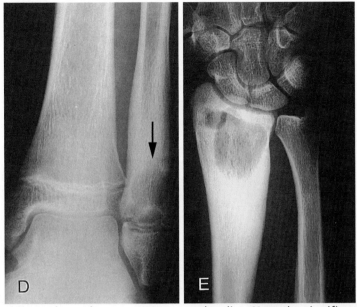

Figure 12-21 (*continued*) with periosteal new bone.
D. Tibia: Small, Prominent Sclerosis. Observe the geographic radiolucent defect in the metaphysis of the distal fibula (*arrow*). There is some thickening of the cortex in the distal fibula and reactive sclerosis adjacent to the lucent defect. **E. Radius: Large, Prominent Sclerosis.** Note the large, circular, radiolucent defect within the subarticular portion of the dis-tal radius. Note the significant reactive sclerosis of bone, with expansion of the cortex and a portion of the medullary canal of the distal radius. After biopsy, *Staphylococcus aureus* organisms were cultured, confirming the presumptive radiographic diagnosis of Brodie's abscess. (Reprinted with permission from **Yochum TR:** *Brodie's abscess of the distal radius.* ACA Council Roent November, 1981.)

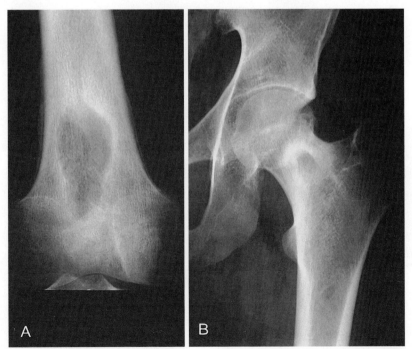

Figure 12-22 **BRODIE'S ABSCESS. A. Distal Femur.** Observe the oval radiolucent defect in the distal metaphysis of the femur. There is a minimal degree of reactive sclerosis surrounding this lesion. **B. Proximal Femur.** Note the large Brodie's abscess in the femoral neck, with an exuberant degree of encapsulating reactive sclerosis about the lucent defect. The similarity to osteoid osteoma in this location is striking. *COMMENT:* Patients with Brodie's abscess can present with the identical clinical signs and symptoms as osteoid osteoma: pain worse at night and remarkable alleviation of pain with the use of aspirin.

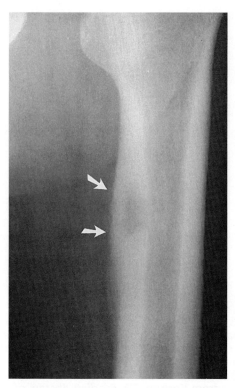

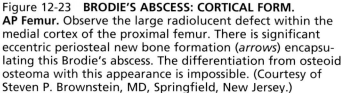

Figure 12-23 BRODIE'S ABSCESS: CORTICAL FORM. AP Femur. Observe the large radiolucent defect within the medial cortex of the proximal femur. There is significant eccentric periosteal new bone formation (*arrows*) encapsulating this Brodie's abscess. The differentiation from osteoid osteoma with this appearance is impossible. (Courtesy of Steven P. Brownstein, MD, Springfield, New Jersey.)

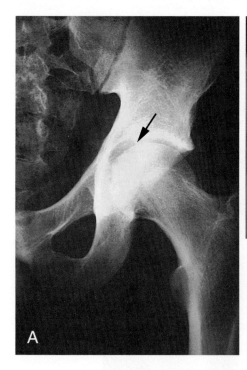

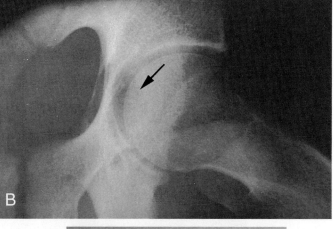

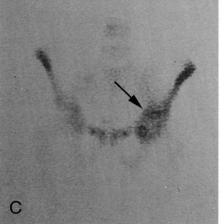

Figure 12-24 BRODIE'S ABSCESS: PELVIS. A. AP Hip. Note the subtle 1-cm geographic lesion in the floor of the acetabulum (*arrow*). **B. Frog-Leg Hip.** Note that the lesion remains subtle but is more discernible (*arrow*). **C. Bone Scan.** Note the increased uptake at the acetabulum. *COMMENT:* This case demonstrates how a bone scan can greatly aid in detecting or excluding bony lesions that may be small or anatomically obscured from view.

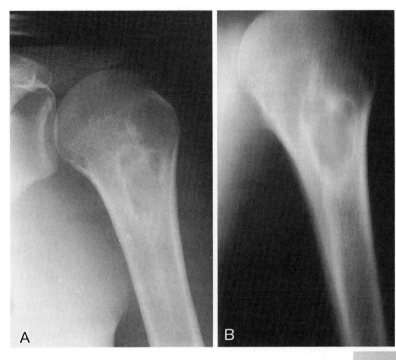

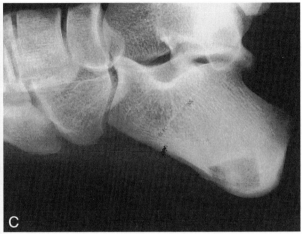

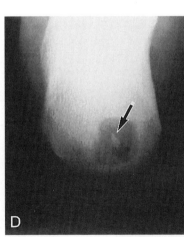

Figure 12-25 **BRODIE'S ABSCESS: UNUSUAL LOCATIONS.**
A and B. Humerus. Note the large radiolucent defect within
the metaphysis of the humerus. Tomographic examination
(panel B) demonstrates a moderate rim of reactive sclerosis
around the abscess. This is an unusual location for Brodie's
abscess. **C and D. Calcaneus.** Observe the large, radiolucent
lesion within the posterior inferior surface of the calcaneus.
A target area of sequestration is noted (*arrow*). **E. Ilium.**
Note the rather large geographic loss of bone density in the
lateral portion of the acetabulum (*arrow*). There is significant

reactive sclerosis about this radiolucent defect. This lesion
should not be confused with a subchondral bone cyst
(geode) because there is no evidence of narrowing of the
lateral weight-bearing compartment of the hip joint or any
presence of degenerative osteophytes. This 32-year-old female presented with localized pain in the area of the hip
joint one month after a severe chest cold. Needle biopsy and
culture of the lesion produced *Staphylococcus aureus* organisms consistent with Brodie's abscess. (Courtesy of
Christopher R. Hart, DC, Melbourne, Australia.)

of a *vascular blush* in the radiolucent nidus on an arteriogram also confirms the diagnosis of osteoid osteoma. (6) Except for the size of the radiolucency in Brodie's abscess, osteoid osteoma and Brodie's abscess cannot be differentiated clinically or by plain films radiologically. (7) Similarly, eosinophilic granulomas share numerous radiographic findings with Brodie's abscess and may be difficult to differentiate. (8) A characteristic MRI finding consistent with subacute osteomyelitis is the *penumbra sign*. (9) On T1-weighted images this sign can be identified by the presence of a high signal intensity lesion (abscess) surrounded by a relatively less hyperintense signal rim. (9) This sign supports the diagnosis of an infectious agent while discrediting the differential of a tumor. (9)

The most effective treatment of Brodie's abscess is surgical. Decompression and curettage of the lesion are most effective in eradicating the abscess; recurrence rates are relatively low. (7)

GARRÉ'S SCLEROSING OSTEOMYELITIS

In 1893 Garré (1) described a peculiar form of chronic, low-grade, diffuse, non-purulent osteomyelitis characterized by a striking absence of viable pathogens on attempted tissue culture. (2) The condition is extremely rare (3) and has been identified only in children and young adults. (4) Some doubt has been raised as to whether the entity actually exists, and little is known about its pathology. (2,5,6) The process is most commonly found in the long tubular bones, where it creates an exuberant degree of fusiform thickening of the bone. The lesion is often cortical with significant ossifying periostitis and reactive new bone formation. No bone destruction or sequestrum is demonstrated. (5) (Fig. 12-26) Moderate noctur-

nal pain is often the chief complaint. (2) On examination a hard bony mass is usually palpable. (4)

CHRONIC OSTEOMYELITIS

The diagnosis and treatment of chronic osteomyelitis often present a dilemma to the physician; however, the prognosis depends heavily on both. (1) Proper identification of the pathogen is essential and contrary to common practice the organism must be isolated from the involved bone(s) and not from non-bone or blood samples. (1) Most commonly, *Staphylococcus aureus* is the organism involved. (2) Chronic osteomyelitis is associated with many complications, including Marjolin's ulcers and **SAPHO** syndrome (**s**ynovitis, **a**cne, **p**ustulosis, **h**yperostosis, and **o**steitis syndrome). (3–6)

The radiographic manifestations of chronic osteomyelitis are dominated by increased density of the involved bone. The single most common site is the tibia, although any bone can be affected. The characteristic radiographic features consist of sclerosis, cortical thickening, periosteal new bone (laminated or solid), areas of destruction, and dense sequestra. (Figs. 12-27 and 12-28) Typically, a long portion of the bone is affected into the diaphysis. Rarely, a soft tissue mass is observed with chronic osteomyelitis, and, if present, it seldom mimics the well-defined margins of a primary soft tissue neoplasm. (7)

Scintigraphy bone scan may be of benefit in the diagnosis (8) as well as in the differentiation of postoperative scar tissue from reactivated infections within the 1st year of surgery. (9) Within this time frame, MRI cannot accurately differentiate scar tissue from infection; however, in the absence of a surgical history,

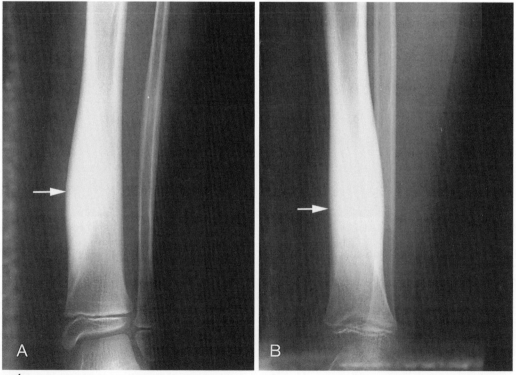

Figure 12-26   GARRÉ'S SCLEROSING OSTEOMYELITIS.
A. AP Tibia. Observe the circumferential thickening of the cortex (*arrow*). **B. Lateral Tibia.** Note that the thickening of the cortex is confirmed (*arrow*). Also, note the characteristic absence of destructive foci.

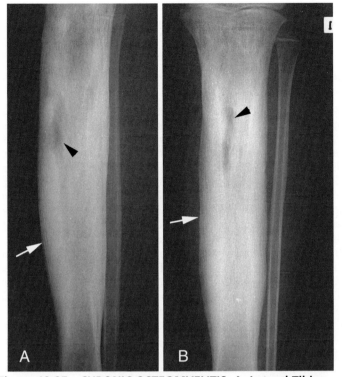

Figure 12-27 **CHRONIC OSTEOMYELITIS. A. Lateral Tibia.** Note that the prominent laminated periosteal new bone has produced circumferential cortical thickening (*arrow*). There has been endosteal reaction that has also contributed to this appearance. Observe the residual destructive focus within the proximal diaphysis (*arrowhead*). **B. AP Tibia.** Note the periosteal new bone (*arrow*) and the destructive lytic focus (*arrowhead*). *COMMENT:* These are characteristic findings of chronic osteomyelitis.

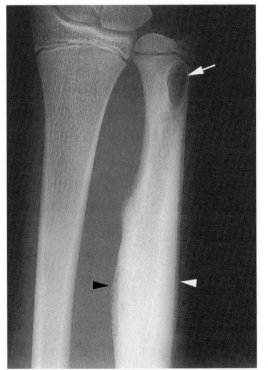

Figure 12-28 **CHRONIC OSTEOMYELITIS. Ulna.** Note the small destructive area within the distal ulna (*arrow*). Prominent periosteal new bone (cloaca) is also present (*arrowheads*).

MRI is more sensitive than bone scan in the identification of low-grade infections. (9) Without a surgical history and in the absence of relevant MRI findings, acute activity of chronic osteomyelitis can virtually be excluded. (9) CT is the modality of choice for visualization of sequestra, cortical erosions, and bony fragmentation. (10)

The choice of drug therapy depends on the organism isolated, but prolonged periods of use are the norm. (11) Owing to frequent fragmentation of the bone, many organisms are separated from the primary site of infection and thus blood supply. (12) This factor renders antibiotic therapy virtually useless to these areas, and surgical débridement is the only treatment option. (12) With advanced stages of bony destruction and fragmentation, surgical stabilization procedures may be necessary. (13)

CHILDHOOD INFLAMMATORY DISCITIS

Childhood inflammatory discitis is separate and distinct from vertebral osteomyelitis. Synonyms for this entity include nonspecific spondylitis, discitis, spondyloarthritis, and childhood intervertebral disc infection. Because these patients do not have a history of vertebral osteomyelitis or an iatrogenic inoculation, a separate pathway must exist for childhood inflammatory discitis. The discal blood supply persisting in individuals up to 20 years of age provides pathogens direct access to the disc. (1) Most authorities believe there is an infectious cause, even though organisms cannot always be isolated. (2) Post-traumatic fragmentation of the cartilaginous endplate has been suggested as a contributing factor. (3) The most common pathogen when cultured is *Staphylococcus aureus.* (2)

The age range of patients presenting with discitis is generally younger than those who present with osteomyelitis. (4) Discitis may occur anywhere from 1 to 16 years of age (5), with a mean of 3 years. (4) Males are more frequently afflicted. The clinical presentation is similar to childhood osteomyelitis but is usually less severe. (4) Constitutional symptoms consisting of a low-grade fever, anorexia, malaise, and irritability are to be expected. The young child with inflammatory discitis often refuses to walk, stand, or sit; the older child complains of back and hip pain. (4) The laboratory investigation shows an elevated ESR with a normal leukocyte count. Most children develop discitis following a variety of head and neck infections, which most commonly originate in the upper respiratory tract.

Radiologic diagnosis is often delayed owing to the latent period of 3–4 weeks before roentgen signs are visible, even though the patient is symptomatic. (6) The most sensitive modality for early diagnosis is by nuclear bone scan; however, MRI and biopsy are usually performed to confirm the diagnosis and to guide treatment. (6,7) MRI will not differentiate pyogenic from tuberculous forms of spondylodiscitis. (8) Common sites of involvement are the lumbar spine (75%) and thoracic spine but rarely the cervical spine. (2) The earliest roentgen sign is disc space narrowing followed by fragmentation and destruction of the adjacent subchondral endplate. As the infectious process progresses, a significant degree of reactive subchondral endplate sclerosis will occur. The diagnosis is usually established by this stage, and antibiotic therapy will alter or halt this process. In some cases reversal of the vertebral bony and disc changes occurred within 34 months of therapy. (9) The posterior elements are usually spared. Occasionally, a mild spinal flexion deformity may occur. It is unusual for ankylosis to develop as a sequela. (2)

SEPTIC ARTHRITIS

General Considerations

Septic arthritis is a known cause of grossly destroyed and disintegrated joints. It affects men and women of all ages, with its greatest incidence being < 30 years of age. (1) Monoarticular involvement is the most common presentation; rarely, multiple joints are involved. (2) The two most common sources of joint contamination are bloodborne pathogens from a distant focus and traumatic direct implantation. Secondary septic arthritis is a well-recognized complication of joint replacement therapy. The natural course of this disease process may be significantly altered by early diagnosis and prompt initiation of effective antibiotic therapy.

Cause

The most commonly isolated microorganism is *Staphylococcus aureus* (3,4), with *Gonococcus* accounting for a majority of cases in patients < 30 years of age. (5) Other commonly found organisms are *Haemophilus,* α- and β-hemolytic streptococci, *Escherichia coli, Salmonella, Pneumococcus, Brucella,* and *Serratia.* (4) Occasionally, *Nocardia,* mycobacterial, and fungal pathogens may also be isolated. Joint aspirates are required to isolate the specific pathogen to initiate specific antibiotic therapy.

Clinical Features

Most patients present with a restricted range of joint motion and function secondary to severe pain and capsular edema. Accompanying symptoms are erythema, acute fever, and occasional chills. The patient will often present with an altered gait if a weight-bearing joint is involved. Restricted range of motion is a common finding in the non-weight-bearing joints. Laboratory findings of elevated ESR, elevated C-reactive protein, leukocytosis with a shift to the left (creating an abundance of premature leukocytes), and positive blood or joint cultures are essential in establishing the diagnosis. The prognosis is generally excellent with early detection and intervention. (3) Antibiotics and joint decompression are the treatments of choice. (6) There have been no direct correlations with the prognostic outcome and the site of the lesion or age of the patient. (2,3)

Pathologic Features

Resnick and Niwayama (7) suggested that during hematogenous spread of infection to a joint the organisms lodge within the vasculature of the synovial membrane, either indirectly from a distant infected source or directly from an adjacent bone infection. Thus infection of the synovial membrane precedes contamination of the synovial fluid. (7) With the accumulation of purulent exudate, capsular distention will occur. This distention may interfere with the normal cartilage nutrition, leading to the death of large numbers of chondrocytes. As the acute inflammatory cells and cartilage cells disintegrate, they release proteolytic enzymes from their cytoplasm, and progressive destruction of the articular surface ensues. Continued joint effusion and distention, coupled with destruction of cartilage and bone, cause eventual dislocation. This is especially true in the hip joint of a newborn but may also occur in the adult hip in an advanced stage of the infective process. Continued use of the joint results in a rapid disintegration from mechanical disturbances, resulting in total loss of articular joint space.

Eventually, the subchondral bone is penetrated and destruction of the articular cortex occurs. Regional hyperemia causes extensive juxta-articular osteoporosis, which is augmented by disuse of the joint. Greater destruction of the bone becomes evident, and a late sequela may be bony or fibrous ankylosis of the joint. (Fig. 12-29)

Rarely, gas formation may be seen in septic arthritis. This gas is usually intra-articular but may also be found in the juxta-articular soft tissue. (8) (Fig. 12-30) The most common offending organisms causing gas production are *Escherichia coli* and *Clostridium perfringens.* (8) The most common cause for gas in the soft tissues near a joint is an open wound communicating with the skin or recent arthrocentesis.

Radiologic Features

The sites of septic arthritis are varied, but the age of the patient, the specific pathogen involved, and the overall host resistance are

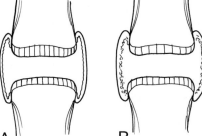

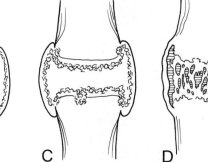

Figure 12-29 SEPTIC ARTHRITIS: SERIAL DEMONSTRATION. A. Normal Synovial Joint. B. Distention. Distention of the joint and synovial membrane. **C. Destruction.** Inflammatory destruction of the articular cartilage and subchondral bone plate as a result of extensive progression of the infection.

D. End Stage. The end stage of complete bony ankylosis following suppurative septic arthritis. (Adapted from **Resnick D, Niwayama G:** *Diagnosis of Bone and Joint Disorders.* Philadelphia, WB Saunders, 1981.)

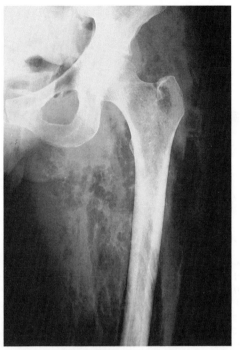

Figure 12-30 **GAS GANGRENE. Thigh.** Observe the extensive radiographic presentation of subcutaneous emphysema (gas) scattered throughout the myofascial planes of the entire visualized portion of the hip and thigh. *COMMENT:* The most common organisms causing gas production are *Escherichia coli* and *Clostridium perfringens.* (Courtesy of Bryan Hartley, MD, Melbourne, Australia.)

influencing factors. (7) The knee, ankle, and hip joints are the most common sites of involvement, accounting for up to 85% of cases. (2) The shoulder, hand, and foot are less often documented locations (9) and typically result from penetrating trauma such as animal or human bites. (10) (Fig. 12-31) Characteristically, changes detected on plain film lag behind the clinical signs. (11) Selective use of ultrasound may isolate intra-articular fluid, which can then be aspirated for microbiologic analysis. Isotopic bone scans can show increased vascular flow and on delayed scans increased uptake of the involved joint as early as 24–48 hr from the onset of symptoms. (Fig. 12-32)

Soft Tissue Alterations

An early sign is distention of the joint capsule by infectious exudate, causing displacement of juxta-articular fat. This is particularly apparent in the hip joint, where deviation of the normal fat folds for the obturator internus, the psoas major, and the gluteus medius is often seen. (12) (Fig. 12-33) An additional early roentgen sign of hip joint disease is *Waldenström's sign.* (12) A measurement is taken from the lateral aspect of *Köhler's teardrop* (the inferior and medial surface of the acetabulum) to the medial margin of the femoral head. A measurement > 11 mm or a difference in measurement > 2 mm compared with the opposite hip is a positive sign and considered clinically significant. (12) (Fig. 12-34) It should be noted that Waldenström's sign is a nonspecific sign of joint effusion and is not pathognomonic of infection. After the exudate builds up in the articular cavity, frank destruction of the cartilage begins. Rapid narrowing of the joint

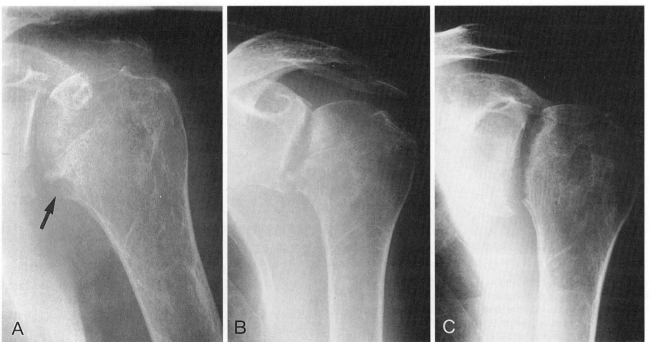

Figure 12-31 **SEPTIC SHOULDER: SERIAL RADIOGRAPHIC PRESENTATION. A. AP Shoulder. Initial Radiograph.** Note the subtle signs of generalized osteoporosis and a radiolucent defect on the medial articular surface of the humerus (*arrow*). There is also the suggestion of a slight symmetric loss of joint space at the glenohumeral articulation.

B. 3-Week Follow-Up. Note the extensive destruction of the articular surface of the humerus, with obliteration of the articular surface. **C. 6-Week Follow-Up.** Note that after antibiotic therapy, progression of the infectious process has occurred. (Courtesy of David P. Thomas, MD, Melbourne, Australia.)

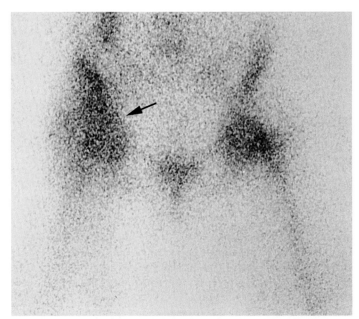

Figure 12-32 **SEPTIC ARTHRITIS. Gallium-67 Scan, Anterior Pelvis.** Note the diffuse uptake at the hip joint (*arrow*). *COMMENT:* The initial plain film was normal and based on a high index of clinical suspicion of an infection, the gallium scan was procured. This case demonstrates the high sensitivity of gallium scans in early infections. Scanning avoids the protracted radiographic latent period of 10 days before plain films will show changes. (Courtesy of Michael A. Fox, MD, Memphis, Tennessee.)

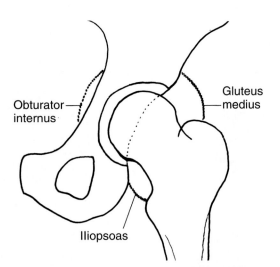

Figure 12-33 **HIP JOINT: NORMAL FAT FOLDS.** With good detailed radiographic examinations, the radiolucent fat folds for the gluteus medius may be seen lateral to the femoral neck; for the iliopsoas, superior to the lesser trochanter; and for the obturator internus, medial to the pelvic brim at the iliopectineal line. *COMMENT:* In patients with septic arthritis of the hip joint, these fat folds may be deviated beyond their normal anatomic positions. (Reprinted with permission from **Guebert GM:** *Tom Smith's arthritis.* ACA Council Roent September, 1981.)

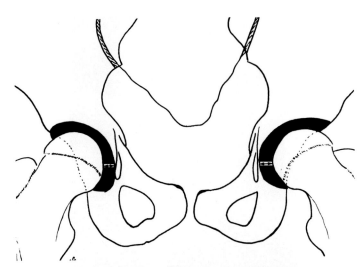

Figure 12-34 **WALDENSTRÖM'S SIGN OF HIP JOINT EFFUSION.** An early sign of septic hip joint disease is an increase in the articular joint space between the femoral head and Köhler's teardrop (the inferior and medial surface of the acetabulum). This measurement is taken from the lateral aspect of Köhler's teardrop to the medial margin of the femoral head; a measurement > 11 mm or a difference in measurement > 2 mm, compared with the opposite hip, is a positive sign and is considered clinically significant. It should be noted that Waldenström's sign is a non-specific sign of joint effusion, is not pathognomonic of infection, and may also occur in post-traumatic and synovial inflammatory cases. (Reprinted with permission from **Guebert GM:** *Tom Smith's arthritis.* ACA Council Roent September, 1981.)

spaces ensues, and complete loss of joint space may occur within a few weeks. (Fig. 12-35) Rarely, gas may be present in the adjacent soft tissue. (8)

Osseous Alterations

The earliest skeletal roentgen sign of septic arthritis is the loss of the normal subchondral cortical bone (subarticular white line). (Fig. 12-36) Radiographs of optimum quality are necessary for demonstrating this sign, along with a high degree of observer suspicion. As the infective process progresses, medullary metaphyseal moth-eaten destruction occurs. If this becomes extensive, it could lead to complete resorption of the articulating ends of the bones. (Figs. 12-37 and 12-38) A laminated periosteal response (extracapsular in origin) may be seen as the destructive lesion disrupts the outer cortex and irritates the periosteum. A late sequela may be complete ankylosis, bony or fibrous, of the affected joint (Fig. 12-39).

As the infection subsides, the articular surface may be remodeled but invariably is left deformed. During healing, remineralization gradually reestablishes discrete bone margins. If the infection has progressed this far, however, one can expect little restoration of articular spacing. (Fig. 12-40)

The time frame in which these roentgen signs and pathologic processes occur is reasonably short in suppurative septic arthritis. (Fig. 12-41) This is in contrast to the extended time sequence so frequently encountered in non-suppurative granulomatous (tubercular) arthritis.

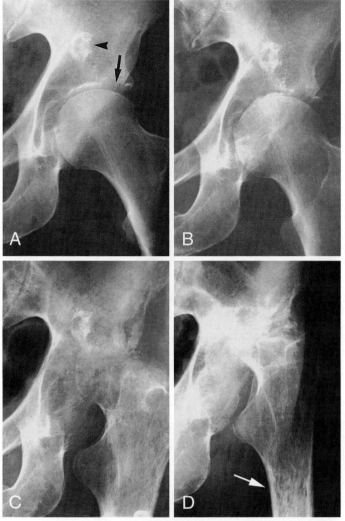

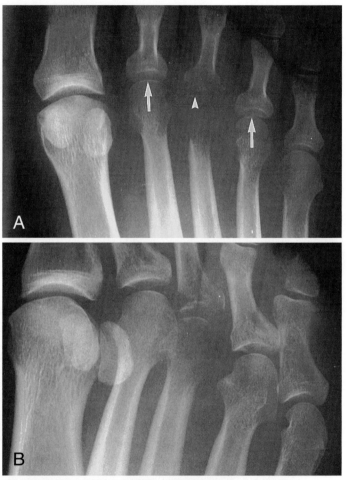

Figure 12-35 SERIAL PROGRESSION OF SEPTIC ARTHRITIS: HIP A. Initial Film. Note that radiographic examination of the hip joint reveals a lytic destructive lesion in the lateral margin of the cortex of the acetabular surface (*arrow*). There is a subtle suggestion of early symmetric loss of the joint space. Of incidental notation is a benign bone cyst (*arrowhead*) present in the supra-acetabular area. **B. 1-Month Follow-Up.** Observe the nearly complete obliteration of the articular joint space, with extensive destruction of the cortical margins surrounding the acetabular rim. **C. 2-Month Follow-Up.** Note the severe resorption of the femoral head, with lateral displacement of the femur from the acetabulum. There is extensive disorganization of the bony structures of the acetabulum and the femoral head. **D. 3-Month Follow-Up.** Note the complete resorption of the femoral head and destruction of the acetabulum. Persistent lateral displacement of the femur from the acetabulum is noted. Of incidental notation, observe the spotty loss of bone density present in the visualized portion of the shaft of the femur as the result of disuse osteoporosis (*arrow*). *COMMENT:* This 25-year-old patient presented with localized pain in the hip joint.

Figure 12-36 EARLY SEPTIC ARTHRITIS. A. PA Foot. B. Oblique Foot. Observe the complete loss of joint space at the third metatarsophalangeal articulation. This loss of bone density is present on both sides of the joint. The early lesion of septic arthritis is loss of the normal subchondral cortical white line (*arrowhead*) in the involved third metatarsal head. Note the normal cortical white line (*arrows*) in the second and fourth metatarsal heads.

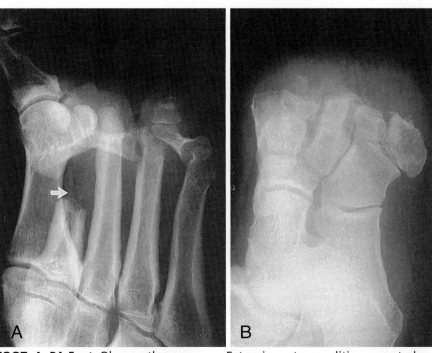

Figure 12-37   DIABETIC FOOT. A. PA Foot. Observe the vascular calcification (*arrow*) between the first and second metatarsal, which is a characteristic complication of long-standing diabetes (Mönckeberg's medial sclerosis). This patient with diabetes had a history of circulatory disturbances. Extensive osteomyelitis warranted surgical removal of the second, third, and fourth toes. **B. Post Amputation.** Note that because the patient's circulatory disturbances and predisposition to osteomyelitis was uncontrollable, a forefoot amputation was eventually required to halt the destructive process.

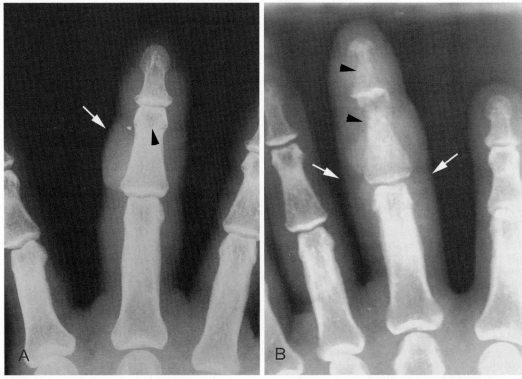

Figure 12-38   SEPTIC ARTHRITIS WITH PROGRESSION. A. Initial Film. Note the prominent soft tissue swelling of the entire digit (*arrow*). Slight bone destruction is evident (*arrowhead*). **B. 1-Month Follow-Up.** Note the marked soft tissue swelling of the entire digit (*arrows*). Moth-eaten destruction of the middle and distal phalanx is evident (*arrowheads*). (Courtesy of Steven P. Brownstein, MD, Springfield, New Jersey.)

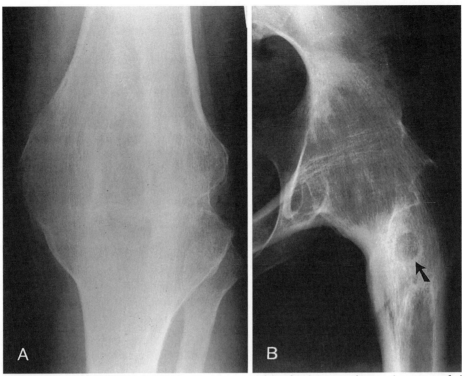

Figure 12-39 **SEPTIC ARTHRITIS: ANKYLOSIS. A. AP Knee.** Note the complete bony ankylosis of the joint between the distal femur and the proximal tibia. This 53-year-old male had septic arthritis of the knee joint 20 years previously. **B. AP Hip.** Note the well-defined radiolucent defect (*arrow*) within the intertrochanteric space of the femur, which was a Brodie's abscess. This elderly veteran had a previous history of septic arthritis of the hip joint, which has healed with total bony ankylosis of the coxal articulation. (Courtesy of Dennis A. Middendorp, DC, Creswick, Victoria, Australia.)

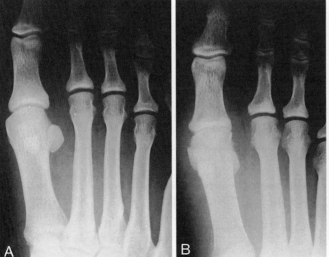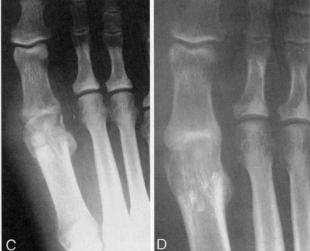

Figure 12-40 **SEPTIC ARTHRITIS OF THE GREAT TOE: A MISDIAGNOSIS. A. Initial Film.** Note that the initial radiographs of the first metatarsophalangeal articulation are normal. **B. 15-Day Follow-Up.** Note the symmetric loss of joint space in the first metatarsophalangeal articulation and destructive lesions. **C. 2-Month Follow-Up.** Note that no further progression of the septic arthritis has occurred; however, significant narrowing of the first metatarsophalangeal joint persists. **D. 4-Month Follow-Up.** Note the partial bony ankylosis as a sequela of the septic arthritis. *COMMENT:* This 32-year-old German female presented to the local physician in a rural community complaining of severe pain in the first metatarsophalangeal articulation. A provisional diagnosis on physical examination was that of septic arthritis, and the patient was referred to the local hospital for definitive diagnosis and follow-up. On admission, the patient was told that her x-rays were normal and that she did not have an infection but, rather, gout. Medication for gout was administered, to which the patient experienced a violent adverse reaction. Finally, because of her persistent pain, follow-up radiographs were taken, which demonstrated the classic signs of septic arthritis. Aspiration of the joint and culturing produced *Staphylococcus aureus* organisms.

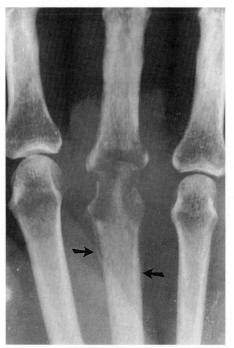

Figure 12-41 SEPTIC ARTHRITIS. PA Hand. Observe the symmetric loss of joint space, with destruction of the cortex of the third metacarpal and the base of its proximal phalanx. The infectious process has caused destruction and resorption of a large portion of the third metacarpal head. Note, also, a small degree of periosteal response in the distal shaft of the third metacarpal (*arrows*). *COMMENT:* The infection followed a penetrating tooth wound incurred during a bar-room fight.

TOM SMITH'S ARTHRITIS

In 1874 Thomas Smith (1), a London physician, published material on postmortem studies of infantile hips that demonstrated osteomyelitis of the proximal metaphyses. Smith noted that bones

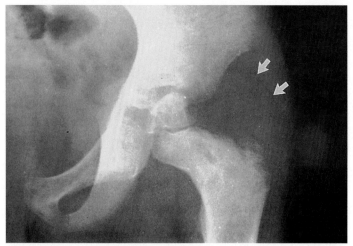

Figure 12-42 TOM SMITH'S ARTHRITIS. AP Hip. Observe the distention of the gluteus medius fat plane (*arrows*) as a result of infectious intracapsular exudate. There is extensive destruction of the metaphysis and the epiphysis of the proximal femur. (Reprinted with permission from **Guebert GM:** *Tom Smith's arthritis.* ACA Council Roent September, 1981.)

that have metaphyses included within the adjacent joint capsule are predisposed to rapid development of septic arthritis. (1,2) The bones that fall into this category are the proximal and distal femur, distal tibia, and proximal and distal humerus. (2) In this anatomic configuration, osteomyelitis can rupture the metaphyseal cortex, enter the articulation, and spread via synovial fluid to the epiphyseal or subarticular end of the bone. This form of septic arthritis has been called Tom Smith's arthritis (1,2) and can be encountered in the hip, knee, ankle, shoulder, and elbow. (Fig. 12-42)

CAPSULE SUMMARY   Septic Arthritis

General Considerations
- Single joint involvement is the rule.
- Most common route of joint contamination is hematogenous spread or direct traumatic implantation.

Cause
- The most frequently isolated organism is *Staphylococcus aureus.*

Clinical Features
- Chills, fever, edema, pain, and redness are often found.
- An elevated ESR and an increase in the white blood cell count occur.
- Altered gait and a painful limp are common in weight-bearing joints.

Pathologic Features
- Purulent exudate creates joint distention.
- Cartilage destruction leads to osseous destruction and loss of joint space.
- Advanced stages may produce dislocation.
- Regional hyperemia leads to juxta-articular osteoporosis.

Radiologic Features
- The knee and hip are the most common sites.
- Joint effusion leads to distortion of the fat folds.
- Positive Waldenström's sign.
- Rapid loss of joint space; loss of the cortical white line and moth-eaten pattern of bone destruction.
- Bony ankylosis rarely occurs.

NON-SUPPURATIVE OSTEOMYELITIS (TUBERCULOSIS)

General Considerations

For nearly 5,000 years tuberculosis was a lethal bone disorder. During the Industrial Revolution, urban overcrowding, malnutrition, and debilitation produced an environment in which tuberculosis became epidemic in the Western world. (1) At the beginning of the 20th century tuberculosis was the leading cause of death in Western society. (2) In previous times there were two modes of infection: inhalation and ingestion. (3) Infection by ingestion was typical for the bovine tubercle bacillus *Mycobacterium bovis,* and this type was responsible for a significant number of the cases of bone and joint tuberculosis.

This form of tuberculosis has largely been eradicated. Nearly all tuberculous infections in the United States are caused by the human strain of *Mycobacterium tuberculosis*.

With the emergence of effective chemotherapeutic agents in the late 1940s and early 1950s for management of tuberculosis, it is now considerably less common in the United States and United Kingdom than in the first half of the 20th century. (4) However, it is estimated that one third of the world's population is a carrier of the bacillus (5), and with the advent of modern travel and the immigration to the Western world of various ethnic groups susceptible to tuberculosis, the condition is still seen with some frequency in the large population centers of the Western countries. (4) More than 10 million people in the United States alone are currently infected. (6) Similarly, in many countries of Asia and Africa, which are characterized by substandard conditions of healthcare, inadequate diet, and even semistarvation, the incidence of skeletal tuberculosis remains high. (4) In addition, evidence accumulates that the organism is developing a degree of resistance to the antibiotics that have been so singularly effective in recent years. (4) Infection of the musculoskeletal system is commonly caused by hematogenous spread of a primary focus within the respiratory tract. The thoracic and lumbar spine are favored skeletal sites. Although once thought to be a disease of childhood, patients of all ages now seem to be susceptible.

Incidence

In 1953, 84,203 cases of tuberculosis were reported in the United States. (7) By 1977 this number was reduced to 30,154 cases, 3,000 of which were fatal. (7) From 1960 to 1970 the case rate per 100,000 population declined from 30.8 to 18.3. From 1971 to 1977 the incidence fell from only 15.8 to 13.9. (7) The incidence of tuberculosis in the United States appears to be stabilizing, with isolated areas of disease still existing among the socioeconomically disadvantaged and among recent immigrants from geographic areas where the disease is still endemic. (8) Because it is considered uncommon, tuberculosis is frequently overlooked in the differential diagnosis of the unknown spinal lesion. (8) This lack of appreciation of spinal tuberculosis contrasts with the large number of papers now appearing on primary spinal bone tumors. (8) These tumors individually and collectively are still much rarer than spinal tuberculosis. (8)

Cause

The most common pathogen isolated is *Mycobacterium tuberculosis*. Accurate diagnosis rests on the recovery of the causative acid-fast pathogen from joint aspirates, tissue exudation, tissue specimens by artificial cultural methods, or animal inoculation.

Clinical Features

Skeletal tuberculosis is estimated to affect only 2% of patients with tuberculosis (9) and probably occurs only in immunodeficient patients after massive exposure to this primarily respiratory pathogen. In individuals such as prepubertal children, debilitated geriatrics, AIDS sufferers, silicosis, lymphoma patients, alcoholics, and drug abusers, tuberculosis often has an accelerated rate of progress. Unlike pyogenic osteomyelitis, tuberculous osteomyelitis tends to arise insidiously and takes a chronic course that can be destructive and resistant to control.

Skeletal tuberculosis is most prevalent in the first three decades and most frequently seen in prepubertal children, though it is exceedingly rare during the 1st year of life. (10) There is no sex predilection. The onset of symptoms is generally insidious and not accompanied by alarming general manifestations such as fever, night sweats, toxicity, or prostration. Pain in the region of the involved joint may be mild at onset and accompanied by a sensation of stiffness. Tuberculous spondylitis presents clinically with an insidious onset of back pain, decreased range of motion, and focal tenderness. This spinal pain may be with or without neurological involvement. The sudden onset of lower limb paraplegia in spinal tuberculosis is referred to as *Pott's paraplegia*. In advanced cases, the patients complain of a pus-draining sinus tract. In children, 70% of patients are ≤ 5 years of age, and the duration of symptoms before treatment averages 1–2 years. (11)

Appendicular tubercular arthritis presents clinically with tenderness, soft tissue swelling, joint effusion, and increased skin temperature around the involved area. As the disease progresses, limitation of joint motion becomes marked because of muscle contractures. Eventually, muscle atrophy and deformity become apparent. Because the knee and hip are the most common sites, patients often develop a limp as a mechanism to protect the involved weight-bearing joint. The articulations of the lower extremities are more frequently involved than are those of the upper extremities.

Pathologic Features

Pathological features are divided into tubercular spondylitis and tubercular arthritis.

Tubercular Spondylitis (Pott's Disease)

Tubercular spondylitis was recognized in ancient times, with descriptions noted for Egyptian mummies dating as far back as 3,000 B.C. (12) The original paper describing this disease was written by Percival Pott (13) in 1779, and the condition is widely known as Pott's disease. It is estimated that the spine is affected in 25–60% of cases of skeletal tuberculosis. (14) The most common sites are the lower thoracic and upper lumbar spine, with L1 being the favored segment of involvement. (14) The concept of vascular dissemination is well established. Most authorities agree that it spreads via the venous pathway of Batson's plexus. (15)

Discovertebral Involvement. The adult intervertebral disc is avascular; therefore, pathogens reach the disc via an alternative route. (Fig. 12-12) Contrary to previous belief, the subchondral vertebral endplate is the earliest site for this infectious focus. Even though disc space narrowing is often the earliest radiographic sign, the initial pathologic focus lies within the anterior vertebral endplate. The infecting organisms travel as emboli via the bloodstream until they block the conducting arterioles or venules. The vascular network of looping redundant vessels at the anterior aspect of the vertebral body creates an opportune environment for organisms to lodge and proliferate. As caseous necrosis ensues, an identifiable lytic vertebral abnormality will be seen in 2–5 months. (16) This weakens the vertebral endplate considerably, creating an alternative mechanism for infectious spread to the disc. (Fig. 12-43) As vertebral collapse ensues, a

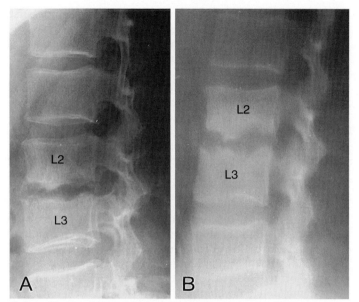

Figure 12-43 DISCOVERTEBRAL INVOLVEMENT (TUBERCU-LOSIS). A. Plain Film, Lateral Lumbar Spine. Observe the narrowing of the disc space between L2 and L3 and resorption of the subchondral cortical vertebral endplate on the inferior surface of L2 and the superior portion of L3. **B. Tomography, Lateral Lumbar Spine.** Note that the tomographic projection demonstrates much more lytic resorption of the vertebral endplates of L2 and L3 than can be appreciated on the plain films. *COMMENT:* Most tubercular infections of the spine involve the discovertebral area, with extension into the vertebral pedicle and neural arch being rare. Most neural arch involvement in tuberculosis is found in tropical climates and occurs in only 2% of the spinal cases of tuberculosis.

herniation of discal material allows contamination of the disc via direct extension. (14) This pathologic process leads to a loss of disc height. (Fig. 12-44) MRI demonstrates the lesion with diminished signal on T1- and increased signal on T2-weighted images. (17)

The entire process is pathologically identical to pyogenic spondylitis; however, tubercular spondylitis is much slower and indolent in its progression. Tubercular extension to the vertebral pedicle and neural arch is rare, occurring in about 2% of spinal cases and being more common in tropical climates. (18,19)

Paravertebral Soft Tissue Involvement. Involvement of the paravertebral soft tissue encompasses abscess formation, subligamentous dissection, and extensive granulomatous formation, which can precipitate paraplegia (Pott's paraplegia).

Abscess Formation. Abscess formation may occur as the infection spreads to the soft tissues. In the cervical spine, anterior spread creates either a retropharyngeal or a retrotracheal abscess, indicated radiographically by an increased retropharyngeal or retrotracheal interspace measurement. (Figs. 12-45 and 12-46) The potential for acute respiratory emergencies exists with retropharyngeal abscess formation owing to direct obstruction or from rupture. (20)

In the thoracic spine the extension is anterolateral, creating necrotizing abscesses that are usually bilateral and large, displacing the paraspinal lines. (Fig. 12-47) Abscess formation in tuberculosis can produce large fusiform soft tissue swelling on frontal radiographs, which appears out of proportion to the degree of osseous and discal destruction. (14)

In the lumbar spine, the anterolateral extension of the infective focus to the psoas muscle is well documented (*psoas abscess*). (21) This represents slowly developing, necrotizing abscess formation, stemming from tuberculous channels that emerge from

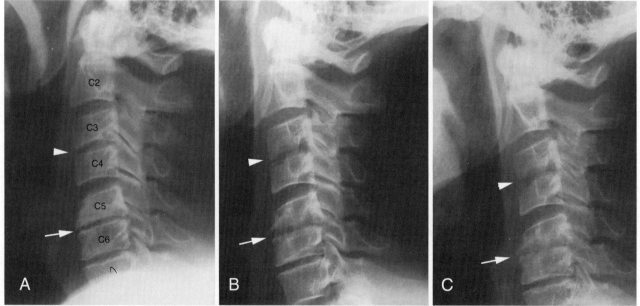

Figure 12-44 TUBERCULOSIS: CERVICAL SPINE WITH PROGRESSION. A. Initial Film. Note that the radiologic findings are non-specific, with loss of disc height at C3, C5, and C6. Note that the endplates are intact. At the sites of infection, there are no diagnostic features (*arrow, arrowhead*). **B. 6-Week Follow-Up.** Observe that signs of infection have developed at the C3–C4 (*arrowhead*) and C5–C6 (*arrow*) disc spaces. Note the characteristic loss of vertebral endplates, which is diagnostic. Slight anterior displacement of the retropharyngeal interspace is evident at C4. **C. 8-Week Follow-Up.** Note that both sites have advanced (*arrowhead, arrow*), as evidenced by the increased loss of the underlying vertebral bodies. (Courtesy of Melvin P. Deutsch, DC, Miami, Florida.)

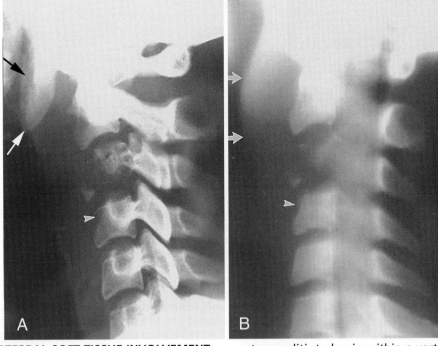

Figure 12-45 **PARAVERTEBRAL SOFT TISSUE INVOLVEMENT.**
A. Abscess Formation. Note that the lateral cervical plain film demonstrates diffuse destruction and collapse of the vertebral body of C3. There is a large retropharyngeal abscess, which has increased the retropharyngeal interspace (RPI) (*arrows*). *COMMENT:* The normal RPI should not be > 7 mm from the anteroinferior tip of the body of C2 to the posterior surface of the pharynx. The measurement in this patient was > 15 mm. Observe the early lytic destruction at the anterosuperior corner of the body of C4 (*arrowhead*). This is the classic site for either suppurative or non-suppurative osteomyelitis to begin within a vertebral segment.
B. Tomography, Tubercular Lesion. Note that the C3 tubercular lesion is clearly defined. The large retropharyngeal abscess (*arrows*), along with the early destructive lesion at the anterosuperior corner of C4 (*arrowhead*), is clearly defined. *COMMENT:* This is an unusual presentation for tuberculosis, without significant disc space narrowing. At first glance, one might consider this to represent a metastatic tumor; however, the presence of the large increase in the RPI does not support that consideration. Most metastatic tumors do not produce large soft tissue masses.

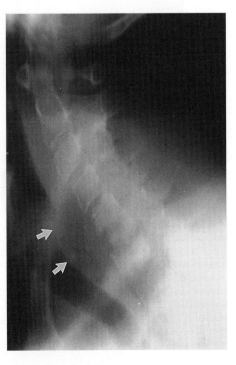

Figure 12-46 **RETROLARYNGEAL ABSCESS. Tomography, Lateral Cervical Spine.** Note the extensive destruction of the C5–C7 vertebral bodies and their respective discs. Note the bulging of the larynx anterior to the C5–C7 segments (*arrows*), measuring 30 mm. This represents a significant increase in the retrotracheal interspace, the normal measurement being no greater than 22 mm from the posterior surface of the larynx to the anteroinferior tip of the body of C6.

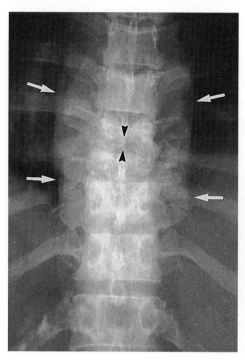

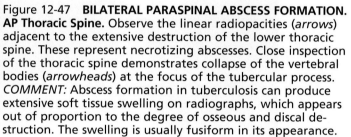

Figure 12-47   **BILATERAL PARASPINAL ABSCESS FORMATION. AP Thoracic Spine.** Observe the linear radiopacities (*arrows*) adjacent to the extensive destruction of the lower thoracic spine. These represent necrotizing abscesses. Close inspection of the thoracic spine demonstrates collapse of the vertebral bodies (*arrowheads*) at the focus of the tubercular process. *COMMENT:* Abscess formation in tuberculosis can produce extensive soft tissue swelling on radiographs, which appears out of proportion to the degree of osseous and discal destruction. The swelling is usually fusiform in its appearance.

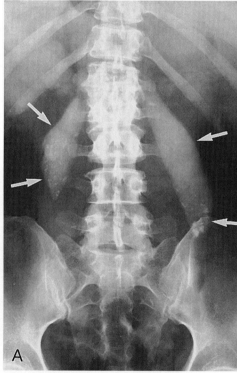

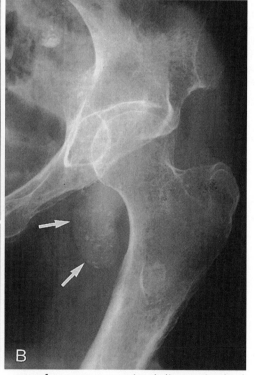

Figure 12-48   **PSOAS ABSCESS. A. AP Lumbar Spine.** Note the bilateral increased density in the area of the psoas muscles. Observe the snowflake, dense type of calcification present throughout both psoas muscles (*arrows*). *COMMENT:* The primary source of the tuberculosis was at the L1 and L2 vertebral segments, where loss of disc height and some destruction of the vertebral bodies can be visualized. **B. AP Hip.** Note the increase in density in the area of the soft tissues about the lesser trochanter (*arrows*) of the proximal femur. This represents the distal extension of a tubercular psoas ab-scess from more proximal disease in the lumbar spine. *COMMENT:* Psoas abscess is most commonly found paraspinally, between L1 and L5. Approximately 5% of tubercular spondylitis patients have associated psoas abscess formation. Calcification is a sign of inactivity of the infectious process and may become quite dense with progressive healing. (Panel A reprinted with permission from **Yochum TR:** *Tuberculosis of L1/L2, with psoas cold abscesses.* ACA J Chiro, 1982. Panel B courtesy of Bryan Hartley, MD, Melbourne, Australia.)

the bone or joint. The abscess may create a draining sinus by dissecting along fascial planes and coming to the surface in the paraspinal region (*empyema necessitatis*) or it may follow the sheath of the psoas muscle and appear in the inguinal region or near the psoas insertion at the lesser trochanter. (Fig. 12-48) The vertebral site shows destruction of the disc and adjacent endplates and vertebral body. The abscess is a collection of caseous necrotic debris. Psoas abscesses may be unilateral or bilateral.

If it remains uncontaminated by pyogenic organisms, the abscess is often the site of precipitation of calcium salts. Tuberculous psoas abscesses calcify in faint amorphous deposits or in a snowflake, dense type of calcification. (22) The appearance of calcification is a sign of inactivity of the infectious process and may become quite dense with progressive healing. The psoas abscess is most commonly found paraspinally between L1 and L5. Approximately 5% of tubercular spondylitis patients have associated psoas abscess formation. (14,21) Non-tuberculous psoas abscesses rarely calcify. (14,21)

Subligamentous Dissection. Subligamentous dissection is an unusual presentation for spinal tuberculosis in which the predominant feature is massive and extensive paraspinal abscess formation, with relatively little osseous involvement. (4) The infectious focus is located at the anterior surface of the vertebral body and the anterior longitudinal ligament. Initially, the disc space is spared as the infection spreads contiguously from one anterior vertebral segment to another. This mode of dissemination is peculiar to tuberculosis and produces a shallow excavation on the anterior aspect of the involved vertebra. (8) Frequently, the anterior concave erosive lesions simulate the effects of aneurysmal pressure or adjacent lymph node erosion, best depicted on CT. (23) (Fig. 12-49) These gouge defects may occur in relation to an abscess at any site in the spine unrelated to aortic pulsations (4) and usually affect three or more spinal segments. In later stages the classical appearance of Pott's disease (disc space narrowing with vertebral collapse) may be expected to develop. (4)

Pott's Paraplegia. A rare complication of Pott's disease is Pott's paraplegia. (22) It represents a life-threatening complication of advanced spinal tuberculosis. Collapse of multiple vertebrae with infectious deterioration of the discs stimulates a growth of considerable granulation tissue. This granulation tissue, coupled with osseous debris (sequestra) from the vertebral bodies, may sufficiently narrow the spinal canal to produce a pressure paraplegia. (Fig. 12-50) (22) Neural arch involvement has a higher risk for

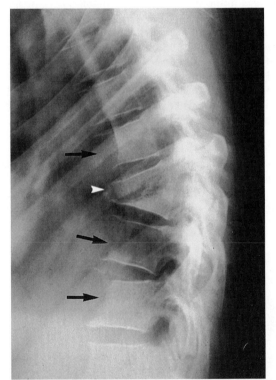

Figure 12-49 **SUBLIGAMENTOUS TUBERCULOSIS. Lateral Thoracic Spine.** Observe the anterior concave erosions (*arrows*) of the lower thoracic segments. There is complete pathologic collapse and destruction of the disc between two thoracic segments (*arrowhead*) as a result of extensive tubercular destruction. Note also the relatively good preservation of disc height at the thoracic segments where there are anterior erosive lesions. *COMMENT:* Subligamentous tuberculosis represents an unusual presentation and form of spread of spinal tuberculosis. The infectious focus is located at the anterior surface of the body and dissects down along the anterior longitudinal ligament. Initially, the disc space is spared as the infection spreads contiguously from one vertebral segment to another. This mode of dissemination is peculiar to tuberculosis and produces a shallow excavation on the anterior aspects of the involved vertebrae. These anterior concave erosive lesions simulate the effects of aneurysmal pressure and have been called *gouge defects*. Usually, three or more spinal segments are involved; in the later stages, the classical appearance of Pott's disease may be expected to develop. (Courtesy of C. H. Quay, MD, Melbourne, Australia.)

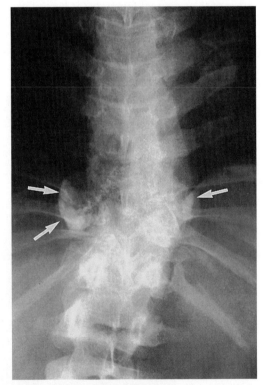

Figure 12-50 **POTT'S PARAPLEGIA. AP Thoracic Spine.** Note the extensive destruction and collapse of multiple lower thoracic segments. Paravertebral abscess formation with calcification (*arrows*) is noted. *COMMENT:* The paraplegia complicating tuberculosis has been referred to as Pott's paraplegia. It occurs as a result of the investment of the dura with granulation tissue and/or pressure applied by liquid abscesses, causing direct mechanical compression. This is a rare complication of spinal tuberculosis (Pott's disease).

cord compression, best shown with MRI. (24) The paraplegia results from the investment of the dura with granulation tissue and/or pressure applied by liquid abscesses, causing direct mechanical compression. Recent research has suggested that patients displaying increased levels of ESR upon evaluation may be more at risk of developing future paraplegia. (25)

Tubercular Arthritis

Tuberculosis involving the weight-bearing appendicular joints is second only to the preferred spinal site. The hip and knee are the most common sites (representing 75% of cases), with the ankle, shoulder, elbow, pubes, and wrist being rarely involved. (4) (Figs. 12-51 and 12-52) Monoarticular involvement is the rule. (14) Most patients are middle-aged or elderly, and many have received multiple intra-articular injections of steroids for a preexisting unrelated joint disorder. (14)

The tubercle bacillus may lodge in the synovium or the metaphyseal portion of the bone. Most tubercular arthritic lesions begin within the metaphysis as an infectious focus with secondary spread to the joint. With this mode of presentation the inflammatory changes in the synovial membrane are extensive, leading to significant early joint effusion. The infected synovial membrane becomes thickened, and granulation tissue spreads to the free surface of the articular cartilage. This interference with the free surface of the articular cartilage affects its nutrition and ultimately leads to its destruction. Early erosions occur involving the portion of the proximal femur that is bare of cartilage but exposed to synovium. Thus the initial erosive lesions may simulate those of early rheumatoid arthritis. As the entire infective process progresses, a non-uniform destruction of the articular surface occurs. As cartilage and bone destruction ensue, sequestrum formation of variable size may occur. This process often involves both surfaces of the joint, leading to the characteristic *kissing sequestrum*. (4,14) (Fig. 12-53)

The increased vascularity of the low-grade tuberculous inflammatory process produces a hyperemic osteoporosis. The degree of osteoporosis is often disproportionate to the extent of the infectious lesion.

Radiologic Features

Tubercular Spondylitis

The spine is the most frequent site of skeletal tuberculosis. The radiographic manifestation of spinal tuberculosis is the appearance of slowly progressing destruction with only minimal reactive changes in the bone. The radiographic latent period for the spine is 21 days, which often delays early diagnosis and treatment. The early roentgen signs consist of a lytic destructive lesion placed in the anterior corner of the vertebral endplate, coupled with a recognizable loss of disc space. (Fig. 12-54)

Easily discerned on the anteroposterior (AP) projection is abscess formation, displacing the paraspinal line. These abscesses are particularly well visualized in the thoracic spine, with the adjacent radiolucent lung providing a sharply contrasted peripheral margin. Paravertebral abscess formation occurs in about half of the adult patients. (22) The lower thoracic–upper lumbar spine is the most common spinal site, with L1 being most prevalent. As an extension of the infectious focus in the lumbar spine, a *psoas abscess* may form. This is seen radiographically as a soft tissue swelling around the destructive spinal lesion. It will be of varied

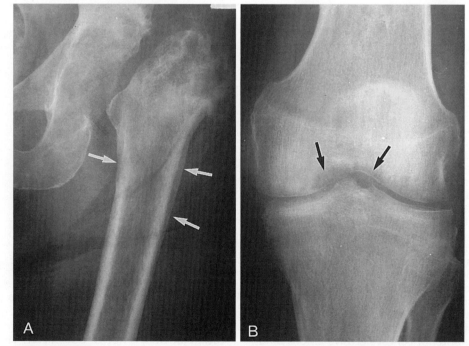

Figure 12-51 **TUBERCULAR ARTHRITIS. A. AP Hip.** Note the extensive resorption of the entire femoral head, with lateral displacement of the femur. Observe the destruction and disorganization of the acetabulum. This is an advanced stage of tuberculosis of the hip. Note the solid periosteal new bone formation on the diaphysis of the proximal femur (*arrows*). **B. AP Knee.** Note the symmetric narrowing of the joint space about the knee articulation. Observe the destruction of the articular cortex of the distal femur (*arrows*). These represent relatively early signs of tubercular arthritis.

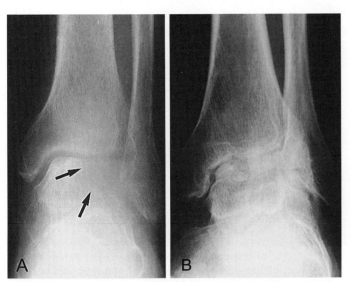

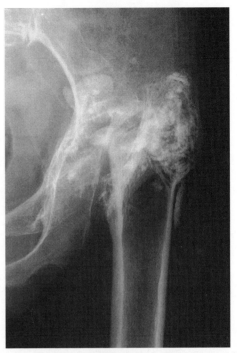

Figure 12-52 **TUBERCULOSIS AT THE ANKLE JOINT. A. AP Ankle: Initial Film.** Note the slight loss of joint space at the ankle mortise between the distal tibia and talar dome. Note the focal destructive area of radiolucency (*arrows*) within the lateral dome of the talus. **B. 6-Month Follow-Up.** Note the significant disorganization of the ankle joint, with calcific debris and near ankylosis.

Figure 12-53 **KISSING SEQUESTRUM: HIP JOINT.** Observe the complete resorption of the femoral head, with extensive destruction of the articular cartilage. Note the lateral displacement of the femur from the acetabulum. There are many bony sequestra scattered throughout the acetabular and femoral head area. An extensive degree of sequestered debris is noted in the area of the greater trochanter. *COMMENT:* The term *kissing sequestrum* has been offered to describe the tubercular process involving both surfaces of the joint, leading to extensive sequestered tubercular debris.

Figure 12-54 **TUBERCULOSIS: EARLY DESTRUCTIVE VERTEBRAL LESION. A. Lateral Cervical Spine.** Note the disc space narrowing between the C6 and the C7 vertebral segments. Observe the early radiographic sign of a lytic destructive lesion placed in the anteroinferior corner of the vertebral endplate of C6 (*arrow*). **B. 3-Month Follow-Up.** Note the further destructive changes of the intervertebral disc, with more destructive changes at the anteroinferior aspect of the corner of the C6 vertebral body (*arrow*). *COMMENT:* On initial observation it could be easy to label the disc space narrowing between the C6 and C7 segments as being degenerative in nature; however, the early destructive lesion at the anteroinferior corner of the body of C6 and the lack of subchondral sclerosis and spondylophyte formation negate that conclusion.

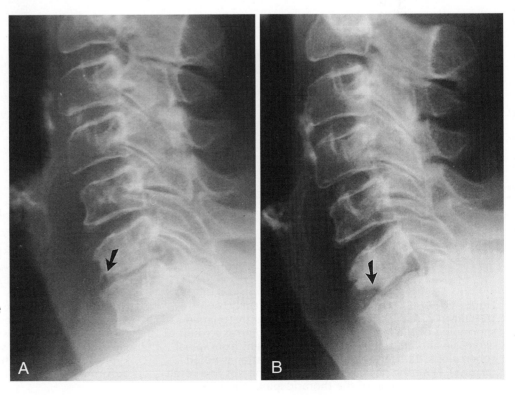

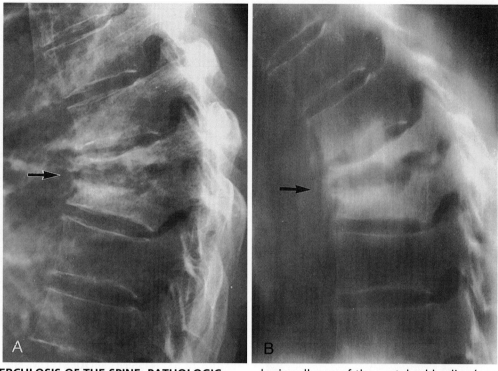

Figure 12-55 TUBERCULOSIS OF THE SPINE: PATHOLOGIC COLLAPSE. A. Lateral Thoracic Spine, Plain Film. B. Lateral Thoracic Spine, Tomography. Note the extensive destruction of two thoracic vertebral segments, with significant patho-logic collapse of the vertebral bodies (*arrows*). Extensive dis-integration of the disc and wedging of the involved verte-brae may predispose to the development of an angular kyphosis or gibbus deformity.

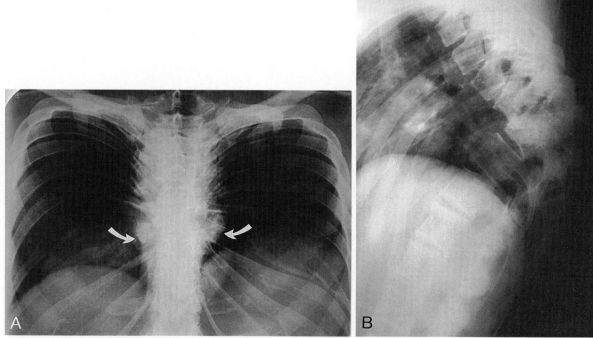

Figure 12-56 EXTENSIVE TUBERCULOSIS: GIBBUS DEFORMITY. A. AP Thoracic Spine. Observe the relative shortening of the length of the thoracic spine as a result of extensive and multiple vertebral involvement from spinal tuberculosis. Paravertebral abscess calcification is noted (*arrows*). Note the peculiar deformity of the ribs as a result of the foreshortening of the thoracic spine. This gives the ribs the appearance of a spider spine. **B. Lateral Thoracic Spine.** Observe the severe angular kyphosis in the lower thoracic spine as a result of multiple vertebral body col-lapse from extensive spinal tuberculosis. This angular kyphosis has been referred to as the classical gibbus deformity of Pott's disease.

size and appear radiopaque on observation. It often assumes a pear-shaped configuration and frequently calcifies.

Eventually, osteolytic destruction of the vertebral bodies occurs. This process weakens the vertebrae to the extent that pathologic collapse follows. (Fig. 12-55) Progressive breakdown of bone, disc disintegration, and vertebral collapse finally result in spinal deformity and obliteration of the intervertebral disc. (22) Wedging of the involved vertebrae is common, with angular kyphosis leading to the development of a gibbus deformity. (Fig. 12-56) The degree of angulation varies with the site and extent of vertebral disease. (14) The angulation is often more acute in the thoracic spine than in the cervical or lumbar regions. (14) It is also more severe when only one or two vertebral segments are destroyed. (14)

Patients with long-standing gibbus deformity secondary to tuberculosis may develop a reversal of the height to width ratio of the vertebral bodies. Normally, weight-bearing lumbar vertebrae in the human are wider than they are tall. In long-standing gibbus deformity, tremendous biomechanical stress is placed on the uninvolved vertebral body immediately caudal to the gibbus.

This stress may alter the appearance of the vertebra, whereby it becomes taller than it is broad. This alteration is found only in those patients in which the growth centers of the vertebral body were not closed at the time the disease affected the thoracic spine. (14) This vertebral alteration has been called the *long vertebra* (26) (Fig. 12-57); it has also been noted in quadriplegic patients, in which case it is referred to as the *tall vertebra*. (27)

The differential diagnosis of tubercular spondylitis includes a wide variety of other infectious and non-infectious disorders. Pyogenic infectious lesions often cannot be differentiated radiographically, and the clinical data are important in the initial diagnosis, whereas joint aspiration is definitive. An insidious and slow onset of back pain (often of several months' duration), a pulmonary infiltrate, previous history, and multiple segment involvement favor the diagnosis of tuberculosis of the spine. Active pulmonary disease is present in 50% of patients with skeletal tuberculosis. (Fig. 12-58)

Scalloping of the anterior surface of the vertebral bodies, which can occur in subligamentous dissection spread of tuberculosis, may also be caused by paravertebral lymphadenopathy owing to metastasis, lymphoma, or myeloma. (14) Occasionally, eosinophilic granuloma of the spine creating a *vertebra plana* can mimic early tuberculosis. (Table 12-2)

Tubercular Arthritis

Tubercular involvement of the appendicular skeleton is not as common as spinal disease. In patients afflicted with skeletal tuberculosis, 50% present with spinal lesions; 30% have hip or knee disease; and 20% are infected at other, lesser known sites

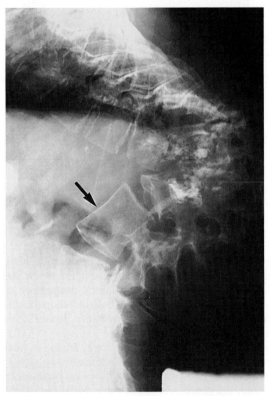

Figure 12-57 TUBERCULAR GIBBUS DEFORMITY: LONG VERTEBRA. Observe the severe lower thoracic–upper lumbar gibbus deformity from spinal tuberculosis. Note the significant increase in height of the L4 vertebral body (*arrow*) in this patient with long-standing deformity. *COMMENT:* Patients with long-standing gibbus deformity secondary to tuberculosis may develop a reversal of the height to width ratio of the vertebral bodies. Normally, weight-bearing lumbar vertebrae in the human are wider than they are tall. In a long-standing gibbus deformity, tremendous biomechanical stress is placed on the uninvolved vertebral body immediately caudal to the gibbus. This vertebral alteration has been called the long vertebra. (Reprinted with permission from **Yochum TR:** *A radiographic anthology of vertebral names.* J Manipulative Physiol Ther 8:2, 1985.)

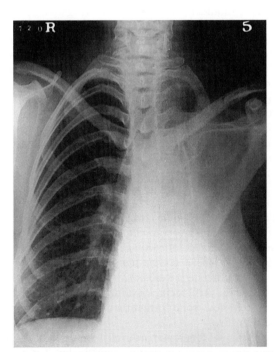

Figure 12-58 PULMONARY TUBERCULOSIS: THORACO-PNEUMOPLASTY. Observe the complete removal of the left lung and ribs two through seven on the left side. In the pre-antibiotic era, the treatment of choice for patients who contracted pulmonary tuberculosis was thoracopneumoplasty.

Table 12-2	Radiologic Signs of Tuberculosis of Bone

Spine
Latent period: 21 days
Early
  Lytic destruction at the anterior subchondral endplate
  Loss of disc height
Late
  Vertebral collapse
  Obliteration of the disc space
  Gibbus formation
    Abscess formation
    Retropharyngeal (cervical spine)
    Paravertebral (thoracic spine)
    Psoas (lumbar spine)
  Multiple segments involved
  Anterior vertebral scalloping (gouge defects)
Extremities
Early
  Joint widening secondary to effusion
  Soft tissue swelling
  Marginal erosions (corner defects)
Late
  Symmetrical obliteration of the joint space
  Destruction of the subcortical bone (white line)
  Moth-eaten osteolytic bone destruction
  Juxta-articular osteoporosis
  Occasional ankylosis

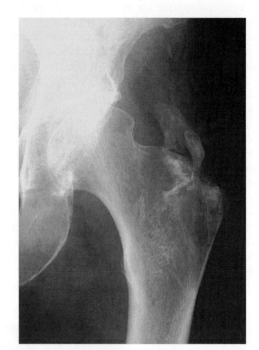

Figure 12-59 TUBERCULOSIS: GREATER TROCHANTER. AP Hip. Observe the fragmentation of the greater trochanter, with some necrotic calcific debris at the base of the trochanter. This is a relatively rare site for tuberculosis of bone.

(pubes, wrist, shoulder, sacroiliac joints). (Figs. 12-59 to 12-63) The knee and hip are the most common appendicular joints involved. Early radiographic signs are joint widening, which is secondary to joint effusion and distention, and soft tissue swelling. This is followed by destruction of the subchondral cortex (*cortical white line*) and a moth-eaten pattern of bone destruction, often on both sides of the joint. (Fig. 12-64) Later, narrowing of the joint occurs as the articular cartilage and bone are destroyed. The entire process is accompanied by juxta-articular osteoporosis, which occurs as a result of hyperemia and disuse atrophy. (Table 12-2)

Often, a triad (*Phemister's triad*) of radiographic findings exists and is characteristic of tuberculous arthritis: progressive and slow joint space narrowing, juxta-articular osteoporosis, and peripheral erosive defects of the articular surfaces. (14) (Fig. 12-65)

Marginal erosions are common, occurring at the corners of the bone, which are bare of cartilage but exposed to the synovial membrane. (14) These corner marginal erosions occur early and may often simulate the erosions of rheumatoid arthritis. (14) Rarely, periostitis will occur, creating a solid or laminated pattern. Periosteal new bone formation is much more common in pyogenic arthritis.

The end stage of tubercular arthritis is fibrous ankylosis of the joint. Bony ankylosis is rare in tuberculosis, but it is a common sequela of pyogenic arthritis. (Fig. 12-66) A peculiar complication of tubercular arthritis in the knee is a focal overgrowth of the medial epiphysis, creating a *megacondyle,* as a result of localized hyperemia. This sometimes mimics a similar appearance of the medial condyle in Still's disease and hemophilia.

Occasionally, tubercular arthritis can affect the sacroiliac joints, creating significant destruction on both sides of the joint. The presentation is usually unilateral. (Fig. 12-67) A *pseudowidening* of the joint, early osteolytic destructive lesions, and eventual ankylosis are the cardinal roentgen signs. Regarding any patient who presents with a unilateral destructive sacroiliac lesion, tuberculosis should always be considered in the differential diagnosis, along with psoriatic arthropathy, Reiter's syndrome, and rheumatoid arthritis.

Tubercular osteomyelitis of the long bones is uncommon. Focal bone destruction, usually in the metaphysis, along with severe osteoporosis, is noted. There is little or no periosteal reaction. Occasionally, the process may resemble pyogenic osteomyelitis, and a definitive diagnosis of tuberculosis often is impossible from plain films alone. Because of the chronicity of the disease, atrophy of surrounding soft tissues ensues. (Table 12-3)

Treatment and Prognosis

The modern standard form of treatment for tuberculosis is chemotherapy. The classic drugs that have been used are isoniazid, ethambutol, and rifampicin. A search for other sites of involvement should be instigated, including the chest, gastrointestinal tract, and genitourinary systems. Management of skeletal tuberculosis includes débridement and arthrodesis. (Fig. 12-68)

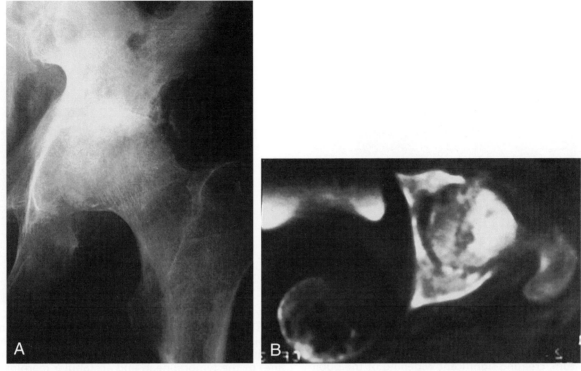

Figure 12-60 **TUBERCULOSIS. A. AP Hip.** Observe the narrowing of the hip joint as a result of destruction of the cartilage and subchondral bone of the acetabulum and femoral head. There is fragmentation and lytic destruction of the femoral head. **B. Axial CT, Hip.** Note the fragmentation and destruction of the femoral head and acetabulum. *COMMENT:* Of patients afflicted with skeletal tuberculosis, 50% present with spinal lesions; 30% have hip or knee disease; and 20% are affected at other, lesser known sites (pubes, wrist, shoulder, sacroiliac joints).

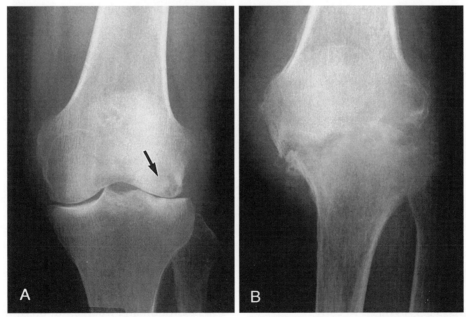

Figure 12-61 **TUBERCULOSIS. A. AP Knee.** Observe the symmetric narrowing of the joint space throughout the knee, a radiographic sign of inflammatory joint disease. There is lytic destruction of the lateral distal condyle of the femur (*arrow*). **B. AP Knee, Follow-Up.** Note the complete disintegration of the joint articulation, with resorption and fragmentation of bone. Spotty disuse osteoporosis is noted in the proximal metaphysis of the tibia.

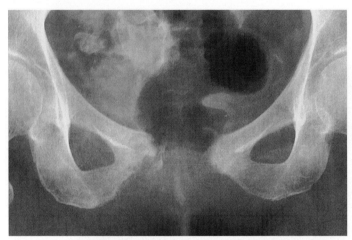

Figure 12-62 **TUBERCULOSIS: PUBIC ARTICULATION. AP Pelvis.** Note the extensive resorption and destruction of the bony architecture, creating significant widening of the pubic articulation. The pubic articulation is a rare location for tuberculosis of bone.

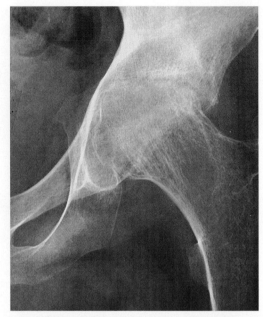

Figure 12-64 **DESTRUCTION OF SUBCHONDRAL CORTEX (CORTICAL WHITE LINE). AP Hip.** Observe the symmetric loss of joint space throughout the entire hip joint. There is extensive resorption of the subchondral cortex (cortical white line) of the femoral head and acetabular margins. These are relatively early signs of tuberculosis of the hip joint. (Courtesy of David P. Thomas, MD, Melbourne, Australia.)

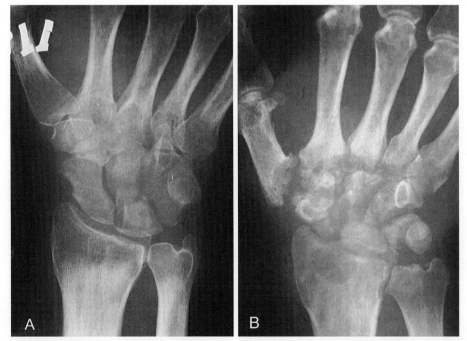

Figure 12-63 **TUBERCULOSIS: PA WRIST. A. Early Involvement.** Observe the significant loss of bone density throughout the visualized carpal bones. The cortical margins of the carpal bones are indistinct as a result of the underlying destruction. **B. Advanced Involvement.** Note the extensive resorption and fragmentation of the carpal bones, including the articulations with the metacarpals (particularly the base of the first metacarpal) and the radiocarpal articulation. (Courtesy of Bryan Hartley, MD, Melbourne, Australia.)

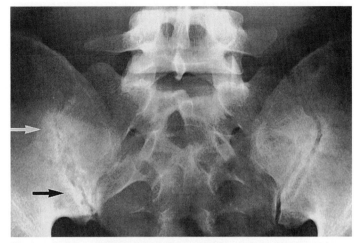

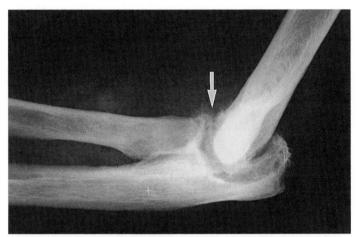

Figure 12-65 **TUBERCULOSIS. Lateral Elbow.** Note the extensive destruction of the elbow articulation. Observe the lytic destruction of the proximal surface of the olecranon and distal humerus, with resorption of the radial head (*arrow*). *COMMENT:* This patient demonstrates Phemister's triad of radiographic findings, characterizing tubercular arthritis: progressive joint space narrowing, juxta-articular osteoporosis, and peripheral erosive defects of the articular surfaces.

Figure 12-67 **TUBERCULOSIS. Sacroiliac Joint.** Observe the extensive destruction and obliteration of the joint articulations of the involved sacroiliac joint (*arrows*). *COMMENT:* Marginal erosion of bone on both sides of the joint, along with minimal subchondral reactive osteitis, characterizes this presentation. Asymmetric facet facings (tropism) at the lumbosacral junction and dysplasia of the first sacral tubercle are incidental findings. Tuberculosis of the sacroiliac joint is usually a unilateral lesion, and the cardinal roentgen signs are those of pseudo-widening of the joint, early osteolytic destructive lesions, and eventual ankylosis. When a patient presents with unilateral destructive sacroiliac signs, tuberculosis should always be considered in the differential diagnosis, along with psoriatic arthropathy, Reiter's syndrome, and rheumatoid arthritis.

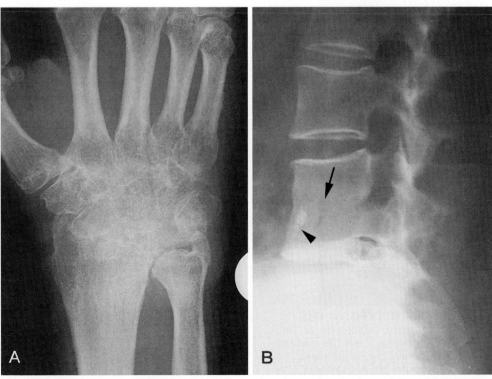

Figure 12-66 **END STAGE TUBERCULOSIS: JOINT ANKYLOSIS.**
A. PA Wrist. Note the ankylosis of all joint compartments.
B. Lateral Lumbar Spine. Note that at the L3–L4 level there has been destruction of the vertebral endplates and intervertebral disc (*arrow*). Note the small area of calcification within a previous psoas abscess (*arrowhead*).

Table 12-3	Comparison of Suppurative Versus Non-Suppurative Osteomyelitis (Tuberculosis)	
Feature	**Suppurative**	**Non-Suppurative (TB)**
Age	Prepubertal	Prepubertal and debilitated geriatric
Clinical features	Fever, acute pain, and swelling; onset and progression is rapid (2 weeks)	Insidious onset; fever, prostration; very slow, relentless progression (months)
Cause	*Staphylococcus aureus*	*Mycobacterium tuberculosis*
Sequestrum formation	Common	Uncommon
Psoas abscess formation	Uncommon	Occurs (5%)
Marjolin's ulcer	Occurs rarely	Does not occur
Sinus formation	Common	Uncommon
Discovertebral disease	Occurs	Most common site
Multiple segmental involvement	Rare	Common
Gouge defects	Do not occur	Occur
Osteoporosis	Moderate	Extensive
Periostitis	Common	Uncommon
Sacroiliac involvement	Rare	Occurs occasionally
End stage	Bony ankylosis	Fibrous ankylosis

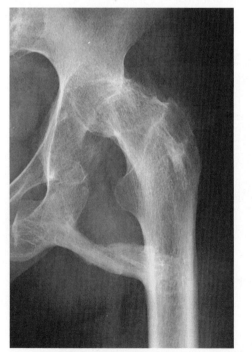

Figure 12-68 TUBERCULOSIS: ARTHRODESIS. AP Hip. Observe the destruction of the femoral head, with partial superolateral displacement of the femur from the acetabulum. There is an osseous bar between the ischium and femoral cortex, representing a fibular strut. *COMMENT:* In the preantibiotic era, the common treatment for tuberculosis of the hip joint was to create an unmovable joint. This allowed the infectious process to run its natural course to full healing.

EXTRASKELETAL MANIFESTATIONS OF TUBERCULOSIS

Scrofula (Mycobacterial Lymphadenitis)

Scrofula is lymphadenopathy in response to a mycobacterial infection. The word has derivatives from Latin and French, meaning "glandular swelling" and "full-necked sow," respectively. (1) Recognition of scrofula as a disease was perhaps first made by Herodotus in 400 B.C., who suggested that those with the "scrofula-like" illness should be isolated from others. (1) Scrofula later became known as *the king's evil* and was said to only be cured by "the royal touch" of monarchs. This ceremonious healing ritual took place in England until the death of King Charles II in 1682. Albucasis, on the other hand, documented surgical excision techniques for treating scrofula as early as A.D. 1000. A professor at Leyden University in the Netherlands was first to link scrofula with pulmonary tuberculosis, and Robert Koch, in 1882, identified the tubercle bacillus. (1)

Lymphadenopathy is the most common extrapulmonary manifestation of tubercular infection, occurring in up to 45% of cases. (1) Isolated lymphadenitis, without pulmonary manifestations, occurs in approximately 35% of patients infected by *Mycobacterium tuberculosis*. (1) The cervical lymph nodes are primarily involved, and the incidence among women is almost twice that of males. (1) Asians, American Indians, and Hispanics have a higher incidence of occurrence, with the disease primarily affecting individuals between the ages of 20 and 40 years. (1)

Scrofula may be completely asymptomatic or constitutional signs of fever, weight loss, and malaise may persist. (1) The most common presentation is the patient who is concerned about a few firm masses palpable in the lateral neck. The patient may reveal that the masses have been slow growing. (2) Unilateral involvement occurs in approximately 60% of cases, and the diagnosis is obtained by needle aspiration. Others advocate that excisional biopsy is required for exact diagnosis. (2) Radiographic evaluation of the chest rarely reveals active pulmonary infection. Cervical radiographs will reveal peripheral calcification of the involved nodes. (Fig. 12-69, *A* and *B*) On occasion, other patterns may be noted, including homogenous or spiculated calcification, making the diagnosis difficult. CT will reveal multiple, low-attenuation node involvement with thick rims of peripheral enhancement. (Fig. 12-69*C*) Occasionally, the walls of the nodes may deteriorate, and several nodes coalesce to form a single necrotic mass, termed a *cold abscess.* Antituberculosis drugs are the treatment of choice; however, excision and drainage of the involved lymph nodes may be required in more complicated cases. (2)

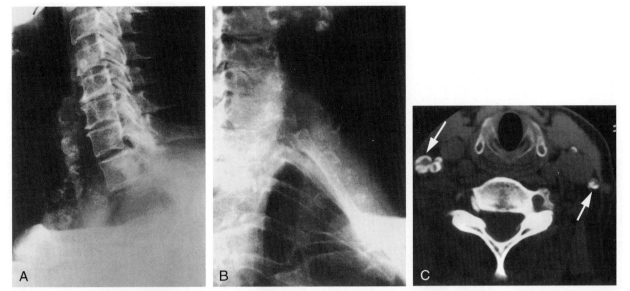

Figure 12-69 **SCROFULA (MYCOBACTERIAL LYMPHADE-NOPATHY): CERVICAL LYMPH NODE CHAIN. A. Lateral Lower Cervical Spine. B. Oblique Lower Cervical Spine.** Observe the circular cystic calcifications affecting a cluster of left-sided lower cervical chain lymph nodes. The peripheral margins of the lymph nodes are densely calcified with a lucent center. **C. Axial CT, Lower Neck.** Observe the bilateral lymph node calcification associated with the tubercular lymphadenopathy (*arrows*). *COMMENT:* Scrofula is a form of bovine tuberculosis affecting and isolated to the cervical lymph nodes. This patient worked on a farm for many years on the plains of Texas and had a history of tubercular lymphadenopathy. (Courtesy of Nancy Hinders, DC, Canyon, Texas, and Ray F. Kilcoyne, MD, Denver, Colorado.)

UNUSUAL PRESENTATIONS OF TUBERCULOSIS

Unusual presentations of tuberculosis are outlined in Table 12-4.

Caries Sicca

In the shoulder joint, the initial tubercular destruction is typically widespread because of the small surface contact area of articular cartilage. Tubercular destruction of the humeral head with multiple large erosive and destructive lesions is called *caries sicca*. This is an old term that is no longer in common usage. (1)

Cystic Tuberculosis

Cystic tuberculosis is a rare form seen mostly in children and young adults, usually in the appendicular skeleton; occasionally a flat bone is involved. (2) Radiographically, the lesions are characterized by symmetric well-defined, round, or oval lytic lesions with little or no periosteal reaction initially. In the untreated case, the lytic lesions can become aggressive and expansile with a laminated periosteal response. (Fig. 12-70) Sequestra are uncommon, and accompanying joint involvement is rare because most of the lesions are diaphyseal or metaphyseal in origin. The differential diagnosis must include polyostotic fibrous dysplasia, enchondromatosis, and eosinophilic granuloma of bone. The prognosis is generally good, particularly with specific chemotherapeutic agents. The lesions appear to be simultaneous in onset and progress and regress in harmony.

Table 12-4	Unusual Presentations of Tuberculosis

Caries sicca: tuberculous erosions of the humeral head.
Cystic tuberculosis: multiple, symmetric, well-defined round or oval lytic lesions of the appendicular skeleton.
Tuberculous dactylitis: tubercular destruction of the short tubular bones of the hand and feet; often called spina ventosa.
Pott's puffy tumor: a tubercular calvarial lesion forming a button sequestrum and a fluctuant cold abscess of the scalp.
Weaver's bottom: tubercular involvement of the subgluteal bursae allowing direct extension to the ischial tuberosity.
Long vertebra: as a result of an extensive gibbus deformity, the vertebra caudal to the gibbus may become taller than it is broad.
Gouge defects: anterior vertebral erosions secondary to subligamentous dissection and spread of the tubercular process.
Kissing sequestrum: represents cartilage and bone destruction leading to complete joint obliteration.
Pott's paraplegia: a pressure paraplegia secondary to collapse of vertebral bodies, extensive granulation tissue, and detached sequestra from the vertebral bodies.
Scrofula: bovine tuberculosis affecting the cervical lymph nodes.

Tuberculous Dactylitis

Tuberculous dactylitis occurs in the short tubular bones of the hands and feet. It is a rare condition (3) that is most commonly seen in children < 5 years of age. (4) It is characterized by multiple lesions of consecutive rather than simultaneous onset. Monostotic involvement is common; however, multiple peripheral lesions occur in 25% of the patients. (5) The typical lesion causes diffuse soft tissue swelling, bone expansion, and thinning of the cortex, so that the description—used long before the days of radiology—of *spina ventosa* (*spina,* "thorn-like"; *ventosa,*

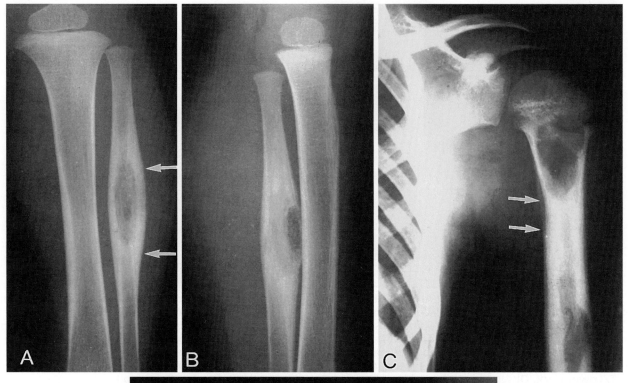

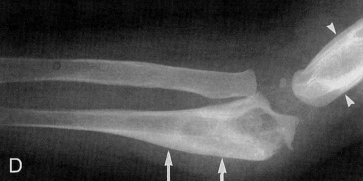

Figure 12-70 CYSTIC TUBERCULOSIS. A and B. Fibula. Observe the large, lytic destructive lesion in the mid-diaphysis of the fibula, with an encapsulating halo of periosteal new bone formation (*arrows*). **C. Proximal Humerus.** Note the large, lytic destructive lesions scattered throughout the visualized metaphysis and diaphysis of the humerus. There is some increase in bone density within the proximal diaphysis. Observe the periosteal new bone formation on the medial metaphyseal cortex of the humerus (*arrows*). **D. Ulna.** Note the extensive lytic destruction of the olecranon and coronoid processes of the proximal ulna. A laminated periosteal new bone formation (*arrows*) is visualized in the metaphyseal area of the ulna. Observe the periosteal new bone forma- tion, creating some enlargement of the distal portion of the humerus (*arrowheads*). *COMMENT:* This rare form of tuber- culosis is seen mostly in children and young adults, usually in the appendicular skeleton but occasionally a flat bone is involved. Radiographically, the lesions are characterized by symmetric, well-defined, round or oval lytic lesions with little or no periosteal reaction initially. In the untreated case, the lytic lesions can become aggressive and expansile, with a laminated periosteal response. The differential diagnosis must include polyostotic fibrous dysplasia, enchondromato- sis, and eosinophilic granuloma of bone. The lesions appear to be simultaneous in onset and progression; they also regress in harmony.

"inflated with air") was particularly appropriate. (6) (Fig. 12-71) Associated joint disease is rare. (6)

Pott's Puffy Tumor

Pott's puffy tumor is a rare calvarial tubercular solitary focus with formation of a button sequestrum and a fluctuant cold ab- scess involving the scalp. (6,7) Its formation is precipitated by the close anatomic relationship of the frontal bone and para- nasal sinuses. (8) Clinically, patients experience frontal scalp swelling, headache, fever, nasal drainage, and sinus tenderness. (7) Neurological symptoms are not uncommon, making this con- dition a serious complication of tuberculosis. (8) Timely surgical and pharmaceutical intervention usually results in a favorable prognosis. (7)

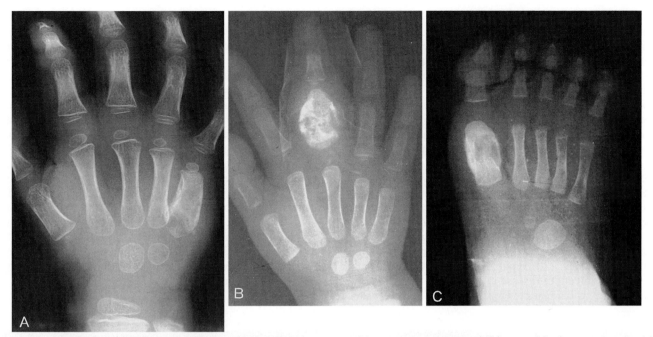

Figure 12-71 TUBERCULOUS DACTYLITIS. A. Hand. Note the fifth metacarpal in this 2.5-year-old patient. **B. Hand.** Note the proximal phalanx of the third digit in this 2-year-old patient. Of incidental notation is some form of a wrap on the patient's involved finger. **C. Hand.** Note the first metatarsal in this 1.5-year-old patient. *COMMENT:* This entity occurs in short tubular bones of the hands and feet and is most common in children, with the greatest incidence < 5 years of age. The typical lesions (as seen here) cause diffuse soft tissue swelling, bone expansion, and thinning of the cortex; thus the description used long before the days of radiology was *spina ventosa*. Associated joint disease is rare. (Courtesy of David P. Thomas, MD, Melbourne, Australia.)

Tuberculous Bursitis (Weaver's Bottom)

The synovial membranes of bursae can be attacked by tuberculosis. Classic sites include the radial and ulnar bursae of the hand and the subdeltoid and subgluteal bursae. (9) Subgluteal involvement was found as an occupational hazard in weavers, caused by continual sliding on benches, and has been called *weaver's bottom.* (6) (Fig. 12-72) The region of the greater trochanter of the femur is a favorite site, with osseous destruction occurring. (10) Late changes of moderate calcification around the deformed trochanter occur as a sign of the infective focus reaching a dormant stage. (11) (Fig. 12-59)

AIDS; HIV Infection

The unprecedented epidemic of AIDS has attracted much publicity and has become the major research focus in recent times. AIDS is currently among the top causes of death across the globe. (12) The responsible retrovirus has been isolated and termed human immunodeficiency virus (HIV), which produces marked deficiency of the T-lymphocyte cells, particularly the T-helper cells. A wide spectrum of disorders has been linked with AIDS, including protozoan infections (*Pneumocystis carinii* pneumonia, *Toxoplasmosis gondii* encephalitis), fungal infections (*Candida albicans* esophagitis–pharyngitis, cryptococcal meningitis), bacterial infections (atypical mycobacteria; *Mycobacterium avium-intracellulare, Mycobacterium kansasii*), viral infections (herpes simplex, cytomegalovirus, progressive multifocal leukoencephalopathy), helminthic infections (ascariasis strongyloides of the intestine), and cancer (Kaposi's sarcoma, lymphoma, oral

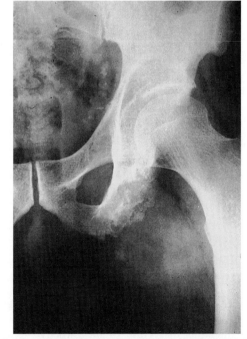

Figure 12-72 TUBERCULOUS BURSITIS: WEAVER'S BOTTOM. Observe the extensive destruction and disorganization of the ischial tuberosity. The pubic and hip articulations show no joint disease. *COMMENT:* The synovial membranes of bursae can be attacked by tuberculosis. One classical site is the subgluteal area, which was found to be an occupational hazard in weavers, caused by continuous sliding on benches. (Reprinted with permission from **Yochum TR:** *Tuberculosis of L1/L2, with psoas cold abscesses.* ACA J Chiro June, 1982.)

and rectal squamous cell carcinoma). (13,14) Owing to the frequent mutations of the virus, current therapies directed toward reproductive suppression of the virus within the cells are becoming less effective. (12) Strategies for developing a vaccine and preventing the initial infection are becoming the mainstream in research and development. (12,15)

Musculoskeletal manifestations of HIV infection are not as common as manifestations in other parts of the body (16) and tend to occur when the disease is relatively advanced. (17) These consist of infections, lymphoma, anemia, Kaposi's sarcoma, polymyositis, and arthritis. (16,18)

Infections can occur in the skin, subcutaneous tissue, muscle, bones, and joints. (17,19) Organisms include S*almonella, Staphylococcus aureus, Mycobacterium, Clostridium,* and *Neisseria.* Pyomyositis is a condition caused by *Staphylococcus aureus,* resulting in a purulent infection of the skeletal muscle. (20) The condition is frequently bilateral and requires antibiotic therapy with surgical drainage. (20) Bacillary angiomatosis is a multisystem bacterial infectious disease in association with cutaneous vascular lesions, which can develop an unusual form of osteomyelitis, causing well-circumscribed osteolytic lesions related to the rickettsia-like organism *Rochalimaea quintana.* (17,21) Tuberculosis often involves the peripheral joints (17,19) but has been noted to involve the spine with an increased incidence among those infected with HIV. (22)

Lymphoma is aggressive and has a poor prognosis. Non-Hodgkin's lymphoma in AIDS patients is > 60 times greater than that in the general population. (17) Together, Kaposi's sarcoma and non-Hodgkin's lymphoma represent the most common malignancies resulting from HIV infection. (23)

Anemia of chronic disease results from hemosiderin-laden marrow, which reduces the marrow signal on MRI examination. (17) Kaposi's sarcoma complicates approximately 15% of AIDS patients and is marked by permeative and moth-eaten foci of bone destruction. Exacerbation of Reiter's syndrome and psoriasis may lead to erosive arthropathy. (17) MRI evaluation of HIV patients with musculoskeletal complaints frequently detects unexpected diseases and aids in the differentiation of neoplastic disorders from infectious disease. (18)

CAPSULE SUMMARY Non-Suppurative Osteomyelitis (Tuberculosis)

General Considerations

- Leading cause of death at the beginning of the 20th century.
- Found in prepubertal children, debilitated geriatrics, AIDS sufferers, silicosis, lymphoma patients, alcoholics, and corticosteroid and drug abusers.

Incidence

- In 1953, 84,203 cases were reported; in 1977, 30,154 cases were reported, 3,000 of which were fatal.
- Tuberculosis is often overlooked in differential diagnosis.

Cause

- *Mycobacterium tuberculosis* is the most common pathogen isolated.
- Two modes of spread exist: inhalation and ingestion.

Clinical Features

- No sex predilection; rare < 1 year of age.
- General symptoms lacking early, insidious onset, chronic course.
- Regional joint pain, decreased range of motion; focal tenderness and swelling are common symptoms.

Pathologic Features

- Pott's disease (tuberculosis of the spine).
- Infective organisms travel as emboli via the bloodstream, lodging in the turbulent flow at the endplate arterioles.
- Earliest site of spinal disease is the anterior subchondral endplate. Disc involvement occurs after endplate destruction.
- Subligamentous dissection of the infective focus occurs down the anterior longitudinal ligament. Anterior vertebral body scalloping occurs, creating gouge defects.
- Abscess formation produces soft tissue swelling that is out of proportion to the degree of bone and discal destruction.
- Retropharyngeal, paravertebral (thoracic spine), and psoas abscess are the common presentations.

- Psoas abscesses frequently calcify in a snowflake, dense pattern; 5% of patients with spinal tuberculosis develop a psoas abscess.
- Pott's paraplegia may complicate extensive spinal involvement.
- Tubercular appendicular arthritis is most common in the hip and knee.
- Cartilage destruction and marginal erosions characterize the pathologic changes of tubercular arthritis.

Radiologic Features

- Spinal tuberculosis is most common at L1, with the lower thoracic and upper lumbar vertebrae also being favored sites.
- 21-day radiographic latent period for Pott's disease.
- Early signs for spine are lytic endplate destruction, loss of disc height, anterior gouge defects, paraspinal swelling (retropharyngeal, retrotracheal, paraspinal line, psoas).
- Advanced signs for spinal involvement are vertebral body collapse, gibbus formation, and obliteration of the disc.
- Long vertebra is found associated with extensive gibbus deformity from tuberculosis.
- Tubercular arthritis is common in the hip and knee.
- Uniform joint space narrowing, early destruction of the subchondral cortex (cortical white line), moth-eaten bone destruction, and juxta-articular osteoporosis are the cardinal roentgen signs of tubercular arthritis.
- Phemister's triad (tubercular arthritis):
  Progressive and slow joint space narrowing.
  Juxta-articular osteoporosis.
  Peripheral erosive defects of the articular surface.

Treatment and Prognosis

- Chemotherapy is quite effective; however, recently it has been shown that the causative organism is becoming somewhat resistant to the modern drug therapy.
- Surgery is seldom necessary.

CAPSULE SUMMARY   Non-Suppurative Osteomyelitis (Tuberculosis) (*continued*)

Unusual Presentations of Tuberculosis

- *Caries sicca:* tubercular destruction of the humeral head with multiple large erosive lesions.
- *Cystic tuberculosis:* a rare form of tuberculosis involving the appendicular skeleton of children. Symmetrical oval lytic lesions are the rule.
- *Tuberculous dactylitis:* occurs most often in the short tubular bones of the hands and feet of children usually < 5 years of age. Sometimes referred to as spina ventosa.
- *Pott's puffy tumor:* a solitary infectious tubercular focus of the calvaria, creating a button sequestrum.

- *Tuberculous bursitis (weaver's bottom):* tuberculous subgluteal bursal involvement with direct extension to the ischial tuberosity.
- *Scrofula:* bovine tuberculosis affecting the cervical lymph nodes.
- *AIDS:* musculoskeletal manifestations not as common as manifestations in other parts of the body and tend to occur when the disease is relatively advanced. These consist of infections, lymphoma, anemia, Kaposi's sarcoma, polymyositis, and arthritis.

SYPHILITIC OSTEOMYELITIS

The incidence of syphilis (lues) has decreased steadily since the early part of the 20th century owing to the advent of penicillin therapy after World War II. However, between 1980 and 1990 there was a reappearance of syphilitic disease. (1) The causative organism, *Treponema pallidum,* is a slender spirochete found in early lesions. Until recently, the standard diagnosis involved the identification of treponemes by using silver staining techniques. Currently, a more accurate assessment using immunofluorescent antigen testing is available. (2) Treponemes are seldom seen in advanced lesions. The basic lesion of syphilis is an angiitis of the vasa vasorum or small arterioles. This endarteritis produces necrosis of the vessel wall, with subsequent infarction of the tissue supplied by the vessel. The end result is a gumma that consists of areas of coagulative necrosis surrounded by an infiltrate of plasma cells and leukocytes. Skeletal syphilis presents as either a congenital or an acquired lesion of bone.

Congenital Syphilis

Congenital syphilis has been on the decline in the United States, with a drop in incidence of 78.2% between 1992 and 1998. (1,3) However, only an estimated 30% of women are screened for syphilis before or during pregnancy. (4) In areas of Africa it is believed that up to 10% of pregnant women have syphilis. (5) The disease is transmitted from the mother to child via the placenta, and the transmission is rare before the 4th month of gestation because the Langhans layer of the chorion presents a barrier to the passage of the pathogen. (6) Spirochetemia in the mother results in intrauterine infection during the 5th or 6th month of pregnancy. In untreated cases, 25% of the fetuses die in utero, and 25–30% die shortly after birth. (7) Of the infected survivors, symptoms usually present within the first 4 months after birth. (8) Up to 40% will develop late symptomatic syphilis. (7) The symptoms are usually quite diverse and may affect any organ system, requiring a high index of suspicion to make the correct diagnosis. (8) The diversity of signs and symptoms seen among symptomatic individuals has prompted many to refer to this disease as the *master*

masquerader. (9) Neonatal congenital syphilis usually lasts into the 2nd year of life.

Radiologic Features

Radiographically, there are three phases of skeletal involvement in congenital syphilis.

Phase 1: Metaphysitis. The first phase is present at birth or shortly thereafter. The lodging of spirochetes beneath the fetal growth plates produces a metaphysitis in which the normal vascular fountain underneath the cartilage is replaced by syphilitic granulation tissue. Bone formation and remodeling in the zone of primary ossification is, therefore, decreased or absent. This process creates radiolucent metaphyseal bands, which may be broad and/or horizontal, occasionally mimicking the lucent bands in leukemia or metastatic disease from neuroblastoma. (10) (Fig. 12-73) These bands often lead to metaphyseal irregularity with fragmentation and infractions, which have been referred to as the *sawtoothed appearance.* (11) These changes occur at the metaphyseal–physis (growth plate) junction and occasionally simulate the appearance of scurvy. (10,11) These metaphyseal abnormalities are often bilateral and symmetrical. Metaphyseal lesions often allow epiphyseal separation, most commonly affecting the upper extremity. The epiphyseal centers are rarely affected because the epiphyseal cartilage is avascular and the organisms are unable to gain access to this region. Therefore, the formation and maturation of cartilage is not affected by the spirochete.

The knees, shoulders, and wrists are the most commonly affected areas. Often, symmetrical erosive defects occur on the medial surfaces of the proximal ends of the tibiae, representing *Wimberger's sign of congenital syphilis.* (12) (Fig. 12-74) The lesions of phase 1 disease generally heal promptly with specific therapy. This usually takes place within 2 weeks and may be complete within 2 months. (13) Spontaneous resolution will occur without treatment, but it is quite slow.

Phase 2: Periostitis. The periosteum may be infiltrated by syphilitic granulation tissue, creating a solid or laminated reaction. The periosteal response is often diffuse and symmetrical, affecting nearly all of the major long bones. Complete remission at this stage can occur with specific treatment. Once again, even

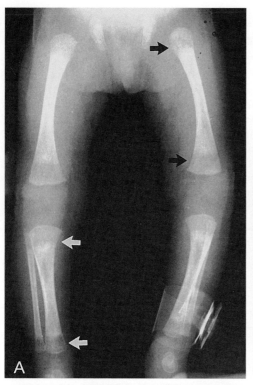

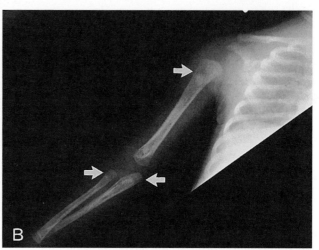

Figure 12-73 CONGENITAL SYPHILIS: SKELETAL INVOLVE-MENT, PHASE 1, METAPHYSITIS (RADIOLUCENT BANDS). A. Lower Extremity. Observe the extensive bilateral radiolucent metaphyseal bands (*arrows*) in both ends of the femora, tibiae, and fibulae. Of incidental notation is a baby identification anklet around the distal tibia and fibula of one leg. **B. Upper Extremity.** Note the extensive radiolucent metaphyseal bands in the proximal humerus, radius, and

ulna (*arrows*). *COMMENT:* The early lesions in phase 1 (metaphysitis) congenital syphilis are those of bilateral radiolucent metaphyseal bands, which may be broad and/or horizontal, occasionally mimicking the lucent bands in leukemia or metastatic disease of neuroblastoma. These bands often lead to metaphyseal irregularity, with fragmentation and infractions that have been referred to as the *sawtooth appearance.*

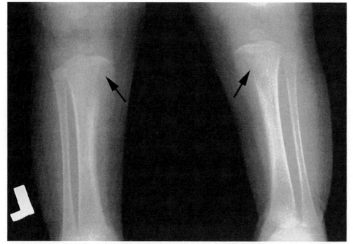

Figure 12-74 CONGENITAL SYPHILIS: WIMBERGER'S SIGN. Note the bilateral destruction at the medial margins of the tibial metaphyses (*arrows*). This is caused by metaphyseal foci of spirochetal infection and is diagnostic for congenital syphilis. (Courtesy of Michael J. Silberstein, MD, St. Louis, Missouri.)

without treatment, spontaneous but slow resolution will occur. (11) (Fig. 12-75)

Phase 3: Osteitis. Infants who have not received therapy or in whom therapy has proven ineffective can develop osteitis. Syphilitic granulation tissue may extend from the metaphysis to the diaphysis, creating an extension of the infectious focus. Reactive sclerosis surrounds the osteolytic lesions, with associated periostitis of the long tubular bones. (Fig. 12-76) Extensive periostitis and cortical overgrowth may create an undulating, dense contour to the long tubular bones. Frequently, both tibiae will be involved, creating the classic *saber shin.* Anterior bowing of the tibia is characteristic, with osteolytic defects (gummata) scattered throughout the bone.

Additional Features

Bilateral painless swellings (syphilitic synovitis) about the joints, especially the knees, in older children have been termed *Clutton's joints.* (14) Contrary to Clutton's original description in 1886, these joints may be warm and painful. (6)

Deformity of the teeth, creating a peg-shaped, hypoplastic, and notched tooth, has been referred to as *Hutchinson's teeth* in congenital syphilis. (15)

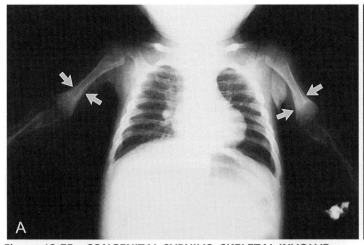

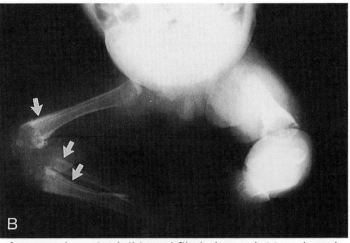

Figure 12-75   **CONGENITAL SYPHILIS: SKELETAL INVOLVE-MENT, PHASE 2, PERIOSTITIS. A. Upper Extremity.** Observe the diffuse periosteal new bone formation about the distal humeri bilaterally (*arrows*). **B. Lower Extremity.** Note the extensive amount of periosteal new bone formation about the femur and proximal tibia and fibula (*arrows*). Metaphyseal irregularity with lytic destruction is noted. The opposite lower extremity is not visualized, as a result of poor patient positioning because of the patient's painful condition. (Courtesy of C. H. Quay, MD, Melbourne, Australia.)

Acquired Syphilis

Skeletal manifestations of acquired syphilis are actually those of tertiary syphilis. The most frequently affected bones are the more superficial portions of the skeleton, which are the skull, tibiae, and clavicles. (11) The predilection for superficial bones is usually attributed to chronic microtrauma and irritation. Fewer than 10% of patients with acquired syphilis ever develop osseous lesions. (16)

Radiologic Features

Radiographic signs of acquired syphilis occur long after the initial infection. The most common sign is proliferative periostitis. (16) This may become extensive, leading to diffuse thickening of both the inner and the outer cortices. Long bone involvement is common, and with advanced disease an alteration in the tubulation of the bone may occur. The pattern of periosteal new bone is generally solid or laminated; however, a more aggressive pattern may occur, leaving a *lace-like* appearance. (Fig. 12-77) The affected segments of the tubular bones will be sclerotic, with lytic gummata occurring in either the cortex or the medullary cavity. Sequestration is rare.

Syphilitic osteomyelitis of the skull is most commonly found in the frontal bone. (17) (Fig. 12-78) The outer table is the target site of destruction. The extent of bone proliferation in the extremities is often greater than in any other condition, except fibrous dysplasia of bone. (18) Tibial involvement is common and usually bilateral. Jaffe (19) stated that the saber shin deformity of acquired syphilis is usually related to *pseudo-bowing* of the tibia, in which the vertical direction of the marrow cavity is unchanged and the outer diameter of the bone is enlarged owing to periosteal proliferation. On the other hand, the saber shin deformity of congenital syphilis is associated with true bowing of the tibia.

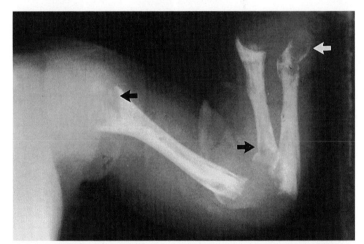

Figure 12-76   **CONGENITAL SYPHILIS: SKELETAL INVOLVE-MENT, PHASE 3, OSTEITIS.** Note the extensive destruction, with metaphyseal (*arrows*) and diaphyseal radiolucencies throughout the humerus, radius, and ulna. Observe the exuberant periosteal overgrowth, with expansile deformity of the bones of the upper extremity. *COMMENT:* Infants who have not received therapy or for whom therapy has proven ineffective may develop osteitis. Syphilitic granulation tissue may extend from the metaphysis to the diaphysis, creating an extension of the infectious focus. Reactive sclerosis often surrounds the osteolytic lesions, with associated periostitis of the long tubular bones. The most frequently involved bone in this stage of the disease process is the tibia, creating the classic *saber shin* anterior bowing deformity.

Although neurotrophic arthropathy (Charcot's joint) is a common sequela of acquired tertiary syphilis, such lesions have no relationship to syphilitic osteomyelitis. (11) Syphilitic granulation tissue does not invade bone in neurotrophic arthropathy; the skeletal findings in this disorder are caused primarily by traumatic joint degeneration. (11)

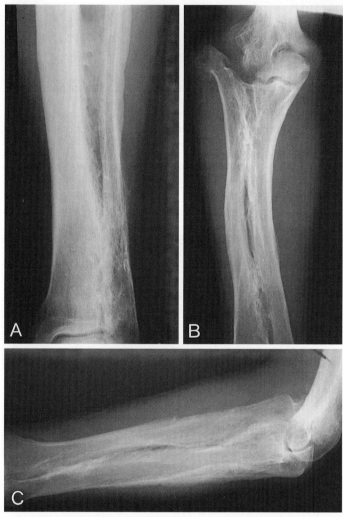

Figure 12-77 ACQUIRED SYPHILIS: SKELETAL INVOLVEMENT. A. Tibia and Fibula. B and C. Radius and Ulna. Observe the extensive proliferative periostitis in the distal tibia, fibula, radius, and ulna, which has created some thickening of both the inner and outer cortices of these bones. This type of periosteal new bone formation in acquired syphilis has been referred to as a *lace-like* pattern. (Courtesy of Bryan Hartley, MD, Melbourne, Australia.)

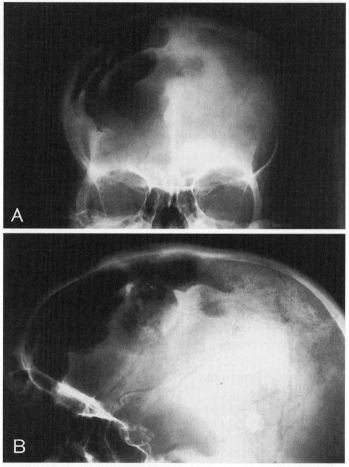

Figure 12-78 ACQUIRED SYPHILIS: FRONTAL BONE IN-VOLVEMENT. A and B. Skull. Observe the scalloped, large lytic lesions scattered throughout the frontal bone in this patient with acquired skeletal syphilis. *COMMENT:* Skull involvement is somewhat rare in syphilis; however, when it occurs, the frontal bone is the target site. Of incidental notation is the approximation of the anterior and posterior clinoids of the sella turcica, creating a bridging appearance. This is a normal variant.

MYCOTIC OSTEOMYELITIS

General Considerations

Most fungal infections of the skeletal system are secondary to a primary infection, either of the respiratory system or from direct extension of an infected devitalized soft tissue focus. Occasionally, hematogenous seeding of skeletal structures may occur. Mycotic osteomyelitis actually represents a very small percentage of all bone infections. There is no characteristic clinical picture to allow adequate differential diagnosis among the varied fungal disorders or tuberculosis. The definitive diagnosis depends on culture studies of synovial fluid or tissue obtained from the local lesion.

The fungi that may affect bone are *Coccidioides, Candida, Aspergillus, Actinomyces, Histoplasma, Cryptococcus (torula), Nocardia,* North and South American *Blastomyces, Sporothrix, Phycomyces (mucor, rhizopus),* and *Monosporium (mycetoma).* Only three of these will be considered in the scope of this text.

COCCIDIOIDOMYCOSIS

Coccidioidomycosis is an infection caused by the fungus *Coccidioides immitis.* In the southwestern United States the disease is endemic, particularly in southern California (San Joaquin Valley), southern Arizona, and New Mexico. (1) The incidence of the disease is sharply increasing, (2,3), especially among the elderly (4) and immunocompromised. (2) Skeletal coccidioidomycosis is usually secondary to respiratory infection. The fungus is an inhabitant of soil and is disseminated through dust. Following spore inhalation, an inflammatory consolidation takes place in the terminal bronchioles. There are two distinct phases of the disease. The primary phase is usually respiratory only, and the secondary phase (dissemination phase) results from bronchial ulceration and aspiration of the infected exudate, or by vascular spread of the pathogens. The clinical presentation may mimic tuberculosis, with multiple systems subject to infection (liver, spleen, lymph nodes, skin, kidneys, bone, and meninges). Most cases in the United States are isolated within the lung, indolent, low grade, and self-limiting. (3,5) However, in the disseminated form it can be serious, with the symptoms varying according to the distribution of the lesions. If widespread dissemination occurs, surgical débridement (6) and/or long-term antifungal therapy is usually prescribed. (7) A successful treatment regime is not based on a curative nature but rather on obtaining a state of remission. (8) The disease is often fatal (2), and with survival, a lifelong risk of recurrence persists. (6,9) Black and Filipino patients seem to have a higher mortality rate than whites affected by coccidioidomycosis. (10)

Radiologic Features

Bone involvement occurs in about 20% of cases of the disseminated form of this disease. (11) The most common bones involved are the spine, pelvis, ribs, and long bones; however, any bone can be a target site. (11) Rarely, the bones of the hand (12) and feet (13) are affected. The infection tends to involve bony prominences, such as the tibial tubercle, medial and lateral malleolus, medial end of the clavicle, trochanters, acromion, patella, calca-

neus, and olecranon. There are no characteristic radiologic criteria to allow definitive differential diagnosis. Radiologically, a well-demarcated lytic destruction occurs early, with some associated laminated periosteal response. (14) In fulminating cases, skeletal lesions tend to be disseminated and a bone scan may help identify the locations of the lesions. (14) Ultimately, cortical disruption occurs, and a moderate degree of sclerosis eventuates usually in the chronic or healing phases. Abscess formation with a draining sinus is common. Joint involvement occurs in approximately 17% of cases, which is more frequent than once thought. (14) When present, joint involvement may simulate tubercular infectious arthritis.

The roentgen signs of spinal coccidioidomycosis include a paraspinal mass (abscess formation) and clearly defined radiolucent lesions in the vertebral body, pedicles, lamina, and adjacent ribs with a relative sparing of the disc spaces. (15) Multiple vertebral involvement is the rule, with vertebral collapse being rare. Contiguous rib involvement is characteristic of this disease, as it presents in the spine. Psoas abscess formation may occur and will occasionally calcify. These psoas abscesses are indistinguishable from those that complicate spinal tuberculosis. The thoracic and lumbar areas are the target spinal sites. The radiographic diagnosis of coccidioidomycosis is only a presumptive one because the lesions often resemble other types of osteomyelitis. Definitive diagnosis must be made by isolation of the pathogen.

ACTINOMYCOSIS

The most common infective agents are *Actinomyces israelii* and *bovis.* These agents are actually bacteria, not fungi, although traditionally they have been considered fungi by most physicians. (1) The pathogens are found in the mouth and bowel of normal individuals and usually cause no harm unless they are lodged in a region of devitalized tissue or penetrate deep into the tissues secondary to an operation or penetrating wound. Recent studies have also suggested that actinomycosis may present as an opportunistic organism secondarily to osteoradionecrosis. (2) There are two major clinical forms of actinomycosis: the *cervicofacial type* and the *chest* and *abdominal* varieties. The abdominal presentation (ileocecal region) is uncommon; however, pulmonary involvement may be found in 15% of the patients. Cervicofacial involvement is the most common clinical presentation, and poor oral hygiene is an associated factor. Since the organisms normally reside in the nasal and oral cavities, the high incidence of face and neck involvement is not surprising. Diagnosis is made by biopsy (2) and the condition requires specific antibiotic therapy with possible surgical debridement. (3)

Radiologic Features

Osseous actinomycosis is usually caused by direct extension from an adjacent long-standing soft tissue infection. Rarely, hematogenous spread acts as the mode of dissemination. An osseous lesion occurs in 15% of cases. (1) The most common bones involved are the mandible, spine, ribs, and pelvis. Mandibular destruction is the most commonly encountered skeletal lesion. This usually follows a tooth extraction or socket infection (4). The characteristic radiographic appearance is that of a lytic destructive lesion, often at the angle of the mandible, with little or no reactive new bone.

Abscess formation and draining sinuses are frequently found associated with the mandibular lesions.

In vertebral column disease the original infective focus often stems from the adjacent retroperitoneal or mediastinal lymph nodes. Several vertebrae are usually involved, with lytic destruction and an occasional area of sclerosis. (4) The intervertebral disc is often spared and of normal height. (4) The thoracic and lumbar spine are favored sites. The neural arch is often involved, and contiguous rib involvement is the rule when the thoracic spine is involved. Paravertebral abscesses may occur (5) but are usually smaller than those of tuberculosis and do not calcify. In some cases the vertebral bodies react like the ribs and thicken by periosteal new bone formation, producing a *"sawtooth"* outline to the vertebral body. (1) Collapse of vertebral bodies and disc space narrowing (common to tuberculosis) are not prominent features of actinomycosis.

MADUROMYCOSIS

Maduromycosis is a chronic granulomatous fungal disease affecting primarily the feet (Madura foot). (1) It is most commonly found in tropical regions, with India having the highest incidence. This is the most common fungal infection to involve the skeletal structures worldwide. (2,3) The usual cause of Madura foot within the United States is *Monosporium apiospermum; Nocardia madurae* and *Nocardia brasiliensis* are the offending agents outside the United States. (4) These organisms are normal inhabitants of the soil. (4) Clinically, a triad of signs and symptoms is typical, consisting of localized swelling, purulent (grain-filled) discharge from sinus tracts, and involvement of the foot. (5,6) This triad is the most common presentation irrespective of the causal agent; however, the infective agent must be identified for appropriate treatment. (7)

Radiologic Features

Direct extension from a soft tissue mycetoma causes osseous involvement. Skeletal involvement occurs after long-standing soft tissue swelling from the pathogens penetrating muscles, tendons, and synovial membranes. (4) The tarsometatarsal region of the foot is the most commonly affected site; rarely, the hand, wrist, arm, or leg may be involved. (4) (Fig. 12-79) The natural course of a mycetoma is progressive and relentless. The early osseous lesions are poorly defined and limited to a few sites. In most cases, the eventual picture is that of widespread lytic destructive lesions. With advanced destruction, a bizarre filiform or undulating deformity of the osseous structures ensues. Fistulae formation is common, whereas periosteal reaction is minimal, and sequestration is rare. In advanced cases nearly all of the bones of the foot may be involved, with diffuse intra-articular osseous ankylosis occurring as a sequela. Very few other disease entities will affect so many bones of the entire foot. Neurotrophic arthropathy, particularly in diabetic patients, may destroy nearly all the tarsal bones, giving a similar appearance. However, with neurotrophic arthropathy, a sclerotic reaction is the predominant radiologic appearance, along with bone destruction and collapse.

MRI of the involved area will reveal a generalized low-intensity signal of the matrix with lesions of high signal intensity interspersed throughout. (8) Within these high signal lesions a small low-intensity focus can be identified, known as the *dot-in-circle sign*. (8) This sign is considered highly specific for mycetoma of the foot. (8)

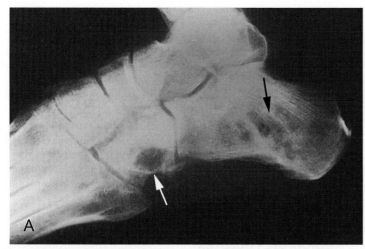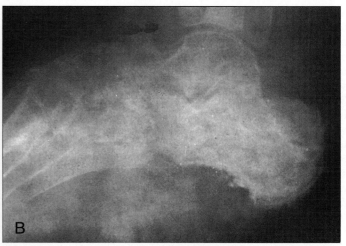

Figure 12-79 **MADURA FOOT. A. Early Phase.** Observe the osteolytic foci within the calcaneus and cuboid (*arrows*). **B. Late Involvement.** Note the advanced destruction of the tarsus and metatarsus regions. Note the undulating surface that at some locations has filiform bone spicules radiating away from the parent bone. These features are characteristic of long-standing mycetoma. *COMMENT:* Madura foot (maduromycosis) is a chronic granulomatous fungal disease primarily affecting the feet. It is most commonly found in tropical regions, with India having the highest incidence. Worldwide, this is the most common fungal infection to involve the skeletal structures. Direct extension from a soft tissue mycetoma causes osseous involvement. (Courtesy of Paul E. Siebert, MD, Denver, Colorado.)

■ References

SUPPURATIVE OSTEOMYELITIS

1. **Bick EM:** *Source Book of Orthopedics.* Baltimore, Williams & Wilkins, 1948.
2. **Rothman RH, Simeone FA:** *The Spine,* ed 2. Philadelphia, WB Saunders, 1982.
3. **Nelaton A:** *Elements de Pathologie Chirurgicale.* Paris, Germer-Bailliere, 1844.
4. **Blockey NJ:** *Osteomyelitis in children.* Equine Vet J 15(1):10, 1983.
5. **Chilton SJ, Aftimos SF, White PR:** *Diffuse skeletal involvement of streptococcal osteomyelitis in a neonate.* Radiology 134:390, 1980.
6. **Resnick D, Niwayama G:** *Diagnosis of Bone and Joint Disorders, Philadelphia.* WB Saunders, 1981.
7. **Gersovich EO, Greenspan A:** *Osteomyelitis of the clavicle: Clinical, radiologic, and bacteriologic findings in ten patients.* Skeletal Radiol 23:205, 1994.
8. **Zvulunov A, Gal N, Segev Z:** *Acute hematogenous osteomyelitis of the pelvis in childhood: Diagnostic clues and pitfalls.* Pediatr Emerg Care 19(1):29, 2003.
9. **Belzunegui J, Rodriguez-Arrondo F, Gonzalez C, et al.:** *Musculoskeletal infections in intravenous drug addicts: Report of 34 cases with analysis of microbiological aspects and pathogenic mechanisms.* Clin Exp Rheumatol May-18(3):383, 2000.
10. **Holzman RS, Bishko F:** *Osteomyelitis in heroin addicts.* Ann Intern Med 75:693, 1971.
11. **Stone DB, Bonfiglio M:** *Pyogenic vertebral osteomyelitis.* Arch Intern Med 112:491, 1963.
12. **Vinas FC, King PK, Diaz FG:** *Spinal aspergillus osteomyelitis.* Clin Infect Dis 28(6):1223, 1999.
13. **Leonard A, Comty CM, Shapiro FL, et al.:** *Osteomyelitis in hemodialysis patients.* Ann Intern Med 78:651, 1973.
14. **Rajbhandari SM, Sutton M, Davies C, et al.:** *"Sausage toe": A reliable sign of underlying osteomyelitis.* Diabet Med 17(1):74, 2000.
15. **Trueta J:** *The normal vascular anatomy of the human femoral head during growth.* J Bone Joint Surg 39B:358, 1957.
16. **Nguyen VD, London J, Cone RO:** *Ring sequestrum: Radiographic characteristics of skeletal fixation pin tract osteomyelitis.* Radiology 158:129, 1986.
17. **Dorland WA:** *The American Illustrated Medical Dictionary,* ed 22. Philadelphia, WB Saunders, 1981.
18. **Saglik Y, Arikan M, Altay M, Yildiz Y:** *Squamous cell carcinoma arising in chronic osteomyelitis.* Int Orthop 25(6):389, 2001.
19. **Smith J, Mello LF, Nogueira Neto NC, et al.:** *Malignancy in chronic ulcers and scars of the leg (Marjolin's ulcer): A study of 21 patients.* Skeletal Radiol 30(6):331, 2001.
20. **McGrory JE, Pritchard DJ, Unni KK, et al.:** *Malignant lesions arising in chronic osteomyelitis.* Clin Orthop 362:181, 1999.
21. **Handmaker H, Leonards R:** *The bone scan in inflammatory osseous disease.* Semin Nucl Med 6:95, 1976.
22. **Gold RH, Hawkins RA, Katz RD:** *Bacterial osteomyelitis: Findings on plain film radiography, CT, MR and scintigraphy.* AJR 157:365, 1991.
23. **Schauwecker DS:** *The scintigraphic diagnosis of osteomyelitis.* AJR 158:9, 1992.
24. **Tang JSH, Gold RH, Bassett LW, et al.:** *Musculoskeletal infection of the extremities: Evaluation with MR imaging.* Radiology 166:205, 1988.
25. **Erdman WA, Tamburro F, Jayson HT, et al.:** *Osteomyelitis: Characteristics and pitfalls of diagnosis with MR imaging.* Radiology 180:533, 1991.
26. **Kleinman PK:** *A regional approach to Osteomyelitis of the lower extremities in children.* Radiol Clin North Am 40(5):1033, 2002.
27. **Capitanio MA, Kirkpatrick JA:** *Early roentgen observations in acute osteomyelitis.* AJR 108:488, 1970.
28. **Murray RO, Jacobson, HG:** *The Radiology of Skeletal Disorders,* ed 2. New York, Churchill Livingstone, 1977.
29. **Goldman AM, Freiberger RH:** *Localized infectious and neuropathic diseases.* Semin Roentgenol 14(1):19, 1979.
30. **Manaster BJ:** *Spondylitis (lumbar spine) due to Brucella abortus. Case report 469.* Skeletal Radiol 17:146, 1988.
31. **El-Desouki M:** *Skeletal brucellosis: Assessment with bone scintigraphy.* Radiology 181:415, 1991.
32. **Talmi YP, Knoller N, Dolev M, et al.:** *Postsurgical prevertebral abscess of the cervical spine.* Laryngoscope 110(7):1137, 2000.
33. **Nolla JM, Ariza J, Gomez-Vaquero C, et al.:** *Spontaneous pyogenic vertebral osteomyelitis in nondrug users.* Semin Arthritis Rheum 31(4):271, 2002.
34. **Buranapanitkit B, Lim A, Geater A:** *Misdiagnosis in vertebral osteomyelitis: Problems and factors.* J Med Assoc Thai 84(12):1743, 2001.
35. **Endress C, Guyot DR, Fata J, et al.:** *Cervical osteomyelitis due to IV heroin use: Radiologic findings in 14 patients.* AJR 155:333, 1990.
36. **Bielicki DK, Sartoris D, Resnick D, et al.:** *Intraosseous and intradiscal gas in association with spinal infection: Report of three cases.* AJR 147:83, 1987.
37. **Kricun R, Shoemaker EI, Chovanes GI, et al.:** *Epidural abscess of the cervical spine.* AJR 158:1145, 1992.
38. **Goodhart GL, Zakem JF, Collins WC, et al.:** *Brucellosis of the spine.* Spine 12:414, 1987.
39. **Madkour MM, Sharif HS, Abed MY, et al.:** *Osteoarticular brucellosis: Results of bone scintigraphy in 140 patients.* AJR 150:1101, 1988.
40. **Guyot DR, Manoli A, Kling GA:** *Pyogenic sacroiliitis in IV drug abusers.* AJR 149:1209, 1987.
41. **Sandrasegaran K, Saifuddin A, Coral A, et al.:** *Magnetic resonance imaging of septic arthritis.* Skeletal Radiol 23:289, 1994.
42. **McHenry MC, Easley KA, Locker GA:** *Vertebral osteomyelitis: Long-term outcome for 253 patients from 7 Cleveland-area hospitals.* Clin Infect Dis 34(10):1342, 2002.

OTHER ASSOCIATED ENTITIES

BRODIE'S ABSCESS

1. **Brodie BC:** *An account of some cases of chronic abscess of the tibia.* Trans Med Chiro Soc 17:238, 1832.
2. **Yochum TR:** *Brodie's abscess of the left ilium.* ACA J Chiro June, 1981.
3. **Jaffe HL:** *Metabolic, Degenerative, and Inflammatory Diseases of Bones and Joints.* Philadelphia, Lea & Febiger, 1972.
4. **Chambler AF, Chapman-Sheath PJ, Pearse MF, Hollingdale J:** *Symmetrical Brodie's abscess.* Postgrad Med J 73(864):660, 1997.
5. **Lopes TD, Reinus WR, Wilson AJ:** *Quantitative analysis of the plain radiographic appearance of Brodie's abscess.* Invest Radiol 32(1):51, 1997.
6. **Lindbom A, Lindvall N, Soderberg G, et al.:** *Angiography in osteoid osteoma.* Acta Radiology 53:377, 1960.
7. **Yochum TR:** *Brodie's abscess of the distal radius* [Roentgen Brief]. ACA Council Roentgenology, February 1981.
8. **Yoshikawa M, Sugawara Y, Kikuchi T, et al.:** *Two cases of pediatric bone disease (eosinophilic granuloma and Brodie's abscess) showing similar scintigraphic and radiographic findings.* Clin Nucl Med 25(12):986, 2000.
9. **Grey AC, Davies AM, Mangham DC, et al.:** *The "pnemumbra sign" on T1-weighted MR imaging in subacute osteomyelitis: Frequency, cause and significance.* Clin Radiol 53(8):587, 1998.

GARRÉ'S SCLEROSING OSTEOMYELITIS

1. **Garré C:** *Üeber besondere formen und folgezustände der akuten infektiosen osteomyelitis.* Bruns Beitr Klin Chir 10:241, 1893.
2. **Aegerter E, Kirkpatrick J:** *Orthopedic Diseases.* ed 4. Philadelphia, WB Saunders, 1975.
3. **Belli E, Matteini C, Andreano T:** *Sclerosing ostemyelitis of Garré periostitis ossificans.* J Craniofac Surg 13(6):765, 2002.

4. **Eswar N:** *Garre's osteomyelitis: A case report.* J Indian Soc Pedod Prev Dent 19(4):157, 2001.
5. **Sutton D:** *A Textbook of Radiology,* ed 2. London, Churchill Livingstone, 1975.
6. **Vienne P, Exner GU:** *Garré sclerosing osteomyelitis* [Trans]. Ortopade 26(10):902, 1997.

CHRONIC OSTEOMYELITIS

1. **Zuluaga AF, Galvis W, Jaimes F, Vesga O:** *Lack of microbiological concordance between bone and non-bone specimens in chronic osteomyelitis: An observational study.* BMC Infect Dis 2(1):8, 2002.
2. **Alonge TO, Ogunlade SO, Fashina AN:** *Microbial isolates in chronic osteomyelitis—A guide to management.* Afr J Med Med Sci 31(2):167, 2002.
3. **Museru LM, Mcharo CN:** *Chronic osteomyelitis: A continuing orthopaedic challenge in developing countries.* Int Orthop 25(2):127, 2001.
4. **McGrory JE, Pritchard DJ, Unni KK, et al.:** *Malignant lesions arising in chronic osteomyelitis.* Clin Orthop 362:181, 1999.
5. **Eyrich GK, Harder C, Sailer HF, et al.:** *Primary chronic osteomyelitis associated with synovitis, acne, pustulosis, hyperostosis and osteitis (SAPHO syndrome).* J Oral Pathol Med 28(10):456, 1999.
6. **Sato T, Indo H, Kawabata Y, et al.:** *Scintigraphic evaluation of chronic osteomyelitis of the mandible in SAPHO syndrome.* Dentomaxillofac Radiol 30(5):293, 2001.
7. **Gulman C, Young O, Tolan M, et al.:** *Chronic osteomyelitis mimicking sarcoma.* J Clin Pathol 56(3):237, 2003.
8. **Guhlman A, Brecht-Krauss D, Suger G, et al.:** *Fluorine-18-FDG PET and technetium-99m antigranulocyte antibody scintigraphy in chronic osteomyelitis.* J Nucl Med 39(12):2145, 1998.
9. **Kaim A, Ledermann HP, Bongartz G, et al.:** *Chronic post-traumatic osteomyelitis of the lower extremity: Comparison of magnetic resonance imaging and combined bone scintigraphy/immunoscintigraphy with radiolabelled monoclonal antigranulocyte antibodies.* Skeletal Radiol 29(7):378, 2000.
10. **Tehranzadeh J, Wong E, Wang F, Sadighpour M:** *Imaging of osteomyelitis in the mature skeleton.* Radiol Clin North Am 39(2):223, 2001.
11. **Greenberg RN, Newman MT, Shariaty S, Pectol RW:** *Ciprofloxacin, lomefloxacin, or levofloxacin as treatment for chronic osteomyelitis.* Antimicrob Agents Chemother 44(1):164, 2000.
12. **Cunha BA:** *Osteomyelitis in elderly patients.* Clin Infect Dis 35(3):287, 2002.
13. **Carek PJ, Dickerson LM, Sack JL:** *Diagnosis and management of osteomyelitis.* Am Fam Physician 63(12):2413, 2001.

CHILDHOOD INFLAMMATORY DISCITIS

1. **Coventry MB, Ghormley RK, Kernohan JW:** *The intervertebral disc: Its microscopic anatomy and pathology.* J Bone Joint Surg 27A:105, 1945.
2. **Boston HC Jr, Bianco AJ Jr, Rhodes KH:** *Disc space infections in children.* Orthop Clin North Am 6:953, 1975.
3. **Alexander CJ:** *The etiology of juvenile spondyloarthritis (discitis).* Clin Radiol 21:178, 1970.
4. **Fernandez M, Carrol CL, Baker CJ:** *Discitis and vertebral osteomyelitis in children: An 18-year review.* Pediatrics 105(6):1299, 2000.
5. **Spiegel PG, Kenglo KW, Issacson AS, et al.:** *Intervertebral disc space inflammation in children.* J Bone Joint Surg 54A:284, 1972.
6. **Wenger DR, Babechko WP, Gilday DL:** *The spectrum of intervertebral disc space infection in children.* J Bone Joint Surg 60A:100, 1978.
7. **Garron E, Viehweger E, Launay F, et al.:** *Nontuberculous spondylodiscitis in children.* J Pediatr Orthop 22(3):321, 2002.
8. **Cusmano F, Calabrese G, Bassi S, et al.:** *Radiologic diagnosis of spondylodiscitis: role of magnetic resonance* [Trans]. Radiol Med (Torino) 100(3):112, 2000.

9. **Brown R, Hussain M, McHugh K, et al.:** *Discitis in young children.* J Bone Joint Surg 83B:1, 2001.

SEPTIC ARTHRITIS

1. **Gillespie R:** *Septic arthritis of childhood.* Clin Orthop 96:152, 1973.
2. **Caksen H, Ozturk MK, Uzum K, et al.:** *Septic arthritis in childhood.* Pediatr Int 42(5):534, 2000.
3. **Chen CE, Ko JY, Li CC, Wang CJ:** *Acute septic arthritis of the hip in children.* Arch Orthop Trauma Surg 121(9):521, 2001.
4. **Borella L, Goobar JE, Summit RL, et al.:** *Septic arthritis in childhood.* J Pediatr 62:742, 1963.
5. **Cucurull E, Espinoza LR:** *Gonococcal arthritis.* Rheum Dis Clin North Am 24(2):305, 1998.
6. **Perry CR:** *Septic arthritis.* Am J Orthop 28(3):168, 1999.
7. **Resnick D, Niwayama G:** *Diagnosis of Bone and Joint Disorders.* Philadelphia, WB Saunders, 1981.
8. **Bliznak J, Ramsey J:** *Emphysematous septic arthritis due to Escherichia coli.* J Bone Joint Surg 58A:138, 1976.
9. **Newman JH:** *Review of septic arthritis throughout the antibiotic era.* Ann Rheum Dis 35:198, 1976.
10. **Murray PM:** *Septic arthritis of the hand and wrist.* Hand Clin 14(4):579, 1998.
11. **Kim PSY, Mierau D, Loback D:** *Septic arthritis of the hip: A case report.* J Can Chiro Assoc 37:151, 1993.
12. **Guebert G:** *Tom Smith arthritis* [Roentgen Brief]. ACA Council Roentgenology, 1981.

TOM SMITH'S ARTHRITIS

1. **Smith T:** *On the acute arthritis of the hip.* St Bartholomew's Hospital Rep 10:189, 1874.
2. **Guebert G:** *Tom Smith arthritis* [Roentgen Brief]. ACA Council Roentgenology, 1981.

NON-SUPPURATIVE OSTEOMYELITIS (TUBERCULOSIS)

1. **Keers RY:** *Pulmonary Tuberculosis—A Journey Down the Centuries.* Balliere Tindall, London, 1978.
2. **Leff A, Lester TW, Addington W:** *Tuberculosis, a chemotherapeutic triumph but a persistent socioeconomic problem.* Arch Intern Med 139:1375, 1973.
3. **Enarson DA, Fujii M, Nakielna EM, et al.:** *Bone and joint tuberculosis: A continuing problem.* Can Med Assoc J 120:139, 1979.
4. **Murray RO, Jacobson HG:** *The Radiology of Skeletal Disorders,* ed 2. New York, Churchill Livingstone, 1977.
5. **Reading AD, Stother IG:** *The painless fracture: Could it be TB?* J R Coll Surg Edinb 43(6):410, 1998.
6. **Silber JS, Whitfield SB, Anbari K, et al.:** *Insidious destruction of the hip by* Mycobacterium tuberculosis *and why early diagnosis is critical.* J Arthroplasty 15(3):392, 2000.
7. **U.S. Department of Health, Education and Welfare; Public Health Service, Center for Disease Control:** *Tuberculosis statistics, State and Cities* [DHEW publication (CDC) 79-8294]. Atlanta, 1977.
8. **Weaver P, Lifeso RM:** *The radiological diagnosis of tuberculosis of the adult spine.* Skeletal Radiol 12:178, 1984.
9. **Ayhan S, Uluoglu O, Demirtas Y, et al.:** *Nonhealing ulcerative mass of the elbow: Do not forget tuberculosis.* Ann Plast Surg 48(5):557, 2002.
10. **Mills TJ, Owen R, Strach EH:** *Early diagnosis of bone and joint tuberculosis in children.* Lancet 2:57, 1956.
11. **Bailey HL, Gabriel M, Hodgson AR, et al.:** *Tuberculosis of the spine in children.* J Bone Joint Surg 54A:1384, 1953.
12. **Zimmerman MR:** *Pulmonary and osseous tuberculosis in an Egyptian mummy.* Bull NY Acad Med 55:604, 1979.
13. **Pott P:** *Remarks on That Kind of Palsy of the Lower Limbs Which Is Frequently Found to Accompany a Curvature of the Spine.* London, J Johnson, 1779.
14. **Resnick D, Niwayama G:** *Diagnosis of Bone and Joint Disorders.* Philadelphia, WB Saunders, 1981.
15. **Heniques CQ:** *Osteomyelitis as a complication in urology, with special reference to the paravertebral venous plexus.* Br J Surg 46:19, 1958.

16. **Hellstadius A:** *Tuberculous necrosis of the entire vertebral body, with negative x-ray findings.* Acta Orthop Scand 16:163, 1946.
17. **Ahmadi J, Bajaj A, Destian S, et al.:** *Spinal tuberculosis: Atypical observations at MR imaging.* Radiology 189:489, 1993.
18. **Bell D, Cockshott WP:** *Tuberculosis of the vertebral pedicles.* Radiology 99:43, 1971.
19. **Mansberg VJ, Rowe LJ, Walker C:** *Atypical case of Pott's disease.* Australas Radiol 35:191, 1991.
20. **Pollard BA, El-Beheiry H:** *Pott's disease with unstable cervical spine, retropharyngeal cold abscess and progressive airway obstruction.* Can J Anaesth 46(8):772, 1999.
21. **Graves UB, Schrieber MH:** *Tuberculous psoas muscle abscess.* J Can Assoc Radiol 24:268, 1973.
22. **Yochum TR:** *Tuberculosis of the L1/L2 motor unit with bilateral psoas cold abscesses* [Radiology Corner]. ACA J Chiro 1982.
23. **Hall FM, Harris AK:** *Osseous sequelae of tuberculous spondylitis as demonstrated by computed tomography: Case report 396.* Skeletal Radiol 15:589, 1986.
24. **Smith AS, Weinstein MA, Mizushima A, et al.:** *MR imaging characteristics of tuberculous spondylitis vs vertebral osteomyelitis.* AJR 153:399, 1989.
25. **Tan SC, Harwant S, Selvakumar K, Kareem BA:** *Predictive factors in the evolution of neural deficit in tuberculosis of the spine.* Med J Malaysia 56(Suppl C):46, 2001.
26. **Schmorl G, Junghans H:** *The Human Spine in Health and Disease,* ed 2 (Am). New York, Grune & Stratton, 1971.
27. **Gooding CA, Neuhauser EBD:** *Growth and development of the vertebral bodies in the presence and absence of normal stress.* AJR 93:388, 1965.

EXTRASKELETAL MANIFESTATIONS OF TUBERCULOSIS
1. **Hanson RA, Thoongsuwan N.** *Scrofula.* Curr Probl Diagn Radiol 31:227, 2002.
2. **Mert A, Tabak F, Ozaras R, et al.:** *Tuberculous lymphadenopathy in adults: A review of 35 cases.* Acta Chir Belg 102(2):118, 2002.

UNUSUAL PRESENTATIONS OF TUBERCULOSIS
1. **Yochum TR:** *Tuberculosis of the L1/L2 motor unit with bilateral psoas cold abscesses* [Radiology Corner]. ACA J Chiro 1982.
2. **Komins C:** *Multiple cystic tuberculosis; review and revised nomenclature.* Br J Radiol 25:1, 1952.
3. **Yoon CJ, Chung HW, Hong SH, et al.:** *MR findings of tuberculous dactylitis: Case report.* Eur J Radiol 29(3):163, 2001.
4. **Resnick D, Niwayama G:** *Diagnosis of Bone and Joint Disorders.* Philadelphia, WB Saunders, 1981.
5. **Herzfeld G, Tod MC:** *Tuberculous dactylitis in infancy.* Arch Dis Child 1:295, 1926.
6. **Murray RO, Jacobson HG:** *The Radiology of Skeletal Disorders,* ed 2. New York, Churchill Livingstone, 1977.
7. **Bambakidis NC, Cohen AR:** *Intracranial complications of frontal sinusitis in children: Pott's puffy tumor revisited.* Pediatr Neurosurg 35(2):82, 2001.
8. **Deutsch E, Hevron I, Eilon A:** *Pott's puffy tumor treated by endoscopic frontal sinusotomy.* Rhinology 38(4):177, 2000.
9. **Mayers LB:** *Carpal tunnel syndrome secondary to tuberculosis.* Arch Neurol 10:426, 1964.
10. **Yamamoto T, Iwasaki Y, Kurosaka M:** *Tuberculosis of the greater trochanteric bursa occurring 51 years after tuberculous nephritis.* Clin Rheumatol 31(5):397, 2002.
11. **McNeur JC, Pritchard AE:** *Tuberculosis of the greater trochanter.* J Bone Joint Surg 37B:246, 1955.
12. **Marcus U, Dittmar MT, Krausslich HG:** *HIV: Epidemiology and Strategies for Therapy and Vaccination.* Inervirology 45:260, 2002.
13. **Wu CM, Davis F, Fishman EK:** *Musculoskeletal complications of the patient with acquired immunodeficiency syndrome (AIDS): CT evaluation.* Semin Ultrasound CT MR 19(2):200, 1998.
14. **Solinger AM, Hess EV:** *Acquired immune deficiency syndrome—An overview.* Semin Roentgenol 22:9, 1987.

15. **Hu DJ, Vitek CR, Bartholow B, Mastro TD:** *Key issues for a potential human immunodeficiency virus vaccine.* Clin Infect Dis 36(5):638, 2003.
16. **Major NM, Tehranzadeh J:** *Musculoskeletal manifestations of AIDS.* Radiol Clin North Am 35(5):1167, 1997.
17. **Steinbach LS, Tehranzadeh J, Fleckenstein JL, et al.:** *Human immunodeficiency virus infection: Musculoskeletal manifestations.* Radiology 186:833, 1993.
18. **Wyatt SH, Fishman EK:** *CT/MRI of musculoskeletal complications of AIDS.* Skeletal Radiol 24(7):481, 1995.
19. **Magid D, Fishman EK:** *Musculoskeletal infections in patients with AIDS: CT findings.* AJR 158:603, 1992.
20. **Al-Tawfiq JA, Sarosi GA, Bushing HE:** *Pyomyositis in the acquired immunodeficiency syndrome.* South Med J 93(3):330, 2000.
21. **Baron AL, Steinbach LS, LeBoit PE, et al.:** *Osteolytic lesions and bacillary angiomatosis in HIV infection: Radiologic differentiation from AIDS-related Kaposi sarcoma.* Radiology 177:77, 1990.
22. **Schinina V, Rizzi EB, Rovighi L, et al.:** *Infectious spondylodiscitis: Magnetic resonance imaging in HIV-infected and HIV-uninfected patients.* Clin Imaging 25(5):362, 2001.
23. **Scadden DT:** *AIDS-related malignancies.* Annu Rev Med 54:285, 2003.

SYPHILITIC OSTEOMYELITIS
1. *Congenital syphilis—United States, 1998.* MMWR Morb Mortal Wkly Rep 48(34):757, 1999.
2. **Rawstron SA, Vetrano J, Tannis G, Bromberg K:** *Congenital syphilis: Detection of Treponema pallidum in stillborns.* Clin Infect Dis 24(1):24, 1997.
3. **Gust DA, Levine WC, St Louis ME, et al.:** *Mortality associated with congenital syphilis in the United States, 1992–1998.* Pediatrics 109(5):E79, 2002.
4. **Frank D, Duke T:** *Congenital syphilis at Goraka Base Hospital: Incidence, clinical features and risk factors for mortality.* P N G Med J 43:121, 2000.
5. **Walker DG, Walker GJ:** *Forgotten but not gone: The continuing scourge of congenital syphilis.* Lancet Infect Dis 2(7):432, 2002.
6. **Curtis BJ, Philpott OS:** *Congenital syphilis.* Med Clin North Am 48:707, 1964.
7. **Thomas EW:** *Syphilis: Its Course and Management.* New York, Macmillan, 1949.
8. **Simmank KC, Pettifor JM:** *Unusual presentation of congenital syphilis.* Ann Trop Paediatr 20(2):105, 2000.
9. **Narain S, Batra B, Abraham SN, Arya LS:** *Symptomatic congenital syphilis presenting at birth.* Indian J Pediatr 68(9):897, 2001.
10. **Cremin BJ, Fischer RM:** *The lesions of congenital syphilis.* Br J Radiol 43:233, 1970.
11. **Murray RO, Jacobson HG:** *The Radiology of Skeletal Disorders,* ed 2. New York, Churchill Livingstone, 1977.
12. **Wimberger H:** *Klinisch—Radiologische diagnostik von rachitis, skorbut und lues congenita im kindesalter.* Ergeb Inn Med Kinderheilkd 28:264, 1925.
13. **Levin EJ:** *Healing in congenital osseous syphilis.* AJR 110:591, 1970.
14. **Clutton HH:** *Symmetrical synovitis of the knee in hereditary syphilis.* Lancet 1:391, 1886.
15. **Hutchinson J:** *Syphilis.* London, Cassell, 1887.
16. **Truog CP:** *Bone lesions in acquired syphilis.* Radiology 40:1, 1943.
17. **Ehrlich I, Kricun ME:** *Radiographic findings in early acquired syphilis: Case report and critical review.* AJR 127:789, 1976.
18. **Edeiken J:** *Roentgen Diagnosis of Diseases of Bone,* ed. 3. Vol 1. Baltimore, Williams & Wilkins, 1981.
19. **Jaffe HL:** *Metabolic, Degenerative, and Inflammatory Diseases of Bones and Joints.* Philadelphia, Lea & Febiger, 1972.

MYCOTIC OSTEOMYELITIS
1. **Forbus WD:** *Coccidioidomycosis: A study of 95 cases of disseminated type, with special reference to the pathogenesis of the disease.* Milit Surg 99:653, 1946.
2. **Vaz A, Pineda-Roman M, Thomas AR, Carlson RW:** *Coccidioidomycosis: An update.* Hosp Pract 33(9):105, 1998.

3. **Nakamura H, Nakamura T, Suzuki M, et al.:** *Disseminated coccidioidomycosis with intra- and paravertebral abscesses.* J Infect Chemother 8(2):178, 2002.
4. **Leake JA, Mosley DG, England B, et al.:** *Risk factors for acute symptomatic coccidioidomycosis among elderly persons in Arizona, 1996–1997.* J Infect Dis 181(4):1435, 2000.
5. **Galgiani JN, Ampel NM, Catanzaro A, et al.:** *Practice guideline for the treatment of coccidioidomycosis. Infectious Diseases Society of America.* Clin Infect Dis 30(4):658, 2000.
6. **Holley K, Muldoon M, Tasker S:** *Coccidioides immitis osteomyelitis: A case series review.* Orthopedics 35(8):827, 2002.
7. **Wrobel CJ, Chappell ET, Taylor W:** *Clinical presentation, radiological findings, and treatment results of coccidioidomycosis involving the spine: Report on 23 cases.* J Neurosurg 95(1 Suppl):33, 2001.
8. **Herron LD, Kissel P, Smilovitz D:** *Treatment of coccidioidal spinal infection: Experience in 16 cases.* J Spinal Disord 10(3):215, 1997.
9. **Oldfield EC III, Bone WD, Martin CR, et al.:** *Prediction of relapse after treatment of coccidioidomycosis.* Clin Infect Dis 25(5):1205, 1997.
10. **Prichard DJ:** *Granulomatous infections of bones and joints.* Orthop Clin North Am 6:1029, 1975.
11. **Dalinka MK, Dinnenberg S, Greendyke WH, et al.:** *Roentgenographic features of osseous coccidioidomycosis and differential diagnosis.* J Bone Joint Surg 53A:1157, 1971.
12. **Huang JI, Seeger LL, Jones NF:** *Coccidioidomycosis fungal infection in the hand mimicking a metacarpal enchondroma.* J Hand Surg 25B:475, 2000.
13. **Fishco WD, Blocher KS:** *Disseminated coccidioidomycosis masquerading as tendinitis.* J Am Podiatr Med Assoc 90(10):508, 2000.
14. **Zeppa MA, Laorr A, Greenspan A, et al.:** *Skeletal coccidioidomycosis: Imaging findings in 19 patients.* Skeletal Radiol 25(4):337, 1996.
15. **Goldman AB, Freiberger RH:** *Localized infectious and neuropathic diseases.* Semin Roentgenol 14(1):19, 1979.

ACTINOMYCOSIS

1. **Goldman AB, Freiberger RH:** *Localized infectious and neuropathic diseases.* Semin Roentgenol 14(1):19, 1979.
2. **Curi MM, Dib LL, Kowalski LP, et al.:** *Opportunistic actinomycosis in osteoradionecrosis of the jaws in patients affected by head and neck cancer: incidence and clinical significance.* Oral Oncol 2000 May;36(3):294–9
3. **Yung BC, Cheng JC, Chan TT, et al.:** *Aggressive thoracic actinomycosis complicated by vertebral osteomyelitis and epidural abscess leading to spinal cord compression.* Spine 2000 Mar 15;25(6):745–8
4. **Nathan MH, Radman WP, Barton HL:** *Osseous actinomycosis of the head and neck.* AJR 87:1048, 1962.
5. **Voisin L, Vittecoq O, Mejjad O, et al.:** *Spinal abscess and spondylitis due to actinomycosis.* Spine 23(4):487, 1998.

MADUROMYCOSIS

1. **Corr P:** *Clinics in diagnostic imagining (26). Madura foot (or mycetoma).* Singapore Med J 38(6):268, 1997.
2. **Davies AGM:** *Bone changes in Madura foot (mycetoma).* Radiology 70:841, 1958.
3. **Arrendondo HG, Ceballos JL:** *Unusual location of mycetoma.* Radiology 78:72, 1962.
4. **Resnick D, Niwayama G:** *Diagnosis of Bone and Joint Disorders.* Philadelphia, WB Saunders, 1981.
5. **Davis JD, Stone PA, McGarry JJ:** *Recurrent mycetoma of the foot.* J Foot Ankle Surg 38(1):55, 1999.
6. **Ten Broeke R, Walenkamp G:** *The Madura foot: An "innocent foot mycosis"?* Acta Orthop Belg 64(2):242, 1998.
7. **Hazra B, Bandyopadhyay S, Saha SK, et al.:** *A study of mycetoma in eastern India.* J Commun Dis 30(1):7, 1998.
8. **Sarris I, Berendt AR, Athanasous N, Ostlere SJ:** *MRI of mycetoma of the foot: Two cases demonstrating the dot-in-circle sign.* Skeletal Radiol 32(3):179, 2003.

Hematologic and Vascular Disorders

13

Lindsay J. Rowe and Terry R. Yochum

HEMATOLOGIC DISORDERS

Numerous blood-related disorders, including various anemias, leukemias, lymphomas, and clotting-deficient diseases (hemophilia), can cause skeletal alterations. Of all the various types of anemias, only those that are chronic and severe will result in radiographically visible osseous changes. Observable skeletal alterations are either related to direct effects of the disorders on the bone marrow or are secondary to complications inherent in the disease. The most notable osseous changes are seen in the congenital hemolytic anemias, especially thalassemia (Cooley's anemia), sickle cell anemia, and hereditary spherocytosis. (1) Chronic iron deficiency anemia produces minor skeletal changes, usually isolated to the skull. (2,3) Leukemia demonstrates characteristic changes largely dependent on age. Hemophilia primarily alters joint function because of recurrent intra-articular hemorrhage. The skeletal manifestations of the lymphomas are discussed in Chapter 11.

SICKLE CELL ANEMIA

General Considerations

Sickle cell disease is a chronic, congenital, and hereditary hemolytic anemia. It was first described in 1910 by Herrick. (1) It is found almost exclusively in black individuals, representing the most common inherited disease among this population. (2) Less commonly, it is seen in certain Mediterranean populations. It is characterized pathologically by an abnormal molecular structure of hemoglobin that, under low oxygen tension, will distort the red blood cell into an elongated, curved, *sickle* configuration. The end result is increased hemolysis, vascular occlusion, and tis-

sue anoxia. The osseous changes are primarily related to infarction, avascular necrosis, marrow hyperplasia, and retarded growth.

Clinical Features

All individuals who possess the sickle cell hemoglobin (Hb) do not necessarily have symptoms or radiographic changes. Usually, only those that are homozygous (Hb SS) have symptoms, whereas those with other genotypes (Hb SA, Hb S-thalassemia) usually remain clinically silent. The disease currently affects an estimated 70,000 Americans. (3)

The onset of clinical signs and symptoms in homozygous patients is usually after 6 months of age, owing to the progressive decrease in levels of fetal hemoglobin (Hb F). (4) Weakness and pallor are usual but non-specific. Episodic abdominal crises, jaundice, acute bone pain, and dactylitis, however, particularly in a black individual, are characteristic clinical findings consistent with intermittent sickle-induced infarctions. (5) It is estimated that affected individuals will have approximately one acute painful episode per year; however, chronic pain syndromes are not uncommon with this condition. (3)

A common symptom in infancy is the so-called *hand–foot syndrome*. This consists of painful swellings of the hands and feet and is the result of either infarction or *Salmonella* infection. (6) In general, there is a predisposition to develop *Salmonella* osteomyelitis, which at times will be bilateral and symmetric. (7,8) Within the skeleton, the major deleterious effect is the development of avascular necrosis of the femoral or humeral heads in 8–13% of cases. (9) The incidence of femoral and humeral head necrosis is equal, but the incidence of postprosthesis failure is as much as 50%. (9) (Fig. 13-1) Owing to the systemic nature of the disease, osteonecrosis is often seen bilaterally. (10) The prevalence of avascular necrosis of the hip increases as the age of the patient and duration of the disease increases. (10) Occasionally, widespread

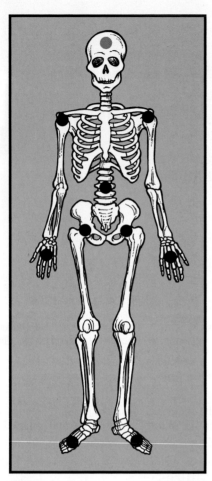

● More common   ● Less common

Figure 13-1   **SKELETAL DISTRIBUTION OF SICKLE CELL ANEMIA.**

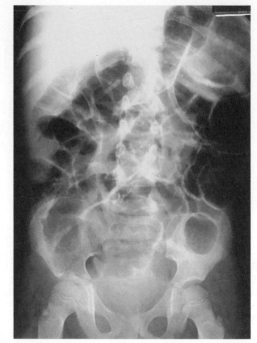

Figure 13-2   **SICKLE CELL ANEMIA: ABDOMINAL CRISIS.** Observe the numerous dilated loops of small intestine that are the result of acute mesenteric thrombosis.

Pathologic Features

The phenomenon of erythrocyte sickling is caused by an abnormal hemoglobin, Hb S. (9) The underlying molecular defect in homozygotes, Hb SS, is owing to the substitution of valine for glutamic acid in the sixth position on the β-globulin chain. (19) In sickle cell hemoglobin C (Hb SC), lysine is substituted for glutamic acid in the sixth position of the β-globulin chain. There are various types of sickle cell disease, based on the gene combination. The true sickle cell individual is homozygous for the sickle cell gene (Hb SS). Other genetic variants of sickle cell disease that may result in bone changes are sickle cell trait (Hb SA), sickle cell hemoglobin C (Hb SC), and sickle cell thalassemia (Hb S-thalassemia). Sickle cell anemia (Hb SS) is found in 1–3% of blacks, and occasional cases in whites have been reported in Greece, Turkey, Italy, and Sicily. (20,21) Sickle cell anemia occurs in 7–9% of black Americans.

The pathologic hallmark of sickle cell anemia is the transformation of a normal-appearing red blood corpuscle to the sickle configuration under local hypoxia. This *sickling phenomenon* results in increased mechanical fragility of the cell itself, increased blood viscosity, stasis, and lowered pH.

The osseous changes in sickle cell hemoglobinopathies occur secondary to marrow hyperplasia, local ischemia, and necrosis. The result is an overall decrease in the number of bony trabeculae, thinning of the cortices, bone death, and growth deformities.

In the developing spine, vascular compromise and regional ischemia result in a unique vertebral body endplate configuration (*fish vertebrae, step-down sign, H vertebra, Reynolds' phenomenon*). (22–25) (Fig. 13-3) Physiologically, the endplates are the vertebral body analogs of a long bone metaphysis, contributing to the development of vertebral height. The central portion of the endplate receives a direct blood supply from branches of the nu-

generalized bone marrow necrosis is evident in patients with sickle cell disease. (11)

With advancing age, compensatory hemopoiesis may result in initial splenic enlargement, usually up to approximately 10 years of age. Later, with progressive infarction and fibrosis, the spleen may completely atrophy, resulting in autosplenectomy. (12) Almost any organ can be involved, with resultant protean clinical symptoms. Cardiomegaly is a common complication in up to 95% of patients, resulting from tricuspid regurgitation in about 50% of cases. (13,14) Most patients reveal pulmonary vasculature complications leading to pulmonary hypertension. (13) Gallstones may be found in up to 65% of patients, owing to hyperbilirubinemia from increased hemolysis. (15,16) More than half of these stones will be visible on plain film examination. (15) Mesenteric vascular thromboses result in acute, severe abdominal pain, the so-called *sickle cell crisis.* (Fig. 13-2) Renal failure from papillary necrosis also occurs. In the brain, infarction of the white and gray matter has been noted, causing both functional and cognitive impairments. (17)

Pain control and blood transfusions are the integral aspects of treatment. (18) Death usually results from infection, visceral infarction, cardiac decompensation, or pulmonary hypertension. (13) Survival beyond 30 years of age in those with the homozygous genotype (Hb SS) is rare.

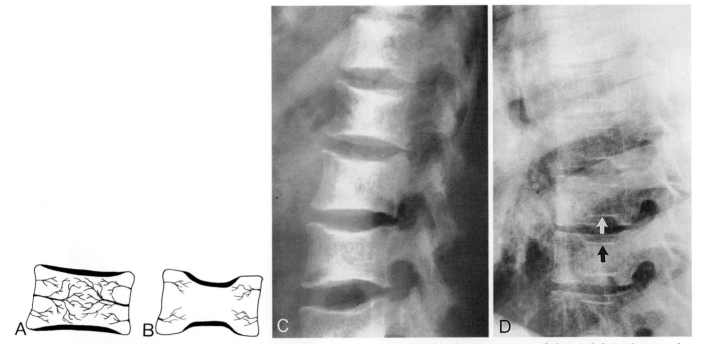

Figure 13-3 SICKLE CELL ANEMIA: SPINAL CHANGES.
A. Normal. Normal circulatory dynamics in a developing vertebral body. **B. After Thrombosis.** Following thrombosis of the central nutrient vessels, central growth is inhibited, producing the characteristic *H vertebra*. **C. Early Changes.** Note that initially, the depression of the endplates is smooth, concave, and shallow. **D. Later Changes.** Observe that later the configuration becomes sharp and more characteristic (*arrows*).

trient artery. At the periphery of the endplates there is a diffuse network of anastomotic perforating vessels. This pattern of vascular distribution and circulatory dynamics results in ischemia of the central endplate zone when the nutrient artery becomes obstructed, such as in a *sickling crisis*. The peripheral vessels, because of their number and anastomoses, allow collateral circulation to develop more easily if they become obstructed. The result is the inhibition of growth of the central endplate zone, culminating in its relative inward displacement. The periphery remains unaffected, contributing to the development of the normal vertebral body height.

Radiologic Features

The pathophysiology of sickle cell anemia correlates closely with the skeletal radiographic manifestations. Essentially, these are related to the effects of marrow hyperplasia, vaso-occlusive phenomena, or complicating osteomyelitis. (4,20,26)

General Characteristics

Marrow Hyperplasia. The extent of marrow hyperplasia determines the degree of osseous changes. Even in the most severe forms of sickle cell disease the marrow response is significantly less than that seen in thalassemia, providing a reliable radiographic differential feature between the two entities. (Fig. 13-4)

Skeletal manifestations include generalized osteopenia, sparse and coarsened trabecular pattern, large vascular channels, widened medullary cavity, cortical thinning, and a loss of the diaphyseal constriction in the small tubular bones. (4) (Table 13-1) In the skull, the osseous changes are limited to the area above the internal occipital protuberance because of the absence of marrow below this point. Skull changes consist of a widened diploic space, granular texture and, in severe cases, a *hair-on-end trabecular pattern.* (27) In the adult a generalized sclerotic pattern may appear in the entire skeleton, except in the spine, owing to chronic endosteal appositional new bone formation. (26,28)

Splenic infarcts, appearing as punctate or amorphous calcific configurations, are seen in up to 30% of patients with sickle cell anemia. (12)

Infarction. The roentgen appearance of infarction depends on the time sequence, location, and extent of the infarction. (Table 13-2) The earliest radiographic sign, especially in the tubular bones of the hands and feet, is initial soft tissue swelling, followed in about 2 weeks by diaphyseal and linear periostitis. (5) Ensuing rarefaction of the involved bone results in a radiologic presentation identical to that of osteomyelitis. Gadolinium-enhanced MRI is unreliable in distinguishing between osteomyelitis and bone infarction. (29) The best method for differentiation is the combined use of technetium and gallium scintigraphy, by which both scans will show focal uptake in the presence of infection in contrast to infarctions, which show uptake of technetium but normal to low uptake of gallium. (30) MRI shows acute infarction as reduced signal on T1- and increased signal on T2-weighted studies. The involvement may be limited to single or multiple bones. Other bones affected include the distal femur, proximal tibia, and distal humerus.

Organized, clearly defined, serpiginous medullary infarcts are sometimes seen. Infarction of an epiphysis, especially of the femoral and humeral heads, is identical to the idiopathic or post-traumatic forms of ischemic necrosis in these locations. Alterations in bone growth result in cupped metaphyses and shortened

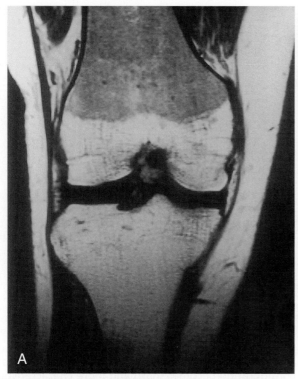

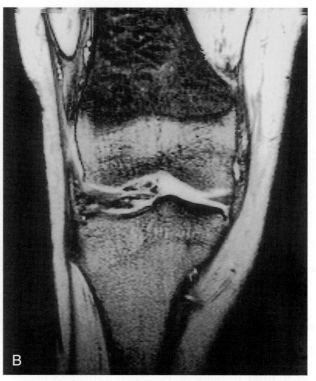

Figure 13-4 SICKLE CELL ANEMIA: MARROW CONVERSION. A. T1-Weighted MRI, Coronal Knee. B. T2-Weighted MRI, Coronal Knee. Note that the low signal intensity seen in the distal femur abutting the metaphysis is abnormal reconversion of red marrow from yellow marrow. *COMMENT:* This 27-year-old sickle cell patient was not a smoker. This marrow conversion was associated with the hemolytic abnormality of sickle cell anemia. (Courtesy of Bruce Bowen, Lehigh Valley MRI, Allentown, Pennsylvania.)

bone length. (5) The tibio-talar slant deformity, owing to closure of the lateral aspect of the distal tibial epiphyses, has also been reported at an incidence of 4% of patients. (31) Protrusio acetabuli may be evident in up to 5% of males and 12% of females. (32)

In the femoral head, ischemic changes are radiographically visible in the homozygous Hb SS form in 8–20% of patients and tends to be bilateral. (9,33,34) Characteristic findings on plain film examination include a subchondral fracture of the weight-bearing surface of the femoral head (*crescent sign*), sharp depression of the articular surface (*step defect*), flattening or irregularity of the weight-bearing surface, and a curvilinear band of involvement of the superior femoral head (*bite sign*). The head will be photopenic on technetium scan even before plain film findings are apparent. CT is useful only in the latter stages, when, in addition to the plain film features, there is loss of the normal star-like pattern (*asterisk sign*) within the femoral head. (9) MRI is extremely sensitive to avascular changes and is the imaging method of choice, showing a low signal on T1- and a high signal on T2-weighted studies. Similar features are seen in afflicted humeral heads.

Osteomyelitis. A peculiar affinity exists for developing *Salmonella* osteomyelitis in patients with sickle cell anemia, with a 100 times increased incidence over the normal population. (7) The exact portal of entry and resulting pathophysiology are unknown. It is hypothesized that infarction in the intestine predisposes pathogens to entry into the circulatory system, with localization into other infarcted areas, such as bone. (8,35) The usual causative organism is *Salmonella paratyphi,* although other Gram-negative pathogens, such as *Escherichia coli* and *Haemophilus influenzae,* have been implicated.

The resultant osteomyelitis is unique; it is often bilateral, symmetric, and diaphyseal in location and exhibits a prominent, *moth-eaten pattern* of destruction and periosteal response. The most common bones involved are the femur, tibia, fibula, humerus, radius, and ulna. Spinal involvement does occur. (Table 13-3)

Table 13-1	Manifestations of Marrow Hyperplasia
Cortical thinning	
Generalized decrease in bone density	
Large vascular channels	
Loss of diaphyseal constriction	
Sparse, coarsened trabecular pattern (honeycomb)	
Widened medullary cavity	

Table 13-2	Manifestations of Infarction
Cortical splitting (bone within a bone)	
Disturbed bone growth	
Epiphyseal necrosis (humeral and femoral heads)	
Linear diaphyseal periostitis	
Organized metaphyseal medullary infarcts	
Patchy areas of lucency and sclerosis	
Soft tissue swelling	

Table 13-3	Manifestations of *Salmonella* Osteomyelitis in Sickle Cell Anemia

Bilateral and symmetric
Diaphyseal location in long bones
Permeative and moth-eaten destruction
Prominent involucrum formation

Table 13-4	Manifestations of Sickle Cell Anemia in the Spine

Common
    Characteristic endplate deformity (fish vertebrae)
    Prominent osteoporosis persisting to adult life
Uncommon
    Enlarged anterior vascular notch
    Intrathoracic extramedullary hemopoiesis
    Rapid vertebral body collapse
    Salmonella spondylitis

Target Sites of Involvement

Long Bones. Depending on the severity of the disease, variable changes in the long bones may be visible. The most prominent alterations include coarsening of the trabecular pattern, patchy medullary sclerosis, bone within a bone appearance of the cortex, laminated or solid periosteal new bone, growth abnormalities, and epiphyseal ischemic necrosis. (4) These changes tend to be widespread and symmetric.

Spine. Alterations in the spine are common and often distinctive. (Table 13-4) The radiographic changes in the vertebrae vary with the stage, intensity, and duration of the disease and are more pronounced as the patient ages. The major diagnostic changes consist of a prominent osteoporotic bone pattern that continues into adulthood and unique vertebral endplate deformities.

Osteoporosis. The radiographic changes of sickle cell osteoporosis are non-specific, except for the childhood onset and persistence with age, despite the diffuse trabecular thickening and endosteal sclerosis of the remaining skeleton. (36) The vertebral centra appear decreased in general density, with a decrease in the number but an increase in the prominence of visible trabeculae. This trabecular accentuation is particularly notable in those oriented vertically. The cortices appear thinned and relatively more prominent than usual.

There are few conditions associated with juvenile or adolescent spinal osteoporosis (e.g., steroid therapy, Cushing's syndrome), aiding in differential diagnosis. The combined findings of spinal osteoporosis and evidence of infarction (sclerosis, deformity, osteochondrosis) make the diagnosis of sickle cell disease likely.

Endplate Deformities. Endplate deformity consists of identical central depressions in the upper and lower endplates of several contiguous vertebral bodies. (Fig. 13-3D) The resultant vertebral configuration is similar to that of certain species of fish and has been referred to as *fish vertebra*. (23) The peripheral endplate maintains its normal flat surface and orientation, but the base of the depression is formed by a similar osseous structure in the same plane. The morphology of this deformity is virtually diagnostic of

thromboembolic phenomena during the growth phase of the vertebral centrum and, therefore, may also be seen in Gaucher's disease or thalassemia. (25,37–39) However, by far the most common cause is sickle cell anemia. This deformity is not commonly seen before the age of 10 years, usually appears before the 3rd decade of life, and is best seen in the thoracic and upper lumbar spines. (7) The endplate deformities should not be confused with osteoporosis, fractures, Schmorl's nodes, or nuclear impressions.

Vertebral Body Collapse. Massive infarction of one or more vertebral bodies has been observed. Usually, there are rapid compressive changes in the vertebral bodies, usually following episodes of ischemic crises. (26,28) Restitution to normal height, however, is not unusual, with only a residual increase in density visible. (40) Early detection and appropriate treatment strategies, including bracing and antibiotics, improve the chances of the restitution. (41) In approximately 14% of cases with vertebral infarction and shortening (collapse), compensatory vertical growth of adjacent vertebra may be seen. (42) This elongated appearance of the vertebral body has been referred to as a *tower vertebra* radiographically. (42)

Miscellaneous Changes. In children the midbody anterior vascular notch may be exaggerated as a reflection of compensatory marrow hyperplasia, best seen in the thoracolumbar region. (43) Signs of *Salmonella* spondylitis are identical to all suppurative spinal infections, with loss of disc height, destruction of the contiguous endplates, vertebral bodies, and soft tissue mass. The presence of intrathoracic extramedullary hemopoiesis is significantly less in incidence than with thalassemia. When present, these soft tissue densities have a lobulated or rounded contour and are located in the posterior mediastinum in the middle and lower thoracic spine. In the abdomen, 30% of homozygous sickle cell patients will exhibit calcification of the spleen. (12) Over half of these will be punctate, the rest being more diffuse or curvilinear in appearance.

CAPSULE SUMMARY   Sickle Cell Anemia

General Considerations

- Chronic, congenital, hereditary hemolytic anemia, characterized by abnormal hemoglobin structure.

Clinical Features

- Homozygous form (Hb SS) most symptomatic.
- Clinical onset usually between 6 months and 2 years—abdominal crises, jaundice, bone pain, avascular necrosis of

femoral and humeral heads, dactylitis (hand–foot syndrome), infections, gallstones, cardiac and renal failure.

Pathologic Features

- Molecular defect in β-globulin chain, where valine is substituted for glutamic acid.
- *Genotypes:* homozygous (Hb SS), trait (Hb SA), hemoglobin C (Hb SC), and thalassemia (Hb S-thalassemia).

(continued)

THALASSEMIA

General Considerations

Thalassemia (Cooley's anemia, Mediterranean anemia) is the world's most common hereditary disorder. (1,2) It is characterized by abnormal hemoglobin synthesis that produces variable degrees of anemia. The first description was by Cooley and Lee in 1925. (3) Most of the early reports were based on individuals of Mediterranean origin, from which the term *thalassemia* ("the sea") has been derived. In addition to its occurrence in Greek and Italian populations, the disease has also been recorded in Turkey, Syria, India, the Philippines, and Thailand; there are also reports in Native Americans and blacks. (4) The different genetic varieties of thalassemia produce a series of disorders known collectively as the *thalassemia syndromes*. However, three general groups have been identified, classified according to the severity of the disease: thalassemia major, thalassemia minor, and thalassemia intermedia. The most severe form is thalassemia major, which has the poorest prognosis. The effects on the skeleton can be severe and manifest radiographically as signs of increased marrow hemopoiesis.

Clinical Features

Of all the genetic varieties, thalassemia major demonstrates the most severe clinical findings (5) Thalassemia minor and intermedia manifest in varying degrees of severity and usually have less serious prognoses, but a wide variety of musculoskeletal system manifestations occur. (6) Most frequently, arthralgia (30%) and low back pain (25%) are the major complaints. (6) The locomotor system is affected in 60% of patients, and scoliosis can be identified in up to 40% of cases. (6) In the major form survival beyond the first few years of life is unusual. Blood transfusions and chelation therapy are the current treatment options available. (1) However, repeated blood transfusions invariably result in hemochromatosis, with subsequent cardiac failure and death by the 2nd or 3rd decade of life. (4) Laboratory studies of the hepatic iron concentration is a reliable indicator in the assessment of total iron stores and hemochromatosis. (7) Recent advances in treatment have increased the survival rate to the 4th decade on average. (8) Currently, newer treatment modalities are under investigation, including gene therapy, bone marrow transfusions, and stem cell transplantation, which may further improve the quality and extent of life in these patients. (1,9)

Physical findings include pallor, lethargy, retarded growth, hepatosplenomegaly, mongoloid facies, maxillary overgrowth (*rodent facies*), and inhibited sexual development. Onset of these abnormalities occurs in the latter part of the 1st year of life. Rarely, epidural extramedullary hematopoietic tissue in the spinal cord can produce spinal cord compression. (10) Laboratory examination reveals a hypochromic microcytic anemia, reticulocytosis, nucleated red blood cells, target cells, and elevated serum bilirubin.

Pathologic Features

The genetic variations producing the abnormal hemoglobins are many. The most severe form (thalassemia major) is an expression of the homozygous genotype, whereas the more clinically benign form (thalassemia minor) is heterozygous. The essential defect is an imbalance in globin chain production (α- and β-chains), which leads to ineffective hemopoiesis, hemolysis, and anemia. (11) Diminished α- and β-chain production are termed α-thalassemia and β-thalassemia, respectively. (12) Thalassemic bone changes are a reflection of overgrowth and overactivity of marrow tissue, which generally is the most severe of all the anemias. In infants and children the entire skeleton is involved because of the presence of red marrow. With increasing age there may be regression of peripheral skeletal changes because the red marrow is normally replaced by fatty marrow. (13) In contrast, the pelvis, spine, and skull may show progression of changes with age. (14)

Pathologic changes in bone relate directly to the erythroid hyperplasia, with marked widening of the medullary cavity, thinning of cortices, expansion in bone diameter, resorption of fine trabeculae, and thickening of remaining trabeculae. Extramedullary hemopoiesis results in hepatosplenomegaly and, in the posterior mediastinal paraspinal soft tissues, the development of hemopoietic masses. CT of these mediastinal masses has shown them to be derived from herniation of expanding bone marrow through the thinned trabeculae of the posterior ribs. (15)

Radiologic Features

Radiographic manifestations are most common and most severe in thalassemia major. (5) The radiograph closely parallels the degree of marrow hyperplasia, which produces characteristic osseous changes. (16) (Fig. 13-5; Table 13-5)

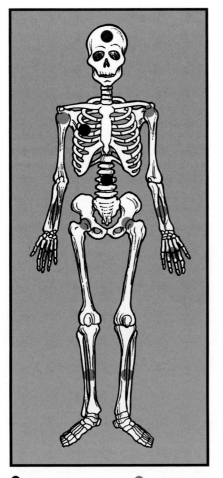

● More common   ● Less common

Figure 13-5 **SKELETAL DISTRIBUTION OF THALASSEMIA.**

Table 13-5	Radiologic Features in Thalassemia

General features
   Coarsened trabecular pattern (honeycomb)
   Cortical thinning
   Expanded bone caliber
   Osteoporosis
   Vascular channel enlargement
   Widened medullary cavity
Special features
   Erlenmeyer flask deformity
   Hair-on-end appearance (skull)
   Persistent spine and pelvis changes with age
   Paraspinal extramedullary hemopoiesis

General Characteristics

Marrow Hyperplasia. Osseous expressions of marrow hyperplasia are generalized cortical thinning, widened medullary cavity, expansion of bone caliber, osteoporosis, coarsened trabecular pattern (honeycomb) (Fig. 13-6), and enlarged vascular channels. (17)

Growth Disturbances. There is a lack of remodeling within long bones, resulting in undertubulation, especially at the diametaphyseal junction. This produces an *Erlenmeyer flask–type* deformity. Premature fusion of a portion of a growth plate may result in shortening and deformity, particularly in the proximal humerus and distal femur. (18) Transverse, linear opacities in the metaphysis are frequent and represent growth arrest lines.

Miscellaneous. Fractures, avascular necrosis, chondrocalcinosis, hemochromatosis, arthropathy, and, occasionally, paraspinal opaque hemosiderin laden lymph nodes may be seen. (19–21)

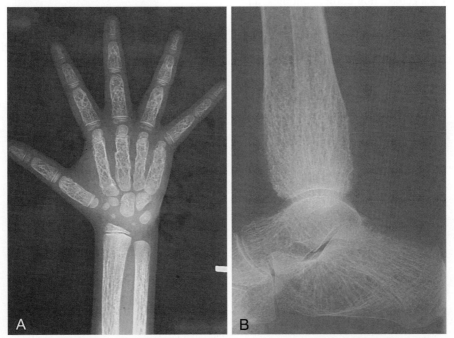

Figure 13-6 **THALASSEMIA: EXTREMITY CHANGES. A. PA Hand and Forearm. B. Lateral Ankle and Leg.** Observe the coarse trabecular pattern (honeycomb) and thin cortices.

Cardiomegaly, hepatosplenomegaly, and paraspinal soft tissue masses (extramedullary hemopoiesis) can also be identified.

Target Sites of Involvement

Long Bones. Manifestations of erythroid hyperplasia are best exemplified in the appendicular skeleton. The medullary cavity is widened, cortices are thinned, and trabeculae are sparse but coarsened (*honeycomb*). (15) Nutrient foramina may be enlarged. (17) Generally, the tubular bones are osteoporotic and lack the normal metaphyseal–diaphyseal concave constriction, at times producing the *Erlenmeyer flask deformity*. Organized medullary infarcts are uncommon, in contrast to sickle cell anemia. Partial premature closure of growth plates may be evident as deformity or alteration in length, especially in the proximal humerus and distal femur. Avascular necrosis of the femoral heads does occur, although it is less common than in sickle cell anemia. (22)

Skull. Of all the anemias, thalassemia creates the most pronounced changes in the skull. In the calvaria, there is a distinct lack of changes below the inferior occipital protuberance owing to the lack of marrow in this area. The frontal bones reveal the earliest and most severe changes. Three patterns of involvement may be visible: granular osteoporosis, widened diploe, and vertical radiating spicules of new bone (*hair-on-end appearance*) with loss of definition of the outer table. (14) (Fig. 13-7) Circumscribed lytic lesions of the calvaria up to 5 cm are occasionally seen. (23) The vascular impressions from the middle meningeal arteries are often enlarged and prominent. (17)

In the facial bones, the effects of erythroid hyperplasia may be severe, a feature rarely seen in sickle cell anemia. The major abnormalities are lack of pneumatization of the frontal, maxillary, sphenoid, and mastoid air cells but not the ethmoids, which remain aerated. (14) The orbits may be displaced laterally, and the upper incisors may be displaced forward, producing malocclusion (*rodent facies*).

Spine. The most prominent changes in the spine consist of osteopenia, coarse vertical trabeculae, thin cortical outlines, and involvement of both the body and neural arch of each segment. These features will also be visible in the sacrum and pelvis. (Figs. 13-8 and 13-9) Slight, generalized concavity of the endplates may be visible, but the discrete, central endplate depression typical of sickle cell anemia is invariably absent. (24) Additional findings may include exaggeration of the anterior body vascular notch, growth arrest lines, enlargement of the dens, and small ring apophyses. (25,26) It is notable that the spinal and pelvic lesions persist and even increase in prominence with increased age, in contrast to regression of the peripheral bone changes. (13) Extramedullary hematopoiesis affecting the spinal cord or nerve roots may exist but is rare. (27–29) MRI and CT examination are essential to assess these lesions. (28,29) On MRI, the mass appears heterogenous on both T1- and T2-weighted images with enhancement on administration of paramagnetic agents. (29)

Chest. Cardiomegaly is a consistent finding. (Fig. 13-10) Posterior mediastinal extramedullary hemopoietic masses will be evident as bilateral opaque paraspinal lobulated masses. (10,15,30,31)

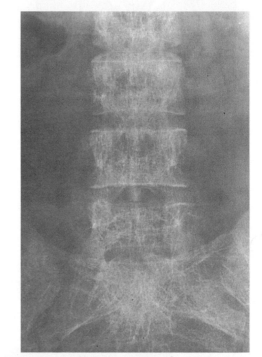

Figure 13-8   **THALASSEMIA. AP Lumbar Spine.** Note that all vertebral components demonstrate the conspicuous *honeycomb* appearance of accentuated trabecular markings.

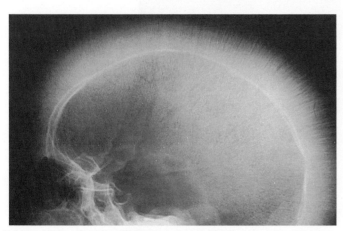

Figure 13-7   **THALASSEMIA. Lateral Skull.** Note the *hair-on-end appearance* that is the result of diploic erythroid hyperplasia.

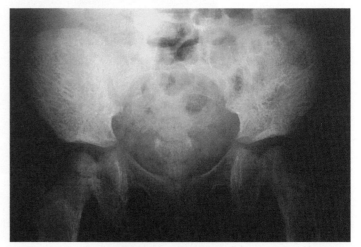

Figure 13-9   **THALASSEMIA. AP Pelvis.** Observe the characteristic coarsened *honeycomb* trabecular patterns.

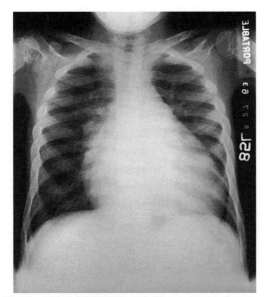

Figure 13-10 **THALASSEMIA. PA Chest.** Note the prominent cardiomegaly, a consistent finding. Note the widened contour of the ribs and coarsened osseous architecture.

Below the diaphragm, the liver and abdominal lymph nodes may be radiopaque owing to hemosiderin deposits. (30) The ribs are widened and osteopenic with a coarsened trabecular pattern. Characteristically, there is a symmetric, bulbous enlargement of the posterior ribs.

CAPSULE SUMMARY   Thalassemia

General Considerations

- Hereditary disorder of hemoglobin synthesis, producing anemia.
- Three forms, classified according to disease severity: major, minor, and intermediate.
- Synonyms: Cooley's anemia and Mediterranean anemia.

Clinical Features

- Onset in last half of first year, with survival beyond 3rd decade rare.
- *Symptoms:* pallor, underdevelopment, organomegaly, altered facies, abnormal blood examination.

Pathologic Features

- *Marrow hyperplasia:* cortical thinning, widened medullary cavity, loss of tubulation, coarse trabeculae (honeycomb), growth disturbances, fractures, chondrocalcinosis, hemochromatosis.

Radiologic Features

- *Spine:* coarse trabeculae, thin cortices, normal endplates.
- *Skull:* the frontal bone shows the earliest and most prominent changes; granular, widened diploe, radiating spicules (hair on end).
- Sinuses obliterated, rodent facies.
- *Chest:* cardiomegaly, posterior mediastinal masses, opaque liver and lymph nodes, rib expansion, coarsened trabeculae.

HEMOPHILIA

General Considerations

Hemophilia is the generic term applied to the group of blood coagulation disorders characterized by a deficiency of specific clotting factors. The two most common bleeding disorders associated with skeletal abnormalities are classic hemophilia (hemophilia A) and Christmas disease (hemophilia B). (1) Both are sex linked, recessive, and inherited. Genetically, the female is the carrier, but usually the disorder manifests clinically only in the male. The radiographic features focus on the effects of hemorrhages within or around bones and joints as well as within visceral organs.

Clinical Features

There are varying degrees of clinical expression of the disease. Mild forms exist that may not demonstrate a significant bleeding tendency. The more severe forms are characterized by spontaneous bleeding or bleeding as a result of minor injuries. (2) The sites of hemorrhage vary, involving all body cavities, tissues, bones, and joints. It is estimated that 80% of the bleeding occurs solely in the joints. (3) Rarely, hematomas occur in the muscle; however, when present loss of function and life-threatening complications are common. (4)

Intraosseous hemorrhage results in a destructive and often expansile alteration, most frequently of the ilium and femur. Articular hemorrhages produce acute and chronic hemarthroses, which subsequently precipitate synovitis and permanent joint changes (hemophilic arthropathy) and are especially prevalent in the weight-bearing joints of the lower extremity. (5) (Fig. 13-11) Injection or radiation synovectomy is the treatment of choice, and chronic arthritic changes are usually inevitable. (5,6) With advancement, total joint replacement is not an uncommon treatment. (7)

Current research is leading toward gene therapy for a viable treatment option in these patients. (5) Few trials of gene transfer therapy have been performed; however, in the limited results, safe and tolerated outcomes have been documented. (8)

Pathologic Features

The basic coagulative defect most commonly is owing to a deficiency of factor VIII (antihemophilic factor; AHF) and results in classic hemophilia A. (9) In hemophilia B there is a lack of factor IX. (9) In the absence of either of these two coagulation factors, the blood-clotting mechanism is rendered non-functional and ineffective, predisposing the patient to severe, uncontrolled hemorrhage.

Within joints, hemophilic hemorrhage, especially when recurrent, initiates a sequence of characteristic alterations. (10,11) Initial bleeding episodes may resolve completely with no sequelae. Repeated hemarthroses, however, eventually precipitate synovial proliferation (*pannus*) and synovial hemosiderin deposition. Articular adhesions and progressive fibrosis of the subsynovium, capsule, and periarticular tissues also occur. (12) Articular cartilage remains resistant to degradation by the synovial pannus for a long time, but eventually marginal erosions and degenerative changes ensue. Within the subarticular bone osteoporosis, cysts,

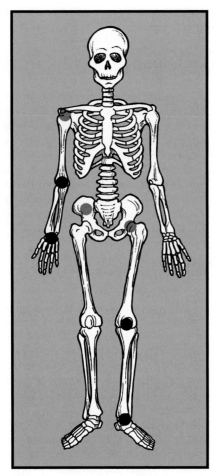

● More common   ● Less common

Figure 13-11 **SKELETAL DISTRIBUTION OF HEMOPHILIA.**

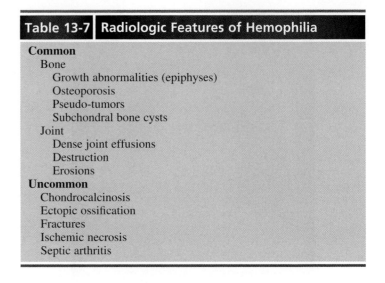

Table 13-7	Radiologic Features of Hemophilia

Common
  Bone
    Growth abnormalities (epiphyses)
    Osteoporosis
    Pseudo-tumors
    Subchondral bone cysts
  Joint
    Dense joint effusions
    Destruction
    Erosions
Uncommon
  Chondrocalcinosis
  Ectopic ossification
  Fractures
  Ischemic necrosis
  Septic arthritis

and epiphyseal overgrowth may be evident. Intraosseous and subperiosteal hemorrhages result in localized bone resorption, expansion, and periosteal new bone formation.

Radiologic Features

Both bones and joints are affected. Joint features are almost always present on reaching adult life. Hemophilic arthropathy progresses through various stages of severity, from the initial episodes of hemarthrosis to total joint disorganization; however, this progression is not absolute and may arrest at any stage. (13) (Table 13-6) The most commonly affected joints are the knee,

Table 13-6	Stages of Hemophilic Arthropathy	
Stage	**Major Radiographic Feature**
I	Soft tissue swelling
II	Osteoporosis
III	Osseous lesions
IV	Cartilage destruction
V	Joint disorganization

ankle, and elbow. Radiographic manifestations of hemophilic bone and joint involvement are distinctive and include dense soft tissue swelling, osteoporosis, subchondral cysts, expansile destructive bone lesions, epiphyseal abnormalities, and joint disorganization. (Table 13-7)

General Characteristics

Soft Tissue Swelling. As a manifestation of hemarthrosis, distension of the skin line, displacement of overlying fascial plane lines, and an increased soft tissue density owing to hemosiderin may be evident. (Fig. 13-12) MRI is useful in depicting synovial hypertrophy, inflammation, fluid accumulation, and loss of articular cartilage. (14,15)
Osteoporosis. Osteoporosis is especially evident within the epiphysis as a manifestation of hyperemia. Later, if the patient becomes inactive, a more generalized decrease in bone density will be evident.
Subchondral Cysts. Beneath the articular cortex, well-demarcated, localized regions of radiolucency represent either escaped synovial fluid or localized hemorrhages. Notably, the articular cortex may be poorly defined. (10)
Expansile Bone Lesions (Pseudo-Tumors). Hemorrhage within bone may result in expansile, geographic lesions simulating a neoplasm (*hemophilic pseudotumor*). (16) (Fig. 13-12) The occurrence of pseudo-tumors is rare, being estimated in only 1–2% of patients. (17) The radiographic manifestations are variable, ranging from a small, benign-appearing lesion to a large, aggressive destruction. (18) The bones most commonly involved are, in order of frequency, the femur, pelvis, tibia, and hand. Pseudo-tumors can also occur in soft tissues, producing a cyst-like lesion, which on T1-weighted and T2-weighted MRI studies is of low to heterogeneous signal intensity. (15,19) The pseudo-tumors are best followed by sonography, to demonstrate resolution or progression. (15) Contrast-enhanced CT shows a hypodense center that peripherally remains isodense with surrounding muscle. (15)
Epiphyseal Abnormalities. In the growing skeleton, chronic hyperemia of the epiphyseal cartilage can produce accelerated growth and maturation of epiphyses. The epiphyses appear bal-

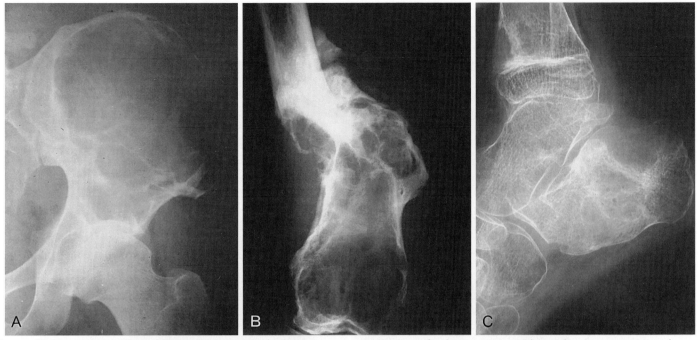

Figure 13-12 HEMOPHILIA: PSEUDO-TUMORS. A. Ilium. B. Femur. C. Calcaneus. Observe the tumor-like expansions of the ilium, femur, and calcaneus that are the result of repeated intraosseous hemorrhage. *COMMENT:* Hemophiliac pseudo-tumors are most common in the ilium but can be found anywhere in the skeleton. The radiographic appearance of an expansile, trabeculated lesion often makes the exclusion of other tumors, such as plasmacytoma, renal, or thyroid metastases and even giant cell tumors, difficult. When located adjacent to a joint, arthritic changes may provide the key differential clue to the diagnosis. (Panel A courtesy of Steven P. Brownstein, MD, Springfield, New Jersey. Panel B courtesy of Gerald A. Fitzgerald, MD, Sydney, Australia.)

looned and enlarged in relation to the adjacent diaphysis, similar to the appearance of juvenile rheumatoid arthritis.

Joint Disorganization. Chronic changes, such as complete loss of joint space, considerable articular fragmentation, sclerosis, osteophytes, and bony misalignment, may become apparent in long-standing hemophilia patients. (20) The similarity to neurotrophic joint disease is striking.

Other Abnormalities. Ischemic necrosis infrequently involves the talus and femoral head. (10) Susceptibility to fractures because of prominent osteoporosis is to be expected and often occurs spontaneously. (21) Ectopic ossification within muscle is most frequent in the pelvic gluteal or hamstring attachments. (22) Chondrocalcinosis has been documented. (23) A predisposition to joint infection is also apparent. (24)

Target Sites of Involvement

The most frequent sites of hemophilic arthropathy are the knee, ankle, and elbow. (3) Bilateral but asymmetric changes are common. In general, intra-articular hemorrhage distal to the elbow and ankle is rare.

Knee. Of all articulations, the knee is the most common site of hemophilic arthropathy. (25) Distinctive radiographic abnormalities include dense articular effusions, prominent epiphyseal osteoporosis, articular irregularity, and subchondral cysts. (Figs. 13-13 and 13-14) All of these findings may be present to varying degrees in the femorotibial and patellofemoral joints. Notably, the joint space is maintained until late in the disease.

The most characteristic alterations focus on the abnormal shape, size, and configuration of the distal femur, proximal tibia, and patella.

- *Distal femur.* The femoral condyles are often grossly enlarged, severely osteoporotic, and exhibit an irregular, flattened contour of their articular weight-bearing surfaces. *Widening of the intercondylar notch* is thought to be related to repeated hemorrhage at the cruciate ligament attachments. (Figs. 13-13A, 13-14A, and 13-15A)
- *Proximal tibia.* The tibial plateau may be flattened, usually with an irregular articular contour. The epiphysis is enlarged and osteoporotic, with a thin cortex and accentuated vertical trabeculae. The proximal fibula exhibits similar abnormalities.
- *Patella.* The inferior pole is sharply attenuated and *squared,* in contrast to the normal tapered apex. (Figs. 13-14B and 13-15B) Repeated hemarthrosis during growth periods inhibits the secondary growth center, resulting in this *squared* configuration. The same appearance of the patella is visible in juvenile rheumatoid arthritis. (26)

Ankle. Radiographic changes at the ankle are frequent. General features include dense swelling, osteoporosis, erosions, irregularity of the articular cortex, and varying degrees of joint space narrowing. (27) The subtalar joint may be fused. Occasionally, premature fusion of the medial tibial epiphysis results in oblique displacement of the tibiotalar joint plane (*tibiotalar*

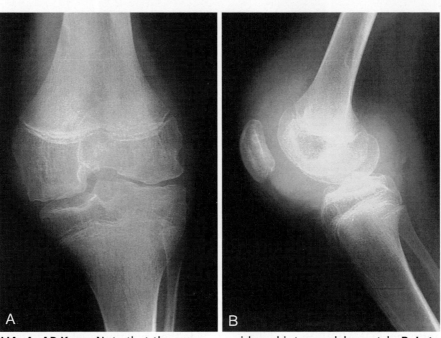

Figure 13-13 **HEMOPHILIA. A. AP Knee.** Note that the overgrowth of the medial condyle has altered the joint orientation. Note the irregular flattened articular contour and widened intercondylar notch. **B. Lateral Knee.** Observe the increase in the periarticular density characterizing hemosiderin deposits from repeated hemarthrosis.

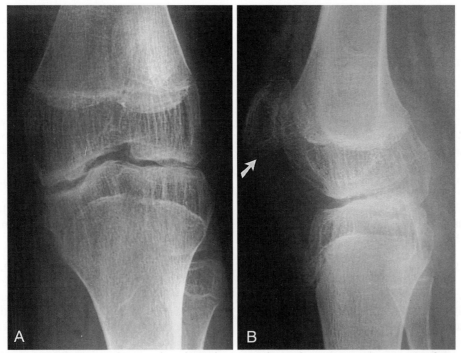

Figure 13-14 **HEMOPHILIA. A. AP Knee.** Observe the altered joint orientation that is caused by overgrowth of the medial condyle, irregular articular surfaces, widened intercondylar notch, and osteoporosis. **B. Lateral Knee.** Note that the inferior pole of the patella is squared and attenuated (*arrow*).

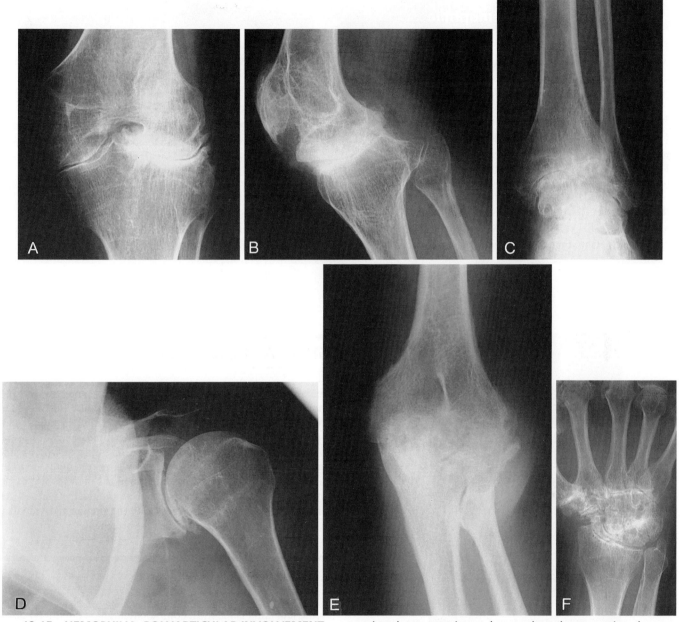

Figure 13-15   **HEMOPHILIA: POLYARTICULAR INVOLVEMENT.**
A and B. Knee. C. Ankle. D. Shoulder. E. Elbow. F. Wrist.
Note that the characteristic features of hemophilic arthropathy are visible in multiple joints in severe, long-standing
cases. Observe the destruction of the articular surfaces,
regional osteopenia, and secondary degenerative changes
(subchondral sclerosis and cyst formation often are congruent with the patient's age). (Courtesy of Jeffry G. Brist, DC,
Minneapolis, Minnesota.)

slant deformity). (Figs. 13-15*C* and 13-16) This deformity is not
specific for hemophilia; it is found in other disorders, including juvenile rheumatoid arthritis, epiphyseal dysplasias, and
neurofibromatosis.

Elbow.   Abnormalities consist of dense effusions with displaced
fat-pads, osteoporosis, and articular erosions. (Fig. 13-15*E*) Enlargement of the radial head may be prominent. Widening of the
radial and ulnar notches, best visualized on the anteroposterior
(AP) view, is a frequent finding.

Other Sites.   No articulation is exempt, and abnormalities can be
found in almost any location. (Fig. 13-15, *A–F*) The hip, shoulder,
hands, and feet can all demonstrate features of hemophilic arthropathy. In the spine, no specific abnormalities are evident, except for
osteoporosis.

CAPSULE SUMMARY   Hemophilia

General Considerations

- A group of disorders characterized by deficiencies of various clotting factors, which predispose the patient to bleeding, especially within joints and, occasionally, within bone.

Clinical Features

- Usually in male patients, with bleeding initiated spontaneously or by minor injury.
- Hemorrhage occurs within joints, especially knee, ankle, elbow.

Pathologic Features

- Most commonly, a lack of factor VIII (classic hemophilia A) or factor IX (Christmas disease, hemophilia B).

- Repeated hemarthrosis precipitates synovial proliferation (pannus), fibrosis, bone erosion, osteoporosis, growth disturbances, late cartilage degeneration.
- Intraosseous hemorrhage may precipitate bone destruction.

Radiologic Features

- Generally produces dense effusions, osteoporosis, erosions, subchondral cysts, growth abnormalities, joint destruction.
- *Joints most commonly affected:* knee, ankle, and elbow; will exhibit distinctive signs.
  Knee: shows enlarged epiphyses, widened intercondylar notch, and squared inferior patella.
  Ankle: may show tibiotalar slant deformity.
- Pseudo-tumors are destructive intraosseous hemorrhages and most commonly occur in the femur and pelvis.

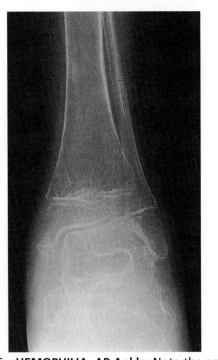

Figure 13-16   HEMOPHILIA. AP Ankle. Note the prominent osteoporosis and alteration of the ankle mortise joint plane (*tibio-talar slant deformity*).

MYELOPROLIFERATIVE DISEASES

This section discusses those entities characterized by the proliferation of particular marrow components. Disorders such as leukemia, lymphoma, polycythemia, myelofibrosis, and mastocytosis fall into this category of bone disease. In this section only leukemia and myelofibrosis will be discussed.

GENERAL CONSIDERATIONS

Leukemia is a malignant disease of the bone marrow and blood characterized by proliferating white blood cells. Various groups are recognized based on age, mode of onset, course, and major cell types. Essentially, those that occur with a rapid onset are classified as being acute and are more common in children, whereas those that begin more insidiously and follow a more lengthy course are called chronic. Histologically, three major cell types are evident: myeloid, lymphatic, and monocytic. Radiologically, various skeletal changes will be evident, especially in younger individuals and in those with more severe disease involvement.

CHILDHOOD LEUKEMIA

Acute leukemia is the most common malignant childhood disease. (1) Together, with the lymphomas, their incidence accounts for approximately 40% of the malignant childhood diseases. (2) The peak incidence is between 2 and 5 years of age. The most common form is the acute lymphocytic type, which is usually fatal within 1 year. Clinically, generalized joint pain, weakness, lethargy, pallor, and loss of appetite are the major symptoms. (3) An elevated erythrocyte sedimentation rate (ESR), lymphadenopathy, splenomegaly, pallor, and general malaise are usually evident on presentation. The definitive diagnosis is made by bone marrow evaluation; however, careful inspection of a peripheral blood smear may reveal excessive or very low white blood cell counts and the presence of immature cell forms.

Radiologic Features

Radiographic osseous changes occur in 50–70% of children with leukemia. (4) The most conspicuous radiologic features are best visualized in the long bones and consist of a generalized osteo-

Table 13-8 | Radiologic Features of Childhood Leukemia

Peak ages 2–5 years
50–70% of cases show abnormalities
Flat and long bones
  Common
    Diffuse osteoporosis
    Radiolucent submetaphyseal bands
    Bone destruction
    Periosteal reaction
  Uncommon
    Growth arrest lines
    Osteosclerosis
    Soft tissue mass (chloroma)
Spine
  Osteoporosis
  Compression fractures
  Radiolucent subendplate bands
Joints
  Juxta-articular osteoporosis
  Effusion
  Soft tissue swelling

porosis, radiolucent submetaphyseal bands, lytic destruction, and periosteal response. (Fig. 13-17; Table 13-8) These changes are identical to those encountered in metastatic neuroblastoma.

Generalized Osteoporosis. In children almost all bones will show a generalized decrease in bone mass owing to the widespread presence of the abnormally proliferating red marrow. Leukemic infiltrates into the marrow cavity precipitate trabecular resorption, seen radiographically as decreased bone density, widened medullary space, and thinning of the cortex.

Radiolucent Submetaphyseal Bands. A submetaphyseal band appears as a linear radiolucent region in the metaphysis beneath and parallel to the opaque zone of provisional calcification at the growth plate. (Fig. 13-18) The best locations to observe these bands are at the distal femur, proximal tibia, proximal humerus, and distal radius. Notably, these occur in a bilateral, symmetric fashion simultaneously and often are the first recognized abnormalities. They represent formation of smaller trabeculae and are also present in neuroblastoma, scurvy, syphilis, and severe systemic diseases. (5) Residual transverse opaque growth arrest lines

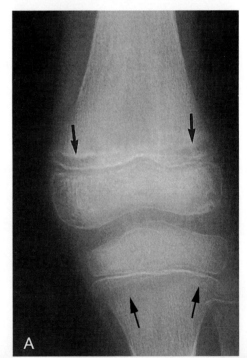
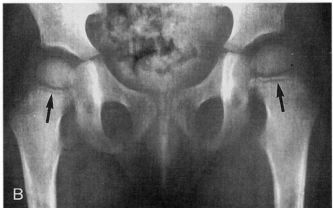

Figure 13-18 **LEUKEMIA: RADIOLUCENT SUBMETAPHYSEAL BANDS. A. AP Knee. B. AP Hips.** Note that submetaphyseal bands (*arrows*) are often the first radiologic signs of childhood leukemia.

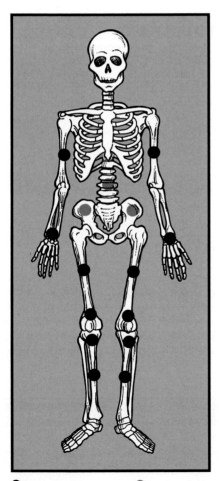

● More common   ● Less common

Figure 13-17 **SKELETAL DISTRIBUTION OF LEUKEMIA.**

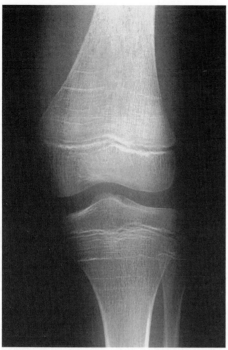

Figure 13-19 LEUKEMIA: GROWTH ARREST LINES. AP Knee. Note the multiple transverse linear opacities within the femur and tibia, which reflect the cyclic repression of bone growth in this child with leukemia.

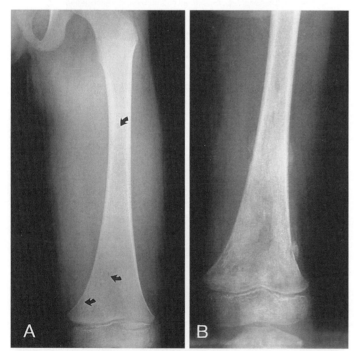

Figure 13-20 LEUKEMIA: BONE DESTRUCTION. A. Early. Observe the discrete metaphyseal and diaphyseal lesions (*arrows*). **B. Later.** Note the more confluent, moth-eaten destruction, with periostitis, mimicking osteomyelitis.

also occur, reflecting cyclic inhibition of enchondral bone growth. (6) (Fig. 13-19)

Bone Destruction. Early in the disease, the pattern of osteolytic destruction consists of small, individual, well-defined medullary lesions that may produce endosteal destruction. (Fig. 13-20) These lytic foci begin in the metaphysis but later involve the diaphysis. Eventually, they coalesce, producing a moth-eaten, mottled effect on bone density. Cortical destruction may accompany these medullary changes. Occasionally, before any osseous or clinical features manifest, a soft tissue mass of leukemic infiltrates, which appears green on gross pathologic examination (*chloroma*), can appear. (7) Late in the disease, sclerosis of the lytic lesions may occur.

Periosteal Response. When present, a periosteal response is seen as a distinctive single or multilayered laminated pattern involving long bone metaphyses and diaphyses. (Fig. 13-20B) Rarely, a spiculated pattern may occur. The presence of a periosteal reaction indicates subperiosteal extension of leukemic cells from the medullary cavity via the Haversian canals.

Other Features. Additional less-common findings include sutural diastasis, articular hemorrhages, effusions, and secondary complications from steroids and other chemotherapeutic regimes. In the spine, osteoporosis, radiolucent sub-endplate bands, and compression fractures are the major findings. (8) MRI has been useful in assessing marrow response to treatment and in detecting relapse by demonstrating altered fat to water ratios; higher fat fractions indicate a good response or remission. (9)

ADULT LEUKEMIA

Adult leukemia most commonly is chronic and is either of the myeloid or the lymphatic variety. Chronic lymphatic leukemia exhibits the most frequent osseous abnormalities. Acute adult leukemia in the majority of patients will not show skeletal lesions because death usually occurs before they develop. Clinically, there is generalized weakness, fatigue, loss of weight, splenomegaly, lymphadenopathy, anemia, and a characteristic blood picture. Currently 75–80% of patients will benefit and enter remission with chemotherapeutic intervention. (1) Unfortunately, up to 50% will relapse. (1)

Radiologic Features

Radiographic osseous changes occur in < 20% of adult leukemia patients owing to the predominance of fatty rather than red marrow in the adult skeleton. As in the childhood forms, the major features include diffuse osteoporosis, radiolucent submetaphyseal bands, lytic destruction, and periosteal response. (Table 13-9) In the spine the diffuse osteoporosis is frequently the initial finding. (2) (Fig. 13-21)

Table 13-9	Radiologic Features of Adult Leukemia
< 20% of cases show abnormalities	
Diffuse osteoporosis (especially of the spine)	
Radiolucent submetaphyseal bands	
Bone destruction	
Periosteal reaction	

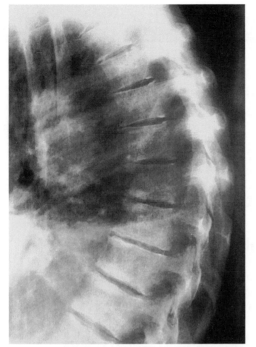

Figure 13-21 **LEUKEMIA. Lateral Thoracic Spine.** Observe the generalized osteoporosis and accentuated trabecular changes in this patient with chronic lymphatic leukemia.

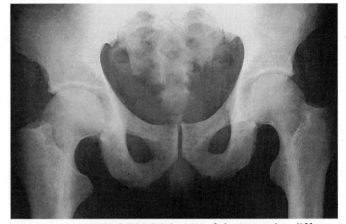

Figure 13-22 **MYELOFIBROSIS. AP Pelvis.** Note the diffuse, mottled sclerosis throughout the pelvis, sacrum, and proximal femora.

MYELOFIBROSIS

General Considerations

Myelofibrosis, also called myeloid metaplasia (1), is a rare hematologic disorder characterized by anemia, leukemic blood changes, and progressive fibrosis of the bone marrow. (2) The cause is unknown; however, it has been shown to occur in association with many autoimmune diseases, including systemic lupus erythematosus. (3) It occurs as a distinct, separate entity but occasionally is found accompanying leukemia or polycythemia vera. Clinically, the disorder affects middle-aged individuals. Fatigue, pallor, gouty symptoms, and generalized bone pain are prominent complaints. On physical examination notable splenomegaly and hepatomegaly are evident. Blood evaluation will demonstrate a normocytic, normochromic anemia, with immature red and white blood cells. A sternal puncture is usually unrewarding; however, an iliac crest biopsy will show the extensive fibrous replacement of the marrow elements. As a sequel to this progressive marrow fibrosis, death is inevitable. (4)

Radiologic Features

The bones commonly involved are those rich in marrow: the pelvis, ribs, thoracic and lumbar spine, skull, femur, and humerus. (5) The major osseous changes in approximately 50% of patients consist of initial osteoporosis later replaced by diffuse sclerosis. (Fig. 13-22; Table 13-10) With progressive sclerosis, the bones initially appear mottled, gradually transforming to become homo-

Table 13-10	Radiologic Features of Myelofibrosis
Middle-aged adults	
Pelvis, ribs, spine, skull, femur, humerus	
Common	
Initial osteoporosis	
Widespread patchy sclerosis	
Diffuse sclerosis	
Massive splenomegaly	
Uncommon	
Periosteal new bone	
Endosteal thickening	
Osteolytic, moth-eaten lesions	
Extramedullary hemopoiesis	

geneously dense. (5,6) At this stage there may be complete lack of definition between the cortex and medullary cavity, suggesting the diagnosis of osteopetrosis, blastic metastasis, Paget's disease, or even fluorosis.

Other osseous features that may be evident include long bone periostitis, endosteal thickening, and osteolytic moth-eaten lesions. In the soft tissues, the most notable feature is massive splenomegaly and, occasionally, posterior mediastinal extramedullary hemopoiesis. (1,7)

Medicolegal Implications

HEMATOLOGIC DISORDERS

- The recognition of hemoglobinopathies and bleeding disorders in predisposed individuals should involve genetic counseling.
- Bleeding disorders such as hemophilia should be treated with extreme care to minimize the risk of soft tissue and intra-articular bleeding.
- Myeloproliferative disorders need to be monitored frequently to assess when sufferers are at greatest risk for secondary infection.

CAPSULE SUMMARY   Myeloproliferative Diseases

General Considerations

- Leukemia, lymphoma, polycythemia, myelofibrosis, mastocytosis.

Leukemia

- Childhood and adult onset, acute and chronic forms.
- *Childhood leukemia:* most common malignancy of children 2–5 years old.
- Osseous diffuse osteoporosis, radiolucent submetaphyseal bands, lytic destruction, periosteal new bone.

- *Adult leukemia:* bone lesions usually in chronic form (20%); same as in the child.

Myelofibrosis

- Fibrous replacement of bone marrow elements.
- Insidious onset in middle age with systemic symptoms; invariably fatal.
- Osseous changes predominantly sclerotic—initially patchy but later diffuse and homogenous.

OSTEONECROSIS

PERSPECTIVES ON OSTEONECROSIS

General Considerations

Osteonecrosis is defined as death of the osseous cellular components and marrow. Many factors have been implicated in precipitating vascular compromise and bone necrosis, including trauma, hemoglobin disorders, alcoholism, and corticosteroid use. There is also a distinct entity with no definite causal agent, which is designated *spontaneous*. Within the skeleton, there is a definite anatomic predisposition for osteonecrosis at the epiphyseal centers, especially in the femoral head, humeral head, and distal femur. (Fig. 13-23) Many synonyms and eponyms are used for these epiphyseal disorders. In addition, the metaphyseal and diaphyseal portions of the long bones are also frequent sites of infarction and necrosis. Despite the many causes and locations of osteonecrosis, common clinical, pathologic, and radiographic features are evident.

Medicolegal Implications

OSTEONECROSIS

- This condition escapes clinical detection and is diagnosed only with bony imaging. Knowledge of the most common sites is essential; these include the femoral and humeral heads, distal femur, and scaphoid.
- High-quality radiographs and adequate views are essential for identifying early and even advanced changes. Equivocal cases may require additional imaging especially CT, MRI, and bone scan.
- Considerable long-term morbidity can follow osteonecrosis, emphasizing the need for early diagnosis and treatment.
- A clear concept of the common causes for osteonecrosis is important for early suspicion of the condition. These include pancreatitis, corticosteroids, alcoholism, and hemoglobin disorders, though the majority of cases are without known cause.

Clinical Features

Clinical manifestations of bone ischemia and infarction are usually non-specific and depend on the cause and location. Epiphyseal osteonecroses become clinically evident, particularly when the articular surface collapses, altering joint function. Before this, symptoms are variable and often absent or relatively minor. This clinical latent period may range from a few weeks up to 1 year in duration. As progressive collapse of the joint surface occurs, greater pain and debility are to be expected. The major physical

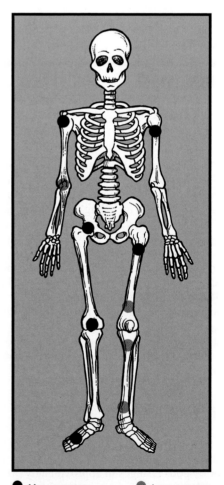

● More common   ● Less common

Figure 13-23   **SKELETAL DISTRIBUTION OF OSTEONECROSIS.** The left side depicts the sites for medullary infarcts.

expressions of epiphyseal necrosis include localized and referred pain, antalgia, reduced and painful ranges of motion, and adjacent muscle atrophy. Metaphyseal and diaphyseal infarcts also exhibit a wide range of presentations, from being completely asymptomatic to acutely symptomatic.

An important integral portion of the clinical examination in osteonecrosis is the isolation of any predisposing condition, of which there are many. (Table 13-11)

Spontaneous. The spontaneous type is the most common category, in which no known cause can be found in association with osteonecrosis. These lesions most frequently involve the femoral capital epiphyses, distal femurs, metatarsal heads, carpal lunate, and the medullary cavity of the metadiaphyseal portions of long bones. Notably, these tend to be isolated abnormalities rather than involving multiple sites, as in other predisposing entities.

Trauma. Fracture, dislocation, and subluxation all may impair circulation to bone, especially the epiphysis. (1) The areas most commonly affected are the intracapsular epiphyses, especially the femoral and humeral heads. Other susceptible sites include the talus and proximal pole of the scaphoid.

Alcoholism. Osteonecrosis is a relatively common phenomenon in chronic alcoholics. The most frequently involved site is the femoral head. Although the mechanism has not been positively identified, fat emboli from a fatty liver and increased marrow fat mass have been implicated. (2,3)

Corticosteroids. The association between corticosteroid therapy, Cushing's disease, and osteonecrosis is well established. The mechanism operative in the induction of osteonecrosis is unknown. However, the release of fat emboli from a fatty liver, microfractures secondary to osteoporosis, and decreased intraosseous blood supply owing to an increased fat cell mass have been implicated (4–6).

Caisson's Disease. Individuals who are removed rapidly from a high pressure environment, such as deep water diving, are predisposed to forming nitrogen bubbles within the blood vessels and precipitating infarction. The bone marrow is histologically predisposed to infarction, owing to its relatively high fat content, because nitrogen exhibits a five times greater affinity for accumulation in fatty tissues. (7) Both epiphyseal and metaphyseal necrosis may occur, often bilateral and extensive. (8)

Gaucher's Disease. A frequent manifestation of Gaucher's disease is osteonecrosis, especially of the femoral heads. (9) This may often be bilateral. The pathogenetic sequence of events leading to osteonecrosis focuses on the mechanical infringement of the marrow sinusoids by the lipid-laden histiocytes. (10)

Hemoglobinopathy. Sickle cell disease, sickle cell trait, and other disorders of hemoglobin structure are potential causes of osteonecrosis. Sickling produces progressive sludging, thrombosis, and eventual infarction, especially in the epiphyses and metadiaphyseal regions. (11) In addition, cortical infarctions in the small bones of the hands and feet in infants are common (*hand–foot syndrome*). (12)

Collagen Diseases. Rheumatoid arthritis and systemic lupus erythematosus have been associated with osteonecrosis. (13,14) Inflammation of the small peripheral blood vessels (vasculitis) promotes the formation of vascular thromboses and tissue infarction. Therapeutic use of corticosteroids in these disorders also increases the likelihood of osteonecrosis.

Radiation. The mechanism operative in radiation-induced osteonecrosis is unknown. Its apparent result is a combination of obliterative endarteritis and cellular death. (15,16) A threshold dose of 3000 rads is necessary to produce osteonecrosis. (15) Doses as low as 300–400 rads can affect epiphyseal bone growth in children. (17)

Pancreatitis. Rarely, pancreatitis may produce fatty emboli that result in infarction of peritoneal and mesenteric fat, brain, kidney, and bone (in frequent). (18–20) These bony infarcts are usually medullary in location. A relationship between pancreatitis and alcoholism may be an additional complicating factor. (21)

Gout. Approximately 30% of patients with gout may demonstrate radiographic evidence of bone infarction. (22) Manifestations include healed metaphyseal–diaphyseal medullary infarcts and osteonecrosis of various epiphyseal centers, especially the femoral heads. The mechanism producing these osseous abnormalities has not been clearly delineated. It may be related to the increased incidence of diabetes mellitus, hypertension, hyperlipidemia, kidney failure, alcohol intake, and small blood vessel disease with basement membrane thickening. (22,23)

Pathologic Features

Epiphyseal Infarction

Pathologic descriptions have largely been derived from examinations of necrotic femoral heads. Intra-articular epiphyses are anatomically predisposed to osteonecrosis because the majority of the blood supply is derived from vessels that penetrate through the joint capsule and lie in a subsynovial position on the external surface of the bone. These vessels are, therefore, susceptible to rupture or compression. Epiphyseal ischemic necrosis is a self-limiting disorder that will eventually heal. The entire process from initial infarction to healed deformity takes a variable time period, from 2 to 8 years. Independent of location, four phases can be considered, even though the transition from one phase to another is both gradual and subtle: *avascular, revascularization, repair,* and *deformity.* (24) (Table 13-12)

Avascular Phase. Obliteration of the epiphyseal blood supply precipitates death of the osteocytes and marrow cells. (25) Subsequently, growth of the involved epiphysis ceases, but the surrounding articular cartilage continues to grow. The involved bone is not weakened and does not show deformity.

Revascularization Phase. Infiltration of new vessels into the necrotic bone results in a twofold response: *deposition* and *resorption.* Deposition occurs at the periphery around the rim of the epiphysis at the chondro-osseous junction as well as centrally.

Table 13-11	Disorders Associated with Osteonecrosis
Unilateral	**Bilateral**
Common	
Spontaneous (idiopathic)	Alcoholism
Surgery	Corticosteroid therapy
Trauma (fracture, dislocation)	Spontaneous (idiopathic)
Uncommon	
Gout	Arteriosclerosis
Hemophilia	Caisson's disease
Infection	Cushing's disease
	Gaucher's disease
	Hemoglobinopathy
	Lupus erythematosus
	Pancreatitis
	Pheochromocytoma
	Rheumatoid arthritis

New bone is deposited directly onto dead bone, thickening the trabeculae and increasing bone density (*creeping substitution*). (25,26) Notably, this new bone formation is easily modeled (biological plasticity) according to stresses on the epiphysis, which accounts for the residual deformity if not appropriately managed.

Table 13-12	Pathologic-Radiologic Correlation in Epiphyseal Ischemic Necrosis
Pathologic Feature	**Radiologic Feature**
Avascular Phase	
Loss of blood supply	Small epiphysis
Bone death	Normal bone density
Cartilage growth	Increased joint space
Low-grade synovitis	Increased joint space
	Capsular swelling
Disuse, hyperemia	Metaphyseal osteoporosis
	Widened growth plate
Revascularization Phase	
Neovascularization	
Periphery	Peripheral sclerotic rim
Center	Homogeneous sclerosis (snowcap)
Subchondral fracture	Crescent sign
Fibrous and granulation tissue (bone resorption)	Clefts and fragmentation
Woven bone	Flattening of surface
Altered biomechanical stress	Widened metaphysis
Repair	
Bone deposition	Reconstitution of epiphysis
Regression of osteoclasis	Disappearance of clefts
Deformity	
Normal bone	Deformed, articular surface

(27) In addition, fracture beneath the articular cortex at the point of maximal stress may occur. Resorption of bone is secondary to phagocytosis, fibrosis, and infiltration by granulation tissue, which produces fragmentation of the involved bone.

Repair and Remodeling Phase. Bone resorption eventually is replaced by bone deposition. As in the necrotic phase, the new bone is easily modeled, and deformity can still be produced, depending on the stresses through the involved bone.

Deformity. After healing, restitution of the epiphysis to its normal configuration occurs in varying degrees. The most important single factor in determining the degree of residual deformity is the compressive forces exerted on the necrotic bone during the revascularization and repair phases. Generally, the closer the deformed shape is to normal, the better the long-term prognosis.

Metaphyseal–Diaphyseal Infarction

The site of metaphyseal–diaphyseal infarction may be cortical or medullary. In the cortex, cellular death is followed by vascular infiltration with absorption and bone deposition. The periosteum is often activated to produce a fine layer of overlying new bone.

Within the medullary cavity a similar sequence of events occurs. The most common location is at the diametaphyseal junction, especially at the distal femur, proximal tibia, and proximal humerus. (28,29) Histologically, a medullary infarct has a central necrotic area confined within a thin, peripheral ischemic zone, which delineates the necrotic bone from the adjacent normal osseous tissue. In the ischemic zone new blood vessels and osteogenic elements may gradually reduce the size of the necrotic area. (27) In those infarcts for which the replacement process ceases the peripheral wall becomes increasingly fibrous and will eventually calcify and ossify. Within the central necrotic area the same fibrosis and calcification process can occur. A rare secondary com-

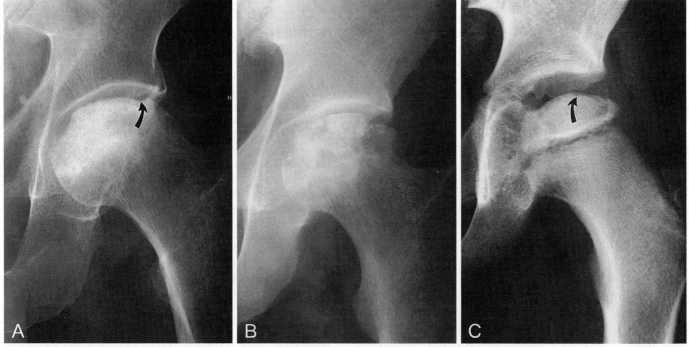

Figure 13-24 **EPIPHYSEAL INFARCTION: GENERAL FEATURES. A. Collapsed Articular Cortex.** Observe the sharp, angular deformity (*arrow*) in the weight-bearing cortex (step defect). Sclerosis of the femoral head is also evident. **B. Epiphyseal Fragmentation.** Note that multiple cystic and linear lucencies produce a mottled, fragmented appearance to the femoral head. This is owing to a combination of fractures, subchondral cysts, and localized repair response. **C. Subchondral Fracture.** Note the thin curvilinear radiolucency (*arrow*) just beneath the weight-bearing articular cortex (crescent sign).

plication is the transformation of the infarct to malignant fibrous histiocytoma (MFH) (30) or fibrosarcoma. (31)

Radiologic Features

Epiphyseal Infarction

Independent of site, epiphyseal ischemic necrosis demonstrates a number of distinctive radiographic signs. (32) (Fig. 13-24; Table 13-13) The time of appearance of these signs depends on the phase

Table 13-13	General Radiologic Features of Epiphyseal Infarction
	Collapse of articular cortex
	Fragmentation
	Mottled trabecular pattern
	Sclerosis
	Subchondral cysts
	Subchondral fracture

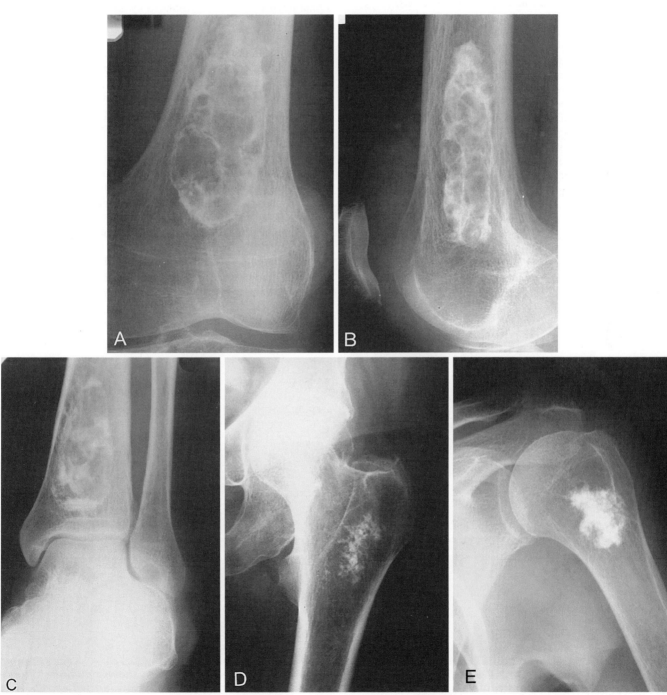

Figure 13-25 **METAPHYSEAL–DIAPHYSEAL INFARCTS. A. and B. Proximal Femur.** Observe the characteristic central location, undulating *serpiginous* contour, and dense calcific margin. **C. Distal Tibia. D. Proximal Femur.** Note that an irregular area of calcification is the only finding. **E. Proximal Humerus.**

of necrosis and repair. Other expressions of ischemic necrosis may occur, depending on the anatomic site affected.

Collapse of the Articular Cortex. Collapse of the articular cortex generally occurs at the region of maximal mechanical stress of the involved cortex and represents a localized impaction fracture of weakened necrotic bone. Displacement of the articular cortex is manifested as a localized loss in the normally smooth articular contour. This may be an angular, step-like defect in a generalized flattened configuration or it may appear as a smooth undulation in the cortex.

Fragmentation. As a manifestation of bone resorption and weakening, radiolucent clefts will be visible traversing the involved bone. The entire epiphysis may even appear almost totally absent because of the large size and number of the clefts.

Mottled Trabecular Pattern. Scrutiny of the trabeculae traversing the ischemic bone demonstrates a thickened, irregular pattern. This is most frequently seen in the revascularization and repair phases and may be an early sign. After resolution of the repair process, the trabecular pattern may be normal in appearance but altered in orientation to accommodate the altered biomechanical stresses through the deformed bone.

Sclerosis. With revascularization new bone is deposited around dead trabeculae, resulting in increased bone density. Three different patterns may be evident. Around the peripheral cortical margin, the density is increased; centrally, a homogenous or patchy increase in density may be evident. In addition, osteoporosis of the adjacent metaphysis may accentuate this increased density.

Subchondral Cysts. Patchy, well-circumscribed rarefactions immediately beneath the articular cortex are frequent. These cystic formations usually localize in the region of greatest articular stress and are identical to those cysts of degenerative joint disease. The most common site at which these cysts are visible is in the femoral capital epiphysis.

Subchondral Fracture. Weakening of the subchondral bone may result in a fracture that separates the articular cortex from the underlying cancellous bone (*rim sign, crescent sign*). This is usually located at the point of maximal articular stress.

Metaphyseal–Diaphyseal Infarction

The bones most frequently involved in a metaphyseal–diaphyseal infarction are the distal femur, proximal tibia, and proximal humerus. Lesions are usually medullary in location. Radiographic features are initially lacking. Isotopic bone scans, however, will demonstrate increased uptake at the site. On MRI, a central high signal intensity zone is surrounded by a serpentine, thin, low signal border. (33) With revascularization, the necrotic bone is first seen as an area of generalized rarefaction, simulating an aggressive neoplasm. Later, as the infarct organizes and develops a peripheral rim of calcification (*mature infarct*), the lesion becomes more clearly delineated. Distinctively, the lesion is longer than it is wide and is usually located toward one end of the involved bone. The peripheral rim is dense, well demarcated, and undulating, creating a *serpiginous* configuration to the lesion. Internally, there may be areas of localized sclerosis. The adjacent cortex is unaffected. (Fig. 13-25) Isotopic bone scans will show increased uptake even in mature infarcts. (Fig. 13-26)

Cortical infarctions are most frequent in the small peripheral tubular bones of the hands and feet, especially in young patients with sickle cell anemia. Within 10 days of the infarction, periostitis and localized foci of rarefaction are present. The cortex may appear split longitudinally. With time, the periostitis increases in thickness and may obliterate the normal diaphyseal constriction, giving the bone a rectangular appearance. Eventually, remodeling will reconstitute the normal bone contour. (Table 13-14)

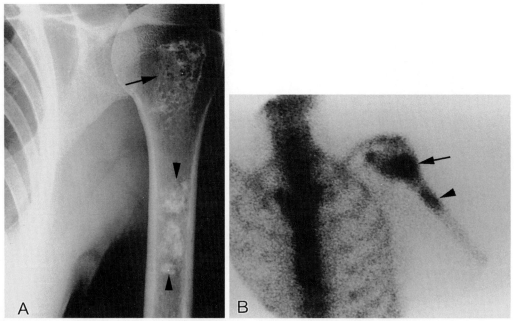

Figure 13-26 METAPHYSEAL–DIAPHYSEAL INFARCTS.
A. Plain Film. Note that two mature infarcts are present, one within the metaphysis (*arrow*), the other within the proximal humeral diaphysis (*arrowheads*). **B. Isotopic Bone Scan.** Note that the delayed technetium scan shows two areas of uptake corresponding to the two sites (*arrow, arrowhead*). (Courtesy of Geoffrey K. Wynn, BAppSc (Chiropractic), Carringbah, Australia.)

Table 13-14	General Radiologic Features of Metaphyseal–Diaphyseal Infarction

Cortical
| Localized rarefaction | Small bones of hands and feet |
| Periosteal response | Split cortex |

Medullary
Central location	Metaphyseal–diaphyseal location
Elongated lesion	Sclerotic, serpiginous contour
Focal internal calcification	Unaffected adjacent cortex

CAPSULE SUMMARY
Perspectives on Osteonecrosis

General Considerations

- Death of bone (osteonecrosis) may occur from unknown or known vaso-occlusive disorders.
- Epiphyses are particularly susceptible to infarction.

Clinical Features

- Depends on location, cause, and extensiveness.
- Epiphyseal necrosis possibly clinically silent until articular collapse occurs.
- Metaphyseal–diaphyseal infarcts often completely asymptomatic.
- *Predisposing factors:* trauma, hemoglobinopathy, Caisson's disease, corticosteroids, collagen disease, radiation, alcoholism, Gaucher's disease, pancreatitis, gout, others.

Pathologic Features

- Epiphyseal infarctions self-limited over 2–8 years, progressing through four phases: avascular, revascularization, repair, deformity.
- Metaphyseal–diaphyseal cortical infarctions characterized by absorption, bone deposition, periostitis.
- Medullary lesions have a central area of necrosis surrounded by a peripheral wall of ischemic and healing tissue.

Radiologic Features

- Epiphyseal osteonecrosis exhibits collapse of articular cortex, fragmentation, sclerosis, mottled trabecular pattern, subchondral cysts, subchondral fracture.
- Cortical infarcts exhibit periostitis and patchy loss of density, usually in small bones of the hands and feet.
- Medullary metaphyseal–diaphyseal infarcts pass through phases: early and late.
- Early lesions can show normal plain films or patchy, moth-eaten destruction.
- Isotopic bone scans will show increased uptake; MRI reveals a central high signal and thin rim of low signal.
- Late (mature) lesions are elongated (longer than they are wide) with a wavy, serpiginous external contour, most commonly found in the distal femur, proximal tibia, and proximal humerus. These can also have increased uptake on isotopic bone scan.

SPONTANEOUS OSTEONECROSIS: FEMORAL HEAD IN ADULTS

General Considerations

Spontaneous (idiopathic) osteonecrosis of the femoral head is defined as bone death of the adult femoral head owing to ischemia of unknown cause. The first detailed description by Freund appeared in 1926. (1) In 1940, Chandler (2) made reference to this disorder as "coronary disease of the hip," which accounts for the eponym Chandler's disease. (3) On occasion this has also been called osteochondritis dissecans of the hip and adult avascular necrosis. Numerous other conditions can precipitate a similar clinical, pathologic, and radiologic presentation in the femoral head. These include alcoholism, trauma, hemoglobin abnormalities, and collagen disease. (Table 13-15)

Clinical Features

There exists a definite (4:1) male predominance. (4) Most individuals present with necrosis between the ages of 30 and 70 years. Bilateral but asymmetric involvement of both femoral heads may be present in as many as 50% of cases. (5) Symptoms initially may be vague and non-specific, consisting of pain in the buttock, groin, thigh, or knee. Usually, there is a gradual increase in intensity of the pain and decreased motion, especially in rotation and abduction. This occurs over several years, precipitating a limping gait and associated muscle atrophy. The initial presentation is commonly misinterpreted as radiating pain from the lumbar spine. (6,7) In the idiopathic form there is a distinct absence of antecedent trauma or known predisposing cause. Treatment is by replacement prosthesis. The use of core decompression has been advocated as a more conservative management alternative in early stages of the disease, although its efficacy is not certain. (8)

Pathologic Features

The pathologic findings vary with the extent of the necrosis; however, in an advanced necrotic femoral head, the alterations are

Table 13-15	Conditions Associated with Osteonecrosis of the Femoral Head	
Unilateral		**Bilateral**
Common		
Spontaneous (idiopathic)		Alcoholism
Surgery		Corticosteroid therapy
Trauma (fracture, dislocation)		Spontaneous (idiopathic)
Uncommon		
Gout		Arteriosclerosis
Hemophilia		Caisson's disease
Infection		Cushing's disease
		Gaucher's disease
		Hemoglobinopathy
		Lupus erythematosus
		Pancreatitis
		Pheochromocytoma
		Rheumatoid arthritis

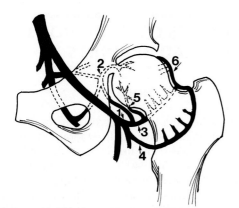

Figure 13-27 VASCULAR SUPPLY: FEMORAL HEAD. There are two sources of blood supply: *profunda femoris* (*1*) and *ligamentum teres* (*2*). From the profunda femoris the circumflex vessels (*3* and *4*) provide the medial and lateral epiphyseal arteries (*5* and *6*). It is probable that the site of precipitating occlusion is at the lateral epiphyseal vessels.

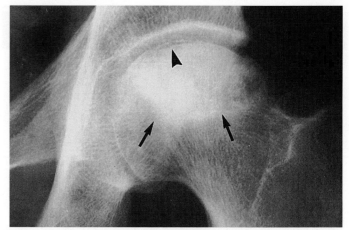

Figure 13-28 AVASCULAR NECROSIS: BITE AND CRESCENT SIGNS. AP Hip. Note the homogeneous increase in density (*snow cap sign*) involving the upper aspect of the head with a curvilinear inferior border (*bite sign*) (*arrows*). Beneath the articular cortex a subchondral fracture (*crescent sign*) can be seen (*arrowhead*).

striking. The necrotic area is distinctively a wedge-shaped region, with the apex directed centrally, involving the anterior superior weight-bearing region. (5) The fovea and inferior femoral head are unaffected. Fibrous tissue intervenes between the necrotic wedge and the sclerotic margin of the adjacent normal bone. Within the necrotic area fissures and cyst-like areas are present. Frequently, the articular cortex and its attached degenerating articular cartilage are separated from the necrotic segment.

Although a number of mechanisms have been proposed, the combination of trauma superimposed on a vulnerable blood supply has been the focus for most investigations. As in the developing femoral head, the adult vascular configuration appears to be susceptible to occlusion specifically involving the lateral epiphyseal and superior retinacular vessels. (9–11) (Fig. 13-27) These structures are responsible for perfusing most of the weight-bearing area of the femoral head, and they freely anastomose with the inferior portion of the head but not with the foveal vessels from the ligamentum teres. This vascular pattern isolates the usual area for necrosis to the anterosuperior aspect of the femoral head.

Radiologic Features

The radiologic manifestations of avascular necrosis of the femoral head are distinctive in location and appearance. (12) (Table 13-16)

Table 13-16	Radiologic Features of Spontaneous Osteonecrosis in the Femoral Head

Anterosuperior location
Cortical collapse (step defect)
Cystic radiolucencies
Degenerative joint disease
Fragmentation
Periosteal bone apposition
Sclerosis (snowcap sign)
Subchondral fracture (crescent, rim sign)
Trabecular alteration
Wedged or semilunar shape (bite sign)

Conventional AP and frog-leg projections must be performed for adequate evaluation. Isotopic bone scans and CT reflect the disease process before changes are visible on the plain film examination. (13) MRI is the most sensitive modality available and can demonstrate changes as early as 1 week after the onset of osteonecrosis, long before plain film abnormalities become detectable. (14)

Location. Characteristic radiographic abnormalities are concentrated to the anterosuperior weight-bearing portions of the head, extending inferiorly in a wedged or semilunar (*bite sign or segmental pattern*) configuration for approximately 1 cm. (15) (Fig. 13-28)

Articular Cortex Collapse. Imperfections in the smooth articular margin of the involved region represent impaction fractures of the underlying necrotic bone, with collapse of the supported cortex. This is a frequent and early radiographic sign and is most commonly visible at the weight-bearing area. Alterations of the cortical contour include a sharp, step-like defect and mild concave undulations. (Fig. 13-29A)

Signs of Degenerative Joint Disease. Altered congruity of the joint surfaces precipitates a loss in joint space, osteophyte formation, increased subchondral bone density, and the formation of subchondral bone cysts. (Fig. 13-29B)

Fragmentation. Within the necrotic zone radiolucent fissures may be visible, isolating variable sizes of bony fragments (Fig. 13-29, B and C). Owing to loss of marrow fat, coronal MRI studies clearly depict the zone of fragmentation as diminished signal on T1- and T2-weighted images. (Fig. 13-30) This follows the typical bite distribution. On MRI at the interface of viable and necrotic bone two opposing lines of high and low signal intensity may be seen (*double line sign*). (16)

Periosteal Bone Apposition. In response to altered biomechanical stress, solid periosteal new bone formation is frequently visible adjacent to the medial surface of the femoral neck (*buttressing*). (Fig. 13-31) This is seen in any disorder that alters the biomechanics of the articulation, including slipped femoral capital epiphysis and degenerative joint disease.

Variable Sclerosis and Radiolucency. A prominent feature is an admixture of varying degrees of sclerosis and cystic radiolucencies, which are limited to the superior weight-bearing portion

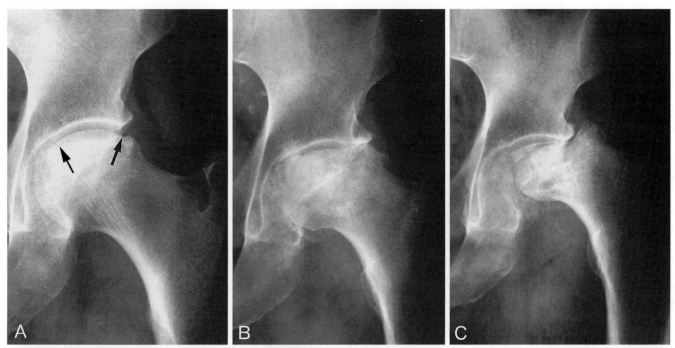

Figure 13-29 **HIP AVASCULAR NECROSIS: PROGRESSIVE ARTICULAR COLLAPSE. A. Initial Film.** Note the two sharp, angular deformities (step defects) at the weight-bearing superior articular cortex (*arrows*). A slight increase in density is visible in the femoral head. **B. 12-Month Follow-Up.** Note that greater collapse is evident. Degenerative changes have also intervened, with loss of joint space and osteophyte formation. **C. 18-Month Follow-Up.** Note that severe collapse and fragmentation have occurred, with considerable lateral displacement of the femur.

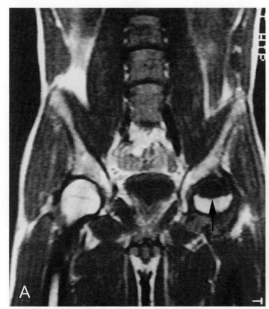

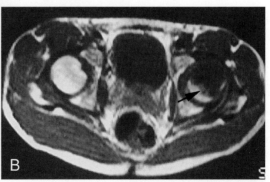

Figure 13-30 **AVASCULAR NECROSIS. A. T1-Weighted MRI, Coronal Pelvis.** Observe the crescent-shaped zone of reduced signal (*arrow*). **B. T1-Weighted MRI Axial Scan, Hips.** Note the clear loss of signal, predominantly on the anterior aspect of the femoral head (*arrow*). Compare these changes with the contralateral normal side. (Courtesy of Steven P. Brownstein, MD, Springfield, New Jersey.)

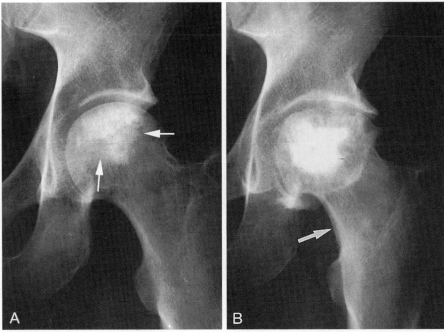

Figure 13-31 **HIP AVASCULAR NECROSIS: PROGRESSIVE COLLAPSE. A. Early Signs.** Note that the only sign is the patchy sclerosis distributed over the femoral head in a semilunar configuration (*bite sign*) (*arrows*). **B. Advanced Signs.** Observe the collapse of the articular surface 6 months later. Note the secondary degenerative joint changes and periosteal buttressing of the medial cortex (*arrow*) from altered mechanical stress.

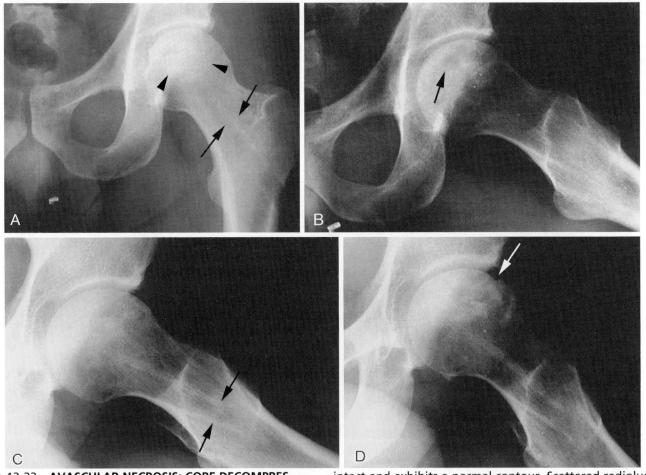

Figure 13-32 **AVASCULAR NECROSIS: CORE DECOMPRESSION. A. AP Left Side, Good Result.** Core decompression was carried out for bilateral idiopathic avascular necrosis with different results. Note the characteristic avascular zone of crescenteric sclerosis (*arrowheads*). Note the tract marking the site of core decompression (*arrows*). **B. Frog Leg, Left Side, Good Result.** Note that the articular cortex remains intact and exhibits a normal contour. Scattered radiolucencies can be identified in the femoral head (*arrow*). It remained unchanged for at least 2 years. **C. Frog Leg, Right Side, Poor Result.** Note the tract for core decompression (*arrows*). **D. Frog Leg, Right Side, Poor Result at 6 Months.** Note the collapse of the articular cortex, as evidenced by the characteristic step defect at the superolateral surface (*arrow*).

of the femoral head. Occasionally, the involved region appears homogeneously sclerotic (*snowcap sign*).

Subchondral Fracture (Crescent or Rim Sign). An arc-like, curvilinear radiolucency directly beneath the superior weight-bearing cortex is a manifestation of a pathologic fracture through the supporting necrotic bone. (Fig. 13-28) This is often best seen in the frog-leg projection or an AP view taken with a traction force of 30–50 lb to the leg approximately 10 sec before and during the exposure, which may allow for nitrogen gas accumulation in the fracture line. (17) MRI can depict a similar finding of a curvilinear zone of high signal intensity within the subchondral bone (MRI crescent sign) before it can be seen on plain film. (16) MRI is also sensitive in demonstrating intraarticular effusion.

Altered Trabecular Pattern. Definition of the traversing trabeculae is frequently disturbed in the necrotic area. Some trabeculae appear thickened and accentuated, whereas others are completely absent, combining to produce a mottled appearance. On CT examination, the normal stellate density of converging trabeculae (*asterisk sign*) becomes partially or totally fragmented. (18)

Although these radiographic features have been described for spontaneous osteonecrosis, other precipitating causes create the same appearance. As a rule, differentiation between the various causes cannot be achieved by radiologic means and must be correlated clinically.

Core Decompression

Core decompression involves removal of a core of bone from the femoral neck into the femoral head. The procedure has the potential to reduce intraosseous hypertension, improve vascular perfusion, and promote healing, although its efficacy is questioned by many. (8) The procedure needs to be performed before subchondral fracture occurs (crescent sign). MRI is the preferred method of assessing the extensiveness and stage of the infarction for appropriate selection for core decompression. (8) Radiographically the radiolucent tract at the decompression site is visible. (Fig. 13-32) (See Chapter 6 for a complete discussion.)

CAPSULE SUMMARY   Spontaneous Osteonecrosis: Femoral Head in Adults

General Considerations

- Osteonecrosis of the femoral head from an unknown cause.
- *Synonym:* Chandler's disease.
- Similar clinical, pathologic, and radiologic features caused by other disorders.

Clinical Features

- Males 4:1, 40–60 years old.
- 50% bilateral.
- Pain, reduced motion, muscle atrophy that is gradually progressive.
- Treated by prosthesis; role of core decompression uncertain.

Pathologic Features

- Necrotic wedge at the anterosuperior aspect of the head, separated by fibrous tissue and sclerotic margin of adjacent normal bone.

- Precipitated by occlusion of lateral epiphyseal and superior retinacular vessels.

Radiologic Features

- AP and frog-leg views required; tomography and bone scan more accurate in early stages.
- *Signs:* location at anterosuperior aspect of the head, curvilinear-semilunar-wedged configuration (bite sign), cortical collapse (step sign), cystic radiolucencies and sclerosis, degenerative joint changes, fragmentation, medial periosteal bone apposition, subchondral fracture (crescent sign), trabecular alterations (asterisk sign).
- Shows increased uptake on bone scan.
- *MRI:* diminished signal on T1-weighted and increased signal on T2-weighted studies.

SPONTANEOUS OSTEONECROSIS: KNEE

General Considerations

Spontaneous osteonecrosis of the knee (SONK) is a disease of unknown origin affecting predominantly the medial condyle of the distal femur in adults. (1) It was first described by Ahlback et al. (1) in 1968. The medial condyle is most frequently affected; infrequently, the lateral condyle is affected, and rarely both simultaneously. (2) The medial tibial condyle is also a rare site for osteonecrosis. (3–5) Osteonecrosis of either the entire patella or its superolateral pole is also rare and has been described following trauma, arthroplasty, and corticosteroids and as an idiopathic phenomenon. (6) The same disorder can be initiated by other known, associated osteonecrotic factors, including steroid therapy, hemoglobinopathies, and transplantation. (7) Acute fracture rarely precipitates the condition. Spontaneous osteonecrosis differs distinctly from adolescent osteochondritis dissecans clinically, pathologically, and radiologically. (8) (Table 13-17)

Clinical Features

Onset is usually after 60 years of age. Females seem to predominate slightly. (8) Characteristically, the acute and sudden onset of pain in the knee cannot be substantiated initially by radiographic examination. No immediate or antecedent trauma is apparently associated with the onset of symptoms. Laboratory examinations are unhelpful. Examination symptoms are localized to the medial aspect of the joint, with sharp tenderness over the medial femoral condyle. A mild effusion may be present. After the initial onset, a gradual increase in the intensity of symptoms occurs, which may

Table 13-17	Differential Features between Spontaneous Osteonecrosis and Osteochondritis Dissecans of the Knee	
Feature	**Spontaneous Osteonecrosis**	**Osteochondritis Dissecans**
Age	40–60 years	< 20
Location	Medial condyle	Medial condyle
	Weight-bearing surface	Non-weight-bearing surface
Cause	Vascular, trauma	Trauma
Plain film		
Flattening	Present	Absent
Collapse	Present	Absent
Sequestration	Present	Present
Loose body	Present	Present
Joint	Degenerated	Normal

become rapidly disabling within a couple of months or remain chronic over 3–5 years.

Prognosis is variable and depends on the stage at detection and the extensiveness of the necrosis. Normal films in symptomatic patients or a small necrotic zone at the time of treatment with restriction of weight bearing may lead to remineralization and resolution with little to no functional limitation. (5,9) Generally, there is progression, with collapse, fragmentation, and loss of joint space, which can rapidly accelerate to produce the appearance of a neuropathic joint. A varus deformity typically develops. When the condylar defect occupies more than 50% of the surface, rapid progression is fairly certain. (10) Total or subtotal arthroplasty is usually indicated in progressive cases.

Pathologic Features

The exact pathogenetic mechanism has not been delineated; however, vascular compromise is certainly focal to the observed pathologic alterations. The role of associated meniscal tears is unclear. (11) Examination of the involved medial femoral condyle reveals necrosis of small fragments of the condyle and collapse of the subchondral bone. Histiocytic bone resorption, granulomatous tissue, and surrounding reactive new bone formation complete the pathologic osseous alterations. (12) The overlying cartilage is discolored and fissured and may even be absent. A detached osteochondral fragment may occur. (8)

Radiologic Features

Initial radiographic examinations after the onset of symptoms are invariably normal, except for some minor age-related, degenerative changes. Before the appearance of plain film changes, isotopic bone scans and MRI evaluations are often characteristic to make the diagnosis. (13,14) Bone scans will demonstrate increased uptake in all phases (flow, blood pool, and delayed) within days after the onset of symptoms. (13) CT scan demonstrates the deformity of the femoral condyle and the necrotic zone to better advantage. The earliest plain film changes can be at 5–6 weeks but generally take months to evolve. (9) In the ensuing weeks and months, progressive changes become visible in the involved femoral condyle. Arthrography commonly shows co-existing tears of the medial meniscus immediately adjacent to the femoral defect. (11)

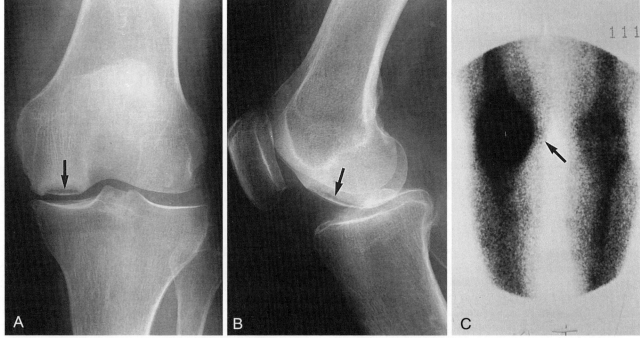

Figure 13-33 SPONTANEOUS OSTEONECROSIS OF THE KNEE: MEDIAL CONDYLE. A. AP Knee. B. Lateral Knee. Note the characteristic step defect at the weight-bearing articular margins of the medial condyle. A distinct linear radiolucency (*crescent sign*) is evident parallel to the involved cortex (*arrows*). The combination of these two findings is diagnostic of this condition. **C. Bone Scan, Knee.** Note the increased uptake in the affected distal femur (*arrow*).

Radiographic manifestations of osteonecrosis include flattening of the articular surface, altered subchondral bone density, osseous collapse, loose bodies, and adjacent articular compartment degenerative changes. (9) (Figs. 13-33 and 13-34; Table 13-18) Attempts to correlate the radiographic appearance with prognosis has led to a staging of the disease process: (5)

- *Stage 1:* Normal plain films, abnormal bone scan or MRI, and symptoms.
- *Stage 2:* Subtle flattening of the femoral condyle.
- *Stage 3:* An area of radiolucency surrounding a sclerotic area in the subchondral bone.
- *Stage 4:* The radiolucency surrounded by a sclerotic halo.
- *Stage 5:* Secondary changes of diminished joint space, sclerosis, osteophytes, and tibial changes.

Altered Articular Contour. The earliest radiographic sign is flattening of the normally convex articular surface. This is most prominent at the weight-bearing surface. As the disease advances, progressive collapse of the subchondral bone may precipitate breaks in the continuity of the articular cortex and more severe depression of the condyle.

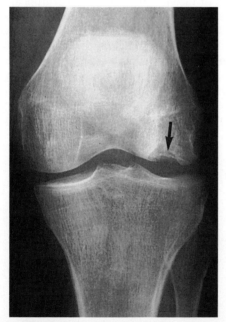

Figure 13-34 **SPONTANEOUS OSTEONECROSIS OF THE KNEE: LATERAL CONDYLE. AP Knee.** Observe the concave defect on the lateral femoral condyle (*arrow*). A reactive halo of sclerosis surrounds the defect.

Table 13-18	Radiologic Features of Spontaneous Osteonecrosis of the Knee

Medial femoral condyle
Weight-bearing surface
Flattened articular contour
Loose bodies
Subchondral sclerosis and lucency
Degenerative joint disease

Altered Subchondral Bone Density. The necrotic zone is identifiable by the isolated sclerotic foci and surrounding fissures, which extend usually < 1 cm into the underlying bone. A linear cleft immediately below and parallel to the involved articular cortex is often visible, representing a subchondral fracture (*crescent sign*). On T1-weighted MRI images there is low signal intensity from the area of necrotic bone owing to the absence of fat, which in half of cases may be bordered at the normal–necrotic bone interface by a linear high signal zone. (14) Early in the disease T2-weighted images may show a slight increase in signal owing to edema, but with progression of the disease, the signal reduces. Isotopic bone scans show localized tracer uptake at the necrotic condylar zone, which may be extensive.

Loose Bodies. Occasionally, intra-articular loose osseous fragments will be visible. These may migrate away from the condyle region and be found anywhere within the joint cavity. Scrutiny of the condyle in the presence of these loose bodies usually reveals the site of origin to be a prominent, excavated concave defect.

Adjacent Articular Changes. As necrosis advances, progressive degenerative changes are frequently observed in approximately one third of cases. (8) These include loss of medial joint space, subchondral bone cysts, sclerosis, and osteophytes. These associated degenerative changes can be rapidly progressive. Calcification within the adjacent menisci, varus deformity, and extensive necrosis may be adverse prognostic indicators, which appear to augment these degenerative changes. (8,15)

CAPSULE SUMMARY
Spontaneous Osteonecrosis: Knee

General Considerations
- Of unknown cause, affecting the medial condyle of the distal femur in adults.
- *Rarer sites:* the lateral femoral condyle, medial tibial condyle, patella.

Clinical Features
- Usually > 60 years of age; sudden onset of knee pain, unassociated with trauma, with gradual deterioration over months.

Pathologic Features
- Osteonecrosis, with resorption, granulomatous tissue, and reactive new bone; the overlying cartilage, degenerated.

Radiologic Features
- Normal plain films at the onset of symptoms; bone scan, and MRI abnormal days after onset.
- *Later progressive changes:* articular cortex flattening and collapse, altered subchondral bone density, loose bodies, articular degeneration.

CAISSON'S DISEASE

General Considerations

Caisson's disease is caused by an accumulation of nitrogen gas bubbles in blood vessels, which act as emboli and precipitate tissue infarction. This phenomenon is most frequently encountered in individuals, such as deep sea divers, who are removed too rapidly from a high pressure environment. Less commonly, rapid removal from low pressure environments, such as in high-altitude flying, may produce a similar condition. The entire syndrome has been called *decompression sickness.* Descriptive terms define the physical manifestations of the acute presentation, such as the *chokes* (respiratory system), the *staggers* (nervous system), and the *bends* (musculoskeletal system).

Specific terms applied to the associated bone and joint abnormalities include dysbaric osteonecrosis, pressure-induced osteoarthropathy, and barotraumatic osteoarthropathy. The bone changes were first described by Bornstein and Plate and, independently, by Bassoe in 1911. (1)

Clinical Features

Potential hazards of sudden atmospheric pressure changes have been well defined; however, increasing recreational, scientific, commercial, and military activities into altered pressure environments have focused renewed, justified attention on the disease. (2–4) As such, the most important clinical feature is to link the presence of signs and symptoms to previous barotrauma. In the acute phase, manifestations include altered neurological status; breathing difficulties; and severe muscle, joint, and bone pain. Later, changes are predominantly related to altered joint function from nitrogen bubble–induced epiphyseal necrosis. The incidence of this ischemic-induced bone disability may be as high as 60% but is most likely to be found in 10–20% of these predisposed individuals. (5) Physical findings of osteonecrosis include progressive joint pain, stiffness, and reduced motion, especially in the hips and shoulders. This frequently occurs bilaterally. Notably, a patient may have osteonecrosis and never have experienced an acute episode of decompression sickness. (2)

Pathologic Features

The histopathologic characteristics of the osseous lesions are consistent with avascular necrosis. (6) The pathogenetic mechanism appears to be the formation of bloodborne nitrogen emboli, which impair tissue perfusion. (3) The origin of these nitrogen bubbles is related to Boyle's law concerning partial pressures of gases with altered atmospheric conditions. Under increased environmental pressure, such as in underwater diving, an individual's tissues become saturated with atmospheric gases. Fatty tissues, such as the bone marrow, spinal cord, and fat storage areas, are capable of absorbing five times more nitrogen than other tissue or blood plasma. (7) Decompression precipitates the dissolved tissue gases, which move back into the bloodstream for expulsion by the pulmonary capillary system. If the decrease in pressure occurs too quickly, nitrogen, in particular, will come out of its dissolved state to form bubbles in the fat-rich tissues, which can then embolize into small capillaries.

Predisposing factors to Caisson's disease include obesity, repeated dysbaric episodes, exposure to greater pressures, and length of time spent in the altered pressure environment. (2,8) In divers the critical depth appears to be > 30 m, below which there is a great increase in observable bone lesions. (1,8)

Localization of nitrogen emboli within bone appears at two locations: fatty marrow and metaphyseal–epiphyseal regions.

Osteonecrosis within the fatty marrow is evidenced by medullary diaphyseal–metaphyseal infarction. At the epiphysis region small end arteries are embolized, precipitating infarction, especially in the femoral and humeral heads. (7)

Radiologic Features

Lesions of dysbaric osteonecrosis may occur unilaterally, bilaterally, or in any combination of sites. A radiologic skeletal survey of an individual suspected of harboring lesions of dysbaric necrosis should include AP views of the heads and proximal shafts of both humeri and femora, as well as AP and lateral views of both knees to include the distal two thirds of the femur and upper one third of the tibia. (9) An important aspect of the radiologic evaluation is the recognition of the long latent period, up to a number of years, before changes may become apparent. (6,7) Lesions can still develop in previously normal areas, with worsening of previously known lesions even after 10 years, despite removal from occupational exposure to high pressure environments. (10)

Radiologically, two types of lesions are apparent based on location: epiphyseal and metaphyseal–diaphyseal. (10)

Epiphyseal Lesions. The epiphyses most commonly involved are the heads of the humerus and femur. The major expressions of epiphyseal involvement are those of avascular necrosis— patchy areas of lucency and sclerosis, curvilinear subchondral fracture (*crescent sign*), and collapse of the articular surface. (Fig. 13-35) These alterations are identical to avascular necrosis precipitated by other causes, including steroid use, hemoglobin disorders, trauma, and the spontaneous variety. In more chronic cases, secondary degenerative joint changes, such as osteophytes and loss of joint space, may be evident.

Metaphyseal–Diaphyseal Lesions. The most apparent change is invariably visible in the medullary cavity of the proximal hu-

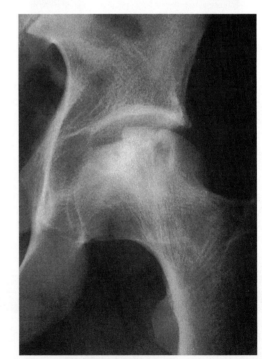

Figure 13-35 CAISSON'S DISEASE. Femoral Head: AP Hip. Note the signs of avascular necrosis: articular collapse (*step defect*), cystic lucencies, and sclerosis. This appearance is identical to the idiopathic form of avascular necrosis.

merus, distal femur, or proximal tibia. The radiologic features are those of a healed, mature, central medullary infarct that is elongated and bordered by a distinctive, dense, undulating sclerotic margin. Internally, an admixture of sclerosis and lucency may be apparent. Additional equivocal lesions that mimic bone islands have been described.

The radiologic diagnosis of Caisson's disease is more likely when multiple medullary lesions are apparent, especially in combination with humeral or femoral head necrosis.

CAPSULE SUMMARY Caisson's Disease

General Considerations

- Characterized by tissue necrosis from nitrogen emboli following too rapid removal from a hyperbaric environment.
- Osseous tissue predisposed to involvement.

Clinical Features

- History of occupational or recreational exposure to altered pressure environments.
- *Acute phase:* neurological, respiratory, and musculoskeletal distress.
- Later changes in bone cause joint pain, especially in the shoulders and hips; seen in 10–20% of patients.

Pathologic Features

- High pressures causing tissue supersaturation with gases, especially nitrogen.
- Rapid removal of high pressure, precipitating formation of bubbles, which act as emboli.
- Fatty tissues with five times the affinity for nitrogen, accounting for involvement of bone.

Radiologic Features

- Epiphyseal lesions most commonly visible in humeral and femoral heads in the form avascular necrosis; lucency, sclerosis, collapse, fragmentation, secondary degenerative joint disease.
- Metaphyseal–diaphyseal lesions characterized by healed mature medullary infarcts; central, elongated, with undulating sclerotic borders; most frequent in proximal humerus, distal femur, proximal tibia.

RADIATION CHANGES IN BONE

General Considerations

The harmful side effects of radiation are well recognized. The first recorded radiation-induced injury was in 1895, just weeks after Roentgen's initial discovery. (1) Known complications to radiation include skin erythema, ulceration, fibrosis, myelopathy, and neoplasia. As a therapeutic agent, radiation in various forms has been applied in the treatment of inflammatory arthritis, skin diseases, and especially in the containment and treatment of neoplasms.

Effects on cartilage and bone inevitably exhibit characteristic radiographic alterations owing to radiation. These changes usually appear after many months or years. Terms relating to radiation-induced osseous changes include radiation osteitis, radiation necrosis, and osteoradionecrosis.

Mechanisms of Skeletal Involvement

Radiation may reach bone by four methods: oral ingestion, intravascular injection, surgical implantation, and external beam application.

Oral Ingestion. The radioactive substances most commonly swallowed and subsequently deposited in bone are radium and strontium. Both appear to act like calcium and subsequently become concentrated within the bone substance. Between 1920 and 1940, radium ingestion accelerated in watchmakers as the demand for luminescent watch faces grew (the radium providing α-particles to bombard the zinc sulfide and produce the illumination). (2) Workers would often use their mouths to moisten the brush and to bring it to a point to more accurately apply the luminescent paint. The paint's deleterious skeletal effects became apparent with the development of sarcomas and fractures. (3,4)

Intravascular Injection. A number of radioactive substances, including radium and thorium, have been used as treatment and as vascular contrast agents. (3) Thorium (thorotrast), in particular, was used between 1930 and the early 1950s as the medium of choice for angiography and, occasionally, myelography. (5–8) It is selectively phagocytosed by the reticuloendothelial (RE) system, especially the liver (70%) and spleen (20%), with only a small amount going to bone (2%). (9) (Fig. 13-36) Complications include anemia, osteomalacia, and bone sarcoma. (10)

Surgical Implantation. The direct implantation of radioactive substances in close proximity to a site of malignancy is occasionally used. (11) (Fig. 13-37)

External Beam Radiation. The most common source of skeletal radiation is from external beam application. Various radiotherapy units use the generation of large amounts of high-energy x-rays. The degree of bone damage is related to dosage, the amount of bone included in the radiation field, the thickness of overlying tissue, and the age of the patient. Radiotherapy of malignant bone metastases typically produces sclerotic conversion of the tumor matrix. (Fig. 13-38)

Pathologic Features

The mechanisms by which bone and cartilage are affected by irradiation are still incompletely known. (12) A combination of retarded cellular division, cell death, cellular transformation, and vascular obliteration is observed. (13) Following irradiation, there is inflammatory reaction of the marrow, with necrosis of the blood-forming elements. Bone cells are all radiosensitive and probably die early. Obliterative endarteritis and periosteal damage further compromise bone perfusion. Superimposed fractures and infections are common. Regeneration is derived from adjacent normal bone by *creeping substitution*— that is, removal of dead bone and deposition of new bone on unresorbed trabeculae. (12)

A single dose of 300–400 rads (Gy) directly applied to the growth plate may temporarily arrest longitudinal growth (12); a dose of 1800–2600 Gy will permanently arrest this growth. Any

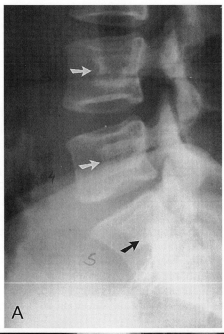

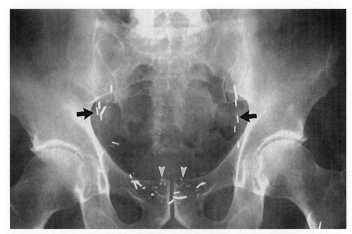

Figure 13-37 **RADIOACTIVE GOLD IMPLANTATION. AP Pelvis.** Observe the multiple vascular clips (*arrows*) from extensive pelvic surgery and the small, round metallic densities (*arrowheads*) of the implants (Whitmore procedure, for carcinoma of the prostate). (Courtesy of William E. Litterer, DC, DACBR, Fellow, ACCR, Elizabeth, New Jersey.)

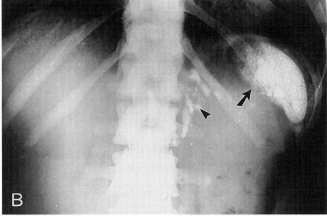

Figure 13-36 **THOROTRAST: SPINE AND SPLEEN. A. Lateral Lumbar Spine.** Note the internal appearance of a small *ghost vertebra* (*arrows*) owing to previous thorotrast injection. Thorotrast, a contrast medium used for diagnostic examinations of viscera, proved toxic and is no longer in use. **B. Spleen.** Note that the spleen (*arrow*) and adjacent lymph nodes (*arrowhead*) are opacified owing to the concentration of thorotrast in those tissues.

skeletal structure in a child that received more than 2000 Gy will show an altered growth pattern (14–16); and within adult bone, cellular death has a 3000–Gy threshold, with definite bone cell death at 5000 Gy. (17,18)

Pathologic changes of irradiated bone include areas of necrosis, marrow fibrosis, and thickened trabecular patterns.

Radiologic Features

General Characteristics

Following the administration of radiation, a radiographic latent period exists before changes will become evident. This is usually at least 3 months and, more commonly, > 6–12 months, depending on the site and type of radiation administered. (12) The general radiologic features consist of altered growth patterns, moth-eaten destruction, patchy sclerosis, trabecular thickening, and periostitis. (Table 13-19) The first phase is osteopenia (postradiation atrophy), followed by trabecular thickening. Irregular areas of lysis and sclerosis are often visible within the cortex. After 2–3 years, small foci of osteolysis gradually enlarge, sometimes reaching 1–2 cm in size, simulating neoplasia.

Complications include epiphyseal avascular necrosis, infection, fracture, and neoplastic change. (12,19) The incidence of radiation-induced sarcoma is < 1–2%. (12) The most common complicating sarcomas of bone are osteosarcoma and, less commonly, fibrosarcoma and that of soft tissue is malignant fibrous histiocytoma (MFH). Complicating sarcoma arises most frequently in the pelvis and shoulder girdle. The most frequent complicating benign tumor is osteochondroma, which occurs in 12–15% of irradiated persons, is usually asymptomatic, is more common in developing long bones, and is uncommon in the spine. (12,20) Radiation-induced spinal osteochondroma usually arises from the posterior elements, especially the spinous process, and is most common in the lumbar spine. (20)

Target Sites of Involvement

Spine. Abdominal neoplasms treated with radiotherapy frequently result in localized vertebral hypoplasia and scoliosis. (15–18,21) This is especially true if the irradiated field is off center and applied to a growing individual. The effect is on the growth of the body, pedicles, and lamina, in combination with fibrosis of the overlying soft tissues.

Radiographic features of radiation applied to a developing spine and pelvis include a mild concave scoliosis with vertebral body hypoplasia, lateral wedging, and endplate irregularity. (15) Occasionally, a *bone within a bone* may be apparent. (22) If the iliac crest epiphysis has been included in the irradiated field, the entire ilium will appear hypoplastic. (Fig. 13-39) The abdominal neoplasms that most commonly may be irradiated include neuroblastoma, Wilms' tumor, and lymphoma. MRI within 1 year of ir-

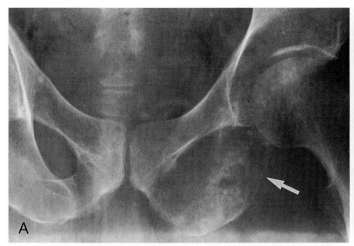
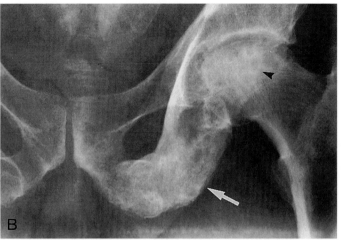

Figure 13-38   **RADIATION THERAPY: PROSTATE METASTASIS. A. Metastatic Lesion.** Note the moth-eaten, destructive lesion throughout the entire ischium (*arrow*). **B. Postradiotherapy.** Note that 1 year after irradiation there has been reconstitu- tion of the bone matrix, which has become sclerotic (*arrow*). Also observe the radiation-induced osteonecrosis of the ad- jacent femoral head (*arrowhead*). (Courtesy of Richard W. Hooke, DC, Dalby, Queensland, Australia.)

radiation will show increased signal owing to marrow replacement with fat. (23) Evidence of radionecrosis includes patchy lucency and sclerosis of the vertebral bodies, pathologic fractures, and the presence of an intravertebral collection of gas (intravertebral vacuum cleft sign). (12,24,25)

Pelvis. A radiologic feature of pelvic radionecrosis is a region of moth-eaten destruction that contains patchy, dense sclerotic foci and trabecular thickening. (Fig. 13-40) Possible additional features include widened sacroiliac joints, femoral head osteo- necrosis, pathologic fractures, and calcified soft tissue masses. Insufficiency fractures of the sacrum may occur in as many as 30% of irradiated female pelves. (12,26) Up to 2% of irradi- ated pelves develop pathologic fractures of the proximal femur. (27) Involvement of the acetabulum can precipitate protrusio acetabuli. (27)

The similarity to Paget's disease is striking, but usually the dis- ease can be excluded because the radionecrosis is more localized, not expanded, and there is normal cortical thickness and normal alkaline phosphatase levels. The most difficult differentiation is that from osseous metastasis, which is excluded on the basis of distant site involvement beyond the irradiated field and elevated alkaline phosphatase levels. (28) The pelvic neoplasms most com- monly irradiated include carcinoma of the cervix, prostate, and urinary bladder.

Mandible. Radiation necrosis of the mandible is a common sequela in the treatment of intraoral neoplasms. It occurs in ap- proximately 30% of patients. (29) Despite this high complication rate, radiotherapy is pivotal in the management of these cancers and greatly alters the long-term prognosis in a positive manner. The mandible is involved more commonly than the maxilla. (30)

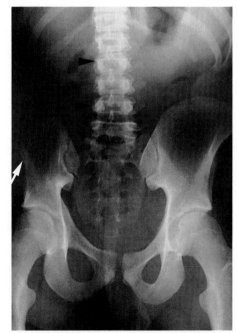

Figure 13-39   **POSTRADIATION PELVIC HYPOPLASIA AND SCOLIOSIS.** Observe the hypoplasia of the ilium (*arrow*) and concave lumbar scoliosis (*arrowheads*). The vertebral bodies are flat and diminished in height. *COMMENT:* The patient received radiotherapy for a left-sided Wilms' tumor. (Courtesy of Anthony M. Richards, BAppSc (Chiro), Dee Why, Australia.)

Table 13-19	Radiologic Features of Radiation Osteonecrosis

Common
    Altered growth patterns
    Bone destruction (cortical, medullary)
    Patchy sclerosis
    Periostitis
    Thickened trabeculae
Uncommon
    Bone resorption
    Epiphyseal avascular necrosis
    Widened sacroiliac joints
    Soft tissue calcification
    Neoplasm (osteosarcoma, fibrosarcoma, osteochondroma)

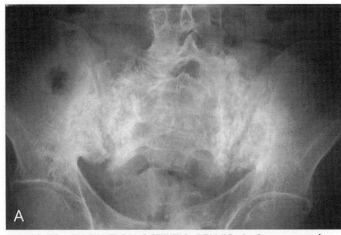
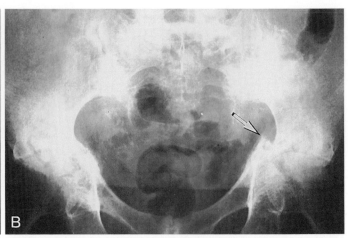

Figure 13-40 RADIATION OSTEITIS: PELVIS. A. Sacrum and Adjacent Pelvis. Note the patchy lucency and sclerosis of the sacrum and adjacent ilium. The sacroiliac joints are slightly widened. This 62-year-old female received irradiation for carcinoma of the cervix. **B. Protrusio Acetabuli.** Observe the increased density in the acetabular regions bilaterally, protrusio acetabuli, and pathologic acetabular fracture (*arrow*). This 50-year-old female received irradiation for carcinoma of the cervix.

Radiologic features consist of moth-eaten destruction, cortical destruction, and possible fracture. Postradiation infection is common owing to decreased salivary gland function and decreased vascularity. The teeth in the area of exposure are removed before the application of radiotherapy.

Shoulder Girdle. The upper ribs, clavicle, scapula, and proximal humerus are frequently irradiated in radiotherapy for carcinoma of the breast. Less than 5% of these patients who have radiotherapy develop radiation-induced changes in the shoulder girdle. (31) Radiologic abnormalities include a moth-eaten type of osteoporosis, patchy reactive sclerosis, bone resorption, and fractures that are painless and slow to heal. (32–34) Occasionally, avascular necrosis of the humeral head may be seen. (Fig. 13-41)

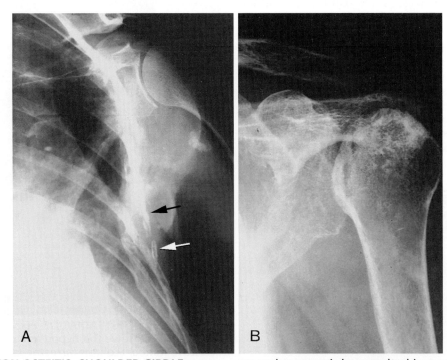

Figure 13-41 RADIATION OSTEITIS: SHOULDER GIRDLE. A. Ribs. Note the osteolysis, fragmentation, and healed rib fractures (*arrows*). The patient had received radiotherapy for breast carcinoma. **B. Humeral Head.** Note that complicating avascular necrosis has resulted in a patchy, sclerotic, and lucent density of the humeral head. Some deformity of the articular surface is evident owing to collapse.

CAPSULE SUMMARY   Radiation Changes in Bone

General Considerations
- Many complications, including soft tissue and bony abnormalities.
- Delayed appearance of bone-related changes.
- *Synonyms:* radiation osteitis, osteoradionecrosis.

Mechanisms of Involvement
- *Oral ingestion:* radium.
- *Intravascular injection:* radium and thorium (thorotrast); retained in RE system, and predisposing patient to sarcoma.
- Surgical implantation.
- *External radiation (radiotherapy):* most common source.

Pathologic Features
- *Altered cell metabolism:* retarded cell division, cell death, and cellular transformation; cell death threshold at 3000 Gy; certain bone cell death at 5000 Gy.

- Vascular obliteration, marrow replacement with fat; heals by creeping substitution.

Radiologic Features
- *General features:* latent period of at least 3 months; altered growth, destruction, sclerosis, periostitis.
- *Complications:* osteonecrosis, infection, fracture, neoplasia.
- *Most common neoplasms:* osteosarcoma, fibrosarcoma, osteochondroma.
- *Spine:* vertebral hypoplasia, arrest lines, endplate irregularities, scoliosis.
- *Pelvis:* hypoplasia, destruction, patchy sclerosis, thickened trabeculae, wide sacroiliac joints.
- *Mandible:* destruction, fracture.
- *Shoulder girdle:* destruction, sclerosis, resorption, fractures.

EPIPHYSEAL DISORDERS

Few entities have had as diverse a terminology as epiphyseal necrosis. Multiple synonyms, such as osteochondritis, osteochondrosis, epiphysitis, aseptic necrosis, and avascular necrosis, represent attempts to classify the disorder according to anatomic site, cause, and pathologic alteration. Further confusion has arisen with the continued use of the many eponyms, reflecting name(s) of the individual(s) who described the disorder in a given epiphysis. (Fig. 13-42; Table 13-20) Careful analysis of each of these epiphyseal abnormalities reveals three major groups: osteonecrosis (primary or secondary), trauma, and confusing growth variations.

Primary and Secondary Osteonecrosis. Primary osteonecrosis is defined as bone death occurring in an epiphysis from an unknown cause. Secondary osteonecrosis is the same condition that occurs from a known cause, such as fracture, sickle cell anemia, corticosteroids, or Gaucher's disease. The most common sites are the femoral heads, humeral heads, distal femurs, metatarsal heads, and carpal lunate.

Trauma. Fragmentation of part of an epiphysis from acute or chronic trauma simulates changes of ischemic necrosis but histologically lacks the characteristic changes. The best examples occur at the tibial tubercle (Osgood-Schlatter disease), medial tibia (Blount's disease), lower pole of the patella (Sinding-Larsen-Johansson disease), and spinal discovertebral junction (Scheuermann's disease).

Growth Variants. Normal variations in ossification within growing epiphyses have inappropriately been attributed to ischemic necrosis. The most common locations for this confusing variation to occur are at the calcaneal apophysis (Sever's disease) and ischiopubic synchondrosis (van Neck's disease).

In general, the most common age group for osteonecrosis is between 3 and 10 years of age. Males tend to be involved more frequently than females, and the disorders may be bilateral at times. Predisposing conditions are many, including thromboembolic disorders, vascular disease, and trauma. Commonly, a specific activity that creates abnormal stresses is associated. Clinical manifestations include localized and referred pain, swelling, reduced range of motion, and muscle atrophy. If the disorder is in a location involved in locomotion, a limp may be evident. Once the disease has run its self-limiting course, deformity of the joint surface and altered joint mechanics may result in chronic pain and disability, while predisposing the patient to premature degenerative joint disease.

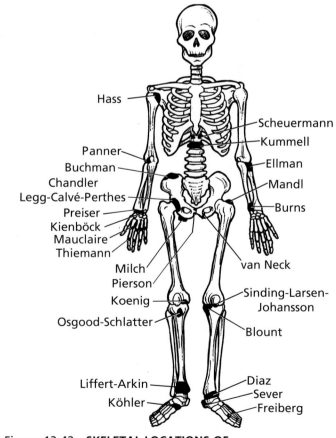

Figure 13-42   **SKELETAL LOCATIONS OF EPIPHYSEAL OSTEONECROSIS.**

Table 13-20	Epiphyseal Disorders		
Region	**Location**	**Synonym**	**Pathophysiologic Mechanism**
Spine			
	Vertebral endplate[a]	Scheuermann's disease	Trauma producing Schmorl's nodes
	Vertebral body, adult	Kümell's disease	Secondary osteonecrosis to trauma
	Child	Calvé's disease	Eosinophilic granuloma
Pelvis			
	Iliac crest	Buchman's disease	Undefined
	Ischial apophysis	Milch's disease	Undefined
	Ischiopubic synchondrosis[a]	van Neck's disease	Normal growth variant
	Symphysis pubis	Pierson's disease	Undefined
Femur			
	Condyles, adult	Spontaneous osteonecrosis	Primary osteonecrosis
	Condyles, child[a]	Koenig's disease, osteochondritis dissecans	Trauma
	Greater trochanter	Mandl's disease	Undefined
	Head, adult[a]	Chandler's disease	Primary osteonecrosis
	Head, child	Legg-Calvé-Perthes disease	Primary osteonecrosis
Patella			
	Primary center	Köhler's disease	Secondary osteonecrosis to trauma
	Secondary center[a]	Sinding-Larsen-Johansson disease	Trauma
Tibia			
	Distal tibia	Liffert-Arkin disease	Secondary osteonecrosis to trauma
	Intercondyloid spines	Caffey's disease	Undefined
	Medial condyle[a]	Blount's disease	Trauma
	Tibial tubercle[a]	Osgood-Schlatter disease	Trauma
Foot			
	Calcaneal apophysis[a]	Sever's disease	Normal growth variant
	Fifth metatarsal base	Iselin's disease	Secondary osteonecrosis or growth variant
	Metatarsal head[a]	Freiberg's disease	Secondary osteonecrosis to trauma
	Navicular[a]	Köhler's disease	Secondary osteonecrosis to trauma or growth variant
	Talus	Diaz's disease	Secondary osteonecrosis to trauma
Humerus			
	Capitellum[a]	Panner's disease	Secondary osteonecrosis to trauma
	Head[a]	Hass's disease	Secondary osteonecrosis to trauma
Radius			
	Radial head	Ellman's disease	Secondary osteonecrosis to trauma
Ulna			
	Distal ulna	Burn's disease	Secondary osteonecrosis to trauma
Hand			
	Complete carpus	Caffey's disease	Undefined
	Lunate	Kienböck's disease	Secondary osteonecrosis to trauma
	Metacarpal heads	Mauclaire's disease	Secondary osteonecrosis to trauma
	Phalangeal base	Thiemann's disease	Secondary osteonecrosis to trauma
	Scaphoid	Preiser's disease	Secondary osteonecrosis to trauma

[a] Most common clinical entities.

EPIPHYSEAL OSTEONECROSIS

Legg-Calvé-Perthes Disease

General Considerations

Legg-Calvé-Perthes disease is the synonym applied to avascular necrosis of the femoral capital epiphysis before closure of the growth plate. It was first recognized in the early 1900s separately by these three investigators. (1–3) The disorder represents true avascular necrosis of bone. It is self-limiting, resolving within 2–8 years but resulting in various degrees of deformity. (4)

Clinical Features

The disorder most frequently affects patients between the ages of 3 and 12 years, with peak incidence in the 5- to 7-year age group. Onset before the age of 4 years exhibits a better overall prognosis. The prognosis worsens with advancing age of onset. (5) A definite male predominance of 5:1 exists. (6) Approximately 10% of the cases entail bilateral involvement, but this is rare in females. The condition is rare in blacks, and there is a familial incidence in 6–12% of cases. (4,7) It has been suggested that with bilateral involvement the pathologic process of one hip does not influence the process of the other. It is believed that each hip develops and progresses through the disease process independently. (8)

The clinical symptom picture includes vague groin pain, occasionally extending down into the anteromedial knee, and a limp. Motion of the involved hip, especially abduction and internal rotation, invariably produces pain, though these symptoms may be intermittent and inconsistent. Chronic cases may exhibit prominent atrophy of the thigh muscles. Previous trauma to the hip is often associated. Specific orthopedic tests, such as the Fabere-Patrick and Trendelenburg tests, may be positive. (4) If the patient is an adult who developed Legg-Calvé-Perthes disease as a child, additional findings consistent with secondary degenerative joint disease may be evident, including diminished and painful ranges of motion, flexion contracture, muscle atrophy, crepitus, a notably shortened limb, and increasing stiffness that is reduced upon walking. (9)

Pathologic Features

The essential pathologic alterations are those consistent with avascular necrosis; however, the primary cause of the vascular disturbance remains obscure. (10) Legg believed trauma to be the cause; Calvé, rickets; and Perthes, infection. Presently, a number of factors have been implicated, including heredity, trauma, endocrine disorders, inflammation, nutrition, and altered circulatory hemodynamics. (4,11,12) Disturbed venous drainage and intraosseous hypertension are important factors. (13) In the majority of cases, the bone age is reduced by 50% of the chronologic age. (14,15)

Intensive investigations into the vascular anatomy of the developing femoral head have identified a vulnerable period between the ages of 4 and 7 years, corresponding to the average age of onset of the disorder. (11) The vascular supply to the femoral head is derived from three primary sources: (*a*) foveal vessels penetrating through the ligamentum teres, (*b*) superior and inferior epiphyseal vessels originating from the medial and lateral circumflex branches of the profunda femoris artery, and (*c*) metaphyseal vessels from the bone marrow. (Fig. 13-43) During the ages of 4–7 years, contributions by the foveal and metaphyseal vessels are negligible, the majority being derived from the epiphyseal vessels, especially the lateral group.

This solitary source of blood vasculature may predispose the patient to ischemic necrosis by not allowing for an alternate collateral supply if these epiphyseal vessels become obstructed. With progressing age, greater contributions are made by the foveal and metaphyseal sources, reducing the vulnerability for developing ischemia. In addition to this growth transition in vascular contribution, the position of these epiphyseal veins and arteries on the surface of the femoral neck in a subsynovial location renders them vulnerable to disruption from fracture, slipping of the epiphysis, intracapsular synovitis, or surgical pinning. (10,16,17)

The observed histopathologic changes as a result of ischemia are complex and dynamic. Essentially, four phases can be identified: *avascular, revascularization, repair, and deformity* phases. (18,19) A double infarction within a short time period appears to be necessary to initiate the full pathologic sequence of events. (20,21) Following death of the osteocytes and bone marrow, there is infiltration of new blood vessels and osteogenic elements. This may be delayed as long as 12 months after the initial infarction. Revascularization precipitates an absorption and deposition process for as long as 4 years. Resorption is characterized by phagocytosis, fibrosis, and formation of granulation tissue. Deposition of new bone occurs by directly overlaying existing dead trabeculae (creeping substitution). (22) Gradually, deposition predominates and the head is remodeled, depending on the epiphyseal stresses during the whole process. Notably, during the necrotic and rebuilding processes, the articular cartilage is invariably not affected. The entire process from initial infarction to residual deformity takes a variable length of time, between 2 and 8 years.

Radiologic Features

Isotopic bone scan may show decreased uptake of the proximal femur before any other changes are identified. (23,24) Ultrasound may show effusion of the joint early in the disease. CT delineates the femoral head changes more clearly and is especially useful in detecting complicating osteochondritis dissecans. MRI facilitates the early diagnosis of osteonecrosis and defines the status of the articular cartilage. (25–27). Plain film studies provide the most common method of early detection and for following progression. Radiologic changes closely parallel the pathologic changes of the disease. (Table 13-21; Fig. 13-44)

Table 13-21	Pathologic-Radiologic Correlation in Legg-Calvé-Perthes Disease
Pathologic Stages	**Radiologic Feature**
Avascular stage (0–12 months)	Capsular distention Increased joint space Lateral femoral displacement (Waldenstrom's sign) Small epiphysis
Revascularization (6 months–4 years)	Flattened, small epiphysis Fragmentation Homogeneous sclerosis (snowcap sign) Increased cortical density (head within a head) Metaphyseal cysts Patchy sclerosis Subchondral fracture (crescent sign) Wide, short femoral neck
Repair and remodeling (1–2 years)	Gradual reconstitution of density and configuration
Deformity	Coxa vara Enlarged head (coxa magna) Flattened head (mushroom deformity, coxa plana) Large greater trochanter

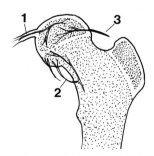

Figure 13-43 BLOOD SUPPLY TO THE FEMORAL HEAD. Two major vessels supply the developing head: ligamentum teres (*1*) and epiphyseal arteries (*2*). It is thought that obliteration of the lateral group (*3*) produces the avascular condition leading to osteonecrosis.

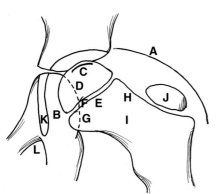

Figure 13-44 EARLY RADIOGRAPHIC SIGNS OF LEGG-CALVÉ-PERTHES DISEASE. *A,* convex distended pericapsular fat lines; *B,* increased medial joint space; *C,* subchondral fracture (crescent sign); *D,* small epiphysis; *E,* linear metaphyseal lucency; *F,* widened growth plate; *G,* medial metaphyseal cyst; *H,* lateral epiphyseal and metaphyseal lucency (Gage's sign); *I,* broad, short femoral neck; *J,* enlarged greater trochanter; *K,* widened teardrop; *L,* small obturator foramen. (Adapted from **Edgren W:** *Coxa plana.* Acta Orthop Scand Suppl 84:1, 1965.)

Soft Tissue Swelling. Evaluation of intra-articular hip effusion is difficult and requires comparison with the contralateral side and careful clinical correlation. Observation of the pericapsular fat lines, especially on the lateral aspect of the femoral neck, will reveal them to be convex rather than exhibit the normal concave contour.

Increased Medial Joint Space. Increase in the width of the medial joint cavity, with an accompanying lateral displacement of the femur (*Waldenström's sign*), is a common early finding. (28) This may be the result of effusion and/or cartilage hyperplasia. (29) Evaluation is performed by measuring the distance between the pelvic teardrop and medial femoral head (*teardrop distance*) and comparing with the other side.

Smaller Obturator Foramen. On the affected side, the obturator foramen may appear strikingly smaller than on the opposing side. (Fig. 13-45*A*) This is owing to a projectional distortion of the pubis and ischium secondary to antalgic flexion, external rotation, and slight abduction of the involved hip. This is not a specific sign of Legg-Calvé-Perthes disease, often being present in any painful condition of the hip.

Small Femoral Head. A reduction in overall size of the femoral head is commonly seen and may be the only radiographic sign

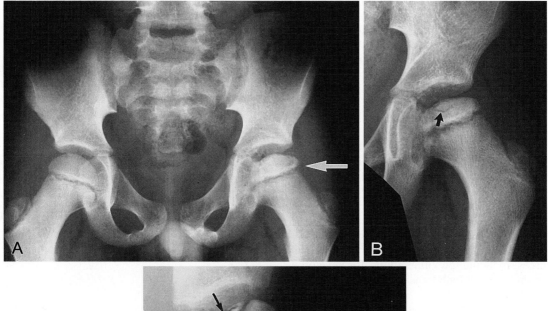

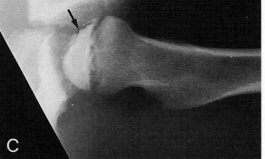

Figure 13-45 LEGG-CALVÉ-PERTHES DISEASE: CHARACTERISTIC FINDINGS. A. AP Pelvis. Note the smaller and more sclerotic femoral head epiphysis (*arrow*). The obturator foramen is also smaller on this side, as an indicator of pelvic rotation from a painful hip. **B. Close-Up, AP Hip.** Note the linear radiolucency in the small femoral head (crescent sign) (*arrow*). The growth plate is wide and irregular. **C. Frog Leg, Hip.** Note the enhancement of the crescent sign owing to the presence of gas produced by the position (*arrow*). Also, observe the homogeneous opacity of the entire epiphysis (*snowcap epiphysis*).

early in the disease. (14) (Fig. 13-45A) Although the disease's true cause has not been delineated, it appears to be the result of a lack of growth because of an impaired blood supply rather than to osseous compression.

Wider Teardrop Size. The widened teardrop is not a reliable singular sign of hip disease but may be seen in combination with other changes. Atrophy of the gluteal muscles on the affected side allows a slight obliquity to occur in the pelvis at the time the radiographic exposure is taken, which projects a widened teardrop contour. (4)

Fragmentation. Radiolucent clefts of various sizes may be visible traversing the epiphysis. The most characteristic is a curvilinear, lucent defect paralleling the superior weight-bearing articulating surface (crescent sign, rim sign). (Fig. 13-45B and C) Nitrogen gas may collect in this subchondral fracture, especially in the frog-leg position, accentuating the lucency, and it is often the first detected osseous change. (14,30) (Fig. 13-45C)

Sclerosis. Increased density within the involved epiphysis is a manifestation of revascularization, where new bone is being deposited directly over dead trabeculae and is, therefore, a radiographic sign of attempted healing. (31) These sclerotic zones on MRI show low signal intensity, and normal density fragments show an intermediate signal. (26) Within the capital epiphysis three patterns of sclerosis may be apparent at any specified time period: peripherally, at the articular cortex, creating a *head-within-a-head appearance;* in patchy, segmented sequestered areas; and as homogeneous sclerosis of the entire epiphysis (*snow-cap appearance*). (Fig. 13-45C)

Metaphyseal Widening and Shortening. The femoral neck frequently is widened transversely and decreased in overall length. In addition, the most lateral cortical margin is often convex rather than the normal concave contour. (32) (Fig. 13-45B) The most likely cause is appositional bone growth by the periosteum and cessation in longitudinal growth at the physis. (4,33)

Metaphyseal Cysts. Metaphyseal "cysts" (defects) are of controversial origin but have been shown to represent displaced uncalcified growth plate cartilage. (10) (Figs. 13-46 and 13-47)

These most commonly are located at the lateral and medial aspects of the neck and simulate a benign neoplasm. (34) Notably, these cystic lesions are found late in the disease and will eventually disappear. A lucent defect at the lateral epiphysis and adjacent metaphysis (*Gage's sign*) may occur early in the disease and may be an indicator of a worse prognosis. (25,32)

Enlarged Greater Trochanter. The greater trochanter occasionally becomes strikingly enlarged. (Fig. 13-48) This is appar-

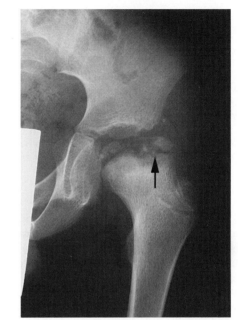

Figure 13-46 **LEGG-CALVÉ-PERTHES DISEASE: METAPHYSEAL CYST.** Note the well-circumscribed region of radiolucency at the lateral metaphyseal margin (*arrow*). *COMMENT:* Such defects are common, transient, and can be confused with more aggressive bone destruction. They represent cartilaginous intrusion from the adjacent physis.

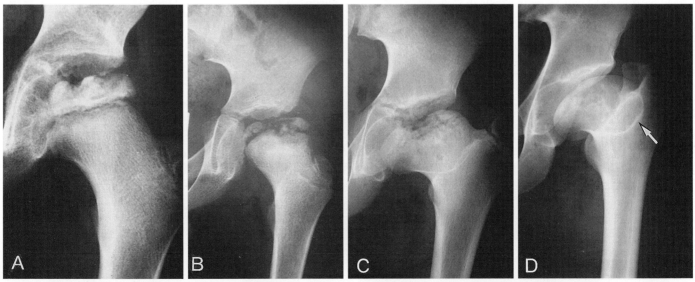

Figure 13-47 **LEGG-CALVÉ-PERTHES DISEASE: PROGRESSIVE CHANGES. A. Initial Study.** Note that after initial fracturing and compression, the necrotic epiphysis progressively breaks up, producing isolated bone fragments. **B. and C. Repair Period.** Observe that as repair occurs the reformed head re- appears in a flattened configuration. Observe the radiolucent metaphyseal cysts and broad, short femoral neck. **D. End Stage.** Note the end stage deformity, in which the head appears enlarged (coxa magna) and grossly flattened (coxa plana or mushroom deformity). A *sagging rope sign* can be seen (*arrow*).

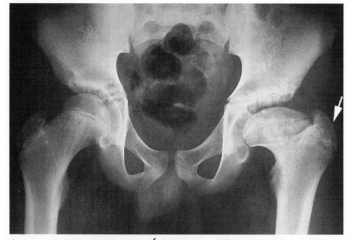

Figure 13-48 LEGG-CALVÉ-PERTHES DISEASE: END STAGE DEFORMITY. Note that the end stage of the disease is readily identified by the flattened femoral head and broad metaphysis (*mushroom deformity*). Also observe the irregular acetabular roof and enlarged, elevated greater trochanter (*arrow*).

ently the result of decreased longitudinal growth of the femoral neck with continued growth of the greater trochanter. (35) Clinically, this elevates the trochanter slightly and impairs the power of the attaching muscles, producing abductor insufficiency and a positive Trendelenburg test. (4)

Other Manifestations. The radiolucent physis may appear widened and irregular, especially on the metaphyseal side. (Fig. 13-49A) (4) Additionally, rather than rounded cystic lesions in the metaphysis, a linear radiolucent submetaphyseal band may be evident. The orientation of the growth plate may become more horizontal than normal. (36) Within the adjacent pelvis, the acetabular roof at its lateral margin is occasionally irregular. On MRI the femoral cartilage at its lateral and medial margins is often hypertrophied and bulging. (26) A late complication seen exclusively in males in < 5% of cases may be the detachment of an osteochondral fragment (osteochondritis dissecans). Similarly, in 5% of cases loss of joint space may occur over 1 year and lead to a stiff and poorly functioning hip (chondrolysis) that may require early

surgical intervention. (37,38) The older the patient at the time of onset of the Legg-Calvé-Perthes disease, the higher the incidence for osteochondritis dissecans. Usually, this occurs at an average of 8 years after the diagnosis of ischemic necrosis. (39)

Following completion of the disease process, the reconstituted femoral head may take on a number of altered configurations. These include an overall enlargement of the head (coxa magnum), flattening of the head (coxa plana), and a combination of flattening and increased transverse dimension (*mushroom deformity*). (Figs. 13-47D and 13-49B)

In addition, there may be a decrease in the femoral angle to < 120° (coxa vara). A concave, curvilinear radiopaque line may be visible superimposed over the metaphysis, caused by the tangential projection of the edge of the deformed femoral head (*sagging rope sign*). (40,41) (Fig. 13-47D) Later in life, superimposed degenerative changes, including loss of joint space, sclerosis, and osteophytes, can occur. (9)

In an adult with a deformed femoral head the main differential diagnosis is congenital hip dysplasia. The most significant differentiating radiologic feature is in the congenital deformity. In congenital deformity there is invariably some degree of accompanying acetabular dysplasia, which is not seen in Legg-Calvé-Perthes disease, and the *sagging rope sign* is absent.

Prognostic Features

Attempts to clarify the most likely outcome for an individual with Legg-Calvé-Perthes disease have isolated a number of key features. (25,36,42) Clinically, the younger the patient at the time of onset, the better the prognosis, especially < 6 years of age. When occurring in adolescents, inadequate epiphyseal remodeling or failure of revascularization frequently occurs, resulting in gross biomechanical alterations and persistent pain in the area. (43) In general, females are likely to experience more complications than are males. If the disease has advanced without appropriate therapy, the prognosis is also worsened. (44) Furthermore, even though the pathologic process of bilateral hip involvement is believed to be independent from side to side, clinical data have revealed an overall worse prognosis for individuals affected bilaterally. (45) The majority of patients will have degenerative joint disease within the affected hip by the 6th or 7th decade of life. (46)

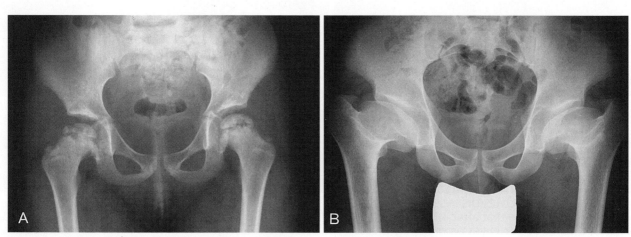

Figure 13-49 LEGG-CALVÉ-PERTHES DISEASE: BILATERAL PRESENTATION. A. Necrotic Phase with Fragmentation. B. Healed Deformities with Mushroom Configurations.

COMMENT: Involvement of both hips occurs in up to 10% of patients.

Radiologic signs signifying a diminished prognosis and a greater *head at risk* include extensive involvement of the femoral capital epiphysis, lateral displacement of the femoral head, necrotic fragments beyond the lateral metaphyseal margin, early closure and horizontal orientation of the growth plate, the presence of an extensive metaphyseal radiolucent defect, and elevation of the greater trochanter. (4,25,36,42,46) (Table 13-22) A prognostic classification (Catterall's classification) based on the concept that the final outcome is proportional to the amount of the epiphysis involved has been shown to be useful but not without limitation. (36,47)

Where there is lateral displacement of the femoral head, there are increasing proportions of the femoral head effectively "uncovered" by the acetabulum. Surgical intervention to help reestablish full "coverage" to improve the long-term prognosis may be performed, including femoral varus derotation osteotomy or a iliac osteotomy (roof procedure) to alter the acetabular angle (theory of containment). (25) (Fig. 13-50) These procedures can often promote spherical remodeling of the cartilage and subsequently the femoral head, enhancing the long-term prognosis; however, these procedures should be limited to more severe cases, as studies have shown that milder cases benefit equally from surgical or conservative measures. (48) MRI allows such changes to be identified and followed. (26,49)

Table 13-22	Head at Risk Features Suggesting Diminished Prognosis
Caterall's groups III, IV	Horizontal orientation of growth plate
Delayed diagnosis	
Early closure of growth plate	Increased age of onset
Elevation of greater trochanter	Lateral displacement of femoral head
Extensive epiphyseal involvement	Lateral epiphysis outside acetabular rim
Females	Severe metaphyseal involvement

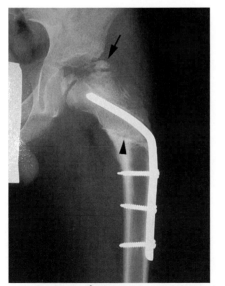

Figure 13-50 LEGG-CALVÉ-PERTHES DISEASE: CORRECTIONAL VARUS OSTEOTOMY. AP Hip. Observe the lack of acetabular coverage of the lateral epiphysis (*arrow*). *COMMENT:* An osteotomy has been performed through the subtrochanteric region of the femur (*arrowhead*). The varus position across the osteotomy site is maintained by the pins and plate. This procedure is performed in an attempt to promote cartilage and femoral head remodeling.

CAPSULE SUMMARY
Legg-Calvé-Perthes Disease

General Considerations
- Synonym applied to avascular necrosis of the femoral capital epiphysis before closure of the epiphyseal plate.

Clinical Features
- Occurs in the 3- to 12-year age group; 5:1 male predominance; 10% bilateral.
- Short history of a painful limp, reduced mobility, muscle atrophy; Trendelenburg test positive.
- Later on, adults develop secondary degenerative joint disease.

Pathologic Features
- *Primary cause obscure:* hereditary, traumatic, endocrine, inflammatory, nutritional, circulatory.
- *Vulnerable vascular period:* 4–7 years of age from solitary epiphyseal vessel supply.
- *Four stages:* avascular, revascularization, repair, deformity.
- Cartilage not affected.
- *Duration of entire process:* 2–8 years.

Radiologic Features
- Isotopic scans cold in early phase before plain film changes; MRI excellent for early detection and identifying status of articular cartilage.
- Soft tissue swelling, smaller obturator foramen, increased medial joint space, small femoral head, wide teardrop, epiphyseal fragmentation, sclerosis.
- Metaphysis wide, short, and cystic; enlarged greater trochanter, head deformities.
- *Prognostic features:* age, sex, prompt diagnosis, radiologic head-at-risk factors, extensiveness, lateral displacement, closed and horizontal growth plate, metaphyseal cyst, elevated greater trochanter, and Catterall's groupings III and IV.
- Treatment of lateral displacement often with correctional osteotomy (femoral, iliac) to promote remodeling of cartilage and femoral head.

Freiberg's Disease

General Considerations

Freiberg's disease is caused by avascular necrosis of a metatarsal head, most commonly the second. Freiberg described the condition in 1914 and is credited with the first analysis. (50,51) He first believed the cause to be directly related to trauma, but later disproved his own theory by making the diagnosis of infarction on a patient without a traumatic history. (52) The terms osteochondrosis, Freiberg's disease, and Köhler's number 2 disease have also been applied. (53) Following collapse of the articular surface, joint incongruity inevitably leads to secondary degenerative joint disease at the involved articulation.

Clinical Features

The disorder is most definitely a disease of the young adolescent female, in a ratio of approximately 5:1. (54,55) Usually, it is first encountered between the ages of 13 and 18 years, with tenderness and pain over the affected joint, usually the second metatarsophalangeal joint, occasionally the third, and rarely any other. The second metatarsal head is involved in as many as 80% of cases. (55) Symptoms may subside gradually and be sharply exacerbated some time later, such as from walking, running, or unusual footwear. Pain, palpable swelling, and mild hyperextension of the digit may be apparent. In an advanced case, palpation will reveal crepitus, stiffness, reduced motion, bony enlargement, and callus formation, which may require surgical intervention. (54,56)

Conservative treatment consists of reduction in activity, cast and crutches until symptoms subside, followed by phased return to activity with metatarsal pads and orthoses. If this fails, excision of the head has been the treatment of choice. (55) Recently, surgical arthroplasty of the deformed head, without complete excision, has shown to provide an excellent prognosis in approximately 77% of cases. (57)

Pathologic Features

The growing metatarsal head epiphysis undergoes avascular necrosis. Although the pathogenesis remains obscure, a displacement at the intervening growth plate may be responsible. (53,58) A congenitally elongated second metatarsal or short first metatarsal (Morton's syndrome) may be additional factors. Following infarction, revascularization results in absorption and bone deposition. Weight bearing on the necrotic bone causes fractures, resultant deformity of the articular cortex, and loose bodies. Secondary degenerative changes and compensatory thickening of the adjacent metatarsal cortex ensue. At surgery there is capsular thickening, synovitis, fragments of cartilage and bone, osteophytes, and fibrocartilage covering the metatarsal surface. (55)

Radiologic Features

A number of radiographic abnormalities are seen in the involved metatarsal head, depending on the stage of the disease. (5) (Figs. 13-51 and 13-52)

Articular Cortex Deformity. The articular margin of the metatarsal head will be minimally flattened. However, this can be a normal finding in some individuals. In more advanced instances, the cortex is completely flat and may even be concave or undulating. After healing, the entire head will appear enlarged and bulbous, as may be the base of the opposing phalanx.

Altered Density. Sclerosis and radiolucent foci within the head are usually visible in the active phase. Occasionally, a radiolucent subchondral fracture paralleling the articular surface can be seen (*crescent sign*). When healed, complete restitution of normal head density will be apparent.

Joint Space. In the active phases, the articular cavity will be wider than normal and may even contain loose bodies derived from the crumbling cortex. Later, as degenerative changes supervene, the joint space will narrow.

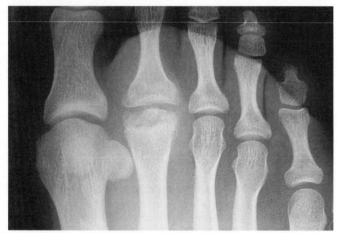

Figure 13-51 FREIBERG'S DISEASE. PA Foot. Note that the second metatarsal head has collapsed, with fragmentation and deformation of the articular cortex.

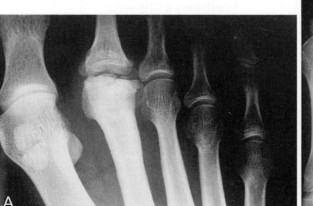

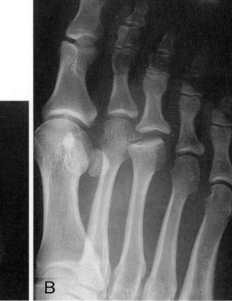

Figure 13-52 FREIBERG'S DISEASE. A. Long-Standing Disease, PA Foot. Note that the second metatarsal head is enlarged and fragmented and shows irregularity of the articular cortex. Also observe the increased density and thickened cortex of the entire second metatarsal, which frequently occurs with a long-standing disease. **B. Healed Disease, Oblique Foot.** Note the flattening deformity at the third metatarsal head.

Metatarsal Shaft. The cortex of the involved metatarsal metaphysis and diaphysis is frequently thickened owing to increased weight-bearing stresses.

Kienböck's Disease

General Considerations

Avascular necrosis of the carpal lunate was first described in detail by Kienböck in 1910. (59) Alternate terms include Kienböck's disease, lunate osteochondrosis, and lunate malacia. It causes major disability as a result of pain and loss of function in the wrists of young, productive patients.

Clinical Features

A definite predilection is apparent in males over females of up to 9:1. (60) The disorder is most commonly observed in the 20- to 40-year age group. A history of previous acute trauma or occupationally excessive hand use, especially of the dominant extremity, may be obtained, but a great many individuals have no known association. (61) Occasionally, the disorder may occur bilaterally. (62,63) Symptoms consist of localized and radiating wrist pain, swelling, and gradually worsening disability. In long-standing cases severe pain, entrapment neuropathy, and degenerative arthritis may complicate the disorder. (64)

Pathologic Features

The histopathologic picture is that of avascular necrosis. Resorption, deposition, fragmentation, and collapse typify the osseous necrosis. The isolation of contributing causes has been inconclusive, although trauma appears to be a prominent factor. Vascular studies of the lunate suggest possible vulnerability. (65,66) A short

ulna (*negative ulnar variance*) is found in up to 75% of cases, which may augment mechanical stresses between the lunate and radius and predispose to vascular impediment. (67)

Radiologic Features

Radiographically, the progression of Kienböck's disease can be staged. In the early stages of the disease (stage I), the radiographic examination may be initially unrewarding for many months. (68) In these circumstances, a bone scan or MRI study will often reveal the necrosis: the bone scan with focal increased uptake and the MRI with diminished signal. (68,69) If the patient has not used the affected hand because of symptoms, disuse osteoporosis of all adjacent bones will accentuate the density of the lunate, which remains normal owing to its lack of blood supply. With progression of the stages, however, a number of signs become evident.

In stage II disease, altered density and compression fracture or collapse ensue. (61) Initially, the entire lunate will be increased in density. Later, with partial fragmentation and collapse, there will be a mixture of lucent and sclerotic areas. Occasionally, a linear subchondral fracture may be evident in the surface opposing the radius. (Figs. 13-53 and 13-54) Flattening, collapse, and irregularity of the articular margin are usually most frequent and severe at the radial surface.

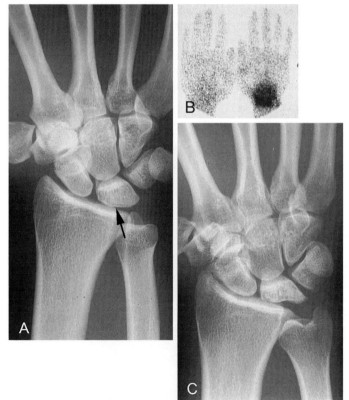

Figure 13-53 **KIENBÖCK'S DISEASE: PROGRESSION. A. Initial Film, PA Wrist.** Observe the subtle subchondral fracture (*arrow*) of the lunate. **B. Bone Scan, Wrist.** Observe the generalized uptake in the wrist. **C. 1-Year Follow-Up, PA Wrist.** Observe the increased density and altered contour of the lunate. *COMMENT:* A 25-year-old male patient presented with wrist pain. Note the negative ulnar variance.

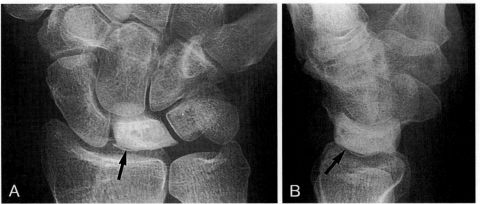

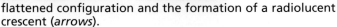

Figure 13-54 KIENBÖCK'S DISEASE. A. PA Wrist. B. Lateral Wrist. Note that the generalized increase in bone density of the lunate is the most striking feature. Observe the overall flattened configuration and the formation of a radiolucent crescent (*arrows*).

In stage III, consisting of further compression and impaction of the necrotic lunate, a diminished overall size of the bone is noted. (Fig. 13-55)

Progression to stage IV entails degenerative changes of the radiocarpal joint and/or the midcarpal joint. (61)

Treatment and Complications

Stage I Kienböck's disease may respond to conservative care, whereas shortening of the radius and/or revascularization of the lunate is usually required in reducing progressive collapse in stage II or III. (61,70) Some clinicians advocate continued conservative care in these stages; however, research has shown mixed results. (71,72) With progression to stage IV, the altered joint congruity and biomechanics precipitate separation of the scaphoid and lunate, with associated secondary degenerative joint disease of the radiocarpal and midcarpal articulations. Treatment at this stage usually requires proximal-row carpectomy with arthrodesis (61) or replacement of the necrotic lunate with a silastic implant. (73) (Fig. 13-56) It is currently accepted today that silicone implants provide only a temporary solution, as complications such as pain and silicone synovitis are inevitable, eventually requiring the implant to be removed. (74) Recent advances in bone grafting allow the surgeon to transfer vascularized bone to the area of necrosis, allowing accelerated healing and a better prognosis for these patients. (68)

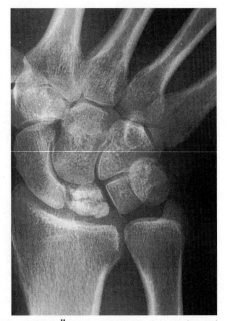

Figure 13-55 KIENBÖCK'S DISEASE. PA Wrist. Observe the increased density, multiple fracture lines, and fragmentation of the lunate.

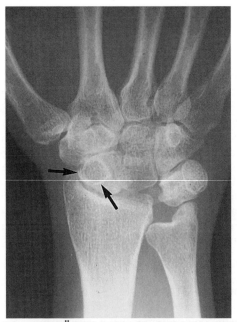

Figure 13-56 KIENBÖCK'S DISEASE: SURGICAL REMOVAL. PA Wrist. Note that the necrotic lunate has been removed. Note the proximal migration of the capitate, rotary subluxation of the scaphoid (*ring sign*) (*arrows*), and the distinctly short ulna (*negative ulnar variance*).

TRAUMATIC EPIPHYSEAL INJURIES

Osgood-Schlatter Disease

General Considerations

Osgood-Schlatter disease is a common, self-limiting, but painful and disabling disorder involving the patellar tendon–tibial tubercle complex in adolescent individuals. The first reports in 1903, made independently by Robert Bayley Osgood and Carl Schlatter, emphasized the apparent close relationship with the onset of the disease and antecedent trauma. (1–3) Subsequent descriptions have erroneously implicated avascular necrosis as the cause of the disease.

Clinical Features

Distinctively, the disease is most frequently encountered in adolescents between 11 and 15 years of age. Males are far more commonly affected than females. An antecedent history of a single violent injury or activity involving repetitive knee flexion and extension movements is usual. (4) Symptoms are typically localized over the tibial tubercle and include pain, tenderness, and soft tissue swelling. In the absence of conclusive radiographic findings, the presence of these symptoms allows the diagnosis to be made. (5) Contraction of the quadriceps muscle against resistance exacerbates the localized pain. The condition is bilateral in 25–50% of cases. (6) The course is chronic and tends to recur over a period of months to several years but usually ceases by the age of 18. Occasionally, symptoms may persist into adulthood.

Pathologic Features

A common misconception is that Osgood-Schlatter disease represents avascular necrosis of the developing tibial tuberosity. The pathologic abnormalities are most consistent with inflammatory changes at the distal patellar tendon. Every case will exhibit increased cellularity, vascularity, intratendinous fibrocartilage, and signs of chronic inflammation. (6) Recent MRI studies support the concept that Osgood-Schlatter disease is primarily a tendinitis.

Some investigators believe that, conversely, there is a partial disruption of the tibial patellar ligament attachment owing to trauma. (7) The combination of the redirected pull of the powerful quadriceps muscle group on the mechanically weak ligament–cartilage attachment at the tibial tuberosity predisposes to this avulsion. (5,8) Depending on the stage of ossification of the tubercle, a piece of cartilage or bone, or both, is displaced, creating a localized inflammatory response. (7,9) Alternatively, heterotopic new bone may form in the inflamed patellar ligament. (10)

Radiologic Features

Radiographic evaluation of the tibial tuberosity for evidence of Osgood-Schlatter disease requires slight alterations in standard

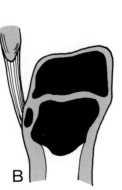
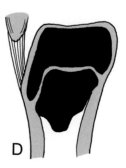
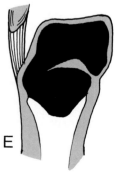
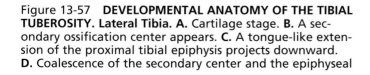

Figure 13-57   DEVELOPMENTAL ANATOMY OF THE TIBIAL TUBEROSITY. Lateral Tibia. A. Cartilage stage. **B.** A secondary ossification center appears. **C.** A tongue-like extension of the proximal tibial epiphysis projects downward. **D.** Coalescence of the secondary center and the epiphyseal extension occurs. **E.** Closure of the proximal epiphysis occurs from the tibial tuberosity, progressing posteriorly. (Adapted from **Ogden JA, Southwick WO:** *Osgood-Schlatter's disease and tibial tuberosity development.* Clin Orthop 116:180, 1976.)

technique. The lateral radiograph is the most diagnostic and should be done of both knees for comparison purposes. In addition, slight internal rotation of the leg about 5° moves the laterally placed tuberosity into its true lateral profile. The assessment of soft tissue changes in conjunction with bony alterations also requires two lateral views to be taken of each knee: one with a lowered peak kilovoltage and one with a higher peak kilovoltage to optimally demonstrate changes in both components. (11)

Developmental variations in the tibial tuberosity often hinder definitive radiographic diagnosis of the condition. (9) (Fig. 13-57) Usually this is overcome by the availability of a lateral comparison view of the opposite side and knowledge of the local development and variations. Significantly, several ossific nodules may develop normally within the developing tubercle and should not be confused with abnormal fragmentation.

The radiologic features include both soft tissue and bony changes. (Table 13-23)

Soft Tissue. The overlying skin contour is displaced from underlying edema. The patellar ligament appears thickened and is poorly defined at its margins, especially closer to its tibial insertion. The adjacent infrapatellar fat-pad may appear blurred at its margin, with obliteration of the inferior angle, and may be increased in density. (11,12) (Fig. 13-58) The three-phase bone scan usually is normal. (6) CT often shows enlargement of the tendon with areas of low attenuation contained. MRI shows a distended infrapatellar bursa, thickening of the tendon, and an increased signal at the insertion site on both T1- and T2-weighted images. (6)

Bone. Bone changes consist of isolated, irregular ossicles, especially toward the anterior aspect of the tibial tuberosity. (13) If no ossicles are present, there may be anterior surface irregularities marking the sites of chondro-osseous avulsion. (8) These are seen better on CT than on MRI. (6) MRI is superior to radiography in the early diagnosis and identification of progression of Osgood-Schlatter disease. (14)

Recently, the MRI findings have been categorized into five stages, consisting of *normal, early, progressive, terminal, and*

Table 13-23	Radiologic Features of Osgood-Schlatter Disease

Technique
  Bilateral, lateral projections (5° medial rotation)
  Low and high kilovolts peak exposures of each knee
  MRI of the patellar tendon
Acute
  Soft tissue
    Displaced overlying soft tissue contour
    Opacified infrapatellar fat-pad
    Thickened, poorly defined patellar tendon
    Increase signal intensity within the patellar tendon on
      T2-weighted images
  Tibial tuberosity
    Irregular anterior contour
    Multiple, irregular isolated ossicles
Healed
  Normal appearance
  Displaced overlying skin contour
  Enlarged, irregular tibial tuberosity
  Persistent free ossicles

healing. (14) In the early stage, MRI signs of marrow edema can be seen in one third of cases with a low signal on T1- and high signal on T2-weighted studies. (6) Progression is noted by the partial avulsion of the secondary ossification center, whereas the terminal stage consists of complete separation. (14) Healing is characterized most significantly by resolution of the soft tissue changes. (Fig. 13-59) Persistence of the ossicles may be asymptomatic but, infrequently, may precipitate persistence of pain into adulthood. (15) (Fig. 13-60) Rarely, genu recurvatum and patella alta may complicate the disorder. (15) It is expected that osseous abnormality will be observable radiographically in an adult who has had previous Osgood-Schlatter disease.

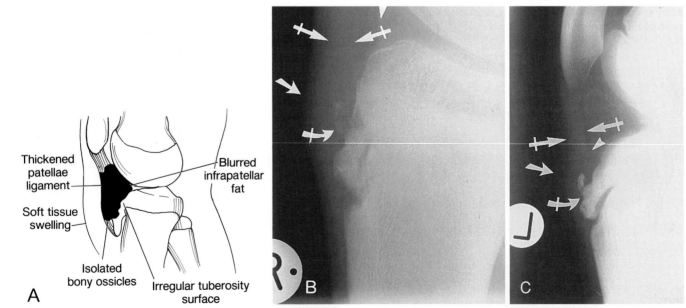

Thickened patellae ligament

Soft tissue swelling

Isolated bony ossicles

Blurred infrapatellar fat

Irregular tuberosity surface

Figure 13-58 OSGOOD-SCHLATTER DISEASE CHARACTERISTIC FEATURES. A. Diagram. B. and C. Lateral Knee. Observe the edema over the tibial tuberosity (*arrows*), blurred infrapatel-lar fat (*arrowhead*), thickened patellar ligament (*crossed arrows*), and fragmentation of the tuberosity (*curved crossed arrows*).

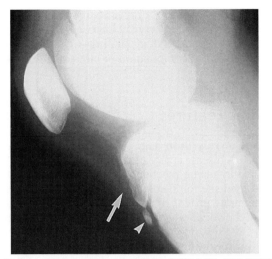

Figure 13-59 **OSGOOD-SCHLATTER DISEASE: INACTIVE PHASE. Lateral Knee.** Note the ossicle at the tibial tuberosity (*arrowhead*), which may coalesce and disappear in adulthood, in this 12-year-old patient with previous Osgood-Schlatter disease. The sharp infrapatellar inferior angle is normal and indicates a lack of adjacent soft tissue edema (*arrow*).

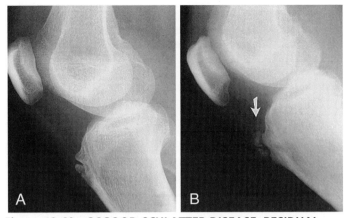

Figure 13-60 **OSGOOD-SCHLATTER DISEASE: RESIDUAL OSSICLES. A. Lateral Knee.** A 25-year-old patient with previous Osgood-Schlatter disease. **B. Lateral Knee.** A 21-year-old patient with previous and now reactivated Osgood-Schlatter disease. Observe the blurred infrapatellar fat (*arrow*), confirming the presence of inflammatory edema. (Courtesy of Ronald Gilbert, DC, Richmond, Virginia.)

CAPSULE SUMMARY
Osgood-Schlatter Disease

General Considerations

- Painful adolescent self-limiting disorder of the tibial tuberosity owing to trauma.
- No evidence of underlying ischemic necrosis.

Clinical Features

- Males, more commonly; 11–15 years of age.
- History of a single violent injury or repetitive flexion–extension movements.
- Pain, swelling, tenderness over the tibial tubercle.

Pathologic Features

- Partial disruption at the patellar ligament–tuberosity attachment, creating localized inflammatory changes.

Radiologic Features

- Requires specific technique: bilateral lateral views with slight medial rotation, using both high and low kilovoltage.
- May be confusing appearance of normal ossicles.
- Displaced skin contour, thickened and indistinct patellar ligament, blurred and opacified infrapatellar fat, isolated irregular ossicles, anterior surface irregularities in the tuberosity.

Scheuermann's Disease

General Considerations

Scheuermann's disease was poorly defined until 1920, when Scheuermann demonstrated radiographically the characteristic vertebral body wedging. (16,17) The disease is a common adolescent disorder that may result in spinal pain and cosmetic deformity and may predispose the patient to thoracic disc herniation and premature degenerative changes. The origin of the disorder is unknown. Early investigators speculated that an ischemic necrosis involving the secondary vertebral ring epiphysis might be the cause; this has since been disproved. (16,18) As such, Scheuermann's disease should not be classified as one of the osteochondroses. Other studies have suggested a wide variety of causes. (19) (Table 13-24) More recent studies implicate traumatic growth arrest and endplate fractures (Schmorl's nodes) during the adolescent growth period as the most likely causal factors. (20) Various synonyms have been applied, including vertebral epiphysitis, juvenile kyphosis, and osteochondrosis juvenilis dorsi.

Clinical Features

The onset of Scheuermann's disease is distinctively within the adolescent period, usually between 13 and 17 years of age. A slight male predominance has been reported, but newer data have suggested a more equal sex distribution. (20,21) The reported incidence may be as high as 8% of the general population (19,20,22–24), representing the most common cause of a structural kyphosis within this age range. (25) There is an increased incidence of the condition within families and among relatives, most likely passed on by an autosomal dominant allele. (26–25) Clinical manifestations are highly variable. Many patients are unaware that they have a deformity and are diagnosed incidentally on routine lateral chest radiographs or on physical examination. The most common spinal regions affected are the middle and lower thoracic areas.

Of those who are symptomatic, pain, fatigue, and defective posture are the main findings. In addition, the individuals tend to occupy jobs that require less activity, exhibit less range of motion, have less strength in trunk extension, and suffer pain more, often distant from their Scheuermann's disease. (28) It is unusual for individuals afflicted with Scheuermann's disease to be predisposed to work injuries or to suffer disability with activities of

Table 13-24	Implicated Causal Factors in Scheuermann's Disease
Avascular necrosis of secondary ring epiphysis
Low-grade infection
Deformity secondary to discal extrusion
Hereditary
Vitamin deficiency
Malnutrition
Endocrine abnormalities
Muscular imbalance
Osteoporosis
Trauma-induced discal extrusion inhibiting growth

Adapted from **Schmorl G, Junghanns H:** *The Human Spine in Health and Disease,* ed 2, trans EF Besemann. New York: Grune & Stratton, 1971.

daily living, athletic pursuits, or diminished self-esteem owing to the deformity.

The increased kyphosis is midthoracic in the majority of cases and is only occasionally present at the thoracolumbar region. The lumbar and cervical lordoses are accentuated, as is the anterior pelvic tilt. The abdomen often appears protuberant. A prominent posterior shift in weight bearing of the upper trunk over the sacral base is frequently observed. Mild scoliosis is often an associated feature. With the patient prone, reduced mobility and almost complete fixation are noted when force is applied in a postero-anterior manner. (29) Direct tenderness by palpation and percussion of the apex spinous processes is commonly elicited. The hamstrings, iliopsoas, and pectoral muscles are frequently hypertonic. (30,31) It is unusual for associated neurological abnormalities to be found, unless complicated by disc herniation or extradural spinal cysts. (32–34)

Conservative management, through exercise and bracing, usually is an effective treatment in association with an early diag-nosis. However, a kyphosis > 75°, curve progression, or neurological deficit may warrant surgical intervention. (21,25)

There will be no laboratory findings. The definitive diagnosis is derived from combination of clinical and radiographic examinations.

Pathologic Features

There are relatively little data published on the pathology of Scheuermann's disease at any stage of its development. Although the exact pathogenetic mechanism has not been clearly delineated, the target site for histologic abnormalities appears to be at the cartilaginous growth plate–bone interface (discovertebral junction) of the vertebral body. (Fig. 13-61) Normally, each vertebral body discal surface is covered by growing cartilage, which is responsible for the development of vertical height of each segment. The peripheral ring epiphysis does not contribute to this vertical dimension but serves as an attachment for the peripheral annulus fibers. (18,35)

Histopathologic studies of the discovertebral junction have not discovered the precise initiating factor in the disorder. However, it appears that the earliest abnormalities are thinning and focal areas of degeneration occurring within the cartilaginous growth plate. (7) Nuclear endplate impressions and swelling of the nucleus pulposus have been implicated but their roles have not been determined. (20,36,37) Following the development of focal necrosis and thinning within the growth plate, herniation of discal substance into the adjacent vertebral body occurs, inhibiting the vertical growth potential. Displacement of the growth plate anteriorly adjacent to the herniation may cause the vertebral body to elongate in its sagittal dimension. The prolapsed disc material consists of annular and nuclear tissue, which may remain localized, extend horizontally beneath the cartilage plate, or even separate the peripheral ring epiphysis (*limbus bone*) from the vertebral body. Notably, there is no evidence of ischemic necrosis.

Developing growth plate-bone interface (discovertebral junction)
↓
Inciting cause (trauma, etc.)
↓
Growth plate thinning and focal degeneration
↓
Distorted, disturbed growth plate
↓
Intrabody discal herniation (Schmorl's nodes)
↓
Loss of disc height
↓
Anterior loss of vertebral body height
↓
Increased fixed kyphosis
↓
Thickened and shortened anterior longitudinal length

Increased cervical and lumbar lordoses

Interbody fusion

Premature degenerative joint disease

Figure 13-61 **PATHOLOGIC SEQUENCE IN SCHEUERMANN'S DISEASE.**

The cumulative effect is to produce multiple intrabody discal extrusions (Schmorl's nodes), anterior vertebral body wedging, irregular endplates, loss of disc height, and a thickened, contracted anterior longitudinal ligament. (38) (Table 13-25) Occasionally, osseous fusion across the involved intervertebral disc spaces can occur. (39)

Radiologic Features

A universal consensus regarding diagnostic criteria is lacking (20); however, the most commonly used definition is a kyphosis owing to at least three contiguous segments, with wedging of 5° or more of each participating vertebral body. (23) Extension of the diagnostic criteria to include irregular endplates, loss of disc height, and an increased kyphosis improves the diagnostic accuracy. (40) The kyphosis is purely thoracic in approximately 75% of patients, with the apex at the T8–T9 region. (20,41) The remaining 25% of cases usually are found in the thoracolumbar area. Cervical involvement is rare. (Fig. 13-62)

The most characteristic radiologic features consist of anterior vertebral wedging, irregular endplates (multiple Schmorl's nodes), and loss of intervertebral disc height. Additional findings may include limbus bones, spontaneous anterior interbody fusion, sagittally elongated vertebral bodies, and mild scoliosis. (Fig. 13-63; Table 13-26) As many as 50% of individuals with Scheuermann's disease may demonstrate spondylolysis in the low lumbar vertebrae and, less commonly, spondylolisthesis. (28,42) At least 50% also will exhibit superimposed degenerative changes in the thoracic spine. (28)

In cases of thoracolumbar Scheuermann's disease, an extremely high association with degenerative phenomena, even in young patients, has been described between the L4 and the

Table 13-25	Pathologic-Radiologic Correlation in Scheuermann's Disease
Pathologic Feature	**Radiologic Feature**
Thin, degenerating growth plate	Decreased anterior body height
	Increased kyphosis
Discal extrusion	Endplate irregularity (Schmorl's nodes)
	Limbus bones
	Loss of disc height
Degenerative changes	Osteophytes

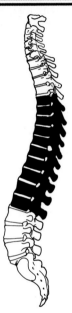

Figure 13-62 **SPINAL DISTRIBUTION OF SCHEUERMANN'S DISEASE.**

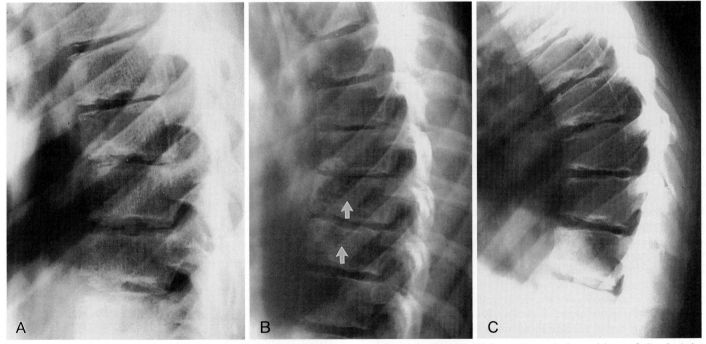

Figure 13-63 **SCHEUERMANN'S DISEASE: THORACIC SPINE. A. Mild Form.** Note the slight anterior wedging, endplate irregularity, and loss of disc height. **B. Moderate Form.** Observe that the changes are more extensive. Observe the increased sagittal dimensions of the vertebral bodies, endplate irregularities (Schmorl's nodes), and loss of disc height. Remnants of the central venous channel can also be seen at multiple levels (*arrows*). **C. Severe Form.** Note that, in addition to the osseous and discal changes, an increase in the kyphotic curvature is evident.

Table 13-26	Radiologic Features of Scheuermann's Disease

Locations
   Midthoracic (75%)
   Thoracolumbar (25%)
Definition
   Anterior wedging (> 5°) of three or more contiguous segments
   Irregular endplates (Schmorl's nodes)
   Loss of disc height
   Increased kyphosis (> 40°)
Additional features
   Anterior interbody fusion
   Fixation of involved curvature
   Increased lumbar and cervical lordoses
   Lumbar spondylolysis
   Irregular growth of ring epiphysis (limbus bones, etc.)
   Mild scoliosis
   Sagitally elongated vertebral bodies
   Persistent venous channels
   Premature degenerative joint disease

L5 levels. The degenerative phenomena consist of disc dehydration (85%), annular tear (67%), narrowing (58%), and herniation (56%). (43,44) It has been suggested that there is an underlying defect of discal integrity that manifests at a young age, and the term *juvenile discogenic disease* has been proposed when the two findings coincide. (43)

Vertebral Body Wedging. The configuration of the affected vertebrae becomes trapezoidal as a manifestation of inhibited growth, particularly on the anterior aspect. The degree of anterior wedging is most prominent at the apex segment and gradually diminishes in each successive segment toward the upper and lower limits of the abnormal kyphosis. In addition, the total sagittal length and the anterior concavity of the vertebral body may be increased.

Irregular Endplates. The degree of endplate irregularities is variable but frequently may be severe enough to be confused with an infectious process. However, careful scrutiny of the irregularities will usually show them demarcated by a sclerotic margin, which is characteristic of a Schmorl's node herniation. These discal-induced endplate imperfections are predominantly located on the anterior two thirds of the vertebral body and are usually most severe at the apical segment.

Ring Epiphysis Abnormalities. Ossification of the ring epiphysis is frequently altered. Instead of the epiphysis being homogeneous and smooth, a fragmented, irregular pattern may be visible. Where extruded discal material isolates the growth center from the underlying body, a persistent, unfused epiphysis remains (limbus bone, Scheuermann's ossicle). Associated during the active phase is the enlargement of the normal step-like defect, where the ring epiphysis eventually develops.

Decreased Intervertebral Disc Height. Approximation of opposing endplates with a diminished discal height is an integral feature of Scheuermann's disease. Notably, there is a more marked loss toward the anterior aspect of the disc. Initially, this diminution is the result of discal extrusion, which is later complicated by premature degenerative loss of resiliency and increasing fibrosis. Infrequently, fusion may be visible across the affected intervertebral disc.

Persistent Venous Channels. Venous channels, vertebral body normal variations, have been reported in almost 25% of individuals with Scheuermann's disease. (45) Radiographically, they will be visible as a thin, linear radiolucency located in the center of the vertebral body and oriented parallel to the endplates. (Fig. 13-63B) The presence of these grooves suggests vertebral body immaturity and is not a definitive feature of the disorder. (18)

Postural Abnormalities. The most apparent abnormality is the marked increase in thoracic kyphosis. (Fig. 13-63C) A measurement of the kyphosis between the upper and lower involved segments (kyphotic angle) of > 40° is abnormal. (40,41) Examination of the remaining spinal areas will show accentuated lumbar and cervical lordoses. If the involvement is localized in the upper lumbar region, the lordosis will be diminished and even reversed. A mild scoliosis is often associated. Flexion and hyperextension lateral projections of the thoracic spine will show almost complete loss of intersegmental mobility. It should be noted that research has shown a broad range of intraobserver and interobserver differences in mensuration outcomes, which should be taken into account during the diagnosis and management of Scheuermann's disease by individual clinicians. (46)

CAPSULE SUMMARY
Scheuermann's Disease

General Considerations

- A spinal disease of unknown cause affecting the adolescent, leading to pain and cosmetic deformity.
- *Synonyms:* juvenile kyphosis and vertebral epiphysitis.

Clinical Features

- Males, 13–17 years of age.
- Most commonly middle and lower thoracic regions.
- Pain, fatigue, defective posture most notable findings.
- Rarely associated with neurologic deficits.

Pathologic Features

- *Site of abnormality:* the discovertebral junction growth plate, especially at the anterior aspect, where thinning and degeneration precipitate intrabody discal herniations, and inhibition of growth.
- No evidence of ischemic necrosis.

Radiologic Features

- No consensus on diagnostic criteria but should include at least three contiguous vertebrae with each wedged at least 5°, irregular endplates, decreased disc height, increased kyphosis.
- *Possible additional findings:* accentuated lumbar and cervical lordoses, mild scoliosis, limbus bones, anterior interbody fusion, persistent venous channels, premature degenerative changes.

Osteochondritis Dissecans

General Considerations

Osteochondritis dissecans is a condition of unknown origin that occurs in children and adolescents and is characterized by a small necrotic segment of subchondral bone. The lesion may heal spontaneously or it may separate and become displaced into the joint cavity, forming an intra-articular loose body. Konig in 1887 gave the condition its name in order to describe the localized inflammatory osteochondritis dissecting away from the underlying bone. (47) Current knowledge suggests that there is no evidence of inflammation and, as such, the term osteochondrosis dissecans is more appropriate. These have been called by various names, including osteochondral defects, osteochondral fractures, transchondral fractures, and osteochondral lesions.

Clinical Features

The most frequent age of onset is between 11 and 20 years. There is a definite male predominance. The most commonly affected location is the knee, followed by the ankle, elbow, and hip. (48) Rare sites of involvement are the first metatarsal head, humeral head, and scaphoid. (Fig. 13-64; Table 13-27) A wide spectrum of clinical manifestations may be evident. Some individuals will be entirely asymptomatic, whereas others will suffer acute pain. Presenting findings may include joint effusion, painful joint motion, clicking, locking, and localized tenderness over the site of osteochondrosis. An antecedent history of acute trauma may be elicited. Usually, the onset is not directly attributable to a single event or group of factors. A hereditary tendency has been evident in some cases involving the knee, especially in shorter-statured

individuals. (49) In general, the treatment goal for osteochondritis dissecans is to preserve a smooth congruity between the opposing articulating surfaces. (50)

Pathologic Features

The exact pathogenetic mechanism has not been clearly delineated (51); however, the prominent role of shearing, rotatory, or tangentially applied forces to the cartilage and subchondral bone appears instrumental in initiating the segmental area of avascular necrosis or separation of fragments. (52,53) (Fig. 13-65) Investigations into subchondral vascular anatomy have been unrewarding in demonstrating an area of susceptible vascular supply.

Examination of the involved location macroscopically reveals a typical appearance. (7) Usually, the overlying cartilage shows a surrounding furrow demarcating a circular or elliptical defect of < 2 cm. The lesion may be firmly or loosely adherent to the underlying bone. Occasionally, there may be fragmentation of the sequestered segment. Microscopically, the loose body is composed of all cartilage or both bone and cartilage (osteochondral loose body). The majority of the overlying cartilage maintains its viability and may continue to proliferate and even calcify, gradually enlarging its overall size. Conversely, the separated bone is wholly necrotic. Individual trabeculae appear thickened with new bone, representing the phenomenon of creeping substitution with attempted healing. (54) The opposing site of origin is covered with fibrous tissue and shows surface osseous metaplasia with deposition peripherally. Interposed between the isolated segment and the adjacent bone, fibrous and fibrocartilaginous tissue is present.

Table 13-27	Locations of Osteochondritis Dissecans
Knee	
Medial condyle, lateral aspect (most common)	
Lateral condyle, inferior aspect	
Patella, medial facet	
Ankle	
Talus, lateral and medial aspects	
Foot	
Metatarsal head	
Shoulder	
Humeral head	
Elbow	
Capitellum	
Wrist	
Scaphoid, proximal pole	
Temporomandibular joint	

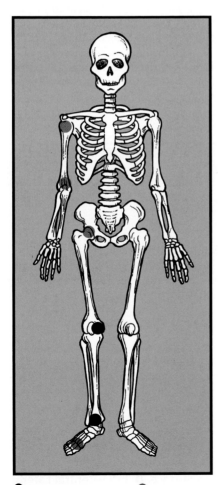

● More common   ● Less common

Figure 13-64 **SKELETAL DISTRIBUTION OF OSTEOCHONDRITIS DISSECANS.**

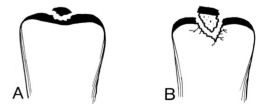

Figure 13-65 **FORMATION OF INTRA-ARTICULAR FRAGMENTS. A. Cartilaginous Only. B. Combination of Bone and Cartilage.** These fragments may be purely cartilaginous or a combination of bone and cartilage. Purely cartilaginous lesions will not be visible on conventional radiographs but are identifiable on arthrography and MRI.

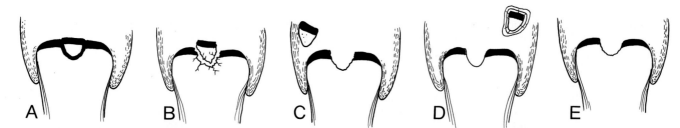

Figure 13-66 **FATE OF SEPARATED INTRA-ARTICULAR FRAGMENTS. A. Reattachment. B. Partial Separation and Displacement. C. Freely Mobile or Embedding into the Synovium. D. Continued Growth. E. Complete Resorption.**

The separated osteocartilaginous lesion has various possible fates: reattachment, displacement embedding into synovium or remaining free in the joint cavity, continued growth, or resorption. (Fig. 13-66) The term *joint mouse* has been used descriptively to identify the ability of the loose body to move elusively from one place to another.

Radiologic Features

Distinctively, two types of osteochondritis dissecans will be visible radiographically, based on whether the separated fragment is in close apposition to its site of origin (in situ) or if it has been separated and displaced. (Table 13-28) In situ types are characterized by the visualization of the separating, arc-like, radiolucent cleft between the underlying bone and resultant fragment. (55) (Table 13-29) This variety may revascularize, eventually reattach, and remain clinically silent. Conversely, the displaced variety is distinctive because of the localized concavity at the site of origin with a distant osteochondral fragment. On occasion, this

displaced osteochondral fragment may be resorbed or undergo enlargement by cartilage growth and calcification.

Target Sites of Involvement

Femoral Condyles. The most frequent site of osteochondritis dissecans is the femoral condyles. The condition may be bilateral in as many as 30% of cases. The medial condyle is affected in approximately 85% of cases. (55,56) The most characteristic location for the osteochondral defect is on the lateral aspect of the medial condyle. (57) Variations in the pattern of medial condyle involvement do occur but are less frequent. (58) (Fig. 13-67) A pathogenetic factor may be an enlarged anterior tibial spine or unusual stress at the attachment of the posterior cruciate ligament. (48) Lateral condylar defects are encountered in up to 15% of individuals and usually involve the central or posterior weight-bearing surface. (59,60) Lateral condylar lesions are generally more symptomatic and rapidly precipitate arthritic degenerative changes when compared with medial condylar lesions. (57) Normal variations in ossification of the articular margins of the femoral condyles can mimic osteochondritis dissecans between the ages of 4 and 12 years. (61)

Table 13-28	Pathologic-Radiologic Correlation in Osteochondritis Dissecans
Pathologic Feature	**Radiologic Feature**
Sequestered, necrotic fragment	Elliptical, dense fragment
Increased bone around defect	Sclerotic, concave border
Interposed fibrous tissue or separation	Radiolucent cleft

Table 13-29	Radiologic Features of Osteochondritis Dissecans
In situ	
Arclike radiolucent cleft	
Opposed and aligned fragment	
Displaced	
Concave defect at site of origin	
Displaced fragment (may resorb)	

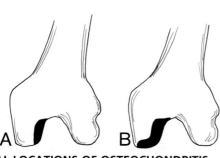
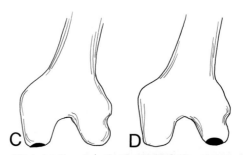

Figure 13-67 **FEMORAL LOCATIONS OF OSTEOCHONDRITIS DISSECANS. A. Classic Medial Condyle, Lateral Aspect (Most Common). B. Extended Classic Medial Condyle, Lateral and Weight-Bearing Surfaces. C. Inferocentral Medial Condyle, Weight-Bearing Surface. D. Inferocentral Lateral Condyle, Weight-Bearing Surface.** (Adapted from **Resnick D, Niwayama G:** *Diagnosis of Bone and Joint Disorders.* Philadelphia, WB Saunders, 1981.)

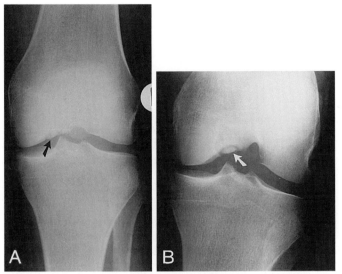

Figure 13-68 OSTEOCHONDRITIS DISSECANS: CLASSIC VARIETY. A. AP Knee. Observe the obscured defect and separated fragment (*arrow*). **B. Tunnel Projection, AP Knee.** Note that the radiologic details are clarified. Observe the in situ location of the fragment and smooth margin of the defect (*arrow*).

Radiographic depiction of osteochondritis dissecans depends on adequate views being taken, which must include the AP, tunnel, and lateral projections. The tunnel view often shows the abnormality when the AP view appears normal. (Figs. 13-68 and 13-69) MRI is useful in determining the activity of the lesion and its clinical significance. On T2-weighted images, an active defect will reveal a high-signal intensity, indicating an acute inflammatory response. (Fig. 13-70) Radiographically, the lesion is characterized by abnormalities at three areas: site of origin, the sequestered fragment, and the interposed zone between origin and fragment. On occasion, secondary degenerative joint disease may ensue.

Site of Origin. The femoral defect is usually concave and < 2 cm in size. Its margin is often sclerotic but may appear frayed and irregular. A sclerotic margin of ≥ 3 mm is associated with instability of the fragment in 50% of cases. (62) With time, the defect will be remodeled, being reduced in its depth to a shallower, more flattened contour. (Fig. 13-71)

Interposed Zone. Between the site of origin and the separated fragment, a radiolucent arc of variable thickness will be visible. With a closely opposed fragment, this radiolucent defect may be barely perceptible and may require tomography for demonstration. MRI can determine (*a*) fragment detachment, by the presence of a smooth high-signal zone; (*b*) partial detachment, in which the high intensity signal is irregular; and (*c*) attachment, by continuity of the signal across the interface. (63) Necrotic bone on MRI shows a decreased signal.

Sequestered Fragment. The separated ossicle is usually oval in shape. Its margins are notably smooth, unless the cartilage has begun to calcify, which may render the surface apparently irregular and even laminated. (Fig. 13-72) Internally, the ossific tissue can be sclerotic and fragmented, while at other times it may appear relatively normal in density and architecture. The most notable feature of the isolated fragment is its ability to be mobile within the joint and be found in a location quite distant from its site of origin. This is the most symptomatic feature of the disorder and requires surgical removal. Lesions < 2 mm are usually stable, whereas those > 8 mm are generally unstable. (62) On isotopic bone scan the greater the uptake, the more likely the fragment is unstable. (62) MRI is reliable for detecting loosening by identifying the presence of fluid between the interfaces and disruption of the overlying cartilage. (62)

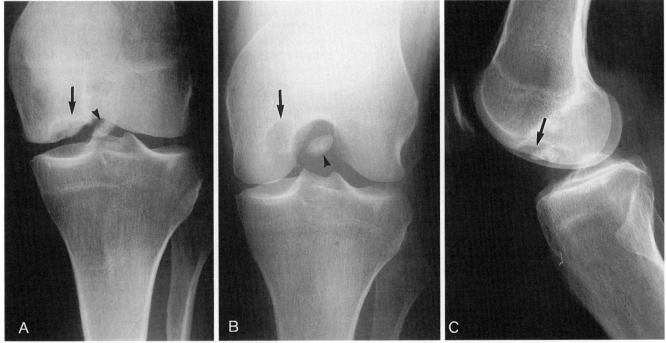

Figure 13-69 OSTEOCHONDRITIS DISSECANS: EXTENDED CLASSIC VARIETY. A. AP Knee. B. Tunnel Projection, AP Knee. Note the displaced fragment in the intercondylar notch (*arrowheads*). The defect exhibits a smooth sclerotic margin (*arrows*). **C. Lateral Knee.** Note the characteristic anterior location on the femoral surface (*arrow*).

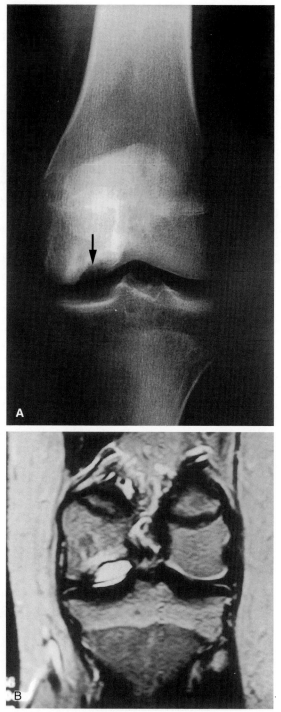

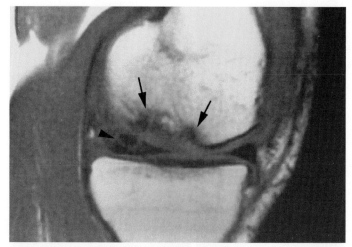

Figure 13-71 OSTEOCHONDRITIS DISSECANS. T1-Weighted MRI, Sagittal Knee. Note that the site of the crater is readily apparent, with areas of low signal intensity coinciding with necrotic bone (*arrows*). Observe the resultant irregular articular surface. A complex grade 3 tear of the posterior horn of the medial meniscus is evident (*arrowhead*), which is a common co-existing finding.

Secondary Degenerative Joint Disease. Osteochondritis dissecans does not necessarily predispose the patient to degenerative articular changes. However, in those individuals who develop osteochondritis dissecans after the growth plates have closed, there is an apparent greater predisposition to developing degenerative joint changes. (59) The pattern of involvement is atypical in that it appears to be premature in onset by approximately 10 years, precipitates a higher incidence of other loose bodies, and tends to involve all three joint compartments of the knee.

Talus. Osteochondral lesions of the talus are relatively frequent, especially in active individuals between the ages of 20 and 40 years. (48) The most common locations involve the dome of the talus at the medial and lateral aspects; central lesions occur occasionally. (64) A minimum of three projections should be applied: AP, 30° oblique, and lateral views. The AP view taken with the foot in plantar flexion enhances the depiction of the lesion. (65) In addition, CT and stress views may be useful, especially in subtle defects. MRI can predict accurately the stability of the fragment; detached fragments exhibit a high intensity, smooth linear signal at the bone–fragment interface, corresponding to fluid, versus a more irregular zone, representing partial attachment with granulation tissue. (66)

Medial Talar Osteochondritis Dissecans. The most common talar region to be involved is the medial surface. (65) The precipitating mechanism appears to be a combination of inversion, rotation, and plantar flexion. The effect is to apply a compressive, shearing force between the posterior lip of the tibia and opposing talar surface, which separates an osteochondral fragment from the medial posterior aspect. (67,68) Radiographically, the lesion may be quite subtle. (69) On AP and oblique views, the defect is visible as a 2- to 5-mm cavity at the medial corner of the talar dome. (70) (Fig. 13-73) Frequently, no imperfection in the smooth articular cortex may be visible, the lesion instead appearing as a well-defined cystic radiolucency 2–5 mm in size. The medial lesion is slightly larger in all dimensions than the lateral defect. Identification of the fragment may be difficult because it is frequently small and flake-like.

Figure 13-70 OSTEOCHONDRITIS DISSECANS: DISTAL FEMUR. A. AP Knee. Observe the subchondral radiolucent defect at the lateral margin of the medial condyle (*arrow*). **B. T2-Weighted MRI, Coronal Knee.** Note the subchondral defect, which shows bright signal intensity and correlates well with the plain film radiograph. The bright signal indicates an acute inflammatory response, suggesting clinical activity. *COMMENT:* Plain film radiographs, including CT studies, do not indicate whether the osteochondritis dissecans lesions are active or inactive. The MRI scan demonstrates focal marrow edema, guiding the clinician to the correct diagnosis of an *active* lesion and to proper patient management. (Courtesy of William J. Droege, DC, St. Louis, Missouri.)

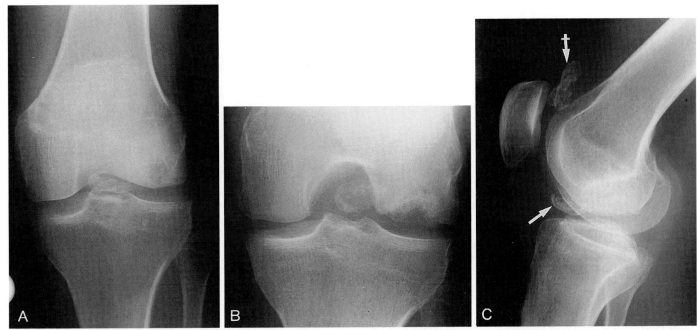

Figure 13-72   **OSTEOCHONDRITIS DISSECANS: MULTIPLE LAMINATED FRAGMENTS, LATERAL CONDYLE. A. AP Knee.** Note the laminated loose body within the intercondylar notch. The site of origin appears as a localized cystic radiolucent area within the lateral condyle. **B. Tunnel Projection, AP Knee.** Note that the surface of the defect is frayed and irreg-ular, which may be the reason for the production of multiple fragments. Note the loose body isolated within the intercondylar notch. **C. Lateral Knee.** Observe the loose body (*arrow*). The laminated calcification (*crossed arrow*) represents synovial chondrometaplasia.

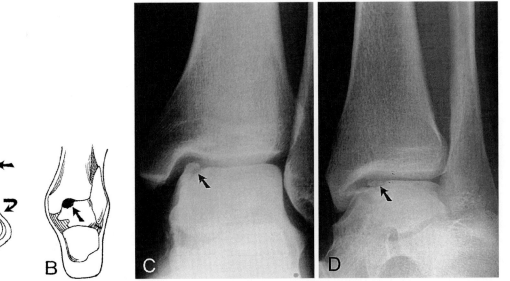

Figure 13-73   **OSTEOCHONDRITIS DISSECANS: MEDIAL TALAR DOME. A. Mechanism of Injury.** A combination of simultaneous plantar flexion, inversion, and rotation pushes the posterior tibial surface into the posteromedial talar dome (*arrows*). **B. Result of Injury.** A separated osteochondral fragment (*arrow*) is the product of this injury. **C. AP Ankle.** Note the small flake of articular bone from the talus (*arrow*). **D. Medial Oblique Ankle.** Note that the demarcation between the separated ossicle and the talus is better defined (*arrow*). (Adapted from **Berndt AL, Harty M:** *Transchondral fractures (osteochondritis dissecans) of the talus.* J Bone Joint Surg 41A:988, 1959.)

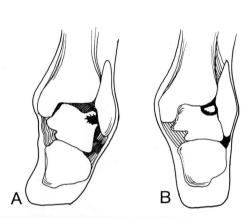

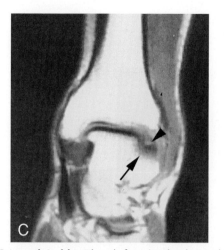

Figure 13-74 OSTEOCHONDRITIS DISSECANS: LATERAL TALAR DOME. A. Mechanism of Injury. Forceful inversion of the ankle pushes the lateral talar margin against the fibula, producing the separated osteochondral fragment. **B. Result of Injury.** The separated fragment is characteristically at the lateral corner of the talar dome. **C. T1-Weighted MRI,**

Coronal Ankle. The defect in the lateral talar dome is well seen (*arrow*). Observe the fragment located within the talar defect (*arrowhead*). (Adapted from **Berndt AL, Harty M:** *Transchondral fractures (osteochondritis dissecans) of the talus.* J Bone Joint Surg 41A:988, 1959.)

Lateral Talar Osteochondritis Dissecans. The major contributing movement is a forceful inversion that compresses the lateral talar border against the adjacent fibula. (69) (Fig. 13-74) When the fibular collateral ligaments are disrupted, there appears to be a greater chance for displacement of the disrupted fragment. On AP and oblique views, the defect is visible as a depression or cystic lucency of 1–2 mm in size. The separated fragment is thin and wafer shaped and often difficult to identify.

Other Sites. Osteochondritis dissecans can involve any joint surface that is traumatized with a shearing-compressive force. However, other than in the femoral condyles and talus, its occurrence is rare.

Hip. The most common location in the hip is the superior weight-bearing surface. A typical lucent concave defect is visible with an isolated fragment. Patients with previous Legg-Calvé-Perthes disease are predisposed to developing osteochondritis dissecans an average of 8 years after the onset of the disease. (71,72)

Patella. The patella is an uncommon site of osteochondritis dissecans. (73) The most likely cause is trauma, but localized vascular compromise may play a role. The usual site is at the medial facet of the patella, best seen on the axial (sunrise) and lateral projections. The concave patellar defect on the lateral view is adjacent to the convexity of the underlying femoral condyle. (74) (Fig. 13-75) Single or multiple fragments may be recognized within the patellofemoral joint space.

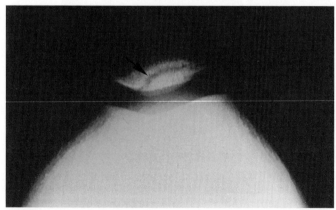

Figure 13-75 OSTEOCHONDRITIS DISSECANS. Skyline Knee Projection, Patella. Note the detached fragment adjacent to the lateral condylar surface (*arrow*). *COMMENT:* Such lesions are often smaller and less obvious than shown here and may consist of a small flake of bone. (Courtesy of Department of Radiology, Childrens Hospital, Denver, Colorado.)

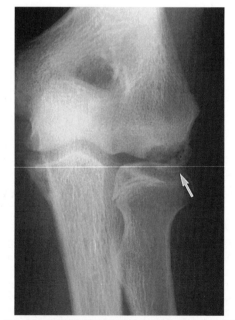

Figure 13-76 OSTEOCHONDRITIS DISSECANS: CAPITELLUM. AP Elbow. Note the separated bony fragment (*arrow*). The site of origin at the capitellum is represented by the cystic rarefaction and the frayed articular margin.

Foot. The most frequent sites in the foot involve the metatarsal heads, especially the first and second. In the second metatarsal, the osteochondral fragment is usually associated with Freiberg's ischemic necrosis. (75) In the first metatarsal, the lesion may be spontaneous or post-traumatic and is best seen on the dorsoplantar view as a small cup-like lucent depression, 1–3 mm, at the apex of the convex articular surface. Identification of the separated fragment may not be possible.

Shoulder. Rarely the humeral head may show a separation of a small subchondral segment at the convex margin opposing the glenoid cavity. This is frequently post-traumatic and may be the early forerunner to complete epiphyseal ischemic necrosis. Anterior dislocation of the humerus may precipitate a small subchondral fragment when the humeral head impacts onto the inferior glenoid rim (*Hill-Sachs lesion*).

Elbow. The capitellum of the humerus is the most common structure of the elbow involved. (76,77) It is particularly com-

mon in Little League pitchers and in children performing other throwing activities. (78) A cystic rarefaction will be visible on the convex surface, which may contain a bony flake of variable size. (Fig. 13-76) Occasionally, the separated fragment will be displaced distal to the capitellum defect, and it is usually more symptomatic. (79) If conservative treatment fails, removal of the fragment, excision of capitellar lesions, fragment fixation and curettage can be expected to reduce pain and improve functional capacity. (78,80)

Wrist. A rare site has been reported at the scaphoid, involving the proximal pole. (81) Trauma appears to have been the cause.

Temporomandibular Joint. Osteochondritis dissecans is a rare finding in the temporomandibular joint. The fragment is usually wholly composed of cartilage, which may calcify, rendering it identifiable on plain film examination. (82) The most definitive method of diagnosis is with MRI, though CT combined with an arthrogram will similarly demonstrate the lesion.

CAPSULE SUMMARY   Osteochondritis Dissecans

General Considerations

- A disorder of adolescence in which a small segment of subchondral bone undergoes ischemic necrosis secondary to trauma or a primary vascular occlusion.
- May heal spontaneously or form a loose body.

Clinical Features

- Occurs between 11 and 20 years, especially in males.
- Most common in the knee and ankle.
- *Variable symptomatology:* asymptomatic, acute pain, swelling, locking.

Pathologic Features

- Shearing, rotatory, or tangentially applied forces are key factors in producing a separated segmental area of subchondral bone and overlying cartilage (osteochondral fragment).
- Bone component may undergo ischemic necrosis.

Radiologic Features

- Dissected fragment may remain in close apposition (in situ) and even reattach.
- In other instances the fragment becomes detached (loose body).
- *Femoral condyles:* most common location of the disorder—85% at medial condyle, 15% at lateral condyle; most common at lateral aspect of medial condyle.
- *Talus:* more common on the medial surface; small lucent areas and separated fragments at corners of the talus.
- *Others:*
  Hip: superior weight-bearing surface and usually following Legg-Calvé-Perthes disease.
  Patella: involves medial facet.
  Foot: first and second metatarsal heads.
  Shoulder: humeral head.
  Elbow: capitellum convex surface.
  Wrist: rarely, lower pole of scaphoid.
  Temporomandibular joint: chondral loose body that may calcify.

GROWTH VARIANTS OF THE EPIPHYSES

Miscellaneous Osteonecroses

Blount's Disease

In 1937, Blount (1) observed a localized disturbance in growth of the medial proximal tibial epiphysis contributing to tibia vara. Two types are identified according to age: *infantile* (1–3 years) and *adolescent* (8–15 years).

The *infantile form* is up to five times more common and appears to be the result of abnormal compressive forces inhibiting

growth at the medial growth plate and not from avascular necrosis. (2,3) The condition is commonly bilateral. Radiographically, the medial epiphysis is wedge shaped, fragmented, or appears absent. (4) The adjacent metaphysis is also depressed and has a beak-like protuberance of rarefied bone oriented medially. (Fig. 13-77) The tibial shaft is in varus position secondary to the metaphyseal–epiphyseal abnormalities.

The *adolescent variety* usually begins between 3 and 15 years of age. It is far less frequent than the infantile variety and is distinctively unilateral. Inhibition of growth secondary to trauma of the medial epiphysis appears to be the origin of this disorder. Radiographically, the medial tibial epiphysis is wedge shaped, the growth plate is locally narrowed, and the diaphysis is angulated medially.

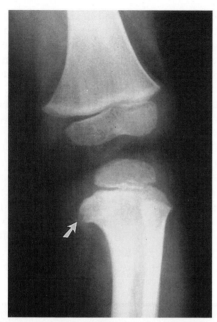

Figure 13-77 BLOUNT'S DISEASE: TIBIA VARA. AP Knee. Note the characteristic depressed and beak-like protuberance at the proximal medial tibial metaphysis (*arrow*). This lesion precipitates a varus deformity of the knee.

Calvé's Disease

In 1925 Calvé (5) advanced the concept that apparent spontaneous collapse of a solitary vertebral body in a child was the result of avascular necrosis. This has since been disproved by biopsy studies, which have demonstrated that the collapse is caused by an eosinophilic granuloma. (6) As such, the term Calvé's disease should not be used.

Diaz's Disease

Apparent idiopathic avascular necrosis of the talus was first described by Diaz in 1928. The disorder is most likely post-traumatic in origin, especially as a result of fractures through the neck of the talus or dislocations. (7,8) Oral corticosteroids and osteotomy for the correction of club foot can also precipitate the lesion. (9) Recently, several authors have suggested an association of talar avascular necrosis with hemophilia. (10) Irrespective of the cause, the talar body, which supports the tibiotalar articulating surface, is the usual site for necrosis to occur.

Radiographic signs appear within 1–3 months after the injury in the form of increased density, patchy radiolucency, and collapse of the articular surface. (Fig. 13-78) Signs following trauma that indicate preservation of the blood supply and unlikely secondary avascular necrosis are (*a*) the simultaneous appearance of disuse osteoporosis in the talus with other bones and (*b*) the early formation of a radiolucent band in the subarticular bone (*Hawkins' sign*). (11) (Fig. 13-79) It has been suggested that osteotomy of the talar neck not be performed on children < 10 years of age to reduce the possibility of Diaz's disease in these individuals. (9)

Hass' Disease

Hass in 1921 first described avascular necrosis of the humeral head. Currently, the humeral head represents the second most

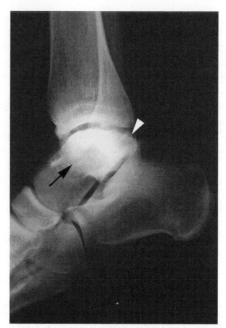

Figure 13-78 AVASCULAR NECROSIS: TALUS. Lateral Ankle. Observe the increased density of the talar dome extending to the articular surface (*arrow*). Collapse of the articular surface is evident with irregularity of the articular margin (*arrowhead*). *COMMENT:* These are characteristic findings for avascular necrosis, the cause in this case being secondary to corticosteroids.

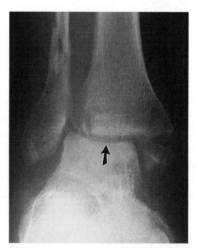

Figure 13-79 HAWKINS' SIGN: TALUS. AP Ankle. Note that after fracture the subchondral talar linear radiolucency (*arrow*) is a good prognostic sign that ischemic necrosis will not likely occur.

common location for avascular necrosis, following the femoral head. (12) As in the femoral head, the vascular supply to the humeral head renders it susceptible to necrosis. (Fig. 13-80) The three major perfusing vessels are the arcuate artery (entering the head in the bicipital groove), branches from the posterior circumflex, and the rotator cuff (which enters at the tendinous insertions of these muscles). (13,14) Obstruction of the muscular insertion supply and arcuate artery will precipitate necrosis. The radiographic findings parallel those in the femoral head, with patchy sclerosis and lucency, curvilinear subchondral fracture

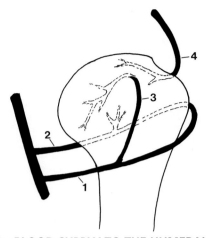

Figure 13-80 **BLOOD SUPPLY TO THE HUMERAL HEAD.** The major vessels are the anterior circumflex artery (*1*), posterior circumflex artery (*2*), arcuate artery (*3*), and rotator cuff arteries (*4*).

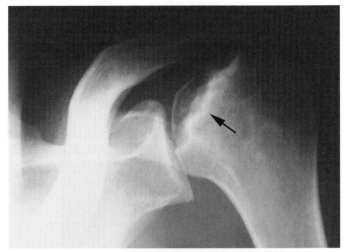

Figure 13-82 **AVASCULAR NECROSIS. Humeral Head.** Note the collapse of the humeral head, with radiolucency, surrounding sclerosis (*arrow*), and irregularity of the articular surface. *COMMENT:* These are characteristic findings for avascular necrosis at this site. The patient was receiving corticosteroid therapy for Crohn's disease.

(*crescent sign*), and depression of the articular cortex. (Figs. 13-81 and 13-82) Osseous collapse is less severe than in the femoral head. The most common predisposing factors are fractures, dislocations, corticosteroids, and hemoglobin disorders. (15) Core decompression procedures and débridement are the treatments of choice early in the disease (15), whereas patients in later stages and those cases involving a greater extent of the humeral head usually require arthroplasty. (16)

Köhler's Disease

In 1908 Köhler first described a disorder with features of avascular necrosis involving the tarsal navicular. (17) Confusion exists as to whether these changes are the result of vascular insufficiency or a normal growth variation because identical-appearing but clinically insignificant changes may be seen bilaterally. (18,19) Diagnosis, therefore, is the combination of localized clinical and radiologic manifestations. Clinically, males are affected predominantly, usually at about 5 years of age. Local pain, swelling, tenderness, and decreased motion are present. (20)

Radiologic expressions in the navicular may show patchy or homogenous sclerosis, collapse, and fragmentation. (21) (Fig. 13-83) The joint spaces are preserved as a reflection of cartilage

non-involvement. Isotopic bone scans show increased or absent uptake, depending on the stage of the disease, and are a useful diagnostic medium in the differentiation from a normal variation in ossification. (22) After healing, reconstitution of the navicular to a normal radiographic appearance and complete resolution of symptoms are to be expected.

Kümmell's Disease

Delayed collapse of a vertebral body subsequent to trauma was described by German surgeon Hermann Kümmell in 1891. (23,24) Various causes have been suggested, including nutritional disturbances, vascular abnormalities, and abnormal healing. The most accepted theory appears to be progression of collapse secondary to additional trauma or from a previously unrecognized fracture. (25,26) This is not an avascular necrosis and is an infrequently encountered entity. Radiologically, following the initial trauma, slight or no signs of vertebral body fracture will be present. Within a period of weeks, rapid and severe compression

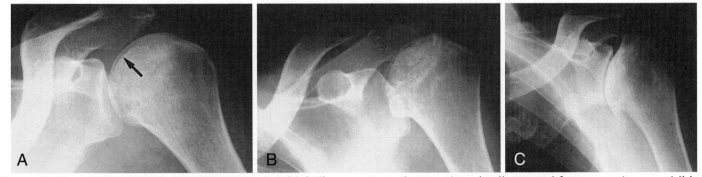

Figure 13-81 **HASS' DISEASE: PROGRESSION. A. Initial Film.** Note the patchy sclerosis and lucency in the humeral head in this 35-year-old female who presented with shoulder pain. A *crescent sign* is also evident (*arrow*). **B. 1-Year Follow-Up.**

Note that continued collapse and fragmentation are visible. **C. 5-Year Follow-Up.** Note that the entire head is deformed, with superimposed degenerative joint disease.

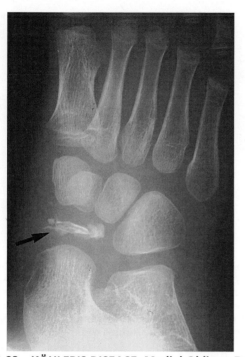

Figure 13-83 **KÖHLER'S DISEASE. Medial Oblique Foot.** Note that the tarsal navicular is collapsed, sclerotic, and fragmented (*arrow*). *COMMENT:* The same appearance can represent a normal growth variation but lacks the clinical features of pain and swelling.

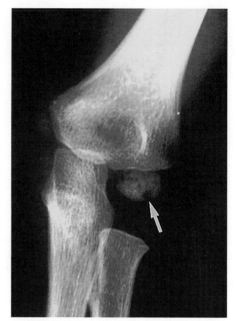

Figure 13-84 **PANNER'S DISEASE. AP Elbow.** Note that the entire capitellum is fragmented with numerous intraosseous cystic and linear areas (*arrow*). The articular surface is also irregular and collapsed. *COMMENT:* This constellation of radiographic findings is characteristic of avascular necrosis involving the entire capitellum.

of the body will occur. (27,28) Ischemic necrosis of the vertebral body as a separate entity is rare and is most commonly associated with thromboembolic disease or corticosteroids. A diagnostic sign of ischemic necrosis is the appearance of the radiolucent vacuum within a collapsed vertebral body (*intravertebral vacuum cleft sign*). (29) Previously, it was suggested that the intravertebral vacuum cleft was always linear in nature; however, recent data have suggested that its appearance is dynamic and may alter in shape and size. (30) Treatment options often include vertebroplasty or stabilization. (30)

Mauclaire's Disease

In 1928, Mauclaire (31) described avascular necrosis of the metacarpal head. This is an uncommon disorder and is most likely post-traumatic in nature (32,33); however, associations with systemic lupus erythematosus and steroid use have been noted. (34) Any of the metacarpals can be affected and progressive collapse of the metacarpal head should be expected; however, spontaneous resolution has been noted. (34) Imaging findings reveal the characteristic signs related to osteonecrosis of any other bone. (34)

Panner's Disease

Avascular necrosis of the capitellum of the distal humerus was first described in 1927 by Panner. (35) Males between the ages of 4 and 10 years are affected almost exclusively. Repetitive trauma, such as in ball-throwing sports, appears instrumental

in precipitating the disease. Localized pain, swelling, stiffness, and flexion contracture may be prominent. Radiologically, the features in the capitellum are comparable to those seen in the femoral capital epiphysis, with sequential sclerosis, fissuring, fragmentation, collapse, and reossification. (36–39) (Fig. 13-84) Distinctively, the entire epiphysis is involved, which distinguishes the condition from osteochondritis dissecans. The trochlear epiphysis less frequently undergoes similar changes. (40) Hyperemia may result in an enlarged radial head and premature epiphyseal fusion. Clinical and radiologic healing is usually evident within 2 years.

Preiser's Disease

In 1910 George Preiser (41) reported necrosis of the entire scaphoid unassociated with fracture; however, scrutiny of his presented cases casts doubt that the disease represents a separate entity because an ununited fracture line is visible. (42) Osteonecrosis of the proximal pole of the scaphoid with and without fracture has been reported. (42) (Fig. 13-85) In the current literature, reports of avascular non-traumatic necrosis of the scaphoid have been idiopathic in nature or associated with metabolic causes. (43)

Sever's Disease

The association between heel pain and irregular ossification of the calcaneal apophysis was first described by Sever in 1912. (44) Later investigations delineated the radiographic apophyseal

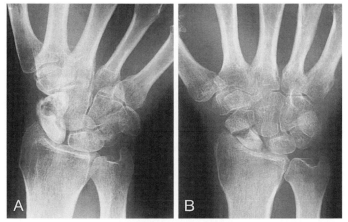

Figure 13-85 **PREISER'S DISEASE. A. PA Wrist, Scaphoid.** Note that the scaphoid is homogeneously increased in density and contains a large subchondral cyst. No definite cause was elicited. **B. PA Wrist, Proximal Pole Scaphoid.** Observe that the proximal pole of the scaphoid is sclerotic. Observe the ununited fracture through the waist of the scaphoid. *COMMENT:* This form of postfracture avascular necrosis is far more common and is not accurately termed Preiser's disease.

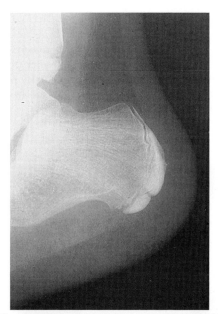

Figure 13-86 **NORMAL CALCANEAL APOPHYSIS VARIANT (SEVER'S DISEASE).** Note that the calcaneal apophysis is densely sclerotic and appears fragmented. *COMMENT:* This is a common growth variation and not the avascular necrosis seen in ambulant children and young adolescents. Typically, it is bilateral but often asymmetric with two or more ossification centers.

irregularities to be a variation in the normal ossification process. (45,46) The apophysis ossifies from several nuclei between the ages of 4 and 10 years and gradually coalesces to form the definitive apophysis. Normally, this apophysis is dense. (47) As such, a fragmented, irregular sclerotic calcaneal apophysis should be considered normal, and the concept of Sever's disease should be eliminated. (Fig. 13-86) Apophysitis as a result of mechanical irritation is the more reasonable diagnosis. (47)

Sinding-Larsen-Johansson Disease

Independent descriptions by Sinding-Larsen in 1921 and Johansson in 1922 delineated an association with pain and osseous fragmentation of the lower patella. (48,49) The syndrome is usually found in males between the ages of 10 and 14 years. Pain, soft tissue swelling, tenderness, limping, and inability to run are the most prominent clinical features. The lesion appears to be related to a traction-induced avulsion of the inferior pole development center or to post-traumatic patella ligament ossification. (50) Osgood-Schlatter disease may co-exist. (51) Radiographically, bone fragments are visible adjacent to the lower pole of the patella, with overlying soft tissue swelling. These fragments may eventually reincorporate into the patella or remain as free ossicles. Clinical resolution usually occurs within 12 months.

Thiemann's Disease

In 1909, Thiemann (52) described an uncommon disorder affecting the epiphyseal centers at the bases of the phalanges of the hands. (52) Although not clearly delineated, the pathogenesis appears to be owing to avascular necrosis, possibly from trauma. (53,54)

Van Neck's Disease

Variations in the appearance of the developing ischiopubic synchondrosis were inappropriately identified by van Neck in 1924 as resulting from avascular necrosis. (55) Correlated pathologic, clinical, and radiologic studies have shown these altered ossification patterns to be a normal variation in the ossification process and not an ischemic necrosis of bone. (56) Radiographically, the opposing ends of the ischium and inferior pubic ramus may be irregular and suggest an expansile destruction of bone. (Fig. 13-87) This developmental variant is usually bilateral but asymmetric.

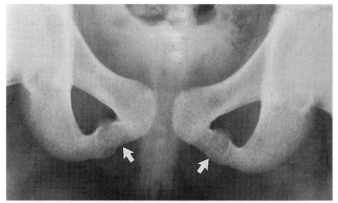

Figure 13-87 **ISCHIOPUBIC SYNCHONDROSIS VARIANT (VAN NECK'S DISEASE). AP Pelvis.** Observe the expansile growth variation bilaterally (*arrows*). It should not be confused with osteonecrosis. *COMMENT:* This was originally thought by van Neck to represent an ischemic necrosis; however, it is a normal developmental variant.

Miscellaneous Sites

Other uncommon possible sites of avascular necrosis include the distal ulna, distal tibia, bilateral carpus, greater trochanter, base of the fifth metatarsal, tibial eminences, primary patellar center, ischial apophysis, iliac crest, radial head, and hallux sesamoid bones. (57–65) (Fig. 13-88)

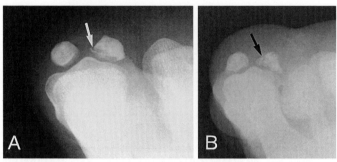

Figure 13-88 HALLUX SESAMOID BONES: AVASCULAR NECROSIS. A. Crescent Sign. Note the linear zone of radiolucency, representing a subchondral fracture, is seen (*arrow*). The remainder of the medial sesamoid is densely sclerotic. **B. Fragmentation.** Observe the medial sesamoid, which is increased in density, compressed in configuration, and exhibits a fracture (*arrow*).

CAPSULE SUMMARY
Miscellaneous Osteonecroses

General Considerations

- Considerable confusion in the nomenclature of epiphyseal disorders.
- *Three general groups:* osteonecrosis (primary, secondary), trauma, growth variations.

Clinical Features

- Usually between 3 and 10 years of age; boys more commonly.
- *Symptoms:* pain, swelling, reduced motion, muscle atrophy.
- Self-limiting disease, but may be a source of disability and premature degenerative joint disease.

Pathologic Features

- *Four basic phases:*
  Avascular: bone death.
  Revascularization: deposition and resorption.
  Repair: deposition, remodeling.
  Deformity: residual altered configuration.
- *Many causes:* trauma, sickle cell anemia, Gaucher's disease, corticosteroids, alcoholism, others.

Radiologic Features

- *Most frequent signs:* collapse of the articular cortex, fragmentation, sclerosis, mottled trabecular pattern, subchondral cysts, subchondral fracture.

■ *References*

HEMATOLOGIC DISORDERS

1. **Moseley JE:** *Skeletal changes in the anemias.* Semin Roentgenol 9(3):169, 1974.
2. **Agarwal KN, Dhar N, Shah MM, et al.:** *Roentgenologic changes in iron deficiency anemia.* AJR 110:635, 1970.
3. **Moseley JE:** *Skull changes in chronic iron deficiency anemia.* AJR 85:649, 1961.

SICKLE CELL ANEMIA

1. **Herrick JB:** *Peculiar elongated and sickle shaped red blood corpuscles in a case of severe anemia.* Arch Int Med 6:517, 1910.
2. **Leong CS, Stark P:** *Thoracic manifestations of sickle cell disease.* J Thorac Imaging 13(2):128, 1998.
3. **Marlowe KF, Chicella MF:** *Treatment of sickle cell pain.* Pharmacotherapy 22(4):484, 2002.
4. **Reynolds J:** *Radiologic manifestations of sickle cell hemoglobinopathy.* JAMA 238:247, 1977.
5. **Cockshott WP:** *Dactylitis and growth disorders.* Br J Radiol 36:19, 1964.
6. **Watson RJ, Burko H, Megas H, et al.:** *Hand-foot syndrome in sickle cell disease in young children.* Pediatrics 31:975, 1963.
7. **Barrett-Connor E:** *Bacterial infection and sickle cell anemia. An analysis of 250 infections in 166 patients and a review of the literature.* Medicine 50:97, 1971.
8. **Hook EW, Campell CG, Weens HS, et al.:** *Salmonella osteomyelitis in patients with sickle cell anemia.* N Engl J Med 257:403, 1957.
9. **Sebes JI:** *Diagnostic imaging of bone and joint abnormalities associated with sickle cell hemoglobinopathies.* AJR 152:1153, 1989.
10. **Mukisi-Mukaza M, Elbaz A, Samuel-Leborgne Y, et al.:** *Prevalence, clinical features, and risk factors of osteonecrosis of the femoral head among adults with sickle cell disease.* Orthopedics 23(4):357, 2000.
11. **Ataga KI, Orringer EP:** *Bone marrow necrosis in sickle cell disease: a description of three cases and a review of the literature.* Am J Med Sci 320(5):342, 2000.
12. **McCall IW, Vidya S, Serjeant GR:** *Splenic opacification in homozygous sickle cell disease.* Clin Radiol 32(6):611, 1981.
13. **Haque AK, Gokhale S, Rampy BA, et al.:** *Pulmonary hypertension in sickle cell hemoglobinopathy: A clinicopathologic study of 20 cases.* Hum Pathol 33(10):1037, 2002.
14. **Falk RH, Hood WB:** *The heart in sickle cell anemia.* Arch Int Med 142(9):1680, 1982.
15. **Flye MW, Silver D:** *Biliary tract disorders and sickle cell disease.* Surgery 72:361, 1972.
16. **Phillips JC, Gerald BE:** *The incidence of cholelithiasis in sickle cell disease.* AJR 113:27, 1971.
17. **Lonergan GJ, Cline DB, Abbondanzo SL:** *Sickle cell anemia.* Radiographics 21(4):971, 2001.
18. **Telen MJ:** *Principles and problems of transfusion in sickle cell disease.* Semin Hematol 38(4):315, 2001.
19. **Williams WJ, Butler E, Ersley AJ, et al.:** *Hematology,* ed 2. New York, McGraw Hill, 1977.
20. **O'Hara AE:** *Roentgenographic osseous manifestations of the anemias and leukemias.* Clin Orthop 52:63, 1967.
21. **Gelpi AP, Perrine RP:** *Sickle cell disease trait in white populations.* JAMA 224:605, 1973.
22. **Ennis JT:** *The radiologic pattern of bone infarction in the hemoglobinopathies.* Br J Radiol 51:71, 1978.
23. **Resnick D:** *Fish vertebrae.* Arthritis Rheum 25(9):1073, 1982.
24. **Reynolds J:** *A re-evaluation of the "fish vertebra" sign in sickle cell hemoglobinopathy.* AJR 97:693, 1966.
25. **Schwartz AM, Homer HJ, McCauley RG:** *"Step-off" vertebral body: Gaucher's disease versus sickle cell hemoglobinopathy.* AJR 132:81, 1979.
26. **Carrol DS, Evans JW:** *Roentgen findings in sickle cell anemia.* Radiology 53:834, 1949.

27. **Sebes JI, Diggs LW:** *Radiographic changes of the skull in sickle cell anemia.* AJR 132 (3):373, 1979.
28. **Legant O, Ball RP:** *Sickle cell anemia in adults.* Radiology 51:665, 1948.
29. **Bonnerot V, Sebag G, de Montalembert M, et al.:** *Gadolinium-DOTA enhanced MRI of painful osseous crises in children with sickle cell anemia.* Pediatr Radiol 24:92, 1994.
30. **Amundsen TR, Siegel MJ, Siegel BA:** *Osteomyelitis and infarction in sickle cell hemoglobinopathies: Differentiation by combined technetium and gallium scintigraphy.* Radiology 153:807, 1984.
31. **Leichtman DA, Bigongiari LR, Wicks JD:** *The incidence and significance of tibiotalar slant in sickle cell anemia.* Skeletal Radiol 3:99, 1978.
32. **Martinez S, Apple JS, Baber C, et al.:** *Protrusio acetabuli in sickle cell anemia.* Radiology 151:43, 1984.
33. **Chung SMK, Ralston EL:** *Necrosis of the femoral head associated with sickle cell anemia and its variants.* J Bone Joint Surg 51A:33, 1969.
34. **Sebes JI, Kraus AP:** *Avascular necrosis of the hip in the sickle cell hemoglobinopathies.* J Can Assoc Radiol 34(2):136, 1983.
35. **Porat S, Brezis M, Kopolovic J:** *Salmonella typhi osteomyelitis long after a fracture.* J Bone Joint Surg 59A:687, 1977.
36. **Murray RO, Jacobson HG:** *The Radiology of Skeletal Disorders,* ed 2. New York, Churchill Livingstone, 1977.
37. **Cassady JR, Berdon WE, Baker DH:** *The "typical" spinal changes of sickle cell anemia in a patient with thalassemia major (Cooley's anemia).* Radiology 89:1065, 1967.
38. **Hansen GC, Gold RH:** *Central depression of multiple vertebral body end plates; a "pathognomonic" sign of sickle hemoglobinopathy in Gaucher's disease.* AJR 129:343, 1977.
39. **Rolfing BM:** *Vertebral end plate depression: Report of two patients without hemoglobinopathy.* AJR 128:599, 1977.
40. **Golding JS, MacIver JE, Went LN:** *Bone changes in sickle cell anemia and its genetic variants.* J Bone Joint Surg 41B:711, 1959.
41. **Emodi JI, Okoye IJ:** *Vertebral bone collapse in sickle cell disease: a report of two cases.* East Afr Med J 78(8):445, 2001.
42. **Marlow TJ, Brunson CY, Jackson S, Schabel SI:** *"Tower vertebra": A new observation in sickle cell disease.* Skeletal Radiol 27(4):195, 1998.
43. **Mandell G, Kricun ME:** *Exaggerated anterior vertebral notching.* Radiology 131:367, 1979.

THALASSEMIA
1. **Rund D, Rachmilewitz E:** *New trends in the treatment of beta-thalassemia.* Crit Rev Oncol Hematol 33(2):105, 2000.
2. **Issaragrisil S:** *Stem cell transplantation for thalassemia.* Int J Hematol 76(Suppl 1):307, 2002.
3. **Cooley TB, Lee P:** *A series of cases of splenomegaly in children with anemia and peculiar bone changes.* Trans Am Pediatr Soc 37:29, 1925.
4. **Modell B:** *Management of thalassemia major.* Br Med Bull 32:270, 1976.
5. **Mosley JE:** *Skeletal changes in the anemias.* Semin Roentgenol 9(3):169, 1974.
6. **Onur O, Sivri A, Gumruk F, Altay C:** *Beta thalassaemia: A report of 20 children.* Clin Rheumatol 18(1):42, 1999.
7. **Angelucci E, Brittenham GM, McLaren CE, et al.:** *Hepatic iron concentration and total body iron stores in thalassemia major.* N Engl J Med 343(5):327, 2000.
8. **Olivieri N:** *Thalassaemia: Clinical management.* Baillieres Clin Haematol 11(1):147, 1998.
9. **Chan LL, Lin HP, Ariffn WA, Ariffin H:** *Providing a cure for beta thalassanemias major.* Med J Malaysia 56(4):435, 2001.
10. **Khandelwahl N, Malik N, Khosla VK, et al.:** *Spinal cord compression due to epidural extramedullary hematopoiesis in thalassemia.* Pediatr Radiol 22:70, 1992.
11. **Williams WJ, Butler E, Ersley AJ et al.:** *Hematology,* ed 2. New York, McGraw-Hill, 1977.

12. **Clarke GM, Higgins TN:** *Laboratory investigation of hemoglobinopathies and thalassemias: Review and update.* Clin Chem 46(8):1284, 2000.
13. **Caffey J:** *Cooley's erythroblastic anemia. Some skeletal findings in adolescents and young adults.* AJR 65(4):547, 1951.
14. **Caffey J:** *Cooley's anemia: A review of the roentgenographic findings in the skeleton.* AJR 78:381, 1957.
15. **Long JA Jr, Doppman JL, Nienhaus AW:** *Computed tomographic studies of thoracic extramedullary hematopoiesis.* J Comput Assist Tomogr 4:67, 1980.
16. **Tunaci M, Tanaci A, Engin G, et al.:** *Imaging features of thalassemia.* Eur Radiol 9(9):1804, 1999.
17. **Lawson JP, Ablow RC, Pearson HA:** *Calvarial and phalangeal vascular impressions in thalassemia.* AJR 143:641, 1984.
18. **Currarino G, Erlandson ME:** *Premature fusion of epiphyses in Cooley's anemia.* Radiology 83:656, 1964.
19. **Dines DM, Canale VC, Arnold WD:** *Fractures in thalassemia.* J Bone Joint Surg 58A:662, 1976.
20. **Winchester PH, Cerwin R, Dische R, et al.:** *Hemosiderin laden lymph nodes. An unusual roentgenographic manifestation of homozygous thalassemia.* AJR 118:222, 1973.
21. **Sella EJ, Goodman AH:** *Arthropathy secondary to transfusion hemochromatosis.* J Bone Joint Surg 55A:1077, 1973.
22. **Orzincolo C, Castaldi G, Scutellari PN, et al.:** *Aseptic necrosis of femoral head complicating thalassemia.* Skeletal Radiol 15:541, 1986.
23. **Orzincolo C, Castaldi G, Bariani L, et al.:** *Circumscribed lytic lesions of the thalassemic skull.* Skeletal Radiol 17:344, 1988.
24. **Cassady JR, Berdon WE, Baker DH:** *The "typical" spinal changes of sickle cell anemia in a patient with thalassemia major (Cooley's anemia).* Radiology 89:1065, 1967.
25. **Mandell GA, Kricun ME:** *Exaggerated anterior vertebral notching.* Radiology 131:367, 1979.
26. **Epstein B:** *The Spine,* ed 4. Philadelphia, Lea & Febiger, 1976.
27. **Alorainy IA, Al-Asmi AR, del Carpio R:** *MRI features of epidural extramedullary hematopoiesis.* Eur J Radiol 35(1):8, 2000.
28. **Tsitouridis J, Stamos S, Hassapopoulou E, et al.:** *Extramedullary paraspinal hematopoiesis in thalassemia: CT and MRI evaluation.* Eur J Radiol 30(1):33, 1999.
29. **Chourmouzi D, Pistevou-Gompaki K, Plataniotis G, et al.:** *MRI findings of extramedullary haemopoiesis.* Eur Radiol 11(9):1803, 2001.
30. **Korsten J, Grossman H, Winchester P, et al.:** *Extramedullary hematopoiesis in patients with thalassemia anemia.* Radiology 95:257, 1970.
31. **Ross P, Logan W:** *Roentgen findings in extramedullary hematopoiesis.* AJR 106 (3):604, 1969.

HEMOPHILIA
1. **Webb JB, Dixon AS:** *Haemophilia and haemophilic arthropathy. An historical review and a clinical study of 42 cases.* Ann Rheum Dis 19:143, 1960.
2. **Kemnitz S, Moens P, Peerlinck K, Fabry G:** *Avascular necrosis of the talus in children with haemophilia.* J Pediatr Orthop B 11(1):73, 2002.
3. **Avina-Zubieta JA, Galindo-Rodriquez G, Lavalle C:** *Rheumatic manifestations of hematologic disorders.* Curr Opin Rheumatol 10(1):86, 1998.
4. **Alcalay M, Deplas A:** *Rheumatological management of patients with hemophilia. Part II: Muscle hematomas and pseudotumors.* Joint Bone Spine 69(5):556, 2002.
5. **Alcalay M, Deplas A:** *Rheumatological management of patients with hemophilia. Part 1: Joint manifestations.* Joint Bone Spine 69(5):442, 2002.
6. **Rodriquez-Merchan EC, Magallon M, Galindo E, Lopez-Cabarcos C:** *Hemophilic synovitis of the knee and elbow.* Clin Orthop 343:47, 1997.
7. **Ishiguro N, Takagi H, Ito T, et al.:** *Rapidly destructive arthropathy of the hip in haemophilia.* Haemophilia 7(1):127, 2001.

8. **Monahan PE, White GC II:** *Hemophilia gene therapy: Update.* Curr Opin Hematol 9(5):430, 2002.
9. **Petrini P:** *Treatment strategies in children with hemophilia.* Paediatr Drugs 4(7):427, 2002.
10. **DePalma AF:** *Hemophilic arthropathy.* Clin Orthop 52:145, 1967.
11. **Mainardi CL, Levine PH, Werb Z, et al.:** *Proliferative synovitis in hemophilia. Biochemical and morphologic observations.* Arthritis Rheum 21:137, 1978.
12. **Rodnan GP, Brower TD, Hellstrom HR, et al.:** *Postmortem examination of an elderly severe hemophiliac, with observations on the pathologic findings in hemophilic joint disease.* Arthritis Rheum 2:152, 1959.
13. **Arnold WD, Hilgartner MW:** *Hemophilic arthropathy. Current concepts of pathogenesis and management.* J Bone Joint Surg 59A:287, 1977.
14. **Yulish BS, Lieberman JM, Strandjord SE, et al.:** *Hemophilic arthropathy: Assessment with MR imaging.* Radiology 164:759, 1987.
15. **Hermann G, Gilbert MS, Abdelwahab IF:** *Hemophilia: Evaluation of musculoskeletal involvement with CT, sonography, and MR imaging.* AJR 158:119, 1992.
16. **Brant EE, Jordan HH:** *Radiologic aspects of hemophilic pseudotumors in bone.* AJR 115:525, 1972.
17. **Ishiguro N, Iwahori Y, Kato T, et al.:** *The surgical treatment of a haemophilic pseudotumour in an extremity: A report of three cases with pathological fractures.* Haemophilia 4(2):126, 1998.
18. **Ahlberg AKM:** *On the natural history of hemophiliac pseudotumor.* J Bone Joint Surg 57A:1133, 1975.
19. **Wilson DA, Prince JR:** *MR imaging of hemophilic pseudotumors.* AJR 150:349, 1988.
20. **Gilchrist GS, Hagedorn AB, Stauffer RN:** *Severe degenerative joint disease. Mild and moderately severe hemophilia A.* JAMA 238:2383, 1977.
21. **Feil E, Bentley G, Rizza CR:** *Fracture management in patients with hemophilia.* J Bone Joint Surg 56B:643, 1974.
22. **Hutcheson J:** *Peripelvic new bone formation in hemophilia.* Radiology 109:529, 1973.
23. **Jensen PS, Putman CE:** *Chondrocalcinosis and haemophilia.* Clin Radiol 28:401, 1977.
24. **Houghton GR:** *Septic arthritis of the hip in a hemophiliac. Report of a case.* Clin Orthop 129:223, 1977.
25. **Handelsman JE:** *The knee joint in hemophilia.* Orthop Clin North Am 10:139, 1979.
26. **Chlosta EM, Kuhns LR, Holt JF:** *The "patella ratio" in hemophilia and juvenile rheumatoid arthritis.* Radiology 116:137, 1975.
27. **Zimbler S, McVerry B, Levine P:** *Hemophiliac arthropathy of the foot and ankle.* Orthop Clin North Am 7:985, 1976.

MYELOPROLIFERATIVE DISEASES

CHILDHOOD LEUKEMIA

1. **Simmons CR, Harle TS, Singleton EB:** *The osseous manifestations of leukemia in children.* Radiol Clin North Am 6:115, 1968.
2. **Parker BR:** *Leukemia and lymphoma in childhood.* Radiol Clin North Am 35(6):1495, 1997.
3. **Carriere B, Cummins-Mcmanus B:** *Vertebral fractures as initial signs for acute lymphoblastic leukemia.* Pediatr Emerg Care 17(4):258, 2001.
4. **Van Slyck EJ:** *The bony changes in malignant hematologic disease.* Orthop Clin North Am 3:733, 1972.
5. **Thomas LB, Forkner CE, Frei E, et al.:** *The skeletal lesions of acute leukemia.* Cancer 14:608, 1961.
6. **Benz G, Brandeis WE, Willich E:** *Radiological aspects of leukemia in childhood. An analysis of 89 children.* Pediatr Radiol 4:201, 1976.
7. **Austin HM:** *Chloroma. Report of a patient with an unusual rib lesion.* Radiology 93:671, 1969.
8. **Epstein BS:** *Vertebral changes in childhood leukemia.* Radiology 68:65, 1957.
9. **Gerard EL, Ferry JA, Amrein PC, et al.:** *Compositional changes in vertebral bone marrow during treatment for acute leukemia: Assessment with quantitative chemical shift imaging.* Radiology 183:39, 1992.

ADULT LEUKEMIA

1. **Burnett AK:** *Acute myeloid leukemia: Treatment of adults under 60 years.* Rev Clin Exp Hematol 6:26, 2002. [Discussion 6:86, 2002.]
2. **Schabel SI, Tyminski L, Holland RD, et al.:** *The skeletal manifestations of chronic myelogenous leukemia.* Skeletal Radiol 5:145, 1980.

MYELOFIBROSIS

1. **Guermazi A, de Kerviler E, Cazals-Hatem D, et al.:** *Imaging findings in patients with myelofibrosis.* Eur Radiol 9(7):1366, 1999.
2. **Gauroncle BA, Doan CA:** *Myelofibrosis, clinical, hematologic and pathologic study of 110 patients.* Am J Med Sci 243:697, 1962.
3. **Pullarkat V, Bass RD, Gong JZ, et al.:** *Primary autoimmune myelofibrosis: Definition of a distinct clinicopathologic syndrome.* Am J Hematol 72(1):8, 2003.
4. **Olipitz W, Behan-Schmid C, Aigner R, et al.:** *Acute myelofibrosis: Multifocal bone marrow infiltration detected by scintigraphy and magnetic resonance imaging.* Ann Hematol 79(5):275, 2000.
5. **Pettigrew JD, Ward HP:** *Correlation of radiologic, histologic and clinical findings in agnogenic myeloid metaplasia.* Radiology 93:541, 1969.
6. **Feldman F:** *Myelosclerosis in agnogenic metaplasia.* Semin Roentgenol 9:195, 1974.
7. **Cromwell LD, Kerber C:** *Spinal cord compression by extramedullary hematopoiesis in agnogenic myeloid metaplasia.* Radiology 128:118, 1978.

OSTEONECROSIS

PERSPECTIVES ON OSTEONECROSIS

1. **Donaldson WF Jr, Rodriguez EE, Shovron M, et al.:** *Traumatic dislocation of the hip in children. Final report by the Scientific Research Committee of the Pennsylvania Orthopedic Society.* J Bone Joint Surg 50A:79, 1968.
2. **Jones JP Jr, Jameson RM, Engelman EP:** *Alcoholism, fat embolism and avascular necrosis* [Abstract]. J Bone Joint Surg 50A:1065, 1968.
3. **Hungerford DS, Zizic TM:** *Alcohol-associated ischemic necrosis of the femoral head.* Clin Orthop 130:144, 1978.
4. **Hill RB Jr:** *Fatal fat embolism from steroid-induced fatty liver.* N Engl J Med 265:318, 1961.
5. **Frost HM:** *The etiodynamics of aseptic necrosis of the femoral head.* In: National Institutes of Health, ed, *Proceedings of the Conference on Aseptic Necrosis of the Femoral Head.* St. Louis, National Institutes of Health, 1964.
6. **Wang GJ, Sweet DE, Reger SI:** *Fat cell changes as a mechanism of avascular necrosis of the femoral head in cortisone treated rabbits.* J Bone Joint Surg 59A:729, 1977.
7. **Kawashima M, Torisu T, Hayahi K, et al.:** *Pathological review of osteonecrosis in divers.* Clin Orthop 130:107, 1978.
8. **Heard JL, Schneider CS:** *Radiographic findings in commercial divers.* Clin Orthop 130:129, 1978.
9. **Amstutz HA:** *The hip in Gaucher's disease.* Clin Orthop 90:83, 1973.
10. **Jaffe HL:** *Metabolic, Degenerative and Inflammatory Diseases of Bones and Joints.* Philadelphia, Lea & Febiger, 1972.
11. **Reynolds J:** *Radiologic manifestations of sickle cell hemoglobinopathy.* JAMA 238:247, 1977.
12. **Watson RJ, Burko H, Megas H, et al.:** *Hand-foot syndrome in sickle cell disease in young children.* Pediatrics 31:975, 1963.
13. **Dubois EL, Cozen L:** *Avascular (aseptic) bone necrosis associated with systemic lupus erythematosus.* JAMA 174:966, 1960.
14. **Smith FE, Sweet DE, Brunner CM, et al.:** *Avascular necrosis in SLE. An apparent predilection for young patients.* Ann Rheum Dis 35:227, 1976.
15. **Dalinka MK, Edeiken J, Finkelstein JB:** *Complications of radiation therapy: Adult bone.* Semin Roentgenol 9:29, 1974.
16. **Woodward HQ, Coley BL:** *The correlation of tissue dose and clinical response in irradiation of bone tumors and normal bone.* AJR 57:464, 1947.

17. **Libshitz HI:** *Radiation changes in bone.* Semin Roentgenol 29:15, 1994.
18. **Gerle RD, Walker LA, Achord J, et al.:** *Osseous changes in chronic pancreatitis.* Radiology 85:330, 1965.
19. **Baron M, Paltiel H, Lander P:** *Aseptic necrosis of the talus and calcaneal insufficiency fractures in a patient with pancreatitis, subcutaneous fat necrosis, and arthritis.* Arthritis Rheum 27(11):1309, 1984.
20. **Immelman EJ, Bank S, Krige H, et al.:** *Roentgenologic and clinical features of intramedullary fat necrosis in bones in acute and chronic pancreatitis.* Am J Med 39:96, 1964.
21. **Lynch MJG, Rappael SS, Dixon TP:** *Fat embolism in chronic alcoholism.* Arch Pathol 67:68, 1959.
22. **Schabel SI, Korn JH, Rittenberg GM, et al.:** *Bone infarction in gout.* Skeletal Radiol 3:42, 1978.
23. **Feldman EB, Gluck FB, Carter AC, et al.:** *Microangiopathy in hyperlipidemia and gout.* Am J Med Sci 268:263, 1974.
24. **Salter RB:** *Experimental and clinical aspects of Perthes' disease. Proceedings of a joint meeting of the American Physicians Fellowship and the Israeli Orthopedic Society.* J Bone Joint Surg 48B(2):393, 1966.
25. **Bobechko WP, Harris WR:** *The radiographic density of avascular bone.* J Bone Joint Surg 42B(3):626, 1960.
26. **Phemister DB:** *Bone growth and repair.* Ann Surg 10:261, 1935.
27. **Phemister DB:** *Changes in bones and joints resulting from interruption of circulation.* Arch Surg 41:1455, 1940.
28. **Bullough PG, Kambolis CP, Marcove RC, et al.:** *Bone infarctions not associated with Caisson disease.* J Bone Joint Surg 47A:477, 1965.
29. **Edeiken J, Hodes PJ, Libshitz HI, et al.:** *Bone ischemia.* Radiol Clin North Am 5:515, 1967.
30. **Mirra JM, Bullough PG, Marcove RC, et al.:** *Malignant fibrous histiocytoma and osteosarcoma in association with bone infarcts. Report of four cases, two in caisson workers.* J Bone Joint Surg 56A:932, 1974.
31. **Furey JG, Ferrer-Torells M, Reagan JW:** *Fibrosarcoma arising at the site of bone infarcts. A report of two cases.* J Bone Joint Surg 42A:802, 1960.
32. **Martell W, Sitterly BH:** *Roentgenologic manifestations of osteonecrosis.* AJR 106(3):509, 1969.
33. **Munk PL, Helms CA, Holt RG:** *Immature bone infarcts: Findings on plain radiographs and MR scans.* AJR 152:547, 1988.

SPONTANEOUS OSTEONECROSIS: FEMORAL HEAD IN ADULTS

1. **Freund E:** *Zur Frage der aseptischen Knochennekrose.* Virchows Arch (Pathol Anat) 261:287, 1926.
2. **Chandler FA:** *Observations on circulatory changes in bone.* AJR 44:90, 1940.
3. **Mankin HJ, Brower TD:** *Bilateral idiopathic aseptic necrosis of the femur in adults: "Chandler's disease."* Bull Hosp Joint Dis 23:42, 1962.
4. **Jaffe HL:** *Metabolic, Degenerative and Inflammatory Diseases of Bones and Joints.* Philadelphia, Lea & Febiger, 1972.
5. **Marcus ND, Enneking WF, Massam RA:** *The silent hip in idiopathic aseptic necrosis. Treatment by bone grafting.* J Bone Joint Surg 55A:1351, 1973.
6. **Cox JM, Hazen LJ:** *Avascular necrosis of the hips.* ACA J Chiro 3:67, 1990.
7. **Thorkeldsen A, Cantillon V:** *Idiopathic osteonecrosis of the hip.* J Manipulative Physiol Ther 16:37, 1993.
8. **Beltran J, Knight CT, Zuelzer WA, et al.:** *Core decompression for avascular necrosis of the femoral head: Correlation between long-term results and preoperative MR staging.* Radiology 175:533, 1990.
9. **Claffey TJ:** *Avascular necrosis of the femoral head. An anatomical study.* J Bone Joint Surg 42B:802, 1960.
10. **Sevitt S, Thompson RG:** *The distribution and anastomoses of arteries supplying the head and neck of the femur.* J Bone Joint Surg 47B:560, 1965.
11. **Trueta J, Harrison MHM:** *The normal vascular anatomy of the femoral head in adult man.* J Bone Joint Surg 35B:442, 1953.

12. **Martell W, Sitterly BH:** *Roentgenologic manifestations of osteonecrosis.* AJR 106(3):509, 1969.
13. **Alvai A, McCloskey JR, Steinberg ME:** *Early detection of avascular necrosis of the femoral head by 99m technetium diphosphonate bone scan: A preliminary report.* Clin Orthop 127:137, 1977.
14. **Brody AS, Strong M, Babikan G, et al.:** *Avascular necrosis: Early MR imaging and histologic findings in a canine model.* AJR 157:341, 1991.
15. **Markisz JA, Knowles RJ, Altchek DW, et al.:** *Segmental patterns of avascular necrosis of the femoral heads: Early detection with MR imaging.* Radiology 162:717, 1987.
16. **Mitchell DG, Rao VM, Dalinka MK, et al.:** *Femoral head avascular necrosis: Correlation of MR imaging, radiographic staging, radionuclide imaging, and clinical findings.* Radiology 162:709, 1987.
17. **Martell W, Poznanski AK:** *The effect of traction on the hip in osteonecrosis. A comment on the "radiolucent crescent line."* Radiology 94:505, 1970.
18. **Dihlmann W:** *CT analysis of the upper end of the femur: The asterisk sign and ischemic bone necrosis of the femoral head.* Skeletal Radiol 8:251, 1982.

SPONTANEOUS OSTEONECROSIS: KNEE

1. **Ahlback S, Bauer GCH, Bohne WH:** *Spontaneous osteonecrosis of the knee.* Arthritis Rheum 11:705, 1968.
2. **Marmor L:** *Osteonecrosis of the knee. Medial and lateral involvement.* Clin Orthop 185:195, 1984.
3. **Houpt JB, Alpert B, Lotem, M, et al.:** *Spontaneous osteonecrosis of the medial tibial plateau.* J Rheumatol 9:181, 1982.
4. **Marmor L:** *Fracture as a complication of osteonecrosis of the tibial plateau.* J Bone Joint Surg 70A:454, 1988.
5. **Lotke PA, Ecker ML:** *Current concepts review. Osteonecrosis of the knee.* J Bone Joint Surg 70A:470, 1988.
6. **LaPrade RF, Noffsinger MA:** *Idiopathic osteonecrosis of the patella: An unusual cause of pain in the knee.* J Bone Joint Surg 72A:1414, 1990.
7. **Bauer GCH:** *Osteonecrosis of the knee.* Clin Orthop 130:210, 1978.
8. **Houpt JB, Pritzker KP, Alpert B, et al.:** *Natural history of spontaneous osteonecrosis of the knee (SONK): A review.* Semin Arthritis Rheum 13(2):212, 1983.
9. **Williams JL, Cliff MM, Bonakdarpour A:** *Spontaneous osteonecrosis of the knee.* Radiology 107:15, 1973.
10. **Lotke PA, Abend JA, Ecker ML:** *The treatment of osteonecrosis of the medial femoral condyle.* Clin Orthop 171:109, 1982.
11. **Norman A, Baker ND:** *Spontaneous osteonecrosis of the knee and medial meniscal tears.* Radiology 129:653, 1978.
12. **Ahuja SC, Bullough PG:** *Osteonecrosis of the knee. A clinicopathological study in twenty-eight patients.* J Bone Joint Surg 60A:191, 1978.
13. **Greyson ND, Lotem MM, Gross AE, et al.:** *Radionuclide evaluation of spontaneous femoral osteonecrosis.* Radiology 142(3):729, 1982.
14. **Pollack MS, Dalinka MK, Kressel HY, et al.:** *Magnetic resonance imaging in the evaluation of suspected osteonecrosis of the knee.* Skeletal Radiol 16:121, 1987.
15. **Watt I, Dieppe PA:** *Medial femoral condyle necrosis and chondrocalcinosis—a causal relationship?* Br J Radiol 56(661):7, 1983.

CAISSON'S DISEASE

1. **Amako T, Kawashima M, Torisu T, et al.:** *Bone and joint lesions in decompression sickness.* Semin Arthritis Rheum 4:151, 1974.
2. **Chryssanthou CP:** *Dysbaric osteonecrosis. Etiological and pathogenic concepts.* Clin Orthop 130:94, 1978.
3. **Kawashima M, Torisu T, Hayahi K, et al.:** *Pathological review of osteonecrosis in divers.* Clin Orthop 130:107, 1978.
4. **Kindwall EP, Nellen JR, Spiegelhoff DR:** *Aseptic necrosis in compressed air tunnel workers using current OSHA decompression schedules.* J Occup Med 24(10):741, 1982.

5. **Jaffe HL:** *Metabolic, Degenerative and Inflammatory Diseases of Bones and Joints.* Philadelphia, Lea & Febiger, 1972.
6. **McCallum RI, Walder DN, Barnes R, et al.:** *Bone lesions in compressed air workers. With special reference to men who worked in the Clyde tunnels 1958 to 1963.* J Bone Joint Surg 481B:207, 1966.
7. **Bell ALL, Edson GN, Hornick N:** *Characteristic bone and joint changes in compressed air workers: A survey of symptomless cases.* Radiology 38:698, 1913.
8. **Ohta Y, Matsunaga H:** *Bone lesions in divers.* J Bone Joint Surg 56B:3, 1974.
9. **Medical Research Council Decompression Sickness Panel:** *Radiological skeletal survey for aseptic necrosis of bone in divers and compressed workers.* Radiography 47(558):141, 1981.
10. **van Blarcom ST, Czarnecki DJ, Fueredi GA, et al.:** *Does dysbaric osteonecrosis progress in the absence of further hyperbaric exposure?* AJR 155:95, 1990.

RADIATION CHANGES IN BONE

1. **Grigg ERN:** *The Trail of the Invisible Light. From X-Strahlen to Radio(bio)logy.* Springfield, IL, Charles C Thomas, 1965.
2. **Janower ML:** *Occupational hazard.* JAMA 190:769, 1964.
3. **Hasterlik RJ, Finkel AJ:** *Diseases of bones and joints associated with intoxication by radioactive substances, principally radium.* Med Clin North Am 49:285, 1965.
4. **Looney WB, Hasterlik RJ, Brues AM, et al.:** *A clinical investigation of the chronic effects of radium salts administered therapeutically (1915–1931).* AJR 73:1006, 1955.
5. **Rondos B:** *Late clinical and roentgen observations following Thorotrast administration.* Clin Radiol 24:195, 1973.
6. **Janower ML, Miettinen OS, Flynn MJ:** *Effects of long-term Thorotrast exposure.* Radiology 103:13, 1972.
7. **Nosik WA, Mortensen O:** *Myelography with thorotrast and subsequent removal by forced drainage, experimental study: Preliminary report.* AJR 39:727, 1938.
8. **Radovici A, Meller O:** *Encephalographie liquidienne par le thorotrast soussarachnoidien.* Ref Neurol 1:479, 1932.
9. **da Silva Horta J:** *Late effects of thorotrast on the liver and spleen and their efferent lymph nodes.* Ann NY Acad Sci 145:676, 1967.
10. **Sindelar WF, Costa J, Ketchan AS:** *Osteosarcoma associated with Thorotrast administration. Report of two cases and literature review.* Cancer 42:2604, 1978.
11. **Deeths TM, Stanley RJ:** *Parametrial calcification in cervical carcinoma patients treated with radioactive gold.* AJR 127:511, 1976.
12. **Libshitz HI:** *Radiation changes in bone.* Semin Roentgenol 29:15, 1994.
13. **Vaughan J:** *The effects of skeletal irradiation.* Clin Orthop 56:283, 1968.
14. **Frantz CH:** *Extreme retardation of epiphyseal growth from roentgen irradiation. A case study.* Radiology 55:720, 1950.
15. **Neuhauser EBD, Wittenborg MH, Berman CZ, et al.:** *Irradiation effects of roentgen therapy on the growing spine.* Radiology 59:637, 1952.
16. **Whitehouse WM, Lampe I:** *Osseous damage in irradiation of renal tumors in infancy and childhood.* AJR 70:721, 1953.
17. **Bragg DG, Shidnia H, Chu FCH, et al.:** *The clinical and radiographic aspects of radiation osteitis.* Radiology 97:103, 1970.
18. **Cade S:** *Radiation-induced cancer in man.* Br J Radiol 30:393, 1957.
19. **Calabro F, Jinkins JR:** *MRI of radiation myelitis: A report of a case treated with hyperbaric oxygen.* Eur Radiol 10(7):1079, 2000.
20. **Cree AK, Hadlow AT, Taylor TKF, et al.:** *Radiation-induced osteochondroma in the lumbar spine.* Spine 19:376, 1994.
21. **Arkin AM, Pack GT, Ransohoff NS, et al.:** *Radiation-induced scoliosis; a case report.* J Bone Joint Surg 32A:401, 1950.
22. **Teplick JG, Head GL, Kricun ME, et al.:** *Ghost infantile vertebrae and hemipelves within adult skeleton from thorotrast administration in childhood.* Radiology 129:657, 1978.
23. **Ramsey RG, Zacharias CE:** *MR imaging of the spine after radiation therapy: Easily recognizable effects.* AJR 144:1131, 1985.
24. **Martin D, Delaollette M, Collignon J, et al.:** *Radiation-induced myelopathy and vertebral necrosis.* Neuroradiology 36:405, 1994.
25. **Malghem J, Maldague B, Labaisse MA, et al.:** *Intravertebral vacuum cleft: Changes in content after supine positioning.* Radiology 187:483, 1993.
26. **Abe H, Nakamura M, Takahashi S, et al.:** *Radiation-induced insufficiency fractures of the pelvis: Evaluation with 99mTc-methylene diphosphonate scintigraphy.* AJR 158:599, 1992.
27. **Deleeuw HW, Pottenger LA:** *Osteonecrosis of the acetabulum following radiation therapy.* J Bone Joint Surg 70A:293, 1988.
28. **Rubin P, Probhasawat D:** *Characteristic bone lesions in post irradiated carcinoma of the cervix—Metastases versus osteonecrosis.* Radiology 76:703, 1961.
29. **Grant BP, Fletcher GH:** *Analysis of complications following megavoltage therapy for squamous cell carcinomas of the tonsillar area.* AJR 96:28, 1966.
30. **Guttenberg SA:** *Osteoradionecrosis of the jaw.* Am J Surg 127:326, 1974.
31. **DeSantos LA, Libshitz HI:** *Adult bone.* In: HI Libschitz, ed, *Diagnostic Roentgenology of Radiotherapy Change.* Baltimore, Williams & Wilkins, 1979.
32. **Dalinka MK, Edeiken J, Finkelstein JB:** *Complications of radiation therapy: Adult bone.* Semin Roentgenol 9:29, 1974.
33. **Meyer JE:** *Thoracic effects of therapeutic irradiation for breast carcinoma.* AJR 130:877, 1978.
34. **Paul LW, Pohle EA:** *Radiation osteitis of the ribs.* Radiology 38:543, 1942.

EPIPHYSEAL DISORDERS

EPHIPHYSEAL OSTEONECROSIS

1. **Legg AT:** *An obscure affection of the hip joint.* Boston Med Surg J 162:202, 1910.
2. **Calvé J:** *Sur une forme particuliere de pseudo-coxalgie greffee sur des deformations caracteristiques de l'extremite superieure du femur.* Ref Chir 30:54, 1910.
3. **Perthes GC:** *Über Arthritis deformans juvenilis.* Dtsch Z Chir 107:111, 1910.
4. **Edgren W:** *Coxa plana: A clinical and radiological investigation with particular reference to the importance of the metaphyseal changes for the final shape of the proximal part of the femur.* Acta Orthop Scand Suppl 84:1, 1965.
5. **Clarke TE, Finnegan TL, Fisher RL, et al.:** *Legg-Perthes disease in children less than four years old.* J Bone Joint Surg 60A:166, 1978.
6. **Murphy RP, Marsh HO:** *Incidence and natural history of "head at risk" factors in Perthes' disease.* Clin Orthop 132:102, 1978.
7. **Wansborough RM, Carrie AW, Walker NF, et al.:** *Coxa plana, its genetic aspects and results of treatment with the long Taylor walking caliper. A long-term follow-up study.* J Bone Joint Surg 41A:135, 1959.
8. **Guille JT, Lipton GE, Tsirikos AI, Bowen JR:** *Bilateral Legg-Calve-Perthes disease: Presentation and outcome.* J Pediatr Orthop 22(4):458, 2002.
9. **McAndrew MP, Weinstein SL:** *A long term followup of Legg-Calvé-Perthes Disease.* J Bone Joint Surg 66A(6):860, 1984.
10. **Ponseti IV:** *Legg-Perthes disease: Observations on pathological changes in two cases.* J Bone Joint Surg 38A:739, 1956.
11. **Trueta J:** *Normal vascular anatomy of the human femoral head during growth.* J Bone Joint Surg 39B:358, 1957.
12. **Wyme-Davies R:** *Some etiologic factors in Perthes' disease.* Clin Orthop 150:12, 1980.
13. **Liu SL, Ho TC:** *The role of venous hypertension in the pathogenesis of Legg-Perthes disease.* J Bone Joint Surg 73A:194, 1991.
14. **Caffey J:** *The early roentgenographic changes in essential coxa plana; their significance in pathogenesis.* AJR 103:620, 1968.
15. **Harrison MHM, Turner MH, Jacobs P:** *Skeletal immaturity in Perthes' disease.* J Bone Joint Surg 59B:37, 1976.

16. **Brodetti A:** *The blood supply of the femoral neck and head in relation to the damaging effects of nails and screws.* J Bone Joint Surg 42B:794, 1960.

17. **Suramo I, Puranen J, Heikkinen E, et al.:** *Disturbed patterns of venous drainage of the femoral neck in Perthes' disease.* J Bone Joint Surg 56B:449, 1974.

18. **Ferguson AB Jr:** *The pathology of Legg-Perthes disease and its comparison with aseptic necrosis.* Clin Orthop 106:7, 1975.

19. **Somerville EW:** *Perthes' disease of the hip.* J Bone Joint Surg 53B:639, 1971.

20. **Inoue A, Freeman MAR, Bernon-Roberts B, et al.:** *The pathogenesis of Perthes' disease.* J Bone Joint Surg 58B:453, 1976.

21. **Jensen OM, Lauritzen J:** *Legg-Calvé-Perthes disease. Morphologic studies in two cases examined at necropsy.* J Bone Joint Surg 58B(3):332, 1976.

22. **Waldenstrom H:** *The first stages of coxa plana.* J Bone Joint Surg 20A:559, 1938.

23. **Gordon I, Peters AM, Nunn R:** *The symptomatic hip in childhood: scintigraphic findings in the presence of a normal radiograph.* Skeletal Radiol 16:383, 1987.

24. **Sutherland AD, Savage JP, Foster BK:** *The nuclide bone-scan in the diagnosis and management of Perthes' disease.* J Bone Joint Surg 62B:300, 1980.

25. **Wenger DR, Ward WT, Herring JA:** *Current concepts review. Legg-Calvé-Perthes disease.* J Bone Joint Surg 73A:778, 1991.

26. **Egund N, Wingstrand H:** *Legg-Calvé-Perthes disease: Imaging with MR.* Radiology 179:89, 1991.

27. **le Pointe HD, Haddad S, Silberman B, et al.:** *Legg-Calvé-Perthes disease: Staging by MRI using gadolinium.* Pediatr Radiol 24:88, 1994.

28. **Phemister DB:** *Bone growth and repair.* Ann Surg 10:261, 1935.

29. **Martel W, Poznanski AK:** *The effect of traction on the hip in osteonecrosis. A comment on the "radiolucent crescent line."* Radiology 94:505, 1970.

30. **Anderson J, Stewart AM:** *The significance of the magnitude of the medial hip joint space.* Br J Radiol 43:239, 1970.

31. **Bobechko WP, Harris WR:** *The radiographic density of avascular bone.* J Bone Joint Surg 42B(3):626, 1960.

32. **Gage HC:** *A possible early sign of Perthes' disease.* Br J Radiol 6:295, 1933.

33. **Robichon J, Desjardins JP, Koch M, et al.:** *The femoral neck Legg-Perthes disease. Its relationship to epiphyseal change and its importance in early prognosis.* J Bone Joint Surg 56B:62, 1974.

34. **Silverman FN:** *Lesions of the femoral neck in Legg-Perthes disease.* AJR 144:1249, 1985.

35. **Barnes JM:** *Premature epiphyseal closure in Perthes' disease.* J Bone Joint Surg 62B:432, 1980.

36. **Catterall A:** *The natural history of Perthes' disease.* J Bone Joint Surg 53B:37, 1971.

37. **Dominguez R, Oh KS, Young LW, et al.:** *Acute chondrolysis complicating Legg-Calvé-Perthes disease.* Skeletal Radiol 16:377, 1987.

38. **Rowe LJ, Ho EK:** *Idiopathic chondrolysis of the hip.* Skeletal Radiol 1996 Feb; 25(2):178.

39. **Goldman AB, Hallel T, Salvati EM, et al.:** *Osteochondritis dissecans complicating Legg-Perthes disease. A report of four cases.* Radiology 121:561, 1976.

40. **Apley AG, Wientraub S:** *The sagging rope sign in Perthes' disease and allied disorders.* J Bone Joint Surg 63B(1):43, 1981.

41. **Clarke NMP, Harrison MHM:** *The sagging rope sign. A critical appraisal.* J Bone Joint Surg 65B(3):285, 1983.

42. **Dickens DRV, Menelaus MB:** *The assessment of prognosis in Perthes' disease.* J Bone Joint Surg 60B(2):189, 1978.

43. **Joseph B, Mulpuri K, Varghese G:** *Perthes' disease in the adolescent.* J Bone Joint Surg 83B(5):715, 2001.

44. **Salter RB:** *The present status of surgical treatment for Legg-Perthes disease.* J Bone Joint Surg 66A(6):961, 1984.

45. **Van den Bogaert G, de Rosa E, Moens P, et al.:** *Bilateral Legg-Calve-Perthes disease: different from unilateral disease?* J Pediatr Orthop B 1999 Jul;8(3):165–8.

46. **Yrjonen T:** *Long-term prognosis of Legg-Calve-Perthes disease: A meta-analysis.* J Pediatr Orthop B 1999 Jul;8(3):169–72.

47. **Katz JF, Siffert RS:** *Capital necrosis, metaphyseal cyst, and subluxation in coxa plana.* Clin Orthop 106:75, 1975.

48. **Hardcastle PH, Ross R, Hamalainen M, et al.:** *Catterall grouping of Perthes' disease.* J Bone Joint Surg 62B:428, 1980.

49. **Zenios M, Hutchinson C, Galasko CS:** *Radiological evaluation of surgical treatment in Perthes' disease.* Int Orthop 25(5):305, 2001.

50. **Freiberg AH:** *Infraction of the second metatarsal bone: A typical injury.* Surg Gynecol Obstet 19:191, 1914.

51. **Freiberg AH:** *The so-called infraction of the second metatarsal bone.* J Bone Joint Surg 8A:257, 1926.

52. **Palamarchuk HJ, Oehrlein CR:** *Freiberg's infraction in a collegiate heptathlete.* J Am Podiatr Med Assoc 90(2):77, 2000.

53. **Smillie IS:** *Freiberg's infarction (Koehler's second disease).* J Bone Joint Surg 391B:580, 1955.

54. **Miller ML, Lenet MD, Sherman M:** *Surgical treatment of Freiberg's infraction with the use of total joint replacement arthroplasty.* J Foot Surg 23(1):35, 1984.

55. **Katcherian DA:** *Treatment of Freiberg's disease.* Orthop Clin North Am 25:69, 1994.

56. **Hoskinson J:** *Freiberg's disease. A review of long-term results.* Proc R Soc Med 67:106, 1974.

57. **el-Tayeby HM:** *Freiberg's infraction: a new surgical procedure.* J Foot Ankle Surg 37:23, 1998.

58. **Gauthier G, Elbaz R:** *Freiberg's infraction: A subchondral bone fatigue fracture. A new surgical treatment.* Clin Orthop 142:93, 1979.

59. **Kienböck R:** *Gber traumatische Malazie des Mondbeins und ihre Folgezustands: Entartungsformen und Kompressionsfrakturen.* Fortschr Geb Roentgenstr Nuklearmed 16:77, 1910.

60. **Simmons EH, Dommisse I:** *The pathogenesis and treatment of Kienböck's disease* [Abstract]. Clin Orthop 105:300, 1974.

61. **Allan CH, Joshi A, Lichtman DM:** *Kienböck's disease: Diagnosis and treatment.* J Am Acad Orthop Surg 9(2):128, 2001.

62. **Taniguchi Y, Tamaki T:** *Bilateral Kienböck's disease.* J Orthop Sci 3(4):216, 1998.

63. **Morgan RF, McCue FC:** *Bilateral Kienböck's disease.* J Hand Surg 8(6):928, 1983.

64. **Beckenbaugh RD, Shives TC, Dobyns JH, et al.:** *Kienbock's disease: The natural history of Kienböck's disease and consideration of lunate fractures.* Clin Orthop 149:98, 1980.

65. **Gelberman RH, Bauman TD, Menon J, et al.:** *The vascularity of the lunate bone and Kienböck's disease.* J Hand Surg 5:272, 1980.

66. **Lee MLH:** *The intraosseous arterial pattern of the carpal lunate bone and its relation to avascular necrosis.* Acta Orthop Scand 33:43, 1963.

67. **Gelberman RH, Salamon PB, Jurist JM, et al.:** *Ulnar variance in Kienbock's disease.* J Bone Joint Surg 57A:674, 1975.

68. **Shin AY, Bishop AT:** *Vascularized bone grafts for scaphoid nonunions and Kienböck's disease.* Orthop Clin North Am 32(2):263, 2001.

69. **Oka Y, Umeda K, Ikeda M:** *Cyst-like lesions of the lunate resembling Kienböck's disease: a case report.* J Hand Surg 26A:130, 2001.

70. **Wiess AP, Weiland AJ, Moore JR, et al.:** *Radial shortening for Kienböck disease.* J Bone Joint Surg 73A:384, 1991.

71. **Delaere O, Dury M, Molderez A, Foucher G:** *Conservative versus operative treatment for Kienböck's disease. A retrospective study.* J Hand Surg 24B:139, 1999.

72. **Salmon J, Stanley JK, Trail IA:** *Kienböck's disease: Conservative management versus radial shortening.* J Bone Joint Surg 82B:820, 2000.

73. **Roca J, Beltran JF, Fairen MF, et al.:** *Treatment of Kienböck's disease using a silicone rubber implant.* J Bone Joint Surg 58A:373, 1976.

74. **Kaarela OI, Raatikainen TK, Torniainen PJ:** *Silicone replacement arthroplasty for Kienböck's disease.* J Hand Surg 23B:735, 1998.

TRAUMATIC EPIPHYSEAL INJURIES

1. **Nowinski RJ, Mehlman CT:** *Hyphenated history: Osgood-Schlatter disease.* Am J Orthop 27(8):584, 1998.
2. **Osgood RB:** *Lesions of the tibial tubercle occurring during adolescence.* Boston Med Surg J 148:114, 1903.
3. **Schlatter C:** *Verletzungen des schnabelformigen Fortsatzes der oberen Tibiaepiphyse.* Bruns Beitr Klin Chir 38:874, 1903.
4. **Woolfrey BF, Chandler EF:** *Manifestations of Osgood-Schlatter's disease.* Am J Pathol 34:803, 1958.
5. **Brower AC:** *The osteochondroses.* Orthop Clin North Am 14(1):99, 1983.
6. **Rosenberg ZS, Kawelblum M, Cheung YY, et al.:** *Osgood-Schlatter lesion: Fracture or tendinitis? Scintigraphic, CT, and MR imaging features.* Radiology 185:853, 1992.
7. **Jaffe HL:** *Metabolic, Degenerative and Inflammatory Diseases of Bones and Joints.* Philadelphia, Lea & Febiger, 1972.
8. **Ogden JA:** *Radiology of postnatal skeletal development.* Skeletal Radiol 11:246, 1984.
9. **Holstein A, Lewis GB, Schulze ER:** *Heterotopic ossification of the patellar tendon.* J Bone Joint Surg 45A:656, 1963.
10. **Crigler NW, Riddervold HO:** *Soft tissue changes in x-ray diagnosis of the Osgood-Schlatter lesion.* Virginia Med 109(3):176, 1982.
11. **Scotti DM, Sadhu VK, Heimberg F, et al.:** *Osgood-Schlatter's disease, an emphasis on soft tissue changes in roentgen diagnosis.* Skeletal Radiol 4:21, 1979.
12. **Hulting B:** *Roentgenologic features of fracture of the tibial tuberosity (Osgood-Schlatter's disease).* Acta Radiol 48:161, 1957.
13. **Mital MA, Matza RA, Cohen J:** *The so-called unresolved Osgood-Schlatter lesion.* J Bone Joint Surg 62A:732, 1980.
14. **Hirano A, Fukubayashi T, Ishii T, Ochiai N:** *Magnetic resonance imaging of Osgood-Schlatter disease: The course of the disease.* Skeletal Radiol 31(6):334, 2002.
15. **Zimbler S, Merkow S:** *Genu recurvatum: A possible complication after Osgood-Schlatter disease.* J Bone Joint Surg 66A:1129, 1984.
16. **Scheuermann HW:** *Kyphosis dorsalis juvenilis.* Ugeskr Laeger 82:385, 1920.
17. **Scheuermann HW:** *Kyphosis dorsalis juvenilis.* Z Orthop Chir 41:305, 1921.
18. **Bradford DS:** *Vertebral osteochondrosis (Scheuermann's kyphosis).* Clin Orthop 158:83, 1981.
19. **Lowe TG:** *Current concepts review. Scheuermann's disease.* J Bone Joint Surg 72A:940, 1990.
20. **Alexander CJ:** *Scheuermann's disease. A traumatic spondylodystrophy?* Skeletal Radiol 1:209, 1977.
21. **Ali RM, Green DW, Patel TC:** *Scheuermann's kyphosis.* Curr Opin Pediatr 11(1):70, 1999.
22. **Dameron TE Jr, Gulledge WH:** *Adolescent kyphosis.* US Armed Forces Med J 4:871, 1953.
23. **Sorensen KH:** *Scheuermann's Juvenile Kyphosis.* Copenhagen, Munksgaard, 1964.
24. **Wassman K:** *Kyphosis juvenilis Scheuermann—An occupational disorder.* Acta Orthop Scand 21:65, 1951.
25. **Lowe TG:** *Scheuermann's disease.* Orthop Clin North Am 30(3):475, 1999.
26. **Linthoudt DV, Revel M:** *Similar radiologic lesions of localized Scheuermann's disease of the lumbar spine in twin sisters.* Spine 19:987, 1994.
27. **McKenzie L, Sillence D:** *Familial Scheuermann's disease. A genetic and linkage study.* J Med Genet 29:41, 1992.
28. **Murray PM, Weinstein SL, Spratt KF:** *The natural history and long-term follow-up of Scheuermann's kyphosis.* J Bone Joint Surg 75A:236, 1993.
29. **Jahn WT, Griffiths JH, Hacker RA:** *Conservative management of Scheuermann's juvenile kyphosis.* J Manipulative Physiol Ther 1(4):228, 1978.
30. **Lamrinudi L:** *Adolescent and senile kyphosis.* Br Med J 2:800, 1934.
31. **Michelle AA:** *Osteochondrosis deformans juvenilis dorsi.* N Y J Med 61:98, 1961.
32. **Bradford DS, Garcia A:** *Neurological complications in Scheuermann's disease. A case report and review of the literature.* J Bone Joint Surg 51A:567, 1969.
33. **Adelstein LJ:** *Spinal extradural cyst associated with kyphosis dorsalis juvenilis.* J Bone Joint Surg 23A:93, 1941.
34. **Yablon JS, Kasdon DL, Levine H:** *Thoracic cord compression in Scheuermann's disease.* Spine 13:896, 1988.
35. **Bick EM, Copel JW:** *Ring apophysis of human vertebra: Contribution to human osteogeny.* J Bone Joint Surg 33A:783, 1951.
36. **Schmorl G:** *Die pathogenese der juvenilen kyphose.* Fortschr Geb Rontgenstrahlen 41:359, 1930.
37. **Schmorl G, Junghanns H:** *The Human Spine in Health and Disease,* ed 2, trans EF Besemann. New York, Grune & Stratton, 1971.
38. **Bradford DS, Moe JH:** *Scheuermann's juvenile kyphosis. A histologic study.* Clin Orthop 110:45, 1975.
39. **Butler RW:** *Spontaneous anterior fusion of vertebral bodies.* J Bone Joint Surg 53B:230, 1971.
40. **Moe JH, Winter RB, Bradford DS, et al.:** *Scoliosis and Other Skeletal Deformities.* Philadelphia, WB Saunders, 1978.
41. **Keim HA:** *The Adolescent Spine.* New York, Grune & Stratton, 1976.
42. **Ogilvie JW, Sherman J:** *Spondylolysis in Scheuermann's disease.* Spine 12:251, 1987.
43. **Heithoff KB, Gundry CR, Burton CV, et al.:** *Juvenile discogenic disease.* Spine 19:335, 1994.
44. **Paajanen H, Alanen A, Erkintalo M, et al.:** *Disc degeneration in Scheuermann's disease.* Skeletal Radiol 18:523, 1989.
45. **Williams HJ, Pugh DG:** *Vertebral epiphysitis: A comparison of the clinical and roentgenologic findings.* AJR 90:1236, 1963.
46. **Statts AK, Smith JT, Santora SD, et al.:** *Measurement of spinal kyphosis: Implications for the management of Scheuermann's kyphosis.* Spine 27(19):2143, 2002.
47. **König F:** *Uber freie Körper in Gelenken.* Dsche Z Chir 27:90, 1887.
48. **Pappas AM:** *Osteochondrosis dissecans.* Clin Orthop 158:59, 1981.
49. **Phillips HO, Grubb SA:** *Familial multiple osteochondritis dissecans. Report of a kindred.* J Bone Joint Surg 67A:155, 1985.
50. **Tatum R:** *Osteochondritis dissecans of the knee: A radiology case report.* J Manipulative Physiol Ther 23(5):347, 2000.
51. **Nagura S:** *The so-called osteochondritis dissecans of Konig.* Clin Orthop 18:100, 1960.
52. **Aichroth P:** *Osteochondral fractures and their relationship to osteochondritis dissecans of the knee. An experimental study in animals.* J Bone Joint Surg 53B:448, 1971.
53. **Milgram JW, Rogers LF, Miller JW:** *Osteochondral fractures: Mechanisms of injury and fate of fragments.* AJR 130:651, 1978.
54. **Chiroff RT, Cooke CP:** *Osteochondritis dissecans: A histologic and microradiographic analysis of surgically excised lesions.* J Trauma 15:689, 1975.
55. **Milgram JW:** *Radiological and pathological manifestations of osteochondritis dissecans of the distal femur. A study of 50 cases.* Radiology 126:305, 1978.
56. **Aichroth P:** *Osteochondritis dissecans of the knee. A clinical study.* J Bone Joint Surg 53B:440, 1971.
57. **Bianchi G, Paderni S, Tigani D, Mercuri M:** *Osteochondritis dissecans of the lateral femoral condyle* [Trans]. Chir Organi Mov Apr-84(2):183, 1999.
58. **Jaberi FM:** *Osteochondritis dissecans of the weight-bearing surface of the medial femoral condyle in adults.* Knee 9(3):201, 2002.
59. **Matthewson MH, Dandy DJ:** *Osteochondral fractures of the lateral femoral condyle. A result of indirect violence to the knee.* J Bone Joint Surg 60B:199, 1978.
60. **Linden B:** *Osteochondritis dissecans of the femoral condyles. A long-term follow-up study.* J Bone Joint Surg 59A:769, 1977.

61. **Caffey J, Madell SH, Royer C, et al.:** *Ossification of the distal femoral epiphysis.* J Bone Joint Surg 40A:647, 1958.

62. **Mesgarzadeh M, Sapega AA, Bonakdarpour A, et al.:** *Osteochondritis dissecans: Analysis of mechanical stability with radiography, scintigraphy, and MR imaging.* Radiology 165:775, 1987.

63. **De Smet AA, Fisher DR, Graf BK, et al.:** *Osteochondritis dissecans of the knee: Value of MR imaging in determining lesion stability and the presence of articular cartilage defects.* AJR 155:549, 1990.

64. **Bauer M, Jonsson K, Linden B:** *Osteochondritis dissecans of the ankle.* J Bone Joint Surg 69B:93, 1987.

65. **Thompson JP, Loomer RL:** *Osteochondral lesions of the talus in a sports medicine clinic. A new radiographic technique and surgical approach.* Am J Sports Med 12(6):460, 1984.

66. **De Smet AA, Fisher DR, Burnstein MI, et al.:** *Value of MR imaging in staging lesions of the talus (osteochondritis dissecans).* AJR 154:555, 1990.

67. **Canale ST, Belding RH:** *Osteochondral lesions of the talus.* J Bone Joint Surg 62A:97, 1980.

68. **Berndt AL, Harty M:** *Transchondral fracture (osteochondritis dissecans) of the talus.* J Bone Joint Surg 41A:988, 1959.

69. **Smith GR, Winquist RA, Allan TNK, et al.:** *Subtle transchondral fractures of the talar dome: A radiological perspective.* Radiology 124:667, 1977.

70. **Runn M, Fazekas EA, Jecker RL:** *Osteochondral lesions of the talus.* J Foot Surg 22(2):155, 1983.

71. **Goldman AB, Hallel T, Salvati E, et al.:** *Osteochondritis dissecans complicating Legg-Perthes disease. A report of four cases.* Radiology 121:561, 1976.

72. **Guilleminet M, Barbier JM:** *Osteochondritis dissecans of the hip.* J Bone Joint Surg 39B:268, 1957.

73. **Edwards DH, Bentley G:** *Osteochondritis dissecans patellae.* J Bone Joint Surg 59B:58, 1977.

74. **Goergen TG, Resnick D, Greenway G, et al.:** *Dorsal defect of the patella (DDP): A characteristic radiographic lesion.* Radiology 130:333, 1979.

75. **Hoskinson J:** *Freiberg's disease: A review of long-term results.* Proc R Soc Med 67:106, 1974.

76. **Roberts N, Hughes R:** *Osteochondritis dissecans of the elbow joint. A clinical study.* J Bone Joint Surg 32B:348, 1950.

77. **Woodward AH, Bianco AJ Jr:** *Osteochondritis dissecans of the elbow.* Clin Orthop 110:35, 1975.

78. **McManama GB, Micheli LJ, Berry MV, et al.:** *The surgical treatment of osteochondritis of the capitellum.* Am J Sports Med 13:11, 1985.

79. **Mitsunanga MM, Adishian DA, Bianco AJ:** *Osteochondritis dissecans of the capitellum.* J Trauma 22(1):53, 1982.

80. **Takeda H, Watarai K, Matsushita T, et al.:** *A surgical treatment for unstable osteochondritis dissecans lesions of the humeral capitellum in adolescent baseball players.* Am J Sports Med 30(5):713, 2002.

81. **Aghasi M, Rzetelni V, Axer A:** *Osteochondritis dissecans of the carpal scaphoid.* J Hand Surg 6(4):351, 1981.

82. **Anderson ON, Datzberg RW:** *Loose bodies of the temporomandibular joint arthrographic diagnosis.* Skeletal Radiol 11(1):42, 1984.

GROWTH VARIANTS OF THE EPIPHYSIS

1. **Blount WP:** *Tibia vara. Osteochondrosis deformans tibiae.* J Bone Joint Surg 19A:1, 1937.

2. **Bathfield CA, Beighton PH:** *Blount disease. A review of etiological factors in 110 patients.* Clin Orthop 135:29, 1978.

3. **Golding JSR, McNeil-Smith JDG:** *Observations on the etiology of tibia vara.* J Bone Joint Surg 45B:320, 1963.

4. **Longenskiold A:** *Tibia vara: Osteochondrosis deformans tibiae. Blount's disease.* Clin Orthop 158:77, 1981.

5. **Calve J:** *Localized affection of the spine suggesting osteochondritis of vertebral body.* J Bone Joint Surg 7A:41, 1925.

6. **Compere EL, Coventry MB:** *Vertebra plana due to eosinophilic granuloma.* J Bone Joint Surg 36A:969, 1954.

7. **Morris HD:** *Aseptic necrosis of the talus following injury.* Orthop Clin North Am 5:177, 1974.

8. **Mulfinger GL, Trueta J:** *The blood supply of the talus.* J Bone Joint Surg 52B:160, 1970.

9. **Huber H, Galantay R, Dutoit M:** *Avascular necrosis after osteotomy of the talar neck to correct residual club-foot deformity in children. A long-term review.* J Bone Joint Surg 84B:426, 2002.

10. **Kemnitz S, Moens P, Peerlinck K, Fabry G:** *Avascular necrosis of the talus in children with haemophilia.* J Pediatr Orthop B 11(1):73, 2002.

11. **Hawkins LG:** *Fractures of the neck of the talus.* J Bone Joint Surg 52A:991, 1970.

12. **Pavelka K:** *Osteonecrosis.* Baillieres Best Pract Res Clin Rheumatol 14(2):399, 2000.

13. **Laing PG:** *The arterial supply of the adult humerus.* J Bone Joint Surg 38A:1105, 1956.

14. **Lee CK, Hansen HR:** *Post-traumatic avascular necrosis of the humeral head in displaced humeral fractures.* J Trauma 21(9):788, 1981.

15. **Hasan SS, Romeo AA:** *Nontraumatic osteonecrosis of the humeral head.* J Shoulder Elbow Surg 11(3):281, 2002.

16. **Hattrup SJ, Cofield RH:** *Osteonecrosis of the humeral head: Relationship of disease stage, extent, and cause to natural history.* J Shoulder Elbow Surg 8(6):559, 1999.

17. **Kohler A:** *Euber eine h äufige bisher anscheinend unbekannte Erkrankung einzelner Kindlicher knochen.* Munchen Med Wochnschr 55:1923, 1908.

18. **Waugh W:** *The ossification and vascularisation of the tarsal navicular and their relation to Köhler's disease.* J Bone Joint Surg 40B:765, 1958.

19. **Williams GA, Cowell HR:** *Köhler's disease of the tarsal navicular.* Clin Orthop 158:53, 1981.

20. **Karp MG:** *Köhler's disease of the tarsal scaphoid. An end-result study.* J Bone Joint Surg 19A:84, 1937.

21. **Weston WJ:** *Köhler's disease of the tarsal scaphoid.* Austral Radiol 22:332, 1978.

22. **McCauley RGK, Kahn PC:** *Osteochondritis of the tarsal navicular. Radioisotopic appearances.* Radiology 123:705, 1977.

23. **Young WF, Brown D, Kendler A, Clements D:** *Delayed posttraumatic osteonecrosis of vertebral body (Kummel's disease).* Acta Orthop Belg 68(1):13, 2002.

24. **Schmorl G, Junghanns H:** *The Human Spine in Health and Disease,* ed 2, trans Besemann. New York, Grune & Stratton, 1971.

25. **Lichenstein L:** *Diseases of Bone and Joints.* St. Louis, CV Mosby, 1970.

26. **Jaffe HL:** *Metabolic, Degenerative and Inflammatory Diseases of Bone and Joints.* Philadelphia, Lea & Febiger, 1972.

27. **Rigler L:** *Kummel's disease. With a report of roentgenologically proven case.* AJR 25:749, 1931.

28. **Brower AC, Downey EF:** *Kummel's disease: Report of a case with serial radiographs.* Radiology 141(2):363, 1981.

29. **Maldague BE, Noel HM, Malghem JJ:** *The intravertebral vacuum cleft. A sign of ischemic vertebral collapse.* Radiology 129:23, 1978.

30. **Osterhouse MD, Kettner NW:** *Delayed posttraumatic vertebral collapse with intravertebral vacuum cleft.* J Manipulative Physiol Ther 25(4):270, 2002.

31. **Mauclaire P:** *Epiphysitis der Metakarpusköpfchen mit Hohlbildung der Hand.* Fortschr Geb Roentgenstr Nuklearmed 37:425, 1928.

32. **Gilsanz V, Cleveland RH, Wilkinson RH:** *Aseptic necrosis: A complication of dislocation of the metacarpophalangeal joint.* AJR 29:737, 1977.

33. **Al'-Katoubi MA:** *Avascular necrosis of the metacarpal heads following renal transplantation.* Br J Radiol 55(649):79, 1982.

34. **Karlakki SL, Bindra RR:** *Idiopathic avascular necrosis of the metacarpal head.* Clin Orthop 406:103, 2003.

35. **Panner HJ:** *An affection of the capitelum humeri resembling Calvé-Perthes' disease of the hip.* Acta Radiol 8:617, 1927.

36. **Klein EW:** *Osteochondrosis of the capitelum (Panner's disease). Report of a case.* AJR 88:466, 1952.

37. **March HC:** *Osteochondritis of the capitellum (Panner's disease).* AJR 51:682, 1944.

38. **Laurent LE, Lindstrom BL:** *Osteochondrosis of the capitelum humeri (Panner's disease).* Acta Orthop Scand 26:111, 1957.

39. **Smith MGH:** *Osteochondritis of the humerus capitelum.* J Bone Joint Surg 46B:50, 1964.

40. **Clarke NMP, Blakemore ME, Thompson AG:** *Osteochondritis of the trochlear epiphysis.* J Pediatr Orthop 3(5):601, 1983.

41. **Preiser G:** *Eine typkische posttraumatische und zur spontanfraktur führende Ostitis des Naviculare carpi.* Fortschr Geb Roentgenstr 15:189, 1910.

42. **Allen PR:** *Idiopathic avascular necrosis of the scaphoid.* J Bone Joint Surg 65B:333, 1983.

43. **de Smet L:** *Avascular nontraumatic necrosis of the scaphoid. Preiser's disease?* Chir Main 19(2):82, 2000.

44. **Sever JW:** *Apophysitis of the os calcis.* NY Med J 95:1025, 1912.

45. **Hughes ESR:** *Painful heels in children.* Surg Gynecol Obstet 86:64, 1948.

46. **Shopfner CE, Coin CG:** *Effect of weight-bearing on the appearance and development of the secondary calcaneal epiphysis.* Radiology 86:201, 1966.

47. **Volpon JB, de Carvalho Filho G:** *Calcaneal apophysitis: A quantitative radiographic evaluation of the secondary ossification center.* Arch Orthop Trauma Surg 122(6):338, 2002.

48. **Sinding-Larsen MF:** *A hitherto unknown affection of the patella in children.* Acta Radiol 1:171, 1921.

49. **Johansson S:** *En forut icke beskriven sjukdom i patella.* Hygiea 84:161, 1922.

50. **Medlar RC, Lyne ED:** *Sinding-Larsen-Johansson disease. Its etiology and natural history.* J Bone Joint Surg 60A:1113, 1978.

51. **Wolf J:** *Larsen-Johansson disease of the patella. Seven new case records. Its relationship to other forms of osteochondritis. Use of male sex hormones as a new form of treatment.* Br J Radiol 23:335, 1950.

52. **Thiemann H:** *Juvenile Epiphysenstorungen.* Fortschr Geb Roentgenstr Nukleurmed 14:19, 1909.

53. **Giedion A:** *Acrodysplasias, cone-shaped epiphyses, peripheral dysostosis, Thiemann's disease, and acrodysostosis.* Progr Pediatr Radiol 4:325, 1973.

54. **Melo-Gomes JA, Melo-Gomes E, Viana-Queiros M:** *Thieman's disease.* J Rheumatol 8(3) 462, 1981.

55. **Van Neck, M:** *Osteochondrite du pubis.* Arch Franco-Belges Chir 27:239, 1924.

56. **Caffey J, Ross SE:** *The ischiopubic synchondrosis in healthy children: Some normal roentgenologic findings.* AJR 76:488, 1956.

57. **Burns BH:** *Osteochondritis juvenilis of the lower ulnar epiphysis.* Proc R Soc Med 24:912, 1931.

58. **Liffert RS, Arking AM:** *Post-traumatic aseptic necrosis of the distal tibial epiphysis.* J Bone Joint Surg 32A:691, 1950.

59. **Mandl F:** *Die Schlatter'sche Krankheit: Als "Systemerkrankung."* Bruns Veitr Klin Chir 126:707, 1922.

60. **Iselin H:** *Wachstumsbeschwerden zur Zeit der Knochernen Entwicklung der Tuberositas metatarsi quinti.* Dtsch Z Chir 117:529, 1912.

61. **Scapinelli R:** *Blood supply of the human patella. Its relation to ischaemic necrosis after fracture.* J Bone Joint Surg 49B:563, 1967.

62. **Orava S, Vintanen K, Typpo T:** *Diffuse osteochondrosis of the patella.* Br J Sports Med 16(3)174, 1982.

63. **Ellman H:** *Unusual affections of the preadolescent elbow.* J Bone Joint Surg 49A:203, 1967.

64. **Taylor JAM, Schultz GD, Hubka MJ:** *Osteonecrosis of the first metatarsal sesamoid: Literature review and case report.* Chiro Sports Med 4:135, 1990.

65. **Taylor JAM, Resnick D:** *Acute foot pain during an aerobics class.* J Musculoskel Med 10(4):81, 1993.

Nutritional, Metabolic, and Endocrine Disorders

14

Lindsay J. Rowe and Terry R. Yochum

OSTEOPOROSIS

Introduction

Osteoporosis is a reduction in bone quantity, with the actual quality of the bone remaining normal. Strictly interpreted, *osteoporosis,* a term introduced by Pommer in 1885, means "increased porosity of bone." (1) This is the most commonly encountered metabolic disease of bone. (2) An all-encompassing term used to describe increased radiolucency in bone is *osteopenia,* meaning "poverty of bone." It does not, however, imply a cause for the decreased bone density. Osteoporosis is classified into three types: generalized, regionalized, and localized. (Table 14-1)

Generalized Osteoporosis. In generalized osteoporosis, bone density is decreased in the majority of the skeleton, especially the axial components of the spine, pelvis, and proximal long bones. A number of conditions predispose an individual to this type of osteoporosis, the most common of which are postmenopausal status and aging.

Regionalized Osteoporosis. Loss of bone density confined to a region or segment of the body, such as an entire limb or portion of a limb, is defined as regionalized osteoporosis. The most typical example is the osteoporosis that follows immobilization of a body part, such as after fracture. Other examples include Sudeck's atrophy and transient regional osteoporosis.

Localized Osteoporosis. Focal losses of bone density affecting a relatively small area of bone are usually the result of local disease such as inflammatory arthritis, neoplasm, or infection.

GENERALIZED OSTEOPOROSIS

Senile and Postmenopausal Osteoporosis

General Considerations

Osteoporosis associated with advancing age in male and female individuals is termed senile osteoporosis, senescent osteoporosis, or old-age osteoporosis. In the female an additional designation used is postmenopausal osteoporosis. These terms encompass the most commonly encountered cause for generalized osteoporosis. The statistics on osteoporosis are staggering: It affects 28 million people in the United States, it causes 1.3 million fractures a year in patients > 45 years of age, and it burdens the economy at an annual rate of $3.8 billion. (1,2) After 35 years of age, bone mass decreases owing to the reduction of osteoblastic differentiation, activity, and life span. (3) This process usually begins earlier and proceeds more rapidly in women from hormonal deprivation that, in turn, stimulates osteoclast activity. (3) The process proceeds at an approximate rate of 1% per year for cortical bone, until approximately 20–40% has been lost by the age of 65. (4,5) Trabecular bone resorbs even faster, at the rate of 2% per year. At menopause, the average rate of bone loss accelerates 10-fold, whereas in the lumbar spine this advances to 20-fold or 6% per year. (6,7)

Clinical Features

Reduction in skeletal mass occurs gradually, becoming clinically observable in the 5th or 6th decade of life in females and in the

Table 14-1	Conditions Associated with Osteoporosis

Generalized
 Majority of skeleton involved, especially axial components
 Common
  Malignant bone disease (multiple myeloma, etc.)
  Senile and postmenopausal osteoporosis
 Others
  Acromegaly
  Alcoholism
  Hemolytic anemia
  Heparin therapy
  Hyperparathyroidism
  Hyperthyroidism
  Idiopathic juvenile
  Steroids (therapy, Cushing's)
Regionalized
 Region of skeleton involved
 Common
  Immobilization
 Others
  Migratory osteoporosis
  Transient osteoporosis
  Sudeck's atrophy
Localized
 Focal involvement
 Common
  Infection
  Inflammatory arthritis
  Neoplasm

6th or 7th decade in males. Women are affected more frequently, with an approximate ratio of 4:1 over men. Approximately 33% of females will be affected by osteoporosis, whereas an estimated 1 in 12 men will develop the disease. (8) After the age of 80 years, the sex ratio equalizes. (9)

Symptomatology related only to the decreased bone mass is variable and frequently absent. The most frequent complications that precipitate pain and disability are spinal compression fractures, increasing thoracic kyphosis, and other fractures of bone—especially the proximal femur, ribs, humerus, and radius. The incidence of hip fractures in women doubles every 5 years after the age of 60 years. (10) The incidence of vertebral fracture in older postmenopausal woman is estimated to be as high as 64% (11) and in relation to osteoporosis accounts for 700,000 fractures per year in the United States. (12) Clinically, many vertebral compression fractures are undiagnosed owing to lack of symptomatology. (13) Physical examination of a patient with osteoporosis complicated by spinal deformity reveals a shortened kyphotic stature and spinal rigidity. The presence of acute compression fractures may be suspected if localized pain is elicited on coughing, sneezing, or straining.

Neurological abnormalities are infrequent in spinal compression fractures, though spinal stenosis from progressive angular deformity within 1 year of fracture should be monitored. (14) A 9-fold increase in the relative risk of death has been estimated in patients with vertebral fractures. (11) Laboratory investigations generally are unrewarding, except for elevated urinary hydroxyproline levels. (15)

Treatment of symptomatic spinal compression fractures has shown favorable results in 78% of patients with vertebroplasty in which cement or acrylic is injected into the collapsed vertebral body. (16) Current surgical vertebroplasty techniques can be per-

formed on an outpatient basis (17); most patients report immediate and substantial results in perception of pain as well as functional capacity. (18,19) The estimated cost of the procedure ranges from $300 to $600, and complications occur in < 1% of surgical procedures performed. (20,21) The most common complication reported to date is nerve root pain, resulting from leakage of the injected material. (18) In general, it has been estimated that 20% patients who have suffered a vertebral fracture related to osteoporosis will experience a subsequent fracture within 1 year. (11)

Pathologic Features

The exact pathogenesis of postmenopausal and senile osteoporosis has not been delineated. Various influential factors have been implicated, such as certain hormones, calcium intake, levels of activity, diet, and age-related involution of osteoblasts and osteocytes. (2)

Histopathologic examination of osteoporotic bone reveals it to be of normal quality but diminished quantity. The cortical bone appears thin. Internally, the trabeculae are also attenuated and sparse. In weight-bearing bones, such as the vertebral bodies, there is preferential resorption of non-essential supporting trabeculae and relative sparing of the major, vertically oriented stress trabeculae. The combination of these trabecular alterations gives the bone a more porous appearance, from which the term osteoporosis is derived.

Assessment

Current literature dealing with non-invasive bone densitometry is characterized by conflicting results and controversy as to which method is most accurate in determining bone status at a particular site. (22)

Radiogrametry. In radiogrametry, the thickness of the cortex is measured in a peripheral bone, typically the second metacarpal, and is calculated against known standards. It measures bone density of the appendicular skeleton but not of the axial skeleton.

Single-Photon Absorptiometry. A single-photon source emits a photon beam that is attenuated as it passes through bone, usually the radius or calcaneus, in single-photon absorptiometry. The density of bone is calculated by the measured transmission count rate. The calcaneus, distal radius, and radial shaft all have about an equal degree of association with vertebral osteoporosis but have high false-negative rates, which makes the technique unreliable. The radiation dose is 2–5 mrad.

Dual-Photon Absorptiometry. In dual-photon absorptiometry, photons are emitted at two different energy levels and are, therefore, not influenced by the thickness of soft tissue. They are applied to the spine and proximal femur. Measurements in the spine relate poorly to those of the proximal femur. Readings are also influenced by osteophytes, sclerosis, facet disease, scoliosis, and vascular calcifications. The radiation dose is 5–15 mrad. Aside from bone density analysis, modern advances of this technique that can deliver high-resolution images have made this modality a useful alternative for the clinical diagnosis and evaluation of vertebral fractures. (13) The major advantage is the relatively low radiation dose. (13)

Quantitative CT. Assessment of bone mineral density with quantitative CT can be performed at any skeletal site; however, it is most commonly used to assess the strength of vertebrae in assessment of fracture risk. (23) A calibration is obtained with a known standard, a *scout scan* is obtained, and a single-photon (or preferably dual-photon) beam is passed through a vertebral body. Density measurements are taken from the calibration phantom and compared with the anterior midvertebral body to calculate the mineral content. Measurements have correlated well with the prevalence of vertebral fracture and have provided an index of fracture risk. The radiation dose is 200–250 mrad.

Other Methods. Alternative methods include neutron activation analysis (extremely accurate, not readily available, and high radiation dose of 300–5000 mrad), dual-energy projection radiography (developing technology and radiation dose of 60–20 mrad), and Compton scattering (accurate, not readily available, and low radiation dose). Micro-MRI techniques, which can visualize the internal architecture of bone, are currently being investigated to assess the biomechanical properties of the bone to resist fracture; however, current drawbacks limit the assessment to the peripheral skeleton and the detection sensitivity is inadequate. (24)

Radiologic Features

General Features. The radiologic abnormalities of osteoporosis closely correlate with the observed pathologic alterations. The major radiographic signs consist of increased radiolucency, cortical thinning, and altered trabecular patterns. In addition, superimposed changes such as fracture and adjacent degenerative arthritis may be evident. (Table 14-2) The degree and type of radiographic abnormalities will depend on the skeletal location.

Increased Radiolucency. The increased radiolucency is purely a reflection of decreased bone mass. At least 30–50% loss of bone tissue must occur before an observable radiographic change becomes evident. (25) The best term to describe this decrease in bone density is *osteopenia.* This generic designation allows for description of the decreased density but does not imply its cause.

As such, osteopenia is also a sign in other disease states that diminish bone mass, such as osteomalacia, hyperparathyroidism, and rickets.

Cortical Thinning. Careful observation of the cortices of the osseous structures will show a generalized thinning, with comparable increase in the marrow cavity size. The cortex of an osteoporotic bone has been described as *pencil thin,* defining its thin and frail appearance. Endosteal scalloping may be visible, especially in the earlier phases. The *metacarpal index assessment* of bone mass uses this parameter of osteoporosis. For this assessment, the combined cortical thickness of the second metacarpal

Table 14-2	General Radiologic Features of Osteoporosis
Increased radiolucency	
Cortical thinning	
Altered trabecular patterns	
Fracture deformity	

Table 14-3	Spinal Manifestations of Osteoporosis
Decreased bone density	
Trabecular changes	
Accentuation of primary trabeculae (pseudo-hemangiomatous appearance)	
Washed-out appearance	
Cortical thinning	
Changes in vertebral shape	
Vertebra plana (pancake vertebra or silver dollar vertebra)	
Wedged vertebra	
Biconcave deformities (fish vertebra)	
Localized endplate deformities	
Schmorl's nodes	

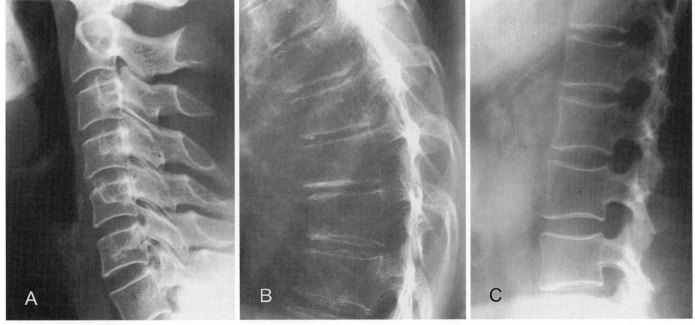

Figure 14-1 **OSTEOPOROSIS. A–C. Spine.** Observe the diminished density of the vertebral bodies and the thinned but relatively prominent cortical endplates. No fracture deformities are evident at this stage.

is normalized with the outer bone diameter at the measuring site. (26) A reduction in the results from normal correlate well with axial bone mass, and the method is favorable with the advent of digital radiographic techniques because an accurate and precise assessment of bone mass can be made from these studies without the use of special imaging procedures. (26)

Altered Trabecular Patterns. Although there is a loss of bone mass, trabecular changes are often radiographically visible. Usually, as trabeculae are resorbed, those that remain appear accentuated, especially along the regions of greatest stress. As the disease becomes more severe, the internal trabecular architecture may be completely lost, giving the bone a *washed-out appearance*.

Target Sites of Involvement

Spine. Spinal manifestations of osteoporosis are frequently distinctive and pronounced. The major features consist of decreased bone density, trabecular changes, cortical thinning, and altered vertebral body shape. (Table 14-3)

Curve Changes. Increased thoracic kyphosis is common in osteoporosis and results from compression fractures, anterior vertebral body remodeling, and loss of disc height. Increased kyphosis or scoliosis increase the risk for compression fractures later in life. (27) Up to 40% of patients with osteoporotic compression fractures have a lumbar or thoracolumbar scoliosis of at least 10°. (28)

Decreased Bone Density. The density, especially of the vertebral body, diminishes in parallel with loss of bone mass. (Fig. 14-1) The radiographic assessment of this diminished density is largely subjective and depends on adequate technologic exposure. A broad indicator is that the internal vertebral body density approaches that of the surrounding soft tissue structures. Fre-

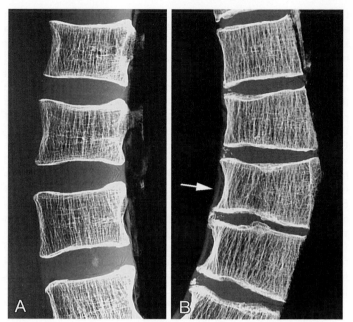

Figure 14-2 **OSTEOPOROSIS: SPECIMEN RADIOGRAPHS, SPINAL TRABECULAR CHANGES. A. Lateral Lumbar Spine.** Note that the trabecular patterns are well seen in each of the lumbar vertebrae. Observe that the vertical struts appear more prominent. **B. Lateral Thoracic Spine.** Observe that similar findings are evident, with the vertical trabeculae distinctively conspicuous. A minimal wedged anterior compression deformity is also present (*arrow*). *COMMENT:* It is this vertical trabecular accentuation that produces the so-called *pseudo-hemangiomatous appearance* of moderately advanced osteoporosis. (Courtesy of Donald Resnick, MD, San Diego, California.)

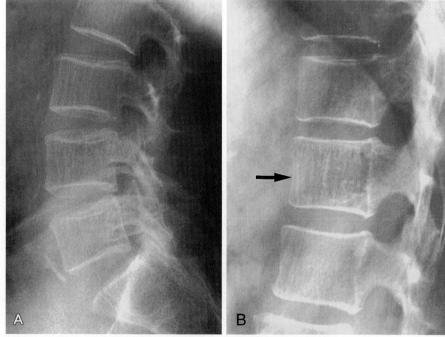

Figure 14-3 **OSTEOPOROSIS: PSEUDO-HEMANGIOMATOUS APPEARANCE. A. Lateral Lumbar Spine Pseudo-Hemangioma.** Observe the accentuated vertical trabecular patterns of multiple segments, producing a *pseudo-hemangiomatous appearance.* This is a manifestation of early to moderate osteoporosis, the appearance being lost in advanced cases. There is loss of the horizontal supports with thickening of the vertical struts. **B. Lateral Thoracolumbar Spine Hemangioma.** Note that this most common benign tumor of the spine presents with strikingly similar accentuated vertical trabecular markings (*corduroy cloth appearance*) but is localized to only one level (*arrow*). (Panel A courtesy of James G. Maxwell, DC, Sydney, Australia.)

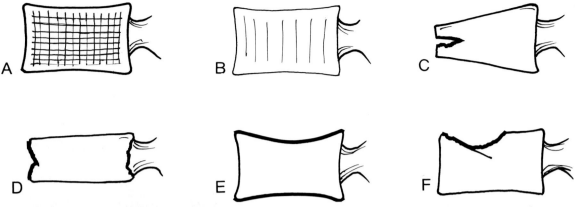

Figure 14-4 **OSTEOPOROSIS: VERTEBRAL BODY CONFIG-URATIONS. A. Normal. B. Normal with Pencil-Thin Cortices. C. Wedge Shape Owing to Anterior Loss of Height. D. Plana** with Both Anterior and Posterior Collapse. E. Biconcave (Fish Vertebra) Owing to Gradual Endplate Depression. F. Angular Endplate Depression from Acute Fracture.

quently, a radiograph calculated on the basis of normal bone density will be overexposed because of the osteoporosis.

Trabecular Changes. Within the vertebral bodies, the vertical trabeculae appear to become increasingly accentuated. This is largely owing to the preferential resorption of the horizontal trabeculae, allowing easier delineation of those remaining. In certain individuals, this may simulate the vertical radiodense striations of hemangioma (*pseudo-hemangiomatous appearance* of osteoporosis). (Figs. 14-2 and 14-3) Osteoporosis can be differentiated because it involves a number of contiguous segments, whereas hemangioma is usually a solitary lesion. In some instances no internal trabeculae may be visible.

Cortical Thinning. The cortical outlines of the vertebral body and neural arch are usually notably thinned. This is best depicted at the vertebral body endplates, which are normally relatively thick.

Changes in Shape. A number of altered vertebral configurations may be evident within an osteoporotic vertebral column. (Fig. 14-4) These are rare in the cervical spine, less common in the upper thoracic spine, and most common in the midthoracic and thoracolumbar regions. It is not uncommon to see all shape types in the one osteoporotic vertebral column. (Fig. 14-5)

Vertebra Plana (Pancake Vertebra). Pancake vertebra is a compression deformity of the vertebral body characterized by a loss in both the anterior and posterior vertical heights, often in multiple segments. (Fig. 14-6) When present, this configuration must be differentiated from a more serious cause, especially metastatic carcinoma and multiple myeloma, by pertinent laboratory

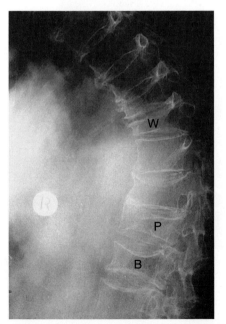

Figure 14-5 **OSTEOPOROSIS: VERTEBRAL BODY SHAPE CHANGES. Lateral Thoracic Spine.** Note that several changes in vertebral body shape can be observed: wedge (*W*), plana (*P*), and biconcave (*B*). Also, the thoracic kyphosis has increased, which is a frequent sequela.

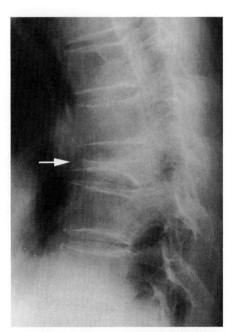

Figure 14-6 **OSTEOPOROSIS: VERTEBRAL BODY PATHO-LOGIC FRACTURE (VERTEBRA PLANA). Lateral Thoracic Spine.** Note the isolated compression fracture at the T8 segment (*arrow*). *COMMENT:* The loss of the posterior and anterior height suggests an underlying pathologic condition for which the differential diagnosis includes multiple myeloma, metastatic carcinoma, other malignancy, and osteoporosis. The diagnosis in this case was osteoporosis. (Courtesy of Melvin P. Deutsch, DC, Miami, Florida.)

investigations. This is an unusual presentation for osteoporosis and, if seen, must arouse the suspicion for these other malignant bone diseases to be the underlying cause for these fractures. MRI does not reliably differentiate between pathologic and osteoporotic fractures. (29)

Wedged Vertebra. Compression deformities that demonstrate loss of the anterior vertebral body height with preservation of the posterior height are termed *wedged vertebrae.* The resultant trapezoidal configuration is diagnostic of this type of compression abnormality and may also be seen at multiple levels (Fig. 14-7). The same shape is also common in traumatic compression fractures of the spine, even those that exhibit normal mineralization. These are most common in the midthoracic and thoracolumbar regions. (27)

Biconcave Deformities (Fish, Codfish, Fish-Mouth, Biconcave, or Hourglass Vertebrae). Central depression of the vertebral body endplates may be apparent at multiple contiguous levels. The endplates show an exaggerated concavity that simulates the vertebral body appearance found in a normal fish. (30,31) (Fig. 14-8) This osseous deformity is the direct mechanical sequela of pressure on the weakened bone from the nucleus pulposus. In the presence of these biconcave deformities, the intervertebral disc spaces are usually of normal height. The same endplate defects frequently accompany other diffuse bone-weakening diseases, such as osteomalacia, Paget's disease, and hyperparathyroidism.

Isolated Endplate Deformities. Frequently, isolated endplate fractures occur peripherally or centrally. Central endplate fractures are most frequent at L1 and L4. (27) These deformities are often depicted only on a single view, such as an oblique, on

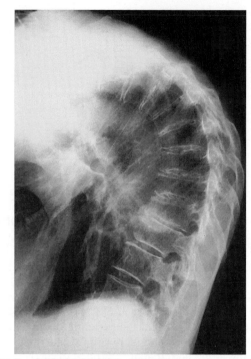

Figure 14-7 OSTEOPOROSIS: SEVERE SENILE KYPHOSIS. Lateral Thoracic Spine. Note the severe postural alteration, which is a complication owing to loss of disc height and anterior wedging of the vertebral bodies. This underlies the physical appearance of the buffalo or dowager's hump deformity.

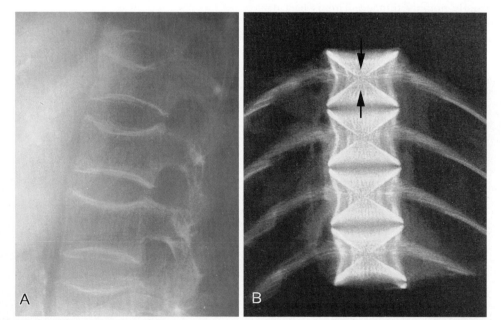

Figure 14-8 OSTEOPOROSIS: BICONCAVE ENDPLATES (FISH VERTEBRAE). A. Lateral Lumbar Spine. Note that the endplates are markedly concave in contour at multiple levels. Note the thin cortices and normal intervertebral disc spaces. This configuration does not occur unless there is loss of vertebral body strength and a normally hydrated nucleus pulposus to exert mechanical deformation of the endplate. **B. Specimen AP Radiography, Alaskan King Salmon Spine.** Note the profile of the endplates can be seen to be deeply depressed centrally, creating an appearance of distinctly biconcave endplates (*arrows*). It is from this striking similarity to the endplate deformities of the osteoporotic vertebral body that the term *fish vertebra* has arisen. (Courtesy of James Heston, DC, Homer, Alaska, and Lee D. Nordstrom, DC, Anchorage, Alaska. Reprinted with permission from **Rowe LJ:** *Fish vertebrae.* J Austr Chiro Assoc 18(3):111, 1988.)

which the endplate is projected into a slightly different plane. Radiographic manifestations consist of an altered orientation of the endplate, sharp offset in continuity, and increased density adjacent to the fracture site.

Schmorl's Nodes. Localized intrabody discal herniations are frequently superimposed on the osteoporotic spinal column. (32) Their appearance is almost identical to those nodes of juvenile onset, although they tend to be smaller and exhibit more irregular borders. Most commonly, these nuclear extrusions occur in the thoracic and upper lumbar spines.

Differential Diagnosis of Compression Fractures. Compression fractures of the spine frequently present diagnostic problems concerning their cause and time of occurrence. Key radiographic signs can often be identified that help solve these dilemmas.

Endplate Deformities. Formation of biconcave endplates (*fish vertebrae*) can be simulated by notochordal remnants (nuclear impressions). Notochordal remnants on the frontal view show a characteristic bilobed endplate configuration (*cupid's bow*), involve the posterior two thirds of the endplate, and on CT scan demonstrate two parasagittal depressions located postero-laterally (*owls' eyes*). Schmorl's nodes are readily excluded by the focal nature and distinctive pit delineated by cortical bone.

Compression Deformities. Traumatic fractures usually exhibit normal bone density and anterior loss of vertebral body height. In more severe trauma, posterior offset is more common owing to a retropulsed fragment or ligamentous instability. Pathologic fractures are often osteopenic, collapsed anteriorly and posteriorly (vertebra plana), and may be associated with pedicle destruction. Vertebra plana containing gas within the vertebral body usually indicates a pathologic cause, including metastatic disease, myeloma, radiotherapy, amyloidosis, or corticosteroid-induced avascular necrosis. (33,34)

Developmental wedge deformity is frequent at T11–L1. Physiological wedging of the thoracic vertebral bodies can be up to 5° at each segment. Multiple anterior Schmorl's nodes frequently increase the sagittal dimension while inhibiting vertical body growth, precipitating a wedged deformity.

Acute and Healed Fractures. Acute fractures often show an area of increased density just beneath the endplate owing to trabecular impaction and later reactive callus. This feature may be present for up to 8–10 weeks postfracture. Offset at the anterior cortex is usually abrupt and angular (*step sign*). In acute thoracic compression fractures, hematoma can be identified by displaced paraspinal lines. In the lumbar spine, air in the small bowel (ileus) may be a clue to an acute fracture. Old fractures lack a zone of sub-endplate density; have no step sign; and usually have adjacent disc degeneration with osteophytes, vacuum phenomenon, and loss of height. Bone scan does not reliably distinguish recent and old fractures < 18 months from the time of trauma. (35) This is best done by MRI. (See Chapter 6.)

Pelvis and Femora. The skeletal components of the pelvis and femur are prominent sites of osteoporosis. Manifestations in these locations are identical to most other sites with decreased bone density, trabecular changes, cortical thinning, and fracture-related deformities. (Fig. 14-9) It should be noted that fractures of the hip are the most serious complication of osteoporosis, and it is estimated that these injuries are increasing in frequency owing to the increasing longevity of the world's population. (36) Approximately 30% of hip fractures occur in males, and the rates of mortality and morbidity appear to be higher when affecting men versus women. (37)

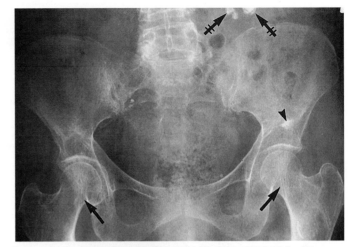

Figure 14-9 **OSTEOPOROSIS: PELVIS AND FEMORA. AP Pelvis.** Observe the thin cortices and relative accentuation of those remaining trabeculae. Within the femoral necks, the principal compressive trabeculae (*arrows*) are enhanced. Of incidental notation are calcified abdominal mesenteric lymph nodes (*crossed arrows*) and a supra-acetabular bone island (*arrowhead*).

Decreased Bone Density. Although there is a widespread rarefaction of the skeletal structures, those areas that are normally thin distinctly reflect the diminishing bone mass. The most prominent sites are the iliac fossae, pubis, supra-acetabular area, femoral neck, and greater trochanter. In these locations, the loss of bone density may simulate destruction from a more aggressive etiology.

Trabecular Changes. Accentuation of the weight-bearing trabeculae is most prominent in the regions between the sacroiliac and the hip joints, as well as in the proximal femur. Analysis of the trabecular pattern of the upper end of the femur is an excellent indicator of the severity of the osteoporosis. (38) (Fig. 14-10) The most readily visible trabeculae consist of three groups:

- *Principal compressive group.* Trabeculae in this group extend from the medial metaphyseal cortex to the superior femoral head and are the major weight-bearing trabeculae. In osteoporosis these appear accentuated and are the last to be obliterated. In the normal patient these trabeculae are the thickest and most densely packed.
- *Secondary compressive group.* Originating adjacent to the cortex, near the lesser trochanter, these trabeculae curve upward and laterally toward the greater trochanter and upper femoral neck. Characteristically, these are thin and widely separated.
- *Principal tensile group.* These trabeculae originate from the lateral cortex, inferior to the greater trochanter, and extend in an arch-like configuration medially, terminating in the inferior portion of the femoral head.

Confluence of these three trabecular groups in the femoral neck forms a triangular region of radiolucency, *Ward's triangle.* (38) In early osteoporosis, radiolucency of this triangle becomes more prominent as the surrounding less-visible trabeculae are resorbed and the bordering groups become more clearly demarcated. With increasing severity, the tensile group regresses from medial to lateral, eventually opening *Ward's triangle* laterally. In advanced

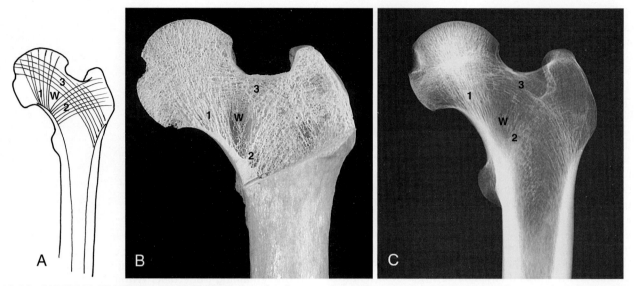

Figure 14-10   NORMAL TRABECULAR PATTERNS. Proximal Femur. A. Diagram. Three major patterns exist: principal compressive group (*1*), secondary compressive group (*2*), and principal tensile group (*3*). The confluence of these trabeculae leaves an area relatively void of structure, *Ward's triangle* (*W*). **B. Specimen Radiograph.** Note that the arrangement of the trabecular bundles can be discerned, defining *Ward's triangle*, which is relatively devoid of bony struts. **C. Specimen Radiograph.** Observe that the corresponding plain film confirms the trabecular orientation and arrangement within the proximal femur and *Ward's triangle*.

osteoporosis, the principal compressive component is the last to be involved and is manifest by a decrease in number and length of individual trabeculae. Eventually, the upper femur may be completely devoid of all trabecular markings.

Cortical Thinning. All cortices of the pelvis and proximal femora are attenuated in thickness and radiographic visibility. The most distinctive locations are the iliac crests, pubic rami, ischia, femoral head, and neck. In severe osteoporosis, the normally sharp demarcation between cortex and medullary cavity may be completely obliterated.

Fracture Deformity. The most frequent sites of fracture involve the pubic rami and proximal femur. (Fig. 14-11) These may occur spontaneously or from incidental trauma. Generally, healing time and quality are not affected, despite the osteoporosis, except in intracapsular fractures of the femoral neck, which may precipitate secondary avascular necrosis of the femoral head. In patients who have both osteoporosis and advanced degenerative joint disease of the hip joint, associated stress fractures occasionally occur through the pubic rami or the medial aspect of the femoral neck.

Degenerative Joint Disease of the Hip. The prevalence of osteoarthritis of the hip is low (< 5%) in the presence of osteoporosis. (39) Conversely, a degenerative hip is associated with a diminished risk for spinal compression fractures.

Additional Skeletal Manifestations. Within the appendicular skeleton the radiographic expressions of osteoporosis are similar to those encountered in the spine and pelvis. The most apparent abnormalities are bone rarefaction, altered trabecular pattern, cortical thinning, and fracture-related deformities. (Fig. 14-12) The most common fractures associated with osteoporosis outside the spine and proximal femora involve the distal radius (Colles' fracture), humeral neck, and ankle malleoli. Attempts to correlate the degree of osteoporosis with changes in the thickness of the cortex of the second metacarpal have shown a reasonable degree of accuracy. (40) In the skull, thinning of the inner and outer tables and generalized loss in density are the only visible features.

Insufficiency Fractures

Clinical Features. Insufficiency fractures occur when the elastic strength of the bone is not sufficient to withstand normal physiological stress. (41) Predisposing bone-weakening disorders

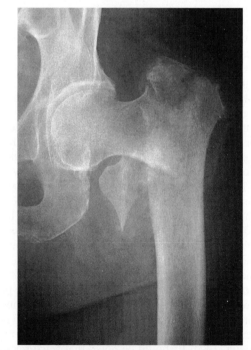

Figure 14-11   OSTEOPOROSIS: INTERTROCHANTERIC FEMORAL FRACTURE. AP Hip. Note the fracture through the intertrochanteric region. *COMMENT:* Fractures of the proximal femur are the most common severe presentation of osteoporosis. Such fractures can occur elsewhere within the proximal femur, including subcapital, midcervical, basocervical, and subtrochanteric locations.

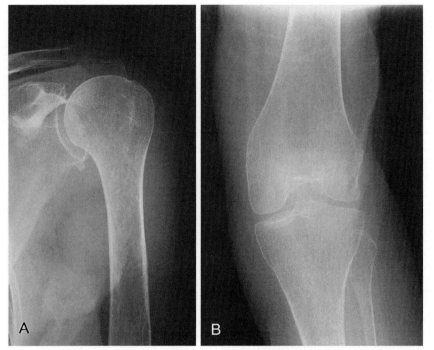

Figure 14-12 OSTEOPOROSIS: EXTREMITY MANIFESTATIONS. A. AP Shoulder. B. AP Knee. Observe the decreased density, trabecular enhancement, and thin cortices.

include osteoporosis owing to any cause (postmenopausal, osteogenesis imperfecta, multiple myeloma, corticosteroid therapy), radiation necrosis, osteomalacia, Paget's disease, and fibrous dysplasia. With respect to osteoporosis, the most common locations for complication from insufficiency fractures are the spine, hip, and distal radius. (1) When affecting the weight-bearing bones of the lower limb, these fractures are frequently bilateral.

Clinically, pain is the major symptom over the fracture site. Because there may be multiple fractures in multiple bones, the diagnosis may not be suspected and found only when a bone scan is obtained. If the cause for the insufficiency fractures is not clear based on history, risk factors, or imaging findings, laboratory examination and, possibly, biopsy may be required for diagnosis. Rest and pain control are the only treatments, and removal of the cause for the bone alteration is rarely possible.

Radiologic Features. Imaging features are the same as stress fractures, with plain film studies frequently unrewarding. When present, the fracture site may be marked by localized periosteal response and transverse opaque zones of callus. Only occasionally a fracture line may be visible. These usually are metaphyseal in location. Such fractures characteristically affect the weight-bearing bones, including metatarsal necks, posterior calcaneum, distal and proximal tibia and fibula at their outer margins, medial neck of femur, and sacral ala. These fractures often are found simultaneously at multiple and symmetrical sites.

Bone scans are the most sensitive imaging modality for demonstrating insufficiency fractures identified by focal increased uptake at the fracture site. CT scan is especially useful for sacral lesions and if doubt arises in the differential diagnosis from underlying pathology.

Sacrum. The most common cause of fracture of the sacrum is senile and postmenopausal osteoporosis with a history of a recent fall onto the buttocks. (42–45) The second most common occurrence is fracture secondary to radiotherapy of the pelvis followed by corticosteroid therapy (rheumatoid arthritis, chronic airways disease), alcohol abuse, multiple myeloma, osteomalacia, osteogenesis imperfecta, and recent hip replacement. (43,44, 46) It is precipitated by the high shear forces through the sacral ala during walking and may coincide with a recent increase in activity. (45)

Onset characteristically occurs after age 65 and afflicts women more than men in a ratio of at least 5:1 or greater. (43,44) Almost 2% of females > 55 years of age with back pain may have a sacral insufficiency fracture present. (44) Increased pelvic tilt is thought to be a predisposing factor. (45) Pain severity is variable, from severely debilitating to relatively asymptomatic. The site of the pain is consistently over the lumbosacral junction, sacrum, or buttocks and is aggravated by weight bearing. Up to 75% of patients have a co-existing insufficiency fracture within the pelvic ring, most commonly of a pubic ramus. (43,44) More than 65% of patients have extrapelvic insufficiency fractures, including the lower ribs, thoracic and lumbar vertebral bodies, and neck of femur.

The most sensitive method of detection is isotopic bone scan. (41–43,45) Three patterns of sacral insufficiency fractures occur based on bone scan appearance: (43,45,47,48)

- *H pattern (butterfly or "Honda" sign).* Bilateral vertical fractures through the sacral ala are connected by a transverse fracture through the S2, S3, or S4 bodies. (49) (Fig. 14-13)
- *I pattern.* A single vertical fracture passes through the sacral ala. This is the most common form of sacral insufficiency fracture in at least 70% of cases. (45) On bone scan the focal linear increased tracer uptake may be misinterpreted as sacroiliitis owing to the proximity of the fracture to the adjacent sacroiliac joint. (44)
- *Arc pattern.* A linear or curvilinear transverse fracture passes horizontally across the sacrum.

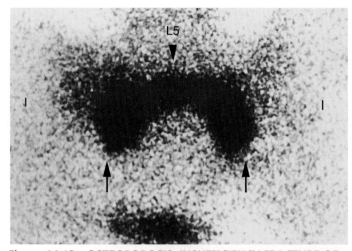

Figure 14-13 **OSTEOPOROSIS: INSUFFICIENCY FRACTURE OF THE SACRUM. Frontal Technetium-99m Isotopic Bone Scan.** Note that the L5 vertebra (*L5*) and adjacent ilium (*I*) are identified. Observe the dense uptake of the isotope within the lateral sacrum as two vertical components corresponding to the sites of fracture (*arrows*). These two vertical fractures are joined centrally by a transverse fracture through the S2 body, signified by the transverse linear uptake zone (*arrowhead*). The combination of these three components produces an H-shaped lesion referred to as the *Honda sign.*

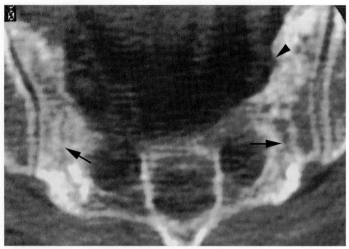

Figure 14-14 **OSTEOPOROSIS: INSUFFICIENCY FRACTURE OF THE SACRUM. CT Axial Scan.** Note the two symmetrically located insufficiency fractures in the lateral sacrum (*arrows*). Note the characteristic cortical offset at the anterior sacral margin (*arrowhead*). These fractures correspond to the vertical fractures depicted on the bone scan in Figure 14-13.

Conventional radiography depicts the fracture in < 5% of cases. (44) This is owing to a low index of clinical suspicion, background osteopenia, non-displaced nature of the fracture zone, low-grade callus formation, overlying obscuring soft tissues, and often an inappropriate view of the sacrum. (44) On the lateral view, there may be offset of the anterior sacral cortex.

Axial CT bone windows clearly identify the fracture zone in > 90% of cases. (44) (Fig. 14-14) Displacement of the anterior cortex of the sacrum within 1 cm of the sacroiliac joint is a reliable feature. Running parallel to the plane of the sacroiliac joint, but lateral to the sacral foramina, the fracture line, or linear sclerosis, may be visible. This is in contrast to traumatic fractures, which usually extend into the foramina or central canal. (44,50)

Transverse components to these fractures will not be detected on axial images. (45)

MRI shows decreased signal intensity on T1-weighted images and increased signal intensity on T2-weighted images. This is especially helpful when the fracture line cannot be seen through the sacral ala and is, therefore, readily overlooked. (51,52)

Pubis. Pubic fractures may occur through the body near the symphysis pubis or in the pubic rami. (53,54) They are most common through the body, are often bilateral, and frequently coexist with insufficiency fractures elsewhere in the pelvic ring, especially the sacral ala. (54) Patchy sclerosis, irregular lysis, disruption of the cortex, and collapse of the articular cortex simulate active neoplastic destruction, especially metastatic disease. (49) (Figs. 14-15 and 14-16) It has been previously referred to as pubic osteolysis.

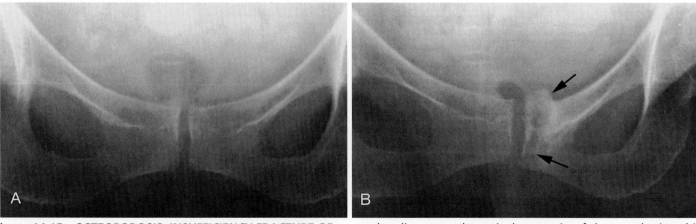

Figure 14-15 **OSTEOPOROSIS: INSUFFICIENCY FRACTURE OF THE PUBIS. A. AP Pubes. Initial Radiograph.** Note that no abnormality is identified, with the pubis bilaterally normal. **B. AP Pubes. Follow-up Radiograph.** Note that a fracture line extends vertically through the body of the pubis immedi- ately adjacent to the articular margin of the symphysis pubis (*arrows*). *COMMENT:* This is a characteristic site for osteoporotic insufficiency fracture and is frequently found in association with similar fractures of the sacrum. (Courtesy of Richard N. Garian, DC, Holliston, Massachusetts.)

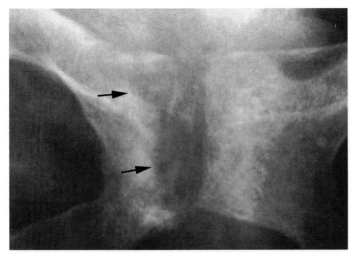

Figure 14-16 **OSTEOPOROSIS: INSUFFICIENCY FRACTURE OF THE PUBIS. AP Pubes.** Note that within the body of the pubis there is a poorly defined zone of rarefaction (*arrows*). Irregularity of the articular margin is also noted. *COMMENT:* In this case, the history was complicated with previous malignancy, and this lesion was initially considered to be a metastatic focus. Bone scan showed this to be a solitary area of uptake. After rest for only 6 weeks, there was some reconstitution of bone and resolution of localized pain.

Other Sites. Fractures are often found simultaneously at multiple and symmetrical sites. The radiographic manifestations are identical to stress fractures.

Sternum. Symptoms of fractures of the sternum include pain and swelling over the upper sternal body. The fracture is most commonly through the upper body of the sternum, transverse, and usually non-buckling in configuration. (55,56) Increased thoracic kyphosis owing to compression fractures > 60° co-exists in more than two thirds of patients. (55,56)

Acetabulum. A hazy, linear sclerotic band is most often visible at the lateral margin of the supraacetabular margin. Some fractures arc parallel to the acetabular cortex medially, at times extending to the pelvic inlet. Up to 20% may be bilateral and often co-exist with other insufficiency fractures of the pelvic ring, including the sacrum and pubis. (56)

Neck of Femur. At the medial femoral neck an indistinct streak of sclerosis may be the only sign passing obliquely upward perpendicular to the axis of the femoral neck. The radiographic signs may also include trabecular interruption, cortical fracture line, endosteal and extracortical callus, and an incomplete fracture line extending through the neck. (57)

Tibia and Fibula. The distal and proximal tibia and fibula at their outer margins are the usual sites of fracture. At the distal tibia, the band of sclerosis lies parallel with the talar dome about 2 cm above the joint line. Proximal tibia and fibula insufficiency fractures often co-exist with significant knee arthritis and are accentuated if a varus–valgus deformity is present.

Posterior Calcaneus. A higher incidence of posterior calcaneus insufficiency fractures is found in diabetes, especially involving the posterior third of the bone. A hazy curvilinear band of sclerosis marks the fracture site, passing obliquely posterior, and upward.

Metatarsal Necks. The most common site of fracture of the metatarsals is at the junction of the shaft and head.

Associated Disorders

Many disorders exhibit generalized skeletal osteoporosis. These are usually conspicuous by their slowly progressive nature and chronic duration.

Congenital Disorders. The major congenital causes are osteogenesis imperfecta, mucopolysaccharidoses, and hemolytic anemias. Idiopathic juvenile osteoporosis is a self-limiting childhood disease characterized by generalized arthritic pain and osteoporosis, especially in the spine. (58)

Vascular Disorders. The most prominent vascular diseases producing generalized osteoporosis are the hemolytic anemias, such as thalassemia and sickle cell anemia.

Nutritional Disorders. Dietary osteopenia may result from a lack of vitamin C (scurvy), vitamin D (rickets), or calcium (osteomalacia) or from excessive vitamin A (hypervitaminosis).

Metabolic and Endocrine Disorders. Hormonal imbalances frequently produce altered bone mass conditions. The most prominent disorders are hyperparathyroidism, hyperthyroidism, and Cushing's disease. Iatrogenic steroid-induced osteoporosis is also a well-documented phenomenon. Pregnancy rarely produces osteoporosis. (59) Large doses of heparin (> 15,000 units/day) also can produce osteoporosis. (60) Alcoholics will demonstrate decreased bone mass. (61)

Neoplastic Disorders. Generalized osteopenia is a frequent manifestation of multiple myeloma, metastasis, leukemia, and other myeloproliferative disorders.

CAPSULE SUMMARY Senile and Postmenopausal Osteoporosis

General Considerations

- Increasing age results in generalized osteoporosis of the entire skeleton.

Clinical Features

- Presentation is typically in the 5th and 6th decades in females by a ratio of 4:1.
- Usually causes pain only when complicated by fracture and deformity, especially in the spine.
- No laboratory findings are useful.

Pathologic Features

- Pathogenesis is unknown.
- Bone quality is normal but deficient in its amount.
- Resorption of cortical and medullary bone results in a thinned cortex and trabecular attenuation.

Radiologic Features

- Assessment remains controversial; methods include radiogrametry, single-photon absorptiometry, double-photon absorptiometry, and quantitative CT; quantitative CT is the most accurate and readily available method that has acceptable radiation dose levels.
- Key signs include increased bony radiolucency, cortical thinning, and altered trabecular patterns.

(continued)

CAPSULE SUMMARY Senile and Postmenopausal Osteoporosis (*continued*)

- *Spine:* demonstrates these findings, in addition to altered vertebral shape (plana, wedged, biconcave endplates, isolated endplate infractions, Schmorl's nodes) and pseudo-hemangiomatous appearance of vertebral bodies.
- *Pelvis and femora:* prone to fractures in the pubic rami and femoral neck. Principal tensile group of trabeculae in the femur is the last to be obliterated.
- *Insufficiency fractures:* sacrum (H, I, and arc patterns), pubis, medial femoral necks, tibia and fibula, calcaneus, and metatarsals.
- *Additional features:* most commonly associated fractures elsewhere involve the distal radius, humeral neck, and ankle malleoli.

REGIONALIZED OSTEOPOROSIS

Reflex Sympathetic Dystrophy Syndrome

General Considerations

Reflex sympathetic dystrophy syndrome (RSDS) is a unique clinical and radiographic entity. Many terms have been applied since its original description in 1864 by Mitchell et al. (1), including post-traumatic osteoporosis, Sudeck's atrophy, acute bone atrophy, and causalgia. Most recently it has been referred to as complex regional pain syndrome to emphasize the multisystem disturbances of the somatic, psychological, and behavioral aspects of the patient's life. (2) Although the mechanism has not been delineated, the syndrome is characterized by an acute onset of a painful regional osteoporosis, usually following trivial antecedent trauma.

Clinical Features

A broad spectrum of clinical signs and symptoms characterizes the syndrome. There appears to be an equal sex distribution, and it is most commonly encountered after 50 years of age. The usual sites of involvement are the hand and shoulder. The most notable feature is the progressive onset of pain, stiffness, swelling, and atrophy at and distal to the site of injury over a 3- to 6-month period. (3) The characteristic changes can usually be classified into three distinct stages: the acute or hyperemic stage, the dystrophic or ischemic phase, and the atrophic stage. (3) The antecedent traumatic event may be apparently trivial or may be enough to cause fracture. Recovery is slow and protracted over many months and may never be complete, with residual atrophy, contracture, and joint stiffness.

Pathologic Features

The pathogenesis of the disease is unclear but appears to be multifactorial because it involves the soft tissues, sensory, motor, vasomotor, and autonomic neurological systems. (2) It is believed to be a reflex overactivity of the sympathetic nervous system that mediates trophic changes in bone and soft tissues in response to external stimulus. (4) Hyperemia of bone augments osteoclastic resorption, which rapidly demineralizes the involved skeletal structures. (5)

Radiologic Features

The most characteristic radiographic change is the rapidity of the appearance and progression of the osteoporosis. Initially, the affected bone appears mottled, as a manifestation of accelerated bone resorption, mimicking the pattern of osteomyelitis. Other manifestations, such as metaphyseal osteoporosis, tunneled cortices, and endosteal resorption may be seen but require fine-detail radiography for demonstration. (6) (Fig. 14-17) Later, the entire bone density is diminished, appearing no different from

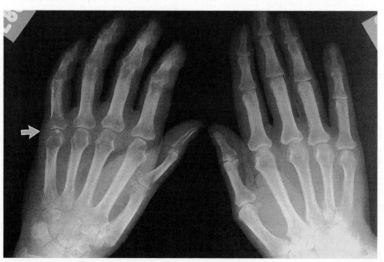

Figure 14-17 REFLEX SYMPATHETIC DYSTROPHY SYNDROME. Bilateral PA Hands. Note the distinct loss of bone density in the affected hand (*arrow*), especially in the periarticular regions of all articulations. Compare this appearance with the normal other side. A minor trauma had been incurred at the wrist 8 weeks previously.

other types of long-standing osteoporosis. Notably, the joint spaces and margins are normal, assisting in differentiating from infection or rheumatoid arthritis. Bone scintigraphy is a useful diagnostic factor in RSDS. (7) Bone scans in true RSDS will always be negative. (7)

Disuse and Immobilization Osteoporosis

Secondary causes of osteoporosis are anticipated to account for up to 50% of the cases diagnosed. (8) The causes are numerous, with the most common causes for regional osteoporosis resulting from traumatic injuries that are immobilized, motor paralysis, and inflammatory lesions of the bones and joints. (9) By natural process, immobilization inhibits osteoblastic activity of bone while osteoclastic-mediated bone resorption is accelerated. (9) Radiographic changes begin to appear after 7–10 days and will be most

extreme by 2 to 3 months. (10) In the acetabulum, the superior cortex appears as a double cortical line (*double cortical line sign*). (11) Changes in the spine and pelvis are less apparent than in the appendicular skeleton.

Therapeutic exercise and electrical stimulation, which increase mechanical stress to the affected area, have shown to be effective treatments. (9) When function is restored to the involved body part, complete restitution to a normal radiographic appearance may be anticipated.

Radiologic features after acute immobilization can be recognized by four patterns of osteoporosis: (Fig. 14-18)

- *Uniform.* All bones involved exhibit a similar degree of bone loss. This is the most common form.
- *Spotty.* Localized circular lucencies predominate, especially within the epiphyseal portions of the bones.
- *Bands.* Linear transverse subchondral or metaphyseal lucent zones.

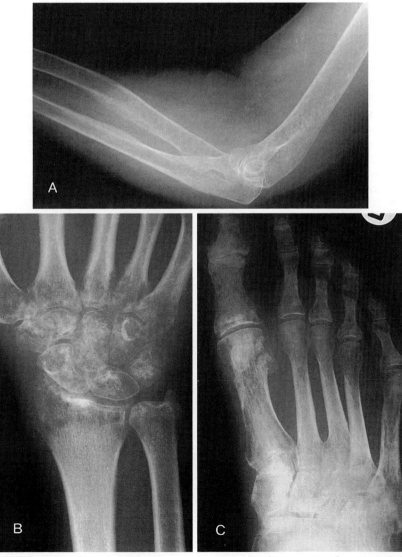

Figure 14-18 **DISUSE OSTEOPOROSIS. A. Lateral Elbow.** Note that the bones are demineralized in a uniform manner following immobilization owing to a cerebrovascular accident. **B. PA Wrist.** Observe the spotty form of disuse osteo- porosis of the wrist after immobilization for an elbow frac- ture. **C. PA Foot.** Note that a similar spotty type of deossifica- tion has occurred after immobilization for an ankle fracture.

• *Cortical.* Lamination or scalloping loss of definition in the outer and inner cortical margins.

Long-standing immobilization, such as from limb amputation or polio, can produce regional osteoporosis owing to reduced mechanical stress. (Fig. 14-19) Polio often exhibits bony underdevelopment as a marker of the childhood neuromuscular illness, which has left the skeleton devoid of muscular and gravitational stress for bone formation. (Fig. 14-20)

Transient Regionalized Osteoporosis

By definition, transient regionalized osteoporosis is used to describe osteoporosis that occurs suddenly, is reversible, affects periarticular bone, and has no associated causal factor. With the advent of MRI, the disorder has also been termed *transient bone marrow edema syndrome.* (12) Two distinct entities have been described as examples of this disorder: *transient osteoporosis of the hip* and *regional migratory osteoporosis.*

Transient Osteoporosis of the Hip

Transient osteoporosis of the hip is a peculiar disorder of unknown origin (13); however, it has been suggested that it actually represents a reversible stage of avascular necrosis. (14) The age of onset is usually between 20 and 40 years, and it is slightly more frequent in males. An association with pregnancy in females has been made dating back to the first documented case in 1959. (15,16) It is interesting that in females the left hip appears be exclusively involved; however, bilateral cases have been documented. (13) The onset is sudden, with pain, antalgia, and a limp. The diagnosis requires close attention to the history in conjunc-

tion with radiographic findings. (17) The clinical course is self-limited, over 3–12 months, with a full recovery expected. (17) Recent studies have shown that administration of bisphosphonates may allow early pain relief, which alternatively allows greater weight-bearing and reduced risk of secondary fracture. (13)

Radiologic features include marked osteoporosis of the femoral head and adjacent, less severe osteoporosis of the femoral neck and acetabulum. The joint space is normal. Isotopic bone scans show increased uptake in the hip region. On T1-weighted MRI studies, the signal is diminished within the femoral neck and head, whereas on T2-weighted images the signal is slightly increased. (18) These MRI signals can extend into the shaft along the primary trabeculae and also involve the acetabulum. Joint effusion often co-exists, though there are no bone erosions, cartilaginous defects, or synovial masses. These marrow changes usually reverse with resolution of the condition. (See Chapter 6.)

Regional Migratory Osteoporosis

Regional migratory osteoporosis is conspicuous by the migration from one joint to another. Middle-aged males are most commonly affected. (14) The most frequent joints are in the lower extremity, especially the knee, ankle, foot, and hip. Concurrent systemic osteoporosis is not an uncommon finding, leading to the hypothesis that regional migratory osteoporosis may simply represent a highly localized and exaggerated process of diffuse osteoporosis. (14) This theoretical situation has been termed a *regional acceleratory phenomena* because it relates to systemic osteoporosis. (14)

Radiologic features include localized osteoporosis of the intra-articular components, which subsequently regresses over approximately a 9-month period only to reappear in another joint. (19)

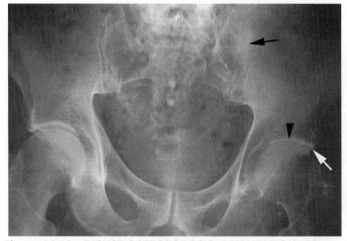

Figure 14-19 DISUSE OSTEOPOROSIS: AMPUTATION. AP Pelvis. Observe that the sacroiliac and hip joint space is narrowed (*arrows*). The cortical margin of the acetabular roof is thinner and less dense than normal (*arrowhead*). Also observe the generalized diminished density of the ilium, ischium, and proximal femur. *COMMENT:* This patient had an above-knee amputation many years earlier, with resultant disuse articular and bone changes. (Courtesy of Donald M. Kuppe, DC, Denver, Colorado.)

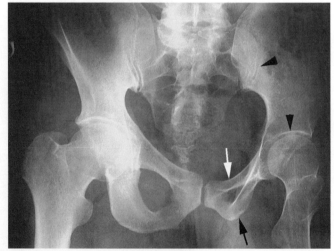

Figure 14-20 DISUSE OSTEOPOROSIS: POLIO. AP Pelvis. Observe the underdevelopment of the femur and particularly the pubis and ischium (*arrows*). Considerable osteoporosis of the entire hemipelvis and proximal femur is also evident. The joint spaces of the hip and sacroiliac joints are also narrowed (*arrowheads*).

CAPSULE SUMMARY Regional Osteoporosis

Reflex Sympathetic Dystrophy Syndrome

General Considerations

- A post-traumatic bone disorder characterized by an acute painful osteoporosis.

Clinical Features

- > 50 years of age.
- History of recent trauma that may have been trivial.
- Progressive pain, swelling, and atrophy distal to the trauma site.

Pathologic Features

- Neurovascular imbalance, promoting osseous hyperemia.

Radiologic Features

- Patchy, mottled osteoporosis.
- Metaphyseal localization.
- Later, more generalized osteoporosis.
- No joint disease.

Disuse and Immobilization Osteoporosis

General Considerations

- Traumatic injuries that are immobilized, motor paralysis, and inflammatory lesions of bones and joints constitute the most common causes.

- Changes appear on plain film after 7–10 days, becoming most extreme by 2–3 months.
- *Four radiologic patterns of disuse atrophy:* uniform, spotty, bands, and cortical lamination or scalloping.

Transient Regional Osteoporosis

General Considerations

- No associated cause.
- Sudden and reversible; affects periarticular bone.
- Two entities.

Transient Osteoporosis of the Hip

- 20–40 years; males predominant.
- Associated with pregnancy in females, left hip exclusively.
- Marked osteoporosis of the femoral head; less severe in femoral neck and acetabulum.

Regional Migratory Osteoporosis

- Males most commonly affected.
- Usually in lower extremities.
- Localized, regressing, migratory osteoporosis.

OSTEOMALACIA

General Considerations

Osteomalacia is a metabolic disorder that alters the quality of bone. It is characterized by a lack of calcium salts being deposited in osteoid tissue. The term *osteomalacia* literally means "soft bones." The condition has also been referred to as *adult rickets*. There are many causes and types of osteomalacia, but most are intimately connected with either calcium, phosphorus, or vitamin D metabolism. (1) (Table 14-4)

Clinical Features

Clinical expressions of osteomalacia are often masked by its varied causes, including intestinal malabsorption syndrome, hypovitaminosis D, and renal osteodystrophy. (2) Enteric malabsorption states such as sprue frequently have abdominal pain, bloating, and diarrhea as their major complaints. However, direct manifestations of osteomalacia include generalized muscle weakness and bone pain on palpation. The most notable features are the resulting deformities, especially in weight-bearing structures such as the pelvis, femur, tibia, and spine.

Biochemically, blood and urine changes are inconstant. Increases in serum parathormone, alkaline phosphatase, and hydroxyproline may occur, whereas calcium and phosphorous concentrations are marginally diminished. (3) When appropriate, the administration of vitamin D and a high calcium diet

Table 14-4	Causes of Osteomalacia and Rickets
Deficiency	
Vitamin D	
Calcium	
Phosphorus	
Dietary chelators	
Absorption	
Gastric abnormalities	
Biliary diseases	
Enteric malabsorption	
Renal tubular	
Proximal tubular lesions	
Proximal and distal tubular lesions	
Distal tubular lesions (tubular acidosis)	
Primary	
Secondary	
Renal osteodystrophy	
Unusual forms and associations	
Fibrous dysplasia	
Neurofibromatosis	
Neoplasm	
Anticonvulsant drugs (Dilantin)	
Hypophosphatasia	

augments osteoid mineralization, as evidenced by healing of the pseudo-fractures. Appropriate treatment protocols are often rewarding, as administration of these supplements may prove to be of benefit within the 1st week of therapy. (3) After 15 months, an increase of bone density of up to 62% may be seen. (3) Residual bone deformities may require corrective osteotomies.

Table 14-5	Alternate Terms for Pseudo-Fractures
Increment fractures Looser lines Milkman's syndrome Umbau zonen	

Table 14-6	Radiologic Features of Osteomalacia
Decreased bone density Coarse trabecular pattern Loss of cortical definition Pseudo-fractures Deformities	

Pathologic Features

Osteomalacia is histologically conspicuous by an abnormal relative increase in uncalcified osteoid that coats the surfaces of trabeculae and linings of the Haversian canals (*osteoid seams*). This histopathologic finding is also seen in other states of high bone turnover. There is a net decrease, therefore, primarily in the quality of the bone as reflected in bone rarefaction and progressive bone deformities.

A frequent associated finding first described by Looser (4) in 1920 and confirmed by Milkman (5) in 1934 is the presence of pseudo-fractures, which are also known by various other terms. (Table 14-5) These are visible both histologically and radiographically. They occur bilaterally and symmetrically as apparent fractures at right angles to the bone margin. It is thought that these are owing to either insufficiency fractures or vascular pulsations acting on the softened bone. (4,6) Histologically, they appear as linear regions of unmineralized osteoid.

Radiologic Features

The structure and density of all osseous components are affected. Frequently, no definitive radiologic diagnosis can be made with-

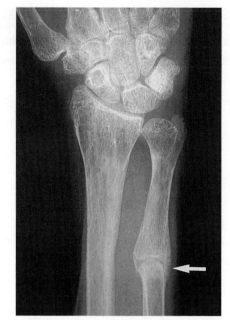

Figure 14-21   OSTEOMALACIA: GENERAL FEATURES. PA Wrist. Note the distinctive malacic changes. Observe the generalized decrease in density, coarsened trabecular patterns, loss of cortical definition, and the pseudo-fracture (*arrow*).

out the appropriate clinical and laboratory support, owing to the non-specific nature of the skeletal changes. However, the major signs of osteomalacia are decreased bone density, coarse trabecular pattern, loss of cortical definition, pseudo-fractures, and deformities. (7,8) (Fig. 14-21; Table 14-6)

Decreased Bone Density. All bones will appear more radiolucent than normal. This is secondary to the diminished bone mineral content.

Coarsened Trabecular Pattern. A decrease in the overall number of bony trabeculae within all bones enhances the contrast of those remaining. As a result, the texture of the spongiosa may appear coarse and mottled.

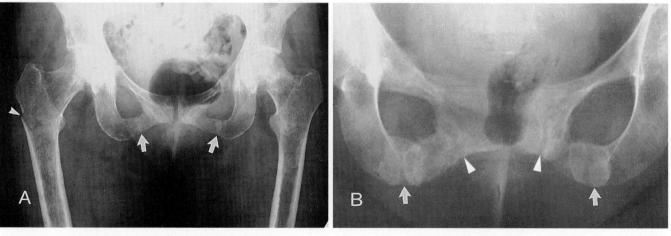

Figure 14-22   OSTEOMALACIA: PSEUDO-FRACTURES. A. AP Pelvis. Note the true subtrochanteric fracture (*arrowhead*) and the pseudofractures (*arrows*) of the pubes. **B. AP Pubis.** Note that the bulbous appearance is caused by callus formation at the pseudo-fracture site (*arrows*). Additional pseudo-fractures can be seen through the body of the pubis (*arrowheads*). (continued)

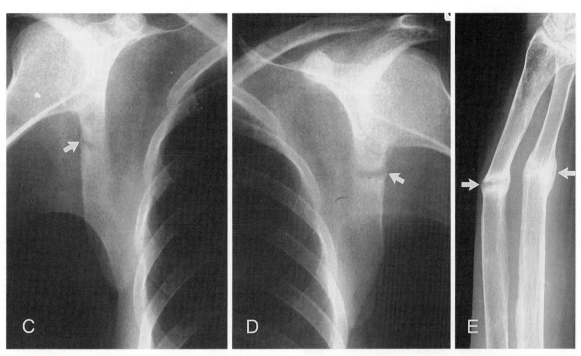

Figure 14-22 (*continued*)   **C and D. Scapular Axillary Borders. E. PA Forearm.** Note the pseudofractures in the radius and ulna (*arrows*). *COMMENT:* These defects are recognized by their bilateral symmetry and perpendicular orientation to the cortex (*arrows*).

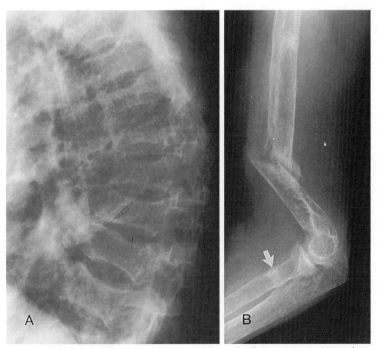

Figure 14-23   **OSTEOMALACIA: DEFORMITY. A. Lateral Thoracic Spine.** Observe the increased biconcave endplate contours. The trabeculae are coarsened. **B. Acute Fracture Lateral Elbow.** Note that after trivial trauma a fracture has occurred through the distal humerus. Note the pseudofracture in the proximal radius (*arrow*).

Loss of Cortical Definition. Close examination of the cortex reveals it to be thinner and altered in structure. Usually, the endosteal surface is blurred and indistinct. In addition, intracortical striations may be evident. (9)

Pseudo-Fractures. Pseudo-fractures are linear radiolucencies that usually occur bilaterally and symmetrically in predictable locations. They are more readily identified in chronic situations owing to the increased width of the defect and increasing sclerosis bordering the lesion. The most common sites for them to occur are the femoral necks, pubic and ischial rami, ribs, and axillary margins of the scapulae. (Fig. 14-22) Bone scintigraphy may be of benefit to aid in the location of these lesions. (10) Pseudo-fractures occur in other bone-softening disorders, including Paget's disease, fibrous dysplasia, rickets, and hyperphosphatasia. (8,11)

Deformities. The majority of the deformities occur in the weight-bearing bones. In the pelvis, inferior displacement of the sacrum produces a triradiate shape to the pelvic canal. Medial acetabular migration forms a protrusio acetabuli deformity. Bowing of the femur and tibia also are seen. In the spine, kyphoscoliosis and increased endplate concavity predominate. A *bell-shaped thoracic cage* has also been described. (12) Acute fracture deformities may also occur. (Fig. 14-23)

CAPSULE SUMMARY   Osteomalacia

General Considerations

- Characterized by a lack of osteoid mineralization leading to generalized bone softening.
- Multiple causes, including lack of intake, diminished absorption, renal disease, and other associations.

Clinical Features

- Muscle weakness, bone pain, and deformities.
- Elevated parathormone, alkaline phosphatase, and hydroxyproline; normal to decreased calcium and phosphorus.

Pathologic Features

- Increased amounts of uncalcified osteoid tissue (osteoid seams).
- *Pseudo-fractures:* probably insufficiency fractures healing with uncalcified osteoid.

Radiologic Features

- Decreased bone density, coarse trabecular patterns, loss of cortical definition, pseudo-fractures, deformities.

RICKETS

General Considerations

Rickets is a systemic disease of the infant and young child. It is the childhood equivalent of osteomalacia in the mature skeleton. In the Western world it is a rare condition; however, evidence of its re-emergence across the world is available. (1,2) The essential pathologic alteration involves deficiencies of vitamin D, calcium, or phosphate. (3)

Clinical Features

The classic vitamin D-deficient presentation develops between 6 and 12 months of age. Symptoms consist of muscle tetany, irritability, weakness, delayed development, small stature, bone deformities and pain, with tetany and pain being the most common. (4) The most notable clinical findings are the soft tissue swellings occurring around the growth plates owing to hypertrophied cartilage. At the anterior rib cage, these are seen as multiple costochondral bumps (*rachitic rosary*). (Fig. 14-24) Clinically, enlargement of the wrists and costocartilage are most suggestive of the disease, with a specificity of 81% and 64%, respectively. (5) Serum evaluations will demonstrate elevated alkaline phosphatase levels, whereas calcium and phosphorus may be normal to slightly diminished. (4)

The causes of rickets are multiple and include inadequate dietary intake of vitamin D (dietary osteopenia), inadequate exposure to ultraviolet radiation, intestinal malabsorption, vitamin D metabolism defects, chronic acidosis, renal tubular defects, aluminum intoxication, and chronic administration of anticonvulsants (Dilantin). Dark-pigmented individuals and infants breastfeed for prolonged periods of time by a multiparous mother appear to be at a greater risk for the development of rickets. (6) Clinicians practicing at higher latitudes should also be more alert to this condition, especially in the winter months, owing to the decreased sun exposure in these areas. (1) Treatment with vitamin D supplementation and increased sunlight exposure usually provide satisfactory results (1); however, renal tubular defects are not cured by the administration of vitamin D and as such are termed vitamin D-resistant (refractory) rickets. Renal osteodystrophy (renal rickets) is the co-existence of rickets and hyperparathyroidism secondary to chronic renal disease. When vitamin D deficiency is the evident cause, it has been recommended that the mother and any siblings of the affected child also be assessed for the hypovitaminosis. (7)

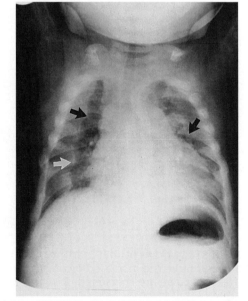

Figure 14-24   RICKETS: RACHITIC ROSARY. PA Chest. Observe the opaque, bulbous indentations of the lung adjacent to the enlarged costochondral junctions (*arrows*).

Pathologic Features

As in osteomalacia, histopathologic examination of rachitic bone demonstrates a decrease in the quantity of calcified osteoid and an increase in uncalcified osteoid (osteoid seams). This lack of mineral content produces the generalized radiolucency evident on the radiograph.

The most important changes occur at the growth plates. In rickets, cartilage cells at the physis grow normally but fail to calcify and degenerate. Consequently, the growth plate is occupied by enlarged masses of overgrown cartilage, widening the region radiographically. (8) Owing to a lack of osteoid mineralization the metaphyseal zone of provisional calcification will also be absent radiographically. The first sign of healing is restitution of this opaque metaphyseal line.

Radiologic Features

Generally, all bones will appear more radiolucent, with coarsened trabecular patterns. The most conspicuous abnormalities will be found at the growth plate regions of long bones. These consist of a widened growth plate with irregular, frayed, and cupped metaphyseal margins (*paintbrush metaphyses*). (9) In addition, no distinct white line of the zone of provisional calcification is visible. (Fig. 14-25) This line reappears on healing and is a useful indicator of a good therapeutic response. (Fig. 14-26) Epiphyses also appear frayed at the borders. Bowing deformities, fractures, decreased bony length, scoliosis, and pseudo-fractures are other notable findings. Bulbous enlargement of the costochondral junctions (*rachitic rosary*) can be seen adjacent to cupped anterior rib ends, which can indent the pleural interface or even the thymic shadow.

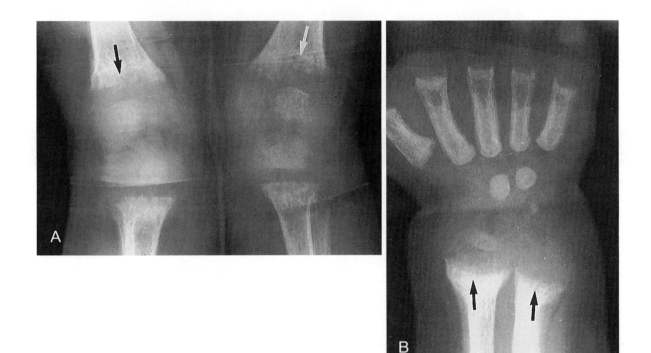

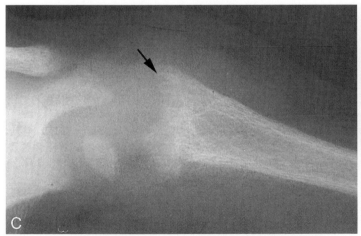

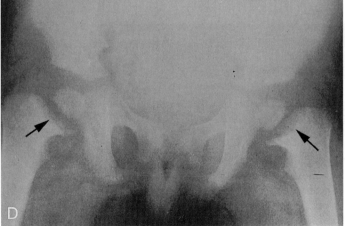

Figure 14-25   **RICKETS: GROWTH PLATE ABNORMALITIES. A. AP Knees. B. PA Wrist. C. AP Shoulder. D. AP Pelvis.** Observe the generalized osteopenia, coarse trabecular patterns, frayed paintbrush metaphyseal margins (*arrows*), a lack of the zone of provisional calcification, and widening of the physis.

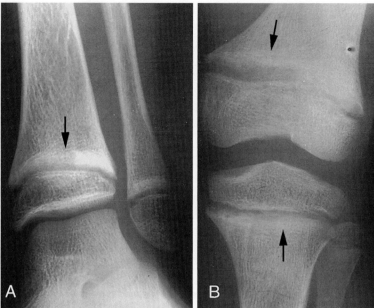

Figure 14-26 RICKETS: HEALING. A. AP Ankle. B. AP Knee. Reconstitution of normal growth at the metaphyseal margin is reflected in the reappearance of the zone of provisional calcification (*arrows*). (Courtesy of Bryan Hartley, MD, Melbourne, Australia.)

CAPSULE SUMMARY   Rickets

General Considerations

- Systemic skeletal disorder owing to a multitude of causes related to the physiology of vitamin D—inadequate dietary intake of vitamin D, inadequate exposure to ultraviolet radiation, intestinal malabsorption, vitamin D metabolism defects, chronic acidosis, renal tubular defects, aluminum intoxication, and chronic administration of anticonvulsants.

Clinical Features

- 6–12 months of age; irritability, tetany, weakness, delayed maturity, deformities, and growth plate swellings.

Pathologic Features

- Growth plate cartilage hypertrophies; fails to mineralize or degenerates; absence of a calcified zone of provisional calcification.

Radiologic Features

- Generalized osteopenia, coarse trabecular changes, widened growth plates, frayed and cupped paintbrush metaphyses, absent zone of provisional calcification; bowing deformities, fractures, decreased bony length, scoliosis, and pseudofractures.

SCURVY

General Considerations

Scurvy (Barlow's disease, hypovitaminosis C) is a disorder associated with a long-term deficiency of vitamin C (ascorbic acid). Its history reaches back to ancient times; however, in 1747, James Lind perhaps performed the first recorded study. (1) He conducted his clinical trial on sea voyagers and concluded that an antiscorbutic effect could be documented consistently with the consumption of oranges and lemons. (1) His research led to the provision of lemon juice to the sea voyagers during his time, and the incidence of scurvy soon became rare among this population. (1) In 1883, Thomas Barlow documented the clinical and pathologic features of the disease affecting infants. (1) Today, it is rare in the Western world, being found almost exclusively in infants between the ages of 8 and 14 months who are fed on pasteurized or boiled milk preparations (infantile scurvy). Occasionally the elderly are affected, when the diet is compromised (adult scurvy). Recent studies have suggested that although true scurvy may be rare, subclinical vitamin C deficiency should be an increasing concern among the general population. (2)

Clinical Features

The preceding period of avitaminosis usually is of at least 4 months' duration before symptoms and skeletal changes become apparent. (3) Infants between the ages of 4 and 18 months are primarily affected. The clinical hallmark of the disorder is the tendency toward spontaneous hemorrhage owing to capillary fragility. Manifestations include cutaneous petechiae, bleeding gums, melena, and hematuria. Other findings include joint swelling, irritability, pain, and a tendency to lie supine and motionless with the thighs abducted (*frog-leg position*). Bulging at the costo-chondral junctions may be evident. Unfortunately, owing to its rare presentation in clinical practice, the initial symptoms of infants with scurvy are sometimes mistakenly diagnosed as child abuse. (4) With laboratory investigations, serum ascorbic acid will be below the normal 0.6 mg/100 mL.

Pathologic Features

Vitamin C is essential to the formation of intercellular substances such as collagen, osteoid, and endothelial linings. In small blood vessels, the deficiency of intercellular cement promotes vascular fragility, as evidenced by the increased occurrence of tissue hemorrhages. Cartilage cells do not proliferate at their normal rate but will still mineralize. Bone cells are also inhibited in their activity, producing generalized osteopenia. (5)

Radiologic Features

A combination of abnormalities occurring at the growing ends of long bones, especially of the lower extremity, represent the most characteristic findings. (5–7) (Fig. 14-27)

- *Osteopenia.* A generalized decrease in bone density will be evident in combination with thinning of the cortex and loss of trabecular definition.
- *Dense zone of provisional calcification (white line of Frankel).* Enhancement of the dense metaphyseal zone of calcified cartilage occurs owing to delayed conversion into bone.

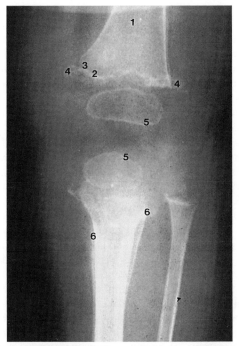

Figure 14-27 **SCURVY. PA Knee.** Note the characteristic changes: generalized osteopenia (*1*), dense zone of provisional calcification (*2*), scorbutic zone (*3*), Pelken's spurs (*4*), Wimberger's sign (ring epiphyses) (*5*), and subperiosteal hemorrhages (*6*).

- *Ring epiphysis (Wimberger's sign).* The peripheral margin of the epiphysis appears dense, whereas the central portion is more radiolucent.
- *Corner (angle) sign.* Irregularity of the metaphyseal margins frequently occurs secondary to infractions of the epiphyseal–metaphyseal junction.
- *Pelken's spurs.* These bony protuberances occur at the metaphyseal margins and extend at right angles away from the shaft axis.
- *Scorbutic zone (Trümmerfeld's zone).* Directly beneath the zone of provisional calcification a radiolucent band may be visible, representing disordered osteoid formation.
- *Subperiosteal hemorrhage.* Extensions of extravasated blood frequently lift the periosteum away from the bone and will later calcify, especially during healing.

These findings constitute the classic signs of infantile scurvy. Such changes are less apparent as the patient ages, which hinders the radiologic diagnosis of the condition. On healing, all changes are reversible on vitamin C therapy, though a single growth arrest line may remain in the metaphysis as a residual of Frankel's line. Following therapy, subperiosteal hematomas rapidly calcify and demarcate. (7)

CAPSULE SUMMARY   Scurvy

Clinical Features

- Hypovitaminosis C (ascorbic acid), which affects mainly infants fed solely on pasteurized milk. Latent period of months.
- Usually aged 8–14 months.
- Spontaneous hemorrhages, swelling, irritability, pain, lying motionless (frog-legged), and costal rosary.
- Serum ascorbic acid < 0.6 mg/100 mL.

Pathologic Features

- Depressed intercellular substance formation, especially in connective tissue, cartilage, and bone.

Radiologic Features

- Osteoporosis, dense zone of provisional calcification, ring epiphysis (Wimberger's sign), corner sign, Pelken's spurs, scorbutic zone (Trümmerfeld's zone), subperiosteal hemorrhages.

HYPERPARATHYROIDISM

General Considerations

Hyperparathyroidism is the general term applied to overactivity of the parathyroid gland, of which there are many causes. The gland's mode of action is primarily related to the release of the strong osteoclastic hormone parathormone (PTH). The skeletal effects are widespread and frequently specific enough for a definitive radiologic diagnosis to be given.

Clinical Features

There are three basic forms of hyperparathyroidism: primary, secondary, and tertiary.

- *Primary hyperparathyroidism.* This is the most common cause of hypercalcemia (1) and may be owing to a parathyroid adenoma (90% of cases), carcinoma, hyperplasia, or ectopic tumors, producing a parathormone type of substance. Characteristically, there are elevated levels of parathormone, hypercalcemia, and hypophosphatemia.
- *Secondary hyperparathyroidism.* This is one of the most common complications of chronic renal disease, allowing for persistent loss of calcium and phosphorous and thus stimulating parathormone release. (2)
- *Tertiary hyperparathyroidism.* In dialysis patients, the parathyroid gland may act independently of serum calcium levels.

A typical clinical profile is that of a woman 30–50 years of age with weakness, lethargy, polydipsia, and polyuria. Females are affected in a ratio of at least 3:1. (3) Owing to hypercalcemia, muscles will be hypotonic and feel weak, whereas in the kidneys calculus formation may be the reason a patient presents for examination. (4) Bone tenderness is common. Serum evaluation will show intermittent hypercalcemia in primary hyperparathyroidism but normal to low in the secondary form. In the presence of bone disease, the alkaline phosphatase levels will be increased. (5) Parathormone concentration will also be elevated, and recent advances in medicine allowing for more accurate assessments have contributed to an increased detection of asymptomatic patients with primary hyperparathyroidism. (1) If successful, surgical removal of the parathyroid gland is curative for primary hyperparathyroidism. (6) To ensure the efficacy of surgical treatment, advanced imaging modalities should be used to accurately locate the gland. (7) Bisphosphonates are currently used to inactivate osteoclastic activity (8), and estrogen therapy may be of benefit in postmenopausal women to reduce the severity of osteoporosis. (6)

Pathologic Features

In primary hyperparathyroidism, elevated parathormone stimulates osteoclastic resorption, liberating calcium and phosphorus into the bloodstream. Phosphorus is more readily excreted and, owing to the constant calcium–phosphorus product, calcium is retained, disturbing homeostasis. (9) The net result is hypercalcemia and hypophosphatemia. In secondary hyperparathyroidism, a combination of calcium loss and abnormal renal vitamin D formation creates continuous hypocalcemia and increases the release of parathormone and bone resorption.

The histopathologic alterations consist essentially of osteoclastic and osteocytic resorption, with fibrous tissue replacement (osteitis fibrosa cystica, Recklinghausen's disease of bone). The bone is decreased in density and exhibits defective lamellar structure and Haversian system development, producing a soft, fragile bone. Occasionally, the accumulations of fibrous tissue containing numerous osteoclastic giant cells produce localized cyst-like destructive bone lesions that appear, on gross examination, brown in color (*brown tumors*). These lesions may undergo hemorrhage, with liquefactive necrosis, and produce cysts. The pathologic hallmark, however, is *subperiosteal bone resorption* of the outer cortex at the insertional points of ligaments and tendons. (5)

Radiologic Features

The radiologic differentiation between primary and secondary hyperparathyroidism is usually not possible. In the era previous to dialysis therapy, brown tumors were more common in the primary form, but they are now found just as commonly in the secondary variety owing to the increased life span of the patient. One notable difference is the greater tendency to produce osteosclerosis in the secondary form.

General Features

Bone. The major changes consist of bone resorption with decreased density, accentuated trabecular pattern, loss of cortical definition, subperiosteal resorption, and brown tumors. (10) Additional infrequently encountered features include pseudofractures, fractures, and deformities.

Subperiosteal Resorption. Stimulation of the inner periosteal layer precipitates bone resorption in predictable locations. This is the single most definitive radiologic sign of hyperparathyroidism. (5) The most characteristic sites include the radial margins of the middle and proximal phalanges of the second and third digits of the hand, medial metaphysis of the humerus and tibia, undersurface of the distal clavicle, trochanters, and tuberosities. This outer cortical erosion produces an irregular, frayed, and *lace-like appearance* of the external bone surface. (Fig. 14-28) In addition, resorption of subarticular bone produces apparently widened joint spaces and osteolysis, particularly at the acromioclavicular, symphysis pubis, and sacroiliac articulations. (11–13) (Fig. 14-29)

Decreased Bone Density. All skeletal structures show diffuse rarefaction. The bones can appear quite granular, as best seen in the skull (*salt and pepper* or *pepper pot skull*).

Accentuated Trabecular Patterns. As non-essential trabeculae are resorbed, those that remain will appear more prominent.

Loss of Cortical Definition. A combination of endosteal, intracortical, and subperiosteal resorption produces a cortex that lacks the normal radiologic borders. The cortex and medullary cavity merge imperceptibly into each other, whereas the outer surface appears blurred and often irregular. Evidence of intracortical resorption within Haversian canals is seen especially in the second metacarpal cortex, where subtle longitudinal striations can be observed.

Subligamentous Bone Resorption. At attachments of ligaments and tendons, focal resorption of cortical bone can be observed. The most frequent sites are at the trochanters, humeral and ischial tuberosities, inferior aspect of the distal clavicle, and inferior surface of the calcaneus.

Brown Tumors (Osteoclastoma). Brown tumors are visible as distinct geographic radiolucencies. They are usually central, slightly expansile, and lightly septated, mimicking a destructive neoplasm. These may heal, as evidenced by their dense sclerotic appearance. The most common sites of occurrence include mandible, pelvis, ribs, and femora, although any bone can be affected. (14) (Fig. 14-30) Brown tumors are usually a marker of primary hyperparathyroidism, though now they can be encountered in the secondary form. Although brown tumors are rare, MRI investigations of brown tumors may reveal a fluid–fluid level. (15)

Joints. A destructive arthropathy—dialysis-related arthropathy (DRA)—involving the axial and appendicular joints can complicate long-term dialysis.

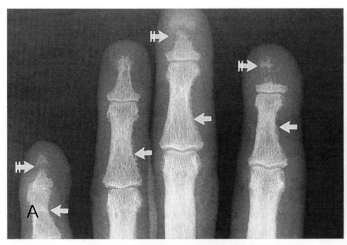
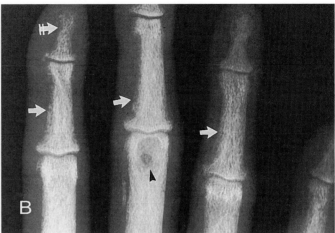

Figure 14-28 **HYPERPARATHYROIDISM: SUBPERIOSTEAL RESORPTION. A and B. PA Hands.** Note the radial margins of the proximal and middle phalanges bilaterally are frayed, irregular, and lace-like (*arrows*) owing to characteristic subperiosteal resorption. Also note the brown tumor (*arrowhead*) and osteolysis of the distal phalanges (*crossed arrows*).

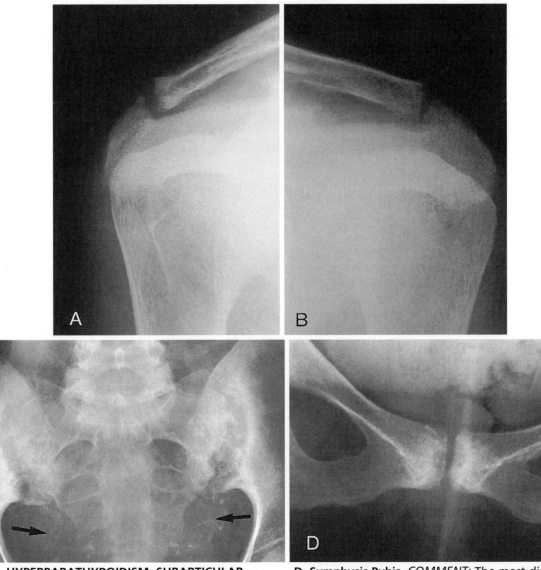

Figure 14-29 **HYPERPARATHYROIDISM: SUBARTICULAR RESORPTION. A and B. Acromioclavicular Joint. C. Sacroiliac Joints.** Note the associated vascular calcification (*arrows*). **D. Symphysis Pubis.** *COMMENT:* The most distinctive features are the widened joint spaces and irregular joint margins. (Courtesy of David P. Thomas, MD, Melbourne, Australia.)

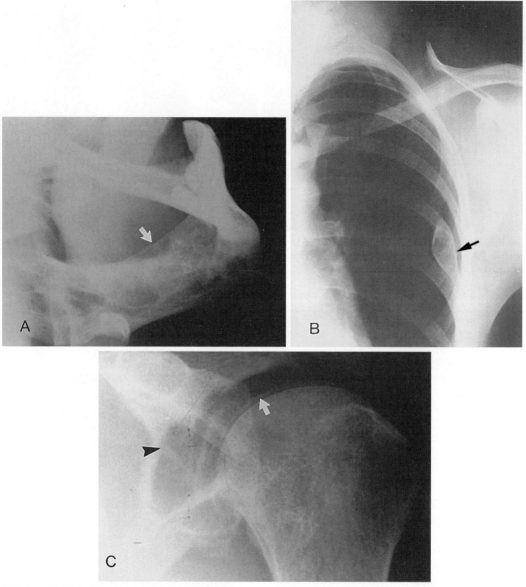

**Figure 14-30   HYPERPARATHYROIDISM: BROWN TUMORS.
A. Mandible. B. Ribs.** Note the tumor-like destructive expansile lesions (*arrows*). **C. Scapula.** Note the geographic expansile lesion (*arrowhead*). Chondrocalcinosis is also visible (*arrow*).

Peripheral Joints. DRA is a chronic, progressive symmetric polyarthropathy involving large and small peripheral joints found in at least 40% of dialysis patients. (16) Features include periarticular cysts and erosions, loss of joint space, loss of the articular surface, and osteopenia. (16,17)

Spine. Dialysis-related spondyloarthropathy (DRSA) develops in 5–15% of patients receiving long-term hemodialysis or peritoneal dialysis and is a component of DRA. (17) It is unusual to have DRSA without concurrent DRA of the hands and wrists. DRSA rarely occurs < 2 years from when dialysis is begun and usually takes 3–5 years. It is most common in the cervical spine and tends to affect multiple levels. Approximately 30% of patients remain asymptomatic, and 20% manifest cord compression, which can be fatal. (17) Deposition of an unusual type of amyloid (β_2-microglobulin) into articular tissues appears to be the common pathophysiological path for spondyloarthropathy.

The radiographic appearance simulates infection or the discovertebral changes of ankylosing spondylitis. Observable changes include narrowing of disc height, subchondral cysts, endplate erosions, collapse and erosion of the contiguous vertebral bodies, facet erosion often with spondylolisthesis (C3–C4 is the most common site), and peridiscal calcification. (17) Exclusion from infection cannot be obtained on plain films. Bone scintigraphy and gallium scans are often cold in DRSA, whereas MRI scans reveal a low to intermediate signal in contrast to the high signal intensity of infection. (17) Rapid progression over months to a year is common.

Soft Tissues. Calcification within subcutaneous, articular, muscular, vascular, and visceral organs is a common finding.

Urinary Tract. Manifestations of hypercalcemia will appear as nephrocalcinosis and renal calculi. This is seen in up to 75% of hyperparathyroidism patients.

Articulations. Calcification of joint cartilages (chondrocalcinosis) is seen in almost 20% of patients with primary hyperparathyroidism. (18,19) This is present most commonly in the knee menisci, as well as the triangular wrist cartilage, shoulders, and hips. (Fig. 14-30*C*)

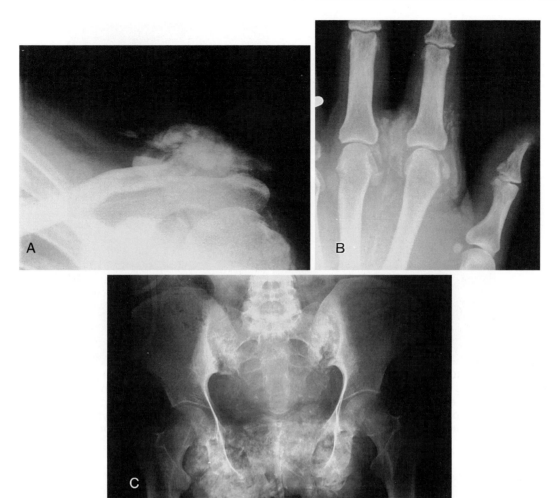

Figure 14-31 **HYPERPARATHYROIDISM: SOFT TISSUE CALCIFICATION. A. Shoulder. B. Hand. C. Pubic Region.** Note the widened sacroiliac joints as a result of subperiosteal resorption. (Courtesy of David P. Thomas, MD, Melbourne, Australia.)

Miscellaneous Tissues. Periarticular structures, such as blood vessels, ligaments, tendons, muscle, and subcutaneous tissues, may exhibit calcification, especially in the secondary form. (20) (Fig. 14-31) Visceral calcification may be seen in the salivary gland, pancreas, lung, and prostate.

Target Sites of Involvement

Hands. Demonstration of subperiosteal resorption is the hallmark of hyperparathyroidism and is first identified in the hands. (21) The most conspicuous locations are at the second and third digits, proximal and middle phalanges, especially on their radial margins. (Fig. 14-28) The outer cortex will appear frayed and irregular. Additional features include generalized deossification with tapering and, at times, complete osteolysis of the distal tufts.
Skull. Diffuse granular deossification produces a mottled appearance to the calvaria (*salt and pepper or pepper pot skull*). (Fig. 14-32) The inner and outer tables lose their sharp definition and cannot be easily seen. Rarely, basilar invagination may occur. A characteristic sign is resorption of the cortical bone (*lamina dura*) surrounding the tooth socket.
Spine and Pelvis. All vertebral segments show generalized deossification and trabecular accentuation. The endplate concavities are frequently increased owing to bone softening. A charac-

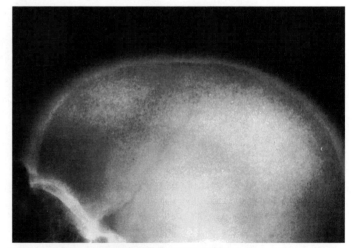

Figure 14-32 **HYPERPARATHYROIDISM. Lateral Skull.** Note the texture of the bone appears granular (*salt and pepper, pepper pot skull*) and the definition of both inner and outer tables has been lost.

teristic alteration is the uniform condensation in the sub-endplate zones of the bodies (*rugger-jersey spine*). (Figs. 14-33 and 14-34) This finding of sub-endplate sclerosis often co-exists with an irregular endplate owing to Schmorl's nodes. Rarely, all bones may

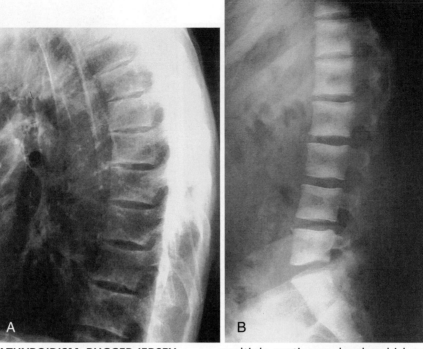

Figure 14-33 HYPERPARATHYROIDISM: RUGGER JERSEY SPINE. A. Lateral Thoracic Spine. Note that the bone density is decreased, the trabecular patterns accentuated, and the endplates slightly increased in concavity. **B. Lateral Lumbar Spine.** Note the prominent linear sub-endplate densities at multiple contiguous levels, which produce this alternating dense–lucent–dense appearance, simulating the transverse bands of a rugby sweater (*rugger jersey spine*). This pattern is distinctive for hyperparathyroidism, though there is similarity to some cases of osteopetrosis.

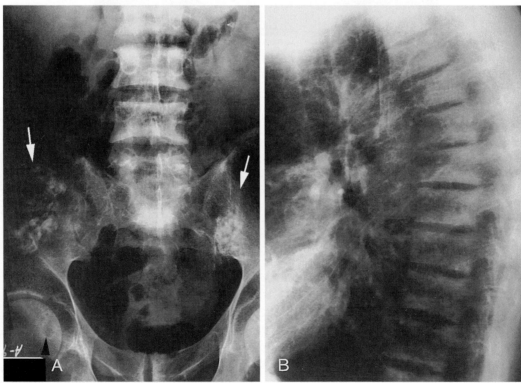

Figure 14-34 HYPERPARATHYROIDISM: RENAL TRANS-PLANTS. A. AP Lumbar Spine. Note that this patient underwent bilateral renal transplantation on separate occasions, which subsequently failed and calcified (*arrows*). Corticosteroid therapy to limit transplant rejection has precipitated bilateral avascular necrosis of the hips; cystic lesions are visible in one femoral head and the other is densely sclerotic (*arrowhead*). Note the prominent sclerosis of the sub-endplate zones in the lumbar spine, reflecting the rugger jersey spine. **B. Lateral Thoracic Spine.** Note the characteristic *rugger jersey spine.* (Courtesy of Scott Keeler, MD, Denver, Colorado.)

become homogeneously sclerotic. (22) Subchondral resorption at the sacroiliac and pubic articulations produces marked apparent widening of these joints and can be readily confused with erosive spondyloarthropathies, such as ankylosing spondylitis. Discovertebral destructive lesions (e.g., DRSA) are most common in the cervical spine and appear identical to infection.

Shoulders. Resorption of the distal clavicle subchondral bone bilaterally is an early and reliable indicator of hyperparathyroidism. The articular surface is indistinct and frayed. The main differential considerations are infection and post-traumatic osteolysis.

CAPSULE SUMMARY
Hyperparathyroidism

General Considerations
- Increased parathyroid activity liberates parathormone, which exerts a strong osteoclastic effect on the skeleton.

Clinical Features
- *Three forms:* primary, secondary, and tertiary.
- Females 3:1, 30–50 years of age.
- Weakness, lethargy, polydipsia, polyuria.
- Elevated alkaline phosphatase and parathormone levels.

Pathologic Features
- Osteoclastic and osteocytic resorption with fibrous tissue replacement (osteitis fibrosa cystica).
- Brown tumors owing to hemorrhagic giant cell proliferations.
- Hallmark is subperiosteal bone resorption.

Radiologic Features
- Bone changes consist of osteopenia, accentuated trabecular patterns, subperiosteal resorption, loss of cortical definition, and brown tumors.
- Joint changes can be present in 40% of chronic dialysis patients owing to amyloid deposition (DRA). periarticular cysts and erosions, loss of joint space, loss of the articular surface, and osteopenia.
- In the spine (most commonly the cervical spine), 5–15% of patients develop a discovertebral destructive process mimicking an infection (loss of endplate, body destruction, loss of disc height) referred to as DRSA.
- Soft tissue changes include nephrocalcinosis, renal calculi, chondrocalcinosis, and calcification in various periarticular tissues and visceral organs.
- *Target sites:*
  Hand: subperiosteal resorption, radial margins of the proximal and middle phalanges of the second and third digits, with acro-osteolysis.
  Skull: salt and pepper, resorption of lamina dura.
  Spine: osteopenia, trabecular accentuation, endplate concavities, rugger jersey spine, widened sacroiliac joints. DRSA manifesting as loss of endplate, vertebral body destruction, and decreased disc height.

HYPERVITAMINOSES

The most frequent hypervitaminoses with osteologic effects are vitamins A and D.

Hypervitaminosis A

Hypervitaminosis A can occur both in adults and in children. Clinically, dermatitis, pruritus, alopecia, and yellowing of the skin may be seen. Hepatosplenomegaly can be present.

Radiologically, the principal feature is solid, periosteal new bone along the shafts of the long bones—notably the femurs, tibia, fibula, metatarsals, humerus, ulna, radius, and metacarpals. Diastasis of the cranial sutures, most marked at bregma, is also common. These sites exhibit increased radioisotope uptake on bone scan and precede plain film changes by weeks. (1) Diffuse osteopenia may be evident as hypervitaminosis A has been shown to stimulate bone resorption. (2)

Hypervitaminosis D

Clinically, the major complaints of hypervitaminosis D are nausea, anorexia, polyuria, and polydipsia. Hypercalcemia is the expected laboratory finding, which has shown to be related to the systemic and dental effects noted. (3) The most characteristic radiologic feature is the extensive calcification in blood vessel walls, kidneys, and periarticular tissues.

ACROMEGALY

General Considerations

In adulthood, excessive growth hormone secretion from a pituitary eosinophilic adenoma produces growth of intramembranous bone tissue and subcutaneous hypertrophy. This is especially prominent in the hands and feet (acral parts), from which the term acromegaly is derived. Excessive production of growth hormone before the closure of the long bone growth centers will manifest as *gigantism.*

Clinical Features

The physical features are characteristic: malocclusion, prominent forehead; thickened tongue; and broad, large hands. Bitemporal hemianopia, headache, and carpal tunnel syndrome are common even before other more obvious stigmata. Acromegalic patients are predisposed to degenerative arthritis, especially of the spine and weight-bearing joints. Median neuropathy is not an uncommon association, often occurring bilaterally as an initial finding. In the past, it was believed that connective tissue and bony overgrowth predisposed patients to the neural compression; however, recent studies have suggested the true cause to consist of edematous changes within the nerve itself. (1) A reduced life span is commonly associated with acromegaly; however, results from genetic research have been promising. (2) Currently, surgical resection of microadenomas and/or radiation therapy are the treatments of choice. (3) Surgical measures, although invasive, provide the most optimal results, with up to 21% of patients being clinically cured. (4,5)

Pathologic Features

The cause of the disease is a growth hormone-producing eosinophilic adenoma of the anterior pituitary gland and, occasionally, hyperplasia of eosinophilic cells. Essentially, growth hormones exert widespread effects on all musculoskeletal tissues. Within bone, the major effect is to activate periosteal appositional new bone, which results in an irregular thickening of the cortex. Ectopic bone formation is enhanced, as evidenced by spurs and other bony excrescences at musculotendinous insertions. Articular cartilage initially proliferates but quickly degenerates. (6) The subcutaneous tissues also undergo hyperplasia and are replaced by increasing amounts of fat.

Radiologic Features

Skin Changes

The usual site for skin changes actually measured is the heel pad thickness. An increase in skin thickness may be visible, especially in the hands and feet, with a heel measurement > 20 mm being suggestive of acromegaly. (7) (Fig. 14-35)

Skull. Many skull changes have been documented; however, the most recognizable include sella turcica enlargement from the pituitary neoplasm, sinus overgrowth, occipital protuberance overgrowth, malocclusion, and widened mandibular angle (pragnathic jaw). (8) (Figs. 14-36 to 14-38)

Hand. Many measurements have been applied to the hand, with variable reliability in the diagnosis of acromegaly; however, the most definitive changes will be seen in bone and joint aberrations.

Bone changes include widened shafts of the phalanges and metacarpals, bony protuberances, and prominent ungual tufts, which may assume a *spade-like appearance*. (8) A reliable indicator is the generalized increase in joint space width owing to cartilage overgrowth. (Figs. 14-39 and 14-40)

Spine. Numerous changes occur in the vertebral column. (9) The dimensions of the vertebra increase in both sagittal and transverse planes, especially in the lumbar spine. The vertical height remains unchanged, resulting in the vertebral bodies appearing flattened and increased in their sagittal dimensions (platyspondyly). Premature degeneration with exuberant osteophytes and widened disc heights complete the most typically observed changes. Occasionally, posterior body scalloping may be observed from dural ectasia. (8,10) The atlantodental interspace

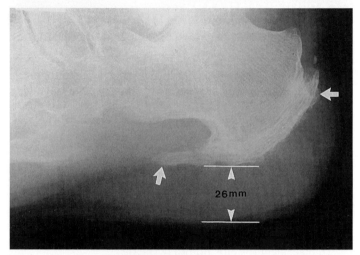

Figure 14-35 ACROMEGALY. Heel Pad. Note that the measurement is 26 mm, well above the normal maximum value of 20 mm. Also observe the hyperostoses often associated in acromegaly (*arrows*).

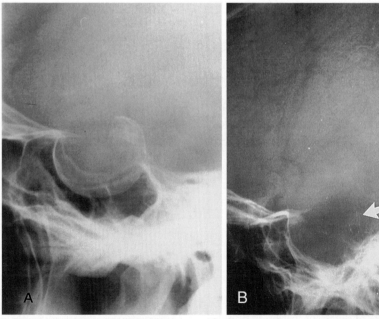

Figure 14-36 ACROMEGALY: SELLA TURCICA ABNORMALITIES. A. Lateral Skull. Note that a generalized concentric expansion (ballooning) of the sella has occurred. **B. Lateral** **Skull.** Note the complete destruction of the floor and posterior clinoids (*arrow*). *COMMENT:* The sella turcica may appear normal, despite the presence of acromegaly.

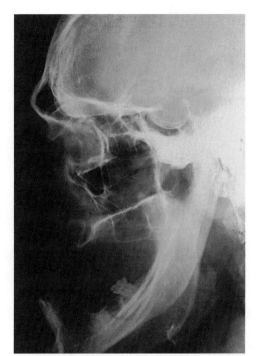

Figure 14-37   **ACROMEGALY: MANDIBULAR CHANGES.** Note that the mandible is elongated, has lost its normal angle, and has produced malocclusion. Observe the expanded sella turcica contour.

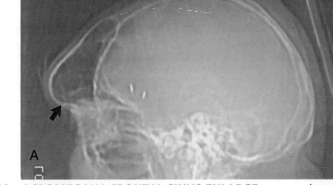

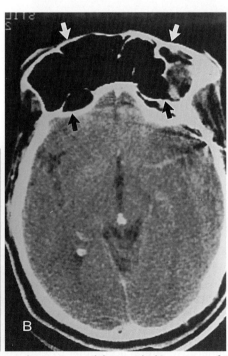

Figure 14-38   **ACROMEGALY: FRONTAL SINUS ENLARGE-MENT. A. Lateral Skull. B. Axial CT, Skull.** Note that gross enlargement has occurred (*arrows*). (Courtesy of Steven P. Brownstein, MD, Springfield, New Jersey.)

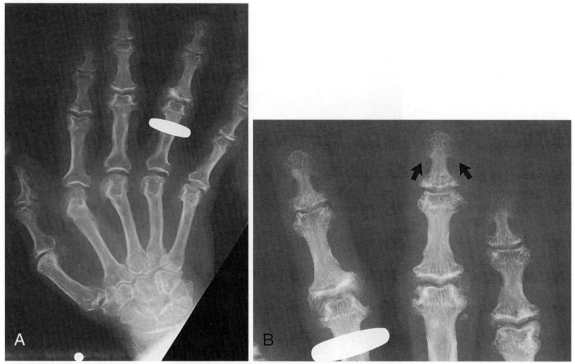

Figure 14-39 ACROMEGALY. A. PA Hand. Note the characteristic features of widened joint spaces and periosteal new bone formation. **B. Close-Up, Distal Tufts.** Note that the distal tufts are classically enlarged, showing the *spade-like deformity* (*arrows*).

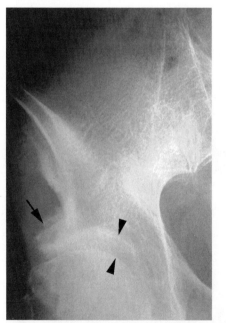

Figure 14-40 ACROMEGALY. AP Hip. Note the widened axial joint cavity, reflecting the overgrowth of intra-articular cartilage (*arrowheads*). Despite this joint widening the weight-bearing superior compartment is narrowed, with evidence of a degenerative lateral acetabular osteophyte (*arrow*). A subchondral cyst can be seen in the femoral head. *COMMENT:* The appearance of degenerative joint changes is common in acromegaly.

may be increased up to 6 mm owing to cartilage overgrowth, not transverse ligament instability. (11) Similar widening of the facet joints can be observed. Hyperostosis of the tips of the spinous processes can be pronounced. (9) Spinal stenosis, although a rare complication, can occur secondary to thickened laminae and articular process with the spinal ligaments thickened and calcified. (12)

CAPSULE SUMMARY   Acromegaly

General Considerations
- Pituitary eosinophilic adenoma secreting growth hormone after the growth plates have fused.

Clinical Features
- Characteristic facial (malocclusion, prominent forehead, thickened tongue) and hand (thick skin) changes.

Pathologic Features
- Activation of periosteal appositional new bone, articular cartilage proliferation, and subcutaneous hyperplasia.

Radiologic Features
- Heel pad > 20 mm.
- *Skull:* sella turcica enlargement, sinus overgrowth, and malocclusion.
- *Hand and foot:* widened shafts, bony protuberances, enlarged distal tufts (spade-like), and widened joint spaces.
- *Spine:* platyspondyly, hyperostoses, widened disc and facet spaces, posterior body scalloping, widened atlantodental interspace.

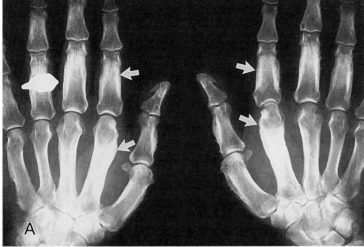

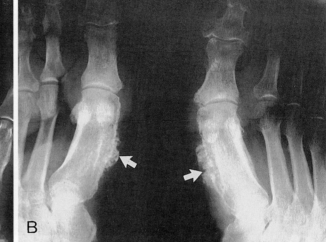

Figure 14-41 **THYROID ACROPACHY. A. PA Hands.** Observe the thick, dense periosteal new bone at the metacarpals and phalanges (*arrows*). **B. PA Feet.** Note that similar changes are seen on the medial surface of the first metatarsal (*arrows*), a distinctively characteristic site for thyroid acropachy of the foot.

THYROID DISORDERS

Three thyroid-related disorders may exhibit skeletal changes: hyperthyroidism, hypothyroidism, and thyroid acropachy.

- *Hyperthyroidism* displays only osteopenia of all bones.
- *Hypothyroidism* in the newborn (cretinism) exerts a considerable growth and developmental-inhibiting factor to the skeleton. Manifestations of cretinism include delayed closure and fragmented epiphyses (*cretinoid epiphyses*), occasional wormian bones, and a wedged thoracolumbar *sail vertebra*. Bilateral slipped capital femoral epiphysis, although rare, has been associated with hypothyroidism and other endocrinopathies. (1)
- *Thyroid acropachy* is an unusual complication to a treated hyperthyroid patient who is now maintaining normal thyroid activity. Only 1% of hyperthyroid patients develop acropachy. (2) Clinically, the patient experiences digital swelling that is painless and progressive. (3) The radiologic findings are virtually diagnostic and consist of periostitis that is thick and dense, usually arising from the radial aspect of the small hand bones. (4,5) Similar changes may be exhibited on the tibial aspects of the foot bones. (Fig. 14-41)

CUSHING'S DISEASE AND STEROID-INDUCED OSTEONECROSIS

Clinical Features

Cushing's disease is produced by the presence of excessive quantities of glucocorticoid steroids released by the adrenal cortex. Occasionally, an anterior pituitary neoplasm may produce the identical clinical feature. Clinically, the patient is obese, especially in the upper thorax and face (*moon face*), and experi-

ences accelerated hair growth and hypertension. Deposition of fat over the upper thoracic spine produces a distinct soft tissue protuberance (*buffalo hump*). Purple striae may be seen on the abdomen and axillae. Fractures of the vertebrae and ribs are common and may be relatively painless.

The same clinical and radiologic picture can be precipitated by the long-term administration of therapeutic corticosteroids. Corticosteroid compounds have been used therapeutically since 1948, with the first iatrogenic effects reported in 1950. (1) A wide range of conditions are treated with corticosteroids on the basis of their potent anti-inflammatory and immunosuppressive actions. Complications in the skeleton include compression fractures of the spine, avascular necrosis, osteopenia, delayed development, infections, destructive arthropathy, impaired healing, tendon rupture, and soft tissue atrophy.

Radiologic Features

The radiologic features revolve around osteopenia, avascular necrosis, and pathologic fractures.

Osteopenia. Cushing's disease and iatrogenic osteopenia show no differences from the more common senile or postmenopausal osteoporosis. Cortices will be thinned, density diminished, and deformities evident. (2,3) In the spine, biconcave endplate configurations are common. Small endplate infractions heal with abundant callus, creating a hazy appearance to multiple endplates. Spontaneous fractures of the vertebrae, ribs, and pubic rami are relatively common. (Fig. 14-42)

Avascular Necrosis (Osteonecrosis). The most common sites of avascular necrosis, in order of incidence, are the femoral and humeral heads, femoral condyles, proximal tibiae, and talus. (Fig. 14-43) If only one femoral head is affected, the contralateral side will similarly be affected in 30–50% of cases. Osteonecrosis is rare in Cushing's disease but common in the therapeutic use of corticosteroids. (4,5) Although reportedly rare in Cushing's disease, the diagnosis of osteonecrosis should not be overlooked, as cases have been documented in which avascular necrosis was the presenting pathology. (6)

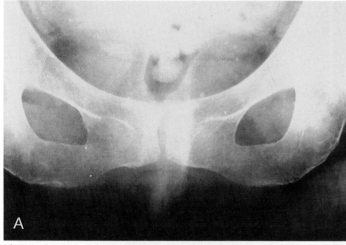

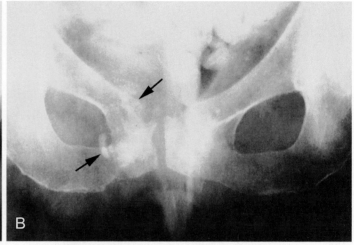

Figure 14-42 **CORTICOSTEROID-INDUCED FRACTURE: PUBIS. A. Initial Study.** Note that this patient with long-standing rheumatoid arthritis and on corticosteroid therapy demonstrates diffuse osteopenia of all skeletal structures, with pencil-thin cortices. **B. 4-Year Follow-Up.** Note an insufficiency fracture has developed through the pubis (*arrows*). No single trauma was involved. (Courtesy of Timothy J. Mick, DC, DACBR, Bloomington, Minnesota.)

The true incidence of steroid-induced avascular necrosis is unknown, though following renal transplant it is approximately 10%. (7) As the dosage level rises and the duration lengthens, the incidence of steroid-induced osteonecrosis increases. Low-dose therapies in renal transplant patients have been shown to reduce the incidence of osteonecrosis to approximately 5%. (8) The average time of onset after beginning a schedule of corticosteroid therapy is 2–3 years.

The mechanism operative in the induction of osteonecrosis is unknown, though the release of fat emboli from a fatty liver, microfractures secondary to osteoporosis, and decreased intra-osseous blood supply owing to an increased fat cell mass have all been implicated. (9) Contemporary consensus supports the theory of fat embolization derived from a fatty liver combined with mechanical deformation and vulnerable blood supply. (10)

Epiphyseal Sites. Features of steroid-induced avascular necrosis are identical to the idiopathic form, though bilateral sites are more commonly owing to the drug. Key signs include subchondral fracture (*crescent sign*) and collapse (*step sign*) as well as patchy sclerosis and lucency of the involved epiphysis. (See Chapter 13.) In the femoral head, this involves the superior weight-bearing segment (*bite sign*); in the humeral head, the superomedial segment; in the medial femoral condyle, the weight-bearing surface; and in the talus, the talar dome. Metaphyseal–diaphyseal infarctions are uncommon.

Vertebral Bodies. In the spine, collapse of a vertebral body owing to avascular necrosis will occasionally occur with collections of nitrogen gas visible within the vertebral body (*intravertebral vacuum cleft sign*). (Figs. 14-44 and 14-45) (11,12) Approximately 50% are found at the thoracolumbar junction (at the T11–L1 levels), with the remainder distributed in the thoracic and lumbar spines; cervical involvement has not been recorded. (13,14) There is usually 25–75% loss of vertebral body height. (13) The presence of the intravertebral vacuum cleft sign is not specific for steroid-induced avascular necrosis; it is also seen in association with osteoporosis, multiple myeloma, metastatic carcinoma, alcoholism, Gaucher's disease, and Kümmell's disease and following radiotherapy. (13–20) It is rarely associated with an infection. (18) The most common cause is osteoporosis (14), though corticosteroids can be more commonly linked in geographic areas such as Thailand, where they are freely available. (21) This should not be confused with an intradiscal vacuum phenomenon, which is found within a degenerative disc. (22) Selective spinal angiography shows absence of vertebral vascularization. (23)

The common pathophysiologic denominator is fracture of the vertebral body in order to allow accumulation of gas within the residual fracture line, which is analogous to the crescent sign of epiphyseal avascular necrosis. The gas is most likely nitrogen derived from fatty marrow, which comes out of solution when the endplates are distracted; this explains why it is more likely to be captured radiographically while the patient is

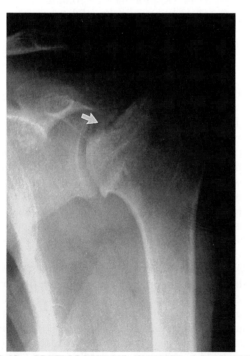

Figure 14-43 **CORTICOSTEROID-INDUCED OSTEONECROSIS. Humeral Head.** Note that the abnormalities (*arrow*) consist of flattening of the surface contour and separation of the articular cortex (*crescent sign*).

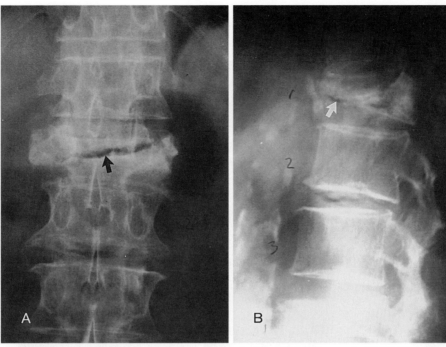

Figure 14-44 **CORTICOSTEROID OSTEONECROSIS: INTRA-VERTEBRAL VACUUM CLEFT SIGN. A. AP Lumbar Spine.** Observe the characteristic intravertebral radiolucent vacuum cleft (*arrow*). **B. Lateral Lumbar Spine.** Note the pathologic fracture at L1. Within it is contained a thin radiolucent wafer of gas (*arrow*). *COMMENT:* The *intravertebral vacuum cleft sign* denotes a number of possible causes but is most often associated with osteoporosis or corticosteroid therapy. (Courtesy of Lawrence A. Cooperstein, MD, Pittsburgh, Pennsylvania.)

supine, when the spine is being placed into slight extension. (12,14,24) The gas can be found in the sub-endplate zone or more centrally.

CT dramatically demonstrates the gas as a low attenuation density within the bony matrix on both axial scans and reconstructions. Changes in appearance occur with time; after hyperextension or traction, gas quickly accumulates, producing the *intrabody vacuum cleft sign.* (13,14) Within 10 min, there is resorption of the gas, which is replaced progressively with fluid. (14) On MRI, the vacuum cleft will appear as a black signal void; later, when fluid accumulates and the gas resorbs, this signal void is replaced by high signal fluid on T2-weighted images. (14,17)

Associated findings include generalized osteopenia of all skeletal structures, adjacent degenerative disc disease, and intervertebral ankylosis. Traction will produce some restitution of vertebral body height and broadening of the radiolucency by 1–4 mm; release of traction will abolish the gaseous collection within 10 min and allow resumption to normal vertebral body height within 24 hr. (13)

Fractures. Fractures are most prevalent in the spine, ribs, and proximal femur.

Spine. Repeated microfractures of the endplate and sub-endplate zones are common in the lower thoracic and upper lumbar spine, which manifest radiographically as abundant callus, especially in the sub-endplate zones, creating a hazy band of sclerosis (*marginal condensation sign*). (1,25) (Figs. 14-46 and 14-47) Biconcave endplates (fish vertebrae) owing to osteopenia are commonly seen. Compression fractures can be wedged (anterior loss of height), plana (anterior and posterior loss of height), or central in morphology.

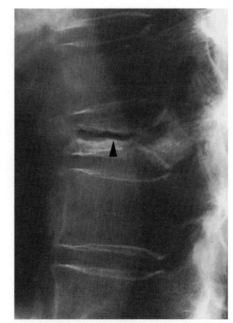

Figure 14-45 **CORTICOSTEROID OSTEONECROSIS: INTRA-VERTEBRAL VACUUM CLEFT SIGN.** Note the pathologic fracture clearly evident at T8, with collapse of the anterior and posterior vertebral body. A sub-endplate linear radiolucent collection of gas can be identified (*arrowhead*). The underlying cause was the long-term use of corticosteroids. (Courtesy of Tyrone Wei, DC, DACBR, Portland, Oregon.)

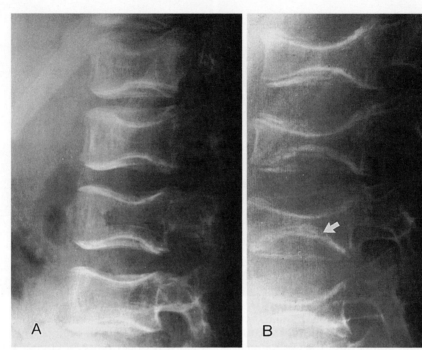

Figure 14-46 **CUSHING'S DISEASE. A and B. Lateral Lumbar Spine.** Note that both examples demonstrate depressed concave endplates owing to the osteopenia. Some loss of end-plate definition is visible (*arrow*), suggesting hypertrophic callus formation.

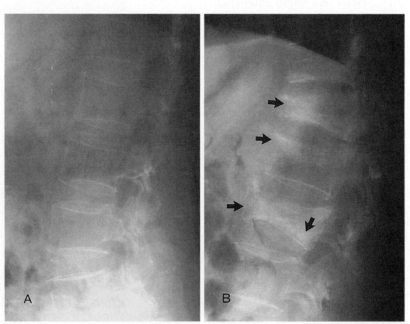

Figure 14-47 **CORTICOSTEROID-INDUCED VERTEBRAL COLLAPSE. A. Pretherapy Lateral Lumbar Spine.** Note the severe diffuse osteoporosis. **B. 3 Months Post-Therapy.** Note that multiple compression deformities are evident. Observe the hazy intrabody density, representing hypertrophic callus formation (*arrows*). *COMMENT:* This 52-year-old female had severe rheumatoid arthritis and had been on corticosteroids for a long time. (Courtesy of Bryan Hartley, MD, Melbourne, Australia.)

Ribs. Multiple fractures can be seen in either the anterior or posterolateral costal segments. Hypertrophic callus at the fracture site is characteristic on healing.

Other Features. Additional manifestations linked to corticosteroid therapy may have radiographic manifestations.

Corticosteroid Arthropathy. A destructive arthropathy may complicate oral or, more commonly, intra-articular administration of corticosteroids. (26,27) Non-steroidal anti-inflammatory drugs (NSAIDs), including phenylbutazone and indomethacin, can also induce the same changes. (1,28) The similarity to a neuropathic joint, which can be rapidly progressive within months, is striking. Fragmentation and collapse of the subchondral bone, sclerosis, and loss of joint space are telltale signs. Gouged-out areas of bone at the articular margins have been compared with animal bites (*bite sign*). (27)

Osteomyelitis and Septic Arthritis. Bone and joint infections are visible. (29) The most common joint for septic arthritis is the knee; the most common implicated organism is *Staphylococcus aureus.*

Tendon and Soft Tissue Injury. Tendon rupture and atrophy of the subcutaneous tissues can follow oral, intra-articular, or intravenous administration of corticosteroids. (30) The drug decreases the fibrous content, reduces its strength, inhibits healing of the injury, delays regeneration, and promotes fatty degeneration and collagen necrosis. (31–33) The most common sites of rupture are the Achilles and patellar tendons. (34,35)

CAPSULE SUMMARY   Cushing's Disease and Steroid-Induced Osteonecrosis

Clinical Features

- Cushing's disease and administration of corticosteroids orally, intravenously, or by intra-articular injection can potentially produce profound changes within the musculoskeletal system.
- Physical manifestations include obesity (moon face, dowager's or buffalo hump, truncal obesity), hirsutism and proximal myopathy, hypertension, and abdominal purple striae. Fractures of the vertebrae and ribs are often painless.
- Skeletal complications include compression fractures of the spine, avascular necrosis, osteopenia, delayed development, infections, destructive arthropathy, impaired healing, tendon rupture, and soft tissue atrophy.

Radiologic Features

- Osteopenia, avascular necrosis, and pathologic fractures.
- *Osteopenia:* thin cortices, diminished density, and deformities.
- *Avascular necrosis (osteonecrosis):* femoral heads (most common, 30–50% bilaterally), humeral heads, femoral condyles, proximal tibiae, and talus. Incidence-dose related, with the average time of onset 2–3 years.
- Mechanism unknown, but fat emboli derived from a fatty liver most accepted explanation.
- *Epiphyseal necrosis:* often bilateral, subchondral fracture (crescent sign), collapse (step sign), patchy sclerosis, and lucency of the involved zone in the epiphysis. Metaphyseal–diaphyseal infarctions are uncommon.

- *Vertebral bodies:* collections of intrabody nitrogen gas (intravertebral vacuum cleft sign). Not specific for avascular necrosis and found in association with osteoporosis, multiple myeloma, metastatic carcinoma, alcoholism, Gaucher's disease, Kümmell's disease, and radiotherapy. Most common cause is osteoporosis.
- Vacuum cleft changes with time; following hyperextension or traction, gas quickly accumulates; after 10 min, it is resorbed and is replaced progressively with fluid. On MRI the vacuum cleft is a black signal void; when fluid accumulates, high signal fluid on T2-weighted images is depicted.
- *Fracture:*
  Spine: most common fractures of various morphologic types; hazy band of sub-endplate sclerosis (marginal condensation sign), biconcave endplates (fish vertebrae), and compression fractures; wedged (anterior loss of height), plana (anterior and posterior loss of height), or central in morphology.
  Ribs: multiple fractures with hypertrophic callus.
- *Other features:* corticosteroid arthropathy; destructive arthropathy similar to a neuropathic joint (rapidly progressive within months, fragmentation, collapse of the subchondral bone, sclerosis, and loss of joint space); gouged-out areas of bone (bite sign).
- *Osteomyelitis and septic arthritis:* knee; the most common implicated organism is *Staphylococcus aureus.*
- Tendon and soft tissue injury, tendon rupture (Achilles, patellar), and atrophy of the subcutaneous tissues.

HEAVY-METAL POISONING

The major metals involved in producing visible radiologic changes are lead, phosphorus, and bismuth. Lead is the most frequent, remaining the most common environmental health problem affecting children living in the United States. (1) Although all cases may not be identified radiographically, it is estimated that currently 1 million preschool-aged American children have elevated blood levels of lead. (2)

Lead may be ingested, inhaled, or implanted. (3,4) (Fig. 14-48) The ultimate consequences of lead exposure are caused by oxidative stress, with children displaying a lower tolerance to any level of exposure. (5,6) Clinical symptoms usually occur abruptly and include abdominal pain, encephalopathy, and disturbances of the nervous system. (7) With chronic exposure to lead, the lungs, blood vessels, testes, sperm, liver, and brain have demonstrated adverse affects (5); however, up to 95% of the lead will deposit in the bone and dentine. (8) Radiologically, the most definitive signs are the linear, transverse densities at the metaphyses (*lead lines*). (9) (Fig. 14-49) The deposition of lead may also precipitate remodeling abnormalities. Phosphorus and bismuth exhibit similar changes.

Workers involved in the polymerization of polyvinyl chloride (PVC) may develop a peculiar form of acro-osteolysis. (Fig. 14-50)

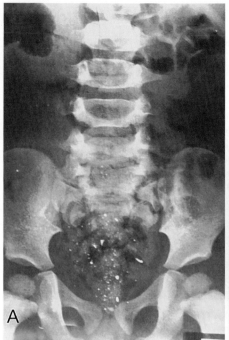

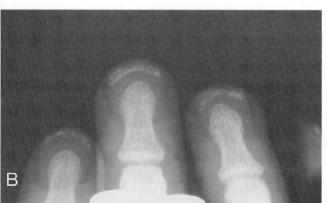

Figure 14-48 **LEAD POISONING. A. AP Abdomen.** Note that the ingested lead-laden paint flakes can be seen in the pelvic basin. **B. Fingertips.** Note that a clue to the origin may be found under the nails. In this patient, persistent scratching of walls covered with lead-containing paint is evidenced by the subungual accumulations.

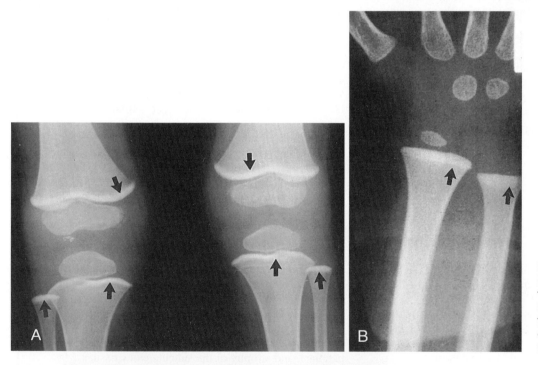

Figure 14-49 **LEAD LINES. A. AP Bilateral Knees. B. PA Wrist.** Note the radiodense metaphyseal bands (*arrows*). Each line corresponds to an episode of systemic intoxication, which in this case was multiple.

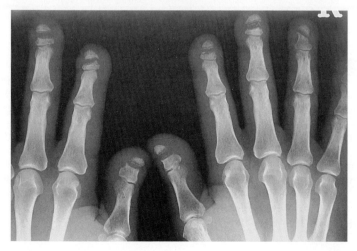

Figure 14-50 **POLYVINYL CHLORIDE TOXICITY. Bilateral Hands.** Note the peculiar osteolytic changes in the distal phalanges.

FLUOROSIS

Chronic ingestion of fluorine (fluorosis) has the potential to produce a spectrum of toxic effects. At 1 ppm the incidence of dental caries may be reduced; 2 ppm or more can precipitate mottled tooth enamel; 8 ppm results in osteosclerosis in 10% of individuals; and > 100 ppm causes growth disturbances, kidney damage, or death. (1) It is most commonly the result of drinking contaminated water in certain geographic areas, especially India and China (endemic fluorosis). (2,3) In the United States, it is estimated that 2% of schoolchildren will be affected, even at the recommended doses of fluorine added to the water. (4) Other causes include industrial and laboratory exposure, fluorine medications, and habitual intake of fluorine-containing wine (wine fluorosis).

The axial skeleton exhibits more marked features than the peripheral skeleton. The key findings are initial osteopenia followed by sclerosis, growth arrest lines, exuberant vertebral hyperostosis, ligamentous calcification, and periostitis. (2) (Fig. 14-51)

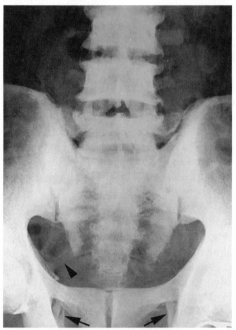

Figure 14-51 FLUOROSIS. AP Pelvis. Note the generalized increase in bone density. Also observe diffuse calcification of multiple ligaments, including the sacrotuberous (*arrows*) and sacrospinous ligaments (*arrowhead*). *COMMENT:* The combination of diffuse osteosclerosis and ligamentous calcifications is virtually diagnostic of fluorosis. (Courtesy of Professor Manorama Berry, MD, All India Institute of Medical Sciences, New Delhi, India.)

HISTIOCYTOSIS X (LANGERHANS' CELL HISTIOCYTOSIS)

Histiocytosis X is a disease of unknown origin that encompasses a wide spectrum of clinical, pathologic, and radiologic features. The hallmark of the disease is an abnormal proliferation of reticuloendothelial cells, predominantly the histiocyte from which the disease derives its name. (1,2) The term histiocytosis X was first proposed by Lichenstein (1) in 1953. In more recent times a name change to Langerhans' cell histiocytosis has been suggested because Langerhans' cell is the major cell type. (3)

The disease is a disorder of immune regulation rather than a neoplastic process and may occur as a solitary lesion, primarily affecting the bones, or be a multisystem entity. (4) The skin is affected in 40% of cases, and in 10% of cases, skin lesions represent the only manifestation. (4) The typical skin manifestations include papules, vesicles, nodules, erosions, ulcerations, crusting, and/or purpura. (4) The disease is generally considered a childhood or juvenile disease but may progress into adult life. (5) In fact, the diagnosis is often not made until the patient reaches adulthood. (5) One case was reported in which the diagnosis was first made when the patient was 61 years old. (6) Patients with multisystem involvement tend to have a worse prognosis when compared with those with solitary bone lesions. Up to 20% of patients with multisystem involvement will reveal disease progression regardless of treatment. (7)

Three entities are encompassed under this term: Letterer-Siwe disease (10%), Hand-Schüller-Christian disease (15–40%), and eosinophilic granuloma (60–80%). Although these are designated as separate entities, they frequently overlap and may transform into each other. The only laboratory findings may be a slightly elevated erythrocyte sedimentation rate (ESR)—20–50 mm at 1 hr—and a slight leukocytosis. (8)

LETTERER-SIWE DISEASE

Letterer-Siwe disease is an acute, fulminating, sometimes fatal disease affecting children < 3 years of age. The child presents critically ill with a high fever, skin rash, bleeding gums, malaise, lymphadenopathy, hepatosplenomegaly, and respiratory symptoms.

Skeletal lesions are infrequent owing to the rapidity of its progression. The most common bone change consists of lytic lesions, often only in the calvaria. Uncommon long bone lesions appear aggressive, with irregular rarefaction of the diaphysis and surrounding laminated periosteal response closely simulating Ewing's sarcoma.

HAND-SCHÜLLER-CHRISTIAN DISEASE

Clinical Features

The lesions of Hand-Schüller-Christian disease are typically isolated to the cranial bones, the eyes, and the pituitary gland. (1) Systemic features of pain, anorexia, weight loss, malaise, lymphadenopathy, hepatosplenomegaly, and respiratory symptoms are common. Painful soft tissue nodules can be felt over the skull. A classic but infrequent triad in < 10% of cases has been associated—

exophthalmus (destruction of orbital walls), diabetes insipidus (pituitary lesion), and lytic skull lesions. The course of the disease is chronic but intermittent. It is occasionally fatal.

Radiologic Features

The radiologic hallmark consists of polyostotic destructive foci in an immature skeleton. These lesions can occur anywhere but are particularly notable in the skull, pelvis, and long bones. Each individual lesion can exhibit a wide spectrum of appearances, from a benign geographic form to a permeative, cortex-destroying malignant process.

In long bones, the initial lesions may consist of multiple lytic defects, some 5–10 mm in size, affecting the entire bone from the diaphysis to the metaphysis and even, on occasion, the epiphysis. These lesions coalesce to create larger defects often marked by endosteal scalloping and *beveling* of the cortex, producing the *hole-within-hole appearance.*

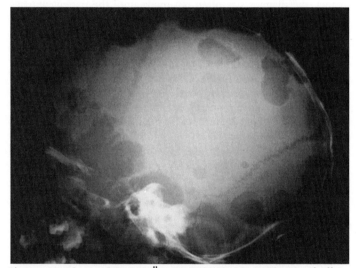

Figure 14-52   HAND-SCHÜLLER-CHRISTIAN DISEASE. Skull. Note the multiple geographic lesions, their confluent nature, and their well-demarcated borders (geographic skull).

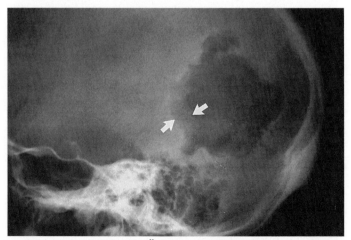

Figure 14-53   HAND-SCHÜLLER-CHRISTIAN DISEASE. Lateral Skull. Note the beveled edge and the hole-within-hole appearance to the lesion (*arrows*).

In the skull, confluence of these individual lesions generates large map-like regions of radiolucency (*geographic skull*), usually with a peripheral *beveled edge* and a *hole-within-hole appearance.* (Figs. 14-52 and 14-53)

EOSINOPHILIC GRANULOMA

Clinical Features

Eosinophilic granuloma is the least severe but most common (60–80%) of all the histiocytoses. (1,2) Peak incidence comes between the ages of 5 and 10 years, and 75% of cases occur in individuals < 20 years of age. (2,3) Symptoms primarily are localized pain and swelling of < 2 months' duration. Eosinophilic granuloma typically lacks the systemic features of Hand-Schüller-Christian or Letterer-Siwe disease. Occasionally, pathologic fracture will be the presenting problem. Vertebral involvement is characterized by pain, and in some cases complicating myelopathy may ensue secondary to cord and nerve root compression. Temporal bone involvement may produce otitis media-like symptoms, and the diagnosis of eosinophilic granuloma should be suspected when patients with suspected otitis media do not respond to traditional medical treatment. (1)

More than 50% of cases involve the skull, mandible (25%), spine (6%), pelvis (20%), and ribs (7%). (4) Of the long bones, the femur (15%), tibia, and humerus (8%) are involved most often. The bones of the hands and feet are affected rarely. (2) Monostotic presentations are three times more common than polyostotic presentations. (2) Monostotic lesions progress to lesions elsewhere in 20% of cases. (5) Pain may be the primary symptom (6), and the diagnosis often requires histopathologic analysis of the lesions as well as the detection of S-100 CD1 antigens on immunohistochemical analysis of the tissues. (1)

Response is usually excellent, with little difference in outcome no matter what method is employed and even without treatment. (3) Radiotherapy or injection into the lesion of corticosteroid can enhance healing of the lesion. Removal by either en-bloc excision or curettage is curative. (7) Chemotherapy is sometimes employed in polyostotic forms. (1) The time for healing to occur is usually 6–24 months; however, reoccurrence may occur and is more common in adults than in skeletally immature patients. (8) Spinal lesions usually do not require treatment, unless the cord is affected.

Pathologic Features

The lesion is composed of proliferating histiocytes (mainly Langerhans' histiocytes) within a granuloma that incites a considerable inflammatory response dominated by eosinophils, from which the name is derived. The Langerhans' cells contain characteristic organelles, termed *Birbeck's granules,* but their function is unclear. (9) A congregation of eosinophils within the granuloma form is termed an *eosinophilic microabscess.* (4)

In the spine, the lesion traditionally was deemed to be the result of avascular necrosis of the vertebral body and was referred to as Calvé's disease. (10) Histopathologic examinations have confirmed the cause to be eosinophilic granuloma. (11)

Radiologic Features

Most lesions are visible on plain films. (2) Once a lesion is isolated, a bone scan may well identify additional lesions. CT and MRI are useful in defining a soft tissue mass (especially in spinal involvement), periosteal response, and characteristics of the lesion.

These lesions are usually solitary and geographic. They are round to oval in shape, have sharply demarcated borders, and exhibit prominent endosteal scalloping, usually with a solid or laminated periosteal response. (12)

Skull and Mandible. A round to oval osteolytic lesion of 1–4 cm is characteristic. (2) It is sharply demarcated and may involve one table greater than the other to produce a double contour (*beveled edge sign,* hole within hole). Within the lesion a central focus of bone may remain isolated, which may be identified only on CT examination (*button sequestrum*). (13) The lesion does not respect suture lines and readily infiltrates into adjacent parts of the calvaria.

In the mandible, pain is the primary symptom in 92% of cases. (14) Radiographically, the lesion is osteolytic, may be expansile, and does not involve the teeth except to leave them displaced and isolated (*floating teeth sign*). Early lesions typically begin in the vicinity of the last molar and enlarge predominantly forward but do not destroy the lower mandibular border. (4)

Spine. More than 50% of cases involve the thoracic spine; 35%, the lumbar spine; and < 15%, the cervical spine. (2) Solitary vertebral involvement is more common, though multiple levels are occasionally involved. With cervical involvement, C2 is the primary target in adults, whereas the middle cervicals are normally affected in children. (15)

The vertebral body is usually involved with relative sparing of the neural arch structures. (10) In contrast, cases have been reported of lesions affecting the posterior arch and lateral masses in the absence of vertebral body involvement; however, this is rare. (16,17) An osteolytic lesion is the expected radiographic appearance. (15)

Neural arch involvement, when present, destroys the internal matrix but preserves the cortical outline, which has been described as a *ghostly appearance.* (18) The most prominent feature in the lumbar and thoracic spine is pathologic fracture, with dramatic loss of vertebral height as thin as 2 mm involving both the anterior and posterior vertebral body surfaces (vertebra plana, *silver dollar vertebra, coin-on-edge vertebra*). (Figs. 14-54 and 14-55) This is rare in the cervical spine. (15) Areas of destruction within the centrum may be observed before collapse. A short-segment kyphosis usually accompanies thoracic vertebral involvement. (11) Paravertebral swelling can be prominent and is more likely to be associated with increased risk to the cord. On CT examination osteolytic destruction can be seen, which simulates aggressive neoplasm; occasionally a sequestrum may be visible.

Bracing is the treatment of choice, and surgical intervention is rarely necessary. (19) Restoration of height with healing is to be expected in at least 90% of cases and can be rapid over 1 year. (3,20) The majority of cases reconstitute to 48–95% of normal height, especially in patients < 15 years of age at the time of onset. (18,11) Residual sclerosis and trabecular accentuation always remain. (21) Rarely, interbody fusion may occur after radiotherapy (22,23), and occasionally there is a bone-within-bone appearance. (23) Healed lesions do not appear to increase the risk for long-term back disability in adulthood. (11)

Pelvis. The ilium is the most frequent component afflicted, especially within the supra-acetabular region. (Fig. 14-56) The lesion can be relatively large, slightly expansile, and usually exhibits a sclerotic beveled edge. Initially, small moth-eaten–permeative,

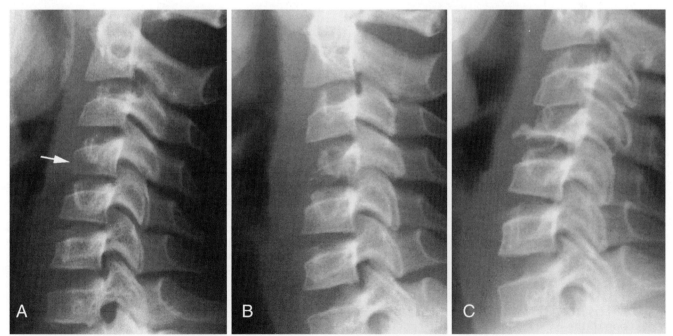

Figure 14-54 EOSINOPHILIC GRANULOMA: 12-YEAR-OLD MALE. Lateral Cervical Spine. A. Initial Film. Observe the subtle destruction of the anterior cortex of the C4 vertebral body (*arrow*). **B. 1-Month Follow-Up.** Note that collapse is now evident, with retropharyngeal swelling. **C. 2-Year Follow-Up.** Observe that the collapse is still persistent. *COMMENT:* This lesion may eventually heal completely and reconstitute to its original height. Radiation therapy, as in this case, may assist in promoting this healing process. (Courtesy of James E. Hether, DC, Marietta, Georgia.)

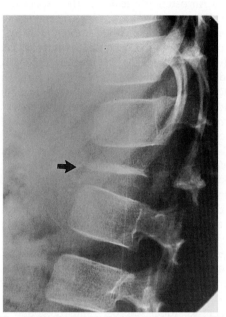

Figure 14-55 **EOSINOPHILIC GRANULOMA: SILVER DOLLAR VERTEBRA. Lateral Lumbar Spine.** Note the extreme flattening of the lumbar vertebral body (*arrow*). Note the disc space is preserved and the posterior arch structures are unaffected. A localized gibbus has occurred with the apex at the collapsed segment.

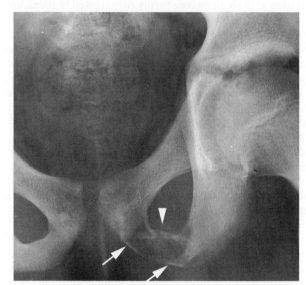

Figure 14-57 **EOSINOPHILIC GRANULOMA. Ischium.** Note the solitary osteolytic lesion within the ischium (*arrows*). A small area of periosteal new bone can be seen (*arrowhead*).

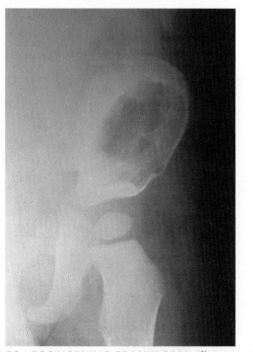

Figure 14-56 **EOSINOPHILIC GRANULOMA. Ilium.** Note that the large lesion of the ilium exhibits the beveled edge with the hole-within-hole appearance. There is some slight expansion laterally, with thinning of the cortex.

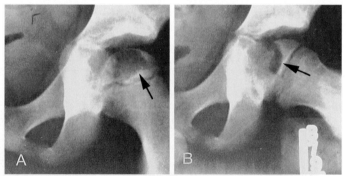

Figure 14-58 **EOSINOPHILIC GRANULOMA: FEMORAL CAPITAL EPIPHYSIS. A. AP Hip.** Note the geographic lesion within the femoral capital epiphysis (*arrow*). It is sharply demarcated with no evidence of matrix calcification. **B. Frog-Leg Hip.** Note that there is no evidence of metaphyseal extension across the cartilaginous growth plate (*arrow*). *COMMENT:* This purely epiphyseal presentation is unusual for eosinophilic granuloma. In this aged patient, if the lesion demonstrated evidence of matrix calcification, chondroblastoma would be the likely diagnosis. (Courtesy of Deborah M. Forrester, MD, Los Angeles, California.)

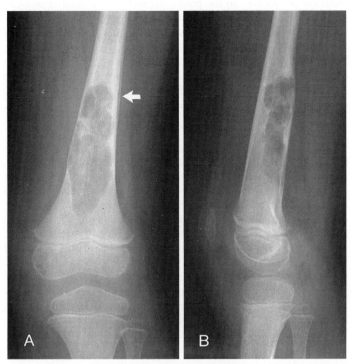

Figure 14-59 **EOSINOPHILIC GRANULOMA. A and B. AP and Lateral Knee.** Note the well-demarcated geographic lesion that has slightly expanded the distal femur. Observe the solid periosteal new bone formation adjacent to the destructive lesion (*arrow*).

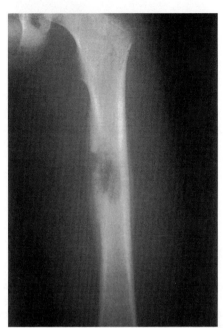

Figure 14-61 **EOSINOPHILIC GRANULOMA: MID-DIAPHYSIS FEMUR.** Note the well-demarcated geographic, moth-eaten lesion, which has produced a slight degree of bone expansion. There is solid periosteal new bone formation seen adjacent to this lytic destructive lesion. *COMMENT:* The geographic, moth-eaten lytic pattern of bone destruction leaves the observer with the question as to whether the lesion is aggressive or benign in nature. The solid periosteal new bone formation is a strong radiographic clue that the underlying lytic process is benign. Eosinophilic granuloma can present with either a geographic (benign-looking) or moth-eaten to permeative (malignant or aggressive-looking) pattern of bone destruction. However, when periosteal new bone formation is produced in a solid pattern, it should be a clue that the lesion is benign. (Courtesy of William J. Droege, DC, CCSP, St. Louis, Missouri, and Joel G. Green, DC, Salem, Massachusetts.)

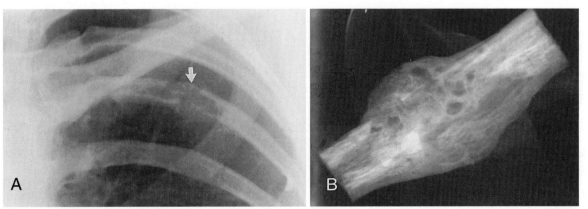

Figure 14-60 **EOSINOPHILIC GRANULOMA: RIB. A. Plain Film.** Note the destructive moth-eaten lesion, extending over some 4 cm (*arrow*). Note how aggressive the lesion appears. **B. Specimen Radiograph.** Observe the moth-eaten pattern of bone destruction and associated periosteal new bone. *COMMENT:* Eosinophilic granuloma often mimics the appearance of Ewing's sarcoma in the ribs.

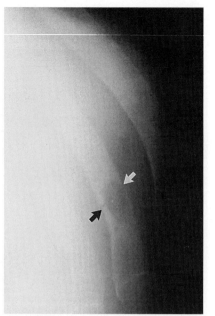

Figure 14-62 EOSINOPHILIC GRANULOMA: RIB PATHOLOGIC FRACTURE. Note that at the anterior end of the tenth rib a 1-cm lytic lesion can be isolated. A pathologic fracture can be discerned traversing the lesion (*arrows*).

multiple lesions may be seen, which rapidly become confluent, producing large geographic defects. Invasion across the triradiate cartilage is unusual. In the pubis, the lesions are smaller and can be associated with a laminated periosteal response along the superior pubic ramus. Ischial lesions similarly may provoke periosteal new bone. (Fig. 14-57)

Long Bones. The femur, tibia, and humerus are involved most often. The bones of the hands and feet are rare sites, as is the fibula. (2,7) The diaphysis is the most common site of involvement (60%). (2,4) Metaphyseal lesions occasionally violate the cartilage growth plate. Epiphyseal foci are rare and mimic chondroblastoma without calcification. (Fig. 14-58)

The lesions tend to be elongated in the long axis of the bone, osteolytic (largely geographic, occasionally moth-eaten–permeative), exhibit endosteal scalloping, cortical thinning, and are slightly expansile. (Figs. 14-59 and 14-60) *Beveling* of the edges and the undulating margin produce a *hole-within-hole appearance.* (4) Periosteal reaction is solid or laminated in about 10% of cases. (2) (Fig. 14-61) Pathologic fracture occasionally occurs. (Fig. 14-62) A moderately enhancing soft tissue mass on CT or MRI is present in < 10% of cases.

Differential Diagnosis. The destructive nature of the lesion makes the diagnosis difficult. The major exclusions are osteomyelitis, Ewing's sarcoma, leukemia, metastatic neuroblastoma, lymphoma, and even fibrous dysplasia.

CAPSULE SUMMARY Histiocytosis X (Langerhans' Cell Histiocytosis)

General Considerations

- A disorder of the reticuloendothelial system characterized by an abnormal proliferation of histiocytes (Langerhans' cell).
- Three entities: Letterer-Siwe disease, Hand-Schüller-Christian disease, and eosinophilic granuloma.

Letterer-Siwe Disease

Clinical Features

- Acute, fulminating, sometimes fatal disease affecting children < 3 years of age.
- Patient presents critically ill with a high fever, skin rash, bleeding gums, malaise, lymphadenopathy, hepatosplenomegaly, and respiratory symptoms.

Radiologic Features

- Skeletal lesions are infrequent; lytic lesions in the calvaria. Uncommon long bone lesions simulate Ewing's sarcoma.

Hand-Schüller-Christian Disease

Clinical Features

- Systemic features of pain, anorexia, weight loss, malaise, lymphadenopathy, hepatosplenomegaly, and respiratory symptoms are common. Painful soft tissue nodules can be felt over the skull.
- Classic triad (< 10% of cases): exophthalmus (destruction of orbital walls), diabetes insipidus (pituitary lesion), and lytic skull lesions.

Radiologic Features

- Polyostotic destructive foci in an immature skeleton.
- Lesions can occur anywhere; skull, pelvis, and long bones most frequent sites.
- Spectrum of appearances; benign geographic form to a permeative, cortex-destroying malignant process.
- Lesions may consist of multiple lytic defects involving the entire bone from the diaphysis to the metaphysis. Coalescence creates larger defects with beveled cortex, producing the hole-within-hole appearance.
- *Skull:* large map-like regions of radiolucency (geographic skull), beveled edge, hole-within-hole appearance.

Eosinophilic Granuloma

Clinical Features

- Least severe but most common (60%) form.
- Most < 20 years of age, peak age between 5 and 10 years.
- Localized pain and swelling of < 2 months' duration; lacks systemic features, occasional pathologic fracture. Complicating myelopathy rare in spinal involvement.
- > 50% involve the skull, mandible (25%), spine (6%), pelvis (20%), and ribs (7%). Long bones: femur (15%), tibia, and humerus (8%) are involved most often.
- Monostotic presentations are three times more common.
- Treatment by radiotherapy, corticosteroid injection into the lesion, excision (en-bloc, curettage), and chemotherapy.

CAPSULE SUMMARY   Histiocytosis X (Langerhans' Cell Histiocytosis) *(continued)*

Pathologic Features

- Proliferating histiocytes (Langerhans' histiocytes) within a granuloma. Incites a considerable inflammatory response dominated by eosinophils.
- Vertebral collapse previously termed Calvé's disease and thought to be an avascular necrosis; histopathologic examinations have confirmed the cause to be eosinophilic granuloma.

Radiologic Features

- Solitary, geographic, round to oval, sharply demarcated borders, exhibit prominent endosteal scalloping, solid or laminated periosteal response.
- *Skull and mandible:* round to oval osteolytic lesion 1–4 cm, sharply demarcated, beveled edge sign, hole-within-hole appearance, button sequestrum, crosses suture lines. Destruction of mandible isolates and displaces teeth (floating teeth sign).
- *Spine:* > 50% involve the thoracic spine, 35% the lumbar spine, and < 15% the cervical spine.

- The vertebral body always involved, with relative sparing of the neural arch structures; pathologic fracture key sign (vertebra plana, silver dollar vertebra, coin-on-edge vertebra). At least 90% reconstitute to 75% of normal height.
- *Pelvis:* ilium (supra-acetabular region); large, slightly expansile, sclerotic beveled edge. Pubic and ischial lesions smaller, usually have a laminated periosteal response.
- *Long bones:* femur, tibia, and humerus most common.
- Diaphysis is the most common site of involvement (60%). Elongated in the long axis of the bone, osteolytic (largely geographic, occasionally moth-eaten–permeative), endosteal scalloping, cortical thinning and slightly expansile, beveling of the edges (hole-within-hole appearance).
- Periosteal reaction is solid or laminated (10%).
- *Differential diagnosis:* major exclusions are osteomyelitis, Ewing's sarcoma, leukemia, metastatic neuroblastoma, lymphoma, and even fibrous dysplasia.

GAUCHER'S DISEASE

Clinical Features

Gaucher's disease is a rare, inborn aberration of lipid metabolism characterized by deficient activity of the liposomal enzyme acid β-glycosidase (β-glucocerebrosidase). (1,2) This results in abnormal accumulation of glycosyl ceramide in the reticuloendothelial cells of the bone marrow, spleen, and liver. (3) In its classic form it is found in the young adult, especially in Ashkenazic Jews. Bone pain is the common complaint, with up to 20% of patients reporting impaired mobility. (1) Splenomegaly, yellowish-brown skin, and scleral pigmentations in a leukopenic patient are highly suggestive of the disorder. (4) On occasion, acid and alkaline phosphatase levels may be raised. (5) Recent studies have suggested an association with gallbladder involvement leading to cholelithiasis. (6)

Three types are recognized: type 1 is the chronic adult form common in Ashkenazic Jews; type 2 is the acute infantile form, with symptoms within 3 months of birth and death within 2 years; type 3 is the subacute juvenile form, with a wide spectrum of presentations. (5) Although skeletal changes are most apparent in the chronic adult form (type 1), a near normal life span can usually be expected. (7) With the use of enzyme-replacement therapy, resolution of skeletal findings has been documented (7); however, it is not a life-long cure. (8). Currently, research is investigating the possible use of gene therapy to prevent or cure this condition. (8)

Pathologic Features

The precise pathophysiologic sequence of skeletal events remains hypothetical. The Gaucher cell is found in the liver, spleen, and bone marrow. It is 20–100 µ in size. It has pale pink cytoplasm on periodic acid-Schiff (PAS), a *crumpled tissue paper cytoplasm,* and lipid and iron deposits. Progressive infiltration and replacement of normal marrow elements by Gaucher cells result in an increased reticulum that acts as a space-occupying lesion, leading to vascular compromise and increased intramedullary pressure followed by marrow necrosis and fibrosis. (9) These marrow changes are thought to precipitate avascular necrosis of the femoral and humeral heads. There is an increased susceptibility to skeletal infection, especially following surgery.

Radiologic Features

Radiologically, the bones are affected by a direct-pressure atrophy of the enlarging cellular mass. The most characteristic features occur in the femur, with avascular necrosis of the head, Erlenmeyer flask deformity, osteoporosis, medullary expansion, and cortical thinning. (9–11) (Figs. 14-63 and 14-64) Individual lytic lesions and periostitis complicate the picture. Degenerative joint disease is common in the hips and knees. CT and technetium bone scans are useful for determining the extent and severity of Gaucher's disease involvement of bone marrow. (5,9) CT demonstrates higher marrow attenuation values owing to increased amounts of fibrotic and calcific replacement. (9) The extent of involvement can be isolated by measuring the marrow attenuation and isolating the interface at which positive values revert to normal negative values. (9) Soft tissue extension beyond the bony confines (Gaucher's cell deposits) may simulate malignancy (12). Bone involvement may rarely be complicated by an intraosseous hemorrhagic cyst. (13)

In the spine, diffuse osteopenia is the characteristic finding. Other spinal manifestations may be collapse of a single or several vertebral bodies with associated kyphosis, endplate step defects similar to that in sickle cell anemia (H-shaped vertebra) (14), biconcave endplates (fish vertebrae), and an intravertebral vac-

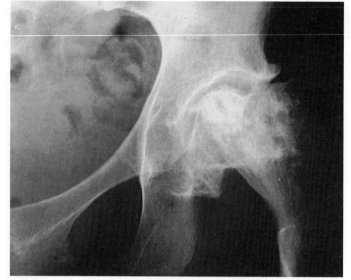

Figure 14-63 GAUCHER'S DISEASE. Femoral Head, AP Hip. Note the collapse, sclerosis, and deformity, which characterize the avascular necrosis. *COMMENT:* These changes are often seen bilaterally in Gaucher's disease. Differentiation from other causes for avascular necrosis as a rule cannot be achieved solely on the basis of the hip radiograph.

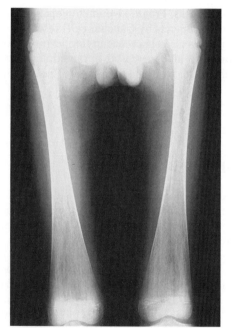

Figure 14-64 GAUCHER'S DISEASE: ERLENMEYER FLASK DEFORMITY. Note the lack of diametaphyseal constriction. *COMMENT:* In a child, this deformity is suggestive of, but not specific for, this disease.

uum cleft sign. (3,15) MRI depicts the vertebral body infiltrated with Gaucher's cells as a high-intensity signal lesion on both T1- and T2-weighted images. (3) MRI also clearly shows spinal cord compression at the site of compression fracture and apex of the gibbus owing to an extradural mass of Gaucher's cell deposits or bone fragments. (3)

CAPSULE SUMMARY Gaucher's Disease

Clinical Features

- Rare, inborn aberration of lipid metabolism; deficient acid β-glycosidase, precipitating accumulation of glycosyl ceramide in the reticuloendothelial cells of bone marrow, spleen, and liver.
- Splenomegaly, yellowish-brown skin, scleral pigmentations, leukopenia, acid, and alkaline phosphatase elevation. Common in Ashkenazic Jews.
- *Three types:*
  Type 1: chronic adult form common in Ashkenazic Jews.
  Type 2: acute infantile form with symptoms within 3 months of birth and death within 2 years.
  Type 3: subacute juvenile form with a wide spectrum of presentations.

Pathologic Features

- Gaucher's cells are found in the liver, spleen, and bone marrow.
- Progressive infiltration and replacement of normal marrow elements by Gaucher's cells; increased reticulum acts as a space-occupying lesion; vascular compromise and increased intramedullary pressure; marrow necrosis and fibrosis.
- Susceptible to skeletal infection, especially following surgery.

Radiologic Features

- Avascular necrosis of the femoral and humeral heads, Erlenmeyer flask deformity, osteoporosis, medullary expansion, cortical thinning, lytic lesions, and periostitis.
- Degenerative joint disease common in the hips and knees.
- *CT:* demonstrates higher marrow attenuation values; able to locate ends of marrow sites; soft tissue extension may simulate malignancy.
- Rarely is complicated by an intraosseous hemorrhagic cyst.
- *Spine:* diffuse osteopenia, pathologic fracture with associated kyphosis, endplate step defects (H-shaped vertebra), biconcave endplates (fish vertebrae), and an intravertebral vacuum cleft sign.
- *MRI:* depicts infiltration as a high-intensity signal lesion on both T1- and T2-weighted images; may show spinal cord compression.

Medicolegal Implications

NUTRITIONAL, METABOLIC, AND ENDOCRINE DISORDERS

- The presence of osteopenia should instigate a search for its cause. This is determined from the combination of history, clinical examination, laboratory data, and imaging features. Osteopenia may be owing to a multitude of causes, including congenital, vascular, neoplastic, drug-related, metabolic, endocrine, and nutritional disorders.
- There should be an attempt made to quantify the degree of bone loss. This may be at a relatively gross level and needs to be placed into the clinical context as to the effects of a proposed therapy.
- Manual therapists need to be aware of the fragility of osteopenic bone and the sites for likely fractures to occur. Techniques may need to be administered in a modified form to minimize the likelihood of iatrogenic complications.

- Childhood dietary osteopenias (scurvy, rickets) need to be recognized early to avoid longer-term morbidity and possibly mortality.
- The osteopenic and osteonecrotic complications of corticosteroid therapy need to be understood and recognized when present. Therapies subsequently administered must be modified according to these complications and appropriate referral pursued.
- In young children with bone pain, radiographs need to be obtained to exclude underlying inflammatory and neoplastic bone disease. Histiocytoses are relatively common in children and need to be considered in the differential diagnosis. Their potentially life-threatening capacity and significant morbidity emphasize the need for early recognition and appropriate treatment.

■ References

OSTEOPOROSIS

1. **Trueta J:** *Studies of the Development and Decay of the Human Frame.* Philadelphia, WB Saunders, 1968.
2. **Lane NE:** *Osteoporosis.* Rheum Dis Clin North Am 20:1, 1994.

GENERALIZED OSTEOPOROSIS

1. **Brunader R, Shelton DK:** *Radiologic bone assessment in the evaluation of osteoporosis.* Am Family Physician 65(7):1357, 2002.
2. **National Institutes of Health, Consensus Panel:** *Consensus development conference on osteoporosis.* JAMA 252(6):799, 1984.
3. **Chan GK, Duque G:** *Age-related bone loss: Old bone, new facts.* Gerontology 48(2):62, 2002.
4. **Ruegsegger P, Dambacher MA, Ruegsegger E, et al.:** *Bone loss in premenopausal and postmenopausal women. A cross-sectional and longitudinal study using quantitative computed tomography.* J Bone Joint Surg 66A:1015, 1984.
5. **Riggs BL, Wahner HW, Melton LJ III, et al.:** *Rates of bone loss in the appendicular and axial skeletons of women.* J Clin Invest 77:1487, 1986.
6. **Firooznia H, Golimbu C, Rafi M, et al.:** *Rate of spinal trabecular bone loss in normal perimenopausal women: CT measurement.* Radiology 161:735, 1986.
7. **Sowers MR, Galuska DA:** *Epidemiology of bone mass in premenopausal women.* Epidemiol Rev 15:374, 1993.
8. **Tuck SP, Francis RM:** *Osteoporosis.* Postgrad Med J 78(923):536, 2002.
9. **Bernstein DS, Sadowsky N, Hegsted DM, et al.:** *Prevalence of osteoporosis in high and low fluoride areas of North Dakota.* JAMA 198:499, 1966.
10. **Greenfield GB:** *Radiology of Bone Diseases,* ed 3. Philadelphia, JB Lippincott, 1980.
11. **Haczynski J, Jakimiuk A:** *Vertebral fractures: A hidden problem of osteoporosis.* Med Sci Monit 7(5):1108, 2001.
12. **Wu SS, Lachmann E, Nagler W:** *Current medical, rehabilitation, and surgical management of vertebral compression fractures.* J Women's Health [Larchmt] 12(1):17, 2003.
13. **Guermazi A, Mohr A, Grigorian M, et al.:** *Identification of vertebral fractures in osteoporosis.* Semin Musculoskelet Radiol 6(3):241, 2002.
14. **Kostuik JP:** *Compression fractures and surgery in the osteoporotic patient.* In: Frymoyer JW, ed, *The Adult Spine.* New York, Raven Press, 1991.

15. **Klein L, Lafferty FW, Pearson OH, et al.:** *Correlation of urinary hydroxyproline, serum alkaline phosphatase, and skeletal calcium turnover.* Metabolism 13:272, 1964.
16. **Gangi A, Guth S, Imbert JP, et al.:** *Percutaneous vertebroplasty: Indications, technique, and results.* Radiographics 23(2):E10-E10, 2003.
17. **Ng PP, Caragine LP Jr, Dowd CF:** *Percutaneous vertebroplasty: An emerging therapy for vertebral compression fractures.* Semin Neurol 22(2):149, 2002.
18. **Hardouin P, Grados F, Cotton A, Cortet B:** *Should percutaneous vertebroplasty be used to treat osteoporotic fractures? An update.* Joint Bone Spine 68(3):216, 2001.
19. **Evans AJ, Jensen MF, Kip KE, et al.:** *Vertebral compression fractures: Pain reduction and improvement in functional mobility after percutaneous polymethylmethacrylate vertebroplasty: retrospective report of 245 cases.* Radiology 226(2):366, 2003.
20. **Fisher A:** *Percutaneous vertebroplasty: A bone cement procedure for spinal pain relief.* Issues Emerg Health Technol 31:1, 2002.
21. **Predey TA, Sewall LE, Smith SJ:** *Percutaneous vertebroplasty: New treatment for vertebral compression fractures.* Am Family Physician 66(4):611, 2002.
22. **Sartoris DJ, Resnick D:** *Osteoporosis assessment: Current and future methods.* Contemp Diagn Radiol 11:1, 1988.
23. **Guglielmi G, Lang TF:** *Quantitative computed tomography.* Semin Musculoskelet Radiol 6(3):219, 2002.
24. **Wehrli FW, Saha PK, Gomberg BR, et al.:** *Role of magnetic resonance for assessing structure and function of trabecular bone.* Topics Magn Reson Imaging 13(5):335, 2002.
25. **Ardran GM:** *Bone destruction not demonstrable by radiography.* Br J Radiol 24:107, 1951.
26. **Nielsen SP:** *The metacarpal index revisited: A brief overview.* J Clin Densitom 4(3):199, 2001.
27. **DeSmet AA, Robinson RG, Johnson BE, et al.:** *Spinal compression fractures in osteoporotic women: Patterns and relationship to hyperkyphosis.* Radiology 166:497, 1988.
28. **Healey JH, Lane M:** *Structural scoliosis in osteoporotic women.* Clin Orthop 195:216, 1985.
29. **Frager D, Elkin C, Swerdlow M, et al.:** *Subacute osteoporotic compression fracture: Misleading magnetic resonance appearance.* Skeletal Radiol 17:123, 1988.
30. **Resnick DL:** *Fish vertebrae.* Arthritis Rheum 25(9):1073, 1982.
31. **Rowe LJ:** *Fish vertebrae: A case report.* J Aust Chiro Assoc 18:111, 1988.

32. **Resnick D, Niwayama G:** *Intravertebral disc herniations: Cartilaginous (Schmorl's) nodes.* Radiology 126:57, 1976.

33. **Malghem J, Maldague B, Labaisse MA, et al.:** *Intravertebral vacuum cleft: Changes in content after supine positioning.* Radiology 187:483, 1993.

34. **Naul LG, Peet GJ, Maupin WB:** *Avascular necrosis of the vertebral body: MR imaging.* Radiology 172:219, 1989.

35. **Ryan PJ, Fogelman I:** *Osteoporotic vertebral fractures: Diagnosis with radiography and bone scintigraphy.* Radiology 190:669, 1994.

36. **Cummings SR, Melton LJ:** *Epidemiology and outcomes of osteoporotic fractures.* Lancet 359(9319):1761, 2002.

37. **Binkley N, Krueger D:** *Osteoporosis in men.* WMJ 101(4):28, 2002.

38. **Singh M, Riggs B, Beabout JW, et al.:** *Changes in trabecular pattern of the upper end of the femur as an index of osteoporosis.* J Bone Joint Surg 52A:457, 1970.

39. **Healey JH, Vigorita VJ, Lane JM:** *The coexistence and characteristics of osteoarthritis and osteoporosis.* J Bone Joint Surg 67A:586, 1985.

40. **Evans RA, McDonnell GD, Schieb M:** *Metacarpal cortical area as an index of bone mass.* Br J Radiol 51:428, 1978.

41. **Pentecost RL, Murray RA, Brindley HH:** *Fatigue, insufficiency and pathological fractures.* JAMA 187:1001, 1964.

42. **Lourie H:** *Spontaneous osteoporotic fracture of the sacrum. An unrecognized syndrome of the elderly.* JAMA 248:715, 1982.

43. **Mathers D, Major G:** *Insufficiency fractures of the sacrum.* Ann Rheum Dis 52:621, 1993.

44. **Weber M, Hasler P, Gerber H:** *Insufficiency fractures of the sacrum. Twenty cases and review of the literature.* Spine 18:2507, 1993.

45. **Leroux JL, Denat B, Thomas E, et al.:** *Sacral insufficiency fractures presenting as acute low back pain. Biomechanical aspects.* Spine 18:2502, 1993.

46. **Cotty P, Fouquet B, Mezange C, et al.:** *Insufficiency fractures of the sacrum.* J Neuroradiol 16:160, 1989.

47. **Ries T:** *Detection of osteoporotic sacral fractures with radionuclides.* Radiology 146:783, 1983.

48. **Balseiro J, Brower AC, Ziessman HA:** *Scintigraphic diagnosis of sacral fractures.* AJR 148:111, 1987.

49. **Rogers LF:** *Radiology of Skeletal Trauma,* ed 3. New York, Churchill Livingstone, 1992.

50. **Denis F, Davis S, Comfort T:** *Sacral fractures: An important problem.* Clin Orthop 227:67, 1988.

51. **Stroebel RJ, Ginsburg WW, McLeod RA:** *Sacral insufficiency fractures: An often unsuspected cause of low back pain.* J Rheumatol 18:117, 1991.

52. **Brahme SK, Cervilla V, Vint V, et al.:** *Magnetic resonance appearance of sacral insufficiency fractures.* Skeletal Radiol 19:489, 1990.

53. **Casey D, Mirra J, Staple TW:** *Parasymphyseal insufficiency fractures of the os pubis.* AJR 142:581, 1984.

54. **DeSmet AA, Neff JR:** *Pubic and sacral insufficiency fractures: Clinical course and radiologic findings.* AJR 145:601, 1985.

55. **Chen C, Chandnani V, Kang HS, et al.:** *Insufficiency fracture of the sternum caused by osteopenia: Plain film findings in seven patients.* AJR 154:1025, 1990.

56. **Cooper KL:** *Insufficiency fractures of the sternum: A consequence of thoracic kyphosis?* Radiology 167:471, 1988.

57. **Dorne HL, Lander PH:** *Spontaneous stress fractures of the femoral neck.* AJR 144:343, 1985.

58. **Nordin BEC, Roper A:** *Post pregnant osteoporosis, a syndrome?* Lancet 1:431, 1955.

59. **Houang MTW, Brenton DP, Renton P, et al.:** *Idiopathic juvenile osteoporosis.* Skeletal Radiol 3:17, 1978.

60. **Griffith CC, Nichols G, Asher JD, et al.:** *Heparin osteoporosis.* JAMA 193:91, 1965.

61. **Dalen N, Feldreich AL:** *Osteopenia in alcoholism.* Clin Orthop 99:201, 1974.

REGIONALIZED OSTEOPOROSIS

1. **Mitchell SW, Morehouse GR, Keen WW:** *Gunshot Wounds and Other Injuries of Nerves.* Philadelphia, JB Lippincott, 1864.

2. **Turner-Stokes L:** *Reflex sympathetic dystrophy—A complex regional pain syndrome.* Disabil Rehabil 24(18):939, 2002.

3. **Kurvers HA:** *Reflex sympathetic dystrophy: Facts and hypotheses.* Vasc Med 3(3):207, 1998.

4. **Fournier RS, Holder LE:** *Reflex sympathetic dystrophy: Diagnostic controversies.* Semin Nucl Med 28(1):116, 1998.

5. **Kozin F, McCarty DJ, Simms J, et al.:** *The reflex sympathetic dystrophy syndrome. I. Clinical and histologic studies: Evidence for bilaterality, response to corticosteroids, and articular involvement.* Am J Med 60:321, 1976.

6. **Genant HK, Kozin F, Bekermann C, et al.:** *The reflex sympathetic dystrophy syndrome. A comprehensive analysis using fine detail radiography, photon absorptiometry, and bone and joint scintigraphy.* Radiology 117:21, 1975.

7. **Driessens M, Dijs H, Verheyen G, Blockx P:** *What is reflex sympathetic dystrophy?* Acta Orthop Belg J65(2):202, 1999.

8. **Fitzpatrick LA:** *Secondary causes of osteoporosis.* Mayo Clinic Proc 77(5):453,2002.

9. **Takata S, Yasusi N:** *Disuse osteoporosis.* J Med Invest 48(3–4):147, 2001.

10. **Jones G:** *Radiological appearances of disuse osteoporosis.* Clin Radiol 20:345, 1969.

11. **Yagan R, Radivoyevitch M, Khan M:** *Double cortical line sign in the acetabular roof: A sign of disuse osteoporosis.* Radiology 165:171, 1987.

12. **Glockner JF, Sundaram M, Pierron RL:** *Radiologic case study. Transient migratory osteoporosis of the hip and knee.* Orthopedics 21(5):600, 1998.

13. **Samdani A, Lachmann E, Nagler W:** *Transient osteoporosis of the hip during pregnancy: A case report.* Am J Phys Med Rehabil 77(2):153, 1998.

14. **Trevisan C, Ortolani S, Monteleone M, Mariononi EC:** *Regional migratory osteoporosis: A pathogenic hypothesis based on three cases and a review of the literature.* Clin Rheumatol 21(5):418, 2002.

15. **Curtis PH Jr, Kincaid WE:** *Transitory demineralization of the hip in pregnancy.* J Bone Joint Surg 41A:1327, 1959.

16. **Beaulieu JG, Razzano D, Levine RB:** *Transient osteoporosis of the hip in pregnancy. Review of the literature and a case report.* Clin Orthop 115:165, 1976.

17. **Crespo E, Sala D, Crespo R, Silvestre A:** *Transient osteoporosis.* Acta Orthop Belg 67(4):330, 2001.

18. **Urbanski SR, De Lange EE, Eschenroeder HC:** *Magnetic resonance imaging of transient osteoporosis of the hip.* J Bone Joint Surg 73A:451, 1991.

19. **Arnstein AR:** *Regional osteoporosis.* Orthop Clin North Am 3:585, 1972.

OSTEOMALACIA

1. **Mankin HJ:** *Rickets, osteomalacia, and renal osteodystrophy.* J Bone Joint Surg 56A:352, 1974.

2. **Reginato AJ, Falasca GF, Pappu R, et al.:** *Musculoskeletal manifestations of ossteomalacia: Report of 26 cases and literature review.* Semin Arthritis Rheum 28(5):287, 1999.

3. **Al-Ali H, Fuleihan GE:** *Nutritional osteomalacia: Substantial clinical improvement and gain in bone density posttherapy.* J Clin Densitom 3(1):97, 2000.

4. **Looser E:** *Über Spaetrachitis und osteomalakie. Klinische, roentgenologische und pathologisch anatomische untersuchungen.* Deutsche Zts Chir 152:210, 1920.

5. **Milkman LA:** *Multiple spontaneous idiopathic symmetrical fractures.* AJR 32:622, 1934.

6. **Steinbach HL, Kolb FO, Gilfillan R:** *A mechanism for the production of pseudofractures in osteomalacia (Milkman's syndrome).* Radiology 62:388, 1954.

7. **LeMay M:** *The early radiological diagnosis of osteomalacia in adults.* Radiology 70:373, 1958.

8. **Steinbach HL, Moetzli M:** *Roentgen appearance of the skeleton in osteomalacia and rickets.* AJR 82:875, 1950.
9. **Meema HE, Meema S:** *Improved roentgenological diagnosis of osteomalacia by microscopy of hand bones.* AJR 125:925, 1975.
10. **Akbunar AT, Orhan B, Alper E:** *Bone-scan-like pattern with 99Tcm(V)-DMSA scintigraphy in patients with osteomalacia and primary hyperparathyroidism.* Nucl Med Commun 21(2):181, 2000.
11. **Fulkerson JP, Ozonoff MB:** *Multiple symmetrical fractures of bone of unresolved etiology.* AJR 129:313, 1977.
12. **Greenfield GB:** *Radiology of Bone Diseases,* ed 3. Philadelphia, JB Lippincott, 1980.

RICKETS

1. **Kaper BP, Romness MJ, Urbanek PJ:** *Nutritional rickets: Report of four cases diagnosed at orthopaedic evaluation.* Am J Orthop 29(3):214, 2000.
2. **Abrams SA:** *Nutritional rickets: An old disease returns.* Nutr Rev 60(4):111, 2002.
3. **McCollum EV, Simmonds N, Becker JE, et al.:** *Studies on experimental rickets: XXI. An experimental demonstration of the existence of a vitamin which promotes calcium deposition.* J Biol Chem 53:293, 1922.
4. **Narchi H, El Jamil M, Kulaylat N:** *Symptomatic rickets in adolescence.* Arch Dis Child 84(6):501, 2001.
5. **Thacher TD, Fischer PR, Pettifor JM:** *The usefulness of clinical features to identify active rickets.* Ann Trop Paediatr 22(3):229, 2002.
6. **Pugliese MT, Blumberg DL, Hludzinski J, Kay S:** *Nutritional rickets in suburbia.* J Am Coll Nutr 17(6):637, 1998.
7. **Nozza JM, Rodda CP:** *Vitamin D deficiency in mothers of infants with rickets.* Med J Aust 175(5):253, 2001.
8. **Mankin HJ:** *Rickets, osteomalacia, and renal osteodystrophy—Part I.* J Bone Joint Surg 56A:101, 1974.
9. **Steinbach HL, Moetzli M:** *Roentgen appearance of the skeleton in osteomalacia and rickets.* AJR 91:955, 1964.

SCURVY

1. **Rajakumar K:** *Infantile scurvy: A historical perspective.* Pediatrics 108(4):E76, 2001.
2. **Akikusa JD, Garrick D, Nash MC:** *Scurvy: Forgotten but not gone.* J Paediatr Child Health 39(1):75, 2003.
3. **Shorhe HB:** *Infantile scurvy.* Clin Orthop 1:49, 1963.
4. **Clemetson CA:** *Barlow's disease.* Med Hypotheses 59(1):52, 2002.
5. **Jaffe HL:** *Metabolic, Degenerative, and Inflammatory Diseases of Bones and Joints.* Philadelphia, Lea & Febiger, 1972.
6. **McCann P:** *The incidence and value of radiological signs in scurvy.* Br J Radiol 35:683, 1962.
7. **Boeve WJ, Martijn A:** *Scurvy. Case report 406.* Skeletal Radiol 16:67, 1987.

HYPERPARATHYROIDISM

1. **Inaba M, Ishikawa T, Imanishi Y, et al.:** *Pathophysiology and diagnosis of primary hyperparathyroidism—Strategy for asymptomatic primary hyperparathyroidism.* Biomed Pharmacother 54(Suppl 1): 7s, 2000.
2. **Jeren-Strujic B, Rozman B, Lambasa S, et al.:** *Secondary hyperparathyroidism and brown tumor in dialyzed patients.* Ran Fail 23(2):279, 2001.
3. **Genant HK, Heck LL, Lanzl LH, et al.:** *Primary hyperparathyroidism. A comprehensive study of clinical, biochemical, and radiographic manifestations.* Radiology 109:513, 1973.
4. **Keating FR Jr:** *Diagnosis of hyperparathyroidism.* JAMA 178:547, 1961.
5. **Pugh DG:** *Subperiosteal resorption of bone. A roentgenological manifestation of primary hyperparathyroidism and renal osteodystrophy.* AJR 66:577, 1951.
6. **Marcus R:** *Diagnosis and treatment of hyperparathyroidism.* Rev Endocrin Metab Disord 1(4):247, 2000.
7. **Sekiyama K, Akakura K, Mikami K, et al.:** *Usefulness of diagnostic imaging in primary hyperparathyroidism.* Int J Urol 10:7, 2003. [Discussion 10:12, 2003.]
8. **Rodan GA:** *Bisphosphonates and primary hyperparathyroidism.* J Bone Miner Res 17(Suppl 2):N150, 2002.
9. **Peacock M:** *Primary hyperparathyroidism and the kidney: Biochemical and clinical spectrum.* J Bone Miner Res 17(Suppl 2): N87, 2002.
10. **Teng CT, Nathan MH:** *Primary hyperparathyroidism.* AJR 83:716, 1960.
11. **Resnick D, Dwosh IL, Niwayama G:** *Sacroiliac joint in renal osteodystrophy: Roentgenographic-pathologic correlation.* J Rheumatol 2:287, 1975.
12. **Resnick D, Niwayama G:** *Subchondral resorption of bone in renal osteodystrophy.* Radiology 118:315, 1976.
13. **Schwartz EE, Lantieri R, Teplick JG:** *Erosion of the inferior aspect of the clavicle in secondary hyperparathyroidism.* AJR 129:291, 1977.
14. **Polat P, Kantarci M, Alper F, et al.:** *The spectrum of radiographic findings in primary hyperparathyroidism.* Clin Imaging 26:197, 2002.
15. **Davies AM, Evans N, Mangham DC, Grimer RJ:** *MR imaging of brown tumour with fluid-fluid levels: A report of three cases.* Eur Radiol 11(8):1445, 2001.
16. **Naidich JB, Karmel MI, Mossey RT, et al.:** *Osteoarthropathy of the hand and wrist in patients undergoing long-term hemodialysis.* Radiology 164:205, 1987.
17. **Stolpen AH:** *Spondyloarthropathy of renal dialysis.* Semin Roentgenol 28:96, 1993.
18. **Dodds WJ, Steinbach HI:** *Primary hyperparathyroidism and articular cartilage calcification.* AJR 104:884, 1968.
19. **Steinbach HL, Gordon GS, Eisenberg E, et al.:** *Primary hyperparathyroidism: A correlation of roentgen, clinical, and pathologic features.* AJR 86:329, 1961.
20. **Hilbish TF, Bartter FC:** *Roentgen findings in abnormal deposition of calcium in tissues.* AJR 87:1128, 1962.
21. **Weiss A:** *Incidence of subperiosteal resorption in hyperparathyroidism studied by fine detail bone radiography.* Clin Radiol 25:273, 1974.
22. **Connor TB, Freijanes J, Stoner RE, et al.:** *Generalized osteosclerosis in primary hyperparathyroidism.* Trans Am Clin Climatol Assoc 85:185, 1973.

HYPERVITAMINOSES

1. **Miller JH, Hayon II:** *Bone scintigraphy in hypervitaminosis A.* AJR 144:767, 1985.
2. **Binkley N, Krueger D:** *Hypervitaminosis A and bone.* Nutr Rev 58(5):138, 2000.
3. **Glunta JL:** *Dental changes in hypervitaminosis D.* Oral Surg Oral Med 85(4):410, 1998.

ACROMEGALY

1. **Jenkins PJ, Sohaib SA, Akker S, et al.:** *The pathology of median neuropathy in acromegaly.* Ann Intern Med 133(3):197, 2000.
2. **Stewart PM:** *Current therapy for acromegaly.* Trends Endocrinol Metab 11(4):128, 2000.
3. **Melmed S, Jackson I, Kleinberg D, Klibanski A:** *Current treatment guidelines for acromegaly.* J Clin Endocrinol Metab 83(8):2646, 1998.
4. **Jane JA Jr, Thapar K, Laws ER Jr:** *Acromegaly: Historical perspectives and current therapy.* J Neurooncol 54(2):129, 2001.
5. **Kaplan FJ, Levitt NS, De Villiers JC, Soule SG:** *Acromegaly in the developing world—A 20-year teaching hospital experience.* Br J Neurosurg 15(1):22, 2001.
6. **Bluestone R, Bywaters EGL, Hartog M, et al.:** *Acromegalic arthropathy.* Am Rheum Dis 30:243, 1971.
7. **Kho KM, Wright AD, Doyle FH:** *Heel pad thickness in acromegaly.* Br J Radiol 43:119, 1970.

8. **Lang EK, Bessler WT:** *The roentgenologic features of acromegaly.* AJR 86:321, 1961.
9. **Woo CC:** *Radiological features of acromegaly.* J Manipulative Physiol Ther 11:206, 1988.
10. **Stuber JL, Palacios E:** *Vertebral scalloping in acromegaly.* AJR 112:397, 1971.
11. **Lin SR, Lee KF:** *Widening of the median atlanto-axial joint in acromegaly.* J Can Assoc Radiol 24:36, 1973.
12. **Parikh M, Iyer K, Elias AN, et al.:** *Spinal stenosis in acromegaly.* Spine 12:627, 1987.

THYROID DISORDERS

1. **Burrow SR, Alman B, Wright JG:** *Short stature as a screening test for endocrinopathy in slipped capital femoral epiphysis.* J Bone Joint Surg 83B:263, 2001.
2. **Nixon DW, Samols E:** *Acral changes associated with thyroid diseases.* JAMA 212:1175, 1970.
3. **Vanhoenacker FM, Pelckmans MC, De Beuckeleer LH, et al.:** *Thyroid acropachy: Correlation of imaging and pathology.* Eur Radiol 11(6):1058, 2001.
4. **Scanlon GT, Clemett AR:** *Thyroid acropachy.* Radiology 83:1039, 1964.
5. **Torres-Reyes E, Staple TW:** *Roentgenographic appearance of thyroid acropachy.* Clin Radiol 21:95, 1970.

CUSHING'S DISEASE AND STEROID-INDUCED OSTEONECROSIS

1. **Murray RO:** *Iatrogenic lesions of the skeleton.* AJR 126:5, 1976.
2. **Curtiss PH, Clark WS, Herndon CH:** *Vertebral fractures resulting from prolonged cortisone and corticotropin therapy.* JAMA 156:467, 1954.
3. **Sissons HA:** *The osteoporosis of Cushing's disease.* J Bone Joint Surg 38B:418, 1956.
4. **Fisher DE, Bickel WH:** *Corticosteroid-induced avascular necrosis.* J Bone Joint Surg 53A:859, 1971.
5. **Madell SH, Freeman LM:** *Avascular necrosis of bone in Cushing's syndrome.* Radiology 83:1068, 1969.
6. **Koch CA, Tsigos C, Patronas NJ, Papanicolaou DA:** *Cushing's disease presenting with avascular necrosis of the hip: An orthopedic emergency.* J Clin Endocrinol Metab 84(9):3010, 1999.
7. **Harrington KD, Murray WR, Kountz SL, et al.:** *Avascular necrosis of bone after renal transplantation.* J Bone Joint Surg 53A:203, 1971.
8. **Lausten GS, Lemser T, Jensen PK, Egfjord M:** *Necrosis of the femoral head after kidney transplantation.* Clin Transplant 12(6):572, 1998.
9. **Wang GJ, Sweet DE, Reger SI:** *Fat cell changes as a mechanism of avascular necrosis of the femoral head in cortisone treated rabbits.* J Bone Joint Surg 59A:729, 1977.
10. **Cruess RL, Ross D, Crawshaw E:** *The etiology of steroid-induced avascular necrosis of bone. A laboratory and clinical study.* Clin Orthop 113:178, 1975.
11. **Maldaque B, Noel H, Malghem J:** *The intravertebral vacuum cleft: A sign of ischemic vertebral collapse.* Radiology 129:23, 1978.
12. **Golimbu C, Firooznia H, Rafii M:** *The intravertebral vacuum sign.* Spine 11:1040, 1986.
13. **Kumpan W, Salomonowitz E, Seidl G, et al.:** *The intravertebral vacuum phenomenon.* Skeletal Radiol 15:444, 1986.
14. **Malghem J, Maldague B, Labaisse MA, et al.:** *Intravertebral vacuum cleft: Changes in content after supine positioning.* Radiology 187:483, 1993.
15. **Gagnerie F, Taillan B, Euller-Ziegler L, et al.:** *Intravertebral vacuum phenomenon in multiple myeloma.* Clin Rheumatol 6:597, 1987.
16. **Schabel J, Moore TE, Rittenberg GM, et al.:** *Vertebral vacuum phenomenon: A radiographic manifestation of metastatic malignancy.* Skeletal Radiol 4:154, 1979.
17. **Naul LG, Peet GJ, Maupin WB:** *Avascular necrosis of the vertebral body: MR imaging.* Radiology 172:219, 1989.
18. **Bielicki DK, Sartoris D, Resnick D, et al.:** *Intraosseous and intra-discal gas in association with spinal infection: Report of three cases.* AJR 147:83, 1986.
19. **Brower AC, Downey EF:** *Kummel disease: Report of a case with serial radiographs.* Radiology 141:363, 1981.
20. **Martin D, Delacollette M, Collignon J, et al.:** *Radiation induced myelopathy and vertebral necrosis.* Neuroradiology 36:405, 1994.
21. **Harveson G:** *Intravertebral vacuum phenomenon.* Clin Radiol 39:69, 1988.
22. **Rowe LJ:** *Vacuum phenomenon.* J Austr Chiro Assoc 18:125, 1989.
23. **Stojanovic J, Kovac V:** *Diagnosis of ischemic vertebral collapse using selective angiography.* Fortschr Geb Rontgenstr Nucklearmed Erganzungsband 135:326, 1981.
24. **Resnick D, Niwayama G, Guerra J Jr, et al.:** *Spinal vacuum phenomena: Anatomical study and review.* Radiology 139:341, 1981.
25. **Resnick D, Niwayama G:** *Osteoporosis.* In: *Diagnosis of Bone and Joint Disorders,* ed 2. Philadelphia, WB Saunders, 1988.
26. **Bentley G, Goodfellow JW:** *Disorganization of the knees following intra-articular hydrocortisone injections.* J Bone Joint Surg 51B:498, 1969.
27. **Miller WT, Restifo RA:** *Steroid arthropathy.* Radiology 86:652, 1966.
28. **Arora JS:** *Indomethacin arthropathy of the hips.* Proc R Soc Med 61:669, 1968.
29. **Tondreau RL, Hodes PJ, Schmidt ER Jr:** *Joint infections following steroid therapy: Roentgen manifestations.* AJR 82:258, 1959.
30. **Sweetman R:** *Corticosteroid arthropathy and tendon rupture.* J Bone Joint Surg 51B:397, 1969.
31. **Salter RB, Murray D:** *Effect of hydrocortisone on musculoskeletal tissue.* J Bone Joint Surg 51B:195, 1977.
32. **Balusubramaniam P, Prathrap K:** *The effect of injection of hydrocortisone into rabbit calcaneal tendons.* J Bone Joint Surg 54B:729, 1972.
33. **Wren RN, Goldner JL, Markee JL:** *An experimental study of the effect of cortisone on the healing process and tensile strength of tendons.* J Bone Joint Surg 36B:588, 1954.
34. **Ismail AM, Balakrishnan MK, Rajakumar MK:** *Rupture of patellar ligament after steroid infiltration.* J Bone Joint Surg 51B:503, 1969.
35. **Halpern AA, Horowitz BG, Nagel DA:** *Tendon ruptures associated with corticosteroid therapy.* West J Med 127:378, 1977.

HEAVY-METAL POISONING

1. **Campbell C, Osterhoudt KC:** *Prevention of childhood lead poisoning.* Curr Opin Pediatr 2(5):428, 2000.
2. **Markowitz M:** *Lead poisoning: A disease for the next millennium.* Curr Probl Pediatr 30(3):62, 2000.
3. **Greengard J:** *Lead poisoning in childhood: Signs, symptoms, current therapy, clinical expression.* Clin Pediatr 5:269, 1966.
4. **Windler EC, Smith RB, Bryan WJ, et al.:** *Lead intoxication and traumatic arthritis of the hip secondary to retained bullet fragments. A case report.* J Bone Joint Surg 60A:254, 1978.
5. **Hsu PC, Guo YL:** *Antioxidant nutrients and lead toxicity.* Toxicology 180(1):33, 2002.
6. **Wigg NR:** *Low-level lead exposure and children.* J Paediatr Child Health 37(5):423, 2001.
7. **Mameli O, Caria MA, Melis F, et al.:** *Neurotoxic effect of lead at low concentrations.* Brain Res Bull 55(2):269, 2001.
8. **Gordon JN, Taylor A, Bennett PN:** *Lead poisoning: Case studies.* Br J Clin Pharmacol 53(5):451, 2002.
9. **Leone AJ Jr:** *On lead lines.* AJR 103:165, 1968.

FLUOROSIS

1. **Resnick D:** *Disorders Due to Medications and Other Chemical Agents.* In: D Resnick, G Niwayama, eds, *Diagnosis of Bone and Joint Disorders,* ed 2. WB Saunders. Philadelphia, 1989.
2. **Wang Y, Yin Y, Gilula LA, et al.:** *Endemic fluorosis of the skeleton: Radiographic features in 127 patients.* AJR 162:93, 1994.

3. **Shortt HE, McRobert GR, Barnard TW, et al.:** *Endemic fluorosis in the madras presidency.* Ind J Med Res 25:553, 1937.
4. **Griffin SO, Beltran ED, Lockwood SA, Barker LK:** *Esthetically objectionable fluorosis attributable to water fluoridation.* Community Dent Oral Epidemiol 30(3):199, 2002.

HISTIOCYTOSIS X
(LANGERHANS' CELL HISTIOCYTOSIS)

1. **Lichenstein L:** *Histiocytosis X.* Arch Pathol 56:84, 1953.
2. **Lieberman PH, Jones CR, Dargeon HWK, et al.:** *A reappraisal of eosinophilic granuloma of bone, Hand-Schüller-Christian syndrome, and Letterer-Siwe syndrome.* Medicine 48:375, 1969.
3. **The Writing Group of the Histiocyte Society:** *Histiocytosis syndromes in children.* Lancet 1:208, 1987.
4. **Chang SE, Koh GJ, Choi JH, et al.:** *Widespread skin-limited adult Langerhans cell histiocytosis: Long-term follow-up with good response to interferon alpha.* Clin Exp Dermatol 27(2):135, 2002.
5. **Muzzi L, Pini Prato GP, Ficarrat G:** *Langerhans' cell histiocytosis diagnosed through periodontal lesions: A case report.* J Periodontol 73(12):1528, 2002.
6. **Becelli R, Carboni A, Gianni C, et al.:** *A rare condition of Hand-Schüller-Christian disease.* J Craniofac Surg 13(6):759, 2002.
7. **Howarth DM, Gilchrist GS, Mullan BP, et al.:** *Langerhans cell histiocytosis: Diagnosis, natural history, management, and outcome.* Cancer 85(10):2278, 1999.
8. **Robert H, Dubousset J, Miladi L:** *Histiocytosis X in the juvenile spine.* Spine 12:167, 1987.

HAND-SCHÜLLER-CHRISTIAN DISEASE

1. **Muzzi L, Pini Prato GP, Ficarrat G:** *Langerhans' cell histiocytosis diagnosed through periodontal lesions: A case report.* J Periodontol 73(12):1528, 2002.

EOSINOPHILIC GRANULOMA

1. **Bayazit Y, Sirikei A, Bayaram M, et al.:** *Eosinophilic granuloma of the temporal bone.* Auris Nasus Larynx 28(1):99, 2001.
2. **David R, Oria RA, Kumar R, et al.:** *Radiologic features of eosinophilic granuloma of bone.* AJR 153:1021, 1989.
3. **Sartoris DJ, Parker BR:** *Histiocytosis X: Rate and pattern of resolution of osseous lesions.* Radiology 152:679, 1984.
4. **Wilner D:** *The Reticuloendothelioses.* In: *Radiology of Bone Tumors and Allied Disorders.* Vol. 2. Philadelphia, WB Saunders, 1982.
5. **McCullough CJ:** *Eosinophilic granuloma of bone.* Acta Orthop Scand 51:389, 1980.
6. **Patil S, Kurdy NM:** *Painless limp as a presentation of pelvic eosinophilic granuloma in a child.* J R Coll Surg Edinb 47(1):418, 2002.
7. **Thijn CJP, Martijn A, Postma A, et al.:** *Histiocytosis X. Eosinophilic granuloma of the fibula. Case report 615.* Skeletal Radiol 19:309, 1990.
8. **Plasschaert F, Craig C, Bell R, et al.:** *Eosinophilic granuloma. A different behaviour in children than in adults.* J Bone Joint Surg 84(B):870, 2002.
9. **Osband ME:** *Histiocytosis X: Langerhans' cell histiocytosis.* Hematol Oncol Clin North Am 1:737, 1987.
10. **Calve J:** *Surune affection particulare de la colonne vertebrale chez l'enfant simulant le mal de Pott. Osteo-chondrite vertebrale infantile.* J Radiol Electrol 9:22, 1925.
11. **Ippolito E, Farsetti P, Tudisco C:** *Vertebra plana. Long-term follow-up in five patients.* J Bone Joint Surg 66A:1364, 1984.
12. **Ochsner SF:** *Eosinophilic granuloma of bone.* AJR 97:719, 1966.
13. **Marioni G, De Filippis C, Stramare R, et al.:** *Langerhans' cell histiocytosis: Temporal bone involvement.* J Laryngol Otol 115(10):839, 2001.

14. **Ardekian L, Peled M, Rosen D, et al.:** *Clinical and radiographic features of eosinophilic granuloma in the jaws: Review of 41 lesions treated by surgery and low-dose radiotherapy.* Oral Surg Oral Med 87(2):238, 1999.
15. **Bertram C, Madert J, Eggers C:** *Eosinophilic granuloma of the cervical spine.* Spine 27(13):1408, 2002.
16. **Geusens E, Brys P, Ghekiere J, et al.:** *Langerhans cell histiocytosis of the cervical spine: Case report of an unusual location.* Eur Radiol 8(7):1142, 1998.
17. **Damry N, Hottat N, Azzi N, et al.:** *Unusual findings in two cases of Langerhans' cell histiocytosis.* Pediatr Radiol 30(3):196, 2000.
18. **Robert H, Dubousset J, Miladi L:** *Histiocytosis X in the juvenile spine.* Spine 12:167, 1987.
19. **Raab P, Hohmann F, Kuhl J, Krauspe R:** *Vertebral remodeling in eosinophilic granuloma of the spine. A long-term follow-up.* Spine 23(12):1351, 1998.
20. **Sherk HH, Nicholson JT, Nixon JE:** *Vertebra plana and eosinophilic granuloma of the cervical spine in children.* Spine 3:116, 1978.
21. **Takahashi M, Martel W, Oberman HA:** *The variable roentgenographic appearance of idiopathic histiocytosis.* Clin Radiol 17:48, 1966.
22. **Green NE, Robertson WW, Kilroy AW:** *Eosinophilic granuloma of the spine with associated neural deficit.* J Bone Joint Surg 62A:1198, 1980.
23. **Poulsen JO, Thommesen P:** *An unusual case of histiocytosis X in the spine.* Acta Orthop Scand 47:59, 1976.

GAUCHER'S DISEASE

1. **Wenstrup RJ, Roca-Espiau M, Weinreb NJ, Bembi B:** *Skeletal aspects of Gaucher disease: A review.* Br J Radiol 75(Suppl 1):A2, 2002.
2. **Patrick DA:** *A deficiency of glucocerebrosidase in Gaucher's disease.* Biochem J 97:17C, 1965.
3. **Hermann G, Wagner LD, Gendal ES, et al.:** *Spinal cord compression in type 1 Gaucher disease.* Radiology 170:147, 1989.
4. **Reich C, Siefe M, Kessler BJ:** *Gaucher's disease: Review and discussion of 20 cases.* Medicine 30:1, 1951.
5. **Tabas JH, Daffner RH, Hartsock RJ, et al.:** *Gaucher disease affecting the skeleton (left femur). Case report 387.* Skeletal Radiol 15:499, 1986.
6. **Rosenbaum H, Sidransky E:** *Cholelithiasis in patients with Gaucher disease.* Blood Cells Mol Dis 28(1):21, 2002.
7. **Kelman CG, Disler DG:** *Metaphyseal undertubulation in gaucher disease: resolution at MRI in a patient undergoing enzyme replacement therapy.* J Comput Tomogr 24(1):173, 2000.
8. **Cabrera-Salazar MA, Novelli E, Barranger JA:** *Gene therapy for the lysosomal storage disorders.* Curr Opin Mol Ther 4(4):349, 2002.
9. **Hermann G, Goldblatt J, Levy RN, et al.:** *Gaucher's disease type 1: Assessment of bone involvement by CT and scintigraphy.* AJR 147:943, 1986.
10. **Levin B:** *Gaucher's disease: Clinical and roentgenologic manifestations.* AJR 85:686, 1961.
11. **Schein AJ, Arkin AM:** *The classic: Hip joint involvement in Gaucher's disease.* Clin Orthop 90:4, 1973.
12. **Hermann G, Shapiro R, Abelwahab IF, et al.:** *Extraosseous extension of Gaucher cell deposits mimicking malignancy.* Skeletal Radiol 23:253, 1994.
13. **Springfield DS, Landfried M, Mankin HJ:** *Gaucher hemorrhagic cyst of bone. A case report.* J Bone Joint Surg 71A:141, 1989.
14. **Schwartz AM, Homer MJ, McCauley RGK:** *"Step off" vertebral body: Gaucher's disease versus sickle cell hemoglobinopathy.* AJR 132:81, 1979.
15. **Hermann G, Goldblatt J, Desnick RJ:** *Kummel disease: Delayed collapse of the traumatized spine in the patient with Gaucher type 1 disease.* Br J Radiol 57:833, 1986.

Report Writing and Risk Management Strategies in Skeletal Radiology

15

Lindsay J. Rowe, Terry R. Yochum, and Chad J. Maola

X rays are like figures in that they are always correct, [but] we may make a mistake in adding up the column of figures and arrive at the wrong answer.
—John Nesbit Scott, 1902

GENERAL CONSIDERATIONS

The formulation of reports in clinical practice is a standard method of documenting a patient's history, examination findings, therapeutic regime, and prognosis. (1) In the practice of skeletal radiology, report writing serves a number of important roles, including (*a*) providing an accurate means of recording findings for use during comparison with previous or later examinations, (*b*) serving as documentation in medicolegal circumstances, (*c*) providing a permanent record in case the radiographs are lost or not immediately available for perusal, (*d*) offering a means of communication with other practitioners and health professionals, (*e*) expediting the management regime by providing a summary of important indications and contraindications for therapy, (*f*) assisting in auditing radiographic quality, and (*g*) providing a database for retrospective research and data collection. (1–8) Up until the first edition of this text in 1987, there was a distinct lack of material on report writing and little on what would be considered a standard style. (4,9–11) Similarly, the art of verbally presenting studies has received little coverage in the literature. (12) Over the past few years there has been increasing scrutiny and numerous publications dealing with aspects of report generation. This increased interest is predominantly aimed at medicolegal risk reduction, which has refocused attention on the whole reporting process. But still the reporting of skeletal studies remains essentially a subjective, personalized procedure, with individuals modifying the report according to their previous training, experience, and needs. The purposes of this chapter are to provide guidelines for the formulation of musculoskeletal imaging reports, review the medicolegal implications of such reports, and summarize risk management strategies.

ENVIRONS AND EQUIPMENT

Reporting Environment

An appropriate environment for performing the interpretation and subsequent reporting is essential. The evaluation of radiographs in circumstances of disruption, noise, or other distractive elements is more likely to result in misinterpretations and in-accurate, incoherent reports. Preferably, the room in which the report is dictated should be isolated from the clinical setting and in an area where the least amount of disturbance will occur, making it conducive to focused concentration. In addition, the room should have the capability for adequately decreasing external light sources.

Equipment

The standard practice uses view boxes, a *hot* (bright) *light,* transcription devices, and computer or file cabinets for report storage. However, with increasing availability of digital radiography and digital **p**ersonalized **a**rchiving **c**ommunication **s**ystems (**PACS**), high-resolution computer screens and large-capacity processing units are now being employed to view and store the images and reports, eliminating the need for film.

Viewing Boxes

The viewing space should be large enough to hold two 43- by 35-cm (14- by 17-inch) radiographs side by side (two-bank view box) and produce a bright, uniform light. Four viewing areas (four-bank view box) of the same dimensions are preferable and should be placed at a height at which interpretation can be done from a seated position.

Hot Light

An indispensable viewing accessory is a single, 100-W bulb (hot light) with a foot pedal–operated rheostat control and a 16-cm opening for illumination. This is used to highlight all overexposed regions of a film and to aid in the delineation of normal anatomic or lesion details. Films observed in this manner must be removed from the light within 5–8 sec; otherwise, the extreme heat generated by the bulb may permanently deform the film.

Reporting and Transcription

There are various methods by which radiographic findings are compiled and transcribed into the typewritten word. Handwritten reporting may be convenient when the volume is low and the reports are short. Checklist (*canned*) methods can be employed when repetitive reporting is involved. (1,2) The most frequently used methods involve verbal dictation with or without voice-recognition technology. The system that is adopted depends on the number and complexity of reports, the necessary capital outlay, and the individual.

Storage

Storage of reports and images is an important legal aspect of any practice. In smaller-volume practices, file cabinets can be used to store hard copies of all information. With computerized transcription techniques, hard copies of reports are often stored in file cabinets in conjunction with electronic file (computer) backups. The computer offers the benefit of being a powerful tool for research, audits, and patient care when the clinician uses special-purpose information and evaluation packages. In high-volume settings using digital technology, PACS will allow for the rapid retrieval and visualization of any previously stored images for reports. (3,4) Modern desktop-publishing techniques make it possible to incorporate selected and annotated images as part of the report. (5)

Digital Radiography

Digital radiography has evolved greatly over the last several years, providing several methods of acquiring images digitally. The use of digital imaging has many advantages in the field of radiography and in clinical practice. For the clinician using digital radiography, this process eliminates the need for dark rooms, processor cleaning, chemicals and their disposal, x-ray film, view boxes, storage of films, repeat x-rays (thus reducing the dosage to patients), and postage to have the films mailed for interpretation. Digital images are traditionally observed on a computer monitor and can be transmitted via the Internet for immediate interpretation by a radiologist. Along with the obvious advantages, the declining cost of digital radiography is making the use of this technology a feasible and practical procedure that will soon become the standard in radiology and private clinical practices. Generally, digital techniques fall into one of two categories: *direct* and *computed* radiography. Both methods offer almost immediate access to image data and are easily integrated into existing workflow systems, such as PACS.

Direct Radiography. Direct radiography (DR) generally refers to capturing an image by exposing radiation directly to a thin silicon or amorphous selenium plate made of individual sensing areas. Images are created by first converting the energy to light through a thin cesium iodide coating (the sensor), made of thousands of pixels. It then captures the light and converts the energy into a high-resolution image. Another method of DR creates images by first converting the radiation to light and then capturing the light with a very sensitive charge-coupled device (CCD). Technologically, DR is the method of choice in radiography owing to its low dose, high speed, and superior resolution. Initially, DR may seem to be a costly method of imaging, but when compared with the film-based high-frequency x-ray systems currently used, the long-term cost effectiveness of DR is substantially greater. (Table 15-1).

Computed Radiography. Computed radiography (CR) is the digital technique most comparable to the traditional film-based procedure. The process exposes a cassette loaded with a CR screen to radiation, which must then be placed into a reader, where it is scanned by laser and transferred into a digital image. Scan times vary but usually take between 15 and 90 sec each. CR is generally referred to as an *interim technology* because of the way it is handled and the time it takes to scan and then erase each image from the screen. CR plates also have a shelf life and need to be replaced periodically. This method produces quality images, but in most cases they are not as good as direct methods. CR has become popular owing to its cost and ease of integration with existing film-based systems.

Table 15-1	Fifteen-Year Cost Analysis: Film-Based X-Ray Versus Direct Radiography						
Film-Based, High-Frequency (100-KHz) X-Ray				**Direct Radiography**			
Purchase		**Five-Year Lease**		**Purchase**		**Five-Year Lease**	
Price	$24,900	Price	$32,370	Price	$49,900	Price	$64,870
60 films/wk/15 years @ $1.10 each	51,480	60 films/wk/15 years @ $1.10 each	51,480			Computer upgrades	5,000
Technician @ $13.00/hr, 3 min/film; developing @ $0.65 each	30,420	Technician @ $13.00/hr, 3 min/film; developing @ $0.65 each	30,420				
100 monthly processor cleanings @ $180.00 each	18,000	100 monthly processor cleanings @ $180.00 each	18,000				
6 processor repairs	6,000	6 processor repairs	6,000				
1 replaced processor	3,600	1 replaced processor	3,600				
Total	$130,400	Total	$137,870	Total	$49,000	Total	$69,870

PLAIN FILM PLACEMENT AND ORIENTATION FOR INTERPRETATION

The placement of radiographs on the viewing area should be done in a standardized procedure. By following a systematic routine in placement and orientation, abnormalities will be more readily identified. (1–4) This is the first step in the interpretation and reporting sequence. (Fig. 15-1)

Spine

Wherever possible all available films of the same spinal region should be viewed simultaneously, with anteroposterior (AP) and lateral side by side, followed by obliques, and then functional studies (flexion–extension).
AP. There is a divergence of opinion as to how AP spinal films should be oriented on the view box. The orthodox method is to place the films as if the patient were being observed from the front, so that the patient's right lies on the observer's left. Other practitioners, especially those involved primarily in the therapy and examination of spine-related complaints, find that films placed as if the patient were being observed from the back are much more practical, so that the patient's right is on the observer's right.
Lateral. Lateral films are best placed as the patient was positioned when the film was taken. A left lateral view should have the apex of a cervical or lumbar lordosis oriented toward the observer's right side. A left marker means that the film was taken with the left side of the patient against the cassette.
Obliques. Preferably, all oblique studies should be placed side to side, for better comparison. It is optimal to place the oblique that shows right-sided structures on the left; therefore, in the cervical spine the right anterior oblique or left posterior oblique should be placed on the left of the interpreter. In the lumbar spine the right posterior and left anterior oblique should be placed on the right side.
Dynamic Views. Placement of dynamic views should be orientated the same as the neutral projection and on the appropriate sides to show the extremes of movement. For example, a left lateral study of the cervical spine should have a flexion view placed to the right and the extension to the left of the neutral view.

Extremities

Preferably all films of the extremities should be viewed simultaneously and generally placed as if viewing the patient from the front. The only exceptions are the hands, wrists, feet, and ankles, which are placed as if looking at the dorsal surface. In addition, films of the hand, wrist, and feet are placed with the digits pointing upward.

Chest

The frontal chest projection should be placed to the left of the lateral study and both films should be viewed simultaneously.
Posteroanterior. Posteroanterior (PA) views are always placed on the view box as if observing the patient from the front. This places the heart to the right of the observer.
Lateral. As with lateral spinal films, lateral chest films are oriented based on patient positioning. The routine procedure in positioning the patient is for a left lateral projection, so that the apex of the thoracic kyphosis would be toward the viewer's left side during interpretation.

Abdomen

Placement of AP abdominal films is as if the patient were being observed from the front; thus, the liver is to the left side of the observer.

Additional Collimated (Spot) Views

For comparison purposes, spot views should be placed alongside the larger film that first delineated the questionable area. Whenever possible, these should be visible simultaneously for proper evaluation.

Comparison Studies

When comparison studies of the same area are available, it is preferable to observe the current films first and isolate any films

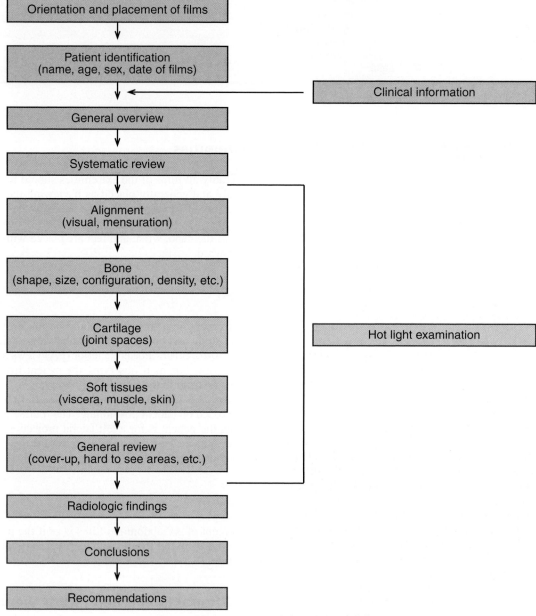

Figure 15-1 **REPORTING FLOW CHART.**

containing areas of abnormality. Subsequently, a sequential retrospective evaluation based on the dates of the films is done, from the more recent to the oldest studies. In these circumstances it may be preferable to make handwritten notes, correlating the dates with the observed changes, before composing the report.

REPORT STRUCTURE AND CONTENT

The structure of the report is an especially personalized procedure; however, there are some basic features that should be included. (1,2) (Table 15-2) Interpretation of the radiographs requires extensive skill and the use of appropriate terminology. The development of an interpretation methodology (*search pattern*) is recommended, so as not to overlook pertinent findings. With repetition the process becomes more rapid and the clinician becomes increasingly more accurate in identifying abnormalities.

Preliminary Information

Stationery. Information in the letterhead should include the name and address of the clinic or individual who is creating the report.
Report Date. The date the report is made should be near the top of the page.

Table 15-2	Essentials of Plain-Film Musculoskeletal Reporting

Preliminary information
  Letterhead information
  Date of report formulation
  Name and address of referring clinician
  Patient information
    Full name
    Address
    Date of birth
    Sex
    File identification
  Examinations performed
    Views submitted
    Dates and location of films taken
  Clinical information
    Chief complaint
    Key clinical findings
    Reason for study
    Numbered summary of pertinent clinical findings, if complex
Report
  Technical factors (kilovoltage, milliamperes, tube–film distance, etc.)—optional
  Radiologic findings
    Descriptive narrative of findings (ABCs)
  Conclusions
    Succinct summary of diagnoses
  Recommendations
    Additional imaging and/or management
    Indications and contraindications to treatment
    Follow-up procedures indicated
  Signature and qualifications

Referring Clinician's Information. If the report is for another clinician, his or her name and address should be placed near the top of the report.
Patient Demographics. The patient's full name, address, date of birth, sex, and file number should be given.
Examination Information. All views that are being submitted for evaluation should be listed, view-by-view, for each anatomic location. Additional information that must be listed here is the location and dates the films were taken. If there is inadequate or unreadable identification, this also should be stated.
Clinical History. Selected important aspects of the presenting complaint, past history, physical examination, laboratory results, and findings from previous examinations should be listed. (3) These details aid the examiner in interpretation because they direct attention to an area for more careful scrutiny and observation and assist in excluding uninvolved structures. (4) Failure to integrate an adequate clinical history and findings diminishes diagnostic accuracy. (5,6) When possible, any abnormality should be related back to the patient's clinical symptoms.

The Report

The report itself is divided into three distinct sections: radiologic findings, conclusions, and recommendations. An optional section may be used to convey technological information.

Technical Information

Inclusion of technical information in the report is optional. Data concerning peak kilovoltage (kVp), milliamperes (mAs), tube–film distance, bucky versus non-bucky, screen type, and gonadal-shielding application can be useful, especially if one considers a later re-evaluation. This part of the report can also be used to calculate the skin radiation dose to the patient. All this information should be kept in an accessible location, even if not part of the final report.

Radiologic Findings

Before beginning to interpret radiographs, it is useful to allow approximately 5 min for light adaptation to occur. Also, while evaluating films, unused view box space is turned off, to reduce unnecessary glare or eyestrain and to improve the ability to detect subtle lesions. (7) It is in this section of the report that the descriptive narration containing the report of findings is made.

Chapter 7 provides guidelines for appropriate terminology for describing various abnormalities. Correct use of terms and an ordered sequence of reporting are essential for accuracy and clarity. (1,8–12) (Table 15-3) This is achieved by means of a systematic method of observation along with the possession of the necessary background in normal radiographic anatomy and signs of disease. (13–15) Most pathologies that are overlooked are missed because of lack of attention to a step-by-step sequential evaluation of normal anatomy and correlation with the pertinent clinical data. (9,16–18) (Fig. 15-1)
General Overview. Make an initial overview of the studies, looking for anything obvious that catches the eye and correlating it on other views. Following this initial inspection for each film, read the identification nameplate, confirming the patient's name

Table 15-3	Summary of Key Terms for Reporting Musculoskeletal Disease

Biomechanical
  Fixation, hypomobility, hypermobility
  Instability
  Misalignment
Congenital
  Hypoplasia, hyperplasia, dysplasia
  Underdeveloped, overdeveloped, maldevelopment
  Agenesis
Trauma
  Fracture: transverse, oblique, spiral, avulsion, pathologic
  Comminution
  Apposition, angulation, displacement, intra-articular
  Subluxation, dislocation
  Non-union, malunion
  Callus
Neoplastic
  Bone destruction: geographic, moth-eaten, permeative
  Position: centric, eccentric
  Periostitis: solid, laminated, spiculated
  Zone of transition: wide, narrow
  Cortical integrity: intact, disrupted, expanded
  Matrix: fibrous, cartilage, osteoid, bone
  Soft tissue mass
  Location: diaphysis, metaphysis, epiphysis
  Distribution: monostotic, polyostotic
Arthritides
  Joint space loss: uniform, non-uniform, ankylosis,
    chondrocalcinosis
  Subchondral bone changes: sclerosis, cysts, osteopenia
  Joint erosions: extra-articular, marginal
  Bony outgrowths: osteophytes, syndesmophytes, hyperostosis
  Periostitis: linear, irregular
  Enthesopathy: erosions, periostitis
  Soft tissue depositions: extra-articular, intra-articular
  Malalignments: subluxations, deformities
Nutritional, metabolic, endocrine
  Osteopenia: osteoporosis, osteomalacia
  Cortical changes: thinning, thickening, erosion
  Trabecular changes: loss, accentuation, thickening
  Soft tissue calcification
Infection
  Bone destruction: geographic, moth-eaten, sequestrum
  Periostitis: solid, laminated (involucrum), Codman's triangle
  Cortex: thickening, destruction (cloaca)
  Articular cortex: preservation, destruction
  Soft tissue planes: displaced, blurred, obliterated

and other demographics. Then identify what projection each film represents. At this stage it is vital to assess each film for technical quality, including exposure, collimation, positioning, motion, phase of respiration, applied markers (erect, supine, right–left, etc.), and artifacts.

Systematic Review. The sequence by which the structures are evaluated depends on what best suits the individual and will frequently vary according to findings. However, adopting a standardized procedure will assist in performing a thorough review of the study. Furthermore, when verbalizing findings over the telephone or presenting a case to other clinicians, such guidelines will provide a more organized discussion of the findings. We have proposed, since the first edition of this text in 1987, the mnemonic **ABCs** as a guide to an ordered, sequential evaluation, which

many have found useful. **ABCs** stands for **a**lignment, **b**one, **c**artilage, and **s**oft tissue. It is important that a flexible use of this approach be adopted, which may be modified depending on a particular case. When a site of abnormality is identified, it should be described completely, which again can be done with the **ABCs** approach. Once this is completed, then the search can be continued to other areas.

Alignment. The first aspect reviewed is the alignment of the skeletal structures. Application of the various mensuration procedures will assist in this part of the evaluation.

In the spine, aspects of spinal curvature, rotation, and other interosseous disrelationships are noted. This part of the examination applies both to static and functional stress studies. Lordotic and kyphotic contours should be assessed in regard to the amount, type, and configuration of the curvature. Using measurement parameters and normal ranges, the investigator can designate the curvatures as hyper, hypo, or normal. (See Chapter 2.) Underlying causes for an altered curve should also be identified.

Scolioses need to be carefully evaluated. (See Chapter 4.) The type of curve should be described (e.g., C, S shape, compensated, uncompensated). The degree of curvature must be measured (*Cobb's method*). The side to which the convexity occurs, the identification of the apical segment, and the degree of rotation within the curve should also be noted. A search for an underlying cause must always be made.

Intersegmental spinal misalignments are common and need to be reported judiciously and in a clinical context. Terminology for vertebral misalignments has been standardized. (19) Designation of the spatial orientation of one vertebra in relation to adjacent segments is called *a listing*. This would include flexion, extension, lateral flexion, rotation, anterolisthesis, retrolisthesis, and laterolisthesis. Spondylolisthesis should be assessed by *Meyerding's classification* as to the grade of slippage or a percentage of slippage. (20) (See Chapter 5.)

In the extremities, relationships of bony components across joints or at fracture sites are integral parts of all radiographic reports. The hand afflicted with rheumatoid arthritis may show a number of misalignments, including ulnar deviation, boutonniere deformities, and zigzag deformities. A full description of a fracture includes a statement about the location, direction, and nature of the fracture line as well as aspects of alignment such as apposition, angulation, and rotation. (21,22) At the hip joint, alignment can be made visually by the continuity of Shenton's and iliofemoral lines. (See Chapter 2.)

Bone. Next, details of the visualized osseous structures are observed. This includes scrutiny of the cortices; medullary trabecular patterns; general density; and the size, shape, and configuration of all bones. In the spine, the key bony landmarks are the vertebral body endplates; vertebral body trabeculae; pedicles; and transverse, spinous, and articular processes. If no osseous abnormality is found, then an appropriate sentence stating this negative finding can be made. For example, if the clinical concern was the presence of fracture that has not been confirmed, then a statement such as "no fracture or dislocation is evident" may suffice. Similarly, the absence of suspected neoplasia could be denoted as "no osseous neoplastic change is radiographically apparent." A generic statement relating that no bony abnormality is present could be "no osseous abnormality has been demonstrated."

Cartilage. Normally, cartilage is not visible on radiographs but instead is manifested by the radiographic joint space. This **C** part of the mnemonic is to remind the observer to look carefully at all joints displayed. In the spine, the joints include the intervertebral disc spaces and the apophyseal, atlantoaxial, neurocentral, and costovertebral articulations. The peripheral joints are readily recognized. Each joint can be assessed for the depth of the joint space, the smooth articular bony cortex, and the bone density beneath the cortex (subchondral bone). The width of the joint cavity reflects the cartilage thickness, with only the small loose joints of the toes or fingers widening owing to effusion. Narrowing of the joint space reflects loss of the articular cartilage and is a sign of arthritis. The articular cortex is thin but is usually clear and sharp in its outline and smooth in contour. Loss of the joint cortex is a key sign of articular disease and may be the result of synovial proliferation, infection, or degenerative synovial cyst (geode). Thickening of the joint cortex can be seen with degenerative joint disease. When reporting about a joint, comments on these features should be made; for a normal joint a relevant statement would be "the joint space is preserved, the articular surfaces are smooth and congruent and of normal density" or "there is no joint abnormality."

Soft Tissue. Although soft tissues may provide many important signs of disease, it is the most commonly overlooked feature on a musculoskeletal radiograph, CT scan, and even MRI study. The visibility of a soft tissue structure predominantly depends on its density, tissue type, and often the presence of encapsulating fat. Skin line displacement can be helpful in identifying a mass or edema. In the extremities, the interspaced fat in the fascial planes can identify the individual muscle bellies; on plain films, the best examples are the pronator quadratus on the lateral wrist view and the supinator fat line on a lateral elbow projection. In the spine, the psoas muscle outline is a key structure, as is the prevertebral soft tissue in the neck. Displaced pericapsular fat in the elbow can be a sign of joint effusion. Additional signs to be searched for include loss of the fascial plane fat, a sign of edema, and displacement of the same fat lines, a sign of adjacent mass and calcification. Perusal of all soft tissues included on the film should be performed. The presence of calcium in abnormalities such as gallbladder and renal calculi, aneurysms of the aorta, and cysts can be diagnostic.

Supplementary Review. On completion of the sequential **ABCs,** a supplemental review must be performed. A number of methods have been proposed by various individuals in an attempt to minimize the possibility of overlooking subtle abnormalities.

- *Review of hard-to-see areas.* On any radiograph there are always details that are usually obscured and difficult to visualize because of anatomic superimposition or because of the projection. Therefore, if an abnormality is present in one of these obscured areas, it is likely to be overlooked without careful scrutiny. (23) This includes those portions of the film that are inherently overexposed or covered by another anatomic structure, such as the view box holding clip, positioning markers, identification plate, and any other obscuring artifact. (Table 15-4)
- *Hot (bright) light examination.* No interpretation is complete without each radiograph being illuminated by the hot light. Examination by this method is especially useful in overexposed areas that are not normally rendered visible on the ordinary view box. In addition, by limiting the field of view, closer inspection of individual details is enhanced. (7,24)
- *Cover-up examination.* This is a useful technique for larger-size radiographs, but it can also be applied to any film. The basic idea is to limit the field of view to a small

Table 15-4	Hard-to-See Review Areas
Cervical spine	Tibial tuberosity
Skull base	Hoffa's fat-pad
Odontoid process	Ankle
Neurocentral joints	Malleoli (3)
Cervicothoracic junction	Talar dome
Prevertebral soft tissues	Anterior process of calcaneus
Trachea	Cuneiforms, cuboid
Lung apices	Subtalar joint
Thoracic spine	Foot
Pedicles	Phalanges
Posterior ribs	Metatarsal heads
Paravertebral lines	Hallux sesamoids
Posterior lung fields	Shoulder
Diaphragms	Lung apex
Posterior costophrenic sulcus	Greater tuberosity
Costotransverse joints	Coracoid and acromion
Lumbar spine	process
Apophyseal joints	Elbow
Pedicles	Fat-pad positions
Pars interarticularis	Radial tuberosity
Lung bases	Olecranon, coronoid fossae
Lower ribs and costal joints	Supinator fat line
Gas patterns	Wrist
Psoas	Scaphoid waist
Pelvis and hips	Scapholunate interspace
Acetabular floor	Hook of the hamate
Iliac crest	Ulnar variance
Sacral foramina	Triangular fibrocartilage
Sacroiliac joints	Metacarpotrapezial joint
Femoral head and neck	Hand
Knee	Distal phalanx
Patellofemoral joint	Metacarpal heads
Intercondylar notch	Metacarpocarpal
Tibial eminences	joints (4–5)

area, inspect it, and move to another portion of the radiograph. The larger the surface area available to be inspected, the more anatomic details that must be examined. A simple way to reduce the observable area is to take a 45- by 37-cm (14- by 17-inch) film envelope, cover the entire film up, and slowly move the envelope down while observing the limited view of the film. In addition to limiting the field, the interpreter's eyes are forced to compare one side with the other, carefully noting individual details. The combination of reduced visual field and augmented visual acuity makes this a useful review method.

- *Other examinations.* Many other methods have been proposed by individuals to enhance visual perception, most of which were "discovered" by personal experience. These methods range from scientific attempts to enhance eye physiology to simple cheating (discussed below). (18)

Fingerprints. One of the simplest "cheating" methods is *Hartley's (25) fingerprint method.* This requires pulling the film off the view box, tilting the radiograph at such an angle that the film surface shines, and looking for fingerprints. The presence of fingerprints in a particular area may disclose an abnormality as a result of the film being previously viewed and the observer's finger pointing out a subtle pathology. Obviously, films do not come out of the processor with accurately placed fingerprints!

Film Tilt. Tilting the film can sometimes be useful because it reduces the field of vision. This is particularly applicable to evaluation of the spinal pedicles, a common site for aggressive neoplastic disease. By slightly tilting a lumbar or thoracic film away from the observer, visual inspection of the pedicle cortices is enhanced, allowing easier comparison with adjacent segments. Almost any structure can be evaluated by this *tilt method*. Also, for traditional films that use two-sided emulsion film, tilt will enhance the parallax differences of each side and may enhance anatomy and any pathologic change.

Magnification. Some have advocated the use of different magnifying devices, most commonly the simple, hand-held lens. This obviously has its greatest advantage when observing fine, individual details, but not during the overall evaluation. Once a questionable area has been isolated, the use of a magnifying glass can help further delineate the characteristics of a possible pathology. Digitized images are readily enlarged by means of computer technology.

Odontoid Identification. One of the more difficult structures to identify is the odontoid process, yet it is a common area of abnormality. A useful method to aid in the scrutiny of this structure is to place a fingertip over the area as closely as possible to where it would be expected to be located. (26) Identification of the atlas anterior tubercle will aid in the correct placement of the finger. Once in place, careful observation of the finger outline is performed and the finger is subsequently removed from the film. Continued attention to the region will often allow the outline of the odontoid to be identified because the size and shape of the finger is quite similar.

Cupped Hand. For increased visual acuity, especially in group circumstances, observing through a cupped hand will additionally reduce unnecessary glare. (27) This *cupped hand method* also enables those who are myopic to enhance their visual range and acuity.

Summarization of Findings. Before developing statements for the conclusion, it is important to summarize and synthesize the findings relevant for formulating diagnoses and relative priorities.

Conclusions

Many radiologists use the term *impression* to label the conclusion section of the report; however, the word *conclusion* is currently the preferred term because it commits the author to succinctly summarize with deductive reasoning the meaning of the described findings and to convey to the clinician their importance. (4) Remember that < 40% of reports are read in full by the treating clinician, with the majority of clinicians focusing only on the conclusion—this stresses the importance of the conclusion section. (28) A point-by-point summary of diagnoses is the desired format. The purpose is to list the most important radiologic findings and diagnoses based on the previous narrative descriptions. These should be short, concise statements using standard and precise terminology. (1,29) Listing of a few selected differential considerations can be useful, but there should be avoidance of long lists.

Recommendations

A short statement or number of statements can be made following the conclusions for the purpose of directing attention to a particularly significant finding or diagnosis. This is an optional component of the report and can be employed at the discretion of the author. This part of the report may address therapeutic implications, contraindications to specific therapies, or suggestions for further evaluation as deemed appropriate. At the end of the report, authors should ascribe their names and qualifications and then add their signature nearby.

REPORT VARIATIONS FOR CT AND MRI

Owing to the inherently more complex modes of image acquisition, a greater number of technical variables and the greater amount of available diagnostic information, CT and MRI reports have to be tailored differently. (1,2)

Computed Tomography

Identification of Images and Information

Significant variations in the format of image display are common, depending on the CT unit and the facility. Despite this, the relevant information provided remains essentially the same. It is recommended to locate the following images and information, before orienting and interpreting the films.

Information Block. Locate the film that is displaying the information on the patient and examination technique. This usually is identifiable as the section that has no anatomic images and instead lists the patient's name, age, clinically relevant data, referring doctor, suspected clinical diagnosis, and examination parameters (e.g., the number of scans and if contrast was used).

Scout Images. A digitally processed frontal or lateral view of the body part being imaged is next identified. On the scout image, lines may or may not be visible representing the site where images were programmed to be obtained. When present, this information is known as the *scan selection technique*. From this, one may then derive the end points of the examination, the number of images taken, the distance intervals between images, gantry (tube) angulation, and areas of interest. Each slice is usually numbered but often not readily decipherable.

Soft Tissue and Bone Windows. Images are usually displayed in two modes, which accentuate particular tissues: a *soft tissue window* and a *bone window*. Most frequently, all soft tissue windows are grouped sequentially on one film, which can be recognized by prominent soft tissue detail and lack of internal bone characteristics. Bone windows are similarly shown on one film, readily identifiable by the visibility of fine bone detail, including trabeculae. It is important to remember these are photographic computations involving only one exposure from which the computer generates two or more images.

Reconstructions. Reconstructions can be obtained in soft tissue or bone windows. Planes of reconstruction are multiple—multiplanar imaging or *multiplanar reconstructions* (MPRs)—but most often are made available in sagittal, coronal, or oblique positions and occasionally three-dimensional images. There is always loss of structural detail on these studies, though with multislice studies, this may be minimal.

Placement and Orientation for Interpretation

Placing films in order can be quite confusing at times and requires a degree of intuitive recognition. Three methods can be employed to assist in hanging the studies in correct order.

- *Film sheets are marked.* Scrutinize each sheet to see if a stick-on number has been applied denoting the sequence of the images.
- *Identify the first and last scans.* By finding where the scan begins and ends, these sheets can be placed first and last with the additional sheets placed between. Usually the information block and scout images are placed immediately before the first image or, less commonly, after the last image, which may assist in locating these scans. If the slice protocols are present and decipherable, the anatomic location of the remaining individual images can be identified by comparison of the numeric markings on the image with those visible on the scout. In addition, a millimetric measurement will be displayed that, when compared with adjacent images, allows deduction of the slice interval employed in the examination.
- *Locate the individual scan number.* This is the definitive way to ensure that the sheets are placed and viewed in correct sequence. There are many numbers on each individual image, which can make it difficult to find the scan number, but it is usually located in the upper left corner, the number changing by one on each successive image.

Preliminary Information

Essentially, the preliminary information of the report remains the same as that used during report writing of plain film radiographs, with one exception: In addition to the current findings listed under clinical information, pertinent positive and negative previous imaging findings (with dates) should be listed, outlining the focus for the CT scan being obtained. Any known reactions to contrast agents should also be described here, giving it the prominence it deserves.

The Report

CT reporting has particular requirements for outlining the imaging protocols used, terminology, and descriptive elements.

Technique Description. Before beginning the narrative of findings it is important to outline details of how the CT study was performed. This could include the anatomic endpoints of the examination, method of image acquisition (*contiguous, selected*), the plane of imaging, reconstructions available, gantry position, windows displayed, and the use of a contrast agent. For example, in a CT scan of the lumbar spine the following introductory statements could be made: "A non-contrast CT study has been performed from L3 to S1, with selected axial images parallel to the intervertebral disc spaces at 3-mm slice thickness at 3-mm intervals. Sagittal reconstructions with bone and soft tissue windows have been obtained."

Terminology. A few terms should be understood and used when appropriate for descriptions. Normal and abnormal tissue densities are described in terms of *attenuation: low attenuation* is when the tissue is of relative lower density, whereas *high attenuation* is when it is a higher density. The density of the visualized tissues can be found in a small square on individual scans displayed in the corner. This is called a *region of interest cursor.* Within the box, the densities are measured and ascribed a number value known as a *Hounsfield unit.* This number is then compared by the computer with a known standard, and a tissue density is derived. A linear

cursor can also be used to measure distances between structures of interest.

Descriptive Narrative of Findings. In all cases, it is imperative to describe the correct anatomic location of abnormalities for clarity of meaning and correlation of the clinical significance of the finding. All CT images are displayed as if the interpreter were viewing the patient axially from the feet toward the head, so that the patient's right is on the interpreter's left. It should be remembered that the scout image should also be analyzed in the same manner as any conventional radiograph for diagnostic information. Many diagnoses can be rendered on this image alone. Evaluation of reconstructions should be done only after the axial images are carefully scrutinized. If an abnormality is found, it is important to state the window and the number of the images on which it occurs. If intravenous or intra-articular contrast has been used, it is important to state its effects on abnormalities.

Magnetic Resonance Imaging

Identification of Images and Information

MRI studies are often complex and contain many individual images. Their display format on film varies according to the facility and magnetic resonance manufacturer. However, much like CT, the relevant information provided remains essentially the same. It is recommended to locate the following images and information, before the orientation and interpretation of the films.

Information Block. Locate the film that is displaying the information on the patient and the examination technique. This can be a separate partition on one page, as in CT, or, frequently, is reproduced onto each page. It contains the patient's name, age, clinically relevant data, referring doctor, suspected clinical diagnosis, examination parameters, and if contrast was used.

Scout (Encoding) Images. Scout images often are not displayed on printed studies but are usually available when studies are interpreted from a computer workstation. They are typically poor-quality images but, if available, should be perused because they frequently include areas outside of the final selected imaging field and occasionally may display unsuspected pathology.

Scan Selection Technique. The scan selection technique is usually the first image on each sheet, which displays the imaging sections obtained. On this image, lines are visible representing the site where images were programmed to be selected. From this one can derive the end points of the examination, the number of scans, the distance intervals between images, field angulation, and areas of interest.

Pulse Sequence Identification. Identifying the pulse sequences can be time-consuming, confusing, and frustrating because each manufacturer and facility uses different terminology and pulse parameters. (See Chapter 6.) The two methods for identification are *visual impression* and *interpreting the printed pulse parameters.* General guidelines for spin-echo imaging can be summarized as follows.

- *T1-weighted images.* Fat is depicted as bright signal, water as an intermediate signal, and cortical bone as low signal. The repetition time (TR) is short (500 msec) as is the echo time (TE) (15 msec) (*short TR–short TE*).
- *T2-weighted images.* Any free water, such as cerebrospinal fluid, joint fluid, and edema, is of high signal.

The TR is long (2500–4000 msec) as is the TE (90 msec).

- *Postgadolinium studies.* These are typically T1-weighted with fat saturation employed to remove the otherwise bright signal of fat that may impair the recognition of a bright signal from contrast enhancement. Look for a +*C* in the corner of each image.
- *Fat saturation.* The subcutaneous and marrow fat is intermediate in signal (gray).

Placement and Orientation for Interpretation

There is no definite order in which the studies need to be interpreted and is an individual choice. The difficulty with MRI is that the number of sequences obtained is often in three or more planes, which results in multiple printed pages of hard-copy film. Standard protocols for spine imaging are displayed in sagittal and axial planes. Extremity studies are usually acquired in a minimum of sagittal, axial, and coronal planes. As a suggestion, find the sequences in the plane that shows the longest sections of the body area first. In the spine, this is usually the sagittal plane, whereas in the extremities it is the coronal plane. Place these same-plane scans alongside each other and then hang the remaining sequences, again grouped by plane. Any postcontrast studies should be placed alongside the same-plane precontrast images.

Initially, it is best to start visual inspection of the study at an image about halfway through the body region because this gives you a reference point where familiar anatomy is displayed. In the spine, for example, this would correspond with the midsagittal image, on which the spinous processes are visible. If the anatomy is not readily recognizable, each individual image is usually marked with a number that can also be identified on the scout images to verify the slice location.

Preliminary Information

As with CT, the preliminary information section of the report remains relatively unchanged from that of plain film imaging, with the exception of clinical information. Here, previous imaging findings and the reason why MRI is being undertaken should be stated. Some institutions will state at this time that the patient consented to the procedure after careful exclusion of contraindications (e.g., cardiac pacemaker).

The Report

MRI, like CT, has specific requirements for describing the imaging protocols used, terminology, and descriptive elements.

Technique Description. The same details as for CT need to be stated, including the anatomic end points of the examination, the plane of imaging, the sequences, and the use of a contrast agent. All sequences are directly obtained and are not reformatted. A sample report on an MRI scan of the lumbar spine could include the following introductory statement: "Non-contrast sagittal and axial T1- and T2-weighted images at 3-mm thickness and 3-mm intervals were obtained from T10 through the sacrum."

Terminology. The key terms for MRI are described in terms of brightness, called *signal: low signal* corresponds to black areas, *intermediate signal* is gray, and *high signal* is white. Increase in

signal (high signal) after intravenous contrast administration is termed *enhancement*. These *signal intensities* are in essence a determination of the available hydrogen protons within the observed tissues. (See Chapter 6.)

Descriptive Narrative of Findings. In all cases, the requirement to describe the correct anatomic location of abnormalities is imperative for clarity of meaning and in correlation of the clinical significance of the finding. If an abnormality is found, it is important to state on which sequence it occurs and the number of images on which it is seen. If intravenous or intra-articular contrast has been used, it is important to state its effects on abnormalities.

RISK MANAGEMENT STRATEGIES IN INTERPRETATION AND REPORT WRITING

Numerous sources of interpretive and reporting errors have been described. (1–4) (Table 15-5) Knowledge of these pitfalls is pivotal in deriving strategies to maximize diagnostic accuracy and clinical impact while minimizing medicolegal risk. (5–7)

Optimum Environs

Suboptimal viewing conditions, such as extraneous light and sources of distraction including telephones, can result in misinterpretations and inaccurate, incoherent reports. Ideally, the reporting area should be remote from general work areas with limited access. Imaging studies should not be sight read other than on proper viewing boxes.

Time Allocation

Adequate time for analysis of the study is imperative to minimize omissions or misjudgments. It is important that a specific time be set aside for performing the interpretations, to reduce the effects of time pressure and allow appropriate time. Imaging studies

Table 15-5	Sources of Interpretive and Reporting Errors
Suboptimal environs	
Inadequate time allocation	
Lack of clarity of content	
Failure to produce a report	
Omission of patient details	
Failure to describe examination details	
Poor and inappropriate terminology	
Misdiagnosis	
Typographical errors	
Failure to suggest appropriate follow-up procedures	
Reporting on poor or inadequate studies	
Failure to inform the treating practitioner	
Failure to enforce confidentiality	
Failure to heed recommendations	
Failure to review previous reports or studies	
Technical inadequacy of the study	
Inappropriate use of second-opinion reviews	
Lack of knowledge	

should be viewed without the patient present to ensure clarity of thought, focused attention to the review process, and to avoid the risk of making inappropriate statements.

Demographic Details

The particulars of each patient should be clearly described, including date of report generation, full name, address, sex, date of birth, referring physician, and clinical facts that may be relevant to the interpretation. (8) This practice ensures that the patient is clearly and correctly identified and the interpretation can be focused to isolate a specific condition. (9)

Targeting Clinical Concerns

Review of the information that the clinician is wishing to gain from the study is important to ensure that the most optimum modality was used and that it was tailored specifically for the clinical problem being investigated. In the report, it is vitally important to address the clinical questions raised in the request. This is especially true if there are no findings to concur with the query, so that the referrer has no doubt that it has been appropriately examined.

Targeting the Recipient's Concerns

Different clinicians require description of specific abnormalities relative to their clinical practice. An orthopedic specialist will have different needs from a vascular specialist and, therefore, will have a different focus for the information. (5) Tailoring the report to address these needs is important and should be considered as the report is formulated. Despite this, every report optimally is all-inclusive, as often these reports will be used by various clinicians, patients, families, and lawyers.

Description of the Study

Providing incomplete details of the study under review is a potential medicolegal trap. Defining what studies were reviewed and when they were taken ensures that the opinions relate only to the film series at hand. It is also important to note any absence of right or left markers. It is often pertinent to make specific comments on the reasons why the study was obtained.

Clarity of Content and Report Structure

The most valued aspect of the report is the clarity of its meaning conveyed in terminology that is understood and comprehended by the referring physician. (5,7,8,10–12) A quality report reflects the credibility of the interpretation and the competence of the author. (2,13) There are seven key points to consider:

Concise Reporting. Long reports are to be avoided. (8) Brevity is the soul of wit. As noted, < 40% of all reports are ever read completely. (14) Reporting a normal examination can be difficult but should clearly convey, with a few concise unequivocal statements, that there are no abnormalities. (12,15)

Correct English. Use of appropriate words, sentence structure, grammar, correct tense, and paragraphing adds a great deal to the

readability and interpretation of the report. (7,16) Minimizing repetitive phrases (e.g., "there is . . .") is encouraged.

Avoid Jargon. Inclusion of radiologic terms, although clear to the author, are frequently not understood by the recipient and should be minimized, if not avoided. When used, their significance should be clarified in the conclusions. (5,16)

Avoid Abbreviations. Abbreviations can be misinterpreted or not understood. In addition, they denote a laziness on behalf of the author, which detracts from the overall credibility of the report. (7)

Quantifying Terminology. If the findings are inconclusive, then the findings need to be qualified by the level of certainty applied to their significance. Examples of qualifying terms are *definite, equivocal,* and *possible.* (16,17) Bland and vague descriptive characterization of abnormalities, if used, should be qualified in the conclusion as to their significance. (17) Grigg (18) reminds us of the fallible nature of radiology and its interpretation by the constant use of hedging terminology and has sarcastically proposed the following be placed at the bottom of each report:

PS: This report does not mention: (1) A few shadows which were not seen because they were not looked at, nor (2) those shadows which may have been looked at but were not seen because of their small size, lack of contrast, or similarly obscuring factors, and certainly not (3) the shadows which (although both looked at and seen) were ignored because the signer of this report has not yet learned what significance, if any, they have!

Standardized Format. Employing a standardized format will improve interpretive accuracy and user understanding and help reduce typographical errors. The major pathology should be addressed early in the report; the description of normal structures should be minimized, except when appropriate; and the normal variations should be mentioned only when there may be possible confusion with a pathology. (5,15)

Measurements. Quantifying any measurements in millimeters, centimeters, or degrees is important for identifying normal, quantifying abnormalities, and providing a basis for future comparisons. (16)

Proofreading. All reports should be run through a word-processing program's spell-checker and manually proofread by the author before being signed and dispatched. (19,20) Look for key terms that may have been misinterpreted or mistyped. Dramatic examples are often those that are prefaced by terms such as *not, no, is,* and *isn't.* (21)

Further Pitfalls

Failure to Produce a Report. Whenever an imaging study is reviewed, a written summary or narrative report should be included in the patient's file. Failure to report on an imaging study is analogous to performing a physical examination but not recording the findings. (22) Significant missed diagnoses in unreported studies do occur (22), and the inference could be made that the study was not interpreted or included in the patient's management. (23) In addition, when a doctor "globally" bills a third-party payer for x-rays, there is a legal obligation for the doctor to include a written radiology report in the patient's file. A global bill to a third-party payer is a request for payment that includes the compensation of a technical fee (taking the films) and a professional fee (interpreting the films). If billed for, failure to incorporate the professional component into the patient's management, by evidence of a written report, constitutes *fraud* and severely jeopardizes the treating physician's practice.

Misdiagnosis (Perceptual Errors). The number of inaccurate diagnoses and missed diagnoses, while hard to establish, is well appreciated in the hospital situation and may be as high as 5–10%. (24,25) One prospective study shows diagnostic error rates of 4–5% for radiologists. (26) The most common reason for a lawsuit, accounting for 80% of such actions with imaging, is diagnostic error. (27–31) Perceptual errors frequently occur with lesions that have poor conspicuity and thus require high technical image quality, adequate projections, and close attention to systematic image review. (31,32) Mistakes can also be owing to failure to recognize a normal variant, failure to continue the search after the first abnormality was found (*"the patient is entitled to more than one disease"*), and failure to detect a lesion at the periphery of the study. (4,9) When a mistake is recognized, the patient should be informed promptly and compassionately with no blame passed to any other person. Careful use of phrases and full documentation of the interactions with the patient must also be documented. (6)

Typographical Errors. Simple errors of number, spelling, or patient details can have serious management and medicolegal implications. (8,19,33) An example may be the description of a fracture or disc lesion in the wrong bone or spinal level. In the spine, the presence of congenital anomalies, especially lumbosacral transitional segments, may lead to assigning the wrong level to a disc lesion, which may subsequently result in surgery at the wrong level. (34) The accidental omission of words such as *no* or the inappropriate designation of right or left can have profound clinical implications.

Technical Adequacy of Studies. Image quality exerts a direct bearing on the ability to render diagnostic opinions. (4,9,35,36) Similarly, an inadequate or inappropriate view detracts greatly from diagnostic interpretations. When a report is being rendered on an inferior quality examination, this should be noted in the report; and in the recommendations, an appropriate strategy to deal with these shortcomings should be addressed. (4) This may include repeating the x-ray with technical alterations, performing additional views, or using an alternative imaging modality.

Communication of the Report

The transmission of the written report to the treating physician may be placed within the film envelope, posted as a separate item, or conveyed by electronic means (such as facsimile or e-mail). (37) However, communication of urgent or significant findings should be done as soon as possible by direct verbal discussion with the physician. (38,39)

Confidentiality

The radiographic report is an integral part of an individual client's record and, as such, must receive the same confidentiality afforded to any part of the doctor–patient relationship. Release of the document should be allowed only after written permission from the patient. The use of electronic communication devices (voice mail, e-mail, fax machines, etc.) may potentially breach confidentiality and should be used with discretion according to the new HIPPA regulations. (37)

Follow-Up Recommendations

When specific recommendations are made regarding the need for follow-up studies, referral for further evaluation, or any other management suggestions, these should be acted on. (37) If the clinician fails to heed such a recommendation, he or she must provide clear, well-documented reasons why this has not been done.

Lack of Knowledge

Educational background, continuing postgraduate training, literature access, and ongoing interaction with peers are vital to maintaining acceptable standards of interpretive skill and ensuring correct judgments regarding the significance of findings. (9,39,40) *The eye doesn't see what the brain doesn't know.* Interpretive error rates are generally inversely proportional to the various levels of education, with the greatest number of errors occurring in students, then residents, non-radiologist specialists, and radiologists, respectively. (29,40–42)

Undergraduate medical and physiotherapy courses teach little to no radiographic interpretive skills. (43) Chiropractors receive a minimum of 300 hr in skeletal radiographic diagnosis and the reporting thereof, especially in their clinical year of schooling. (44) Resident radiologists are often left to their own means to construct reports or are largely influenced by the department in which they interact.

Review of Previous Reports

Significant information may be found in at least 60% of previously rendered reports. (9,45) Review of these may uncover important information or help direct the present interpreter to examine for a specific problem. However, care must be taken: if the previous reports contain errors, they may bias the interpretation of the current study and lead to a repeated (*alliterative*) error. (32)

Comparison with Previous Studies

A reasonable attempt to obtain previous radiographs and reports, if available, is recommended. (46,47) Whenever a comparison study is available, the new report should include an assessment of the comparative radiographs as they relate to the present investigation. It is suggested that, when prior studies are numerous, comparison with the most recent studies may be the most useful. (47) Given the inherent errors that occur in imaging interpretation, all studies should be personally reviewed and any available reports should not necessarily be construed as accurate.

SECOND-OPINION SPECIALTY RADIOLOGY REVIEWS

Second opinions assist in many aspects of radiologic interpretation. (1,2) By seeking second opinions the chances of a perceptual error are significantly reduced. This process of *risk sharing* is especially beneficial when there is a complicated history, previous malignancy or surgery, lack of therapeutic response, and when multimodality imaging is to be reviewed. Radiologists with a specialty interest and bias in their practices to multimodality musculoskeletal imaging demonstrate the highest interpretive accuracies. (3) In medicine, the consultant musculoskeletal radiologist fulfills this role; whereas in chiropractic the diplomate in radiology—DACBR (United States); FCCR (Canada)—performs this function. (4–7) For non-radiologists who perform their own primary interpretations on imaging studies, they are solely responsible for making accurate interpretations and correct diagnoses. When studies are performed and interpreted elsewhere, the interpretive and medicolegal responsibilities will be shared. Second-opinion reviews are encouraged in a number of situations. (Table 15-6)

Complicating History. So-called *red flag* indicators often associated with medically significant underlying disease, such as previous neoplasia, trauma, fever, chills, weight loss, drug or alcohol abuse, long-standing use of corticosteroids, and a history of surgery, are potential reasons for seeking a second review.

Abnormal Clinical Examination Findings. Discovery of a mass, neuromotor deficit, or deformity may raise suspicion of an underlying abnormality that may need further collaboration.

Failure to Respond to Therapy. Failure to respond to the recommended therapy may point to a misdiagnosis, missed diagnosis, or subtle abnormal finding that had been overlooked. After a second review, decisions can often be made as to the appropriate test or imaging modality that may elucidate a reason for the patient's unresponsiveness.

Unexplained Deterioration of the Condition. When a patient continues to deteriorate, this can point to the evolution of a serious disease process or a complication such as pathologic fracture. A second review of the available imaging may allow explanation of the deterioration.

Confirming the Practitioner's Interpretation. Certainty of radiographic findings translates into more effective decision making about patient care and directs follow-up imaging.

Establishing a Diagnosis. Confirmation of a patient's condition at times relies solely on radiographic depiction. A specialty consultation will help ensure the correct diagnosis is made and that an unsuspected diagnosis is not overlooked. It will also address the need for confirmatory testing.

Improving Interpretation Skill. Careful scrutiny of radiographs by a practitioner, correlation with the clinical picture, and then confirmation by second opinion empowers the practitioner with greater knowledge, insight, and experience. The rapport subsequently developed with the second reviewer will facilitate future problem solving.

Interpreting Equivocal Findings. Not infrequently, appearances on a particular image may be of concern, especially when the clinical scenario warrants suspicion of abnormality. These may be in the form of artifacts, normal variations, or unusual manifestations of a common problem such as osteoarthritis. Clarification with a second review is especially useful to help differentiate these from significant findings, which may include fractures, infections, and neoplasia.

Use of Complex Multimodality Imaging. Many different studies may be performed at varying time intervals, especially in therapeutically resistant cases. It is often appropriate for a retrospective correlative review to be performed to seek a missed abnormality or identify subtle findings.

Medicolegal Support. When there is known litigation or third-party involvement, confirmation of findings is vital for establishing the status of the studies being reviewed.

Table 15-6	Indications for a Second-Opinion Radiologic Review

Complicating history
    Previous neoplasia, trauma, fever, rigors, weight loss, drug or
      alcohol use, surgery
Abnormal clinical examination findings
    Discovering a mass, neuromotor deficit, or deformity
Failure to respond to therapy
    Misdiagnosis, an overlooked or subtle abnormal finding
Unexplained deterioration
    Developing serious disease process
    Iatrogenic complication
Confirming the practitioner's interpretation
    Developing clinical certainty and appropriateness of therapy
Establishing a diagnosis
    Confirming a patient's condition
    Directing follow-up imaging and other tests
Improving interpretation skills and education
    Obtaining greater knowledge, insight, and experience
Interpreting equivocal findings
    Differentiating among significant and insignificant findings
Use of complex multimodality imaging
    Correlating findings
Medicolegal support
    Known litigation or third-party involvement

CONCLUSIONS

Compiling radiologic reports is an integral part of clinical and radiologic practice. Developing skill in their formulation requires providing an adequate environment, equipment, staff, interpretive skill, and knowledge base. An absolute awareness of the errors inherent in the interpretation of all imaging studies, no matter who performs the interpretation, is vitally important. Potential errors in interpretation charge all treating practitioners with the responsibility to interpret every set of studies personally. Clinicians should not assume that any available report is accurate and thus must formulate their own reports, reflecting their own interpretation. A failure to provide a report or provision of an inaccurate report is a legal liability.

Date: October 7, 2000
Patient: Oscar Dalmatia
Address: Akademy Units
                  Swiftgate Street
                  Abermain, New South Wales, Australia
Sex: Male
Age: 69 years (D.O.B.: 11-10-30)
File Number: K9-007
Examinations: Lumbar spine: anteroposterior, lateral (10-5-2000)
Clinical Findings: Back pain, worse at night, unresponsive to therapy

Radiologic Findings

Lumbar Spine (Weight Bearing)

- The lumbar lordosis is mildly reduced, with no intersegmental weight-bearing-induced instability.

- The internal bony trabecular architecture at the L1 and L3 vertebral bodies has been lost, and there is poor definition of the anterior and posterior cortical margins as well as the superior and inferior endplates. Both segments show destruction of at least the left pedicles. Pathologic collapse of the L1 vertebral body has occurred, with decreased anterior and posterior heights.

- A more subtle decrease in bone density at the L2 vertebral body is thought to be present, though both pedicles are intact and there is no evidence for pathologic collapse.

- The intervertebral disc spaces are all of normal shape, size, and configuration. No definite facet disease is displayed.

- No soft tissue abnormality is present.

Conclusions

1. Aggressive osteolytic destruction of the L1 and L3 vertebrae. The L2 segment may also be involved. Features are consistent with osteolytic metastatic carcinoma.

2. Pathologic fracture of the L1 vertebral body.

Recommendations

These bony changes are consistent with bone malignancy, most likely metastatic in nature. The most likely primary sites for osteolytic carcinoma are lung, colon, and thyroid. The differential diagnosis may include multiple myeloma.

Further investigation is required. MRI is suggested to examine the spinal canal for impending cauda equina compression; an isotopic bone scan will assess the extent of skeletal involvement. CT scan of the chest and abdomen will be of assistance for further staging and identifying the primary site of origin.

Dr. Lindsay J. Rowe
MAppSc (Chiro), MD
DACBR, FCCR, FACCR, FICC, FRANZCR
Consultant Radiologist

Report Commentary

This report structure follows the classical ABCs format. The findings were not prioritized in order of clinical importance. In this case, in which signs of bone malignancy are present, it is a justifiable criticism that description of these findings should have been first and the statements relating to the alignment, joints, and soft tissue placed later.

The alignment statement relates to the status of the lumbar lordosis and the presence of displacement between the vertebral segments. The comment on the absence of weight-bearing instability is relevant because, if present, would signify a high probability for neurologic dysfunction and the urgent clinical need for neurosurgical assessment.

In the description of the bony changes there is a great deal of detail because in this case they are the most important part of the report. There is particular attention to the signs of malignancy

Figure 15-2, *A* and *B*

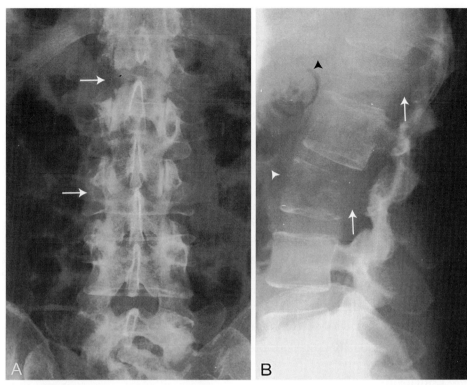

Figure 15-2 **OSTEOLYTIC METASTATIC CARCINOMA. A. AP Lumbar.** Observe the loss of the reading left pedicles of L1 and L3 (*arrows*). **B. Lateral Lumbar.** Note the dramatic loss of bone architecture within the vertebral bodies at L1 and L3 (*arrowheads*). Also, both levels show loss of the normal pedicle outlines (*arrows*). More subtle osteolysis is present at L2. Complicating pathologic fracture with loss of the anterior and posterior vertebral body height is present at L1.

at the L1 and L3 vertebra, with an accurate resume of the altered anatomic components. The changes at the L2 level are less definite and have been described accordingly; they will be elucidated on follow-up imaging. Inclusion of the comment on disc height retention is appropriate as this is an important negative finding to exclude infection as a cause for the osteolysis.

Close observation of the upper sacrum shows a spina bifida occulta of the S1 segment, which in the context of the malignancy has been electively omitted from the report; this is appropriate because it has no clinical relevance. Similarly, the statement on the status of the lumbar lordosis could have been left out. These two findings in another clinical setting, for example, of uncomplicated back pain, may have more relevance and as such should be included in the report.

Date: May 7, 2002
Patient: Robyn Cunningham
Address: 1 Ocean Headland Road
                   Hamilton Island, Queensland, Australia
Sex: Female
Age: 52 (D.O.B.: 5-7-1950)
File Number: 2077
Examinations: Right hip: anteroposterior (5-6-2002)
Clinical Findings: Bilateral peripheral joint pains, now increasing bilateral hip stiffness

Radiologic Findings

Right Hip

- A single frontal projection study is available for review, which limits the interpretation.

- Medial and axial migration of the femoral head is present, with displacement of the acetabular floor into the pelvic inlet (protrusio acetabuli).

- Diffuse osteopenia of all skeletal structures is apparent. The femoral head cortex is smooth and convex with no evidence of collapse. There are numerous subtle subchondral cysts in the femoral head. No definite fracture is evident on this limited study.

- The joint space shows uniform loss throughout the entire hip articulation. The visualized lower sacroiliac joint shows no abnormality.

- No soft tissue abnormality is present.

Conclusions

1. Diffuse and generalized osteopenia of the hemi pelvis and proximal femur.

2. Chronic inflammatory arthritis of the hip joint with secondary protrusio acetabuli.

Recommendations

The described changes are most likely the result of rheumatoid arthritis. Other less likely differential possibilities include psoriatic arthritis and atypical degenerative joint disease.

Confirmation of the diagnosis should be made by careful clinical examination and further radiographs, as required, of the other hip, hands, feet, and cervical spine. Additional oblique views of the right hip would be suggested for more complete analysis. There is no evidence for complicating osteonecrosis or acute or insufficiency fracture on this single film study; MRI and nuclear bone scan would be more sensitive for their detection.

Lindsay J. Rowe
MAPPSc (CHIRO), MD
DACBR, FCCR, FACCR, FICC, FRANZCR
CONSULTANT RADIOLOGIST

Report Commentary

The lead-in statement has underlined that a bare minimum radiographic study is available, which limits the interpretation. This was reinforced in the recommendations section, in which an additional oblique film has been requested. These are important facts to report because assessing an inadequate study will result in missed diagnoses and serves to remind the referring clinician of this short-coming.

The report has been tailored to follow the ABCs format because the case lends itself to this standard layout. The tandem alignment problems are the medial migration of the acetabular floor and femoral head, which appear to be linked with a common pathologic process. The recognized background osteopenia provides the clue to a long-standing, inflammatory, and probably immobilizing disease. Careful description of the loss in joint space identifies that there is a generalized loss of intra-articular cartilage, which typically excludes a mechanical degenerative arthropathy and indicates an inflammatory cause. Combining these features prioritizes rheumatoid arthritis as the most likely diagnostic consideration.

Figure 15

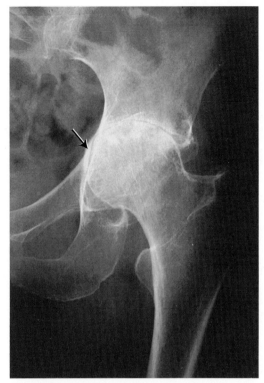

Figure 15-3 **RHEUMATOID ARTHRITIS. AP Hip.** Note the medial displacement of the acetabular floor (protrusio acetabuli) with a uniform loss of hip joint space (*arrow*). Generalized osteopenia is evident, with cortical thinning and loss of trabecular detail.

Recommending further plain films may be redundant because it is most likely, given the usual chronic course of rheumatoid arthritis, that previous studies would be available. It would be more pertinent to request these for comparative review to assess disease progression and the appearance of complications. It is these secondary problems that are likely to be more important for the current presentation, which is why they have been listed and why relevant, more sensitive investigations have been suggested.

Date: July 9, 2001
Patient: Wayne Minter
Address: 1 Thredbo Way
                   Thredbo, New South Wales, Australia
Sex: Male
Age: 39 years (D.O.B.: 1-10-1961)
File Number: 33333
Examinations: Right wrist: posteroanterior, lateral (7-9-2001)
Clinical Findings: Fall onto outstretched hand while skiing, pain and swelling

Radiologic Findings

Right Wrist

- A comminuted and impacted fracture is present in the distal radius, with some loss of length. A separated fragment is visible at the dorsal articular margin of the radius. There is dorsal angulation of the distal fragment.

- A fracture has also occurred through the ulnar styloid process.

- The carpal bones are intact and there is no evidence of dislocation.

- Associated prominent soft tissue swelling is present.

- Joint spaces are preserved.

Conclusions

1. Impacted Colles'-type fracture of the distal radius.

2. Fracture of the ulnar styloid process.

Recommendations

Reduction of the fracture deformity and appropriate immobilization are required.
   Postreduction and follow-up progress radiographs at 1, 6, and 10 weeks are suggested.

Lindsay J. Rowe
MAppSc (Chiro), MD
DACBR, FCCR, FACCR, FICC, FRANZCR
Consultant Radiologist

Report Commentary

The ABCs format has been employed but in compiling the report on this routine fracture, the author intuitively combined them into a sequence of statements that describe the primary abnormalities, especially the bony abnormalities and the misalignments. By describing the fracture components accurately, the author assists the involved clinicians in deciding if and how the deformities can best be reduced and provides a baseline for comparison with progressive healing. Important negative statements have been included to assess any associated fractures or dislocations that may have been overlooked.

In the conclusions, the use of a synonym (*Colles' fracture*) is usually discouraged as it assumes knowledge of what the term means and is open to misinterpretation. However, in common conditions, such as in this case, the use of a common synonym is generally not considered unusual and does in fact succinctly summarize the findings. The inclusion of the term *impacted* draws attention to an important feature that requires attention during treatment.

Recommending sequential studies is commonly employed in fracture management to assess stability, fragment position, and signs of healing and to recognize complications, such as malunion and non-union.

Figure 15-4, *A* and

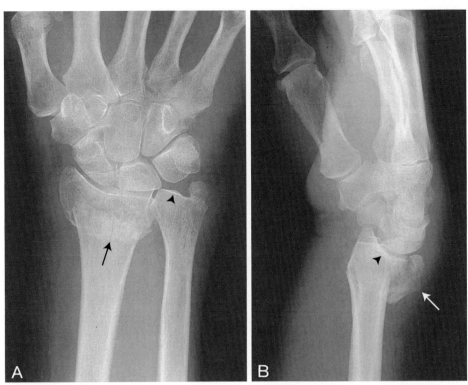

Figure 15-4   COLLES' FRACTURE. A. PA Wrist. Note the site of fracture impaction of the radius, which is visible as cortical disruption and an increase in density transversely (*arrow*). Observe that the head of the ulna lies distal to the articular surface of the radius (positive ulnar variance) owing to the impaction (*arrowhead*). **B. Lateral Wrist.** The separated dorsal fragment is readily visible (*arrow*). The plane of the ular surface of the radius is tilted dorsally (*arrowhead*). tissue swelling is manifested by the generalized increase periarticular density and a lack of fat planes, such as th ventral pronator quadratus fat line.

Date: January 23, 1999
Patient: Jezebel Brown
Address: Fystenborgvej 9999
                Skjern, Denmark
Sex: Female
Age: 25 (D.O.B.: 9-11-73)
File Number: K99-007
Examinations: Thoracic spine: lateral (1-10-99)
Clinical Findings: Chronic interscapular pain; poor posture; possible anomaly

Radiologic Findings

Thoracic Spine

- No frontal projection is available for review, which limits full assessment of the thoracic spine.

- The thoracic kyphosis is increased most marked from T6 to T10.

- At the T6–T10 levels there is marked anterior wedging of the vertebral bodies. The endplates at the anterior two thirds of these segments show marked irregularity. The ring epiphyses remain unfused.

- The adjacent intervertebral discs from T6 to T10 are narrowed.

- The paravertebral soft tissues cannot be assessed without a frontal projection.

Conclusions

1. Scheuermann's disease of the thoracic spine between T6 and T10.

2. Increased thoracic spine kyphosis.

Recommendations

This deformity is usually managed non-surgically, unless it becomes rapidly progressive. Occasionally, there may be associated arachnoid cysts or even thoracic disc herniations, which can give rise to various neurologic sequelae. In addition, involvement of the lumbar spine can lead to spinal stenosis and lumbar pars defects (spondylolysis).

MRI would be the optimum non-invasive study to identify these abnormalities of the thoracolumbar spine. It is also strongly suggested that an anteroposterior projection be obtained to allow more complete review of the thoracic spine.

Lindsay J. Rowe
MAppSc (Chiro), MD
DACBR, FCCR, FACCR, FICC, FRANZCR
Consultant Radiologist

Report Commentary

This case was reviewed for a second opinion, and only the lateral thoracic film was submitted. As in Case Study 2, the single film limits the interpretation and poses increased medicolegal risks. When the study has been technically compromised by a lack of images or poor image quality, it is important to state this in the report.

The standard ABCs format has been employed, which succinctly states the findings in a logical sequence. Because this case was reviewed for a second opinion, the recommendations section was extended, especially in terms of disease associations that may not be known by the referring physician and the most optimum imaging method to employ if they need to be excluded. In addition, the lack of an anteroposterior projection is reinforced as representing an inadequate study.

Figure 15-5

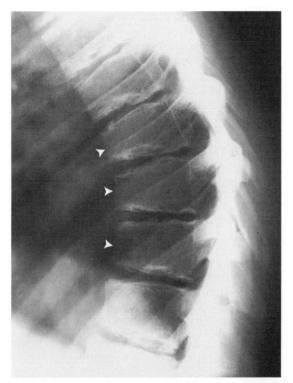

Figure 15-5   **SCHEUERMANN'S DISEASE. Lateral Thoracic.**
Observe that the most notable findings are the increased
kyphosis, irregular endplates, anterior vertebral wedging
(*arrowheads*), and reduced disc space heights.

Date: January 23, 2002
Patient: Edgar Baxter
Address: 77 Tapanui Drive
                   Heriot, New Zealand
Sex: Male
Age: 60 years (D.O.B.: 9-12-1941)
File Number: RR#2
Examinations: Cervical spine: anteroposterior open mouth, lateral, right and left obliques
                   (1-22-2002)
Clinical Findings: Lower neck pain, left C6 radicular symptoms

Radiologic Findings

Cervical Spine

- In the neutral position, the cervical lordosis is reversed with the apex at the C4 level.

- No bony abnormality is present. No cervical rib is visualized.

- Multilevel degenerative disc disease is present at C4–C5, C5–C6, and C6–C7, with loss of disc height and osteophytes. Neurocentral joint (joints of von Luschka) arthrosis is present at these levels bilaterally and is most severe at C6–C7. The related intervertebral sagittal dimension of the foramina is narrowed bilaterally and is most severe on the left side at C6–C7. The narrowest spinal canal is at C5, with a measurement of 14 mm.

- At the C3–C4 level, a 2-mm anterolisthesis is apparent, secondary to severe facet arthrosis. Additional levels of facet arthrosis are identified at C2–C3 and C7–T1.

- The trachea is midline, and the lung apices are normally aerated. The prevertebral soft tissues are of normal thickness.

Conclusions

1. Kyphosis of the cervical spine.

2. No bony abnormality.

3. Multilevel degenerative disc disease at C4–C5, C5–C6, and C6–C7.

4. Bilateral foraminal stenosis secondary to neurocentral joint arthrosis at C4–C5, C5–C6, and most marked on the left side at C6–C7.

5. Facet arthrosis at C2–C3, C3–C4, and C7–T1, more severe on the left side.

6. Degenerative spondylolisthesis at C3–C4.

Recommendations

The constellation of findings described is consistent with degenerative disc and facet disease. Consideration to sagittal stress views in flexion and extension would be suggested to evaluate for intersegmental instability, especially at the degenerative spondylolisthesis at C3–C4. There is foraminal stenosis on the left side from C4 to C7 and is most prominent at C6–C7, which may correlate with the clinical findings.

   MRI would be useful to delineate the presence of this stenosis or disc herniation. Analysis of the spinal cord for myelopathy or other abnormality can also be made at this time.

Lindsay J. Rowe
MAppSc (Chiro), MD
DACBR, FCCR, FACCR, FICC, FRANZCR
Consultant Radiologist

Report Commentary

This case demonstrates the difficulties in reporting degenerative joint disease, which is common but also often bears no relationship to clinical findings. The most challenging aspect of these reports is to describe the abnormalities in adequate detail while keeping it of reasonable length and being mind-

Figure 15-6, A-

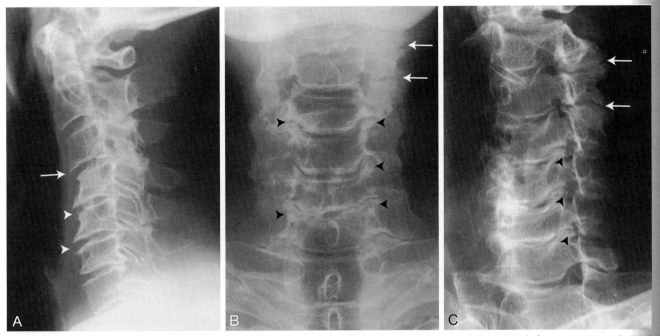

Figure 15-6 **MULTILEVEL DEGENERATIVE DISC DISEASE: CERVICAL SPONDYLOSIS. A. Lateral Cervical.** Note the reversed lordosis, multilevel degenerative disc disease (*arrowheads*), and degenerative spondylolisthesis at C3 (*arrow*). **B. AP Lower Cervical.** Observe that the neurocentral joint (joints of von Luschka) arthrosis can be assessed by the bulbous shape of the uncinate processes (*arrowheads*). The facet arthrosis, especially on the left at C2–C3 and C3–C4, can also be identified (*arrows*). **C. Left Anterior Oblique Cervical.** Note the ventral encroachment into the C5–C6, C6–C7, and C7–T1 foramina by neurocentral (von Luschka) osteophytes (*arrowheads*) and dorsally from facet osteophytes at C2–C3 and C3–C4 (*arrows*).

ful to highlight any feature that is of greater clinical relevance. In this example, an all-embracing, succinct statement has been used to cover the three levels of disc disease rather than dealing with each individual level. Many would argue that it is more accurate to report each disc individually; and, in some cases, especially one with medicolegal implications, this would be true. Such reports are often necessary because of the number of levels with abnormalities, but they can be long and complex. With CT and MRI this segmental approach to reporting is more useful because of the higher incidence of significant abnormalities not appreciated on plain film studies.

Employing a straight ABCs approach in this case requires flexibility in its use. Initially, the cervical curve can be analyzed, followed by an osseous review. In association with the loss of disc height, there are bony changes such as osteophytes, and it is pertinent to provide some insight into some soft tissue effects, such as foraminal encroachment and the size of the central canal. In addition, when the facet joints are being assessed there is loss of joint space, osteophytes, and encroachment into the adjacent foramina as well as a misalignment, which may be clinically relevant. This flexible ABCs format is the preferred approach because it allows the integration of all information at one site and for simpler conversion into the clinical setting.

When there are extensive degenerative changes even in peripheral joints, it is important that the conclusion summarizes them clearly to assist the clinician ascribing significance to the findings. The recommendations are especially important to highlight potentially correlative findings with the clinical findings and what additional imaging may be useful to confirm these suspicions.

Date:	January 3, 2002
Patient:	John Zapitello
Address:	5555 Grand Avenue
	St. Paul, Minnesota, USA
Sex:	Male
File Number:	#66666
Age:	30 years (D.O.B.: 10-12-71)
Examinations:	Lumbar spine: anteroposterior, lateral (12-12-1999); CT Scan: L3–S1 (12-18-1999)
Clinical Findings:	Weightlifter and active sportsman; lower back and left leg pain

Radiologic Findings

Lumbar Spine
Plain Film Examination (Erect)

- The lumbar lordosis is reduced. A 2-mm retrolisthesis is present at L4 upon L5.

- The vertical trabeculae at the anterior L5 vertebral body appear accentuated without visible cortical thickening, sclerosis, or expansion. The remaining bony structures are unremarkable.

- At the L4 level, there is approximately 25% loss of intervertebral disc height without osteophyte formation. At the posteroinferior margin of the L4 vertebral body, a curvilinear area of calcification is evident.

- The remaining intervertebral disc spaces, T12–L5, are of normal shape, size, and configuration. No definite abnormality of the facet or sacroiliac joints.

- No soft tissue abnormality is defined.

CT Scan (L1–L3)

- *Technique:* Sequential and contiguous axial images were performed parallel to the endplates of the L3–L5 disc spaces at 5-mm intervals, with bone and soft tissue windows available for review. Multiplanar reconstructions in sagittal and coronal planes were performed along with three-dimensional images.

- *L3–L4:* No bony abnormality, disc bulge, or herniation is present. The central and lateral canals are capacious with no stenosis. Facet joints are normal.

- *L4–L5:* At the posteroinferior margin of the L4 vertebral endplate, a focal bony depression is present with posterior displacement of the vertebral rim. This bony fragment contacts and effaces the anterior thecal sac. The L5 lateral recesses bilaterally are narrowed, with compression of the L5 nerve roots. Both L4 nerve roots exit without impingement. A focal hemangioma is confirmed at the anterior third of the L5 vertebral body, with coarsened trabeculae and contained low attenuation fat. No evidence of pathologic fracture or extension into the spinal canal is present.

- *L5–S1:* No bony abnormality, disc bulge, or herniation is present. The central and lateral canals are capacious with no stenosis. Facet joints are normal.

Conclusions

1. Lumbar hypolordosis.
2. Posterior Schmorl's node at the posterior inferior margin of the L4 vertebral body with displacement of the adjacent vertebral ring.
3. Compression of the ventral thecal sac and narrowing of the lateral recesses bilaterally with compression of the L5 nerve roots.
4. Loss of intervertebral disc height at the L4 level.
5. Focal hemangioma of the anterior third of the L5 vertebral body.

Recommendations

The rim lesion at L4 is well documented in the literature as a cause for nerve compression, which may or may not require surgical intervention. The time of onset of the L4–L5 lesion cannot be assessed based on the observed findings and modalities used. MRI may elucidate bone marrow edema, providing evidence for a recent and active lesion.

Figure 15-7, A–C

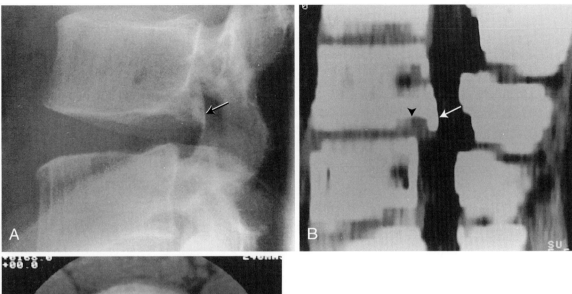

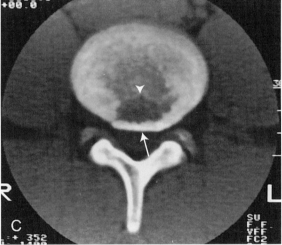

Figure 15-7 **POSTERIOR SCHMORL'S NODE WITH DISPLACED VERTEBRAL RIM. A. Lateral Lumbar.** Note the curvilinear calcification extending from the posterior inferior margin of the L4 vertebral body (*arrow*). **B. CT, Lateral Lumbar Spine Reconstruction.** Note that the posterior calcification seen on the plain film is clearly depicted (*arrow*), as is the focal depression representing a marginal intra-osseous (Schmorl's) node (*arrowhead*). **C. CT, Axial L4.** Note that the Schmorl's node exists as the low attenuation defect in the posterior vertebral body margin (*arrowhead*), with the separated posteriorly displaced vertebral rim shifted into the central canal (*arrow*).

Lindsay J. Rowe, CONSULTANT RADIOLOGIST

Report Commentary

A common problem in musculoskeletal radiology is that more than one pathologic entity is identified, which may or may not be relevant. The definite bony abnormality at the single L4 vertebra presents little difficulty in reporting its features and conforms to a classical presentation of this entity. The radiologist attached relevant references to the report to provide the referring clinician with further information on the condition.

The incidental finding of a hemangioma at the L5 vertebral body presents a number of reporting problems. Initially, the plain films were obtained and reported normal. On second opinion, the review identified evidence of the rim lesion, and a CT scan was arranged to confirm the diagnosis. The hemangioma recognized on the plain film was not reported on the CT. The CT was reviewed again as a second opinion, and the hemangioma was authenticated. The patient became frustrated by these circumstances and turned to the Internet to find information; he discovered numerous references noting that these lesions may be responsible for significant neurologic problems. This accounts for the report specifically stating its relatively distant location and lack of apparent complications to help satisfy the patient of the relative clinical insignificance of this finding.

The case highlights how conflicting reports can lead to misdiagnosis and why all previous reports need to be reviewed. Inconsistent reports often lead to medicolegal conflict as well as creating clinical uncertainty. When an abnormality is identified, even if it is thought to be of little clinical relevance it remains paramount to describe it accurately and ascribe a relative importance to the finding. Additional imaging, especially MRI, often helps clarify these circumstances. When multimodality imaging has been used, it is vital that all studies are retrospectively reviewed at one time to correlate all findings.

Date: May 15, 2002
Patient: Patricia Masanz
Address: 2323 Santa Monica Boulevard
                   Santa Monica, California, USA
Sex: Female
Age: 34 years (D.O.B.: 8-7-67)
File Number: 77777
Examinations: Lumbar spine: plain films: anteroposterior, lateral (4-15-2002); CT scan: L3–S1 (4-24-2002); MRI scan: T12–S3 (5-2-2002)
Clinical Findings: Severe back pain, normal neurology

Radiologic Findings

Lumbar Spine

Plain Film Examination

- An antalgic lateral list of the lumbar spine to the right is present without intersegmental rotation.

- No bony abnormality is evident. A prominent broad-based indentation is at the inferior endplate of the L5 vertebral body as a variant of normal (nuclear impression, notochordal persistency). The intervertebral disc spaces are preserved. The facet and sacroiliac joints are normal.

- No soft tissue abnormality.

CT Scan (L3–S1)

- *Technique:* Sequential and contiguous axial images were performed parallel to the endplates of the L3–L5 disc spaces at 5-mm intervals, with bone and soft tissue windows available for review. Multiplanar reconstructions in sagittal and coronal planes were performed.

- *L3–L4, L4–L5:* No bony abnormality, disc bulge, or herniation is present. The central and lateral canals are capacious with no stenosis. Facet joints are normal.

- *L5–S1:* No bony abnormality. Diffuse concentric disc bulging is present, which abuts the ventral thecal sac but causes no compression of the exiting L4 or L5 nerve roots. Facet joints are normal.

MRI Scan

- *Technique:* Sagittal and axial T1- and T2-weighted images were performed.

- The conus is of normal signal and size, terminating at the L1–L2 disc space.

- *T12–L4:* The disc spaces are normally hydrated and of normal height. There is no disc herniation or canal stenosis (central/lateral). All nerve roots exit without compression and demonstrate no abnormality. Bony elements are of normal signal. No fracture or pars defect is evident. Paraspinal soft tissues are unremarkable.

- *L5–S1:* The intervertebral disc shows diminished signal from dehydration. Posterior bulging of the intact annulus has occurred, which contains a focal area of high signal intensity (high intensity zone-HIZ). Bony elements are of normal signal with no fracture or pars defect evident. Paraspinal soft tissues are unremarkable.

Conclusions

1. Diffuse symmetric bulging and diminished signal at the L5–S1 disc from degenerative disc dehydration.

2. The focal intra-annular high signal may represent a partial-thickness tear with associated granulation tear.

3. No central or lateral canal stenosis. No nerve root compression.

Recommendations

The specificity for correlative clinical pain syndromes with a high intensity zone remains controversial. Confirmatory study is possible with provocational discography, which can reproduce the patient's symptom complex. This may be especially helpful if surgery is being contemplated.

Figure 15-8, A–C

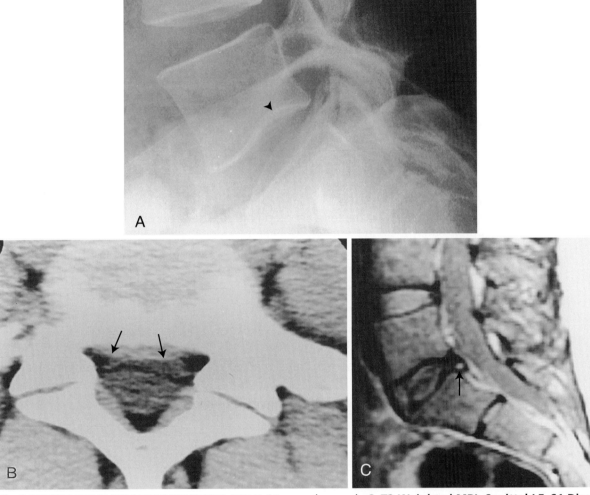

Figure 15-8 **DEGENERATIVE DISC DEHYDRATION AT L5–S1: ANNULAR TEAR. A. Lateral Lumbar.** Note that the L5–S1 disc space is maintained. The L5 inferior endplate exhibits a normal-variant prominent nuclear impression (*arrowhead*). **B. CT, Axial L5–S1 Disc.** Observe the concentric disc bulge as a soft tissue density, which extends beyond the bony margin (*arrows*). **C. T2-Weighted MRI, Sagittal L5–S1 Disc.** Note that the internal matrix of the L5–S1 disc is of intermediate signal (gray) compared with L4, as a sign of dehydration. Within the posterior annular fibers there is focal high signal (HIZ), which is covered posteriorly by an intact outer annular layer (*arrow*).

Lindsay J. Rowe
MAppSc (Chiro), MD
DACBR, FCCR, FACCR, FICC, FRANZCR
Consultant Radiologist

Report Commentary

As in Case Study 5, the plain film and CT studies show non-specific common findings of dubious significance, in this case a dehydrated, bulging disc. The entity still requires an adequate description, despite its common, usually asymptomatic occurrence. The same applies to the normal endplate variation of nuclear impression, which, while well known and of no known significance, may lead to some confusion with fracture or osteoporotic deformity.

Note that in both CT and MR descriptions a segmental approach has been employed, which assists the clinician in the analysis of each site and in determining any clinical correlates. The finding in the L5–S1 disc on MRI of a focal high signal is a controversial finding, and it is difficult to ascribe its importance. It is important to try to assign a level of certainty in the report, whenever possible, to any abnormal findings and to offer a method for confirming or negating their significance. In the presented case, a provocational discogram has been suggested as the only reliable method for elucidating its role as a focus in the genesis of the symptom complex.

Date: April 24, 2001
Patient: Ryan James
Address: 1 South Seward Avenue
                  Auburn, New York, USA
Sex: Male
File Number: 88888
Age: 42 years (D.O.B.: 12-7-58)
Examinations: Left hip: anteroposterior (3-14-2001); CT scan (3-19-2001); Bone scan (3-23-2001)
Clinical Findings: Left hip pain for 4 years, getting worse

Radiologic Findings

Left Hip

Plain Film Examination

- Within the greater trochanter a geographic loss of bone density is identified. This lesion measures approximately 2 cm in diameter. Multiple fine septations can be seen traversing the lesion.

- The cortex is intact but thinned internally with some slight expansion apparent. There is suggestion of matrix calcification at its inferior margin.

- No periosteal new bone formation.

CT Scan

- *Technique:* Sequential axial non-contrast images at 3-mm slice thickness at 2-mm intervals were obtained. Bone and soft tissue windows with coronal reconstructions were calculated.

- The cortex is intact and demonstrates marked endosteal scalloping. Some matrix calcification is noted inferiorly.

- No periosteal new bone or soft tissue mass is present.

- No pathologic fracture is depicted.

Nuclear Bone Scan

- *Technique:* A triphasic flow, blood pool, and delayed study were performed.

- Flow and blood pool studies are unremarkable.

- On the delayed study, marked tracer uptake is apparent throughout the greater trochanter region. There is no appreciable uptake beyond the radiologic margins.

- No other bony lesions are present.

Conclusions

1. Geographic lesion 2 cm in size involving the greater trochanter of the left femur.

2. The differential diagnosis includes enchondroma, giant cell tumor, fibrous dysplasia, or other benign skeletal tumor.

Recommendations

The most likely diagnosis for these bony changes is a benign bone tumor. Infection is unlikely.
   There should be immediate follow-up for further evaluation and management. A bone biopsy is required.

Lindsay J. Rowe
MAppSc (Chiro), MD
DACBR, FCCR, FACCR, FICC, FRANZCR
Consultant Radiologist

Figure 15-9, A

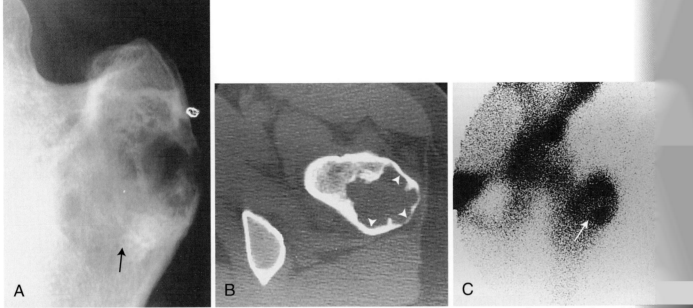

Figure 15-9 **ENCHONDROMA: PROXIMAL FEMUR. A. AP Hip.** Note the well-circumscribed lesion in the greater trochanter and extending into the adjacent femoral neck and upper shaft (*arrow*). **B. CT, Axial Proximal Femur.** Note that the lesion demonstrates endosteal erosion without ruption of the cortex (*arrowheads*). No definite matrix can be determined. **C. Bone Scan, Proximal Femur.** Obse the increased uptake coinciding with the lesion (*arrow*).

Report Commentary

This report structure could not follow the classic ABCs format owing to the focused projection on the area of interest. The plain film and CT images do not depict any joint articulations, making it impossible to comment on the alignment and cartilaginous aspect of the ABCs format. Thus, the absence of the report containing statements on these components is justifiable. On the other hand, a statement on soft tissue integrity should have been included, even with the limited amount of soft tissues visualized.

The plain film and CT descriptions of the bony changes encompass great detail because this is the major area of interest in this case. There is particular attention given to the structure of the tumor, which will aid in the ruling of the benign or malignant nature of this lesion. Yet again, a statement emphasizing the lack of soft tissue changes could have been beneficial in making this decision. In this report, the retrospective review of all the modalities used, including the nuclear bone scan, has demonstrated the importance of correlating findings to narrow the diagnosis.

Date: August 23, 2001
Patient: Minnie Minor
Address: Sibley Manor
Maynard Street
St. Paul, Minnesota, USA
Sex: Female
Age: 74 years (D.O.B.: 12-7-26)
File Number: 999999
Examinations: Left knee: anteroposterior, lateral, intercondylar, tangential (5-7-2001, Met Center Hospital); MRI: T1-weighted coronal and sagittal, T2-weighted coronal and axial, short tau inversion recovery coronal, three-dimensional gradient echo sagittal (8-23-2001)
Clinical Findings: Persistent knee pain over 3 months now worsening, plain film studies normal

Radiologic Findings

Left Knee
Plain Film Examination

- There is no weight-bearing-induced deformity or femorotibial subluxation.

- Bone density appears mildly decreased without destructive focus.

- The joint spaces are preserved. A small joint effusion is evident in the suprapatellar pouch.

MRI Scan

- *Technique:* T1-weighted coronal and sagittal, T2-weighted coronal and axial with fat saturation, short tau inversion recovery (STIR) coronal with fat saturation and three-dimensional gradient echo sagittal sequences were performed.

- There is a transverse linear fracture with a second oblique fracture component extending into the medial tibial condyle, best delineated on the coronal T1-weighted sequence (Sequence 2, Image 7). The STIR coronal study confirms the inflammatory nature of the fracture, with fluid at the fracture site and surrounding localized bone marrow edema (Sequence 4, Image 8). No bone destruction, marrow disease, or soft tissue mass is present. There is a joint effusion.

- No intra-articular derangement is demonstrated, with intact cruciate ligaments and menisci. There are no loose bodies. The extensor mechanism shows no abnormality.

Conclusions

1. Fracture of the proximal tibial metaphysis with edema and joint effusion. In the absence of acute trauma, the appearances are those of insufficiency fracture.

Recommendations

Assessment of bone density for evidence of osteoporosis with dual-energy x-ray absorptiometry (DEXA) would be suggested. A bone scan may be indicated if other pain sites are present to identify other sites of insufficiency fracture. Assessment of history for factors associated with osteopenia, such as corticosteroid use, and an orthopedic and endocrinologic consultation would be relevant.

Lindsay J. Rowe
MAppSc (Chiro), MD
DACBR, FCCR, FACCR, FICC, FRANZCR
Consultant Radiologist

Report Commentary

The plain film was essentially normal, other than a small effusion. However, important negatives—especially the absence of degenerative joint disease and osteonecrosis—were noted. The standard ABCs format has been followed.

Musculoskeletal MRI examinations usually use thin-section multiple sequences and generate up to a couple of hundred images. Frequently, only a few images are diagnostically important, and the

Figure 15-10, A–C

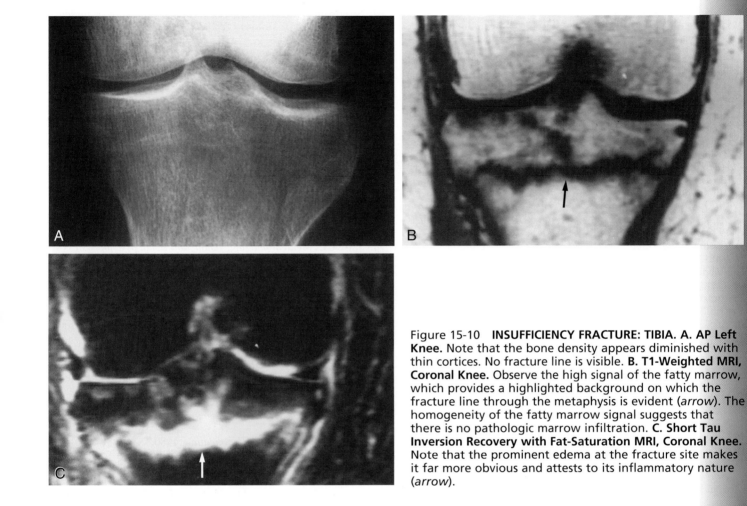

Figure 15-10 **INSUFFICIENCY FRACTURE: TIBIA. A. AP Left Knee.** Note that the bone density appears diminished with thin cortices. No fracture line is visible. **B. T1-Weighted MRI, Coronal Knee.** Observe the high signal of the fatty marrow, which provides a highlighted background on which the fracture line through the metaphysis is evident (*arrow*). The homogeneity of the fatty marrow signal suggests that there is no pathologic marrow infiltration. **C. Short Tau Inversion Recovery with Fat-Saturation MRI, Coronal Knee.** Note that the prominent edema at the fracture site makes it far more obvious and attests to its inflammatory nature (*arrow*).

method for reporting these requires a numbering system by sequence and image number. Placement of a sticker or marking with a removable pencil on the crucial images is often done.

When analyzing musculoskeletal MRI scans, the clinician can use an ABCs format with reasonable accuracy, but a more flexible approach is suggested based on anatomic structures. In the knee as described, this would include the bones, ligaments, menisci, articular cartilage, tendons, joint fluid, and synovium. Describing the changes sequence by sequence is not suggested because this is confusing to the reader, who doesn't usually possess knowledge of these findings. It is preferable to be intuitive and to correlate the abnormal findings on each sequence and present them in a succinct manner.

The finding of an acute fracture is readily described in terms of signal changes and location. Early in the interpretation of the MRI studies, one should examine a water-sensitive study (T2-weighted, STIR, or proton density) with fat saturation, preferably in a long anatomic plane, because this augments edema-fluid, which is a common marker of the active sites of disease. Using these locations, the radiologist can make a correlation with more anatomically sensitive sequences (T1-weighted or three-dimensional gradient echo studies) and structural derangements can be identified.

The recommendations section gives the opportunity to confirm the suspicion for underlying osteoporosis with complicating fracture. DEXA has been suggested as the most sensitive and readily available test to exclude the most common cause for pathologic fracture in this age group. A bone scan has been introduced to consider if there are more generalized symptoms to identify other remote sites of insufficiency fracture. The clinician has been also been prompted to review for osteopenic factors, such as corticosteroid use, which are common causes.

■ References

GENERAL CONSIDERATIONS

1. **Cassidy JD, Mierau DR, Nykoliation JW, et al.:** *Medical-chiropractic correspondence.* J Can Chiro Assoc 29(1):29, 1985.
2. **Conley RN, Nicholson DL:** *How to Avoid a Malpractice Suit* [Roentgen Brief]. ACA Council Roentgenology, 1983.
3. **Phillips RB:** *Plain film radiology in chiropractic.* J Manipulative Physiol Ther 15:47, 1992.
4. **Taylor JAM:** *Writing radiology reports in chiropractic.* J Can Chiro Assoc 34(1):30, 1990.
5. **Chapman-Smith D:** *Referral letters and written reports.* Chiro Rep 6(2):1, 1992.
6. **Ewing CL:** *Medicolegal radiology.* Radiology 63:673, 1954.
7. **Hirtle RL:** *Chiropractic malpractice.* ACA J Chiro 35, 1987.
8. **Saxton HM:** *Should radiologists report on every film?* [Editorial]. Clin Radiol 45:1, 1992.
9. **Etter LE:** *Glossary of Words and Phrases in Radiology, Nuclear Medicine and Ultrasound,* ed 2. Springfield, IL, Charles C Thomas, 1970.
10. **Friedman PJ:** *Radiologic reporting: Structure* [Editorial]. AJR 140:171, 1983.
11. **Friedman PJ:** *Radiologic reporting: The hierarchy of terms* [Editorial]. AJR 140:402, 1983.
12. **Squire LF:** *On the art of presenting films at conferences.* Radiol Clin North Am 9:149, 1971.

ENVIRONS AND EQUIPMENT

1. **Choplin RH, Boehme JM, Cowan RJ, et al.:** *Computerized radiologic reporting system.* Radiology 150:345, 1984.
2. **Hunter TB, Boyle RR:** *The value of reading the previous radiology report* [Letter]. AJR 150:697, 1988.
3. **Haug PJ, Ranum DL, Frederick PR:** *Computerized extraction of coded findings from free-text radiologic reports. Work in progress.* Radiology 174:543, 1990.
4. **Gillespy T:** *Advanced applications of personal computers in the radiologist's office.* Radiographics 13:163, 1993.
5. **Rowberg AH, Price TD:** *The need and user requirements for integrating images with radiology reports.* Proc Annu Symp Comput Appl Med Care 163, 1991.

PLAIN FILM PLACEMENT AND ORIENTATION FOR INTERPRETATION

1. **Swensson RG, Hessel SJ, Herman PG:** *Omissions in radiology: Faulty search or stringent reporting criteria.* Radiology 123:563, 1977.
2. **Butt WP:** *Interpreting the spinal x-ray. 1.* Br J Hosp Med 40:46, 1988.
3. **Butt WP:** *Interpreting the spinal x-ray. 2.* Br J Hosp Med 40:124, 1988.
4. **Stoker DJ:** *Interpreting the skeletal x-ray.* Br J Hosp Med 40:143, 1988.

REPORT STRUCTURE AND CONTENT

1. **Taylor JAM:** *Writing radiology reports in chiropractic.* J Can Chiro Assoc 34(1):30, 1990.
2. **Friedman PJ:** *Radiologic reporting: Structure* [Editorial]. AJR 140:171, 1983.
3. **Duke JS:** *What a consultant wants to know from a GP.* Practice Manag 85, 1986.
4. **Orrison WW, Nord TE, Kinard RE, et al.:** *The language of certainty: Proper terminology for the ending of the radiologic report.* AJR 145:1093, 1985.
5. **Renfrew DL, Franken EA, Berbaum KS, et al.:** *Error in radiology: Classification and lessons in 182 cases presented at a problem case conference.* Radiology 183:145, 1992.
6. **Doubilet P, Herman P:** *Interpretation of radiographs: Effect of clinical history.* AJR 137:1055, 1981.
7. **Baxter B, Ravindra H, Normann RA:** *Changes in lesion detectability caused by light adaptation in retinal photoreceptors.* Invest Radiol 17:394, 1982.

8. **Friedman PJ:** *Radiologic reporting: The hierarchy of terms* [Editorial]. AJR 140:402, 1983.
9. **Swensson RG, Hessel SJ, Herman PG:** *Omissions in radiology: Faulty search or stringent reporting criteria.* Radiology 123:563, 1977.
10. **Revak CS:** *Dictation of radiologic reports* [Letter]. AJR 141:210, 1983.
11. **Berlin L:** *Malpractice issues in radiology. Radiology reports.* AJR 169:943, 1997.
12. **Berlin L:** *Alliterative error.* AJR 174:925, 2000.
13. **Butt WP:** *Interpreting the spinal x-ray. 1.* Br J Hosp Med 40:46, 1988.
14. **Butt WP:** *Interpreting the spinal x-ray. 2.* Br J Hosp Med 40:124, 1988.
15. **Stoker DJ:** *Interpreting the skeletal x-ray.* Br J Hosp Med 40:143, 1988.
16. **Tuddenham WJ:** *Visual search, image organization, and reader error in roentgen diagnosis.* Radiology 78:694, 1962.
17. **Morrish HF, Messenger OJ:** *Medicolegal encounters in Canadian radiology.* Can Assoc Radiol J 41:259, 1990.
18. **Jaffe CC:** *Medical imaging, vision, and visual psychophysics.* Med Radiogr Photogr 60(1):1, 1984.
19. **Peterson DH:** *Chiropractic terminology: A report.* Am Chiro Assoc J 68, 1988.
20. **Wiltse LL, Winter RB:** *Terminology and measurement of spondylolisthesis.* J Bone Joint Surg 65A:768, 1983.
21. **Pitt MJ, Speer DP:** *Radiologic reporting of orthopedic trauma.* Med Radiogr Photogr 58:14, 1982.
22. **Pitt MJ, Speer DP:** *Radiologic reporting of skeletal trauma.* Radiol Clin North Am 28:247, 1990.
23. **Kundel HL, Revesz G:** *Lesion conspicuity, structured noise, and film reader error.* AJR 126:1233, 1976.
24. **Baxter B, Normann RA, Ravindra H:** *The effect of extraneous light on lesion detectability. A demonstration.* Invest Radiol 18:105, 1983.
25. **Hartley B:** *Personal communication,* 1980.
26. **Kanizsa G:** *Subjective contours.* Sci Am 234:48, 1976.
27. **Oestrich AE:** *Use of the cupped hand for improved viewing of radiographs.* Radiology 143:563, 1982.
28. **Clinger NJ, Hunter TB, Hillman BJ:** *Radiology reporting: Attitudes of referring physicians.* Radiology 169:825, 1988.
29. **Berlin L:** *Malpractice issues in radiology. Communication of the significant but not urgent finding.* AJR 168:329, 1997.

REPORT VARIATIONS FOR CT AND MRI

1. **Friedman PJ:** *Radiologic reporting: Structure* [Editorial]. AJR 140:171, 1983.
2. **Albertyn LE. Reporting:** *The neglected aspect of the new imaging modalities.* Austral Radiol 35:340, 1991.

RISK MANAGEMENT STRATEGIES IN INTERPRETATION AND REPORT WRITING

1. **Conley RN, Nicholson DL:** *How to avoid a malpractice suit* [Roentgen Brief]. ACA Council Roentgenology, 1983.
2. **Taylor JAM:** *Writing radiology reports in chiropractic.* J Can Chiro Assoc 34(1):30, 1990.
3. **Chapman-Smith D:** *Referral letters and written reports.* Chiro Rep 6(2):1, 1992.
4. **Sellers T:** *Diagnostic or non diagnostic?* Am Chiro Assoc J 22:65, 1988.
5. **Albertyn LE. Reporting:** *The neglected aspect of the new imaging modalities.* Austral Radiol 35:340, 1991.
6. **Berlin L:** *Malpractice issues in radiology. Admitting mistakes.* AJR 172:879, 1999.
7. **Ridley LJ:** *Guide to the radiology report.* Austral Radiol 46:366, 2002.
8. **Berlin L:** *Malpractice issues in radiology. Communication of the significant but not urgent finding.* AJR 168:329, 1997.
9. **Renfrew DL, Franken EA, Berbaum KS, et al.:** *Error in radiology: Classification and lessons in 182 cases presented at a problem case conference.* Radiology 183:145, 1992.

10. **Fischer HW:** *Better communication between the referring clinician and radiologist.* Radiology 146:845,1983.
11. **LaFortune M, Broton G, Baudouin JL:** *The radiological reports: What is useful for the referring physician?* Can Assoc Radiol J 39:140, 1988.
12. **McLoughlin RF, So CB, Gray RR, Brandt R:** *Radiology reports: How much descriptive detail is enough?* AJR 165:803, 1995.
13. **Cassidy JD, Mierau DR, Nykoliation JW, et al.:** *Medical-chiropractic correspondence.* J Can Chiro Assoc 29(1):29, 1985.
14. **Clinger NJ, Hunter TB, Hillman BJ:** *Radiology reporting: Attitudes of referring physicians.* Radiology 169:825, 1988.
15. **Friedman PJ:** *Radiologic reporting: Structure* [Editorial]. AJR 140:171, 1983.
16. **Revak CS:** *Dictation of radiologic reports* [Letter]. AJR 141:210, 1983.
17. **Berlin L:** *Malpractice issues in radiology. Pitfalls of the vague radiology report.* AJR 174:1511, 2000.
18. **Grigg ERN:** *The Trail of the Invisible Light.* Springfield, IL, Charles C Thomas, 1965.
19. **Ewing CL:** *Medicolegal radiology.* Radiology 63:673, 1954.
20. **Tuddenham WJ:** *Visual search, image organization, and reader error in roentgen diagnosis.* Radiology 78:694, 1962.
21. **Martin LFW:** *The language of the radiology report: A response.* AJR 176:1597, 2001.
22. **Saxton HM:** *Should radiologists report on every film?* [Editorial]. Clin Radiol 45:1, 1992.
23. **Stone PC, Hilton CF:** *Medicolegal aspects of emergency department radiology.* Radiol Clin North Am 30:495, 1992.
24. **Pringle RG:** *Missed fractures.* Injury 4:311, 1972.
25. **de Lacey G, Barker A, Harper J, et al.:** *An assessment of the clinical effects of reporting accident and emergency radiographs.* Br J Radiol 53:304, 1980.
26. **Siegle RL, Baram EM, Reuter SR, et al.:** *Rates of disagreement in imaging interpretation in a group of community hospitals.* Acad Radiol 5:148, 1998.
27. **Hirtle RL:** *Chiropractic malpractice.* ACA J Chiro 35, 1987.
28. **Morrish HF, Messenger OJ:** *Medicolegal encounters in Canadian radiology.* Can Assoc Radiol J 41:259, 1990.
29. **Vincent CA, Driscoll PA, Audley RJ, et al.:** *Accuracy of detection of radiographic abnormalities by junior doctors.* Arch Emerg Med 5; 101, 1988.
30. **Berlin JW, Berlin L:** *Radiographic errors: When and why do we make them? How can we eliminate or minimize them? Do they constitute malpractice?* Contemp Diagn Radiol 24(7):1, 2001.
31. **Berlin L, Hendrix RW:** *Perceptual errors and negligence.* AJR 170:863, 1998.
32. **Berlin L:** *Alliterative error.* AJR 174:925, 2000.
33. **Hunter TB:** *Radiologic reports: Structure and review* [Editorial]. AJR 142:647, 1984.
34. **McCulloch JA, Waddell G:** *Variation of the lumbosacral myotomes with bony segmental anomalies.* J Bone Joint Surg 62B:475, 1980.
35. **Hopper KD, Rosetti GF, Edmiston RB, et al.:** *Diagnostic radiology peer review: A method inclusive of all interpreters of radiographic examinations regardless of specialty.* Radiology 180:557, 1991.
36. **Levin DC:** *The practice of radiology by nonradiologists: Cost, quality and utilization issues.* AJR 162:513, 1994.
37. **Kline TJ, Kline TS:** *Radiologists, communication and Resolution 5: A medicolegal issue.* Radiology 184:131, 1992.
38. **Berlin L:** *Malpractice issues in radiology. Radiology reports.* AJR 169:943, 1997.
39. **Berlin L:** *Malpractice issues in radiology. Communication of the urgent finding.* AJR 166:513, 1996.
40. **Taylor JAM, Clopton P, Bosch E, et al.:** *Interpretation of abnormal lumbosacral spine radiographs.* Spine 20:1147, 1995.
41. **Rhea J, Potsaid M, Deluca S:** *Errors of interpretation as elicited by a quality audit of an emergency radiology facility.* Radiology 132:277, 1979.
42. **Halvorsen JG, Kunian A:** *Radiology in family practice: a prospective study of 14 community practices.* Fam Med 22:112, 1990.
43. **Scheuger SR:** *Introduction to critical review of roentgenograms.* Phys Therapy 68:1114, 1988.
44. **Inglis B:** *New Zealand Royal Commission on Chiropractic.* New Zealand Government Printer, 1979.
45. **Hunter TB, Boyle RR:** *The value of reading the previous radiology report* [Letter]. AJR 150:697, 1988.
46. **Berlin L:** *Possessing ordinary knowledge.* AJR 172:879, 1999.
47. **Berlin L:** *Must radiographs be compared with all previous radiographs, or only with the most recently obtained radiographs.* AJR 174:611, 2000.

SECOND-OPINION SPECIALTY RADIOLOGY REVIEWS

1. **Vincent CA, Driscoll PA, Audley RJ, et al.:** *Accuracy of detection of radiographic abnormalities by junior doctors.* Arch Emerg Med 5:101, 1988.
2. **Halvorsen JG, Kunian A:** *Radiology in family practice: A prospective study of 14 community practices.* Fam Med 22:112, 1990.
3. **Taylor JAM, Clopton P, Bosch E, et al.:** *Interpretation of abnormal lumbosacral spine radiographs.* Spine 20: 1147,1995.
4. **Taylor JAM:** *Writing radiology reports in chiropractic.* J Can Chiro Assoc 34(1):30, 1990.
5. **Saxton HM:** *Should radiologists report on every film?* [Editorial]. Clin Radiol 45:1, 1992.
6. **Craig JOMC:** *The Knox lecture: Radiology and the law.* Clin Radiol 40:343, 1989.
7. **Rose JF, Gallivan S:** *Plain film reporting in the UK.* Clin Radiol 44:192, 1991.

Radiographic Artifacts 16

Terry R. Yochum and Lindsay J. Rowe

INTRODUCTION

Since the early days of radiology, artifacts have appeared on radiographs. Actually, the first radiograph ever taken had an artifact present, a metallic ring on the patient's hand. Artifacts are a common cause of repeat radiographs; they often occur in unexpected places, with many peculiar internal objects being detected. Without a complete history, many unusual artifactual shadows cannot be adequately identified. This chapter is presented in atlas format, using a pictorial review of various artifacts. Few radiologic interpretation texts show any artifacts, despite their common occurrence. This fact provided the impetus for us to add this atlas to the book. No attempt at an in-depth discussion of the production or physics behind radiographic artifacts is intended in this chapter because the technical aspects are thoroughly covered in other texts. (1–4)

Adherence to detail, especially in patient preparation, factor selection, positioning, and darkroom technique, using state-of-the-art equipment, will reduce the chances for producing artifacts.

TECHNICAL

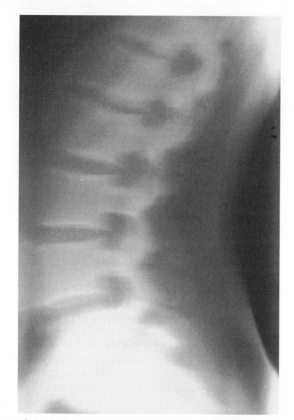

Figure 16-1 **MOTION PROBLEMS. Lateral Lumbar.** The image unsharpness was caused by patient movement.

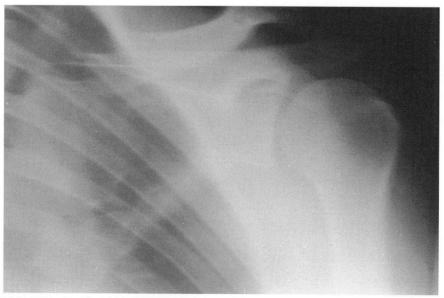

Figure 16-2 **MOTION PROBLEMS. AP Shoulder.** Patient motion blurred the final image of this shoulder. *COMMENT:* Motion is the greatest cause of image unsharpness on the final radiograph. (Courtesy of Felix G. Bauer, DC, DACBR(Hon), Sydney, Australia.)

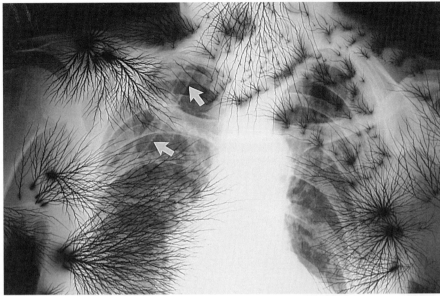

Figure 16-3 **STATIC ELECTRICITY. PA Chest.** This chest radiograph demonstrates a characteristic appearance of static electricity. Superimposed over the right upper thorax is a drainage tube (*arrows*).

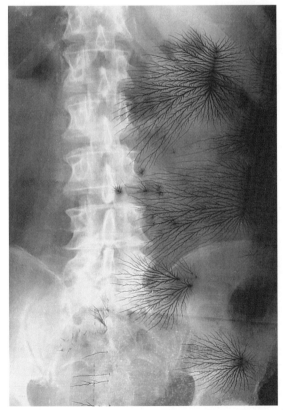

Figure 16-4 **STATIC ELECTRICITY. AP Lumbar.** The black streaks are static electricity markings on the radiograph. (Courtesy of Kenneth E. Yochum, DC, St. Louis, Missouri.)

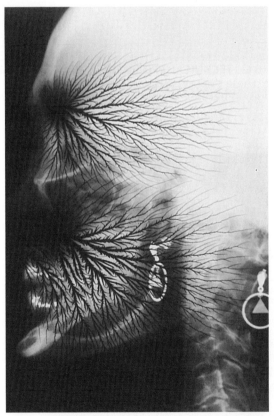

Figure 16-5 **STATIC ELECTRICITY. Lateral Cervical Skull.** The lightning-like black densities represent static electricity. *COMMENT:* This might make quite an advertisement for headaches. The metallic devices are earrings, which should always be removed when doing an x-ray examination of the skull or cervical spine.

TECHNICAL, *continued*

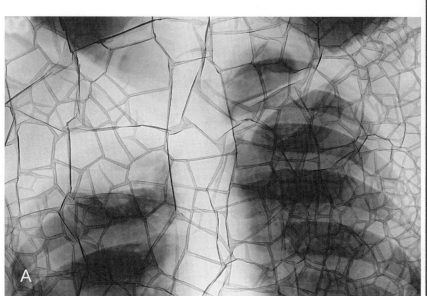

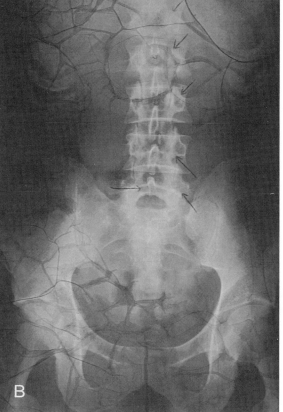

Figure 16-6 **TECHNICAL PROBLEMS. A. PA Chest. B. AP Lumbar.** These radiographs demonstrate a wrinkling of the film emulsion because of shrinkage of the film base over many years in storage. This process has been called *reticulation*. On panel A, note the opacity of the right lung apex secondary to thoracopneumoplasty.

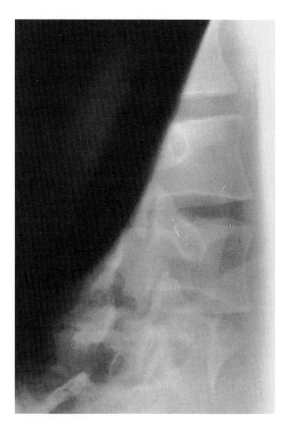

Figure 16-7 **DEVELOPMENT PROBLEMS. Oblique Lumbar.** The black area represents light exposure on the radiograph, which occurred sometime during the development process.

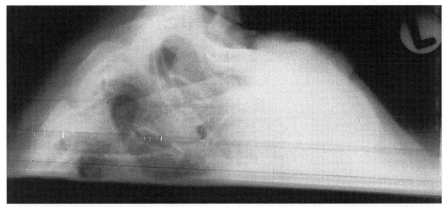

Figure 16-8 **DEVELOPMENT PROBLEMS. Lateral Cervico-Thoracic.** The lower portion of this radiograph was struck by light after the film was exposed to x-ray. *COMMENT:* This usually occurs as the film is entering the automatic processor and someone accidentally turns on the lights or opens the darkroom door too soon.

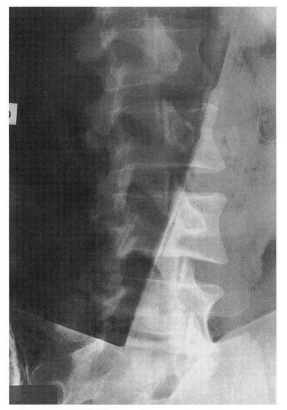

Figure 16-9 **DEVELOPMENT PROBLEMS. Oblique Lumbar.** The darkened area over this oblique lumbar radiograph is caused by two films overlapping in the development procedure. *COMMENT:* This may occur if insufficient time is allowed between feeding film through the automatic processor.

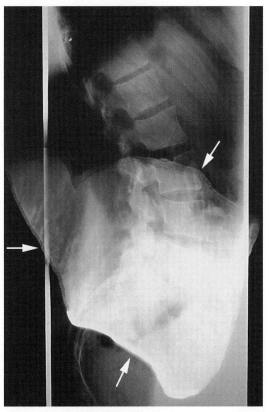

Figure 16-10 **DEVELOPMENT PROBLEMS. Lateral Lumbar.** The artifact on the radiograph represents an area where two radiographs became attached to each other in the manual developing process (*arrows*). This has been called a *kissing defect.* (Courtesy of Felix G. Bauer, DC, DACBR(Hon), Sydney, Australia.)

TECHNICAL, *continued*

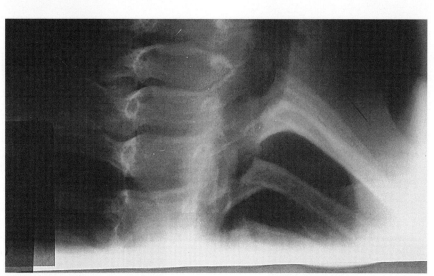

Figure 16-11 **DEVELOPMENT PROBLEMS. Oblique Upper Thoracic.** The gray area on the lower portion of this oblique radiograph was not developed because of the low level of developer solutions in the manual developing tank.

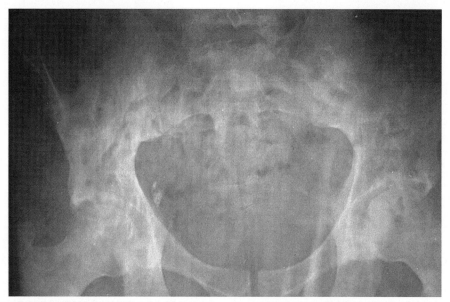

Figure 16-12 **DEVELOPMENT PROBLEMS. AP Pelvis.** These mottled streak-like densities occurred in the manual processing of this film from lack of proper agitation of the developer during the developing process.

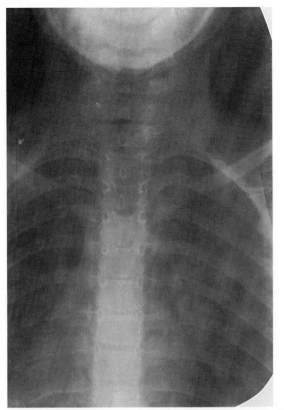

Figure 16-13 **DEVELOPMENT PROBLEMS. AP Thoracic.** The washed-out image was caused by exhausted developer solution. *COMMENT:* This occurs when the developer oxidizes or has been replenished with water rather than with fresh chemicals. (Courtesy of Felix G. Bauer, DC, DACBR(Hon), Sydney, Australia.)

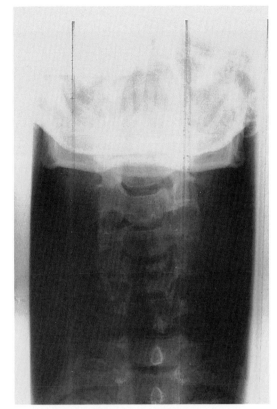

Figure 16-14 **DEVELOPMENT PROBLEMS. AP Lower Cervical.** The abnormal marks represent artifacts from dirty rollers in an automatic film processor.

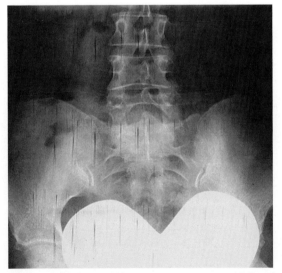

Figure 16-15 **DEVELOPMENT PROBLEMS. AP Pelvis.** The streaked marks represent a processing artifact from the crossover deflector guides in the automatic processor. The radiopaque heart-shaped structure is an ovarian gonadal shield that was positioned too low.

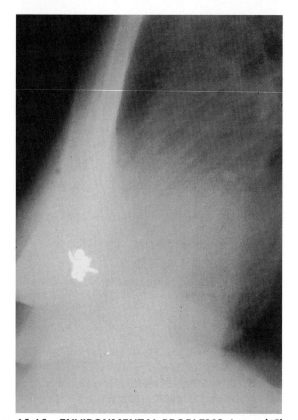

Figure 16-16 **ENVIRONMENTAL PROBLEMS. Lateral Chest.** This is a very unusual artifact; a bee was trapped inside the cassette, blocking the luminescence of the screen in this area. *COMMENT:* Other more common objects, such as slivers of paper, may cause a similar radiopaque artifact. We hope you have gotten the *beeline* on this case. (Courtesy of Richard T. Coade, MIR, DC, Kempsey, Australia.)

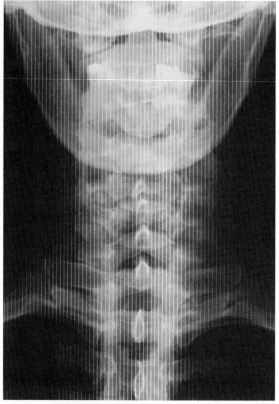

Figure 16-17 **TECHNICAL PROBLEMS. AP Lower Cervical.** The vertical radiopaque lines represent grid lines. This occurs when the grid does not move during the exposure because of a nonfunctioning bucky mechanism or a short exposure time.

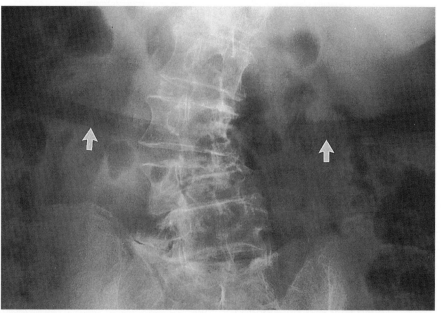

Figure 16-18 **PATIENT PROBLEMS. Lumbar Spine.** The broad radiolucent stripe across the abdomen (*arrows*) represents compression of the fat across the waistline by the patient's undergarment. *COMMENT:* This can be avoided by having the patient remove all undergarments and wear an examination gown when being radiographed through the abdomen. (Courtesy of Donald M. Kuppe, DC, Denver, Colorado.)

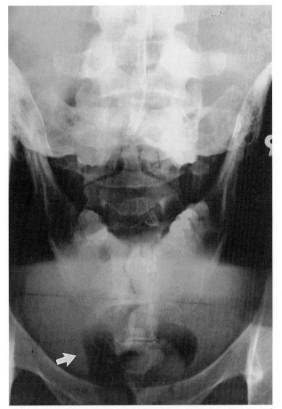

Figure 16-19 **TECHNICAL PROBLEMS. AP Open Mouth and AP Pelvis.** This film shows a double exposure of an AP open mouth and AP lumbosacral projection. *COMMENT:* Note the tampon above the pubic rami (*arrow*). (Courtesy of one of our students, Melbourne, Australia.)

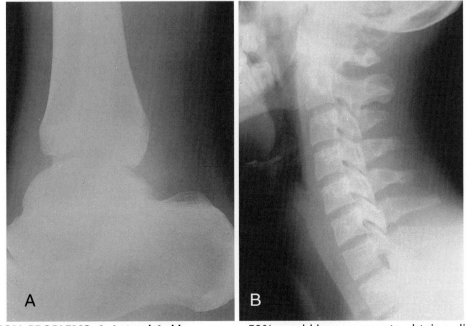

Figure 16-20 **TECHNICAL PROBLEMS. A. Lateral Ankle. B. Lateral Cervical.** Both films were underexposed. An increase in the milliamperage seconds (mAs) by approximately 50% would be necessary to obtain a diagnostic film; the kilovoltage peak (kVp) should not be altered.

TECHNICAL, *continued*

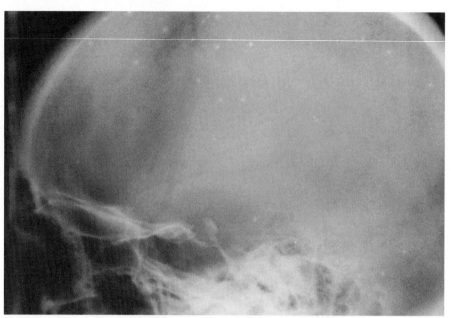

Figure 16-21 **TECHNICAL PROBLEMS. Lateral Skull.** The white, circular areas scattered throughout the skull depict screen artifacts. These represent areas within the screen where the phosphor is no longer adequate and illumination is not occurring properly. *COMMENT:* It is time to replace these screens.

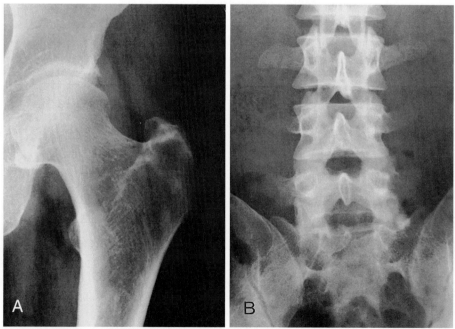

Figure 16-22 **TECHNICAL PROBLEMS. A. AP Hip. B. AP Lumbar.** The blurred appearance of the bony trabeculae in the area of the greater trochanter is the result of poor film–screen contact. Similar blurred areas are seen scattered throughout the lumbar spine, as a result of underlying poor film–screen contact. (Courtesy of John A. M. Taylor, DC, DACBR, Seneca Falls, New York.)

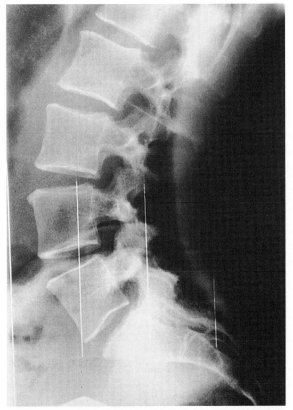

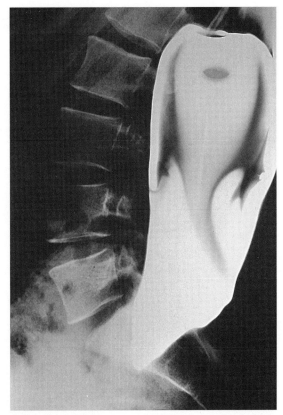

Figure 16-23 **DEVELOPMENT PROBLEMS. Lateral Lumbar.** The white lines seen on this radiograph are scratches from the crossover racks during automatic processing. (Courtesy of John A. M. Taylor, DC, DACBR, Seneca Falls, New York.)

Figure 16-24 **DEVELOPMENT PROBLEMS. Lateral Lumbar.** This is a large *kissing* artifact, which occurs when two films stick together during the developing process. (Courtesy of Felix G. Bauer, DC, DACBR(Hon), Sydney, Australia.)

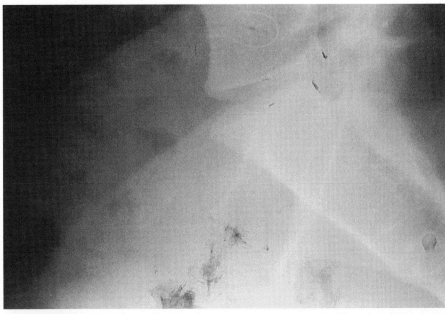

Figure 16-25 **TECHNICAL PROBLEMS. Lateral Lumbosacral.** The blackened, smudge-like areas on the lower aspect of the film represent fingerprints. *COMMENT:* During the development process the film should be handled at the corners; otherwise such fingerprint artifacts will occur. (Courtesy of John A. M. Taylor, DC, DACBR, Seneca Falls, New York.)

TECHNICAL, *continued*

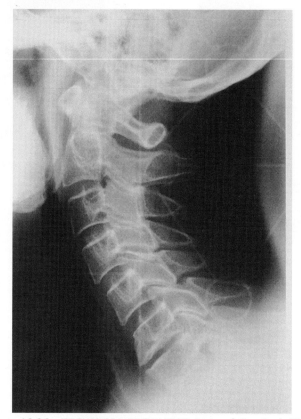

Figure 16-26 **TECHNICAL PROBLEMS. Lateral Cervical.** The peculiar circular and linear radiopaque densities have occurred as a result of the cassette being placed in the cassette chamber backward. (Courtesy of John A. M. Taylor, DC, DACBR, Seneca Falls, New York.)

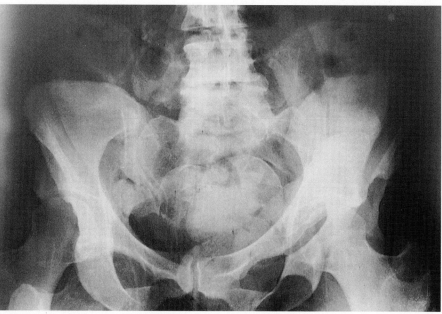

Figure 16-27 **DOUBLE EXPOSURE. AP Pelvis.** The peculiar appearance of the radiograph is the result of a double exposure. (Courtesy of Beverly L. Harger, DC, DACBR, Portland, Oregon.)

THERAPEUTIC

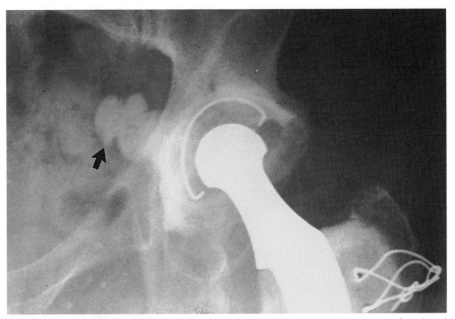

Figure 16-28   **POST-JOINT REPLACEMENT. AP Hip.** This patient has undergone a hip joint replacement procedure from which some of the acrylic bone cement (*arrow*) leaked into the pelvic basin. (Courtesy of Richard W. Jackson, DO, St. Louis, Missouri.)

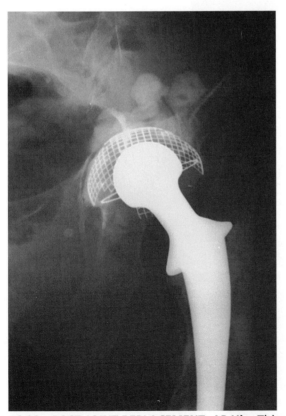

Figure 16-29   **POST-JOINT REPLACEMENT. AP Hip.** This patient has had a total hip replacement with a metallic prosthesis. (Courtesy of John M. Bauler, DC, Clovis, New Mexico.)

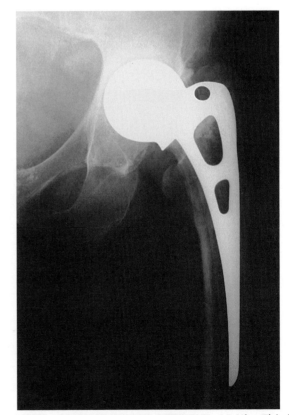

Figure 16-30   **POST-JOINT REPLACEMENT. AP Hip.** This is a Moore's hip prosthesis.

THERAPEUTIC, *continued*

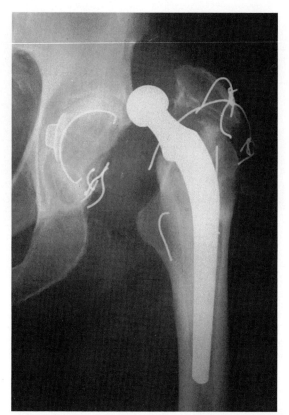

Figure 16-31   **POST-JOINT REPLACEMENT. Hip.** This patient's prosthetic hip has luxated and some of the wires have broken.

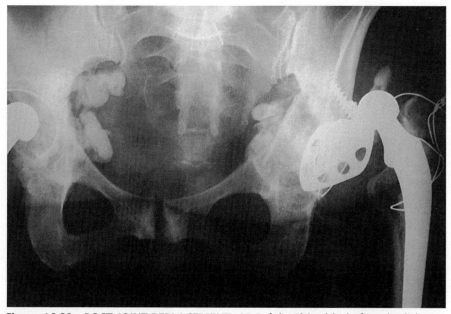

Figure 16-32   **POST-JOINT REPLACEMENT. AP Pelvis.** This elderly female dislocated her hip prosthesis after a recent fall. (Courtesy of David B. Taylor, DC, Joliet, Illinois.)

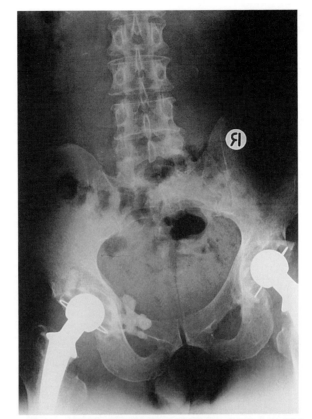

Figure 16-33 **POST-JOINT REPLACEMENT. AP Pelvis.** This patient has had a bilateral total hip replacement. The radiopaque densities adjacent to the left acetabulum represent leaking of acrylic bone cement.

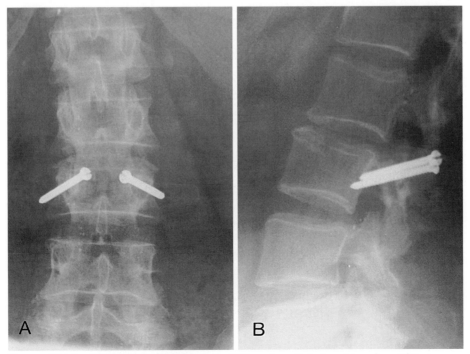

Figure 16-34 **POST-ARTHRODESIS. A. AP Lumbar. B. Lateral Lumbar.** This patient underwent arthrodesis with threaded screws through the inferior facets of L2 and into the pars and pedicles of L3.

THERAPEUTIC, *continued*

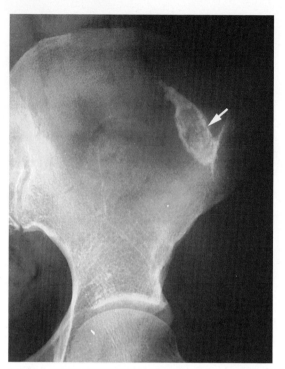

Figure 16-35   **POST-INJECTION. AP Hip.** This calcified injection granuloma (*arrow*) is in the soft tissues of the buttocks.

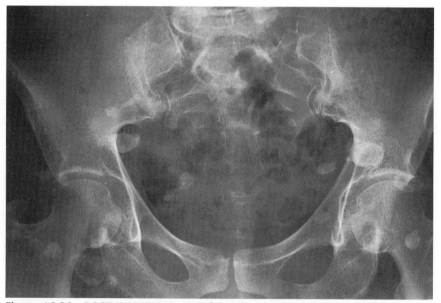

Figure 16-36   **POST-INJECTION. AP Pelvis.** The circular calcific densities represent sites of vitamin B$_{12}$ injections in the buttocks (injection granulomas).

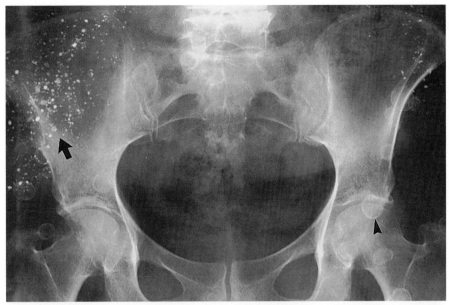

Figure 16-37   **POST-INJECTION. AP Pelvis.** There are two forms of artifacts on this pelvic radiograph. The metallic densities are the sequelae of heavy metal injections for syphilis (*arrow*). The calcific cystic densities are injection granulomas (*arrowhead*). (Courtesy of Richard A. Bergeron, DC, Golden, Colorado.)

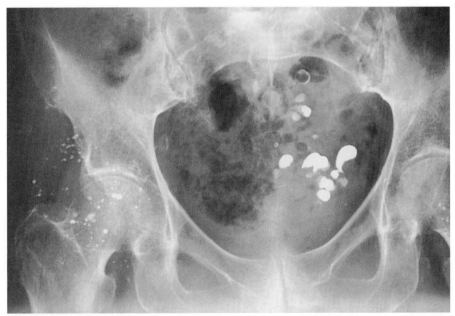

Figure 16-38   **POST-INJECTION. AP Pelvis.** The radiopaque densities about the hip joint and in the buttocks represent injection sites with metallic residuals. The radiopaque densities in the pelvic basin represent residual barium in diverticula of the sigmoid colon. (Courtesy of Beverly L. Harger, DC, DACBR, Portland, Oregon.)

THERAPEUTIC, *continued*

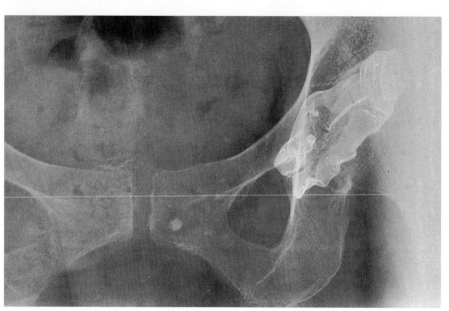

Figure 16-39 **SURGICAL MATERIAL. AP Pelvis.** The radi-opaque density represents a wire mesh substance called *tan-* *talum,* a non-corrosive, malleable metal used for making prosthetic appliances.

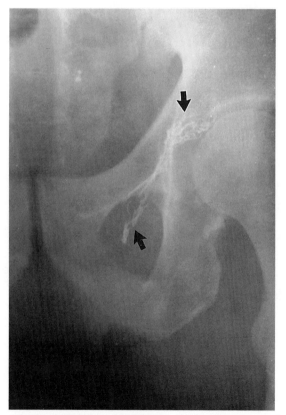

Figure 16-40 **SURGICAL MATERIAL. AP Pelvis.** The metallic densities (*arrows*) represent residual surgical material from repair of an inguinal hernia.

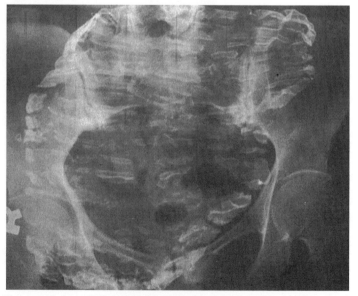

Figure 16-41 **SURGICAL MATERIAL. AP Hip.** The fragmented radiopaque densities represent surgical gauze (tantalum mesh) left within the abdomen. (Courtesy of Terry D. Sandman, DC, DACBR, Chicago, Illinois.)

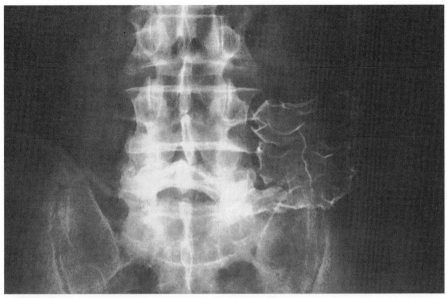

Figure 16-42 **SURGICAL MATERIAL. AP Pelvis.** This is tantalum wire mesh, which was used to repair abdominal hernias years ago.

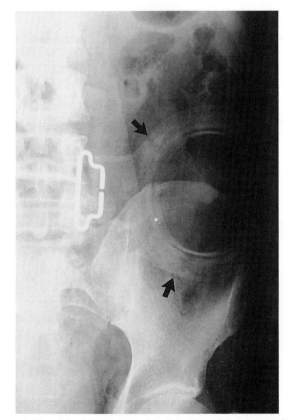

Figure 16-43 **COLOSTOMY BAG. AP Hip.** This patient had his colon removed for ulcerative colitis; the artifact present is a colostomy bag (*arrows*).

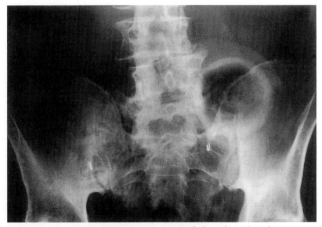

Figure 16-44 **BLADDER BAG. AP Pelvis.** The circular radiopaque density represents a bladder bag. (Courtesy of Paul E. Price, DC, Erie, Denver, Colorado.)

THERAPEUTIC, *continued*

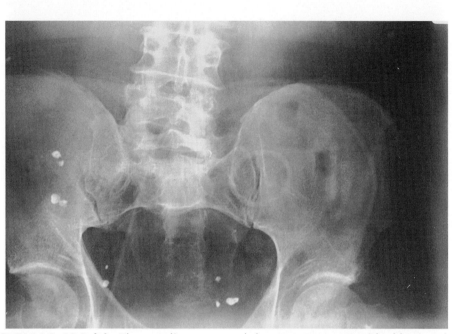

Figure 16-45 **COLOSTOMY BAG. AP Pelvis.** The peculiar spherical artifactual radiopacity represents a colostomy bag. The scattered radiopaque densities in the opposite lower abdomen represent residual barium in diverticula of the colon. (Courtesy of Beverly L. Harger, DC, DACBR, Portland, Oregon.)

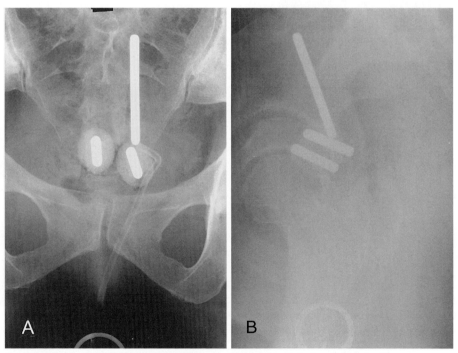

Figure 16-46 **CANCER TREATMENT. A. AP Pelvis. B. Lateral Pelvis.** These metallic artifacts are radium implants used in the treatment of carcinoma of the cervix.

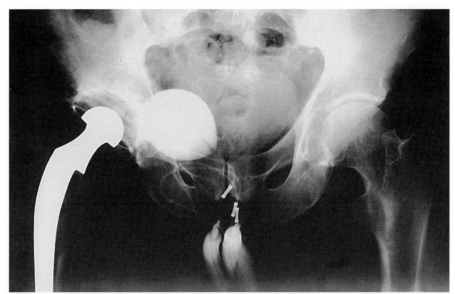

Figure 16-47 **IMPOTENCE PUMP. AP Hip.** This male patient has a metallic hip prosthesis. The device seen in the groin and scrotal region is a surgically implanted mechanical pump used in cases of impotence. (Courtesy of Kenneth E. Yochum, DC, St. Louis, Missouri.)

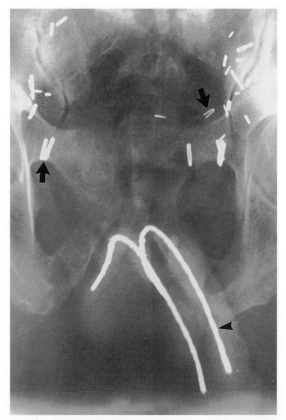

Figure 16-48 **THERAPEUTIC DEVICE. AP Pelvis.** This 62-year-old male had a prostatectomy; the remnant surgical clips are present (*arrows*) as well as a penile implant for impotence (*arrowhead*). (Courtesy of John K. Hyland, DC, DACBR, DABCO, Denver, Colorado.)

THERAPEUTIC, *continued*

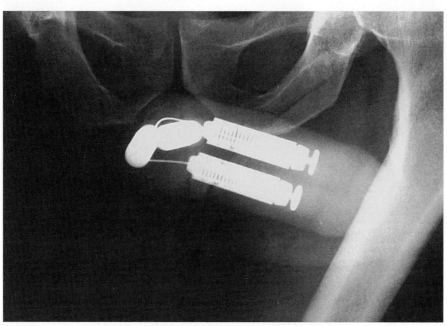

Figure 16-49 **PENILE IMPLANT. AP Pelvis.** This patient has a mechanical impotence pump within the penis. (Courtesy of Jerry Collyer, RT(R), Denver, Colorado.)

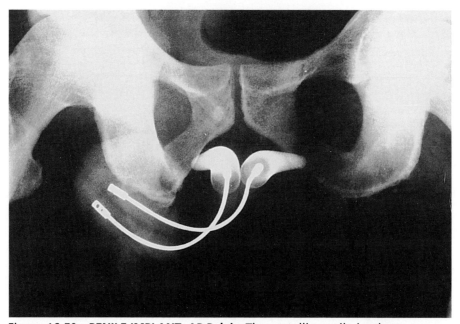

Figure 16-50 **PENILE IMPLANT. AP Pelvis.** The metallic penile implants are used to treat impotency. (Courtesy of John A. M. Taylor, DC, DACBR, Seneca Falls, New York.)

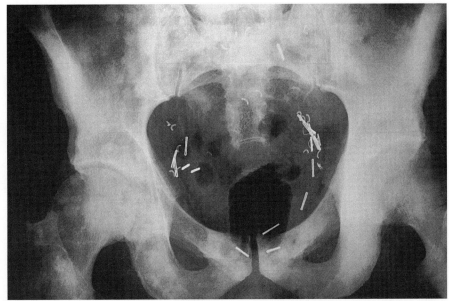

Figure 16-51   **SURGICAL MATERIAL. AP Pelvis.** The metallic surgical clips are the densities left after this patient had a prostatectomy for carcinoma. Note the typical blastic metastatic lesions scattered throughout the pelvis and femora. (Courtesy of Gary E. Spears, DC, Denver, Colorado.)

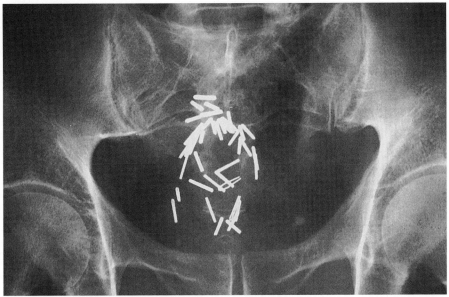

Figure 16-52   **SURGICAL MATERIAL. AP Pelvis.** This 60-year-old male patient has had a colonic resection for carcinoma of the sigmoid colon. The metallic clips are the results of the surgery. (Courtesy of Donald M. Kuppe, DC, Denver, Colorado.)

THERAPEUTIC, *continued*

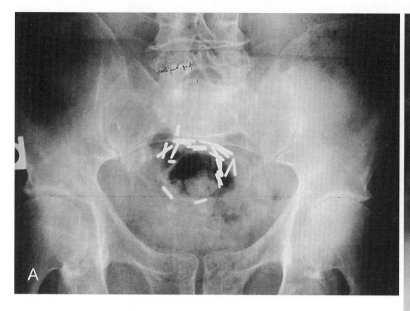

Figure 16-53 **SURGICAL MATERIAL. A. AP Pelvis. B. Lateral Sacrum.** The metallic clips anterior to the sacrum represent residual surgical clips for colon resection. (Courtesy of Beverly L. Harger, DC, DACBR, Portland, Oregon.)

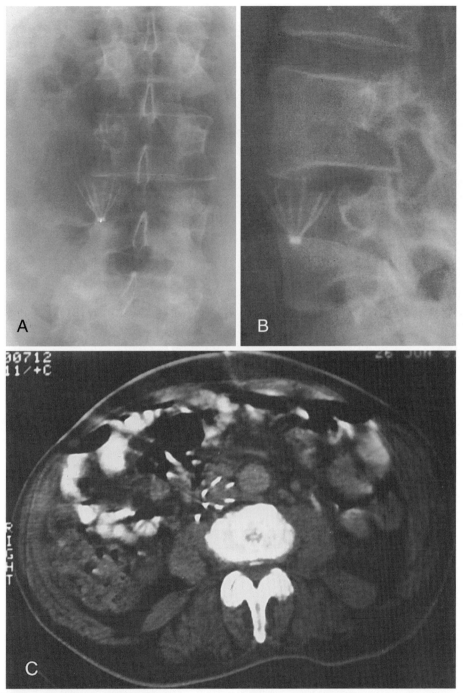

Figure 16-54   **IVC UMBRELLA FILTER. A. AP Lumbar. B. Oblique Lumbar.** The metallic artifact represents an umbrella filter in the inferior vena cava (IVC), used to catch blood clots. **C. CT, Axial Abdomen.** This CT scan of another patient shows an IVC filter in place. *COMMENT:* These filters are used in patients with a long-standing history of thrombophlebitis. (Panels A and B courtesy of Nathaniel S. Wirt, PhD, DC, and Gary M. Guebert, DC, DACBR, St. Louis, Missouri. Panel C courtesy of Steven P. Brownstein, MD, Springfield, New Jersey.)

THERAPEUTIC, *continued*

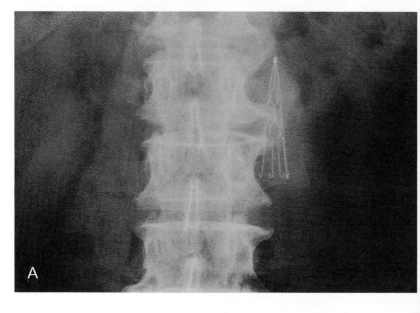

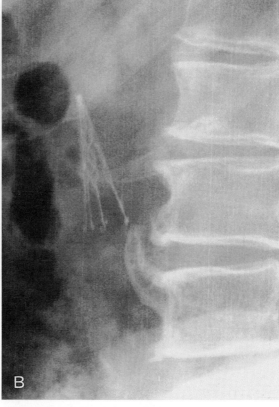

Figure 16-55 **IVC UMBRELLA FILTER. A. AP Lumbar. B. Lateral Lumbar.** This metallic umbrella filter is placed in the inferior vena cava to capture emboli from the lower extremities in patients with thrombophlebitis. (Courtesy of John C. Slizeski, DC, Denver, Colorado.)

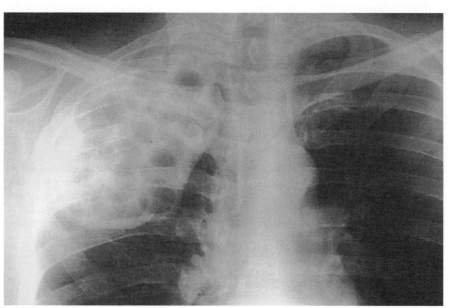

Figure 16-56 **PLOMBAGE PROCEDURE. PA Chest.** A right upper lobectomy for tuberculosis has been performed; the tissue was replaced with implanted lucite balls, referred to as a *plombage procedure. COMMENT:* This technique was employed to reduce mediastinal shift and maintain anatomic relationships within the chest. (Courtesy of William E. Litterer, DC, DACBR, Fellow, ACCR, Elizabeth, New Jersey.)

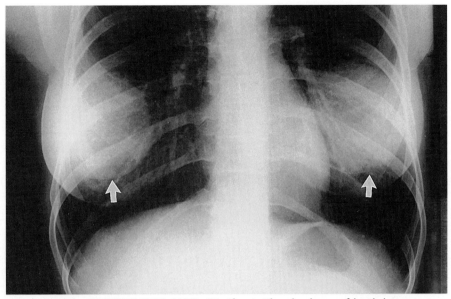

Figure 16-57 **SILICONE IMPLANTS. PA Chest.** The shadows of both breasts appear very dense because of the presence of silicone implants (*arrows*).

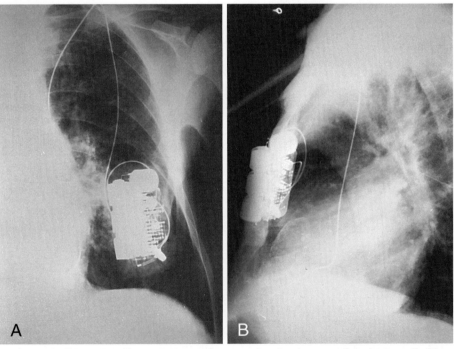

Figure 16-58 **CARDIAC PACEMAKER. A. PA Chest. B. Lateral Chest.** This metallic artifact is a subcutaneously placed pacemaker in the anterior chest wall. (Courtesy of M. Bruce Farkas, DO, J.D., Chicago, Illinois.)

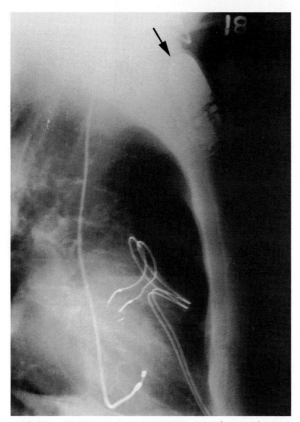

Figure 16-59 **CARDIAC PACEMAKER. PA Chest.** There is a cardiac pacemaker (*arrow*) in the subcutaneous tissues of the anterior chest wall. The string-like radiopacities represent the cardiac leads from the pacemaker. (Courtesy of Donald Resnick, MD, San Diego, California.)

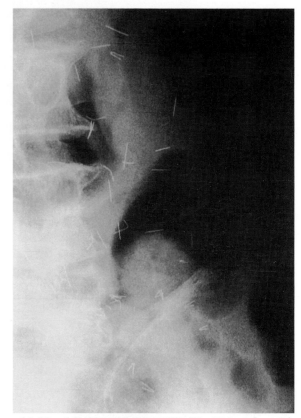

Figure 16-60 **ACUPUNCTURE NEEDLES. AP Lumbar.** Observe the multiple radiopaque densities scattered throughout the subcutaneous tissues. These represent broken-off acupuncture needles in a patient who has had many acupuncture treatments. (Courtesy Ian Chen, MD, San Francisco, California.)

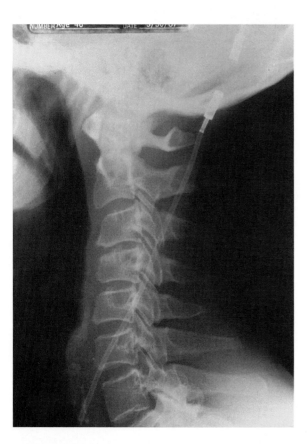

Figure 16-61 **CSF SHUNT. Lateral Cervical.** A plastic tube can be seen passing obliquely within the soft tissues of the neck from the skull into the thorax and eventually to the abdominal cavity. This is referred to as a *ventriculoperitoneal shunt*, used to manage high-pressure hydrocephalus by redirecting cerebrospinal fluid produced in the lateral ventricles of the brain into the peritoneal cavity where it is resorbed.

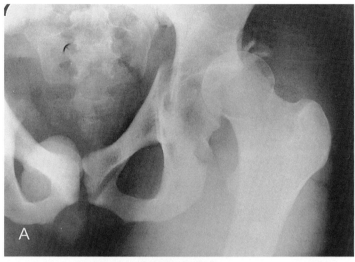

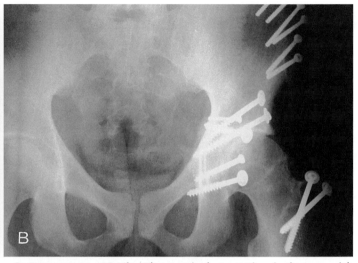

Figure 16-62 **SURGICAL MATERIAL. A. Presurgery AP Hip.** This young football player was tackled, which caused a fracture of the acetabulum and dislocation of the femur.

B. Postsurgery AP Hip. The surgical correction is shown, with multiple screw fixations. (Courtesy of James C. Wagner, DC, Denver, Colorado.)

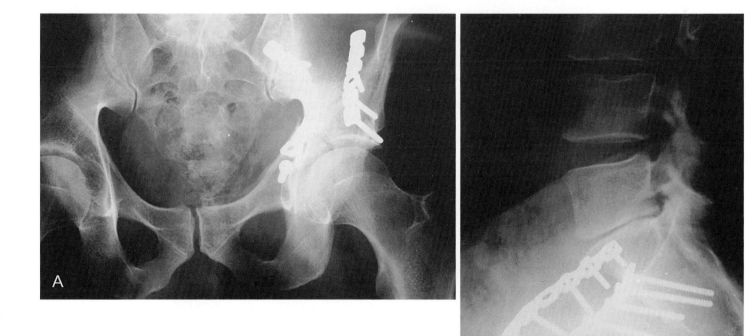

Figure 16-63 **FRACTURED ACETABULUM: SURGICAL MATERIAL. A. AP Hip. B. Lateral Lumbar.** This patient was in an automobile accident and sustained a fractured acetabulum and ilium. The surgical screw fixation was successful in the treatment of this patient. *COMMENT:* Patients with these types of injuries are often destined to develop premature degenerative osteoarthritis of the hip as a post-traumatic sequela.

THERAPEUTIC, *continued*

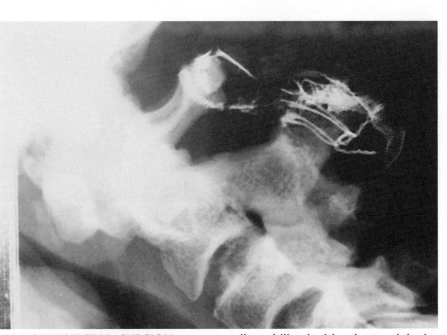

Figure 16-64 **TRANSVERSE LIGAMENT TEAR: SURGICAL MATERIAL. Lateral Cevical Flexion.** This patient had a history of atlantoaxial instability owing to disruption of the transverse ligament after a motor vehicle accident. This was surgically stabilized with atlantoaxial wires (Gallie's procedure). Seen here, the wires have since broken, rendering the upper cervical complex once again unstable. (Courtesy of Richard Edmonds, BAppSc (Chiro), Melton, Australia.)

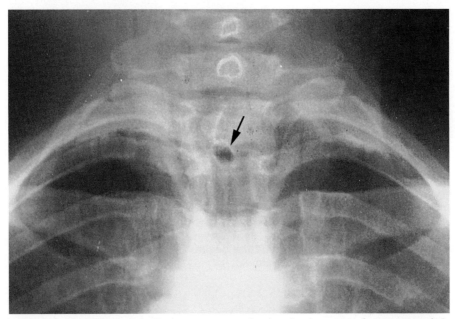

Figure 16-65 **STOMA: SURGICAL MATERIAL. PA Chest.** There is a peculiar circular radiolucent area seen at the T2–T3 level (*arrow*). This represents the stoma in a patient who has had surgery for cancer of the throat. (Courtesy of George E. Springer, DC, Clearwater, Florida.)

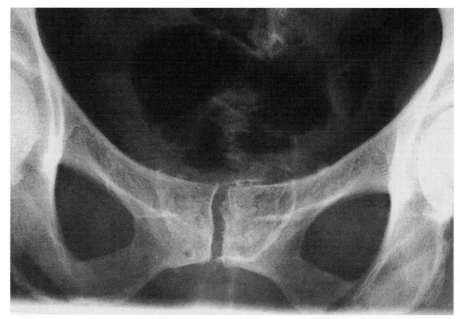

Figure 16-66 **PHARMACEUTICAL MATERIAL. AP Pubes.** The peculiar radiopaque oval density seen outlining the rectum represents zinc oxide, from chronic abuse of suppositories.

(Courtesy of Jeffrey R. Thompson, DC, DACBR, Houston, Texas, and David Jones, DC, Spokane, Washington.)

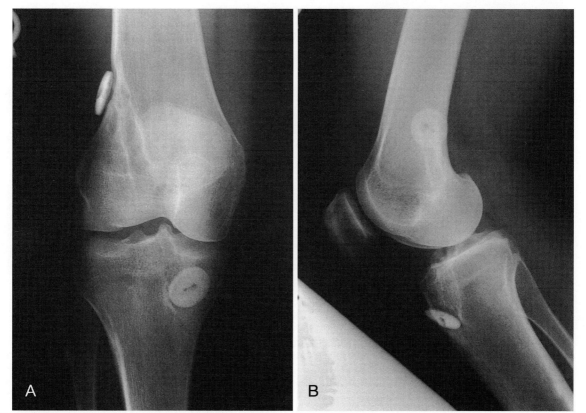

Figure 16-67 **SURGICAL MATERIAL. A. AP Knee. B. Lateral Knee.** The radiopaque button-like densities represent the areas of securing the surgical synthetic replacement for the anterior cruciate ligament. Notice that there is a curvilinear density tracking through the bone, making a passageway for the reconstructed synthetic anterior cruciate ligament. (Courtesy of Tyrone Wei, DC, DACBR, Portland, Oregon.)

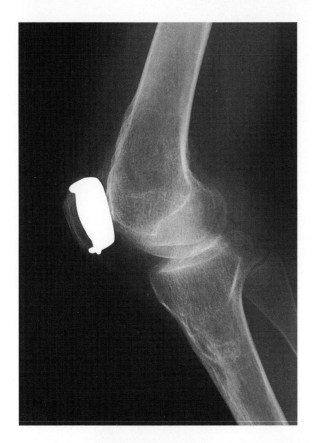

Figure 16-68   **PROSTHETIC PATELLA. Lateral Knee.** This patient had a previous fracture of the patella with subsequent retropatellar degenerative disease, creating an unstable joint. A prosthetic metallic patella has been inserted to stabilize the knee. (Courtesy of William E. Litterer, DC, DACBR, Fellow, ACCR, Elizabeth, New Jersey.)

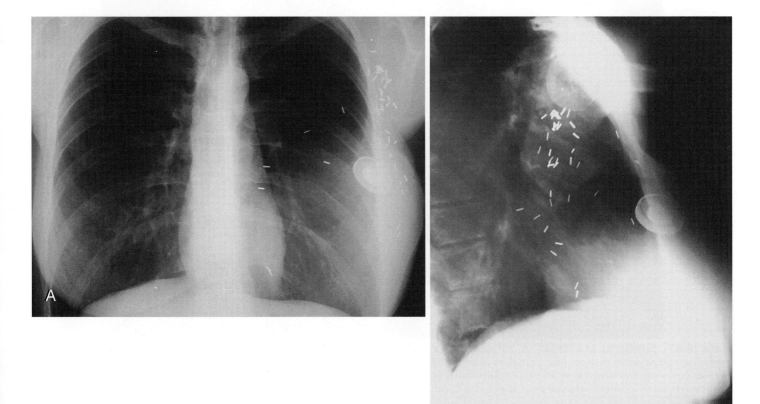

Figure 16-69   **MASTECTOMY AND BREAST RECONSTRUCTION. A. PA Chest. B. Lateral Chest.** The multiple surgical sutures and circular artifacts are the result of a partial mastectomy and breast reconstruction.

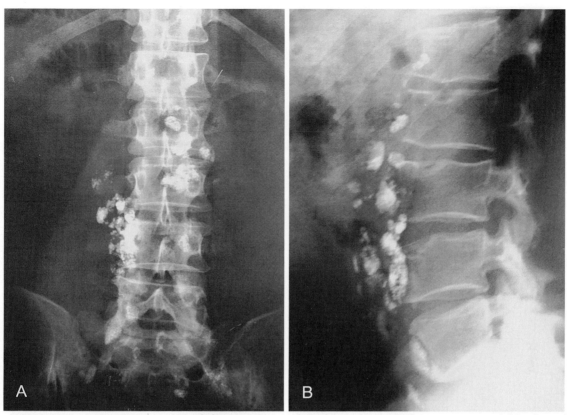

Figure 16-70 **HODGKIN'S LYMPHOMA. A. AP Abdomen. B. Lateral Abdomen.** There is residual contrast from a recent lymphangiogram present in the retroperitoneal lymph nodes in a young patient who has been diagnosed with Hodgkin's lymphoma. Retained contrast material in these lymph nodes for an extended period suggests underlying organic pathology. (Courtesy of Richard M. Nuzzi, DC, Boulder, Colorado.)

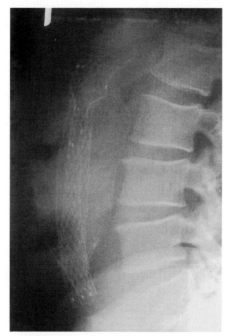

Figure 16-71 **SURGICAL MATERIAL: ABDOMINAL AORTIC ANEURYSM. Lateral Abdomen.** Observe the calcified abdominal aortic aneurysm. Treatment of the aneurysm was performed by inserting a graft to lessen the likelihood of rupture. This patient has done well postsurgically. (Courtesy of Anne P. Odenweller, DC, Baton Rouge, Louisiana.)

THERAPEUTIC, *continued*

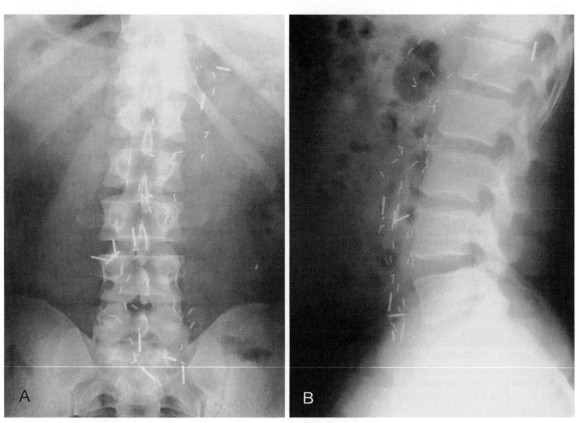

Figure 16-72 **HODGKIN'S LYMPHOMA. A. AP Abdomen. B. Lateral Abdomen.** There are multiple scattered metallic surgical clips in the area of the retroperitoneal lymph nodes from T12 through the lumbosacral junction. These represent the sequelae from surgical treatment for Hodgkin's lymphoma. (Courtesy of Richard L. Green, DC, Boston, Massachusetts.)

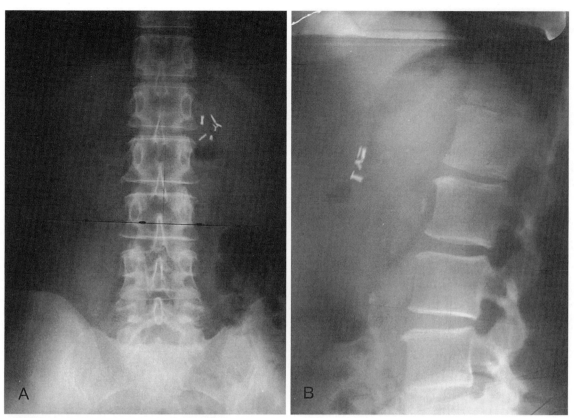

Figure 16-73   **CHOLECYSTECTOMY CLIPS. A. AP Abdomen. B. Lateral Abdomen.** Observe the cholecystectomy clips in the right upper quadrant of the abdomen. (Courtesy of Ralph E. Brewer, DC, Denver, Colorado.)

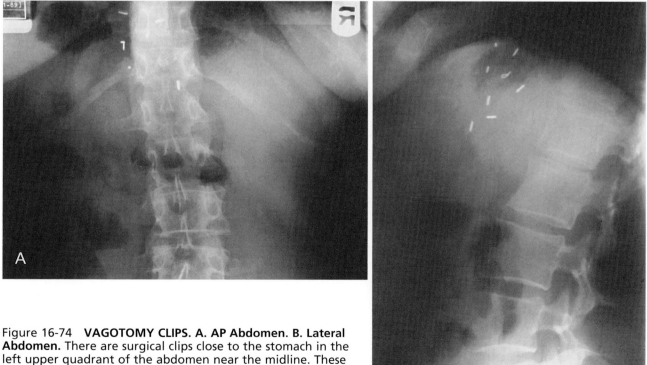

Figure 16-74   **VAGOTOMY CLIPS. A. AP Abdomen. B. Lateral Abdomen.** There are surgical clips close to the stomach in the left upper quadrant of the abdomen near the midline. These represent vagotomy clips in a patient who had a history of chronic ulcers. (Courtesy of George E. Springer, DC, Clearwater, Florida.)

THERAPEUTIC, *continued*

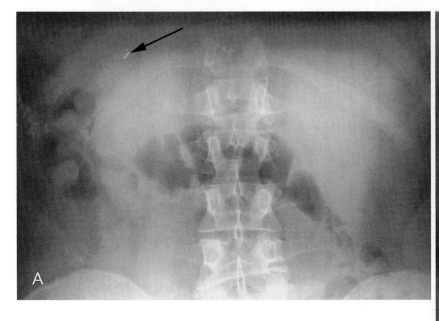

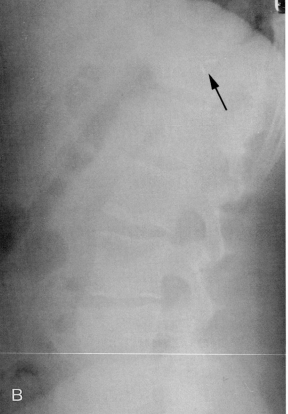

Figure 16-75   **SPLENECTOMY CLIPS. A. AP Abdomen. B. Lateral Abdomen.** There are surgical clips in the posterior aspect of the left upper quadrant of the abdomen (*arrows*). These represent splenectomy clips. There is an old fracture of the L4 vertebral body. **COMMENT:** This patient underwent severe trauma to the spine and abdomen with a ruptured spleen, which led to splenectomy. (Courtesy of George E. Springer, DC, Clearwater, Florida.)

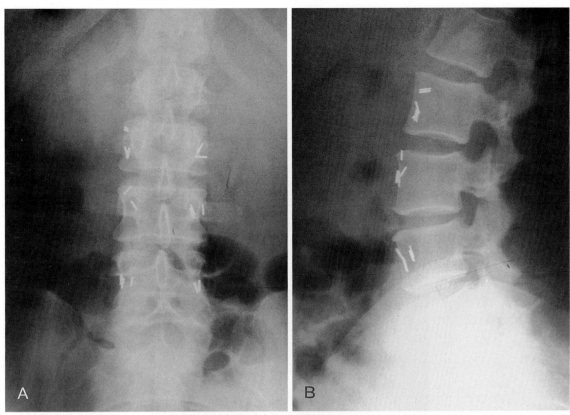

Figure 16-76 **SYMPATHECTOMY CLIPS. A. AP Lumbar. B. Lateral Lumbar.** Surgical clips are present bilaterally from L3 through S1. These represent the remnants of a sympathec- tomy, which was performed on this patient for severe Raynaud's phenomenon. (Courtesy of Eugene Ver Meer, DC, Denver, Colorado.)

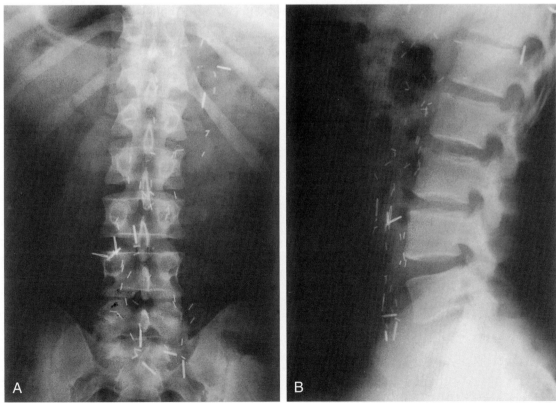

Figure 16-77 **HODGKIN'S LYMPHOMA. A. AP Lumbar. B. Lateral Lumbar.** There are bilateral surgical metallic clips in this patient who has Hodgkin's lymphoma. (Courtesy of Richard L. Green, DC, Boston, Massachusetts.)

THERAPEUTIC, *continued*

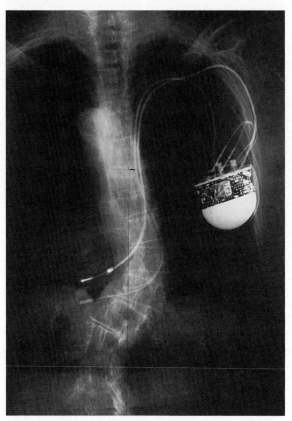

Figure 16-78 **CARDIAC PACEMAKER. PA Chest.** There is a cardiac pacemaker present in the subcutaneous tissues of the anterior chest wall with appropriate cardiac leads in place. (Courtesy of Paul Van Wyk, DC, Denver, Colorado.)

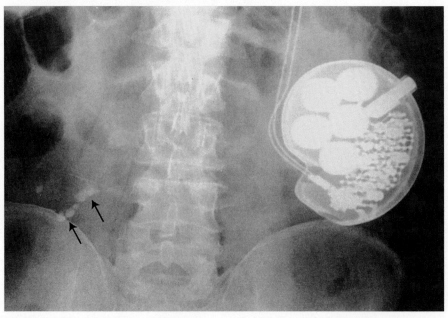

Figure 16-79 **CARDIAC PACEMAKER. AP Lumbar.** There is a cardiac pacemaker present in the subcutaneous tissues of the abdomen. Of incidental notation are some calcified abdominal lymph nodes present in the lower abdomen (*arrows*).

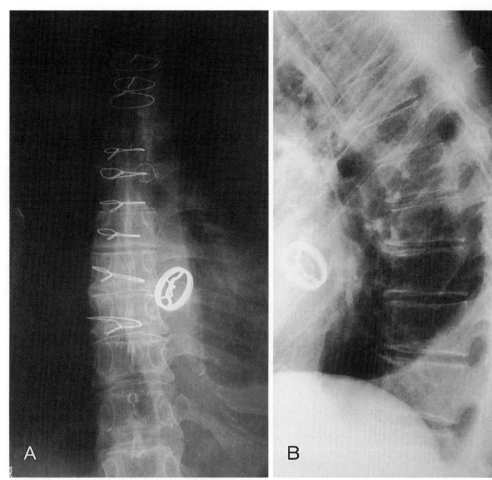

Figure 16-80   **PROSTHETIC MITRAL VALVE. A. AP Thoracic. B. Lateral Thoracic.** There is a prosthetic mitral valve seen on both radiographs. Observe the surgical sternal sutures used to close the chest wall following thoracotomy. (Courtesy of James M. Kolodziej, DC, Denver, Colorado.)

THERAPEUTIC, *continued*

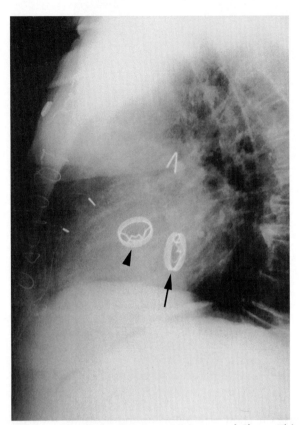

Figure 16-81 **DOUBLE HEART VALVES. Lateral Chest.** This patient has prosthetic mitral (*arrow*) and aortic (*arrowhead*) valves. There are surgical clips within the chest and wire sutures in the area of the sternum from the thoracotomy procedure. (Courtesy of Donald Resnick, MD, San Diego, California.)

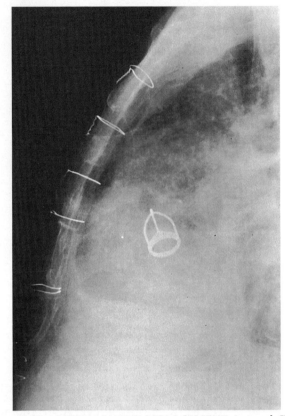

Figure 16-82 **MITRAL VALVE REPLACEMENT. Lateral Chest.** A prosthetic mitral valve is seen. Observe the surgical sternal sutures used to close the chest from thoracotomy. (Courtesy of William E. Litterer, DC, DACBR, Fellow, ACCR, Elizabeth, New Jersey.)

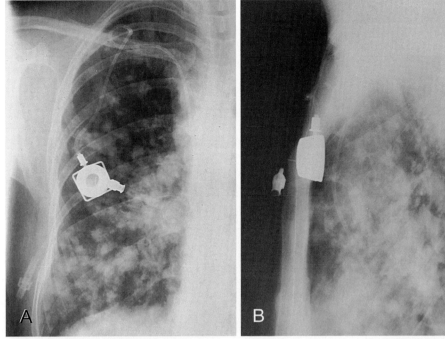

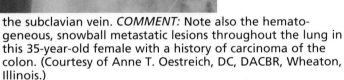

Figure 16-83 **HICKMAN INFUSION CATHETER. A. PA Chest. B. Lateral Chest.** This subcutaneously placed metallic device represents a Hickman continuous infusion catheter. This is used for administering time-released chemotherapy to cancer patients, providing an intravenous route without repeated intravenous injections. The catheter is deposited into the subclavian vein. *COMMENT:* Note also the hematogeneous, snowball metastatic lesions throughout the lung in this 35-year-old female with a history of carcinoma of the colon. (Courtesy of Anne T. Oestreich, DC, DACBR, Wheaton, Illinois.)

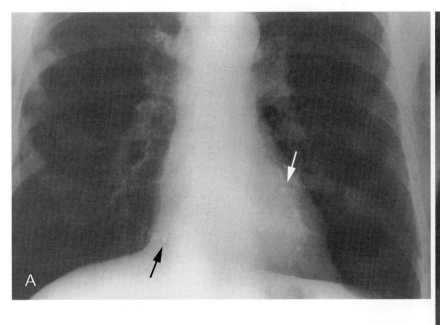

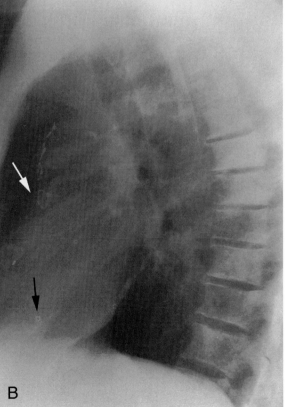

Figure 16-84 **CORONARY BYPASS: SURGICAL MATERIAL. A. PA Chest. B. Lateral Chest.** Observe the metallic densities in and about the cardiac silhouette (*arrows*). These represent the residuals of surgical intervention for coronary bypass. Notice also that the ribs and thoracic spine demonstrate an ill-defined radiopacity with altered trabeculae, representing prostatic metastatic carcinoma. (Courtesy of Gregory W. Peterson, DC, Denver, Colorado.)

THERAPEUTIC, *continued*

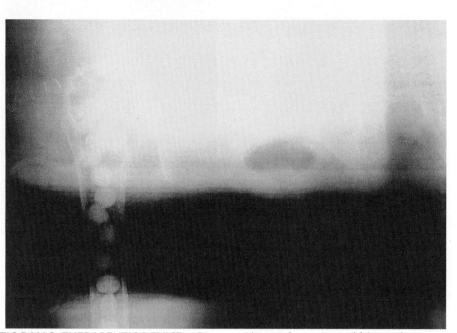

Figure 16-85 **ANTIBIOTIC BALLS: THERAPEUTIC DEVICE. AP Femur.** The circular radiopaque densities present within the shaft of the femur represent antibiotic balls, which are used for prevention of osteomyelitis. *COMMENT:* This patient is going to have a total hip replacement, and these have been packed in the femoral shaft before the final placement of the prosthesis.

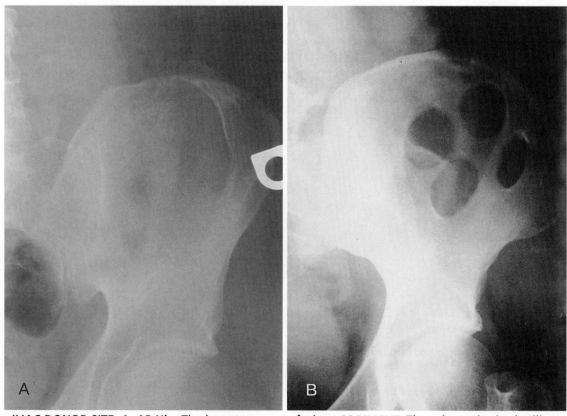

Figure 16-86 **ILIAC DONOR SITE. A. AP Hip.** The lucent deformity is a post-traumatic sequela from a surgical donor site. **B. AP Hip.** The four radiolucent holes in the ilium represent a surgical donor site for a patient who required a spinal fusion. *COMMENT:* These lucencies in the ilium should not be confused with any underlying organic pathology. The surgical history is important in the complete evaluation of any patient.

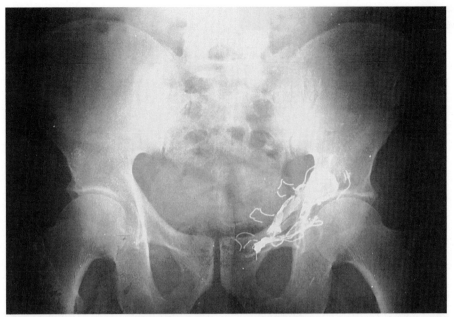

Figure 16-87 **INGUINAL HERNIA: SURGICAL MATERIAL. AP Pelvis.** The metallic densities present in the inguinal area represent surgical repair for an inguinal hernia. The surgical wire mesh is present to inhibit hernia recurrence.

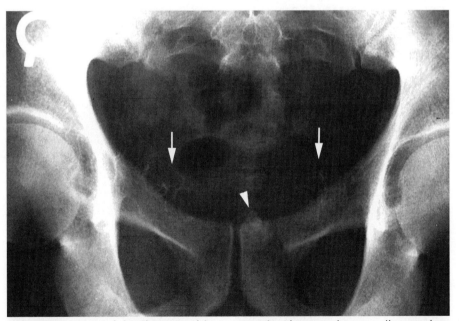

Figure 16-88 **SURGICAL MATERIAL. AP Pelvis.** There are bilateral surgical wires in the area of the inguinal canal (*arrows*), representing the remnants of inguinal hernia repair. Also noted are small, granular calcifications present in the prostate gland (*arrowhead*). (Courtesy of W. B. Champion, DC, Wainwright, Alberta, Canada.)

THERAPEUTIC, *continued*

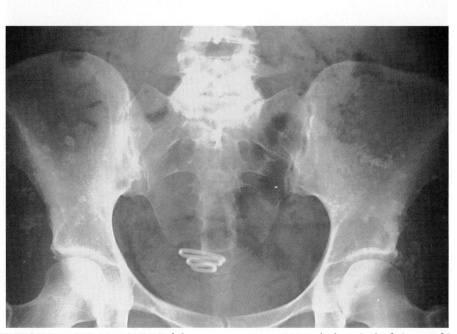

Figure 16-89 **POST-INJECTION GRANULOMAS. AP Pelvis.**
There are multiple cystic calcifications present in the muscles of the buttocks, representing injection granulomas. These most often occur in patients who receive multiple injections over an extended period of time. Of incidental notation is a metallic intrauterine device within the pelvic basin. (Courtesy of Lynton G. F. Giles, DC, PhD, Townsville, Queensland, Australia.)

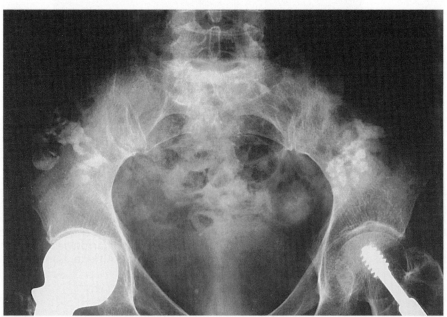

Figure 16-90 **POST-INJECTION GRANULOMAS AND POST-JOINT REPLACEMENT. AP Pelvis.** The dense radiopaque calcifications seen superimposed over both ilia are in the soft tissues of the buttocks and represent injection granulomas. There has been a total hip replacement on the patient's right, and a metallic rod stabilization pin placed in the left femur for previous fracture of the femoral neck. (Courtesy of Mark W. Terry, DC, DABCO, Centralia, Illinois.)

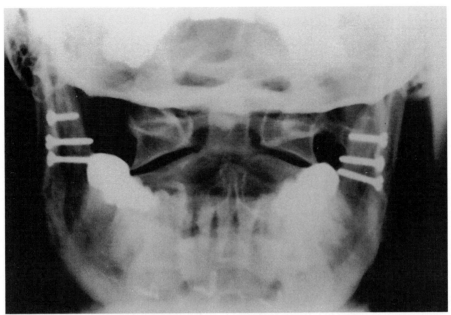

Figure 16-91   **MANDIBLE FRACTURE: SURGICAL REPAIR. AP Open Mouth.** This patient had a previous bilateral fracture of the mandible, which has been surgically repaired with screw fixation. (Courtesy of Kevin J. Determan, DC, Rapid City, South Dakota.)

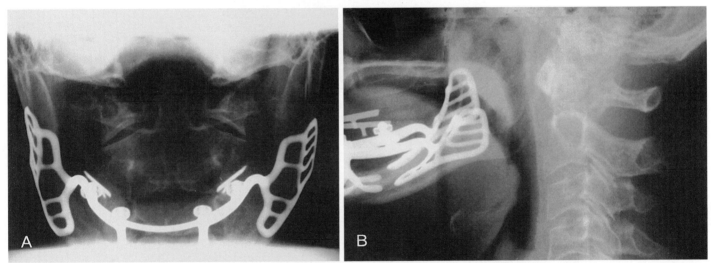

Figure 16-92   **MANDIBULAR PROSTHESIS. A. AP Open Mouth. B. Lateral Cervical.** This patient has had a severe bilateral comminuted fracture of the mandible. In order to reconstruct the mandible, sophisticated, wired prosthetic implants have been placed. (Courtesy of Gregory W. Peterson, DC, Denver, Colorado.)

THERAPEUTIC, *continued*

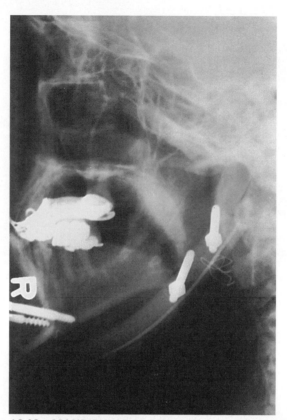

Figure 16-93 **MANDIBULAR PROSTHESIS. Lateral Mandible.** This patient has a mandible prosthesis following resection of the mandible for a malignant tumor. (Courtesy of James J. Holland, DC, DABCO, Carmichael, California.)

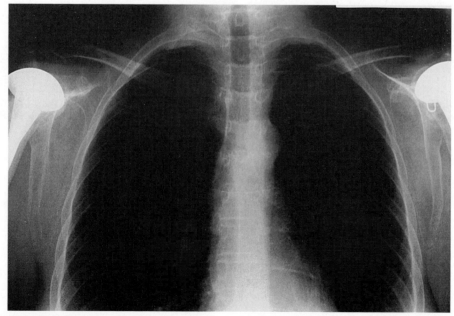

Figure 16-94 **POST-JOINT REPLACEMENT. PA Chest.** There have been bilateral total shoulder replacements with prosthetic humeral heads. Notice the tapering of the distal clavicles with resorption of bone and overall osteopenia consistent with this patient's long-standing rheumatoid arthritis. The shoulder replacements occurred as a result of extensive rheumatoid arthritis at both glenohumeral articulations. (Courtesy of Brian A. Howard, DC, MD, Charlotte, North Carolina.)

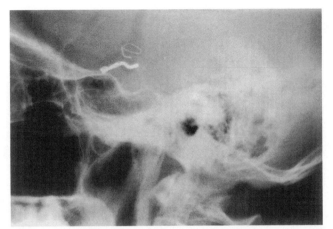

Figure 16-95 **INTERNAL CAROTID ANEURYSM REPAIR: SURGICAL MATERIAL. Lateral Skull.** There is metallic postsurgical material in the suprasellar area. These are the sequelae from previous surgical intervention for the treatment of an internal carotid artery aneurysm. (Courtesy of Steven J. Gaunya, DC, Southbridge, Massachusetts.)

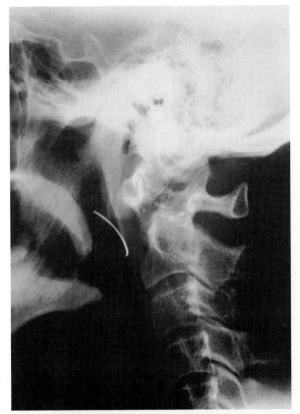

Figure 16-96 **POST-TONSILLECTOMY: SURGICAL MATERIAL. Lateral Cervical.** There is a surgical hook present in the area of the oropharynx, which had broken off during a tonsillectomy procedure years ago. This patient, incidentally, also has an os odontoideum with atlantoaxial subluxation of C1 upon C2. (Courtesy of Gary E. Spears, DC, Denver, Colorado.)

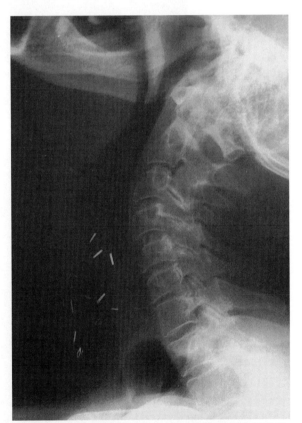

Figure 16-97 **THYROIDECTOMY: SURGICAL MATERIAL. Lateral Cervical Extension.** Observe the metallic clips present anterior to the lower cervical spine, which represents surgical intervention for removal of the thyroid gland (thyroidectomy). (Courtesy of Paul Van Wyk, DC, Denver, Colorado.)

THERAPEUTIC, *continued*

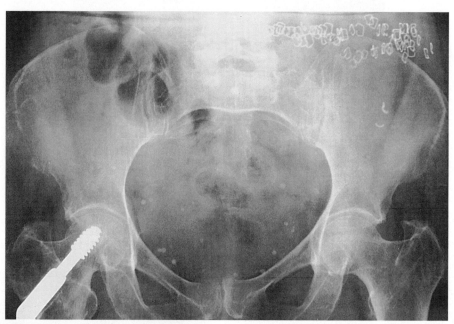

Figure 16-98 SURGICAL MATERIAL. AP Pelvis. The surgical metallic clips in the abdomen are from a previous laparotomy. There has also been a metallic screw fixation device placed within the left hip. (Courtesy of Beverly L. Harger, DC, DACBR, Portland, Oregon.)

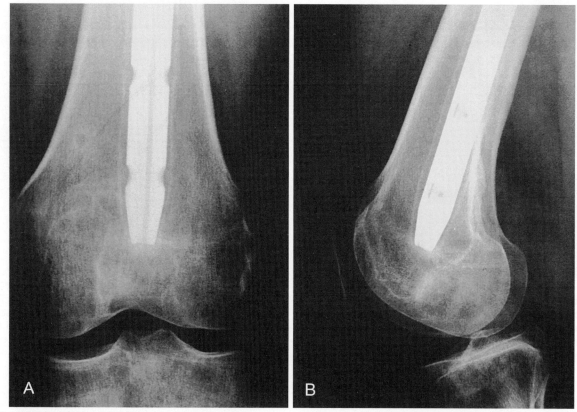

Figure 16-99 INTRAMEDULLARY ROD. A. AP Femur. B. Lateral Femur. The distal aspect of an intramedullary rod is visualized in the lower femur. Observe the radiolucent tracking appearance adjacent to the metallic rod, suggesting that there is some instability of the rod itself. (Courtesy of Michael S. Barry, DC, DACBR, Denver, Colorado.)

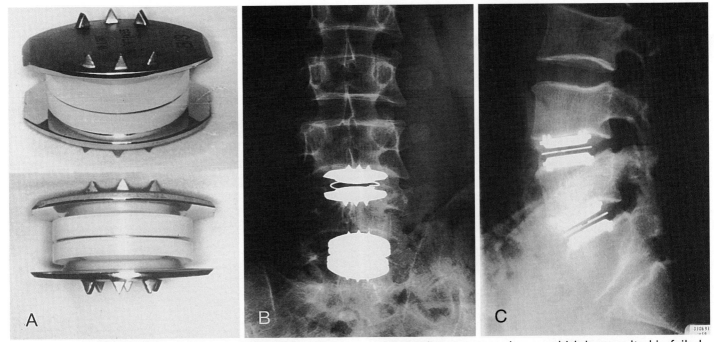

Figure 16-100   **DISC REPLACEMENT. A. Link Charité Prosthesis. B and C. Link Charité Prosthesis, Lumbar Spine.** The Link Charité intervertebral disc replacement prosthesis was designed for use between the lumbar vertebrae. This modular system is based on the low-friction principle and consists of two endplates made of a cobalt–chromium alloy, together with a sliding core. This unique implant permits near normal physiologic movements of the lumbar segments. Indications for such a prosthesis may be vertebral segmental instability, which is either singular or multiple, and postdiscectomy syndrome, which has resulted in failed back syndrome. The preservation of anatomic function using this endoprosthesis may be a more favorable alternative to spinal fusion. The implants are available in various sizes, together with special instruments for the implantation. This implant is MRI compatible. *COMMENT:* These implants are used throughout Europe, primarily in Germany and France, and have met with great therapeutic success. (Courtesy of Siegfried Brunner, Link America, Inc., Denville, New Jersey.)

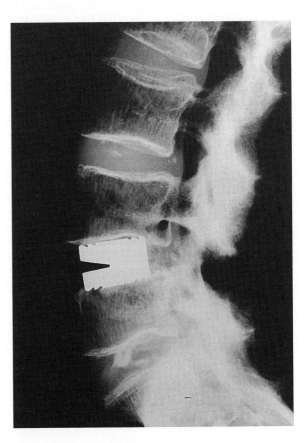

Figure 16-101   **DISC REPLACEMENT. Lumbar Spine Specimen Radiograph.** A Danek disc prosthesis has been implanted at the L4–L5 level in this anatomic specimen. The prosthesis is made of stainless steel and is MRI compatible. (Courtesy of Kenneth A. Pettine, MD, Loveland, Colorado.)

THERAPEUTIC, *continued*

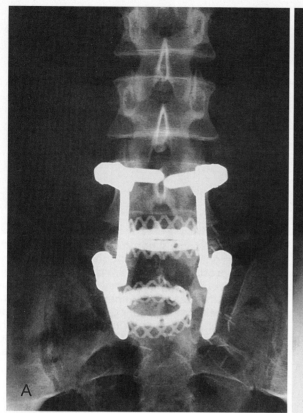

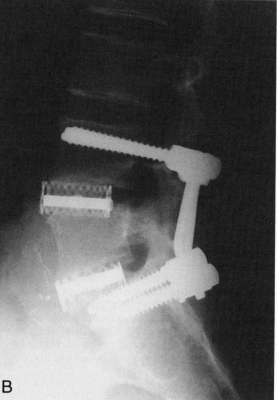

Figure 16-102   **ARTHRODESIS: MOSS CAGE. A. AP Lumbar. B. Lateral Lumbar.** This patient has had a 360° anterior and posterior spinal fusion. A Moss cage has been placed within the L4/L5 and L5/S1 disc space. This cage is made of titanium and serves to resist torsion and rotational forces, helping ensure fusion. The cage is filled with allograft decalcified bone in the hope that irritation of the cage on the vertebral end-plates will generate a reactive change to secure vertebral fusion. There has been a posterior pedicle fixation with screws in place. The metallic clips anterior to the lumbar vertebrae represent vascular clips and are a sequela from the previous surgical intervention. (Courtesy of Kenneth A. Pettine, MD, Loveland, Colorado.)

SURGICAL

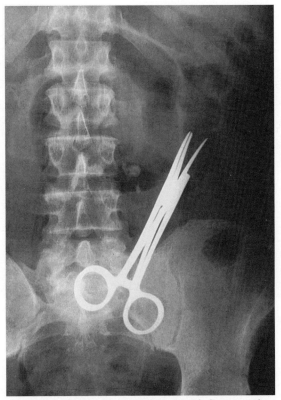

Figure 16-103 **SURGICAL MISHAP. AP Abdomen.** These surgical clamps were left in the abdomen of a patient after surgery for appendicitis.

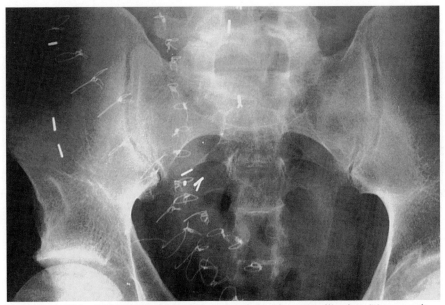

Figure 16-104 **SURGICAL SUTURES. AP Pelvis.** The metallic densities are the result of surgical sutures. (Courtesy of Kenneth E. Yochum, DC, St. Louis, Missouri.)

SURGICAL, *continued*

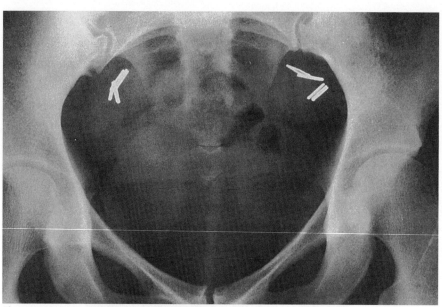

Figure 16-105 **POST-CONTRACEPTIVE SURGERY. AP Pelvis.** These metallic clips represent a tubal ligation.

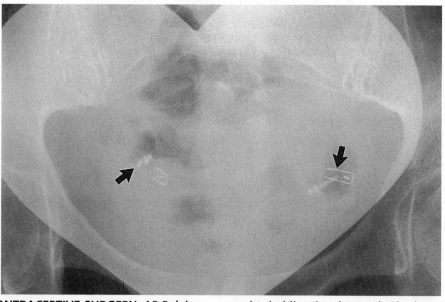

Figure 16-106 **POST-CONTRACEPTIVE SURGERY. AP Pelvis.** The small, metallic clips are the surgical remnants of bilateral tubal ligation (*arrows*). The heart-shaped object is a copper and aluminum ovarian shield.

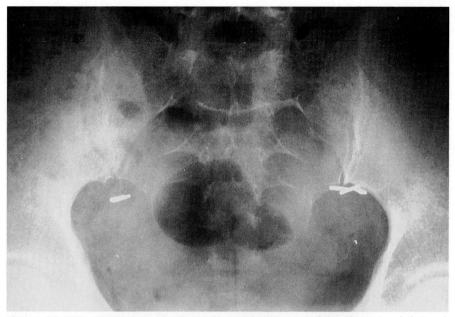

Figure 16-107 **POST-CONTRACEPTIVE SURGERY. AP Pelvis.** There are bilateral metallic tubal ligation clips identified. (Courtesy of Craig Reese, DC, Boulder, Colorado.)

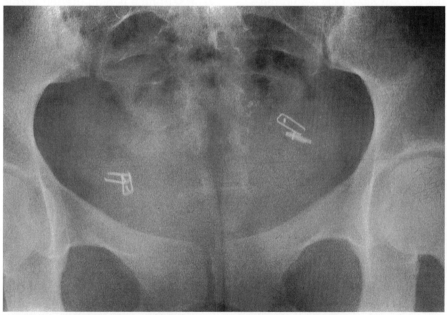

Figure 16-108 **POST-CONTRACEPTIVE SURGERY. AP Pelvis.** There are metallic tubal ligation clips identified bilaterally within the pelvic basin. (Courtesy of Paul Van Wyk, DC, Denver, Colorado.)

SURGICAL, *continued*

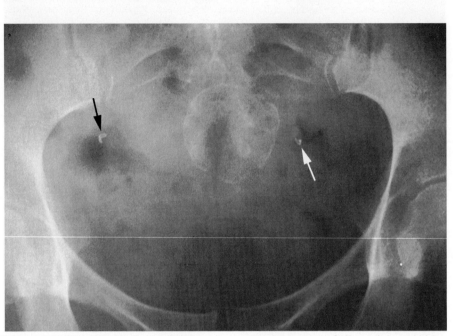

Figure 16-109 **POST-CONTRACEPTIVE SURGERY. AP Pelvis.** There are metallic densities present bilaterally within the pelvic basin, representing tubal ligation clips (*arrows*). In the central portion of the pelvic canal is a large, calcific density, representing a benign uterine fibroid. (Courtesy of Douglas W. Kuhns, DC, Lamar, Colorado.)

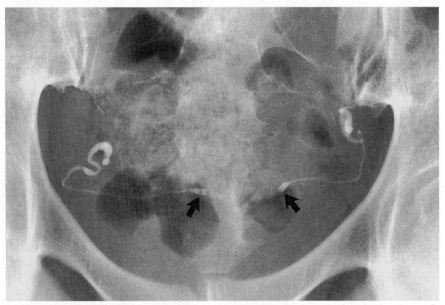

Figure 16-110 **POST-CONTRACEPTIVE SURGERY. AP Pelvis.** The opacified oviducts are filled with silicon and contrast medium. This is a contraceptive procedure. Note the small metallic tip (*arrows*), which allows for elective removal at a later time. (Courtesy of Richard A. Bergeron, DC, Golden, Colorado.)

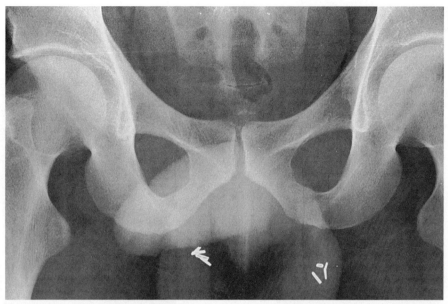

Figure 16-111 **VASECTOMY CLIPS: POST-CONTRACEPTIVE SURGERY. AP Pelvis.** These surgical clips represent a bilateral vasectomy. (Courtesy of Donald E. Freuden, DC, DABCO, Denver, Colorado.)

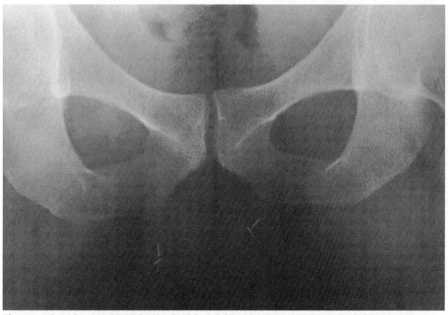

Figure 16-112 **VASECTOMY CLIPS: POST-CONTRACEPTIVE SURGERY. AP Pelvis.** There are metallic sutures noted bilaterally in the area of the proximal scrotum, representing vasectomy clips.

SURGICAL, *continued*

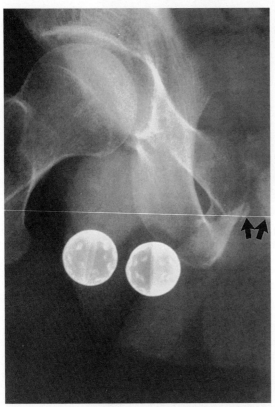

Figure 16-113 POST-HERNIA REPAIR. Frog-Leg Hip. This 35-year-old male presented with low back pain. At age 5 he had surgical repair of a bilateral scrotal hernia. He is presently sterile and impotent and was unaware that his testicles had been removed and replaced with prosthetic devices. On close inspection of the prosthesis, it is noted that they are actually ocular implants rather than testicular. Because of the significant androgen imbalance, there is a delay in closure of the secondary growth centers of the inferior pubic rami (*arrows*). (Courtesy of Donald E. Freuden, DC, DABCO, Denver, Colorado.)

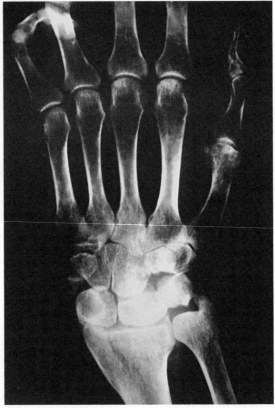

Figure 16-114 POST-TRANSPLANT SURGERY. PA Hand. Note the thumb is on the ulnar side of the hand. This female patient initially suffered a stroke, rendering one hand non-functional. Later, the normal extremity suffered a severe mutilating injury, which was treated by transplanting the stroke-affected hand.

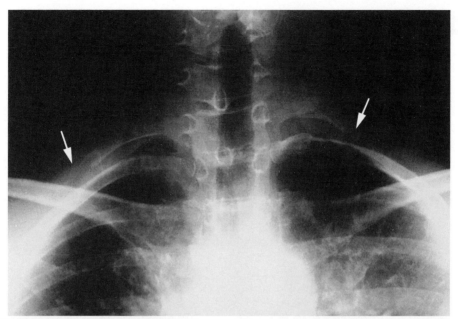

Figure 16-115   **FIRST RIB RESECTION: POST-THERAPEUTIC SURGERY. PA Chest.** There has been bilateral surgical removal of the anterior and lateral portions of the first ribs (*arrows*). This procedure was performed in an attempt to reduce persistent symptoms of thoracic outlet syndrome.

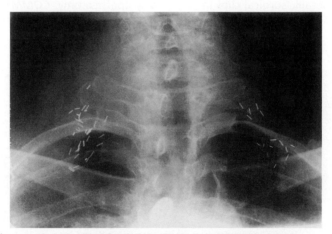

Figure 16-116   **THORACIC OUTLET SYNDROME: POST-THERAPEUTIC SURGERY. PA Chest.** This patient has had bilateral complete surgical removal of the first ribs. Observe the postsurgical metallic clips in the area of the first ribs. This surgery was performed to reduce the symptoms of bilateral thoracic outlet syndrome. (Courtesy of Luke F. MacKinnon, DC, Fort Mill, South Carolina.)

SURGICAL, *continued*

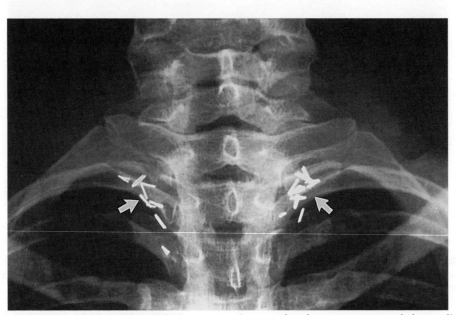

Figure 16-117 **SYMPATHECTOMY: POST-THERAPEUTIC SURGERY. AP Thoracic.** There are metallic surgical clips in the paraspinal area adjacent to T2 (*arrows*). This patient had Raynaud's phenomenon, and these clips are the remnants of a sympathectomy. *COMMENT:* Scleroderma patients with Raynaud's phenomenon are often treated the same way.

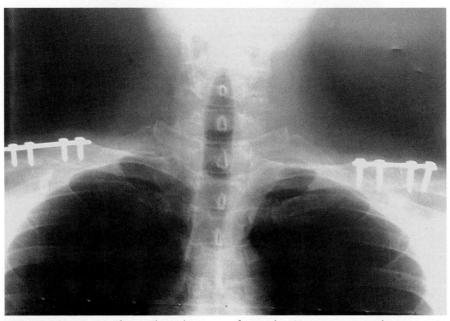

Figure 16-118 **POST-FRACTURE REPAIR. PA Chest.** There has been bilateral metallic bar and screw fixation of both clavicles. *COMMENT:* It is quite unusual to reduce fracture–dislocations of the clavicle with metallic devices. This radiograph was performed > 40 years ago and represents an older approach to the treatment of fractured clavicles. (Courtesy of Jon Paul Carmichael, DC, Denver, Colorado.)

FOREIGN BODIES OR SUBSTANCES

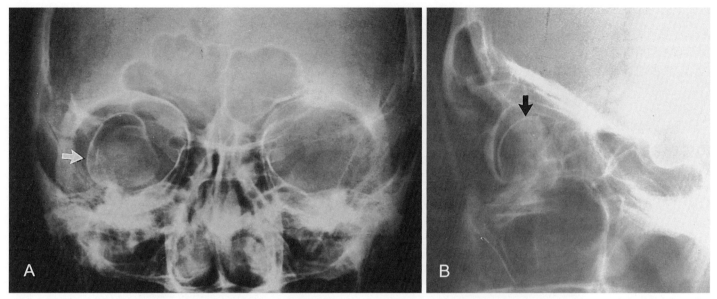

Figure 16-119   **COSMETIC DEVICE: GLASS EYE. A. PA Skull. B. Lateral Sinus.** The halo rim of intraorbital radiopacity (*arrows*) represents a glass eye.

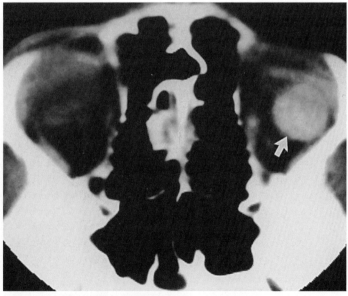

Figure 16-120   **COSMETIC DEVICE: GLASS EYE. Axial CT: Orbits.** The circular radiopacity seen in this CT is a glass eye (*arrow*). (Courtesy of Steven P. Brownstein, MD, Springfield, New Jersey.)

FOREIGN BODIES OR SUBSTANCES, *continued*

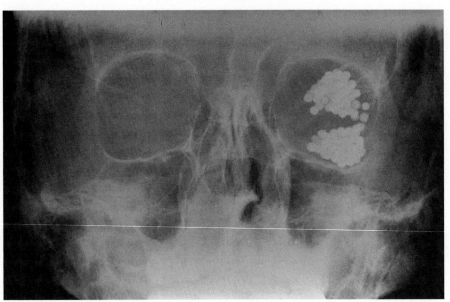

Figure 16-121   **COSMETIC DEVICE: ORBITAL IMPLANTS. PA Skull.** The circular metallic densities represent orbital im- plants in a patient with an artificial eye. (Courtesy of Tyrone Wei, DC, DACBR, Portland, Oregon.)

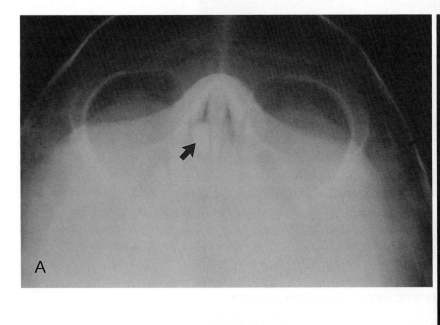

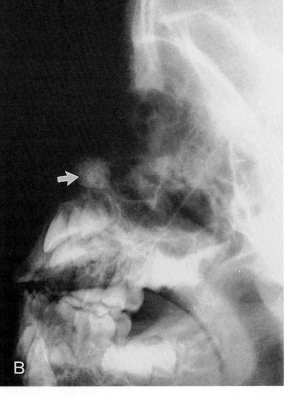

Figure 16-122   **FOREIGN BODY: PEANUT. A. AP Water's. B. Lateral Sinus.** This young patient has a peanut lodged within the nasal cavity (*arrows*).

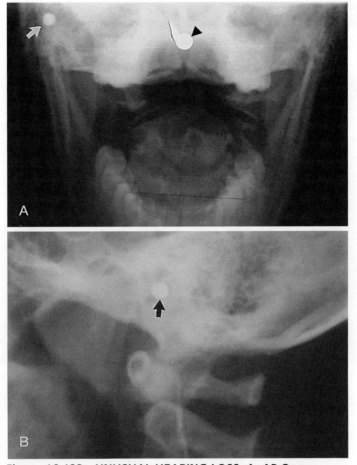

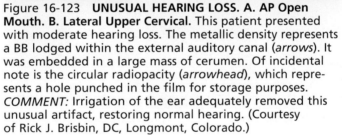

Figure 16-123 **UNUSUAL HEARING LOSS. A. AP Open Mouth. B. Lateral Upper Cervical.** This patient presented with moderate hearing loss. The metallic density represents a BB lodged within the external auditory canal (*arrows*). It was embedded in a large mass of cerumen. Of incidental note is the circular radiopacity (*arrowhead*), which represents a hole punched in the film for storage purposes. *COMMENT:* Irrigation of the ear adequately removed this unusual artifact, restoring normal hearing. (Courtesy of Rick J. Brisbin, DC, Longmont, Colorado.)

FOREIGN BODIES OR SUBSTANCES, *continued*

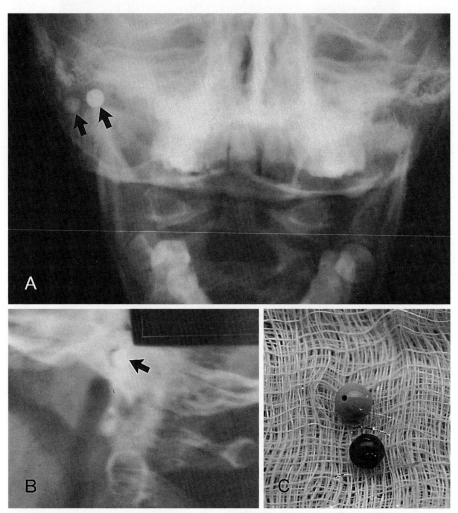

Figure 16-124 UNUSUAL FOREIGN BODY. A. AP Open Mouth. B. Lateral Upper Cervical. This 9-year-old boy presented to a chiropractor complaining of headaches and a stiff neck. His mother had recently noted that the child was not responding to verbal commands and that for the past 5 years the boy had answered the phone with his right hand and put it to his left ear. The boy had been having learning problems, especially with reading. Radiographs revealed two circular radiopacities in the right external auditory canal (*arrows*). Otoscopic examination confirmed their presence, and after a warm water irrigation of the ear, two wooden beads were evacuated. (Courtesy of John C. Slizeski, DC, Denver, Colorado.)

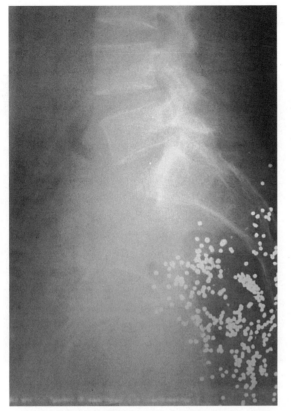

Figure 16-125 **BUCKSHOT. Lateral Lumbar.** This patient was shot while deer hunting. The pellets are within the soft tissues of the buttocks. (Courtesy of Barton W. Dukett, DC, Bigelow, Arkansas.)

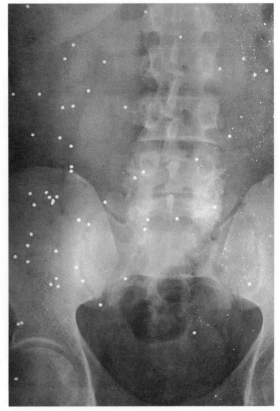

Figure 16-126 **BUCKSHOT. AP Pelvis.** The multiple metallic densities represent buckshot in a patient who was shot. (Courtesy of Stanley S. Kaplan, DC, DABCO, Cocoa Beach, Florida.)

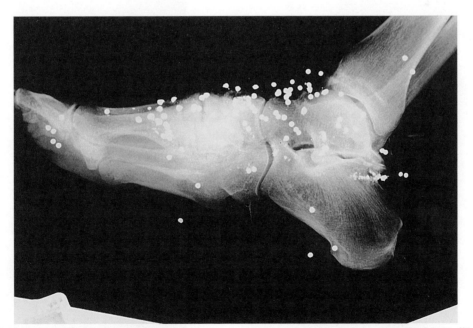

Figure 16-127 **TRAUMA. Lateral Foot.** This patient had inadvertently shot himself in the foot during a hunting excursion, and the multiple, rounded metallic densities represent BBs. (Courtesy of Tim A. Vavarik, RT, Denver, Colorado.)

FOREIGN BODIES OR SUBSTANCES, *continued*

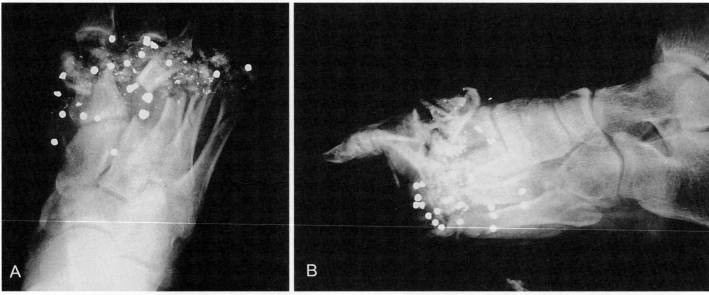

Figure 16-128 TRAUMA. A. PA Foot. B. Lateral Foot. This patient was hunting with some friends, had a terrible fall, and shot himself in the foot. Observe the fracture fragmen-tation of all of the metatarsals. The metallic densities represent buckshot. (Courtesy of Tim A. Vavarik, RT, Denver, Colorado.)

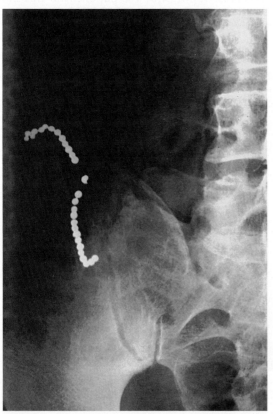

Figure 16-129 APPENDIX: ACCIDENTAL INGESTION. AP Abdomen. Buckshot pellets lie within the appendix subsequent to the ingestion of wild game, which had been shot. The lead pellets lodged in the blind sac of the appendix in the right lower quadrant.

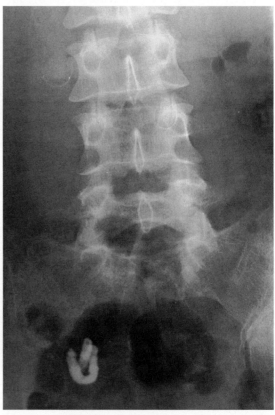

Figure 16-130 APPENDIX: BARIUM. AP Abdomen. The curvilinear radiopacity is barium that has been retained within the appendix following a barium enema. Occasionally, it may be retained for months.

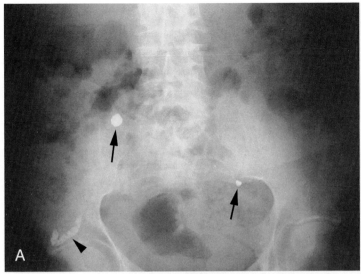 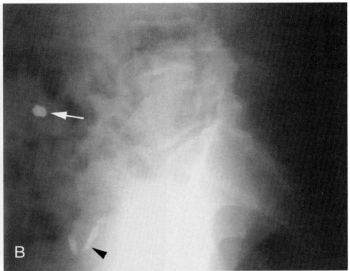

Figure 16-131   **RETAINED BARIUM. A. AP Pelvis. B. Lateral Lumbar.** There are circular areas of radiopacity representing contrast retained in the diverticulae of the lower colon (*arrows*). Additional contrast medium is seen in the appendix (*arrowheads*). *COMMENT:* These are upright films, and this patient has visceroptosis with a low-lying appendix. (Courtesy of Ronald A. Dahl, DC, Loveland, Colorado.)

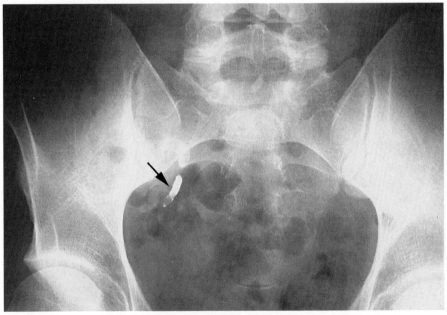

Figure 16-132   **BARIUM IN THE APPENDIX. AP Pelvis.** There is residual contrast within the vermiform appendix (*arrow*).

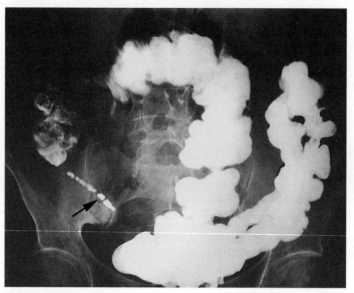

Figure 16-133 **BARIUM EDEMA. AP Abdomen.** This is residual barium in the colon following a recent barium enema examination. Note the appendix, which is opacified (*arrow*). (Courtesy of John A. M. Taylor, DC, DACBR, Seneca Falls, New York.)

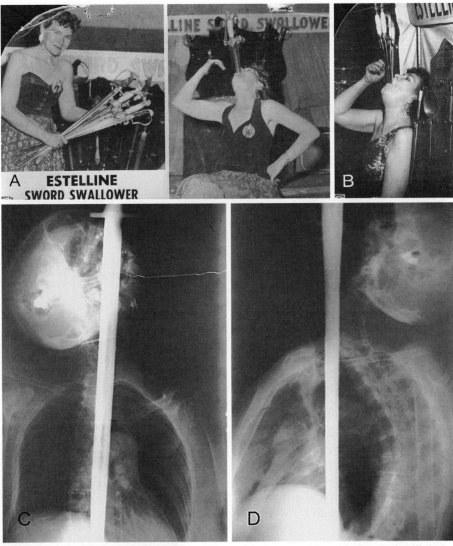

Figure 16-134 **OCCUPATIONAL HAZARD. A and B. The Patient. C and D. Neck and Thorax.** This patient presented to a chiropractor complaining of a stiff neck. She was a sword swallower, so no wonder her neck hurt! The swords pass along her esophagus and enter the fundus of the stomach.

(Courtesy of Franklyn J. Rethwill, DC, Eugene, Oregon. Special thanks to Appa L. Anderson, DC, DACBR, Fellow, ACCR, Portland, Oregon, for her help in obtaining this interesting case.)

FOREIGN BODIES OR SUBSTANCES, *continued*

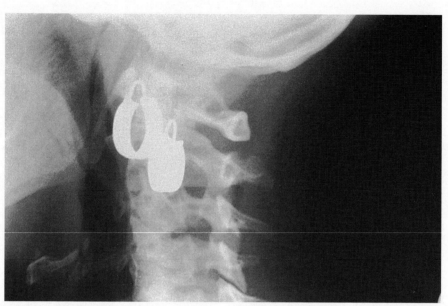

Figure 16-135 **JEWELRY. Oblique Cervical.** These circular artifacts are earrings, which should have been removed before the x-ray examination. (Courtesy of Felix G. Bauer, DC, DACBR(Hon) Sydney, Australia.)

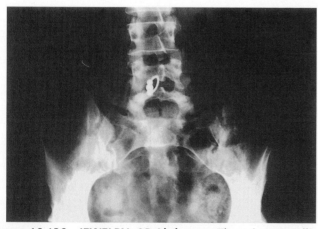

Figure 16-136 **JEWELRY. AP Abdomen.** There is a metallic ring inserted in the patient's umbilicus, seen superimposed in the area of L4 and L5. (Courtesy of Eric A. Schluter, DC, Tulsa, Oklahoma.)

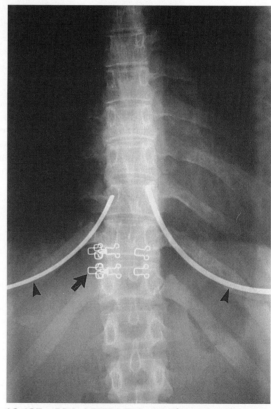

Figure 16-137 **BRA ARTIFACTS. AP Thoracic.** The metallic clips (*arrow*) and ring supports (*arrowheads*) are in the patient's bra, which should have been removed before the radiographic examinations.

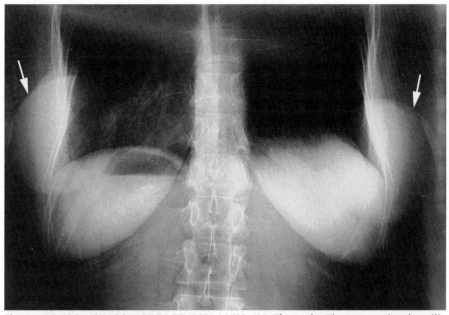

Figure 16-138 **SILICON BREAST IMPLANTS. AP Thoracic.** There are circular silicone implants (*arrows*) present in both breasts. (Courtesy of Ralph E. Brewer, DC, Denver, Colorado.)

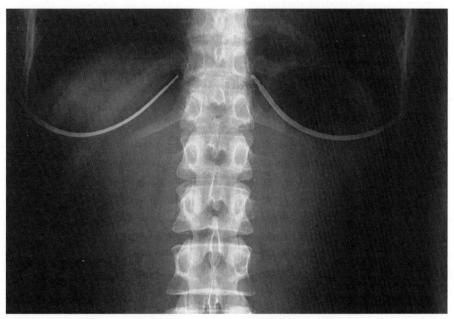

Figure 16-139 **BRA ARTIFACT. AP Lumbar.** The curvilinear, ring-like supports represent metal within the patient's bra. This should have been removed before the radiographic examination. (Courtesy of George E. Springer, DC, Clearwater, Florida.)

FOREIGN BODIES OR SUBSTANCES, *continued*

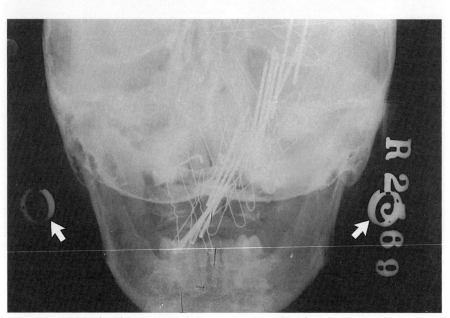

Figure 16-140   **JEWELRY. AP Open Mouth.** This patient did not remove her earrings (*arrows*) or hairpins for the radiographic examination. *COMMENT:* Jewelry should always be removed before radiographic examination of the head or neck area.

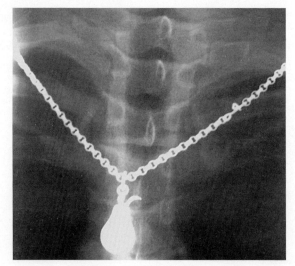

Figure 16-141   **JEWELRY. PA Chest.** The metallic device is the patient's necklace. *COMMENT:* All metallic artifacts that the patient is wearing should be removed before radiographic examination.

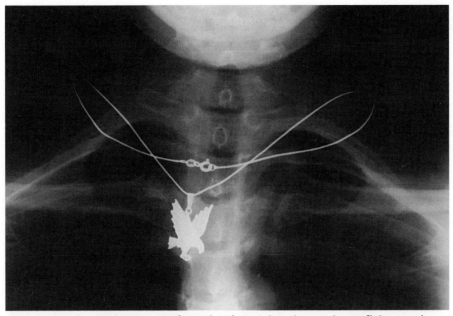

Figure 16-142 **JEWELRY. AP Thoracic.** The patient is wearing a flying eagle metallic necklace.

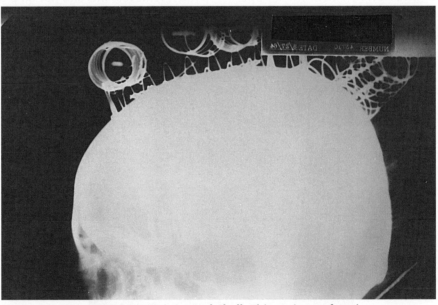

Figure 16-143 **HAIR ROLLERS. Lateral Skull.** This patient refused to remove her hair rollers before radiographic examination, which has produced this bizarre appearance.

FOREIGN BODIES OR SUBSTANCES, *continued*

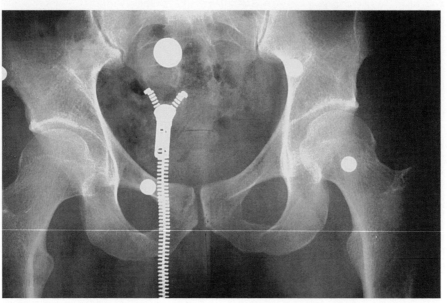

Figure 16-144 **CLOTHING ARTIFACT. AP Pelvis.** These zipper and button artifacts illustrate the importance of having a patient remove pants and put on a gown before performing a radiographic examination of the low back and pelvic area.

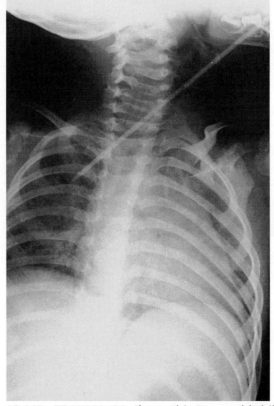

Figure 16-145 **TRAUMA. PA Chest.** This 2-year-old child fell in his mother's sewing room and drove a knitting needle through his throat into the thorax. (Courtesy of David P. Thomas, MD, Melbourne, Australia.)

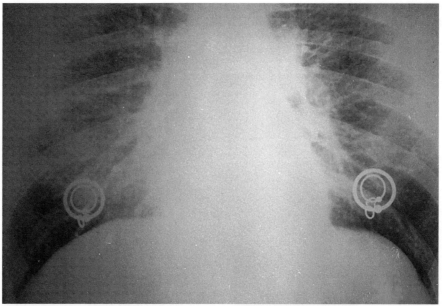

Figure 16-146   **JEWELRY. PA Chest.** These metallic rings were placed through the nipples of the breasts in a patient who was an exotic dancer. (Courtesy of Marshall N. Deltoff, DC, DACBR, Toronto, Canada.)

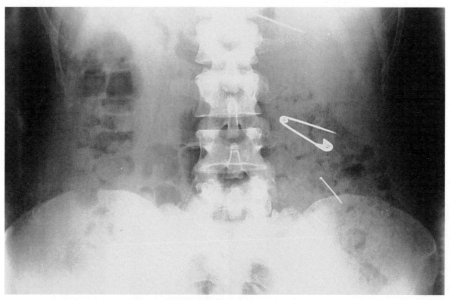

Figure 16-147   **ACCIDENTAL INGESTION. AP Abdomen.** This patient has swallowed some pins, one of which is an open safety pin. Do you think this patient will get the point?

FOREIGN BODIES OR SUBSTANCES, *continued*

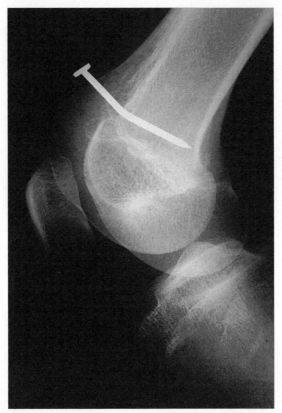

Figure 16-148   **TRAUMA. Lateral Knee.** This patient fell onto some boards from a high position, driving a nail into his leg. (Courtesy of Gerald A. Fitzgerald, MD, Sydney, Australia.)

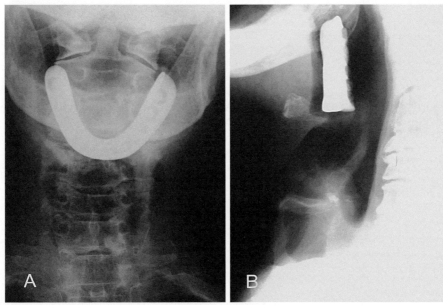

Figure 16-149   **ACCIDENTAL INGESTION. A. AP Open Mouth. B. Lateral Cervical.** This unfortunate 80-year-old veteran was left unattended in a hospital corridor, where his roller-bed turned over. He experienced immediate dyspnea and dysphagia from swallowing his dentures!

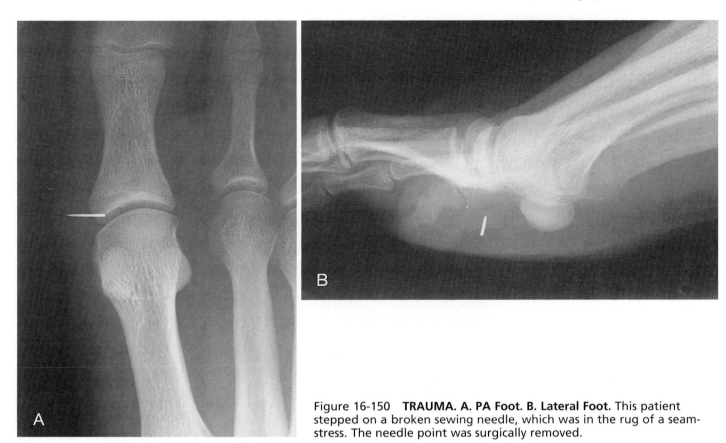

Figure 16-150   **TRAUMA. A. PA Foot. B. Lateral Foot.** This patient stepped on a broken sewing needle, which was in the rug of a seamstress. The needle point was surgically removed.

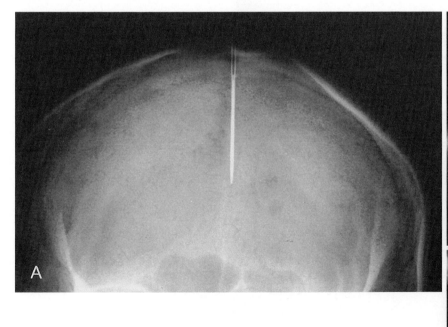

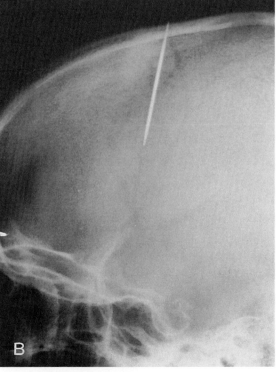

Figure 16-151   **TRAUMA. A. PA Skull. B. Lateral Skull.** This is a 32-year-old psychiatric patient who drove this needle into his own skull.

FOREIGN BODIES OR SUBSTANCES, *continued*

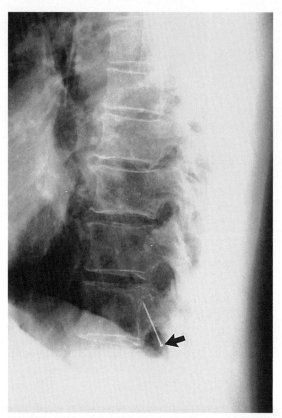

Figure 16-152 **PIN ARTIFACT. Lateral Chest.** This pin is in the soft tissues of the thorax, not within the lung (*arrow*). The patient fell on a number of pins.

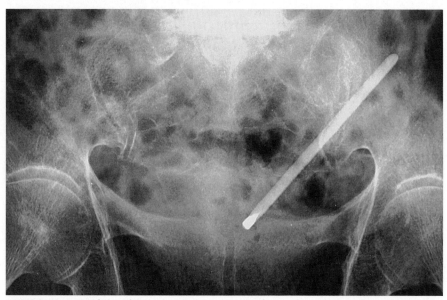

Figure 16-153 **RECTAL ARTIFACT. AP Pelvis.** This is an oral thermometer that has been placed in an inappropriate cavity of a male patient. (Courtesy of Bryan Hartley, MD, Melbourne, Australia.)

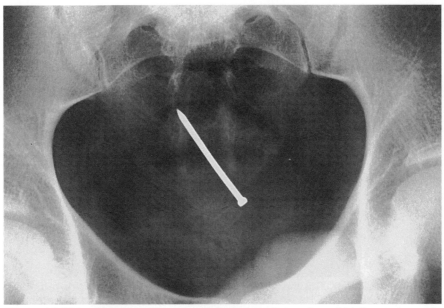

Figure 16-154 **RECTAL NAIL. AP Pelvis.** This nail was found in the rectum of this patient after he noticed blood in the stool.

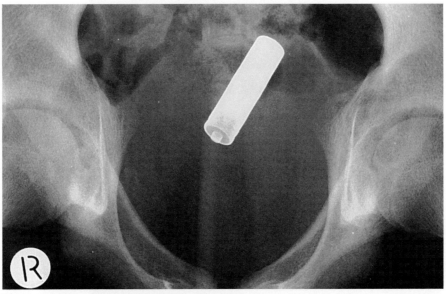

Figure 16-155 **RECTAL BATTERY. AP Pelvis.** This metallic artifact represents a flashlight battery within the rectum. (Courtesy of David P. Thomas, MD, Melbourne, Australia.)

FOREIGN BODIES OR SUBSTANCES, *continued*

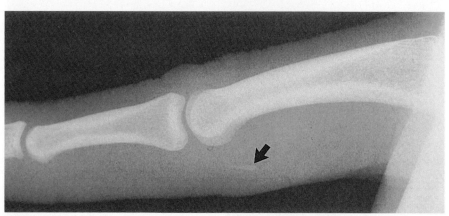

Figure 16-156   **SNAKE FANG. Lateral Finger.** This patient presented with pain and swelling in his finger. He recalled being bitten in the reptile house at the Melbourne Zoo, his place of employment. This radiopaque density (*arrow*) was surgically removed and turned out to be a snake fang. (Courtesy of Paul G. Staerker, DC, Perth, Australia.)

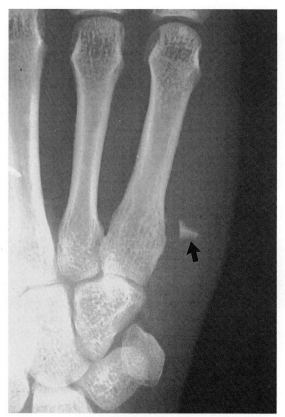

Figure 16-157   **GLASS ARTIFACT. PA Hand.** This patient presented with localized pain after a fall on some glass. The radiopaque foreign body is a sliver of glass in the soft tissues of the hand (*arrow*).

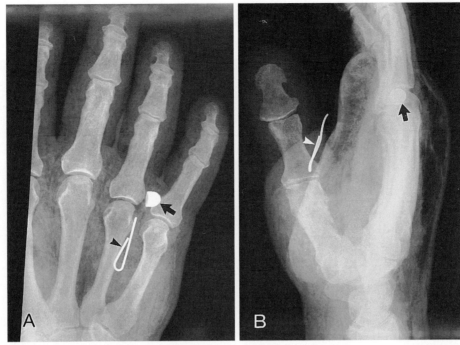

Figure 16-158   **BULLET ARTIFACT. A. PA Hand. B. Lateral Hand.** Observe the two metallic densities representing a bullet head (*arrows*) and a point of entry marker (*arrowheads*). Note the subcutaneous emphysema (air in the soft tissues) diffusely distributed throughout the soft tissues of the entire hand.

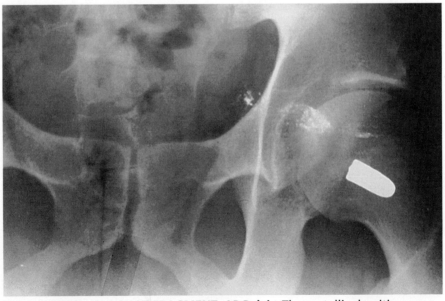

Figure 16-159   **GUNSHOT FRAGMENT. AP Pelvis.** The metallic densities represent a bullet head and debris following a gunshot wound. These artifacts were lodged in the soft tissues of the groin.

FOREIGN BODIES OR SUBSTANCES, *continued*

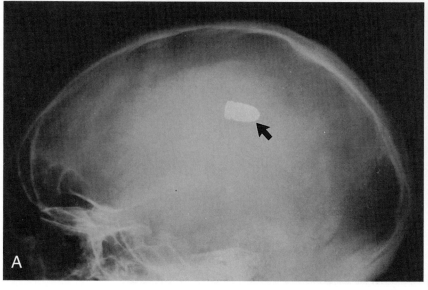

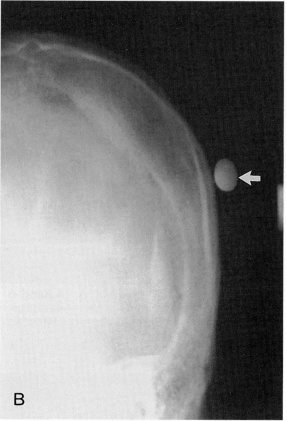

Figure 16-160 **TRAUMA. A. Lateral Skull.** In the region of the cranium a single bullet can be identified, which appears to be lodged in an intracranial location (*arrow*). **B. AP Towne's Skull.** This view reveals that the bullet is actually lodged within the scalp in an extracranial location (*arrow*). **COMMENT:** This case demonstrates the necessity of having two views at 90° degrees to each other in order to localize any lesion. (Courtesy of M. Bruce Farkas, DO, J.D., Chicago, Illinois.)

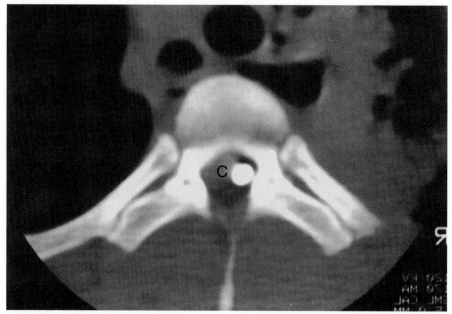

Figure 16-161 **TRAUMA. CT, Axial Thoracic.** There is a metallic bullet lodged within the spinal canal, which has deviated the spinal cord (*C*). Despite its location and distortion of the spinal cord, the individual suffered no permanent long-term neurologic deficits. (Courtesy of Geoffrey Hodies, DC, Oakland, California.)

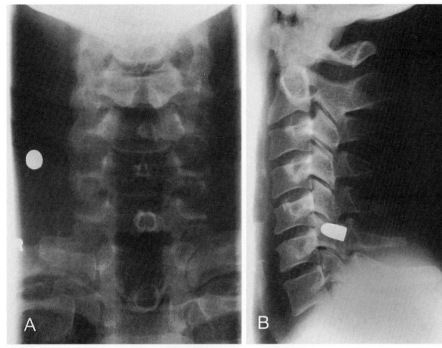
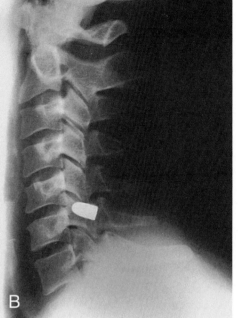

Figure 16-162 **TRAUMA. A. AP Lower Cervical. B. Lateral Cervical.** The head of a bullet is seen lodged in the soft tissues adjacent to the C6–C7 segments in the left side of this patient's neck. (Courtesy of John C. Slizeski, DC, Denver, Colorado.)

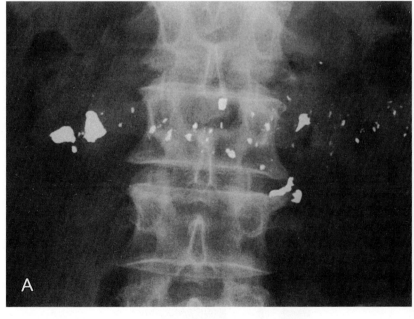
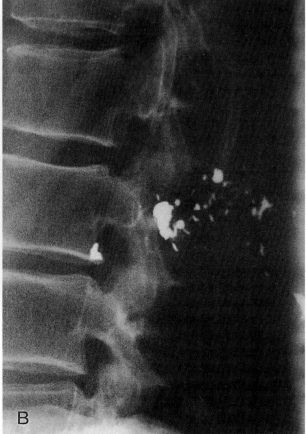

Figure 16-163 **SHRAPNEL. A. AP Lumbar. B. Lateral Lumbar.** The shrapnel fragmentation is left from a dumdum soft-nosed bullet. This patient was shot in Wehrmacht while retreating from the advancing Russians in World War II. (Courtesy of Mahinder Lall, BSc(Hon), MSc, DC, Melbourne, Australia.)

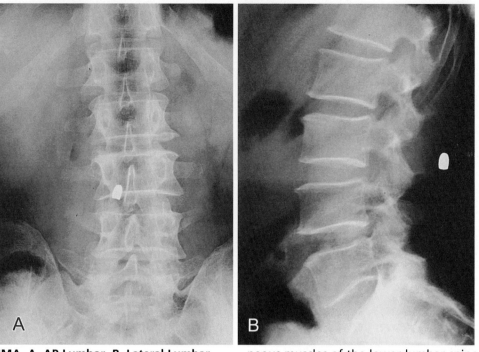

Figure 16-164 TRAUMA. A. AP Lumbar. B. Lateral Lumbar. A metallic bullet head is seen embedded in the subcuta- neous muscles of the lower lumbar spine. (Courtesy of Felix G. Bauer, DC, DACBR(Hon), Sydney, Australia.)

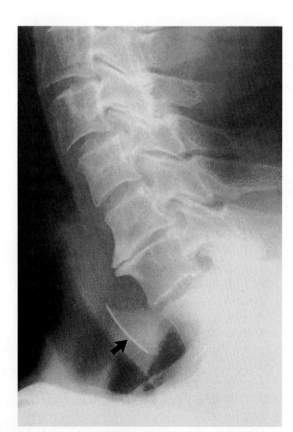

Figure 16-165 ACCIDENTAL INGESTION: EGGSHELL. Lateral Cervical. This patient swallowed an eggshell, which is seen as the thin curvilinear radiopacity anterior to C7–T1 (*arrow*). This was surgically removed. (Courtesy of David P. Thomas, MD, Melbourne, Australia.)

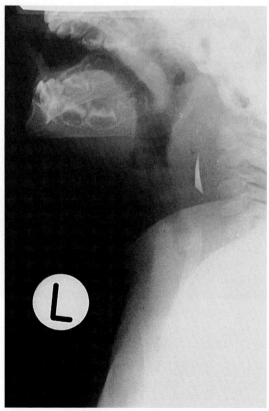

Figure 16-166 ACCIDENTAL INGESTION: CHICKEN BONE. Lateral Cervical. This young child has swallowed a chicken bone, which is lodged in the cervical esophagus anterior to the C4–C5 area. (Courtesy of David P. Thomas, MD, Melbourne, Australia.)

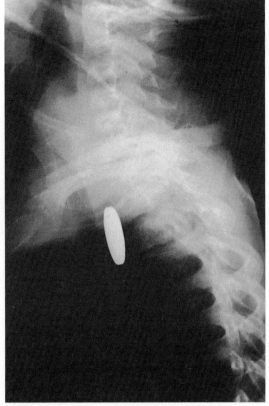

Figure 16-167 **ACCIDENTAL INGESTION: COIN. Lateral Cervico-Thoracic.** This metallic artifact is an ingested coin, which is lodged in the patient's esophagus. (Courtesy of David P. Thomas, MD, Melbourne, Australia.)

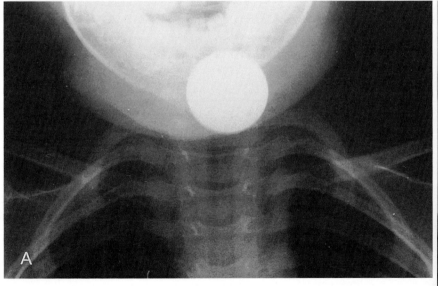

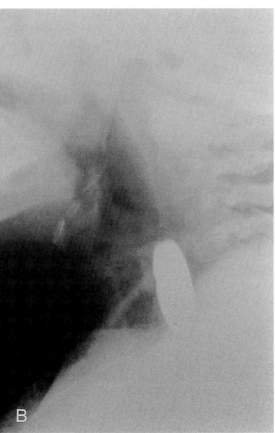

Figure 16-168 **ACCIDENTAL INGESTION: COIN. A. AP Lower Cervical. B. Lateral Cervical.** This young patient has swallowed a coin, which is lodged in his esophagus. (Courtesy of Bryan Hartley, MD, Melbourne, Australia.)

FOREIGN BODIES OR SUBSTANCES, *continued*

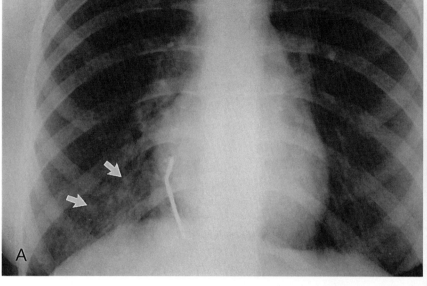

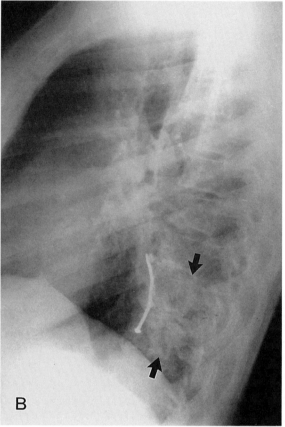

Figure 16-169 **ACCIDENTAL INGESTION: NAIL. A. PA Chest. B. Lateral Chest.** This carpenter accidentally swallowed this bent nail, which has lodged in a lower lobe bronchus. Note the streaky radiopacities in the adjacent right lower lobe representing localized pneumonitis (*arrows*).

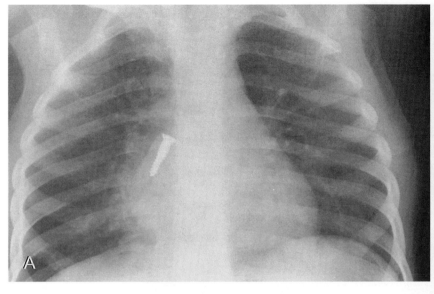

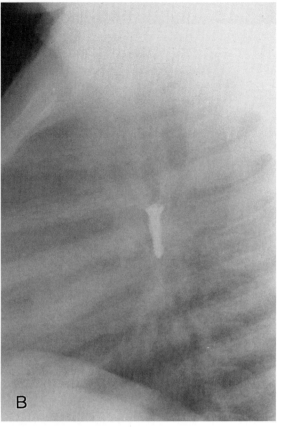

Figure 16-170   **ACCIDENTAL INHALATION. A. PA Chest. B. Lateral Chest.** While playing, this small child inhaled a metallic screw. It is lodged in the right main stem bronchus. (Courtesy of Bryan Hartley, MD, Melbourne, Australia.)

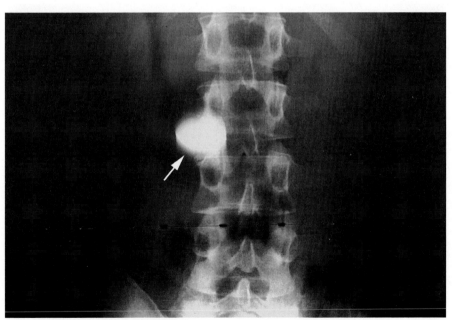

Figure 16-171   **ACCIDENTAL INGESTION: COIN. AP Abdomen.** The circular radiopaque area (*arrow*) represents a quarter that has been swallowed by this patient and is now in the gastric antrum. (Courtesy of Tyrone Wei, DC, DACBR, Portland, Oregon.)

FOREIGN BODIES OR SUBSTANCES, *continued*

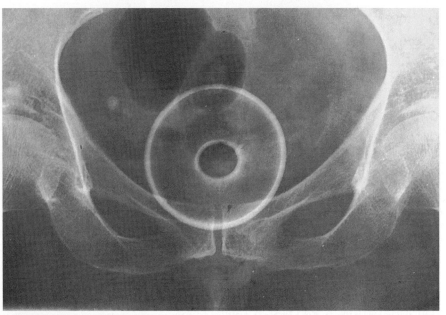

Figure 16-172 **PESSARY: THERAPEUTIC DEVICE. AP Pelvis.** This circular-shaped artifact is a pessary, a supportive device for a prolapsed uterus. (Courtesy of Kenneth E. Yochum, DC, St. Louis, Missouri.)

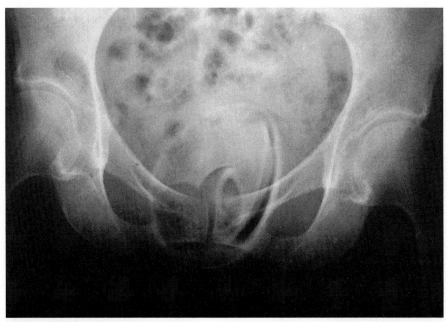

Figure 16-173 **PESSARY: THERAPEUTIC DEVICE. AP Pelvis.** The peculiar egg-like density seen in the area of the pubic articulation is a pessary, a supportive device for a prolapsed uterus. (Courtesy of George R. Phillips, DC, Casper, Wyoming.)

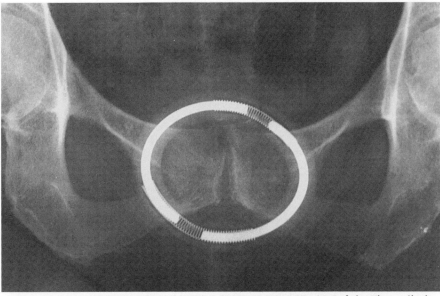

Figure 16-174   **DIAPHRAGM: CONTRACEPTIVE DEVICE. AP Pelvis.** The coiled artifact is a contraceptive device—a diaphragm. (Courtesy of William J. Droege, MSc, DC, CCSP, St. Louis, Missouri.)

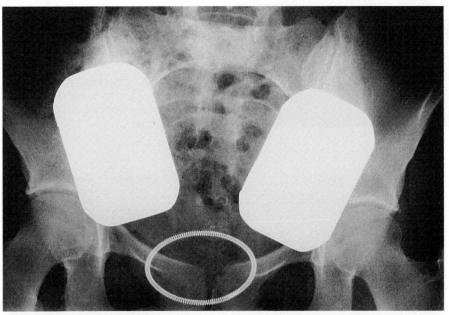

Figure 16-175   **DIAPHRAGM AND OVARIAN SHIELDS. AP Pelvis.** The metallic coil-like structure seen in the area of the pubic rami represents a diaphragm, a contraceptive device that covers the cervix. The two rectangular radiopaque densities represent lead shields for the ovaries. (Courtesy of John A. M. Taylor, DC, DACBR, Seneca Falls, New York.)

FOREIGN BODIES OR SUBSTANCES, *continued*

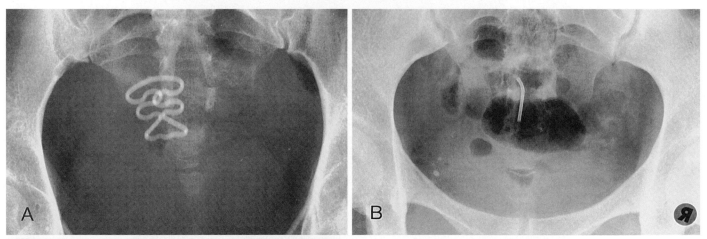

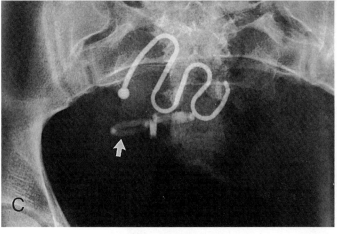

Figure 16-176 **CONTRACEPTIVE DEVICES. A–C. AP Pelvis.** These metallic artifacts represent intrauterine devices (IUDs). Note that there are two IUDs (*arrow*) within the patient shown in panel C.

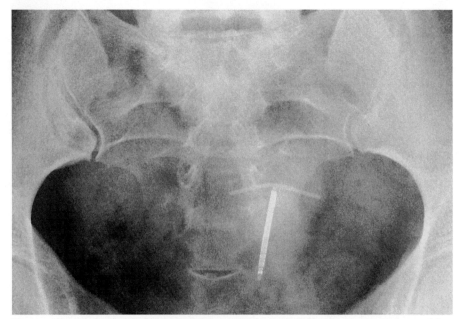

Figure 16-177 **IUD CONTRACEPTIVE DEVICE. AP Pelvis.** There is a T-shaped intrauterine device (IUD) within the uterus. (Courtesy of John A. M. Taylor, DC, DACBR, Seneca Falls, New York.)

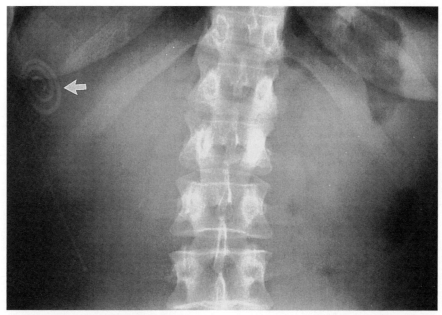

Figure 16-178   **CONTRACEPTIVE DEVICE. AP Abdomen.** This female patient presented with low back pain. By coincidence, an intrauterine device (IUD) was found under the right hemidiaphragm (*arrow*). Apparently, the IUD had ruptured the uterine wall and migrated to this unusual location. (Courtesy of Keith H. Charlton, DC, and Robert D. Maxwell, BAppSc (Chiro), Brisbane, Australia.)

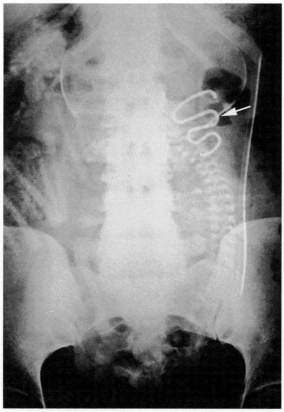

Figure 16-179   **CONTRACEPTIVE DEVICE. AP Abdomen.** This radiograph demonstrates a breech presentation of a fetus. It is also of interest that there is an intrauterine device (*arrow*) present within the distended uterus, which obviously did not impede this pregnancy. (Courtesy of John A. M. Taylor, DC, DACBR, Seneca Falls, New York.)

FOREIGN BODIES OR SUBSTANCES, *continued*

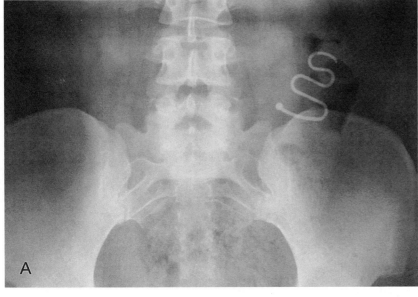

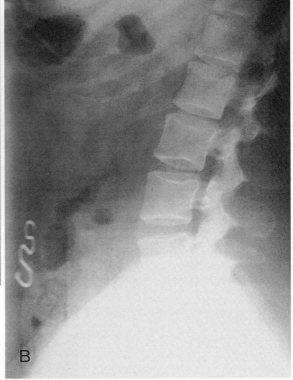

Figure 16-180 **CONTRACEPTIVE DEVICE. A. AP Pelvis. B. Lateral Lumbar.** This 34-year-old patient had a grabbing pain in her side as a result of a ruptured uterus. Note the metallic intrauterine device, which has left the confines of the uterus. (Courtesy of Brent D. Owens, DC, DABCO, Waldorf, Maryland.)

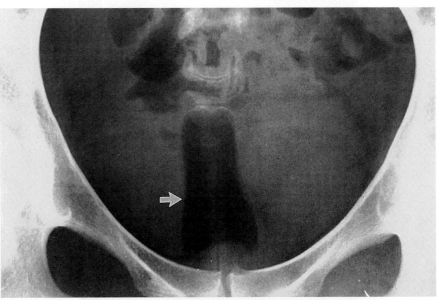

Figure 16-181 **PERSONAL HYGIENE. AP Pelvis.** The rectangular radiolucent image is a tampon in the vagina of this patient (*arrow*). (Courtesy of Donald E. Freuden, DC, DABCO, Denver, Colorado.)

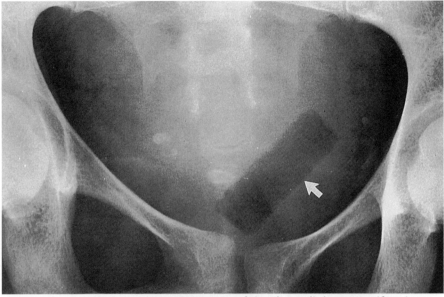

Figure 16-182 **PERSONAL HYGIENE. AP Pelvis.** The radiolucent artifact is a tampon in the vagina (*arrow*). (Courtesy of Douglas R. Petty, DC, Evergreen, Colorado.)

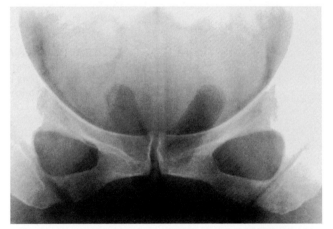

Figure 16-183 **PERSONAL HYGIENE: TWO TAMPONS. AP Pelvis.** There are two tampons present within the vaginal vault. *COMMENT:* The tampon is radiolucent because it has not absorbed any blood at this time. Once it is engorged with blood, it will merge with the water density of the bladder and will not be visualized. (Courtesy of Terry L. Sweet, DC, and A. C. Kuersten, DC, Grand Junction, Colorado.)

FOREIGN BODIES OR SUBSTANCES, *continued*

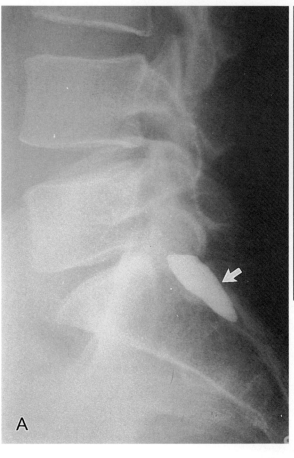

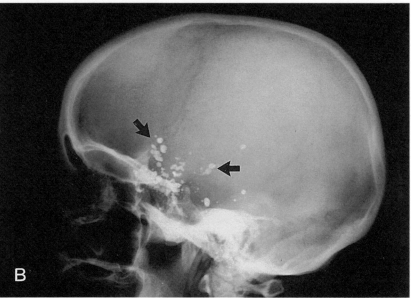

Figure 16-184 **CONTRAST MATERIAL. A. Lateral Lumbar. B. Lateral Skull.** The radiopaque substance remains from a previous myelographic examination (*arrows*). This is the older, oil-based contrast medium, *Pantopaque*, which is a known irritant to the meninges, often inducing an arachnoiditis, creating chronic back pain and headache. This medium will be absorbed at the rate of only 1 cc per year. The new water-soluble medium (Metrizamide) is resorbed and excreted through the urinary tract with no residuals remaining.

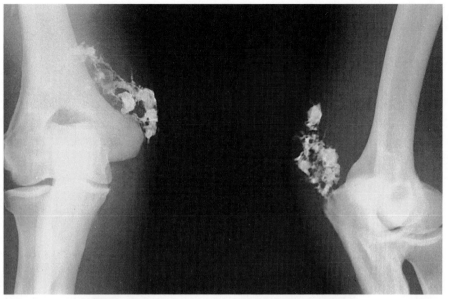

Figure 16-185 **CONTRAST MATERIAL. Elbow.** This is contrast material retained within the soft tissues of the elbow from a previous arthrogram. (Courtesy of Bryan Hartley, MD, Melbourne, Australia.)

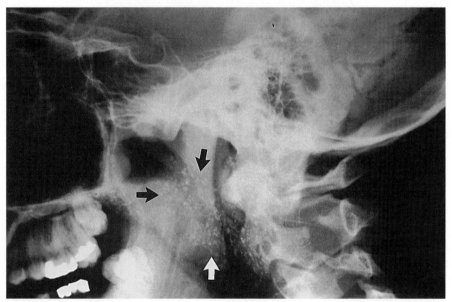

Figure 16-186 **PAROTID GLAND CONTRAST. Oblique Cervical.** The scattered radiopacities represent residual contrast media in the parotid gland following a contrast examination (sialogram) (*arrows*).

FOREIGN BODIES OR SUBSTANCES, *continued*

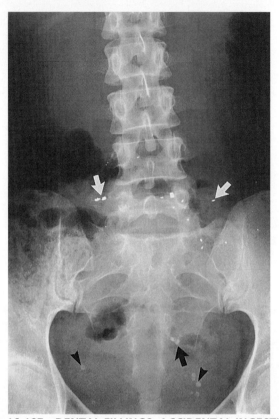

Figure 16-187 **DENTAL FILLINGS: ACCIDENTAL INGESTION. AP Lumbar.** The radiopaque densities scattered throughout the bowel represent metal fillings (*arrows*). This patient had visited her dentist in the morning to have a cavity filled and then saw her chiropractor later that day, at which time he took a set of low back radiographs. These artifacts should not be confused with the phleboliths within the pelvic inlet (*arrowheads*).

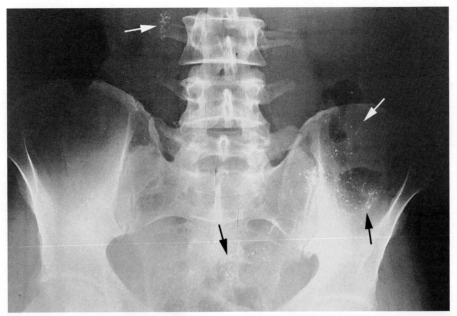

Figure 16-188   **DENTAL FILLINGS: ACCIDENTAL INGESTION. AP Pelvis.** There are multiple areas of scattered radiopacities seen throughout the bowel (*arrows*). These metallic densities represent swallowed shavings from fillings associated with this patient's visit to her dentist the morning that the radiographs were taken. (Courtesy of Beverly L. Harger, DC, DACBR, Portland, Oregon.)

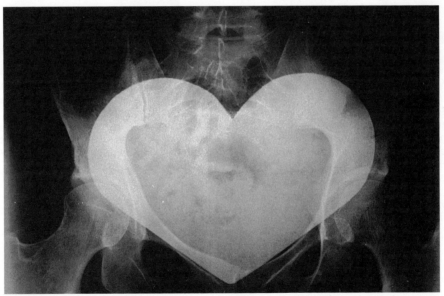

Figure 16-189   **OVARIAN SHIELD. AP Pelvis.** This is a see-through, heart-shaped ovarian shield. It is made of copper and aluminum and reduces the primary radiation dose to the ovaries significantly, without total obliteration of osseous detail. (Courtesy of John R. Nolan, DC, Wanganui, New Zealand.)

FOREIGN BODIES OR SUBSTANCES, *continued*

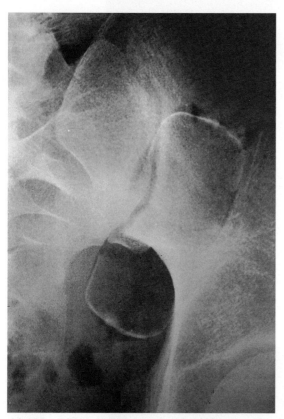

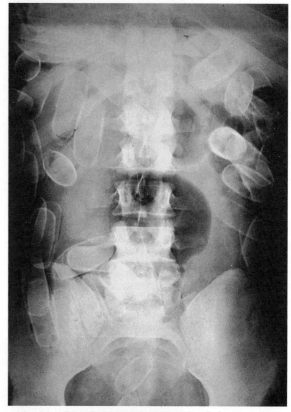

Figure 16-190 DRUG SMUGGLING. AP Abdomen. This rectangular density is within the distal descending colon. It represents two condoms filled with heroin, which this patient swallowed when he boarded his flight in Bombay, India. Upon arrival in Melbourne, Australia, customs officials checked the traveler and, after examination, took an abdominal radiograph. *COMMENT:* This appearance has been reported as the *double condom sign.* If these condoms had ruptured, the individual would have been at high risk of dying of acute heroin toxicity. (Courtesy of Bryan Hartley, MD, Melbourne, Australia.)

Figure 16-191 DRUG SMUGGLING. AP Abdomen. There are > 50 condoms within this patient's gastrointestinal tract. This has created the *double condom sign. COMMENT:* This is the smuggler's way of transporting heroin within condoms, which have been double tied, wrapped, and swallowed. (Courtesy of Kathleen H. King, DC, DACBR, San Francisco, California.)

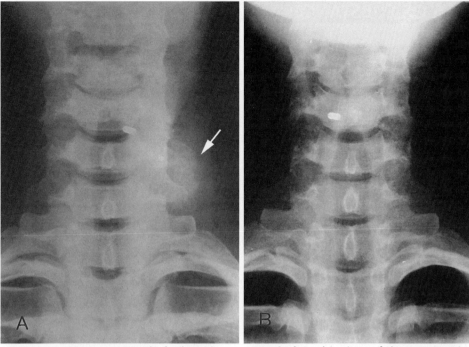

Figure 16-192 **HAIR ARTIFACT. AP Lower Cervical.** There is a questionable radiopaque density (*arrow*) seen to the right of the C6–C7 vertebral segments. Initial observation might suggest the possibility of an osteoblastoma or aneurysmal bone cyst of the neural arch at this level. However, observe the metallic densities seen near the midline. **B. AP Lower Cervical.** In this view of the same patient, a similar metallic density is seen near the midline; however, no pathology is seen at the C6–C7 level. This represents a hair artifact (pony-tail). It is clear on the follow-up image that no abnormality in the C6–C7 bony elements is present. (Courtesy of Michael P. Newmann, DC, Miami, Florida.)

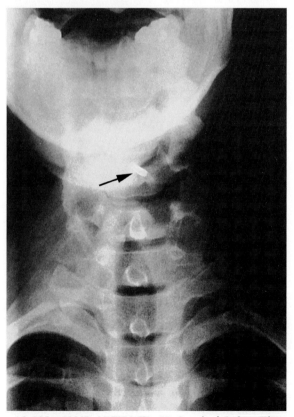

Figure 16-193 **HAIR ARTIFACT. AP Cervical Spine.** There is a metallic hair clip (*arrow*) seen on this lower cervical film. (Courtesy of John A. M. Taylor, DC, DACBR, Seneca Falls, New York.)

FOREIGN BODIES OR SUBSTANCES, *continued*

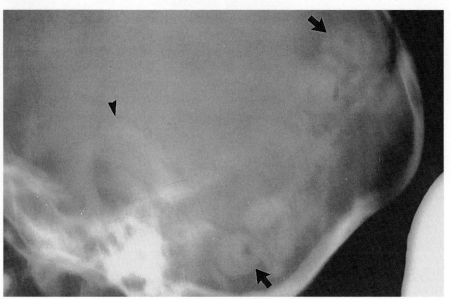

Figure 16-194   **HAIR ARTIFACT. Lateral Skull.** These circular artifacts are hair fasteners with colored plastic balls (*arrows*). The pinna of the ear is also noted (*arrowhead*). (Courtesy of Marshall N. Deltoff, DC, DACBR, Toronto, Canada.)

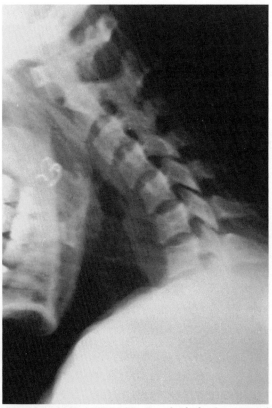

Figure 16-195   **HAIR ARTIFACT. Cervical Flexion.** Braids in the hair of this patient created these streak-like densities. (Courtesy of Joseph W. Howe, DC, DACBR, Fellow, ACCR, Los Angeles, California.)

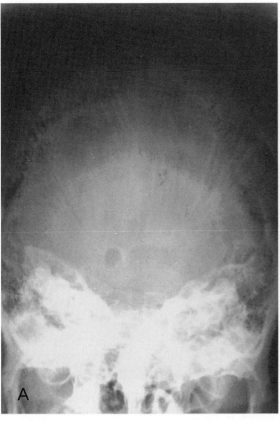

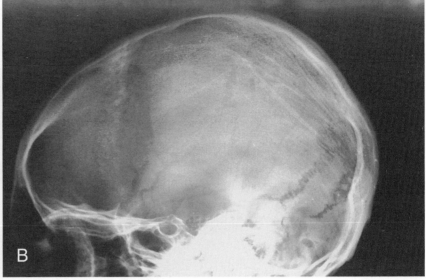

Figure 16-196 **HAIR ARTIFACT. A. AP Towne's Skull. B. Lateral Skull.** The linear, radiolucent, streak-like densities are caused by the patient's very greasy hair.

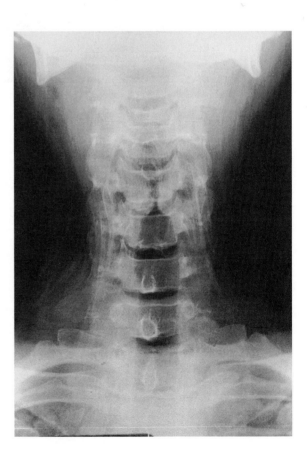

Figure 16-197 **HAIR ARTIFACT. AP Lower Cervical.** The peculiar, strand-like appearance superimposed on the spine and in the paravertebral space represents a hair artifact. This patient had very long, thick hair, which created this artifact. (Courtesy of Beverly L. Harger, DC, DACBR, Portland, Oregon.)

FOREIGN BODIES OR SUBSTANCES, *continued*

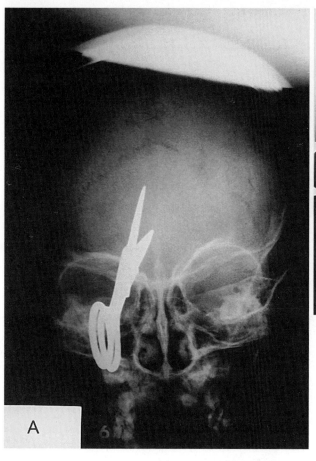

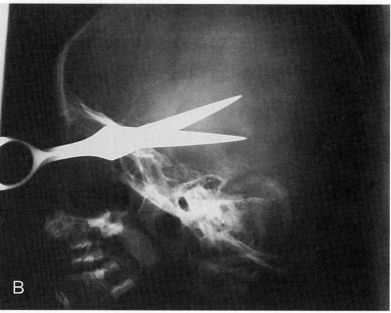

Figure 16-198 **TRAUMA. A. PA Caldwell's Skull. B. Lateral Skull.** While playing with his older brother, this 2-year-old child fell from the upper tier of a bunk bed onto a piercing set of scissors. Oddly enough, this child's accident caused no brain damage. These were the emergency room radiographs upon admission to the hospital. The scissors were removed and the patient has had no neurological deficit. (Courtesy of Gary D. Schultz, DC, DACBR, Los Angeles, California.)

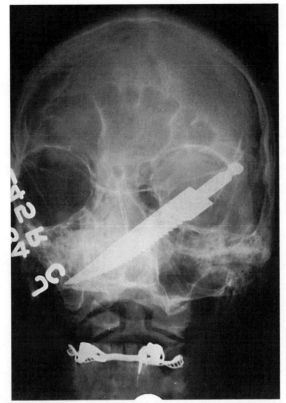

Figure 16-199   **TRAUMA. PA Caldwell's Skull.** This patient had a knife run through his nasal cartilage in a domestic quarrel. It was removed in the emergency department of a hospital, where he received only three sutures. (Courtesy of William E. Litterer, DC, DACBR, Fellow, ACCR, Elizabeth, New Jersey.)

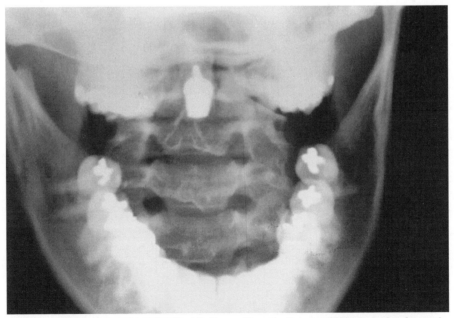

Figure 16-200   **DENTAL WORK. AP Open Mouth.** Dental fillings and a frontal upper false tooth can be seen. (Courtesy of John A. M. Taylor, DC, DACBR, Seneca Falls, New York.)

FOREIGN BODIES OR SUBSTANCES, *continued*

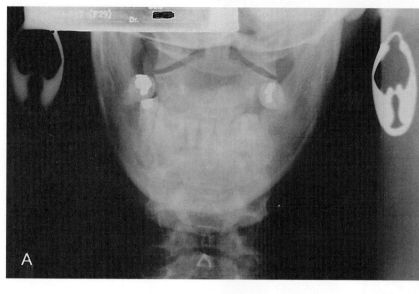

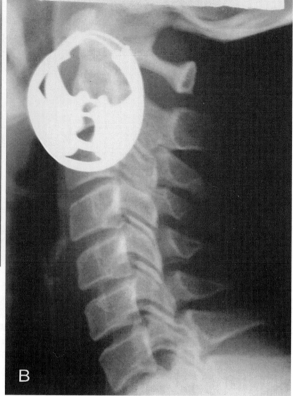

Figure 16-201   **JEWELRY. A. AP Open Mouth Skull. B. Lateral Cervical.**
These huge earrings are seen on both views. They inhibit the doctor's
ability to interpret the C1, C2, C3 area on the lateral radiograph.
COMMENT: All earrings should be removed when any radiographic
examination of the cervical spine is performed. (Courtesy of John A. M.
Taylor, DC, DACBR, Seneca Falls, New York.)

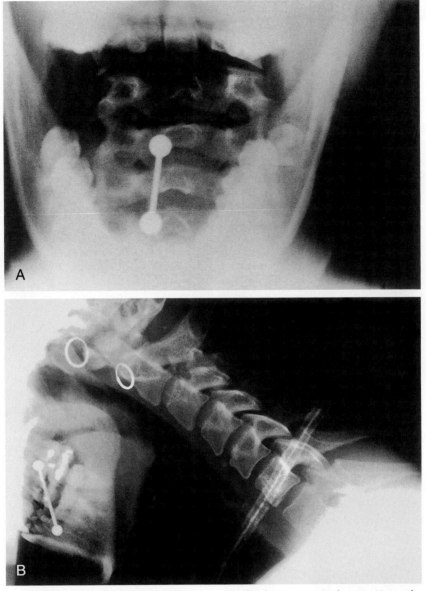

Figure 16-202   JEWELRY. A. AP Open Mouth. The metallic artifact is associated with a tongue piercing. **B. Lateral Cervical Flexion.** Circular metallic earrings are seen superimposed on the upper cervical spine, along with a necklace in the lower cervical area. Note the tongue artifact. *COMMENT:* All metallic devices should be removed whenever possible in any radiographic examination. (Courtesy of Douglas R. Petty, DC, Evergreen, Colorado.).

FOREIGN BODIES OR SUBSTANCES, *continued*

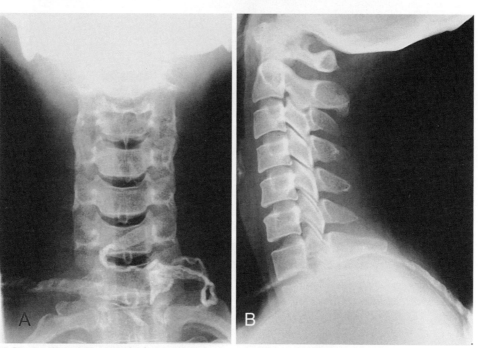

Figure 16-203 **ARTIFACT. A. AP Lower Cervical. B. Lateral Cervical.** The peculiar worm-like, radiopaque structures seen at the cervico-thoracic junction represent a clothing artifact. (Courtesy of John A. M. Taylor, DC, DACBR, Seneca Falls, New York.)

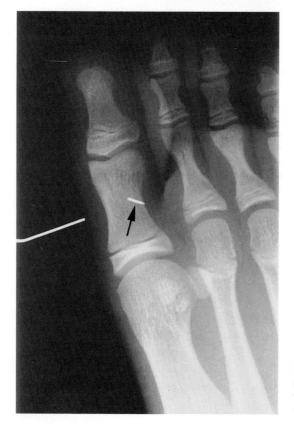

Figure 16-204 **TRAUMA. PA Toes.** There is a broken needle (*arrow*) in the soft tissues of this patient's great toe. The other long, metallic marker, which was outside of the patient, helped identify the pin-point area of pain. (Courtesy of John A. M. Taylor, DC, DACBR, Seneca Falls, New York.)

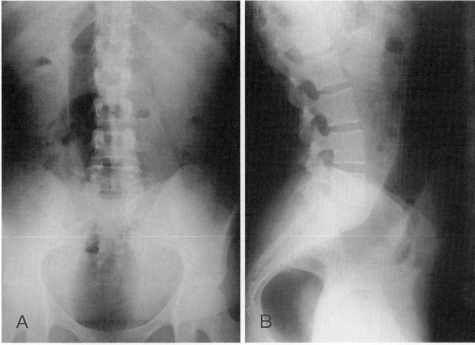

Figure 16-205   **SEXUAL DEVICE. A. AP Pelvis. B. Lateral Lumbar.** There is a peculiar tubular radiolucent structure within the rectum and lower colon. This is a phallic device placed within the rectum and sigmoid colon. *COMMENT:* Follow-up radiographic examination the next day showed this device to have been removed. (Courtesy of Tyler J. Hammell, DC, Chamberlain, South Dakota.)

FOREIGN BODIES OR SUBSTANCES, *continued*

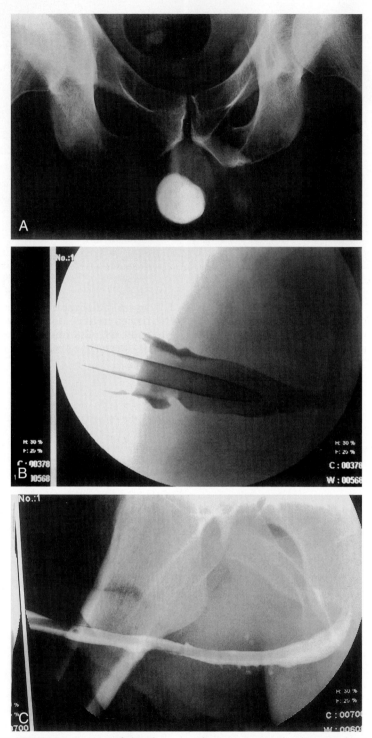

Figure 16-206 **BALL POINT PEN ARTIFACT. A. AP Pelvis.** The circular area of radiopacity in the region of the proximal scrotum represents a foreign body within the urethra. This was identified as a ball point pen. The laminar area of radiopacity around this pen represents dystrophic calcification of the spongy body of the penis, which is referred to as the *corpus spongiosum* (the cavernous body surrounding the urethra). **B. Retrourethrogram.** The pen can be seen within the urethra. **C. Voiding Retrourethrogram.** Contrast outlines the urethra where the foreign body has been removed; however, there are pseudo-diverticula occurring off the inferior wall of the urethra as a result of long-standing altered mechanical pressure in this area. *COMMENT:* This foreign body had been present within the urethra for 40 years. At the age of 12, this patient inserted the pen up his urethra. It caused little to no symptoms until recently, when he developed some pressure and signs of infection in the area of the penis. This was successfully surgically removed. (Courtesy of Kenneth J. McCabe, MD, and Joyce D. Schroeder, MD, Department of Radiology, University Hospital, Denver, Colorado.)

MISCELLANEOUS

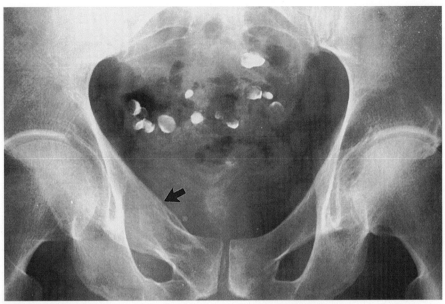

Figure 16-207   **SIGMOID TICS: BARIUM. AP Pelvis.** The radi-opaque circular densities are the residuals of a barium enema examination contained within sigmoid diverticula. Observe the healed and deformed superior pubic ramus fracture (*arrow*).

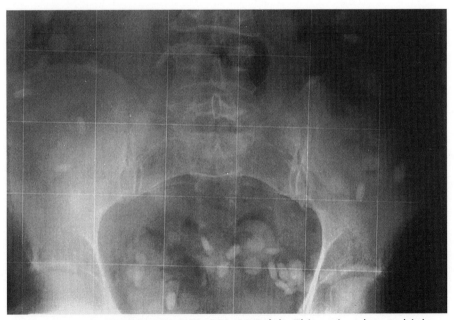

Figure 16-208   **UNDISSOLVED TABLETS. AP Pelvis.** This patient has multiple undissolved pills within the bowel.

MISCELLANEOUS, *continued*

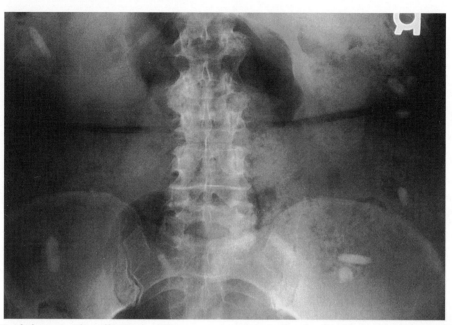

Figure 16-209 **PILLS. AP Abdomen.** The elliptical radiopaque densities scattered throughout the abdomen represent undissolved tablets. (Courtesy of Paul Van Wyk, DC, Denver, Colorado.)

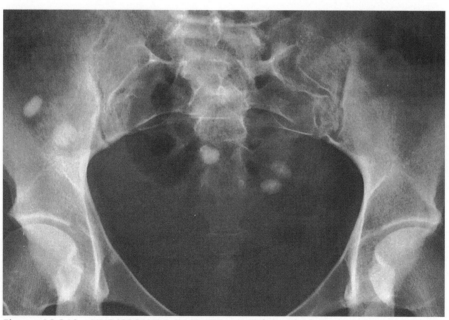

Figure 16-210 **UNDISSOLVED TABLETS. AP Pelvis.** There are numerous, round radiopaque densities present in the lower bowel, representing undissolved tablets.

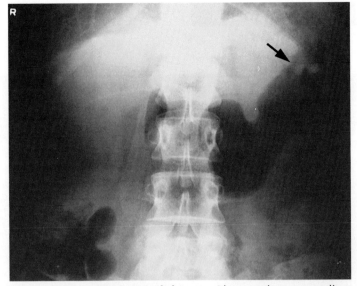

Figure 16-211   **PILLS. AP Abdomen.** Observe the two undissolved tablets (*arrow*) present in the fundus of the stomach.
COMMENT: The stomach can be outlined with air to include
the gastric antrum, lesser curvature, and proximal duodenum.

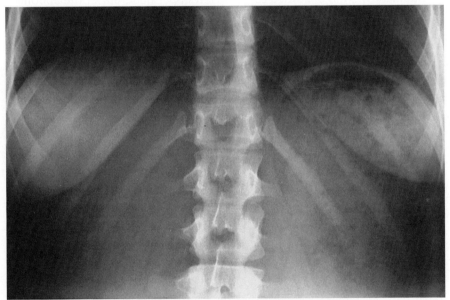

Figure 16-212   **FOOD. AP Abdomen.** The unusual air and
water density under the left hemidiaphragm represents food
substances in the stomach mixed with air. (Courtesy of David
E. Friedman, DC, Denver, Colorado.)

MISCELLANEOUS, *continued*

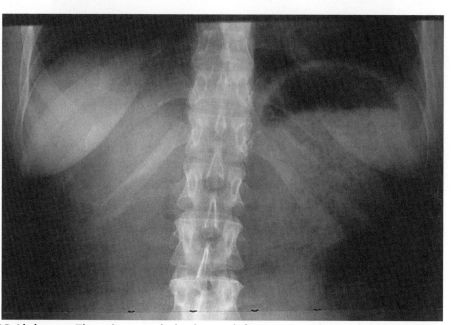

Figure 16-213   FOOD. AP Abdomen. There is a mottled collection of radiolucency with mixed radiopacity seen in the left upper quadrant of the abdomen. This represents air mixed with retained food substances within the stomach.

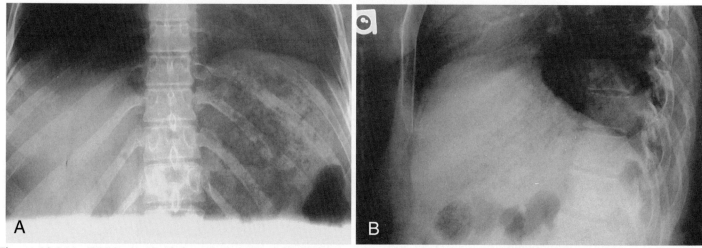

Figure 16-214   FOOD. A. AP Abdomen. B. Lateral Abdomen. The mottled radiolucent and radiopaque density in the left upper quadrant of the abdomen seen on both AP and lateral projections represents a mixture of air and retained food substances in the gastric fundus and antrum.

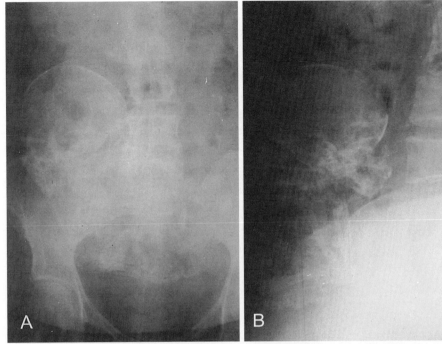

Figure 16-215   FETAL REMAINS. A and B. Pelvis. This is a calcified dead fetus, sometimes called a *lithopedion,* or *stone baby.* COMMENT: The patient is a 49-year-old woman who has refused surgical removal for religious reasons. Because she has either a bicornuate uterus or an ectopic peritoneal pregnancy, she has been able to bear seven additional children with the lithopedion in place, including two sets of twins! There was no history of abscess formation or other symptoms related to this peculiar set of circumstances. (Courtesy of Allison M. Henson Jr., DC, Alexandria, Virginia.)

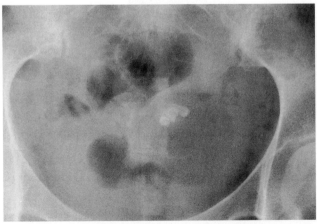

Figure 16-216   OVARIAN DERMOID CYST. AP Pelvis. Well-formed teeth are seen in this young patient's dermoid cyst of the ovary. A clearly defined area of radiolucent fat is seen adjacent to the teeth, which is part of the cystic growth. COMMENT: These dermoid cysts must be surgically removed. (Courtesy of Hal Grass, DC, Denver, Colorado.)

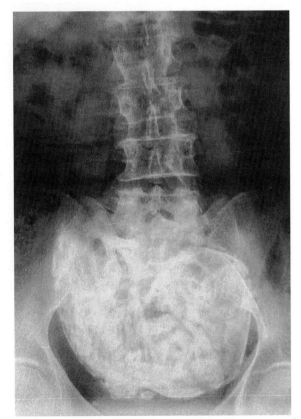

Figure 16-217   FETAL REMAINS. AP Pelvis. There is a calcified dead fetus (*lithopedion*) within the pelvic basin. (Courtesy of Darrell English, DC, Devine, Texas.)

MISCELLANEOUS, *continued*

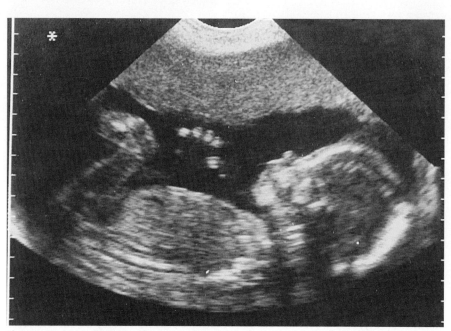

Figure 16-218 **FETUS. Ultrasound, Pelvis.** There is a fully formed normal fetus seen on this diagnostic ultrasound image.

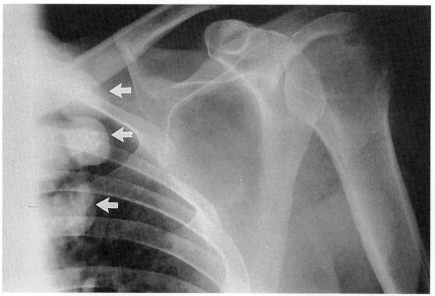

Figure 16-219 **ANATOMIC OVERLAP. AP Shoulder.** The radiopaque densities in the upper lung fields represent the distal digits of the patient's hand (*arrows*). Initially, this was thought to represent a lung abnormality. (Courtesy of Thomas P. Molyneux, BAppSc (Chiro), DACBR, Melbourne, Australia.)

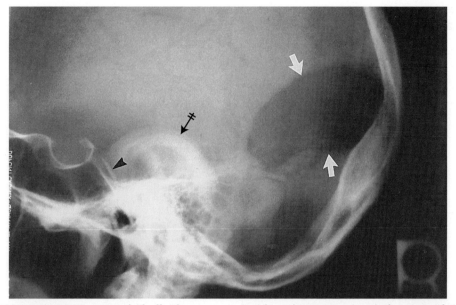

Figure 16-220 **SURGICAL REMNANTS. Lateral Skull.** The sharply circumscribed radiolucent area in the occipital bone represents a surgical entrance site and not a true pathologic lesion (*arrows*). *COMMENT:* History of the patient is often essential for the proper identification of various artifacts. Of incidental notation is calcification of the petroclinoid ligament (*arrowhead*), which is a normal physiologic calcification and is of no clinical significance. Also note the prominent pinna of the ear (*crossed arrow*). (Courtesy of John C. Slizeski, DC, Denver, Colorado.)

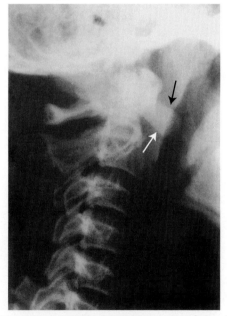

Figure 16-221 **ANATOMIC OVERLAP. Lateral Cervical.** This patient has a prominent lower ear lobe (*arrows*). (Courtesy of Joseph A. Young, DC, Texarkana, Texas.)

MISCELLANEOUS, *continued*

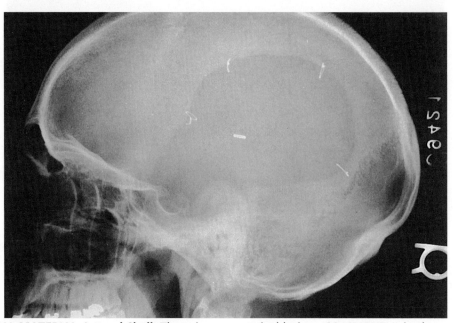

Figure 16-222 **SURGICAL MATERIAL. Lateral Skull.** There is a circumscribed radiolucent area in the temporal bone. The surrounding metallic sutures tip off the fact that this is a surgical lesion. *COMMENT:* It is always important to get an adequate history of the patient in order to identify any pathologies or artifacts.

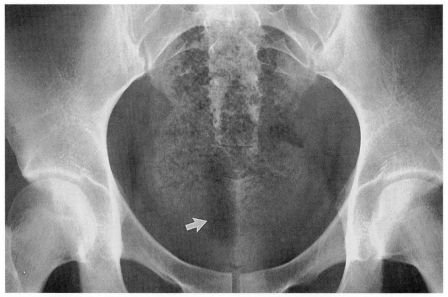

Figure 16-223 **FECAL MATTER. AP Pelvis.** The granular, mottled radiolucent densities anterior to the sacrum are gas intermixed with fecal material. Also note the tampon seen just above the pubic rami (*arrow*). (Courtesy of Donald E. Freuden, DC, DABCO, Denver, Colorado.)

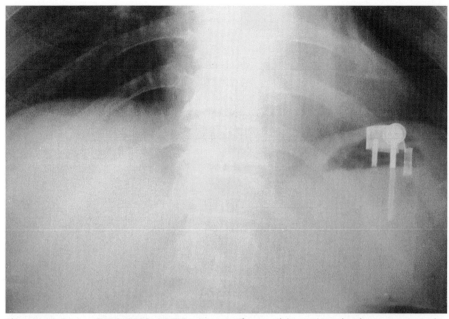

Figure 16-224   **CLOTHING ARTIFACT. PA Chest.** This patient had not removed his shirt and within the pocket was a cigarette lighter. (Courtesy of David E. Friedman, DC, Denver, Colorado.)

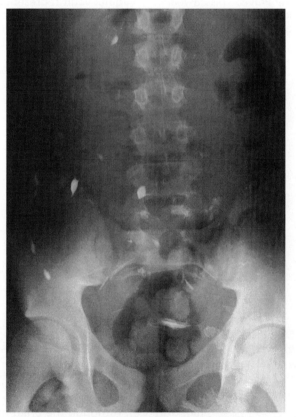

Figure 16-225   **RETAINED BARIUM. AP Pelvis.** This patient had previous abdominal surgery for rupture of the bowel. The scattered radiopaque densities represent residual contrast in the peritoneal cavity, which had not been fully resorbed. (Courtesy of Claudia G. Chapman, DC, Covington, Tennessee.)

MISCELLANEOUS, *continued*

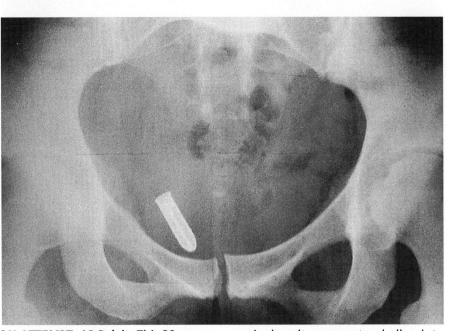

Figure 16-226 **ABORTION ATTEMPT. AP Pelvis.** This 28-year-old woman presented with lower back, abdominal, and groin pain. The peculiar rectangular radiopacity within the vaginal vault represents a ball point pen top. This was a self-induced abortion attempt. (Courtesy of Donald L. Wood, DC, Grand Prairie, Alberta, Canada.)

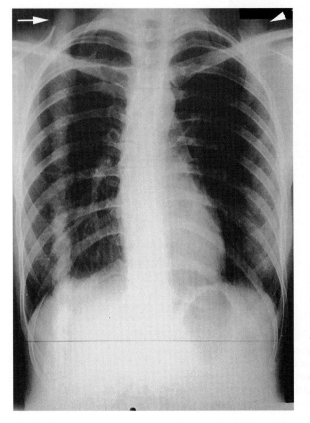

Figure 16-227 **HAIR ARTIFACT. PA Chest.** The patient's hair braids are superimposed on the lung fields. The braids were concealed by the patient's gown and were not apparent to the radiographer. The right braid was anterior to the chest, in contact with the image receptor (*arrow*); the left braid was draped over the posterior chest (*arrowhead*) (increased object–film distance). Although the braid on the right side of the chest is seen clearly, the braid artifact on the left side of the radiograph simulates a unilateral grid cutoff, owing to the increase in image blur associated with an increased object–film distance. (Reprinted with permission from **Cullinan AM, Cullinan JE:** *Producing Quality Radiographs,* ed 2, Philadelphia, JB Lippincott, 1994.)

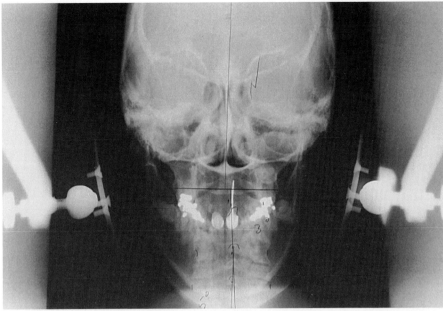

Figure 16-228 **EQUIPMENT ARTIFACTS. AP Open Mouth.** The visible metallic head-restraining devices (head clamps) are used in some upper cervical analysis technique systems. (Courtesy of Beverly L. Harger, DC, DACBR, Portland, Oregon.)

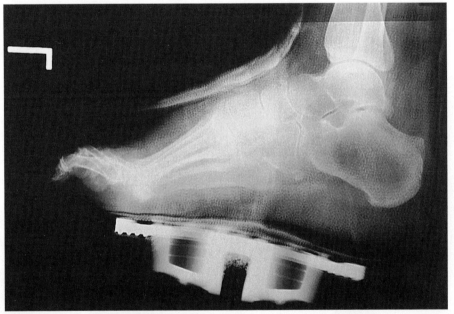

Figure 16-229 **WALKING CAST: POST-FRACTURE. Lateral Foot.** This patient, who had sustained a fracture at the base of the fifth metatarsal, is in a walking cast. (Courtesy of John A. M. Taylor, DC, DACBR, Seneca Falls, New York.)

MISCELLANEOUS, *continued*

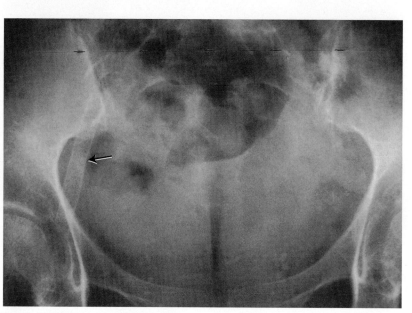

Figure 16-230 **FEMORAL STENT: SURGICAL MATERIAL. AP Pelvis.** This 70-year-old patient has diffuse atherosclerotic disease and has been a smoker for 55 years. The patient had a femoral artery bypass, and a stent (*arrow*) has been placed within the iliac artery. (Courtesy of Ronald M. Spallone, DC, Denver, Colorado.)

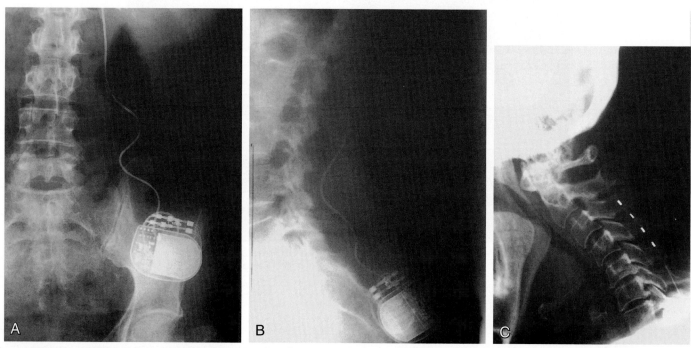

Figure 16-231 **SPINAL CORD STIMULATOR. A. AP Pelvis. B. Lateral Lumbar. C. Lateral Cervical Flexion.** There is a dorsal spinal cord stimulator implanted in the subcutaneous tissues of the upper buttocks. The metallic leads to the dorsal cord can be identified in both the lumbar and cervical spinal areas. (Courtesy of Kevin J. LaLonde, DC, Duxbury, Massachusetts.)

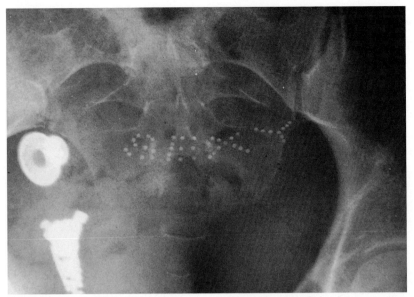

Figure 16-232   **CLOTHING ARTIFACT. AP Pelvis.** A metallic zipper and button artifact from the patient's blue jeans can be seen. Of particularly interest is the word *sexy* projected over the area of the lower sacrum. This metallic artifact was part of this female patient's underwear. (Courtesy of Mark Baker, DC, Chicago, Illinois.)

■ *References*

1. **Sweeney RJ:** *Radiographic Artifacts: Their Cause and Control.* Philadelphia, JB Lippincott, 1983.
2. **Buschong SC:** *Radiologic Science for Technologists—Physics, Biology, and Protection,* ed 2. St. Louis, CV Mosby, 1980.
3. **Sherman R, Bauer F:** *X-ray X-pertise—From A to X.* Fort Worth, TX, Parker Chiropractic Research Foundation, 1982.
4. **Guebert GM, Pirtle OL, Yochum TR:** *Essentials of Diagnostic Imaging.* St. Louis, CV Mosby, 1995.

A Radiographic Anthology of Vertebral Names* 17

Terry R. Yochum, Bryan Hartley, David P. Thomas, and Gary M. Guebert

The material in this chapter formed the basis for the first scientific exhibit ever accepted for display at the Radiological Society of North America (RSNA) by a chiropractor or from the country of Australia. The exhibit was displayed in Chicago in November 1982 and was titled "By Their Names You Will Know Them." The exhibit was honored by receiving an RSNA Honorable Mention Citation.

INTRODUCTION
ANTHOLOGY OF NAMED VERTEBRAE

CONCLUSION
ACKNOWLEDGMENT

REFERENCES

INTRODUCTION

"Since biblical times in the Tower of Babel men have ceased to speak a universal language. This is particularly true in the healing arts where the use of medical jargon frequently prevents physicians from communicating accurately." (1)

*Reprinted by permission of the *Journal of Manipulative and Physiological Therapeutics* Vol 8, No 2, June 1985.

Before the turn of the twentieth century many radiologists appreciated this difficulty and used their imagination to overcome it. The literature has thus become replete with descriptive appearances, for example, "names." Benjamin Felson stated: "A (sic) name saves time, helps you to remember the sign, and advertises it. A sobriquet selected should be appropriate and on target." (2) A total of 88 such named vertebrae have been extracted from the literature. With so many names from scattered sources, we thought it helpful to collate them in a single presentation.

A short description is given when appropriate, and the anatomic and pathogenic reasons for the appearances are briefly considered. A list of conditions associated with each named vertebra, when appropriate, accompanies the descriptive paragraph. The named vertebrae are presented in alphabetical order.

Accessory Transverse Process Sign. This term denotes lack of continuity of the transverse process with the lumbar vertebra. This floating transverse process, when associated with absence of the ipsilateral pedicle shadow at the same level, is an additional supportive roentgen sign of a congenital origin.

 Pedicle agenesis in the lumbar spine (3)

Bamboo Spine (Poker Spine). This refers to the appearance seen in an anteroposterior (AP) projection of the lumbar spine. The appearance is the result of symmetrical bridging of multiple intervertebral disc spaces by marginal syndesmophytes. (Fig. 17-1)

 Ankylosing spondylitis (4)
 Psoriatic arthritis (5)
 Enteropathic spondylitis (5)
 Reiter's syndrome (6)
 Following poliomyelitis (occasionally) (7)

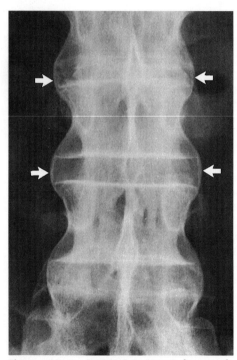

Figure 17-1 BAMBOO SPINE (arrows). Ankylosing spondylitis.

Barrel-Shaped Vertebra. This vertebra is seen in the lateral projection. Owing to complete resorption of the anterosuperior and inferior body margins and reactive midbody osteitis, the anterior contour assumes a convex contour. (Fig. 17-2)

 Ankylosing spondylitis (8)

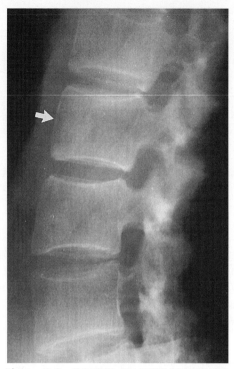

Figure 7-2 BARREL-SHAPED VERTEBRA (arrow). Ankylosing spondylitis. (Courtesy of Gerald A. Fitzgerald, MD, Sydney, Australia.)

Beaked Vertebra (Notched or Hooked Vertebra). This anomaly is seen in the lateral projection. Anterosuperior vertebral body notching leads to kyphosis. (9)

 Achondroplasia (9)
 Diastrophic dwarfism (9)
 Spondyloepiphyseal dysplasia (9)
 Trisomy 21 syndrome (Down's syndrome or mongolism) (9)
 Werdnig-Hoffman syndrome (familial spinal muscular atrophy) (9)
 Trauma (battered child, non-accidental trauma syndrome) (9)
 Hypothyroidism (9–11)
 Mucopolysaccharidosis I (Hurler's syndrome) (9)
 Mucopolysaccharidosis IV (Morquio's syndrome) (9)
 Phenylketonuria (9)

Biconcave Lens Vertebra. This vertebra is seen in the lateral projection. It is the result of softening of the vertebra, which becomes narrow in the center after weight bearing begins. (Fig. 17-3)

 Osteogenesis imperfecta (12)

Blind Vertebra. This vertebra is seen in the AP projection and is a direct result of bilateral destruction of the pedicles. (Fig. 17-4)

 Osteolytic metastatic carcinoma (13)

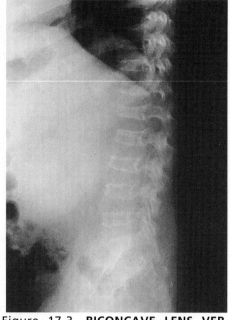

Figure 17-3 BICONCAVE LENS VERTEBRA. Osteogenesis imperfecta.

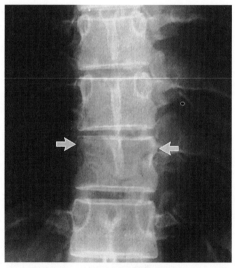

Figure 17-4 BLIND VERTEBRA (arrows). Osteolytic metastatic carcinoma.

Bone within a Bone. This may be seen in both AP and lateral projections, as well as in the oblique view. (Fig. 17-5)

 Normal infants (14)
 Cleidocranial dysplasia (12)
 Osteopetrosis (12)
 Progressive diaphyseal dysplasia (12,15)
 Following radiotherapy for Wilms' tumor (10,12,16)
 Gaucher's disease (17)
 Oxalosis (18)
 Paget's disease (10,14)

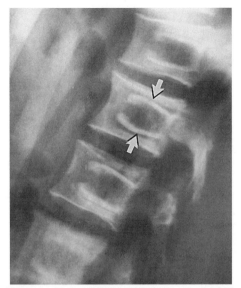

Figure 17-5 **BONE WITHIN A BONE** (*arrows*). Osteopetrosis.

Bottle-Like Vertebra. This is seen in the thoracic spine in the lateral view, on which the posterior portions of the intervertebral disc spaces appear widened compared with the central portion of the body. (Fig. 17-6)

  Hypothyroidism (10)

Bowline of Brailsford (Gendarme's Cap, Inverted Napoleon's Hat). This vertebra is seen in the AP projection of the L5 vertebra, on which the caudally displaced vertebral body represents a curved density below the level of the sacral base. (1) (Fig. 17-7)

  Spondylolisthesis (types III and IV)

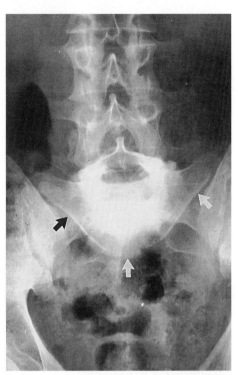

Figure 17-7 **BOWLINE OF BRAILSFORD** (*arrows*). (Reprinted with permission from **Yochum TR:** *A radiographic anthology of vertebral names.* J Manipulative Physiol Ther 8:87, 1985. Courtesy of Bruce F. Walker, DC, and C. Alison Hogg, MD, Melbourne, Australia.)

Bullet-Nosed Vertebra. This is caused by wedging of the anterior aspect of the vertebral body, resulting in a kyphosis. (Fig. 17-8)

  Achondroplasia (11)
  Myelomeningocele (19)

Butterfly Appearance. This abnormality is seen in elderly patients in the AP view. It is the result of bone softening, which allows protrusion of disc material into the weakened adjacent vertebral endplates.

  Paget's disease (10)

Butterfly Vertebra. There are two types of butterfly vertebra. (20)

  Type I (or double-D) depends on the persistence of a sagittal cleft and is seen in the AP view. (Fig. 17-9) Type II (or double-wedge) depends on the persistence of

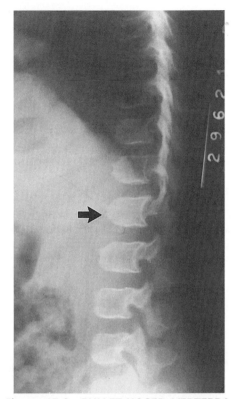

Figure 17-8 **BULLET-NOSED VERTEBRA** (*arrow*). Achondroplasia. (Courtesy of Paul E. Siebert, MD, Denver, Colorado.)

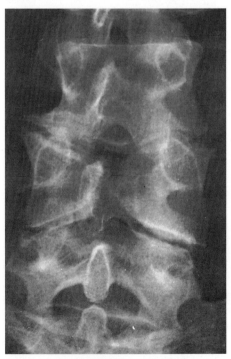

Figure 17-9 **BUTTERFLY VERTEBRA.** Congenital midline defect.

both sagittal and coronal clefts and is seen in the AP and lateral views.

Charcot Spine (5). See *Jigsaw Vertebra.*

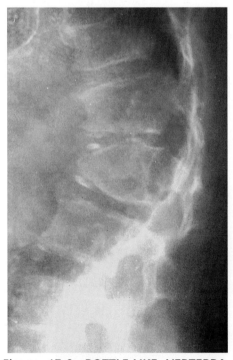

Figure 17-6 **BOTTLE-LIKE VERTEBRA.** Hypothyroidism (cretinism). (Reprinted with permission from **The Center for Devices in Radiological Health, the FDA, and the American College of Radiology:** *The Learning File, Skeletal Section, SK-508.*)

Clover Leaf Vertebra. This is seen in the vertebral bodies and is arranged like clover leaves. Globular radiolucencies become surrounded by densities of calcium.

Rickets (less acute stage) (21)

Codfish Vertebra. This is seen in the lateral projection. There is increased concavity with a smooth curvature of the superior and inferior vertebral margins owing to bone softening.

Osteomalacia (22)

Coin-on-End Vertebra (Silver Dollar, Vertebra Plana, Wafer-Thin Vertebra). This appearance is the result of compression of the vertebral body. Uniform density is noted, and it is wider than normal in both sagittal and coronal planes. (Fig. 17-10)

Eosinophilic granuloma (23)

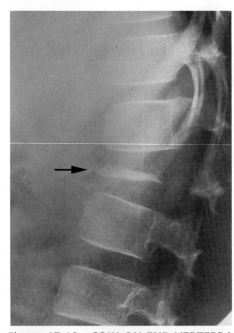

Figure 17-10 COIN-ON-END VERTEBRA (*arrow*). Eosinophilic granuloma.

Corduroy Cloth Vertebra (14) (Honeycomb Appearance [10], Striated Vertebra [13]). This represents an accentuation and thickening of the vertically oriented trabeculae of the vertebral body. (Fig. 17-11)

Intraosseous hemangioma (10,13,14)

Corner Vertebra (Step-Off Vertebra). This is the result of an anterolateral defect in the vertebral body and is seen in the lateral view. It may give rise to kyphoscoliosis. (24)

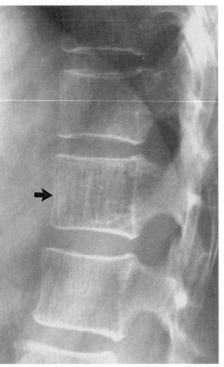

Figure 17-11 CORDUROY CLOTH VERTEBRA (*arrow*). Intraosseous hemangioma.

Cupid's Bow Contour. This vertebra is seen in the AP view of the lower lumbar spine, where the inferior endplates of the L3–L5 bodies frequently have paired parasagittal upward concavities. (Fig. 17-12)

Normal variant (25)

Cupped Vertebra (9) (H Vertebra [15]). This is the result of central depression in the endplate that occurs with an abrupt transition to the

more normal periphery. Usually best seen in the lateral view, but may also be seen in the AP view. (Fig. 17-13)

Gaucher's disease (11,17)
Hereditary spherocytosis (11,17)
Sickle cell anemia (11,17)
Thalassemia (11,17)

Dog Spine. This is seen in the lateral view when the AP dimension of the body is reduced and thus there is relative increase in the posterior vertical measurement. The spine assumes a posteriorly curved appearance, simulating that seen in a dog's spine.

Ependymoma (10)

Double Contour Spine. This anomaly has a similar appearance to a bone within a bone. It is produced by the same process.

Infantile cortical hyperostosis (26)

Double Spinous Process Sign. On the conventional AP view of the cervical spine, one can identify a double shadow of the spinous process owing to caudal displacement of the avulsed fragment. (Fig. 17-14)

Clay shoveler's avulsion fracture (27)

Empty Vertebra. This is seen in the AP view of the spine. Horizontal fractures through both pedicles and transverse processes produce a horizontal lucent defect that is projected over the body of the involved vertebra. (Fig. 17-15)

Chance (lap seat belt) fracture (1)

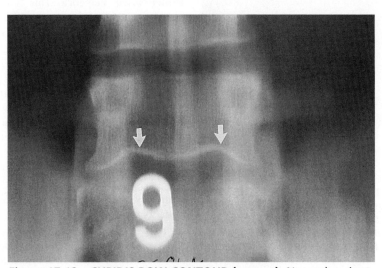

Figure 17-12 CUPID'S BOW CONTOUR (*arrows*). Normal variant.

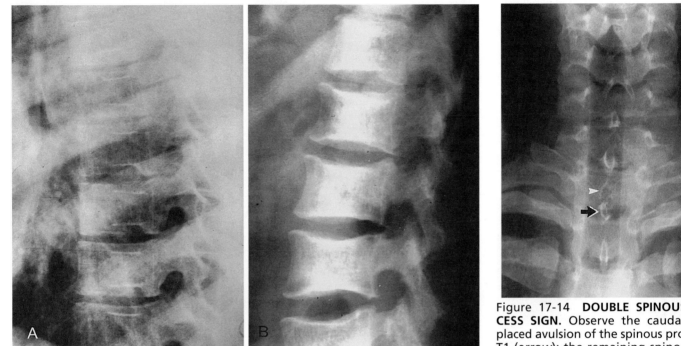

Figure 17-13   **THE CUPPED VERTEBRA. A and B.** Sickle cell anemia. This is also known as the H vertebra.

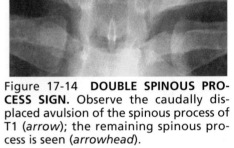

Figure 17-14   **DOUBLE SPINOUS PROCESS SIGN.** Observe the caudally displaced avulsion of the spinous process of T1 (*arrow*); the remaining spinous process is seen (*arrowhead*).

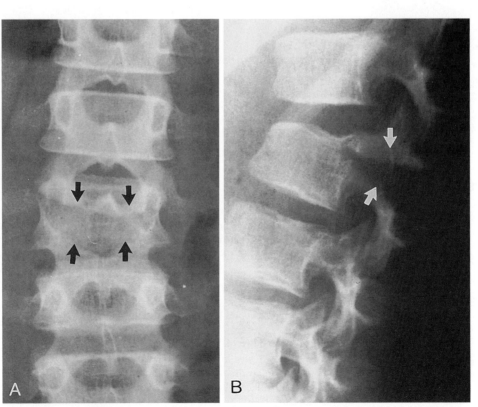

Figure 17-15   **EMPTY VERTEBRA (*arrows*). A and B.** Lap seat belt fracture (Chance's fracture).

Fish Vertebra (Codfish Vertebra, Fishbone Vertebra, Hourglass Deformity). The shape of the vertebral body conforms to upward and downward bulging of the intervertebral disc. This simulates the vertebral shape found in fish. (Fig. 17-16)

Hyperparathyroidism (primary and secondary) (26)
Neurofibromatosis (26)
Juvenile idiopathic osteoporosis (28)
Rickets (28)
Hand-Schüller-Christian disease (28)
Sickle cell anemia (29)

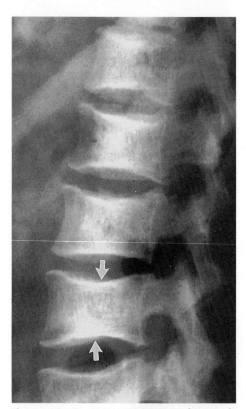

Figure 17-16   **FISH VERTEBRAE (arrows).** Sickle cell anemia.

Fishbone Vertebra. See *Fish Vertebra*.

Flame-Shaped Vertebra. This vertebra is seen on the lateral view of the spine. The superior and inferior vertebral endplates taper to form a central beak. (Fig. 17-17)

Mucopolysaccharidosis IV (Morquio's syndrome) (28)

Frame-Like Vertebra. This occurs when the vertebral bodies have an osteosclerotic border with a relatively radiolucent center.

Idiopathic hypercalcemia of infancy (10,12)

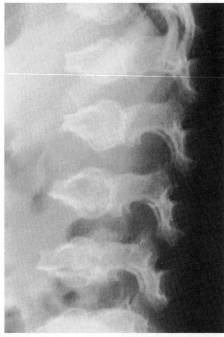

Figure 17-17   **FLAME-SHAPED VERTEBRA.** Morquio's syndrome. Note the characteristic middle beaking.

Frog Head Vertebra. This anomaly is a result of an anterior compression fracture of the vertebral body and is best seen in the lateral view.

Trauma (28)

Gendarme's Cap. See *Bowline of Brailsford*.

Ghost Vertebrae Sign. This sign is best seen on the lateral radiograph. It demonstrates radiopaque densities of infantile vertebrae within the adult vertebral body. (Fig. 17-18)

Intravenous thorotrast administration (30)

Goose-Neck Deformity (Swan-Neck Deformity). This is caused by dislocation or subluxation of the cervical vertebra and is seen on the lateral view. It is associated with progressive thoracic kyphosis and compensatory cervical hyperlordosis. (Fig. 17-19)

Postoperative (following extensive laminectomy) (22,31)

H Vertebra. See *Cupped Vertebra*.

Heaping-Up Vertebra (4) (Pear-Shaped Vertebra [11]). This is seen in the lateral view and is the result of an accumulation of bone at the posterior aspect of the superior and inferior vertebral endplates. (Fig. 17-20)

Spondyloepiphyseal dysplasia tarda (4,11)

Honeycomb Appearance (10). See *Corduroy Cloth Vertebra*.

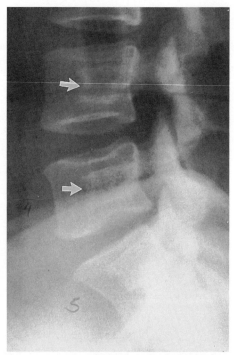

Figure 17-18   **GHOST VERTEBRAE (arrows).** Intravenous thorotrast administration.

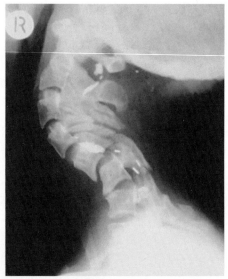

Figure 17-19   **GOOSE-NECK DEFORMITY.** This anomaly is seen after extensive laminectomy for neurofibromatosis.

Hooked Vertebra. See *Beaked Vertebra*.

Hourglass Deformity. See *Fish Vertebra*.

Hourglass Vertebra. In this appearance, the endplates are compressed by upward and downward protrusion of the intervertebral disc material in the midportion of the body of the vertebra, above and below. It is best seen on an AP projection. (Fig. 17-21)

Senile osteoporosis (28)

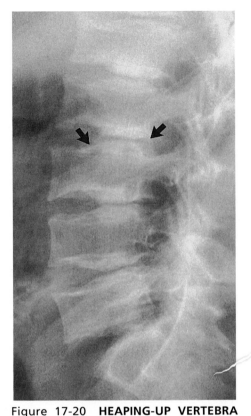

Figure 17-20   **HEAPING-UP VERTEBRA** (*arrows*). Spondyloepiphyseal dysplasia tarda. (Courtesy of John R. Nolan, DC, Wanganui, New Zealand.)

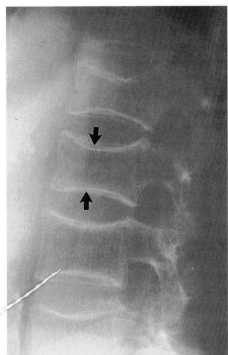

Figure 17-21   **HOURGLASS VERTEBRA** (*arrows*). Osteoporosis.

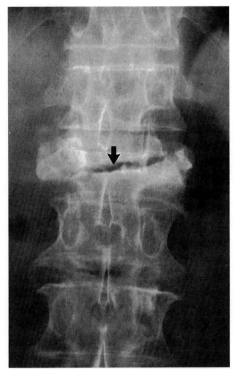

Figure 17-22   **INTRAVERTEBRAL VACUUM CLEFT SIGN** (*arrow*). Steroid-induced ischemic necrosis in a patient with long-standing rheumatoid arthritis. (Courtesy of Lawrence A. Cooperstein, MD, Pittsburgh, Pennsylvania.)

Intravertebral Vacuum Cleft Sign. The radiographic appearance of a gaseous cleft within a transverse separation of the vertebral body in a patient with vertebral collapse defines this appearance. (32) It is best seen in extension and may disappear in flexion. (Fig. 17-22)

   Ischemic vertebral collapse (32,33)

Inverted H Vertebra. See *Inverted U Vertebra.*

Inverted Napoleon's Hat. See *Bowline of Brailsford.*

Inverted U Vertebra (Inverted H Vertebra). This is seen in the AP view of the spine and is caused by flattening of the vertebral body superimposed on the well-mineralized posterior elements.

   Thanatophoric dwarfism (14)

Ivory Vertebra. This is a uniformly radiopaque vertebral body. (Fig. 17-23)

   Osteopetrosis (6)
   Fluorosis (6)
   Lymphoma (6)
   Myelosclerosis (6)
   Paget's disease (6)
   Osteoblastic metastases (6)

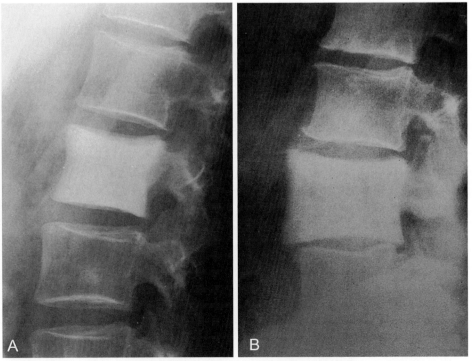

Figure 17-23   **IVORY VERTEBRA. A. Osteoblastic Metastasis (Prostate). B. Paget's Disease.** (Courtesy of Joseph W. Howe, DC, DACBR, Fellow, ACCR, Los Angeles, California.)

Jigsaw Vertebra (34) (Tumbling Building Block Spine [5], Charcot Spine [5]). This vertebra is the result of fragmentation of a vertebra as seen in a neurotrophic process. (Fig. 17-24)

Neurotrophic arthropathy (34)

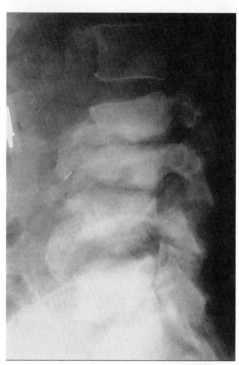

Figure 17-24 **JIGSAW VERTEBRA.** Neurotrophic arthropathy. This patient has tabes dorsalis. (Courtesy of Lawrence T. Sellers, DC, DACBR, Portland, Oregon.)

Keel-Shaped Vertebra. This is seen in the lateral view and is caused by anterior wedging of the vertebral body.

Metatrophic dwarfism (11)

Kissing Spine. In this condition, there is increased lordosis with obliteration of the interspinous ligaments, so that the tips of the spinous processes become contiguous. (Fig. 17-25)

Baastrup's disease (35)

Lattice-Like Appearance. See *Soap Bubble Vertebra.*

Limbus Vertebra. This is seen on the lateral view and represents separation of the ring apophysis of the vertebra from the vertebral body. (Fig. 17-26)

Scheuermann's disease (11)
Trauma (11)

Long Vertebra. This appearance is best seen on the lateral projection. It is caused by an increase in the vertical height of the vertebral body in compensation for a severe thoracic gibbus. (Fig. 17-27)

Spinal tuberculosis (28)

Lozenge-Shaped Vertebra. The vertebral bodies are small and flat, and there are widened intervertebral disc spaces.

Hypophosphatasia (newborn) (10)

Notched Vertebra. This is seen on the lateral view. An enlarged and persistent notch is present on the anterior aspect of the vertebral bodies where the vascular channels enter.

Normal infant spine (12)
Sickle cell anemia (36)

Occipital Vertebra. This results from the failure of the most caudal portion of the C1 vertebrae to fuse with the occiput. (10)

One-Eyed Vertebra (14) (Winking-Owl Vertebra [37]). Seen on the AP radiograph of the spine, this vertebra represents unilateral pedicle destruction. (Fig. 17-28)

Osteolytic metastatic carcinoma (14)

Pear-Shaped Vertebra (11). See *Heaping-Up Vertebra.*

Pedicle Sign. This radiographic sign is used to differentiate multiple myeloma from osteolytic metastases. Because myeloma primarily involves the red marrow, it usually causes vertebral body destruction without pedicle destruction. Therefore, pedicle destruction without vertebral body involvement suggests metastatic carcinoma. (Fig. 17-29)

Multiple myeloma (37)

Picture-Frame Vertebra (14) (Window-Like Vertebra [10]). This is caused by cortical thickening around an expanded vertebral body. (Fig. 17-30)

Paget's disease (10,14)

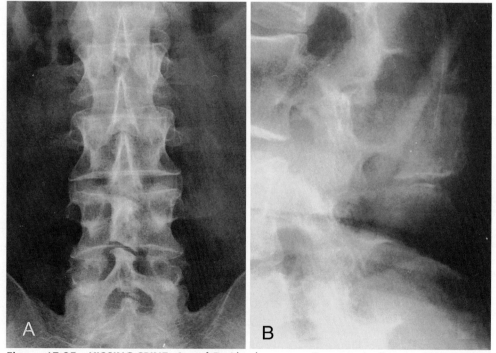

Figure 17-25 **KISSING SPINE. A and B.** Also known as Baastrup's disease. (Courtesy of George E. Springer, DC, Clearwater, Florida.)

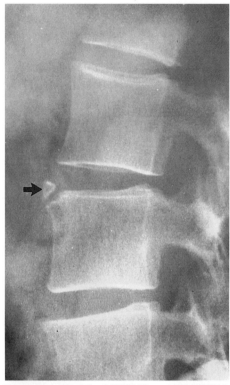

Figure   17-26   **LIMBUS   VERTEBRA** (*arrow*). Trauma.

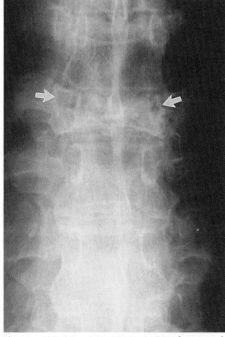

Figure 17-27   **LONG VERTEBRA (*arrow*).** Tuberculosis.

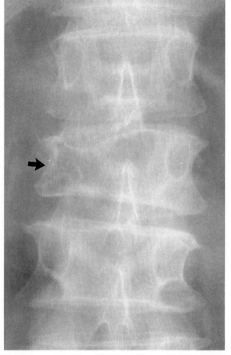

Figure   17-28   **ONE-EYED   VERTEBRA** (*arrow*). Osteolytic metastatic carcinoma.

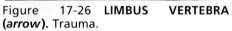

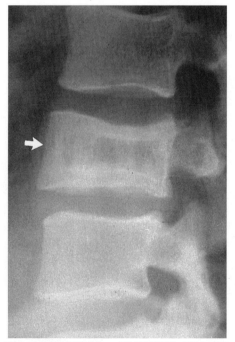

Figure 17-29   **PEDICLE SIGN (*arrows*).** Multiple myeloma.

Figure   17-30   **PICTURE-FRAME VERTEBRA (*arrow*).** Paget's disease.

Pig Snout Vertebra. This is seen on the oblique radiograph of the lumbar spine. It represents a congenital malformation of the transverse process, creating an unusual deformity similar in appearance to the nose of the Scotty dog. (Fig. 17-31) This appearance was named by Dr. William E. Litterer. (38)

Normal variant (38)

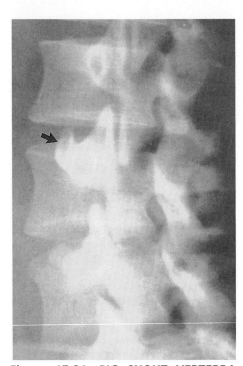

Figure 17-31 **PIG SNOUT VERTEBRA** (*arrow*). Normal variant. (Reprinted with permission from **Keats TE:** *Atlas of Normal Roentgen Variants That May Simulate Disease,* ed 3. Chicago, Year Book Medical, 1984. Courtesy of William E. Litterer, DC, DACBR, Fellow, ACCR, Elizabeth, New Jersey.)

Poker Spine. See *Bamboo Spine.*

Railroad Track Spine. This anomaly is seen on the AP view of the lumbar spine when the apophyseal periarticular ligaments are heavily calcified or ossified. (Fig. 17-32)

Ankylosing spondylitis (10)

Rat Tail Deformity. This appearance is caused by extensive apophyseal ankylosis in the cervical spine. (Fig. 17-33)

Juvenile rheumatoid arthritis (39)

Rugger Jersey Spine. There is osteosclerosis of the superior and inferior endplates with a relatively lucent central portion. The horizontally striped rugby football jerseys were those

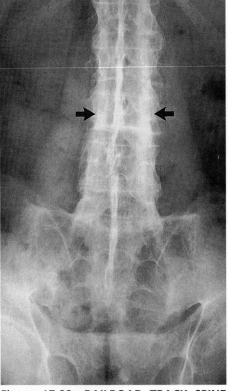

Figure 17-32 **RAILROAD TRACK SPINE** (*arrows*). Ankylosing spondylitis.

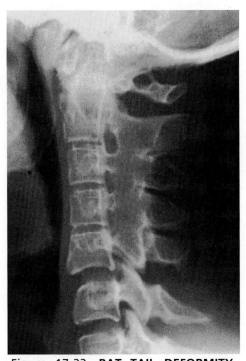

Figure 17-33 **RAT TAIL DEFORMITY.** Juvenile rheumatoid arthritis. Observe the complete ankylosis of the facets from C2 through C5.

of University College Hospital, London, with which the original describer was associated. (40) (Fig. 17-34)

Hyperparathyroidism (primary and secondary) (40,41)

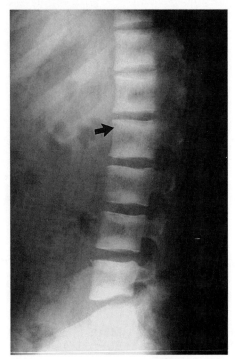

Figure 17-34 **RUGGER JERSEY SPINE** (*arrow*). Hyperparathyroidism.

Sail Vertebra. This is seen on the lateral view of the upper lumbar vertebra. A wedge or hook shape on the anterior surface of the affected segment is seen. (Fig. 17-35)

Achondroplasia (14)
Mucopolysaccharidosis I (Hurler's syndrome) (14)
Mucopolysaccharidosis IV (Morquio's syndrome) (14)
Cretinism (14)

Sandwich Vertebra. This is the result of a uniform increase in the density of the superior and inferior endplates with a relative lucency of the midportions. It can be seen best on the lateral view. (Fig. 17-36)

Osteopetrosis (10,11,14)

Scalloped Vertebra. This vertebra is seen on the lateral view as an exaggerated concavity of the dorsal surface of the vertebral body. (Fig. 17-37)

Normal variant (6,42)
Achondroplasia (6,41)
Ehlers-Danlos syndrome (6,42)
Hydatid disease (6,42)

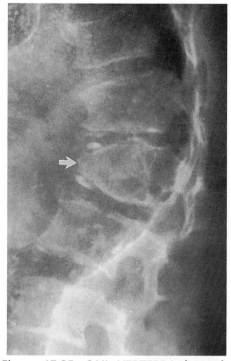

Figure 17-35   **SAIL VERTEBRA (*arrow*).** Cretinism. (Reprinted with permission from **The Center for Devices in Radiological Health, the FDA, and the American College of Radiology:** *The Learning File, Skeletal Section, SK-508.*)

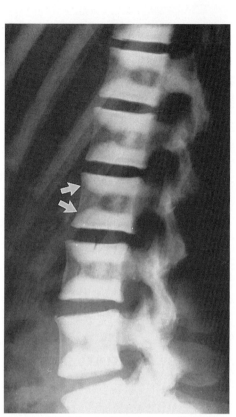

Figure 17-36   **SANDWICH VERTEBRA (*arrows*).** Osteopetrosis.

Lipoma (6,42)
Meningioma (6,42)
Dermoid tumors (6,42)
Mucopolysaccharidosis IV (Morquio's syndrome) (6,42)
Marfan's syndrome (6,42)
Metatrophic dwarfism (6,42)
Osteogenesis imperfecta (6,42)
Neurofibromatosis (6,42)
Ependymoma (6,42)
Syringomyelia (6,42)
Mucopolysaccharidosis I (Hurler's syndrome) (6,42)
Acromegaly (6,42)

Scotty Dog Appearance. This is visualized on the oblique lumbar projection. The ear of the dog is the superior articular facet; the nose, the transverse process; the eye, the pedicle; the forefoot, the inferior articular process; the body, the lamina; the neck, the pars interarticularis; and the spinous process, the tail. This represents normal anatomic landmarks. (Fig. 17-38)

Pars interarticularis defect (18)
Trauma (18)

Scimitar Sacrum. This is a bulging of the arachnoid dural complex that produces a curvilinear defect on the anterior aspect of the sacral canal and resembles a curved Turkish sword.

Myelomeningocele (16)

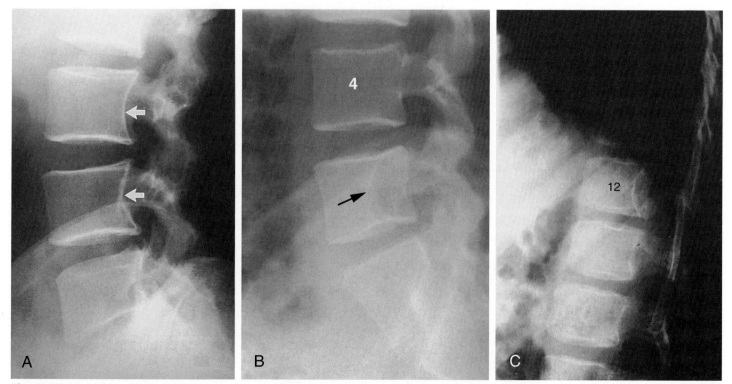

Figure 17-37   **SCALLOPED VERTEBRA. A. Neurofibromatosis (*arrows*). B. Neurofibroma of L5.** Note the posterior vertebral body erosion (*arrow*). **C. Ependymoma of T12.**

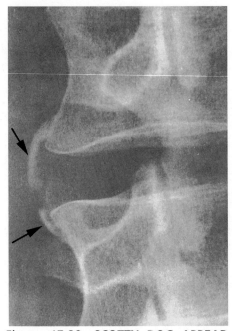

Figure 17-38 **SCOTTY DOG APPEAR-ANCE.** This is a normal radiographic landmark (see text for details). Of incidental notation is a non-marginal syndesmophyte (*arrows*) affecting the vertebral bodies anteriorly. These spurs are characteristic of the seronegative spondyloarthropathies (this patient has psoriasis).

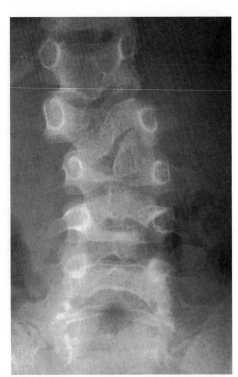

Figure 17-39 **SCRAMBLED SPINE.** Hemivertebrae.

Scrambled Spine. This appearance is the result of multiple congenital anomalies in one area of the spine. (Fig. 17-39)

    Block vertebra (43)
    Hemivertebra (43)
    Butterfly vertebra (43)

Shiny Corner Vertebra. This is caused by reactive osteitis at an anterior corner of the vertebra. (Fig. 17-40)

    Ankylosing spondylitis (8)

Silver Dollar Vertebra. See *Coin-on-End Vertebra.*

Soap Bubble Vertebra (Honeycomb Appearance, Lattice-Like Appearance). Numerous channel-like areas of permeative destruction are seen throughout the vertebral body on both views.

    Actinomycotic infection (6,37)

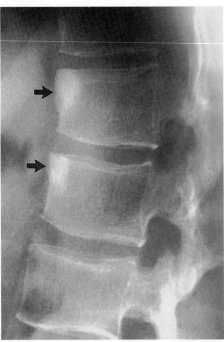

Figure 17-40 **SHINY CORNER VERTEBRA (*arrows*).** Ankylosing spondylitis. (Courtesy of Miriam E. Minty, DC, Perth, Australia.)

Square Vertebra. This is caused by cortical expansion of the anterior aspect of the affected vertebra, as seen on the lateral view. (Fig. 17-41)

    Paget's disease (6)

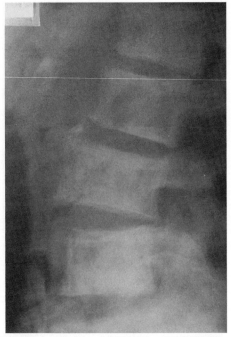

Figure 17-41 **SQUARE VERTEBRA.** Paget's disease of L4 and L5.

Squared-Off Vertebra. This appearance is caused by loss of the normal anterior concavity of the vertebra and is best seen on the lateral projection. (Fig. 17-42)

    Normal variant (6,19)
    Turner's syndrome (6,19)
    Ankylosing spondylitis (6)
    Psoriatic arthritis (6)
    Reiter's syndrome (6)
    Rheumatoid arthritis (6)

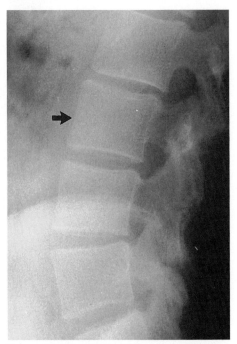

Figure 17-42 **SQUARED-OFF VERTEBRA (*arrow*).** Ankylosing spondylitis.

Step-Off Vertebra. See *Corner Vertebra.*

Striated Vertebra (13). See *Corduroy Cloth Vertebra.*

Swan-Neck Deformity. See *Goose-Neck Deformity.*

Tall Vertebra. Relative increase of the height of the vertebral bodies is seen in hypotonia. Lack of muscular stimulation results in diminished growth of the posterior and lateral appendages of the vertebra.

> Trisomy 21 (Down's syndrome) (44)
> Rubella syndrome (44)
> Neurotrophic disorders (44)

Tongue-Shaped Vertebra. This is seen on the lateral view at the thoracolumbar junction, where the vertebrae have endplates that taper to an anterior beak.

> Cretinism (11)

Tower Vertebra (45). Compensatory growth in height gives this vertebra its vertically elongated appearance. It is seen adjacent to shortened vertebrae that suffered impaired growth owing to sickle cell anemia. More than one tower vertebra may exist next to the compressed segments. (45) The long vertebra of tuberculosis and tall vertebra of the post-paretic patient closely resemble the radiographic appearance of this abnormality.

> Sickle cell disease (45)

Tumbling Block Spine (5). See *Jigsaw Vertebra.*

Two-Eyed Scotty Dog. This is seen best on the oblique lumbar radiograph. The second eye of the Scotty dog is created by an unusually prominent mammillary process.

> Normal variant (46)

Vertebra Plana. See *Coin-on-End Vertebra.*

Wafer-Thin Vertebra. See *Coin-on-End Vertebra.*

Wafer-Like Vertebra. This is best seen on the lateral projection and is the result of complete flattening of the vertebral bodies, with associated widened intervertebral disc spaces.

> Thanatophoric dwarfism (47)

Wasp Waist Vertebra. This is best seen on the lateral view and is the result of anterior indentation at the site of the remnant disc in a congenital block vertebra. (12) (Fig. 17-43)

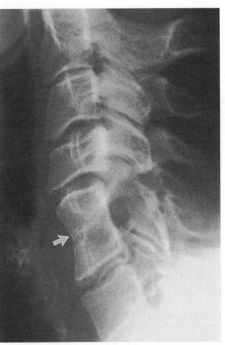

Figure 17-43   WASP WAIST VERTEBRA (*arrow*). Congenital block vertebra. (Courtesy of John R. Nolan, DC, Wanganiu, New Zealand.)

Wedge Vertebra. This vertebra is seen on lateral or AP views and is caused by the loss of anterior bone height, which may be the result of a compression injury or softening.

> Isolated hemivertebra (with advanced spinal deformity) (10)

> Compression injury (8)
> Scheuermann's disease (12)
> Osteomyelitis with collapse (12)
> Myelomeningocele (occasionally) (19)
> Neoplastic infiltration (primary and secondary) (12)

Window-Like Vertebra. See *Picture-Frame Vertebra.*

Winking-Owl Vertebra (48). See *One-Eyed Vertebra.*

Wrinkled Vertebra. This is seen on the AP or lateral view and is a result of softening of the vertebral body, which results in partial collapse of the anterior aspect. (Fig. 17-44)

> Multiple myeloma (10)

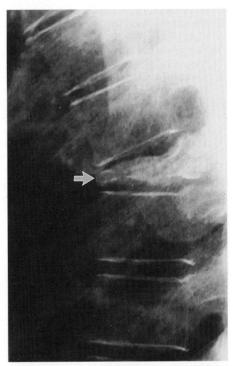

Figure 17-44   WRINKLED VERTEBRA (*arrow*). Multiple myeloma.

CONCLUSION

Although many people do not advocate a pictorial approach to skeletal radiology, many such terms are in use in the current radiologic literature. We believed it would be interesting to collect as many of these as possible to create a list that may be used as a reference to help solve difficult diagnostic problems.

"Then shall our names . . . Familiar in his mouth as household words, Be in their flowing cups remembered." (**Shakespeare,** ***Henry V***)

Although we have diligently searched the literature in the preparation of this chapter, we realize there may be unintentional omissions. We would greatly appreciate notification of any such omissions, so that we can prepare a more complete list at some time in the future.

ACKNOWLEDGMENT

Special thanks to John H. Wilson, JP, MA, AAIM, for his editorial assistance in the preparation of this chapter.

References

1. **Gehweiler JA, Osborne RL, Becker RF:** *The Radiology of Vertebral Trauma.* Philadelphia, WB Saunders, 1980.
2. **Felson B:** *Chest Roentgenology.* Philadelphia, WB Saunders, 1973.
3. **Stelling CB:** *Anomalous attachment of the transverse process to the vertebral body: An accessory finding in congenital absence of a lumbar pedicle.* Skeletal Radiol 6:47, 1981.
4. **Aegerter E, Kirkpatrick J:** *Orthopedic Diseases,* ed 4. Philadelphia, WB Saunders, 1975.
5. **Forrester DM, Brown JC, Nesson JW:** *The Radiology of Joint Disease,* ed 2. Philadelphia, WB Saunders, 1978.
6. **Reeder M, Felson B:** *Gamuts in Radiology.* Cincinnati, OH, Audiovisual Radiology of Cincinnati, 1975.
7. **Teplick JG, Haskin ME:** *Roentgenologic Diagnosis: A Compliment in Radiology to the Beeson and McDermott Textbook of Medicine,* ed 3. Philadelphia, WB Saunders, 1976.
8. **Dihlmann W:** *Current radiodiagnostic concept of ankylosing spondylitis.* Skeletal Radiol 4:179, 1979.
9. **Swischuk LE:** *The beaked, notched or hooked vertebra.* Radiology 95:661, 1970.
10. **Epstein BS:** *The Spine: A Radiological Text and Atlas,* ed 4. Philadelphia, Lea & Febiger, 1976.
11. **Murray R, Jacobson H:** *The Radiology of Skeletal Disorders,* ed 2. Edinburgh, UK, Churchill Livingstone, 1977.
12. **Meschan I:** *Analysis of Roentgen Signs in General Radiology.* Vol 1. Philadelphia, WB Saunders, 1973.
13. **Wackenheim A:** *Radiodiagnosis of the Vertebra in Adults.* New York, Springer-Verlag, 1983.
14. **Greenfield GB:** *Radiology of Bone Diseases,* ed 3. Philadelphia, JB Lippincott, 1980.
15. **Mottram ME, Hill HA:** *Diaphyseal dysplasia.* AJR 95:162, 1965.
16. **Epstein B:** *The Vertebral Column: An Atlas of Tumor Radiology.* Chicago, Year Book Medical, 1974.
17. **Schwartz AM, Homer MJ, McCauley RG:** *"Step-off" vertebral body: Gaucher's disease versus sickle cell hemoglobinopathy.* AJR 132:81, 1979.
18. **Edeiken J, Hodes PJ:** *Roentgen Diagnosis of Diseases of Bone,* ed 2. Vol 1. Baltimore, Williams & Wilkins, 1978.
19. **Ozonoff MB:** *Pediatric Orthopedic Radiology.* Philadelphia, WB Saunders, 1979.
20. **Cane P:** *Butterfly vertebrae.* Br J Radiol 31:503, 1958.
21. **Oppenheimer A:** *Ricketts of the spinal column.* Clin Radiol 8:332, 1939.
22. **Rothman R, Simeone F:** *The Spine.* Vol 2, Philadelphia, WB Saunders, 1975.
23. **Feldman F:** *Miscellaneous localized conditions: A whirlwind review of the "oh my aching back" syndrome.* Semin Roentgenol 14(1):58, 1979.
24. **Moe J, Winter R, Bradford D, et al.:** *Scoliosis and Other Spinal Deformities.* Philadelphia, WB Saunders, 1978.
25. **Deitz GW, Christinsen EE:** *Normal "cupid's bow" contour of lower lumbar vertebrae.* Radiology 121:577, 1976.
26. **Macleod W, Douglas D, Mahaffy R:** *Infantile cortical hyperostosis.* Clin Radiol 16:269, 1965.
27. **Cancelmo JJ:** *Clay shoveler's fracture: A helpful diagnostic sign.* AJR 115:540, 1972.
28. **Schmorl G, Junghans H:** *The Human Spine in Health and Disease,* ed 2. New York, Grune & Stratton, 1971.
29. **Reynolds J:** *A re-evaluation of the "fish vertebra" sign in sickle cell hemoglobinopathy.* AJR 97:693, 1966.
30. **Teplick JG, Head GL, Kricun ME, et al.:** *Ghost infantile vertebrae and hemipelves within adult skeleton from Thorotrast administration in childhood.* Radiology 129:657, 1978.
31. **Sim FH, Svien HJ, Bickel WJ, et al.:** *Swan neck deformity following extensive cervical laminectomy.* J Bone Joint Surg 56A:564, 1974.
32. **Bhalla S, Reinus WR:** *The linear intravertebral vacuum sign of benign vertebral collapse.* AJR Am K Roentgenol 179(6):1563, 1998.
33. **Maldague BE, Noel HM, Malghem JJ:** *The intravertebral vacuum cleft: A sign of ischemic vertebral collapse.* Radiology 129:23, 1978.
34. **Feldman F, Johnson AM, Walter JF:** *Acute axial neuropathy.* Radiology 111:1, 1974.
35. **Rissanen PM:** *"Kissing spine" syndrome in the light of autopsy findings.* Acta Orthop Scand 32:132, 1962.
36. **Riggs W, Rockett J:** *Roentgen chest findings in childhood sickle cell anemia: A new vertebral finding.* AJR 104:838, 1968.
37. **Jacobson HG, Poppel MH, Shapiro JH, et al.:** *The vertebral pedicle sign: A roentgen finding to differentiate metastatic carcinoma from multiple myeloma.* AJR 80:817, 1958.
38. **Keats TE:** *Atlas of Normal Roentgen Variants That May Simulate Disease,* ed 3. Chicago, Year Book Medical, 1984.
39. **Feldman F:** *Radiology, Pathology and Immunology of Bones and Joints: A Review of Current Concepts.* New York, Appleton-Century-Crofts, 1978.
40. **Dent CE, Hodson CJ:** *General softening of bone due to metabolic causes. Radiologic changes associated with certain metabolic bone diseases.* Br J Radiol 27:605, 1954.
41. **Vaughn BF, Walters MNI:** *Sclerotic banded vertebra (rugger jersey spine).* Austral Radiol 7:87, 1963.
42. **Mitchell GE, Lourie H, Berne AS:** *The various causes of scalloped vertebra with notes on their pathogenesis.* Radiology 89:67, 1967.
43. **Wilkinson RH, Strand RD:** *Congenital anomalies and normal variants.* Semin Roentgenol 14(1):7, 1979.
44. **Gooding CA, Neuhauser EBD:** *Growth and development of the vertebral bodies in the presence and absence of normal stress.* AJR 93:388, 1965.
45. **Marlow TJ, Brunson CY, Jackson S, Schabel SI:** *"Tower vertebra": A new observation in sickle cell disease.* Skeletal Radiol 27(4):195, 1998.
46. **Resnik CS, Smithson LV, Bradshaw JA, et al.:** *The two-eyed scotty dog: A normal anatomic variant.* Radiology 149:680, 1983.
47. **Paul L, Juhl J:** *The Essentials of Roentgen Interpretation,* ed 3. Hagerstown, Maryland, Harper & Row, 1972.
48. **Macnab I:** *Backache.* Baltimore, Williams & Wilkins, 1977.

Masqueraders of Musculoskeletal Disease

18

Lindsay J. Rowe and Terry R. Yochum

"Things are seldom what they seem, skim milk masquerades as cream"
—Gilbert & Sullivan's H.M.S. Pinafore

INTRODUCTION

Musculoskeletal conditions are the underlying cause for the presenting complaints of most patients who are seen by a clinician in a musculoskeletal-related practice. Because of this, a particular bias toward a musculoskeletal diagnosis may certainly develop over time because the preponderance of cases actually prove to be of this origin. The purpose of this chapter is twofold: First, to remind the practitioner that a number of conditions, some minor and others quite serious, can mimic the clinical presentation of musculoskeletal disease while others may have an atypical presentation resembling that of common musculoskeletal disease. Second, to provide a brief summary of the more relevant masqueraders involving the head, soft tissues of the neck, thorax, abdomen, and lower extremities. With those objectives in mind, we have given this chapter the title "Masqueraders of Musculoskeletal Disease." In keeping with the earlier editions of *Essentials of Skeletal Radiology,* the plain film findings are emphasized when applicable and other imaging modalities are provided when appropriate. The approach of this chapter differs dramatically from other chapters in this text by following an anatomic format and by using a cat-

egorical and condition-specific discussion of the various pathologies. In addition, the information included for each entity is abbreviated to include only the most pertinent facts.

This chapter is by no means intended to be a comprehensive compilation of disorders; thus, the material content for each entity is in synoptic form. The text provides only the most relevant clinical and imaging features of the entities discussed. When more information or detail regarding a certain condition is required, a more comprehensive text, dedicated to that specialized area of study, should be consulted.

THE HEAD: MASQUERADERS OF MUSCULOSKELETAL DISEASE

Common musculoskeletal complaints emanating from the intracranial contents include headache, neck pain and stiffness, limb pain, and neurological dysfunction. Additional clues to the presence of significant brain disease may be elicited with a more detailed history and physical examination. The list of possible conditions that have been implicated in these complaints is long; the most common and important are presented here.

INTRACRANIAL HEMORRHAGES

Intracranial hemorrhage is a relatively common cause for acute neurological dysfunction and arises from many entities including trauma, hypertension, arterial disease, aneurysms, arteriovenous malformations, and tumors. The three key imaging correlates in hemorrhage are location, age of the bleed, and determining the cause. (1) Establishing these often requires correlating findings of CT, MRI, and, occasionally, angiography.

Hemorrhages are classified according to the anatomic site of blood accumulation: extradural (epidural), subdural, subarachnoid, intracerebral, and intraventricular. Regardless of location, extravasated blood undergoes a series of chemical changes that causes imaging findings to vary according to the time elapsed from the bleeding event until imaging is performed. (Table 18-1) For CT and MRI purposes, hemorrhagic events are described as hyperacute (4–6 hr), acute (12–48 hr), subacute (2–7 days), and chronic. (2,3) Tomography is seldom used owing to the availability of CT.

Hyperacute and acute hemorrhage is best imaged with CT because it is most sensitive to the detection of early bleeds and allows easiest and fastest image acquisition. (4) The role of MRI in intracranial bleeding events is nonetheless critical and rapidly expanding. A brief overview of MRI findings that occur in the evolution of the acute through the chronic stages of hemorrhage follows.

MRI studies of intracranial hemorrhage produce a spectrum of appearances based on the stage of hemoglobin degradation. (4,5) (Table 18-1) For the first 24 hr, extravasated blood cannot be easily discerned. It responds in the same way to the magnetic field of the scanner and therefore has the same signal properties as (i.e., is *isointense* with) the surrounding brain. During this period, MRI findings are limited to edema. Over time oxyhemoglobin becomes methemoglobin, which does respond differently to the magnetic field than does the surrounding tissues because of its paramagnetic properties.

The most paramagnetic phase (when detection is greatest) occurs in the subacute period, 3–14 days after the event. During this time methemoglobin produces high signal on T1-weighted studies. Subsequent conversion of methemoglobin to hemosiderin results in low MRI signal on all pulse sequences and typically occurs first around the periphery of a hemorrhagic site. (1,3) MRI remains the most sensitive method in determining the cause for the hemorrhage, allowing demonstration of an underlying mass lesion and identification of other smaller co-existing mass lesions of metastases and features of arteriovenous malformations. Magnetic resonance angiography (MRA) is also rapidly replacing angiography for depicting aneurysms. (6,7)

Epidural (Extradural) Hemorrhage

The dura of the cranium is actually the periosteum of the inner table of the skull. Epidural (extradural) hemorrhage (EDH) causes an accumulation of blood between the inner table and the firmly adherent dura. Epidural bleeding is typically from an arterial source, often a branch of the middle meningeal artery. The most anatomically vulnerable site is over the squamous portion of the temporal bone, which is thin and has branches of the middle meningeal artery embedded in the inner table. The most common cause of bleeding is direct skull trauma with associated skull fracture. (3,6)

Clinical Features. The presentation may be that of headache, confusion, irritability, and history of a temporary loss of consciousness. EDH is the nemesis of the unwary—a quick recovery from the initial injury effects may be followed within hours by a classic *lucid interval,* during which only headache or other minimal symptoms occur. The patient later goes to sleep and, unless monitored, fails to regain consciousness owing to gradually increasing intracranial pressure, which leads to compromised brainstem function as the result of the mass effect of the hemorrhage. Death may ensue in up to 10% of cases. (8)

Imaging Features. Skull radiographs may show fracture; however, close inspection of CT bone windows at the site of hematoma will demonstrate a fracture in 95% of cases. (9) On CT examination the acute blood is hyperdense. A classic lentiform (i.e., *lens-like* or *biconvex*) shape occurs owing to the firm adherence of the dura to the inner skull table. (Fig. 18-1) Depending on the size of the hematoma, mass effect may cause local displacement of brain tissue or more massive shifting of cranial contents (*midline shift*). If intracranial pressure builds sufficiently, the brainstem may be forced downward into the foramen magnum (*coning* of the brainstem).

Treatment of EDH consists of surgical evacuation of the hematoma and achieving hemostasis of the bleeding site once it has been identified. Follow-up CT studies often show localized gliosis of the underlying cortex as low attenuation changes and focal atrophy. (1,4)

Subdural Hemorrhage

In subdural hemorrhage (SDH), blood accumulates between the dura and outside of the arachnoid layer. In contrast to EDH, bleeding sources in SDH are usually venous, following disruption of the bridging subdural veins. (10) The most common mechanism is a shearing force that tears subdural veins when intracranial contents shift during trauma. The elderly are predisposed to SDH because of brain atrophy, which allows for a greater magnitude

Table 18-1	MRI Appearance of Hemorrhage					
				Weighting		
Phase	Timing	Location	Hemoglobin	T1	T2	Comments
Hyperacute	< 24 hr	Intracellular	Oxyhemoglobin	Isointense	High	CT most sensitive
Acute	1–3 days	Intracellular	Deoxyhemoglobin	Isointense	Low	CT most sensitive
Subacute, early	3–6 days	Intracellular	Methemoglobin	High	Low	T1 high signal
Subacute, late	7–13 days	Extracellular	Methemoglobin	High	High	T1 high signal
Chronic, center	> 14 days	Extracellular	Hemachromes	Isointense	High	—
Chronic, rim	> 14 days	Intracellular	Hemosiderin	Low	Low	Gradient echo sensitive

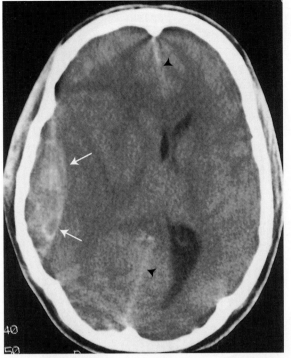

Figure 18-1   EPIDURAL HEMORRHAGE. CT, Axial Head. Note the sharply marginated density abutting the inner table of the temporal bone indicating an acute hemorrhage (*arrows*). Observe the characteristic biconvex shape of the blood accumulating in the extradural (epidural) space. The hematoma and cerebral edema produce a midline shift to the left, with bowing of the falx (*arrowheads*) and compression of the lateral ventricle. *COMMENT:* This type of hemorrhage is usually associated with a co-existing fracture that lacerates a branch of the middle meningeal artery.

of brain movement from lesser degrees of trauma. Laceration of the arachnoid membrane can also cause a similar injury if cerebrospinal fluid (CSF) leaks into the subdural space without hemorrhage (*subdural hygroma*).

Clinical Features. In young patients, high-velocity trauma is the most common mechanism. A frontoparietal location is typical. Between 10% and 15% are bilateral and up to 50% have concurrent intracerebral hemorrhage, brain contusion, and shearing brain injury. (7,11) Isolated subdural bleeds have a mortality of 20% and mortality can be as high as 60–90% when associated with intracerebral injury. (12) Confusion, headache, seizure, and upper motor neuron abnormalities are the most common features in acute cases. In the elderly, acute SDH is often found superimposed on chronic subdural hemorrhage. In non-accidental injury in children (shaken baby syndrome), bilateral SDH or SDH in the falx are characteristic findings. (13)

Imaging Features. The characteristic CT finding is a crescent or sickle-shaped mass with a concave inner border. (4) (Fig. 18-2) The internal density varies according to the time interval since the initiating event. Generally, the masses are hyperdense in the first 7 days and then become progressively lower in density after the initiating event. During 1–3 weeks postbleeding the blood

becomes isodense with the brain and may need to be outlined with intravenous contrast. After 3 weeks the fluid is typically hypodense. (3,7) Repeated episodes of bleeding, especially in the elderly, may lead to a hypodense fluid collection with a *hematocrit effect* as the cellular components settle into a layered appearance. Compression of the adjacent brain is evidenced by loss of the sulci, displacement away from the collection, and a small ipsilateral lateral ventricle. (1,7)

Subarachnoid Hemorrhage

Blood between the arachnoid and pia (subarachnoid space) is most commonly the result of a ruptured intracranial aneurysm but can be seen following trauma. Such subarachnoid hemorrhage (SAH) most commonly affects vessels forming or immediate branching from the circle of Willis. Because bleeding occurs into the CSF space, the presence of blood elements on CSF examination (*spinal tap*) is diagnostic.

Clinical Features. Confusion, photophobia, headache, and seizure are the most common clinical features. The classic presentation is acute onset of severe headache, often described as "the worst headache of my life." A less severe event may have occurred within the previous 1–3 days, described as a *sentinel bleed*. Although more classically associated with infectious meningitis, nuchal rigidity may also be seen with bleeding into the subarachnoid space. (5,6,14) This entity is discussed more completely later in this chapter (see "Aneurysms"). Hydrocephalus often complicates SAH because the blood elements in the CSF obstruct the resorptive capacity of the arachnoid granulations. Complicating hydrocephalus is a poor prognostic indicator

Imaging Features. CT studies in the first 24 hr detect at least 90% of SAH, although the changing nature of extravasated blood makes most bleeds undetectable on CT after 3 days. (15) Axial images show high-density blood that pools in the basal cisterns, following the course of the cerebral arteries at the circle of Willis. Extensive blood accumulation can form a five-sided (pentagonal) shape. (4,7) (Fig. 18-3) With aneurysms, the area of accumulation of SAH may have localizing value for the site of origin. Additional common sites where SAH is visible is in the Sylvian fissure, tentorium, and posterior falx. MRI is relatively insensitive for detection of acute SAH owing to the poor paramagnetic properties of oxyhemoglobin found in acutely extravasated blood. (2,3)

Intracerebral Hemorrhage

Bleeding into the brain parenchyma occurs from a ruptured vessel, usually an artery or capillary, though occasionally a vein. The incidence of underlying tumor in intracerebral hemorrhage is 1–5%. (16)

Clinical Features. Acute collapse, confusion, photophobia, headache, and seizure are the most common features. The most common cause is hypertension (essential, malignant, eclampsia) but intracerebral hemorrhage can be seen with tumors, vascular disease, arteriovenous malformation, aneurysm, and trauma. Up to two thirds of hypertensive hemorrhages occur in the basal ganglia secondary to ruptured microaneurysms (Charcot-Bouchard aneurysms). (17) Other sites include the

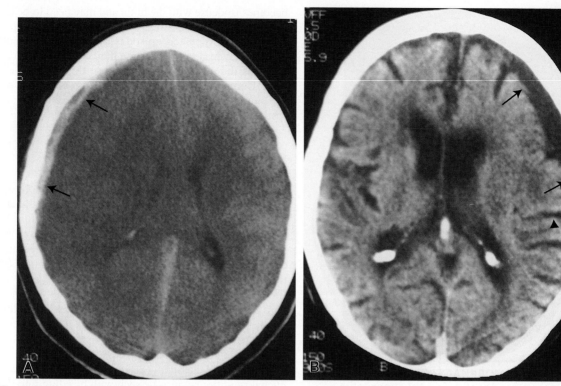

Figure 18-2 SUBDURAL HEMORRHAGE. A. Acute Subdural Hemorrhage, Young Patient, CT, Axial Head. Observe the dense, thin, lens-like collection of subdural hemorrhage (*arrows*) paralleling the concave inner table of the parietal bone. **B. Chronic Subdural Hemorrhage, Elderly Patient, CT, Axial Head.** Note the low-density fluid collection, which is exerting some mass effect on the adjacent cerebral cortex (*arrows*). The darker and widened sulci of the brain indicate atrophy, commonly found in the more chronic residual form of the hemorrhage (*arrowhead*). *COMMENT:* This type of hemorrhage results from disruption of the perforating veins that traverse the subdural space and often follows severe head trauma in the young or mild trauma in the elderly. The appearance of the hemorrhage on CT changes with time—it is initially dense, then isodense with the brain, and subsequently hypodense.

thalamus (15%), pons (10%), and cerebellum (5%). (17) Rupture of the ventricular walls—intraventricular hemorrhage (IVH)—occurs in about 50% of cases and is a poor prognostic indicator, especially if there is blood in the fourth ventricle. The clinical course is variable, though 25% of patients will die within 48 hr. (3) Perinatal hemorrhage of the newborn is more common in premature babies, hypoxia, and traumatic and multiple births. These are best imaged with transcranial ultrasound through the patent fontanelles. (2,3)

Imaging Features. CT studies typically show a solitary round, high-density lesion of variable size, usually located in the basal ganglia. The high attenuation is primarily owing to protein in the hemorrhage rather than hemoglobin. (18) There is frequently a rim of low-attenuation edema, mass effect onto adjacent structures, and generalized hemispheric edema. (Fig. 18-4) With resolution, the density gradually reduces to become hypodense over 10–20 days. (4,5,7) Contrast injection will usually produce *ring enhancement* of the lesion for at least 3 months after the hemorrhagic event. Old hemorrhagic foci produce low-attenuation areas, as a result of gliosis, which may contain fluid and produce a *porencephalic cyst.* Communication of such cysts with the ventricular system may result from periventricular hemorrhage. (3,6) MRI studies of intracerebral hemorrhage produce a spectrum of appearances based on the stage of hemoglobin degradation. (4,5) (Table 18-1)

Diffuse Axonal Injury

Diffuse axonal injury (DAI), rupture of nerve axons, can occur following trauma and is usually accompanied by torn small arteries, resulting in focal *petechial* hemorrhages.

Clinical Features. There is usually a loss of consciousness at the time of trauma. The mechanism is usually caused by rotational or acceleration–deceleration forces. Axonal shear-strain injury following trauma ruptures the nerve fibers and results in retraction bulbs and loss of nerve function. (10) DAI is a factor in post–head injury syndromes.

Imaging Features. Initial CT scans are frequently normal, with findings seen in < 20–50% of cases. (12) Delayed scans, 1–3 days after injury, may show abnormalities, more frequently consisting of small high-density lesions at the gray–white interfaces of the frontal lobes, corpus callosum, and upper brainstem. (19) MRI T2-weighted scans are more sensitive and show small high signal foci. Functional MRI may be useful in locating the anatomic sites of neural dysfunction in post–head injury syndromes. (3,6)

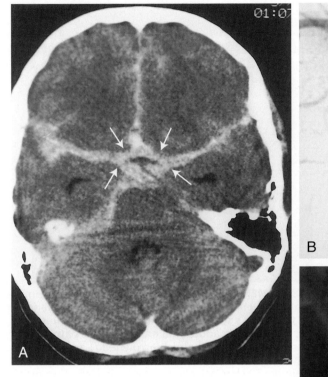

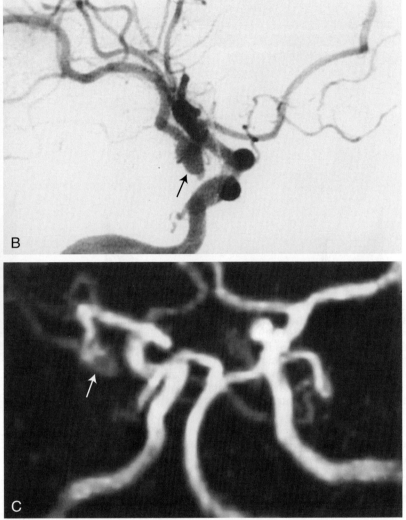

Figure 18-3 **SUBARACHNOID HEMORRHAGE WITH CIRCLE OF WILLIS ANEURYSM. A. CT, Axial Head.** Acute blood lies within the subarachnoid space surrounding the branches of the circle of Willis, creating the classic pentagonal shape (*arrows*). The anterior midline collection lies in the interhemispheric fissure, laterally within the Sylvian fissure and posteriorly over the tentorium. **B. Digital Subtraction Angiogram, Cerebral.** Contrast, injected after selective catheterization of the internal carotid artery, clearly identifies the aneurysm (*arrow*). **C. Three-Dimensional Time-of-Flight MRA, Cerebral.** The aneurysm within the middle cerebral artery is visible as a localized outpouching (*arrow*). *COMMENT:* MRA is a non-invasive modality that can be used to identify aneurysms in high-risk patients. It is, however, a flow-dependent study, and those aneurysms with thrombus or slow flow may not be demonstrated.

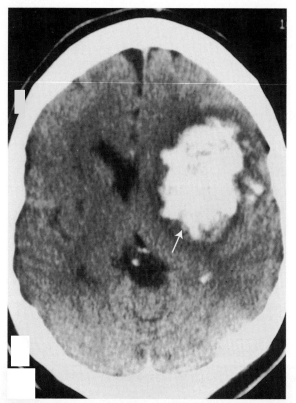

Figure 18-4 INTRACEREBRAL HEMORRHAGE, BASAL GANGLIA, CT, Axial Head. Note the localized, high-attenuation hematoma within the region of the basal ganglia (*arrow*). *COMMENT:* Spontaneous intracerebral hemorrhage, often associated with hypertension, most commonly involves the basal ganglia. When found outside this location, the probability of other causes—including hemorrhagic tumor, arteriovenous malformation, and amyloid angiopathy—increases.

INTRACRANIAL INFECTIONS

Meningitis

Infection of the meninges is the most common intracranial infection. Meningitis can be divided into three general categories: acute pyogenic, lymphocytic, and chronic. (1)

- *Acute pyogenic meningitis.* This form is usually bacterial in origin, and the specific pathogen varies with age. In neonates, group B streptococcus, *Escherichia coli*, and *Listeria* predominate; in children under 7 years of age, *Haemophilus influenzae* is common; and in older children and young adults, *Neisseria meningitides* is the most common cause. Adult bacterial meningitis is most often the result of *Streptococcus pneumoniae*. The infection is characterized by a purulent exudate that fills the subarachnoid space and can be complicated by hydrocephalus, vasospasm, infarction, cerebritis, abscess, and ventriculitis. (2,3)
- *Lymphocytic meningitis.* Enterovirus (echovirus and coxsackievirus) makes up 50–80% of the cases and tends to be self-limiting. There are no imaging findings.
- *Chronic meningitis.* The most common pathogens include

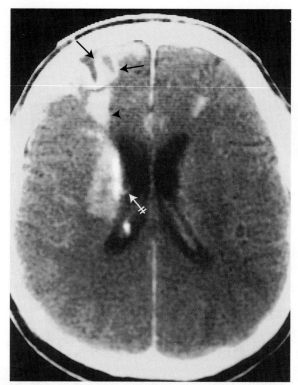

Figure 18-5 MENINGITIS. CT, Axial Head. After the administration of intravenous contrast there is localized enhancement of the brain's surface, characteristic of meningitis (*arrows*). Observe the additional enhancement within the brain parenchyma (encephalitis) (*arrowhead*) and ventricular surface (ventriculitis) (*crossed arrow*). *COMMENT:* Non-contrast images are relatively insensitive in detecting meningitis. The phenomenon of contrast enhancement is the result of the capillaries becoming increasingly permeable, which allows the intravenous contrast to extravasate into the interstitial space. This can be seen in a number of conditions, including infection, tumor, infarction, radiation, trauma, and demyelinating disease.

Mycobacterium tuberculosis (TB), *Coccidioidomycosis immitis*, and *Cryptococcus neoformans*. While relatively uncommon, there is a predisposition to involving the base of the brain. (3,4)

Clinical Features. Headache, fever, and neck stiffness are the characteristic triad of clinical findings. The classic signs of meningitis include flexion of the knees and hips when the neck is flexed (Brudzinski's sign) and the inability to straighten the knee when the leg is elevated (Kernig's sign). Viral meningitis results in less severe symptoms. Three patterns of presentation have been documented. In 25% of cases there is a fulminant and often life-threatening onset over 24 hr. (5,6) Up to 50% of cases will develop meningitis more progressively, over 1–7 days; the infection is associated with respiratory symptoms. Less than 20% of patients have an onset over 1–3 weeks. (3,4) Lumbar puncture may provide the diagnosis, with leukocytosis, elevated protein, low glucose, Gram stain, and culture-grown pathogenic colonies. (3)

Imaging Features. CT scan is often normal in the early phases. (7) The use of intravenous contrast is imperative for diagnosis when there may be enhancement of the meninges. (Fig. 18-5)

Non-specific signs may also include hydrocephalus. MRI T1-weighted postcontrast studies are the most sensitive method for detection. (8)

Encephalitis

Diffuse brain parenchymal inflammation can be caused by a wide spectrum of pathogens but is most commonly of viral origin. Pathogens include herpes simplex, arthropod-borne disease, and non-viral agents (e.g., toxoplasmosis). Additional causes include AIDS, Creutzfeldt-Jakob disease, and acute disseminated encephalomyelitis (ADEM). (4)

Clinical Features. There is a spectrum of presentations, depending on the underlying agent, ranging from acute, fulminating disease to an indolent, chronic course. The diagnosis often remains elusive and requires CSF, blood studies, imaging, and even biopsy.

Herpes simplex is the most common cause of encephalitis, characterized by rapid onset of confusion, seizures, fever, and headache. (6) The mortality rate may be as high as 50–70%, and survivors suffer significant morbidity. (6) It reaches the brain by retrograde spread from the orofacial superficial infection along the olfactory and trigeminal nerves and remains latent within the Gasserian ganglion. (6)

Imaging Features. Herpes simplex encephalitis typically involves the limbic system—including the temporal lobes, insula, subfrontal, and cingulate gyri—with petechial hemorrhages, necrosis, and lymphocytic infiltrations. (9) In the early stages CT studies are frequently normal. Later, low-density changes within the temporal lobes and heterogeneous gyriform or patchy enhancement with contrast are typical. MRI is more sensitive than CT, especially in the early stages. On T2-weighted studies, high signal is present in the temporal lobes, cingulate gyrus, and insular cortex with sparing of the adjacent putamen. Postcontrast enhancement of these same regions is common. (2,10)

Cerebral Abscess

Purulent brain infection is relatively uncommon, but early diagnosis and treatment are important for reducing mortality.

Clinical Features. Purulent brain infection may occur secondary to hematogenous spread from an extracranial site or directly from infection of the meninges, mastoid, or frontal sinuses. Headache, fever, and confusion are common; mortality is up to 50%. (3) A sequence of changes occurs in the infected brain parenchyma, beginning with acute cerebritis as a diffuse infiltrate with edema (*early cerebritis; 3–5 days*) and progressing to central necrosis with a peripheral rim of inflammatory change (*late cerebritis; 5–14 days*). (11) A well-defined capsule of collagen and elastin forms after 2 weeks (*early capsule phase*) surrounding a liquefactive core; after months the capsule becomes thicker and mature (*late capsule phase*). (11) Resolution slowly occurs with shrinkage of the abscess cavity. The frontal and parietal lobes at the corticomedullary junction are the most common sites of involvement.

Imaging Features. The phase of the infection governs the imaging signs. Generally, cerebritis images as high signal on T2-weighted studies, with poorly defined enhancement of the involved area. (Fig. 18-6) After progression to capsule formation *ring enhancement* occurs; the capsule is often thinner toward the ventricle and thicker toward the cortical surface. (11) Compli-

cations include satellite abscesses, ventriculitis, meningitis, and choroid plexitis. Contrast studies will show enhancement of these structures. (4,5)

Parasitic Infection

Numerous parasites can infect the brain. These include toxoplasmosis, cysticercosis, schistosomiasis, and echinococcosis.

Clinical Features. Toxoplasmosis can occur as a primary infection or in combination with HIV. Cysticercosis is caused by the ingestion of pork that contains *Taenia solium*. The worm resides in the small intestine and sheds eggs that hatch larvae and bore through the wall to disseminate hematogenously. Up to 60–90% of cases will have the disease in the brain. (6)

Imaging Features. Toxoplasmosis involves the basal ganglia and cerebral hemispheres and causes a mass-type lesion with peripheral nodular ring enhancement and a central focus of enhancement (*target lesion*). Multiple lesions are common. Cysticercosis of the brain (neurocysticercosis) in the acute phase is visible on MRI and CT as small focal-enhancing lesions with surrounding edema. A small mural nodule may be visible, which represents a scolex. Later they will calcify, which is more obvious on CT. In peripheral muscle the cysticerci encyst and calcify as 1- to 3-mm round to oval shapes (*rice grains* or *cigar shaped*), with the long axis orientated along muscle fascial planes. (3,4,10)

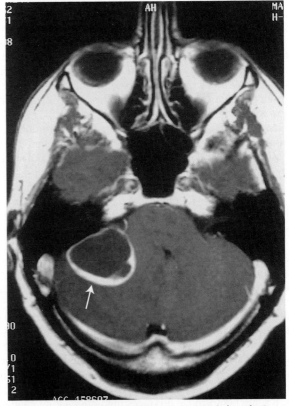

Figure 18-6 CEREBELLAR ABSCESS. T1-Weighted, Contrast-Enhanced MRI, Axial Brain. A ring-enhancing lesion is present within the right cerebellar hemisphere (*arrow*). No enhancement of the adjacent meninges is present. *COMMENT:* Contrast enhancement is not specific for tumor and is also found in infections, inflammation, traumatic injuries, and postradiation therapy.

INTRACRANIAL TUMORS

Tumors are a relatively uncommon pathology of the brain in adults but in children are the most common solid mass. This bimodal age distribution also correlates with different tumor types and locations. Posterior fossa tumors are the most common lesions in children (medulloblastoma, pilocytic astrocytoma, ependymoma, hemangioblastoma), whereas supratentorial gliomas (glioblastoma) and meta-stases predominate in adults. (1,2)

Musculoskeletal Symptoms. A broad spectrum of clinical signs and symptoms occur in the presence of a brain tumor, for example, neurological deficits (weakness, paralysis, paresthesia) of the limbs or face, altered behavior, seizure activity, loss of memory, early morning vomiting, and visual and speech disturbances. (3) Headaches are the main musculoskeletal association, which may be the result of complicating hemorrhage, hydrocephalus, or dural irritation. The headache may be non-specific, but key features such as increasing severity, unrelenting nature, and early morning wakening with headache may arouse suspicion for intracranial tumor. (3) Torticollis may be found, especially with posterior fossa tumors, secondary to altered tonic neck reflexes. The triad of increasing severity of headache, vomiting, and neurological deficit is a marker of an intracranial mass. (3,4)

Imaging Signs. Although each tumor type may have variable findings, the key imaging signs on CT and MRI can be summarized by the following six basic findings. (2,5)

* *Mass lesion.* Tumor tissue creates localized enlargement at the site of origin, which compresses adjacent structures (*mass effect*), displacing structures away from the mass and changing the normal surface contours locally (*effacement*). The imaging density of the mass relative to normal tissue may be the same (isodense, isointense), greater (high attenuation, high signal), or less (low attenuation, low signal). (4,6,7)
* *Edema.* Increased local water content at the tumor site is a common finding, owing to two mechanisms: cytotoxic and vasogenic edema. (2,3) Cytotoxic edema is usually caused by ischemia, which increases intracellular water as a result of a breakdown in the cellular membrane transport mechanisms (e.g., $Na^+–K^+$ pump), precipitating net osmotic flow into the cell. Vasogenic edema occurs from increased vessel permeability from tumor vessels lacking a basement membrane, altered gap junctions, inflammatory mediators, and other mechanisms. On CT, edema creates decreased attenuation in the brain, especially of the white matter (*pseudo-pod sign*), gyral swelling, sulcal effacement, and mass effect onto adjacent structures. (1,5)
* *Hemorrhage.* Tumors that are more heavily vascularized, rapidly growing, angioinvasive, and undergoing necrosis are prone to complicating hemorrhage. This may occur in as many as 15% of brain tumors and includes high-grade astrocytoma, pituitary adenoma, and leukemia as well as metastases from the kidney, thyroid, and melanoma. (2) On CT acute hemorrhage produces high-attenuating changes in acute bleeds, evolving over 7–10 days to low-attenuating fluid. The MRI findings of hemorrhage are more variable, with the progressive breakdown of hemoglobin (see introduction to "Intracranial Hemorrhages"). (1,2) (Table 18-1)
* *Necrosis.* Variable degrees of unviable tissue occur in brain tumors, and this is recognized as a sign of aggressive behavior. On CT signs of tumor necrosis are low-attenuation center, lack of enhancement, calcification, and cyst formation; cysts may have fluid or fluid–fluid levels from previous hemorrhage. On MRI the necrotic tissue usually remains low in signal on both T1- and T2-weighted studies, does not enhance with gadolinium, and reveals internal fluid. (3,7) The fluid may be purely high signal on T2-weighted studies or may contain signs of previous hemorrhage, including layering of cellular debris and hemoglobin degradation products of variable intensity, depending on their age. (1)
* *Calcification.* The presence of calcification may occur secondary to necrosis or as a result of neoplastic formation. Tumors that may contain calcium include meningioma, oligodendroglioma, astrocytoma, and craniopharyngioma. (2,4)
* *Enhancement.* The phenomenon of increased tissue attenuation on CT or MRI signal after the administration of intravenous contrast agent (CT, iodinated contrast; MRI, gadolinium) is referred to as *enhancement*. The pathophysiologic basis for contrast enhancement is essentially the result of a combination of increased vascularity and increased vascular permeability, which allows the intravascular contrast agent to leak into the extravascular space and accumulate in the adjacent interstitium. It occurs both within the tumor and within the normal edematous tissue interface. Contrast enhancement is not specific for tumor and occurs in infection, trauma, infarct, radiotherapy, and any inflammatory condition. (3,5) The phenomenon of ring enhancement, by which there is contrast accumulation predominantly in the periphery of a lesion, reflects the lack of internal vascularity, usually from necrosis and the inflammatory peripheral interface with normal tissue. (4,5)

Astrocytoma

Arising from astrocytes within the central nervous system (CNS), astrocytoma is the most common primary malignant brain (75% of cases) and spinal cord tumor. (5) Of variable growth potential, it can also be the most rapidly progressive tumor, producing death within a short time of diagnosis.

Clinical Features. Astrocytoma most commonly occurs in adults between 20 and 40 years of age. (5) The incidence of location is proportional to the amount of white matter present; the most common locations are above the tentorium (*supratentorial*) in the parietal, frontal, or temporal lobes. In children, it most commonly arises in the posterior fossa, involving the cerebellum or brainstem; is more benign in its clinical course; and has a specific histologic appearance, in which the astrocytes exhibit fine filiform hair-like processes (*pilocytic astrocytoma*). Its biological activity covers a spectrum ranging from low to high grade, based on the degree of cellularity, necrosis, and neovascularization. (5) Grade 1 astrocytoma (low grade) is the most benign, in which there is an absence of necrosis or neovascularization. Grade 2 (anaplastic) is based on cellular atypia without necrosis; whereas grade 3 (glioblastoma multiforme) is the most malignant (neovascularization and necrosis are demonstrated). (2,6,8)

The most common scenarios of presentation are increasing frequency and severity of headaches; seizures; stroke-like episodes; personality changes; and motor and sensory deficits of the face, throat, and limbs. (2,8)

Imaging Features. MRI remains the premier imaging modality in the detection, differential diagnosis, surgical planning, and follow-up of astrocytoma. CT with contrast enhancement is often the first study to detect the tumor in acute presentations and has a high sensitivity for detection, approaching that of MRI. (Fig. 18-7) On non-contrast CT the lesion is often obscured by the surrounding white matter vasogenic edema, evidenced by enlargement of the subcortical extensions (pseudo-pod appearance). (6,7) Commonly there is midline shift and compression of adjacent structures (mass effect), especially the ventricles. Low-density changes within the tumor that fail to enhance are the result of necrosis and cyst formation. When high density is seen it is usually because of hemorrhage. (7,9) On contrast administration, the peripheral tumor edge is highlighted as an irregular rim (ring enhancement). The presence of cystic change, vivid enhancement, hemorrhage, and edema are features of higher-grade tumors.

MRI features parallel those of CT, including edema, midline shift, mass effect, and cystic cavities (which may have fluid–fluid levels from previous hemorrhage and peripheral enhancement). (5)

Meningioma

Meningioma, usually a benign tumor, is the most common primary non-glial CNS neoplasm arising from meningothelial cells (arachnoid cap cells) within the meninges. It is the most common extra-axial brain tumor and makes up 15–18% of adult primary intracranial tumors. (5)

Clinical Features. The age range for this tumor is 35–70 years, with a peak at 45 years. In patients < 50 years of age, females predominate at approximately 3:1; in patients > 50 years, there is a 1:1 gender involvement. (10) Less than 10% of cases are symptomatic, with seizures, hemiparesis, visual defects, headaches, and nerve palsies. The anatomic distribution parallels the venous sinuses, confluence of sutures, and arachnoid granulations. Almost 50% involve the cerebral hemispheres near the coronal suture and falx; 20% occur at the sphenoid ridge and 10% in the posterior fossa. (2,5) Up to 12% occur in the spine. (2,5)

Four histologic types are described: The two benign forms are fibroblastic and transitional; the more aggressive types are meningothelial and angioblastic. (2,5) Calcification is common within *psammoma* bodies. Known associations include neurofibromatosis (type II), radiotherapy, and sex hormone–related conditions (e.g., perimenopause and breast cancer); size may increase during pregnancy. Treatment is by resection, with a 3–7% recurrence rate in benign forms increasing to 75% in anaplastic varieties. (11)

Imaging Features. Plain film findings may include hyperostosis of the adjacent bone that may extend to the outer table, parenchymal calcification, prominent dural membrane ossification, and prominent vascular grooves. (2,4) On non-contrast CT 75% of tumors are hyperdense, with 25% exhibiting some form of matrix calcification. On contrast CT there is intense homogeneous enhancement of the tumor mass and occasionally of the contiguous dura (*dural tail*). (5) (Fig. 18-8) On MRI T1- and T2-weighted images the lesion is typically isointense with gray matter (isointense meningioma). Encasement of the internal carotid artery, especially at the cavernous sinus, may render it only partially resectable. Internal vascularity can be seen with flow voids, and there is often peritumoral edema. Gadolinium enhancement is vivid and dural extension (dural tail) is seen more commonly. (2) Angiography shows a vascular mass that often derives most of its blood supply from the external carotid artery. (1,5)

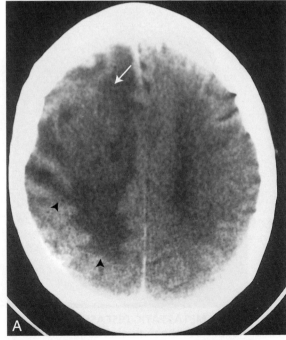
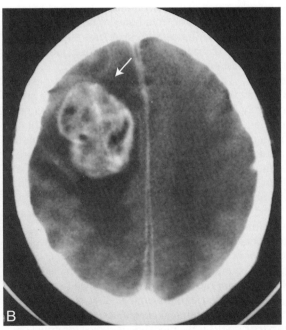

Figure 18-7 **ASTROCYTOMA. A. Non-Contrast CT, Axial Head.** Observe the tumor, which is relatively inconspicuous within the deep white matter of the frontal lobe (*arrow*). The adjacent edema is extensive and is the most prominent abnormal feature (*arrowheads*). **B. Contrast-Enhanced CT,** **Axial Head.** After intravenous contrast the tumor shows peripheral ring enhancement and more internal heterogeneous perfusion owing to necrosis (*arrow*). *COMMENT:* Astrocytoma is the most common primary intra-axial brain neoplasm.

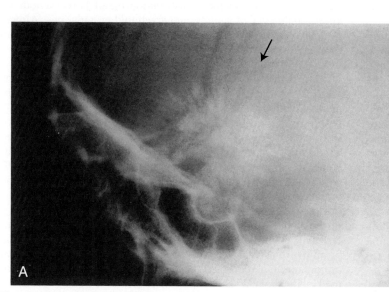

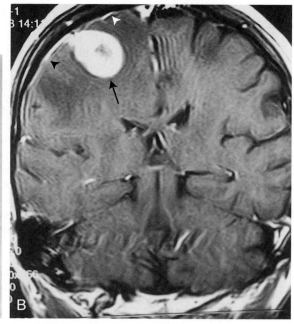

Figure 18-8 **MENINGIOMA. A. Lateral Skull.** Observe the dense, spiculated calcification anterior to the sphenoid and adjacent to the planum sphenoidale (*arrow*). **B. Contrast-Enhanced, T1-Weighted MRI, Coronal Brain.** Note the readily identifiable smoothly marginated and vividly enhancing tumor (*arrow*). In addition, there is characteristic enhance-ment of the adjacent dura (dural tail) (*arrowheads*). *COMMENT:* Although 25% of meningiomas will exhibit radiologically detectable calcification, this is usually only on CT; few are visible on plain film radiographs. It is the most common non-glial (extra-axial) tumor of the brain.

Metastatic Tumors

Secondary tumors to the brain are most commonly derived from hematogenous dissemination and less commonly by direct extension through the skull foramina or from bone lesions. They occur within the brain parenchyma (intra-axial) in at least 80% of cases and less commonly involve the leptomeninges (extra-axial). (5,12) They account for at least one third of all brain tumors. (5,12)

Clinical Features. Tumors of the lung, breast, and gastrointestinal and genitourinary tracts constitute the majority of cases. Prostate cancer rarely spreads to the brain. The most common primary site is the lung. Melanoma is the most common cause of brain metastases in young patients and is the most common lesion to present with hemorrhage. Lesions can be asymptomatic or produce seizures, motor weakness, or sensory changes. Tumors of the frontal lobes can manifest with personality changes. The majority occur above the tentorium but can occur anywhere. Insidious presentations are less common than acute presentations of delirium, vomiting, headache, altered consciousness, and seizures owing to secondary hemorrhage within the lesion as well as edema. Posterior fossa metastases may produce cerebellar signs; headaches; and neck symptoms, such as torticollis, pain, and muscle spasms. Solitary brain metastases may be removed surgically in the absence of any evidence of disseminated disease. Multiple brain lesions are not usually surgical candidates. (3,4)

Imaging Features. MRI is the modality of choice for initial detection, identifying additional subtle lesions, surgical planning, and characterizing complications such as hemorrhage and compression effects. CT for a patient with known malignancy or in the acute setting remains a commonly used procedure. (12) Use of intravenous

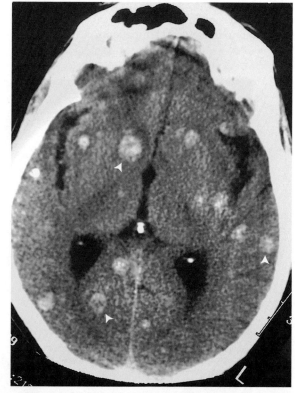

Figure 18-9 **METASTATIC DISEASE. Contrast-Enhanced CT, Axial Head.** Note the multiple round enhancing lesions present throughout both cerebral hemispheres (*arrowheads*). *COMMENT:* The most common causes for cerebral metastases are carcinomas of the lung and breast. In this case, the primary site was a melanoma of the leg excised 9 years previously.

contrast is necessary for both MRI and CT examinations to ensure the high sensitivity and specificity that both these modalities are capable of, especially for detection of small lesions. (1,2,8)

Intra-Axial Metastases. Intra-axial tumors are usually round and of variable size, exhibit a peripheral halo of vasogenic edema, displace adjacent structures (mass effect), and are typically found at the gray–white matter junction. On administration of contrast, there is characteristic ring enhancement of the tumor. (Fig. 18-9) Complicating hemorrhage on CT shows high attenuation; MRI sequences demonstrate variable signal changes, depending on the hemoglobin degradation status of the hemorrhage. (4–6) (Table 18-1)

Leptomeningeal Metastases. Dissemination to the brain membranes without parenchymal involvement occurs in < 10% of cases and remains a difficult, often overlooked imaging diagnosis. The key finding is postcontrast enhancement of the meninges on both CT and MRI, although MRI displays superior sensitivity. Meningeal enhancement patterns range from diffuse with normal thickness to diffuse with increased thickness to more nodular, irregular thickening. (Fig. 18-9) Solitary meningeal-based metastases is an uncommon presentation. (1)

Miscellaneous Brain Tumors

Many other tumors occur in the brain and their complete description lies outside the focus of this chapter. However, they can produce musculoskeletal symptoms, depending on their location, similar to astrocytoma, metastatic disease, and meningioma.

Posterior Fossa Tumors. Tumors of the posterior fossa can involve the cerebellum, brainstem, and cranial nerves (III–XII) and have a greater incidence in children. (13) The most common musculoskeletal presentations include headache (often mistaken for migraine), torticollis, neck spasms, and pain. The four most common tumors of the posterior fossa in children are pilocytic astrocytoma, medulloblastoma, ependymoma, and hemangioblastoma. (4,13) MRI is the modality of choice for diagnosis, presurgical planning, and post-treatment assessments. (4,13) (Fig. 18-10)

Cerebellopontine Angle Tumors. The two most common lesions in the cerebellopontine angle are meningioma and acoustic neuroma. Characteristic findings are sensorineural hearing loss and tinnitus. Long tract signs in the extremities may occur if the tumor is of sufficient size. Widening of the internal auditory me-

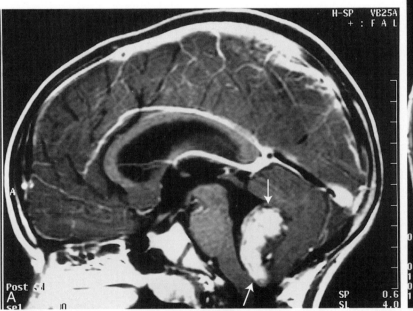

Figure 18-10 **MEDULLOBLASTOMA. A. Contrast-Enhanced, T1-Weighted MRI, Sagittal Brain.** Observe the vividly enhancing lesion within the fourth ventricle (*arrows*). **B. Contrast-Enhanced, T1-Weighted MRI, Axial Brain.** Note that the enhancing tumor mass occupies the vermis and extends into the fourth ventricle (*arrows*), causing obstructive hydro-

cephalus with dilatation of the temporal horns of the lateral ventricles. *COMMENT:* Posterior fossa tumors are most common in children. The differential diagnosis includes pilocytic astrocytoma, ependymoma, and hemangioblastoma. Clinical symptoms of tumors in this region are headaches, unsteady gait, and torticollis.

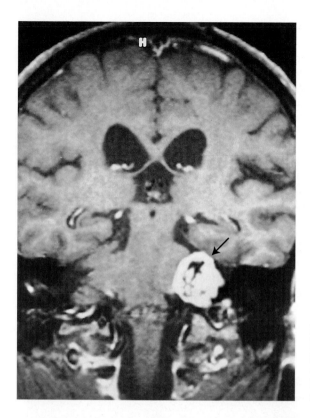

Figure 18-11 **ACOUSTIC NEUROMA. Contrast-Enhanced, T1-Weighted MRI, Axial Brain.** Note the localized fusiform enlargement within the acoustic nerve, indicating an acoustic neuroma (*arrow*).
COMMENT: Acoustic neuroma is the most common tumor of the cerebellopontine angle and is usually associated with ipsilateral tinnitus and sensorineural deafness.

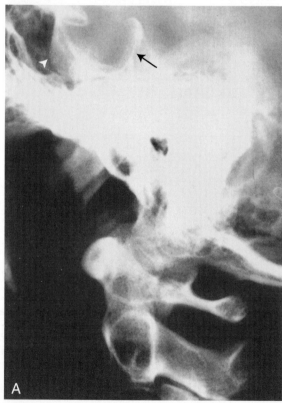

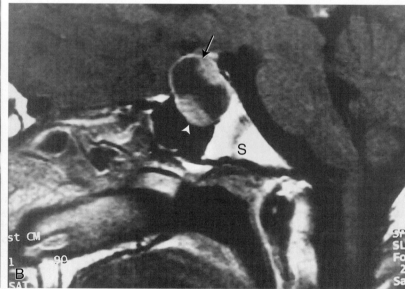

Figure 18-12 **PITUITARY MACROADENOMA. A. Lateral Cervical.** Observe the uniform enlargement of the pituitary fossa (*arrow*) with a soft tissue density extending into the posterior aspect of the sphenoid sinus (*arrowhead*). **B. Contrast-Enhanced, T1-Weighted MRI, Sagittal Brain.** A macroadenoma is present within the pituitary fossa, extending above the sella (*arrow*). Note the pressure erosion into the posterior aspect of the sphenoid sinus (*arrowhead*) anterior to the body of the sphenoid (*S*). *COMMENT:* The patient presented with cervical spine pain after a motor vehicle accident and was experiencing visual field hemianopia caused by long-standing compression of the optic nerve at the chiasm from this pituitary macroadenoma. The finding of an enlarged pituitary fossa on plain film radiographs leads to the investigation using MRI.

atus may be seen on CT, along with an enhancing mass lesion. (1,2) MRI with contrast has superior sensitivity in identifying small lesions without bone erosion, demonstrating focal enlargement and enhancement of the acoustic nerve. (2,4) (Fig. 18-11)

Pituitary Gland Tumors. Various cell types occur in pituitary gland tumors, depending on their lobe of origin; each exhibits specific stain characteristics on histopathology (chromophobe, acidophilic, basophilic). These tumors are usually slow growing, producing mass effect symptoms, especially on the optic chiasm. Hemianopia, headaches, or endocrine disorders constitute the majority of presentations. Many cases are discovered during CT or MRI for other clinical reasons. Enlargement and erosion of the sella turcica margins are often absent or minimal, so plain film examination is of limited value. Imaging is best performed with MRI in all three planes, precontrast and postcontrast. (3,7)

Pituitary gland tumors are described according to their size: Those > 5 mm are *macroadenomas,* and smaller tumors are *microadenomas.* (Fig. 18-12) Microadenomas require dynamic scanning after contrast injection over 30–60 sec; the normal background pituitary enhances whereas the tumor does not. Spontaneous hemorrhage into the tumor is occasionally observed (*pituitary apoplexy*) (4,5)

VASCULAR DISORDERS

Stroke

The word *stroke* is a generic term that encompasses many disorders that impair blood flow within the brain. The term dates back to antiquity when an afflicted person appeared to be suddenly and inexplicability struck down, as if by a "stroke" from God. It is the third leading cause of death in the United States, after myocardial infarction and cancer. (1,2) Imaging plays a pivotal role in the diagnosis and differential diagnosis and in guiding its subsequent management.

Synonyms. Cerebrovascular accident (CVA), apoplexy, cerebral infarction.

Clinical Features. The vascular causes of stroke include infarction (80%), hemorrhage (15%), vasospasm from subarachnoid hemorrhage (4%), and venous sinus thrombosis (1%). (3) Each type of stroke displays its own demographics and clinical and imaging findings.

Non-Hemorrhagic Stroke (Infarction). Infarction is the most common cause of stroke. There are numerous causal mechanisms, but the majority of cases are the result of atheromatous disease of the extracranial vessels (especially the carotid arteries) or small intracerebral arterioles and of cardiogenic emboli. Depending on which artery is occluded the perfused territory undergoes variable degrees of infarction, along with necrosis and a surrounding critically ischemic zone (*penumbra*). (4,5) An embolus in a proximal larger vessel (40–50% of cases) affects a larger territory of infarction, whereas a smaller arteriole occlusion (25% of cases) produces small, focal *lacunar* infarcts. Secondary hemorrhage into a recent infarct (hemorrhagic conversion, reperfusion hemorrhage) may occur in 5–15% of cases and tends to appear 1–3 days after infarction. (1)

Hemorrhagic Stroke. The causes of hemorrhagic stroke include hypertension (40–60%), amyloid angiopathy (15–25%), arteriovenous malformation (15%), bleeding disorders, and anticoagulants. (1,3) Hypertensive bleeds are most commonly the result of rupture of small vessels or microaneurysms (Charcot-Bouchard aneurysms) and usually occur in the putamen, globus pallidus, external capsule, thalamus, and pons.

Vasospasm. Secondary vasospasm of the cerebral arteries is the leading contributor to the morbidity and mortality of hemorrhagic stroke . (6) It most commonly occurs 4–12 days after subarachnoid hemorrhage and may occur in up to 75% of cases; but all are not symptomatic. Ischemic defects from vasospasm are symptomatic in about 30% of cases. (1,4)

Imaging Features. At initial presentation, CT is performed because of its high sensitivity and specificity in the identification of hemorrhage, a finding that significantly affects initial stroke management. It also rapidly allows identification of non-vascular causes, such as tumor, vascular malformation, and subdural hematoma, which collectively account for < 2% of cases. (1,7) MRI examination is more sensitive in predicting the ischemic penumbra and identifying acute infarction in the presence of a normal CT study. Angiography is preserved for determining underlying pathology, such as aneurysm in the presence of hemorrhage, and can be used to guide interventional procedures, such as selective intracranial thrombolysis, angioplasty, and placement of endovascular coils in aneurysms. (1,4)

Non-Hemorrhagic Stroke (Infarction). In infarction CT is most commonly performed first, but examination findings will be normal in up to 60% of cases within the first 4 hr. (Fig. 18-13) Combining intravenous injection with rapid CT thin slice acquisition, a perfusion study can be obtained that will show the ischemic territory in the absence of any structural change. This

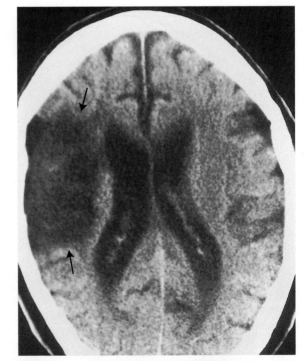

Figure 18-13 NON-HEMORRHAGIC INFARCT, CT, Axial Head. Note the well-demarcated region of low attenuation in the right parietal lobe that extends across the gray–white matter interface (*arrows*). There is no mass effect, midline shift, or volume loss of the right lateral ventricle. *COMMENT:* This scan was obtained 3 days after the onset of symptoms. This patient's initial head CT was normal. The latency period of infarct detection by CT in patients with non-hemorrhagic stroke is 2–3 days. Early changes are best detected with MRI.

can also be used to direct early intervention for thrombolysis of the occlusion. (8,9) Within the first 12 hr the earliest signs are a hyperdense middle cerebral artery (*dense MCA sign*), loss of definition of the lentiform nucleus, and blurring of the gray–white interface at the insula (*insular ribbon sign*). (8,10)

Over the ensuing 3 days from the initial infarction low-density changes occur in a typical wedge-shaped area that reflects the involved vascular territory, usually traversing the gray–white interface. Mass effect with effacement of the overlying sulcal spaces also helps identify the lesion. Use of contrast is not helpful in differentiation from tumor, as both will show enhancement. After 3 months encephalomalacic changes occur with volume loss, cystic gliotic cavities (*porencephalic cysts*), and sulcal widening. (1,8,10)

MRI studies also reflect these sequential changes but with more accuracy in identifying acute infarcts, in establishing if the lesion is acute or chronic, in defining the area of ischemic penumbra, and in differential considerations. In the acute phase, diffusion-weighted images can allow diagnosis as early as 15 min from the time of onset. Other acute signs occurring within the first 3 days include high signal of the infarcted zone on T2-weighted sequences, intravascular-meningeal-parenchymal enhancement, and sulcal effacement. (1,5) Chronic changes may include high T2-weighted signal fluid-filled cavities and low signal intensity areas of hemosiderin if bleeding occurred. Lacunar strokes are round, well-defined lesions that appear hypodense on CT or as high signal lesions on T2-weighted MRI pulse sequences. Typical locations include the internal capsule, basal ganglia, and thalami. (4)

Hemorrhagic Stroke. At the site of acute hemorrhage, high density occurs on CT imaging and variable altered signal changes are seen on MRI (see "Intracranial Hemorrhages").

Vasospasm. Following subarachnoid hemorrhage, both standard angiography and MRA can show marked vessel narrowing caused by vasospasm. Segmental or generalized effects may be seen. This phenomenon peaks at around day 4 after hemorrhage and may not be evident initially. This complication is often associated with marked territorial infarction and is treated aggressively with vasodilator medications and, when available, endovascular angioplasty.

Arteriovenous Malformations

Intracranial vascular malformations include arteriovenous malformations (AVMs), capillary telangiectasia, cavernous hemangioma (cavernoma), and venous angioma. The venous angioma is the most common form encountered. These are congenital lesions characterized by a nidus of tortuous and dilated vessels with dilated feeding arteries and draining veins. There are no intervening capillaries. Two basic types occur: parenchymal (pial) and dural.

Synonyms. None.

Clinical Features. AVMs are congenital lesions characterized by a lack of capillaries. The parenchymal type is more common, and 85% are supratentorial in location. (1,11,12) Up to 2% may be multiple. Almost 25% will become symptomatic before 15 years of age although most patients present in the 20- to 40-year age range. (11,12) Symptoms include acute hemorrhage, seizures,

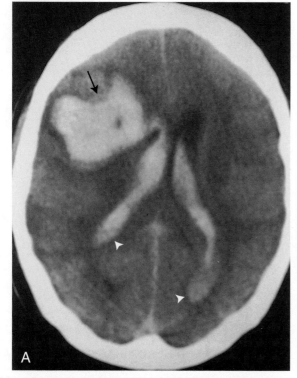

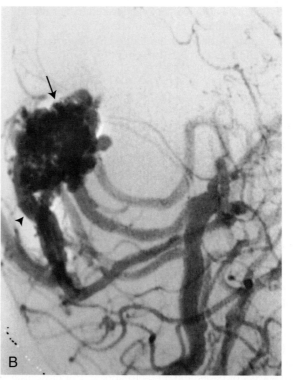

Figure 18-14 **ARTERIOVENOUS MALFORMATION. A. Peripheral Intracerebral Hemorrhage, CT, Axial Head.** Observe the high-density hematoma situated peripherally in the deep white matter of the frontal lobe (*arrow*). Note the intraventricular extension of the bleed (*arrowheads*). **B. Digital-Subtraction Cerebral Angiogram.** Note the arteriovenous nidus, evident as a dense collection of tortuous, engorged vessels (*arrow*). A dilated feeder vessel is demonstrated (*arrowhead*). *COMMENT:* Arteriovenous malformation (AVM) is one of the most common causes for intracerebral hemorrhage in a young person and may be suspected in a normotensive, peripheral bleed. MRA is the most sensitive non-invasive modality for AVM detection before hemorrhage occurs.

headache, steal syndromes, and focal neurological deficits. The risk of hemorrhage is estimated at 2–4% annually. With every hemorrhagic event, the risk of death is approximately 30%, with a further 25% patients suffering long-term morbidity. (11,13) Smaller AVMs may carry a higher level of risk for hemorrhage because the feeding arteries have higher pressures. Other factors linked with hemorrhage include central venous drainage pattern, periventricular location, and the presence of co-existing aneurysm. Flow-related aneurysms occur in the feeding arteries or within the nidus in 8–12% of cases.

Cavernous angioma (*cavernoma*) are discrete lesions characterized by endothelial-lined sinusoidal spaces. More than 80% are supratentorial. The estimated risk for hemorrhage is < 1% per year. *Venous angiomas* are usually asymptomatic, with a very low incidence of hemorrhage. (14,15)

Imaging Features. CT studies without contrast can be strikingly normal in the presence of an AVM, with occasional subtle calcification (25–30%) or a localized increased in density. (13) On contrast CT the nidus will enhance and the dilated arteries and veins are frequently visible. On the MRI T2-weighted studies the nidus and associated vessels will show prominent flow voids (*salt and pepper*), and there may be signs of hemorrhage in various stages of evolution. Surrounding gliosis will demonstrate high signal on T2-weighted sequences. MRA is useful for showing the nidus and associated vascular changes. (16) Angiography shows the nidus, feeding arteries, and venous drainage and may be the only method for demonstrating an associated aneurysm. (5,14,17) (Fig. 18-14)

Cavernoma is a round, well-circumscribed lesion with cystic spaces. On CT these produce focal, round lesions (around 1 cm in size) that show vivid enhancement. MRI is the technique of choice; the lesion is often surrounded by a low signal rim of hemosiderin on gradient echo sequences. *Venous angioma* shows only a dilated draining vein without a nidus or arterial feeders. It is a benign vascular malformation, most commonly seen in the frontal lobe or cerebellum. (2,5)

Aneurysms

Focal dilatation of an intracranial artery is a relatively common pathology of the brain that can occur secondary to numerous diseases. Known causes include infection (*mycotic aneurysm*) and in tandem with arteriovenous malformation, vasculitis, and hypertension (*Charcot-Bouchard aneurysm*). The most common type is the *berry aneurysm,* found typically in or adjacent to the circle of Willis, either as an idiopathic phenomenon with familial clustering or secondary to other diseases.

Synonyms. None.

Clinical Features. Aneurysms of the intracranial circulation are relatively common, with a population prevalence estimated at 2–9%. (18) It is estimated that first- and second-degree relatives have a 4–7 times higher risk of aneurysmal development. They are rare under 20 years of age. The rupture rate per year for those with aneurysm is 1–3%, with a slightly higher incidence occurring in women. (19) The peak incidence for rupture

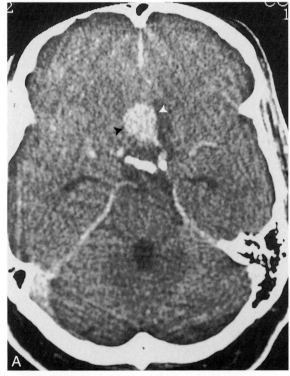

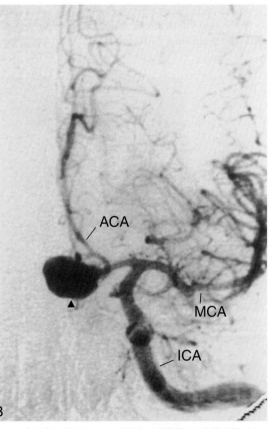

Figure 18-15 **ANTERIOR COMMUNICATING ARTERY ANEU-RYSM. A. Contrast-Enhanced CT, Axial Head. B. Digital-Subtraction Cerebral Angiogram.** The aneurysm rapidly fills with contrast (*arrowheads*) originating from the anterior communicating artery. *ACA,* anterior cerebral artery; *ICA,* in-ternal carotid artery; *MCA,* middle cerebral artery. *COMMENT:* This is one of the most common sites for intracranial aneurysm. Clinically this patient presented with chronic frontal headaches. The lesion was initially identified on a sinus CT study.

is in the 5th and 6th decades of life. At least 20–30% of patients will have more than a single aneurysm. Other implicated risk factors include hypertension (including eclampsia), smoking (3 times risk), alcohol (2–4 times risk), physical activity, polycystic kidneys, Marfan's syndrome, and a family history. (18) Once a rupture has occurred the chance for rebleed is 30–50% within 3–4 weeks; the highest risk is within the first 24 hr, with an associated mortality rate of 50%. (19)

Aneurysms of the intracranial circulation are acquired, not congenital, lesions. The term *berry aneurysm* is frequently applied based on the macroscopic appearance of a saccular outpouching. At the aneurysm neck there is absence of the muscular wall and internal elastic lamina. These aneurysms occur in or near the circle of Willis at vascular bifurcation points; 90% are derived from the carotid branches and 10% from the vertebrobasilar system. (18) The sites of occurrence are the anterior communicating arteries, origin of the posterior communicating arteries, and bifurcation of the middle cerebral arteries. Aneurysms > 2.5 cm in diameter are designated *giant aneurysms* and have a higher incidence of rupture. (18,20) When rupture occurs, blood extravasates into the subarachnoid space, sometimes intracerebrally and occasionally into the ventricles. Aneurysms account for 75% of non-traumatic subarachnoid bleeds, with the second most common cause being arteriovenous malformations. (18)

Presentation patterns fall into four general categories: sudden severe onset with early death, sudden severe onset with survival and variable neurological deficits, neuro-ophthalmic signs, and as an incidental finding on brain imaging. Many patients experience the sudden, spontaneous onset of severe headache often described as the "worst headache of my life." Common associated findings include neck and suboccipital pain, neck rigidity, photophobia, nausea, and vomiting. Differentiation from acute mi-

graine can be difficult. Careful history taking may reveal that within the preceding few days the patient experienced a less severe headache and mild symptoms secondary to a small, self-limiting rupture of the aneurysm, referred to as a *sentinel bleed.* Neuro-ophthalmic signs include third nerve palsy, dilated unreactive pupil, and visual field loss secondary to pressure from the aneurysm on the associated cranial nerves coursing near the circle of Willis. (2,17) Up to 8–12% of patients will die before receiving medical attention. Between 40 and 70% of those who survive initially will either die or suffer significant disability. (18) Elective surgery has a morbidity rate of 4% and mortality rate of 1%. (18) Placement of endovascular coils delivered from percutaneous intravascular catheters are being employed as alternatives to surgery with similar results.

Imaging Features. Plain films that include the skull base may show erosion of the posterior clinoids or curvilinear parasellar calcification. Detection of an aneurysm may occur incidentally, in the investigation of headache or visual disturbance, or following rupture. The CT detection of aneurysms is based on peripheral calcification and high-density clot, with demonstration of the aneurysmal lumen on contrast examination. (Fig. 18-15) Rapid scanning with infused intravenous contrast can allow for three-dimensional CT–angiography images to be reconstructed. CT scanning within 24 hr of bleeding is the imaging technique of choice for identifying subarachnoid hemorrhage, with a sensitivity approaching 90%. (5,17)

MRI is relatively insensitive to the detection of acute hemorrhage. (4,7) To identify the aneurysm, cerebral angiography remains the gold standard; MRA as a non-invasive examination may not be able to locate aneurysms < 2–3 mm, those containing clot, or those in the presence of vasospasm. (7) MRA, however, is a useful non-invasive screening tool for individuals with established risk

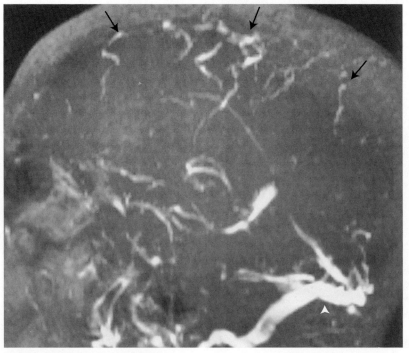

Figure 18-16   SUPERIOR SAGITTAL SINUS THROMBOSIS. Magnetic Resonance Venogram, Sagittal Brain. Note that this single maximum intensity projection image shows no flow within the superior sagittal sinus (*arrows*). Flow is present in the transverse sinus draining into the sigmoid (*arrow-* *head*). *COMMENT:* This phenomenon of sinus thrombosis is being increasingly recognized as a cause of headache. Procoagulative disorders, dehydration, tumor, and trauma can all precipitate the thrombosis.

factors. MRA has 95% sensitivity for aneurysms > 3 mm in size; smaller aneurysms reduce the sensitivity to as low as 70%. (1,7)

Venous Sinus Thrombosis

Occlusion of the intracranial veins is an underdiagnosed potentially life-threatening condition that has become increasingly recognized with the use of MRI in the investigation of headache. (21)
Synonyms. None.
Clinical Features. There is a wide spread of age and clinical findings in this condition. Known precipitants include local disease such as mastoiditis, sinusitis, trauma, and tumor. Systemic disorders such as dehydration, blood dyscrasia, migraine patients, oral contraceptives, amphetamines, pregnancy, coagulopathy, collagen, and inflammatory bowel disease have been implicated. At least 25% remain idiopathic. (5) The superior sagittal sinus is the single most common site followed by the transverse, sigmoid, and cavernous sinuses. Occasionally other veins, such as the cortical branches, can be involved, but rarely in isolation. Treatment is anticoagulation.
Imaging Features. Non-enhanced CT may show high-density blood along the course of the involved sinus. On contrast studies, the thrombus creates a filling defect surrounded by an enhancing sinus wall, which in the superior sagittal sinus creates the *empty delta sign.* (22) Cortical hemorrhages are sometimes visible (venous cortical infarcts), which occur in a non-arterial territorial distribution. MRI findings of the thrombus depend on its age and stage of hemoglobin degradation; the most diagnostic sign occurs with subacute thrombosis (days 3–14) because methemoglobin is visible as high signal on T1-weighted studies. (22) Although magnetic resonance venogram (MRV) is prone to flow artifact error, it remains the graphical method of choice. (Fig. 18-16) Chronic thromboses are low in signal and may show collateral drainage veins at the site. (4,5)

THE NECK: MASQUERADERS OF MUSCULOSKELETAL DISEASE

The presentation of neck pain can be a problematic issue for clinicians. There are many disorders of this region that can mimic bone and joint disorders. Imaging often plays a crucial role in diagnosis and appropriate management.

VERTEBRAL ARTERY

Tortuous Vertebral Artery

Synonyms. Dolicoarterial loop (of Danziger) and vertebral artery ectasia or dilatation.
Clinical Features. Age-related vertebral arterial wall thinning and elongation precipitates dilatation and ectasia, generally without sufficient hemodynamic flow deficits to cause symptoms. (1) However, when symptoms do occur from this altered blood flow to the hindbrain they are often bizarre and clinically confusing. (2–4) This clinical picture has been described as the Barre-Lieou syndrome and often includes headache, dizziness, nystagmus, and sub-

occipital pain as well as nausea and vomiting. (2–4) Occasionally these changes allow pulsatile transmission to adjacent bony structures, which may produce extrinsic bony erosion (Hadley's erosive defect) first described by Hadley in 1958. (2–4) An astute diagnostician may recognize the erosive defect on cervical plain films, usually obtained for other clinical reasons. The majority are unilateral. (5) Symptoms may occur if there is radicular compression or, rarely, if pathologic fracture results from extensive bone erosion. (6,7) Pregnancy may precipitate radicular symptoms. (8) Bilateral atherosclerotic occlusion of the carotid arteries may precipitate vertebral artery dilatation as a compensatory mechanism for maintaining cerebral perfusion. Vertebral tortuosity can be a predisposing factor in dissection of the vertebral artery; therefore, it is important to examine the plain film findings before rendering any spinal manipulation or physical therapies for the cervical spine. (1,9)
Imaging Features. The characteristic plain film findings are enlargement of the transverse foramen, with pedicle and posterolateral vertebral body erosion expanding the intervertebral foramen. Extrinsic bone erosion is most commonly seen in the midcervical segments, usually at C4–C5, with erosion of the C4 pedicle and body. (2,3,6,10–12) The second most common site is C3–C4, followed by C2 as the third most common. (2,3,6,10–12) At C2, these erosions can occasionally be identified on routine frontal and lateral radiographs as a discrete, sharply demarcated radiolucent defect in the region of the axis transverse process and extending into the pedicle and beneath the articular surface of the atlantoaxial joint. (2–4) (Figs. 18-17–18-20)

In the midcervical spinal segments, erosion of the pedicle is the dominant feature, with widening of the intervertebral foramen. Erosion of the vertebral body occasionally can be seen on the frontal view as a well-defined lucent defect in its lateral margin. CT is the best method for showing the erosive defects and allowing differential diagnostic decisions to be made to exclude other causes for pedicle erosion. (5,13) MRA is the non-invasive method of choice for confirming the presence of a tortuous vertebral artery, though diagnostic angiography is often used. (5,13) A complete loop may be seen on these angiographic studies and is referred to as a *dolicoarterial loop.* (14)

The differential diagnosis of an enlarged intervertebral foramen from pedicle erosion or destruction includes neurofibroma, meningioma, meningocele, and bone tumor (aneurysmal bone cyst, osteoblastoma, lytic metastatic disease). (12) Congenital absence of the pedicle is another cause to consider. Pedicle erosion related to a dolicoarterial loop or increased vertebral artery flow may also occur secondary to underlying vascular conditions, including arteriovenous malformation, pseudoaneurysm, aortic coarctation, subclavian steal syndrome, and carotid obstruction. (6,12,14)

Vertebral Artery Dissection

Synonyms. Vertebral artery syndrome (VAS), vertebral artery hematoma, and Babinski-Mageotte syndrome.
Clinical Features. Dissection of the vertebral artery is an uncommon vascular disorder of the neck characterized by varying degrees and patterns of vertebral artery wall disruption with hematoma formation. Musculoskeletal symptoms of occipital headache and cervico-occipital neck pain do occur. Secondary neurological complications may occur owing to ischemia of the CNS in areas normally perfused by the vertebrobasilar circulation. Severity ranges from mild, transient effects to catastrophic, irreversible neurological damage or death. The onset of neurological

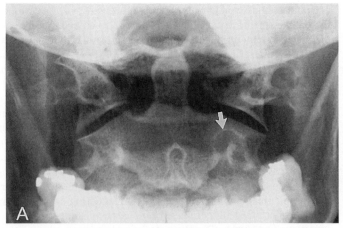

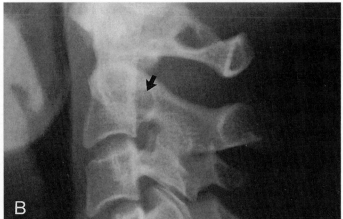

Figure 18-17　**VERTEBRAL ARTERY TORTUOSITY WITH ERO-SIVE DEFECT OF THE AXIS. A. AP Open Mouth.** Observe the well-defined, circular defect adjacent to the pedicle and transverse foramen of the axis (*arrow*). **B. Lateral Cervical Spine.** The circular erosion of the transverse foramen is clearly identified (*arrow*). This characteristic plain film appearance is frequently overlooked. *COMMENT:* This 32-year-old female complained of mild suboccipital headaches. The relationship of her clinical symptoms to the radiographic findings is unclear.

changes typically occurs within hours to days after dissection but can be delayed as long as 14 days. (15,16) Approximately 4% of ischemic strokes in young adults occur from cervical artery dissection; of those, two thirds involve the internal carotid arteries and one third, the vertebral arteries. (15,17) Vertebral artery dissection may occur either with a known precipitant or without definable cause or event (*spontaneous dissection*). The vertebral artery is composed of four divisions: (18)

- *Proximal (V1).* From the subclavian origin (ostium) to the C6 transverse foramen.
- *Intraforaminal (V2).* The vertical course from C6 to C2 within the transverse foramina.
- *Atlantoaxial (V3).* The upward and lateral course from C2 to C1 transverse foramina, then curving posterior and medial to the lateral masses to pierce the atlanto-occipital membrane and dura to the foramen magnum.

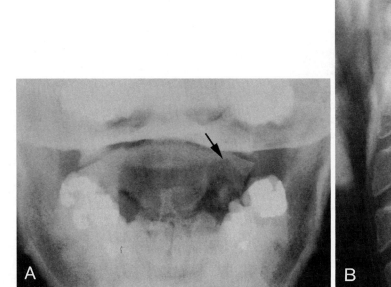

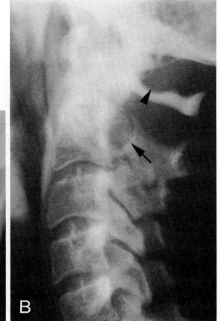

Figure 18-18　**VERTEBRAL ARTERY TORTUOSITY WITH LARGE EROSIVE DEFECT OF THE ATLAS AND AXIS. A. AP Open Mouth.** Note the prominent, well-defined, circular defect adjacent to the pedicle and transverse foramen of the axis (*arrow*). Compare this appearance with the contralateral normal side. **B. Lateral Cervical Spine.** Observe the clearly identified greatly expanded axis transverse foramen (*arrow*). Also note the accentuated concavity at the atlas posterior arch (*arrowhead*) created by a pressure erosion phenomenon from the tortuous vertebral artery. *COMMENT:* This young female presented with headaches and postural vertigo that could be provoked by hyperextension and rotation of the neck. (Courtesy of Robert J. Longenecker, DC, DACBR, Dallas, Texas.)

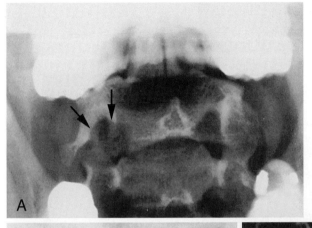

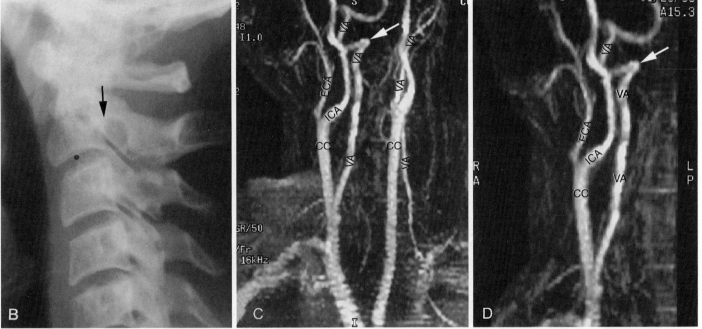

Figure 18-19   **VERTEBRAL ARTERY TORTUOSITY WITH HADLEY'S EROSION OF THE AXIS. A. AP Open Mouth. B. Lateral Cervical Spine.** Note the discrete, sharply demarcated, radiolucent defect in the region of the axis transverse process and extending into the pedicle and the inferior aspect of the articular surface of the atlantoaxial joint (*arrows*). **C. MRA, Coronal Neck. D. MRA, Oblique Neck.** Note that the right vertebral artery (*VA*) is larger than the left throughout its course. The right vertebral artery is tortuous and dilated (*arrows*) at the site corresponding to the osseous erosions seen on the plain films. The common carotid (*CC*), internal carotid (*ICA*), and external carotid arteries (*ECA*) are also visualized. *COMMENT:* This 38-year-old female consulted a chiropractor for discomfort in her upper neck. MRA is the best non-invasive imaging modality for investigating the course and structural details of the craniovertebral vasculature, especially of the vertebrobasilar system. In the case of tortuosity demonstrated here, MRA graphically demonstrates the underlying vascular abnormality. (Courtesy of Daniel L. Perkins, DC, Denver, Colorado.)

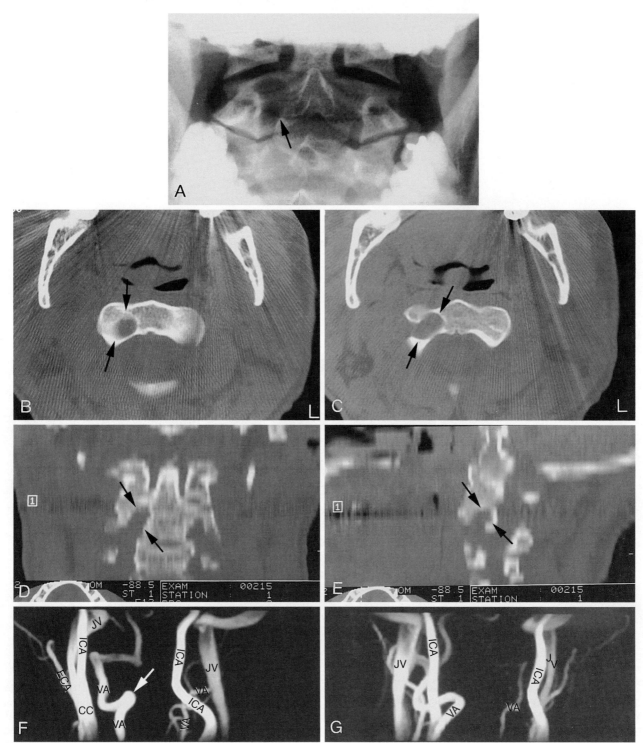

Figure 18-20   **CORRELATIVE IMAGING OF VERTEBRAL ARTERY TORTUOSITY WITH EROSION OF THE AXIS. A. AP Open Mouth.** Note the characteristic radiolucent defect near the C2 pedicle body junction (*arrow*). **B and C. CT, Axial C2.** Sequential images confirm the extension of the erosion from the C2 transverse foramen into the vertebral body immediately inferior to the articular surface of the atlantoaxial joint (*arrows*). **D. Coronal Reformatted CT, C1–C2. E. Sagittal Reformatted CT, C1–C2.** Observe that the contiguous nature of the defect, which arises from the transverse foramen, is confirmed (*arrows*). **F and G. MRA, Oblique and Coronal Neck.** Note that the vertebral arteries (*VA*) are asymmetric in caliber, with the right being larger than the left. At the level of the axis corresponding to the bony erosion, the vertebral artery is dilated and tortuous (*arrow*). *CC,* common carotid

artery; *ICA,* internal carotid artery; *ECA,* external carotid artery; *JV,* jugular vein. *COMMENT:* This 44-year-old female complained of chronic cervical spine pain, which initiated cervical radiographs. Familiarity with this appearance is important to practitioners of manual therapy because it represents a potential risk factor in the development of vertebro-basilar neurological syndromes and, as such, may preclude these therapies from being administered. In addition, the differential diagnosis of the plain film examination findings may include benign neural arch tumors (e.g., aneurysmal bone cyst, osteoblastoma), malignant arch tumors (e.g., lytic metastasis), and neural canal tumors (e.g., neurofibroma, meningioma). (Courtesy of James L. Quayle, MD, Englewood, Colorado, and the Chronic Neck Pain Study, Foundation for Chiropractic Education and Research.)

- *Intracranial (V4).* From the foramen magnum to the lower pons where it joins the opposite vertebral artery to form the basilar artery. (19–21)

The most common site of dissection is between the atlas and the axis (V3). (15,17) Less common sites are the point of arterial entry into the transverse foramina at the C6 level and at the C4 and C5 levels. (15,17) Intradural dissections (V4) occur in 14% of cases. Because this portion of the artery lacks an external elastic lamina, has a thinner adventitia, and contains fewer elastic fibers in the tunica media, associated subarachnoid hemorrhage is common. (22)

Spontaneous Dissection. The frequency of spontaneous vertebral artery dissection is one third that of spontaneous internal carotid dissection. (15) It is less common than dissections linked to known causes. The most common symptoms are the sudden onset of ipsilateral occipital or upper neck headache and brainstem ischemia, especially the lateral medullary (Wallenberg) syndrome. (15) Females, most commonly in the 3rd–4th decades of life, make up 60% of cases. (15) Up to 80% occur between 30 and 50 years of age. (23,24) At least two thirds involve the segment between the atlas and axis (V3) with 20% extending intradurally (V4). (15) Up to 60% will have multivessel dissection of either the contralateral vertebral or one or both internal carotid arteries. (15) Hypertension is common, with estimates approaching 50%. Fibromuscular hyperplasia is present in approximately 15%, often in the renal artery. Arteritis and cystic medial necrosis are additional implicated associations. (25) The contributions of smoking, migraines, and birth control pills remain unclear. The prognosis associated with spontaneous dissection is good and 90% are expected to make an excellent recovery; those associated with subarachnoid hemorrhage have a guarded prognosis. (15,26)

Dissection Secondary to Disease or Trauma. More than 60 causes have been linked with dissection secondary to disease or trauma and include a wide spectrum of entities. (27) (Table 18-2) The literature has focused on the very rare manipulation-induced vertebral artery injury. This wide coverage in the literature would appear more related to the devastating outcome than the actual frequency of the event. Many of these cases involve chiropractors because they administer most of the manipulative therapy used today. Several published reports have erroneously attributed vertebral artery injury to "chiropractic manipulation," when the manipulation was actually administered by another type of practitioner (medical physician, physiotherapist, osteopath, naturopath) or even a layperson. (24,27) In fact, approximately 50% of all cases of vertebral artery stroke following manipulation have been performed by non-chiropractors. (24,27) In several of these instances the level of training, skill, and experience of the person administering manipulation undoubtedly played a role in the unfortunate outcome.

Another confounding factor for evaluating the association between manipulation and vertebral artery injury is the likely possibility that at least some cases reported as manipulation-induced are in fact spontaneous dissections in progress. Doppler studies have shown that no changes in blood flow generally occur after manipulation. (28) Experimental data suggest that elongation forces on the vertebral artery during manipulation are < 50% of that experienced during normal physiological movements. (29) The incidence for manipulation-induced dissection is rare, and estimates range from 1 in 1–2 million neck treatments to as high as 1 in 400,000 and 1 in 120,000. (24,27,30,31) As is true for

Table 18-2	Pathogenesis of Vertebral Artery Injury
Activities of daily living	Exercises
None (spontaneous)	Football
Ceiling and wall painting; overhead work	Star gazing
Hanging out the wash	Swimming
Physiologic neck motions	Tai chi
Sexual intercourse	Wrestling
Sleeping	Yoga
Sneezing, coughing, nose blowing	**Vascular diseases**
	Atherosclerosis
Iatrogenic	Arteritis
Anesthesia and surgery	Cystic medial necrosis
Childbirth	Fibromuscular hyperplasia
Dental work	**Related disorders**
Diagnostic angiography	Atlantoaxial instability
Epistaxis control	Anomalous vertebral artery size and course
Hairdressing (barber's chair/ beauty parlor syndrome)	Cervical fractures and dislocations
Cervical manipulation	Fascial bands arising from the cervical muscles
Neck extension radiography	Hypertension
Recreational drugs (marijuana)	Marfan's and Ehlers-Danlos syndromes
Resuscitation	Neurofibromatosis
Sports and recreation	Occipitalization
Aircraft watching	Odontoid anomalies
Amusement park rides	Polycystic kidneys
Archery (bow hunters' syndrome)	Rheumatoid arthritis
Athletics	Syphilis
Basketball	Seizure
Bicycle riding	Trauma
Break dancing	Vertebral segmentation anomalies
Driving	

Modified from **Terrett AGJ:** *Current Concepts in Vertebrobasilar Complications Following Spinal Manipulation.* Des Moines, IA, NCMIC Publications, 2001.

spontaneous dissection, the most common site of involvement is the atlantoaxial segment (V3). (15,17) Several different kinds of vascular events have been reported as possible complications to manipulation, including the following:

- Vasospasm.
- Formation of an intramural or subintimal hematoma.
- Intimal tear (with or without wall dissection), which may extend to the adventitial layer to form a pseudo-aneurysm.
- Full-thickness wall rupture.
- Embolus formation.

The effects are usually distal, in the supplied territory of the brainstem, cerebellum, thalamus, and occipital lobes. Dissection may extend along the length of the artery and occlude exiting branches (posterior inferior cerebellar, anterior spinal, pontine). Hematomas cause luminal narrowing and reduced flow, resulting in ischemia, whereas intimal damage can act as a nidus for thrombus formation and embolic phenomena. Rarely, an arteriovenous fistula may occur after significant trauma. (19,21)

Mechanical factors that may be instrumental in the pathogenesis of these vertebral arterial injuries have been isolated. (27)

- *Atlantoaxial rotation.* At least 45–50° of rotation occur between the atlas and axis. The artery (V3) is fixed within the transverse foramina. The adventitia is continuous with the periosteum, imparting longitudinal stretch, torque, and shear stresses during atlantoaxial rotation. The artery on the contralateral side to rotation is at greatest risk for these forces.
- *Atlanto-occipital membrane.* The vertebral artery penetrates the membrane as it courses posteriorly behind the lateral mass. The ligament shares direct attachment with the arterial adventitia, which could potentially exert mechanical stresses to the vessel wall. (32) Whether or not calcification at the margin (posterior ponticle) increases the risk for injury remains conjectural.
- *Second ventral ramus.* During rotation, the ventral ramus of the second cervical vertebra can compress the vertebral artery but is an unlikely cause for injury. (33)
- *Atlantoaxial muscles.* Compression of the vertebral artery between the atlas and axis transverse foramina by the intertransversarii or obliquus capitis inferior can occur. (34)
- *C3 articular process.* Rotation may cause the ipsilateral vertebral artery to be impinged by contact with the anterior aspect of the C3 superior articular process as the axis rotates posteriorly.
- *Osteoarthritis.* The radiographic demonstration of degenerative disc disease, neurocentral joint osteophytes, and facet arthritis has not been shown to be a reliable risk factor in elderly patients for vertebral artery dissection. (35) Despite this low-sensitivity radiographic finding, cases are recorded of vertebral artery compression from neurocentral (von Luschka) joint osteophytes, usually at C4–C5 or C5–C6, with symptoms provoked on ipsilateral head rotation. (36)
- *Myofascial bands.* Anomalous attachment or fibrous bands of the longus colli and scalenus anticus muscles, especially at C6, can cause significant occlusion of the vertebral artery on head rotation. (37)
- *Anomalous vertebral arteries.* Tortuosity and dilatation may render the artery more susceptible to injury. (38) Asymmetry in the size of the vertebral arteries is common. The largest diameter vessel is designated as the *dominant* vessel because it supplies more blood to the vertebrobasilar circulation. Only 8% of vertebral arteries are symmetrical in size; the left is dominant in 51% and the right in 41% of cases. (39) One vessel is virtually absent in up to 10% of cases. (40) A dissection, stenosis, or occlusion of the dominant artery can produce greater neurological sequelae. (18,36,37,41) Vertebral anomalies—including odontoid variations, block vertebrae, Klippel-Feil syndrome, occipitalization, and basilar impression—are associated with anomalous vertebral arteries. In 5–8% of individuals the vertebral arteries do not join at brainstem; one vertebral artery continues as the basilar artery and the other continues as the posterior inferior cerebellar artery (*PICA termination*). (18,36,42–46)

Manifestations of vertebrobasilar ischemia (VBI) are characterized by the *five Ds* (**d**izziness, **d**iplopia, **d**ysarthria, **d**ysphagia, and **d**rop attacks) and the *three Ns* (**n**ausea, **n**umbness, and **n**ystagmus). (27) Numerous screening physical examination tests have been proposed to test the sufficiency of the ver-

tebrobasilar circulation before manipulation (Maigne's, Houle's, and DeKleyn's vertebrobasilar tests). These procedures involve positioning the head and neck in extension and rotation in an attempt to decrease blood flow in one vertebral artery, thereby challenging the sufficiency of the contralateral side. Although none of these tests has demonstrated significant sensitivity or specificity in identifying patients at risk for manipulation-induced vertebral artery injury, they are still recommended as part of a premanipulation screening examination. (18,24,47) There are no diagnostic tests or imaging procedures that will accurately identify the patient at risk. (24,27)

Prompt and accurate diagnosis are important for treatment of vertebral artery dissections. Anticoagulant therapy is given for extracranial dissections but is problematic for intradural lesions. (15)

Imaging Features. Understanding the course and anatomy of the vertebral artery is a key point in properly identifying and locating a vertebral artery dissection.

An imaging strategy to identify these dissections centers around MRA because it allows simultaneous assessment of the intracranial contents for hemorrhage, infarction, and detection of the dissection. Although angiography continues to be used in many centers, it is an invasive test that carries a 1–3% risk for inducing stroke and worsening a vertebral dissection.

Plain Film. There are few reported findings on plain film radiography of vertebral artery disease, and no specific findings for vertebral artery dissection or occlusion. Dilatation and tortuosity may enlarge the transverse foramen, which is especially visible at the axis. (Figs. 18.17–18.20) The intervertebral foramen may also appear enlarged owing to pedicle thinning. The predictive value of degenerative disc disease or facet or neurocentral joint disease relative to vertebral artery disease is extremely low. It is rare for calcified atheroma to be visible on plain film studies.

Plain film simulators of vertebral artery calcification include calcification in the lateral wings of the thyroid cartilage, stylohyoid ligament, and atlanto-occipital membrane. The lateral wings of the thyroid cartilage extend superiorly at C4–C6 bilaterally and diverge from the midline. Calcification of the stylohyoid ligament (*Eagle's syndrome*) is often bilateral and travels an oblique course anteromedially from the styloid process to insert at the lesser cornu of the hyoid bone. Calcification posterior to the atlas lateral mass in the margin of the oblique occipital membrane (*pons posticus*) marks the point of passage of the vertebral artery over the atlas posterior arch and is not within the vessel wall. (19–21) (See Chapter 3.)

CT. Non-intravenous contrast studies offer no diagnostic information, except in a dilated tortuous vertebral artery. (48) Post-intravenous contrast CT may show obstruction from thrombosis or mural hematoma, a thin contrast column with a thickened vessel wall, contrast within the vessel wall, or an intimal flap. (49,50) A rapid arterial-phase helical acquisition can allow three-dimensional images to be formed. Examination of the posterior fossa contents may detect subarachnoid hemorrhage as high-density fluid around the basal cisterns surrounding the brainstem in intradural (V4) dissections. (15) Infarctions will show low attenuation parenchymal defects in the cerebellum or brainstem.

Ultrasound. Signs of dissection can be shown on ultrasound, including increased outside diameter of the artery, thickened wall, decreased pulsatility, intravascular echoes, stenosis, or occlusion. Ultrasound is reliable in demonstrating vertebral artery flow; however, its efficacy as a screening test for identifying those at risk for vertebral artery dissection has not been demonstrated owing to high false-positive and false-negative values. Up to 5% of asymptomatic individuals will have < 10% flow in the contralateral artery at more than 45° of rotation. (51)

Angiography. Angiography remains the gold standard for investigation of the vertebral artery, but is rapidly being replaced by MRA because of advances in technology. This test is invasive and carries a complication rate for stroke of 1–3%. (15,19,20,44) Placement of the catheter successively in both vertebral and internal carotid arteries from transfemoral percutaneous access allows depiction of each vessel as well as assessment of the dynamic effects of neck rotation. The most characteristic signs of vertebral dissection are a gradual decrease in luminal size with occlusion (*flame sign*), a section that is generally narrowed (*string sign*), an area with superimposed localized outpouchings (*pearl sign*), a localized eccentric filling defect, a double lumen, and a thin linear filling defect attached to the wall representing an intimal flap. (19,44) (Fig. 18-21) Localized saccular pseudo-aneurysms or true

aneurysms are occasionally demonstrated at the sites of dissection. More than three quarters of cases at follow-up angiography will have a normal-appearing artery. (15,19,20)

MRA and MRI. MRA remains the non-invasive method of choice for initial diagnosis and follow-up examinations for dissection of the vertebral artery. Demonstration of hypoplasia or developmental narrowing may assist in modifying treatments, including spinal manipulative therapy. (52) The key imaging signs are luminal narrowing, occlusion, demonstration of thrombus as high signal on T1-weighted images, increased external diameter of the vessel, and aneurysms. (Fig. 18-22) Often, the dissection is best detected on the source partition images used for the generation of MRA images.

The additional benefit of MRI is visualization of the brain and brainstem, allowing simultaneous examination for signs of vertebrobasilar infarction with sensitivity exceeding that of CT examination. High-signal changes on T2-weighted studies and diffusion-weighted images mark the sites of acute infarction. Progress and documentation of dissection resolution can be accurately obtained with MRI and MRA. (18,22)

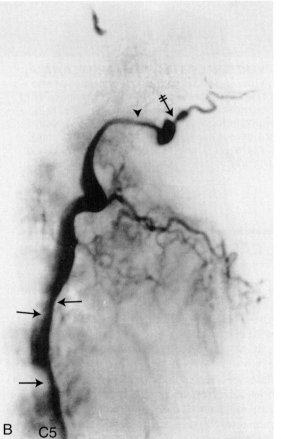

Figure 18-21 VERTEBRAL ARTERY DISSECTION, ANGIOGRAM. A. Unsubtracted, Lateral Neck. Note that the bony structures are visible to allow orientation of the anatomy. Observe the irregular outline of the vertebral artery as it courses from C5 cephalically through the C1 region (*arrows*). This appearance contrasts the normal smooth margin of the vessel and is related to hematoma within the tunica media. This produces external compression of the lumen. **B. Subtracted, Lateral**

Neck. With the bones removed from the image the detail of the vertebral artery is highlighted. Note the corkscrew appearance (*arrows*). The intramural component shows marked tapering (*arrowhead*), and there is occlusion of the basilar artery (*crossed arrow*). *COMMENT:* This is an example of a longitudinal dissection of the vertebral artery. Short segment dissections will have similar but more localized changes. (Courtesy of Anne C. Heller, MD, Manchester, England.)

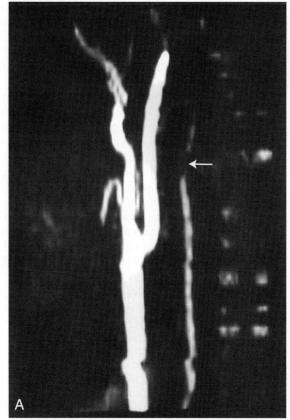
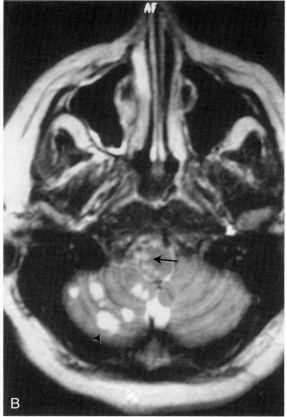

Figure 18-22 VERTEBRAL ARTERY DISSECTION. A. MRA, Coronal Neck. Flow in the vertebral artery ceases at the C3 level (*arrow*). The common, internal, and external carotid arteries demonstrate normal flow. **B. T2-Weighted MRI, Axial Brain.** Multiple high-signal (white) foci are present within the right cerebellar hemisphere (*arrowhead*) and lateral medulla (*arrow*). These represent small embolic infarcts from vertebral artery dissection. *COMMENT:* MRA is the technique of choice for determining dissection because it is non-invasive, has high sensitivity and specificity, and allows for simultaneous evaluation of brain involvement. It is particularly well suited for screening patients for vertebral artery anomalies and reassessing those with known dissection to document recanalization and resolution of the occlusion.

INTERNAL CAROTID ARTERY DISSECTION

Synonyms. Carotid artery dissection (CAD), internal carotid artery intramural hematoma.

Clinical Features. Internal carotid artery dissection (ICAD) occurs when blood extrudes into the vessel wall, with or without intimal tearing. ICAD has been recorded in patients from 11 to 74 years of age; however, 70% occur between the ages of 35 and 50 years. (1) Males are affected in 50–55% of cases. (1,2) ICAD accounts for at least 25% of strokes under 45 years of age, but only 3% of all strokes over all ages. (3) The internal carotid is the most common artery in the neck to develop dissection and is involved at twice the rate as vertebral artery dissections. (1) Dissection of the neck vessels involves a single internal carotid artery (ICA) in 50% of cases, a single vertebral artery in 20%, simultaneous bilateral carotid and vertebrals in 15%, bilateral carotids in 10%, and bilateral vertebrals in 5%. (1,2)

The clinical triad of anterior neck pain, stroke, and Horner's syndrome is highly suggestive of the condition, especially in younger patients. Other indicators for ICAD are transient ischemic attack (45%), cerebral infarction (33%), ipsilateral headache, neck or head pain (16%), pulsatile tinnitus (4%), monocular blindness, and an asymptomatic bruit (2%). (1) There is a high prevalence of Horner's syndrome (oculosympathetic paresis), reported in as many as 50% of cases. This is explained by the compressive effects of the hematoma on the sympathetic plexus within the artery wall that innervates the face and eye. (4)

Many causes have been reported, although a large percentage of cases have no direct attributable event or definable disease and are referred to as *spontaneous dissections.* (1,5) (Table 18-3) The time interval from the occurrence of the dissection to the onset of symptoms (*lucid interval*) is variable, from hours to a few days. (1) Predisposing risk factors are similar to vertebrobasilar dissections, including fibromuscular hyperplasia (15%), cystic medial necrosis, Marfan's syndrome, familial history, smoking (47%), migraine (11%), hypertension (36%), drug abuse, pharyngeal infections, and severe or minor trauma. Examples of trivial traumatic incidents involving hyperextension and rotation are coughing, brushing of teeth, nose blowing, and sporting activities (such as tennis, skiing, boxing, basketball, volleyball, football, and bowling). (1) Manipulation of the cervical spine has been implicated in < 10 reported cases of ICAD. This usually occurs at the

Table 18-3	Associations with Carotid Artery Injury
Activities of daily living	**Vascular diseases**
None (spontaneous)	Atherosclerosis
Brushing teeth	Arteritis
Nose blowing	Cystic medial necrosis
Violent coughing	Fibromuscular hyperplasia
Iatrogenic	Fragmentation of elastic
Diagnostic angiography	fibers
Cervical manipulation	**Medical diseases**
Sports and recreation	Hypertension
Basketball	Marfan's and Ehlers-Danlos
Bowling	syndromes
Football	Neurofibromatosis
Marching	Syphilis
Skiing	Trauma—penetrating and
Tennis	blunt
Volleyball	Whiplash

Modified from **Hart RG, Easton JD:** *Dissections of cervical and cerebral arteries.* Neurol Clin 1(1):155, 1983.

level of the atlas transverse process and typically affects younger persons. (4,6–15)

The prognosis is generally good, with only 5% mortality from brain infarction. Recurrent transient ischemic attacks (TIAs) are common with Horner's syndrome, persisting for months or permanently. Treatment is usually conservative; intravenous heparin is used initially and then long-term anticoagulation is started. Endovascular stents are occasionally employed when aneurysm or an intimal flap is evident. Recurrence is uncommon and estimated at 1% per year. (16)

Imaging Features. There are no plain film findings for ICAD. MRA, diagnostic angiography, and ultrasound can all play a role in diagnosis. (2,16,17) The advantage of MRI examination is that the brain can be assessed at the same time, identifying peripheral shower sites of embolic infarction, visible in at least 15% of ICAD. (1) MRA is the technique of choice as the first-line investigation for ICAD and to document its course for progression, recanalization, and subsequent co-existent involvement of other neck vessels. (Fig. 18-23) Three locations are recognized as the most common sites of dissection: near the carotid bifurcation, at the atlantoaxial segment, and within the petrous portion of the temporal bone. (18,19) Imaging findings depend on the area of involvement, as noted below.

Juxta-Bifurcation. Juxta-bifurcation is the most common type and begins about 2 cm distal to the common carotid bifurcation, continuing for a variable distance distally. On angiography and MRA, various morphological signs have been described (2,16,17):

- *String sign.* The lumen remains patent throughout its length, but is narrowed and may be irregular in contour.
- *Flame sign.* The lumen tapers distally and eventually disappears as a result of the extrinsic compression formed by the hematoma in the tunica media.
- *Double lumen sign.* Two lumens are present; the pseudo-lumen demonstrates delayed flushing of the contrast.

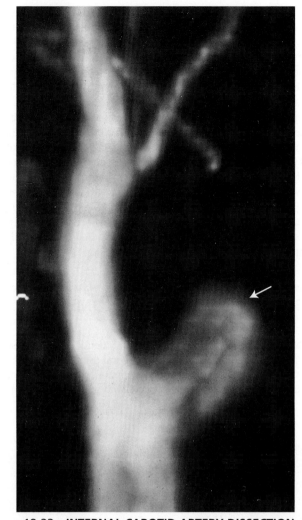

Figure 18-23   INTERNAL CAROTID ARTERY DISSECTION. MRI Angiogram, Coronal Neck. Observe that there is no flow beyond the origin of the internal carotid artery (*arrow*), caused by circumferential compression of the lumen. *COMMENT:* MRA is the procedure of choice for investigating internal carotid artery dissection (ICAD) and for documenting its progression. In addition, co-existent involvement of other neck vessels and any embolic complications in the brain can be identified. This bifurcation site is the most common location for ICAD.

- *Pseudo-aneurysm.* Localized, short-segment dilatation of the lumen.
- *Flap sign.* A thin linear filling defect is visible where the intimal layer has separated away from the tunica media; this is useful in localizing the origin of the dissection.
- *Spiral (corkscrew) sign.* The dissection often winds spirally around the vessel as it extends distally.

Axial MRI studies show the narrowed eccentric lumen, wall hematoma with high signal on T1-weighted images owing to methemoglobin of the subacute hemorrhage, and an increase in the overall outer diameter of the artery. (2,16,17) The hematoma lies on the convex side of the vessel and is often seen to "spiral" around the vessel distally. (1,17)

Atlantoaxial Segment. Dissection at the atlantoaxial segment most commonly happens in the upper ICA adjacent to the transverse processes of the atlas and axis as a sequelae of hyperextension and rotational injury. (6) Imaging shows a short-segment hematoma of the posterior vessel wall that expands the vessel external diameter and narrows the lumen. A localized aneurysm is sometimes seen. (6)

Petrous Segment. The least frequent lesions occur in the petrous segment and usually follow skull base fractures, although the fracture may or may not involve the carotid canal. Extension of the aneurysm into the intracavernous and supraclinoid ICA may occur. The demographics differ, typically occurring in the 2nd decade of life, with headache and the onset of a stroke within minutes. Massive stroke is the rule, with a poorer prognosis. On angiography, tapered narrowing or abrupt occlusion occurs. T1-weighted MRI studies exhibit definitive findings, including high-signal wall hematoma as two parallel lines (*railway tracks*). (17,20,21)

SUBCLAVIAN STEAL SYNDROME

Synonyms. Steal syndrome, steal phenomenon, Harrison-Smyth syndrome, reversed (paradoxical) vertebral artery flow syndrome.

Clinical Features. In 1829 Harrison recorded the importance of the vertebral artery flow when the subclavian artery is occluded proximal to the vertebral artery branch. (1) The result is retrograde blood flow from the vertebrobasilar circulation caudally through the vertebral artery, supplying the upper extremity via the distal portion of the subclavian. Because blood is "stolen" from the posterior circulation of the brain, the term *subclavian steal* is applied to this phenomenon. When symptomatic, the term *subclavian steal syndrome* (SSS), coined by Fisher in 1961, is applied. (2)

The majority of patients with vertebrobasilar steal do not have symptoms. Components of classic SSS involve characteristic features of vertebrobasilar ischemia: the *five Ds* (**d**izziness, **d**rop attacks, **d**iplopia, **d**ysarthria, and **d**ysphagia) and the *three Ns* (**n**ausea, **n**umbness on one side, and **n**ystagmus). (3) Upper limb claudication on activity often affects the hand more than the arm or forearm. The physical signs are loss of the ipsilateral radial pulse, a difference in right to left brachial systolic blood pressure readings > 20 mm Hg, and occasionally a neck bruit. *Drop attacks* and dizziness may be induced with the arm swinging test (i.e., repetitive active circumduction of the ipsilateral upper extremity). (4,5)

The classic description of the pathophysiology is a stenosis, usually high grade or total occlusion, proximal to the origin of the vertebral artery. On the left side this is within the subclavian, anywhere from the aortic arch to the ostium of the vertebral artery. Right-sided lesions occur within the subclavian artery distal to the common carotid takeoff but proximal to the vertebral artery branch. The left side is involved in a ratio of 3:1 compared with the right side. (6) It has been demonstrated in 6% of asymptomatic cervical bruits. (7) There is a slight male predominance,

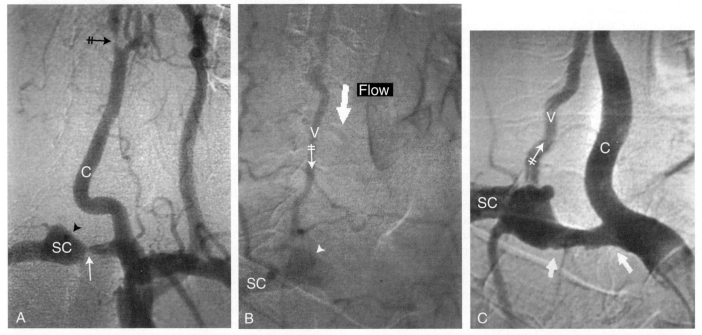

Figure 18-24 RIGHT-SIDED SUBCLAVIAN STEAL SYNDROME. A. Initial Digital-Subtraction Angiogram, Right Subclavian. Observe the focal stenosis (*arrow*) with poststenotic dilatation (*arrowhead*) of the subclavian (*SC*) artery. Note the lack of vertebral artery opacification compared with the normal common carotid artery (*C*). There is co-existent stenosis at the origin of the internal carotid artery (*crossed arrow*). **B. Delayed 15-Sec Digital-Subtraction Angiogram, Right Subclavian.** On the 15-sec postinjection image note the retrograde filling of the vertebral artery (*V*) (*crossed arrow*). The vertebral artery origin can be seen just distal to the poststenotic dilatation of the subclavian artery (*arrowhead*). **C. Postangioplasty Digital-Subtraction Angiogram, Right Subclavian.** After endoluminal angioplasty there is a significant increase in the size of the lumen (*white arrows*) and restitution of normal antegrade flow in the vertebral artery (*crossed arrow*). *COMMENT:* Many subclavian steal cases remain asymptomatic unless there is co-existing occlusive disease of the carotid artery. This patient was symptomatic, presenting with upper extremity claudication and syncopal episodes initiated by upper body (limb) exercises. (Courtesy of Arjith DeSilva, MBBS, FRANZCR, Newcastle, New South Wales, Australia.)

with the average age of symptom onset early in the 6th decade of life. It accounts for < 3% of all extracranial occlusions. (8,9)

The most common cause for subclavian steal is atherosclerosis, which accounts for at least 95% of cases. (7) Less frequent causes are coarctation, arch and great vessel anomalies, aneurysms (especially dissecting type), radiation or surgical fibrosis, apical lung tumor, and inflammatory arteritis. Of those that become symptomatic, at least 80% will have a significant stenosis or occlusion elsewhere in the common or internal carotid artery. (7) Known associations include coronary artery disease (present in 27–65%) and smoking (present in 78–100% of cases). (10)

Different types of subclavian steal have been described: (1,6,10)

- *Asymptomatic subclavian steal.* Continuous reversed flow is present but without symptoms, even with activity. This is the most common form, accounting for at least 60% of cases.
- *Activity-induced symptomatic subclavian steal.* Usually this occurs on a background of continuous reversed flow, with symptoms induced on limb activity.
- *Occult steal syndrome.* Normal antegrade vertebral artery flow is present at rest, reversing with activity and producing symptoms.
- *Continuous symptomatic subclavian steal.* Symptoms are present both at rest and with activity.
- *Partial steal syndrome.* Retrograde flow is present only in the systolic cardiac phase and reverts to the normal antegrade in diastole. This is not symptomatic.
- *False steal.* High-pressure contrast agent injection during angiography can occasionally induce contralateral retrograde vertebral artery flow as an artifact.

Imaging Features. On plain film studies of the neck, chest, or shoulder, calcified atheroma may be seen over the course of the subclavian artery, but this finding is not sufficiently sensitive or specific for the diagnosis of SSS. Occasionally on plain film or CT, enlargement of the transverse foramina bilaterally may be seen as an indicator of vertebral artery dilatation secondary to increased flow; however, this can also be seen as a normal variant and in bilateral carotid occlusions. The most sensitive tests are ultrasound and angiography. Dynamic-contrast MRA has also been used as a non-invasive alternative. (4,11)

Ultrasound is the best non-invasive test for showing retrograde vertebral artery flow, either at rest or after exercise. The direction of flow can be displayed anatomically, graphically, and numerically on Doppler studies. In addition, by applying a blood pressure cuff above systolic for 5 min on the affected limb and observing the vertebral artery flow, the reversal may be shown on cuff removal owing to limb hyperemia. (12,13) For cases initiated by atherosclerotic disease, identifying the offending atheroma is technically more difficult because of the superimposed bony anatomy that may deter adequate visualization.

Angiography is the gold standard for identification of atheromatous occlusion. (Fig. 18-24) This is performed initially by an arch aortogram and followed by selective studies of the subclavian artery. Delayed images following contrast injection over 30–60 sec may be required to show the reversed downward flow in the vertebral artery. The atheroma or alternative causes for the contralateral subclavian stenosis can usually be identified, although selective studies may be necessary for full characterization. Deployment of angioplasty balloons and stents can be performed in symptomatic cases.

STYLOHYOID LIGAMENT OSSIFICATION

Synonyms. Eagle's syndrome, styloid-stylohyoid syndrome, elongated styloid process, styloid syndrome, styalgia.

Clinical Features. Bone formation within the stylohyoid ligament is a relatively frequently observed radiologic finding that, on rare occasions, has been linked with neck-related symptoms. Ossification of the ligament was first described anatomically in 1652 by Marchetti (1,2) and was first described radiologically by Dwight in 1907 (1); in the late 1940s the relationship to clinical symptoms was alluded to by Eagle, whose name has become inexorably associated with the anomaly (Eagle's syndrome). (3,4)

Anomalies of the styloid process and stylohyoid ligament are seen on < 2% of radiographs and are present at 4% of autopsies. (1,4,5) Embryologically, cartilaginous elements are present between the second and the third branchial arches, which represent the styloid process, stylohyoid ligament, and lesser cornu of the hyoid (collectively, Reichert's cartilage). Nonetheless, this ossification occurs as a developmental variation rather than cartilage degeneration. (2,5) In some animals it is a normal structure, referred to as the *epihyal bone*. (5) Anatomically, the styloid process lies between the internal and external carotid arteries, is immediately adjacent to the pharyngeal wall in the palatine fossa, and serves as the attachment of three muscles. (5) When ossified it can be palpated both transorally in the palatine fossa and behind the mandible. The ligament acts as a suspensory support for the hyoid bone and provides a fulcrum for sagittal rotation during swallowing.

Given the common occurrence of ossification in the population, the true incidence of symptomatic cases is not known. Of all cases observed radiologically, very few will be proven to have symptoms related to this ossified ligament. (6) Dentists often suggest the diagnosis, as it permeates their literature and is well shown on panoramic radiography of the jaws (*orthopantomograph;* OPG). Ossification can be seen in patients as young as 18–22 years and appears to become more prominent and common with progressive age. There is no gender predominance.

Symptomatic stylohyoid bone formation generally occurs after the 4th decade, and findings may include dysphagia, throat discomfort, otalgia, headache, and, rarely, glossopharyngeal neuralgia. (5,7) These may occur without a distinct precursor event but have been more commonly described as beginning after a tonsillectomy. This so-called classic stylohyoid syndrome following tonsillar removal in the presence of ossification causes the stylopharyngeus muscle to distort the pharynx superiorly and laterally, causing the glossopharyngeal nerve to be stretched over the bony bar, resulting in dysphagia. (5,8) An additional symptom complex is pain arising from carotid artery compression (*carotodynia*) with anterolateral neck pain, especially on neck rotation. The resultant discomfort may be erroneously attributed to lymphadenopathy.

Thickness of the ossification rather than its length appears to be more important in symptom production. (2,7) The common depiction on imaging of apparent "joints" along the length of the ossification should not be confused with fracture and are not related to symptoms. These *pseudo-articulations* are filled with cartilage. (1) Thick ossification occurs with an increased frequency in diffuse idiopathic skeletal hyperostosis (DISH), though symptoms have not been described in instances of these tandem lesions. Fracture has not been documented. Treatment in selected refractory symptomatic cases is transoral removal. (5) Stylohyoid ligament ossification does not appear to be a contraindication to cervical spine manipulation, although careful technique selection is required to reduce rotation and avoid a possibly painful direct

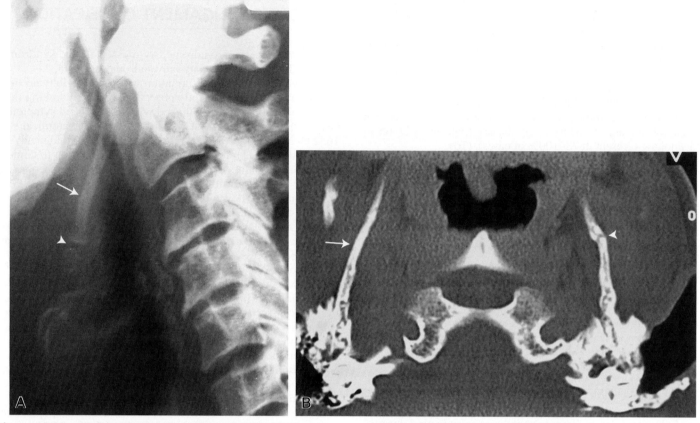

Figure 18-25 STYLOHYOID LIGAMENT OSSIFICATION.
A. Lateral Cervical Spine. Observe the well-corticated linear ossification extending obliquely in the anterior portion of the upper neck (*arrow*). There is a cleft distally (*arrowhead*) that has isolated a smaller ossicle. **B. CT, Axial Head.** Note the bilateral ossification of the ligament, extending from the temporal bone and coursing laterally to the pharyngeal wall.

On the right side the bony bar is virtually continuous (*arrow*), whereas the contralateral side exhibits a pseudo-joint (*arrowhead*). *COMMENT:* These ossifications are common and rarely symptomatic (Eagle's syndrome). On plain film radiographs this should not be confused with vascular calcification, especially of the vertebral artery, which rarely, if ever, is radiographically evident.

contact over the ligament. (5,9) There are no published reports citing the condition as a risk factor for carotid dissection, despite the close anatomical associations.

Imaging Features. Ossification is readily identified on plain film studies of the neck and mandible and is virtually always bilateral but usually asymmetrical. (Fig. 18-25) Ligamentous ossification may take three different patterns: continuous elongation uninterrupted over > 25 mm but unattached to the hyoid (uncommon), continuous elongation with attachment to the hyoid (uncommon), and segmental ossifications over its length separated by apparent joints (common). (5) The thickness of the ossification usually is < 5 mm, but can be variable up to the extreme of 25 mm. (2) Ossification is evident, with an outer cortex and marrow containing medullary cavity.

The normal styloid process arises just medial to the mastoid process on the temporal bone and projects anteriorly and inferiorly, usually not exceeding 25 mm in length. The anteroposterior (AP) open mouth radiograph shows the medial angulation of the styloid, anticipating the subsequent course of the stylohyoid ligament. (5) Panoramic radiography of the jaw depicts the ossification clear of the mandible, beginning laterally at the skull base and passing medially to the hyoid. Lateral or oblique views show the ossification extending anteriorly from near the mastoid process and coursing across the retropharyngeal soft tissues to the lesser cornu of the hyoid. In the more common segmented forms, differentiation from fracture is indicated by the typically bulbous

and smooth adjoining ends of the individual segments. CT scans of the neck also will show the ossification and its anatomic relationships to the carotid artery and pharyngeal wall. (10)

GRISEL'S SYNDROME

Synonyms. Distension luxation of the atlas, spontaneous hyperemic dislocation of the atlas, non-traumatic (spontaneous) atlantoaxial dislocation, *maladie de Grisel*, and *enucleation de l'atlas et torticollis*.

Clinical Features. Spontaneous subluxation (or rarely, dislocation) of the atlas after infection of the pharynx is an uncommon entity, usually occurring in children. (1,2) In 1830, Bell recorded the first case in association with a pharyngeal syphilitic ulcer. (3) In 1930 Grisel described two cases complicating nasopharyngeal infection. (4) The usual time of onset of the atlantoaxial instability following the infection varies from 1 day to weeks, although at least 50% will present within 7–10 days of the initiating pharyngeal inflammation. (4,5) Atlantoaxial instability secondary to rheumatic fever may be delayed for years, however. (6) The most common presentation is that of a painful torticollis. History of an upper respiratory infection is common; however, fever and other signs of infection are frequently resolved. Additional findings include neck pain and stiffness. Signs of cord compression are rare.

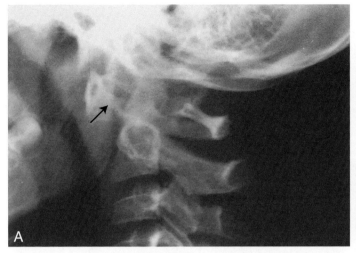 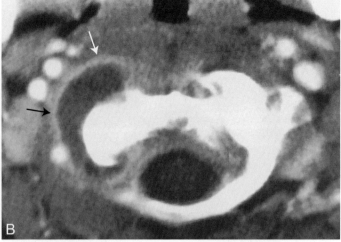

Figure 18-26 GRISEL'S SYNDROME. A. Lateral Cervical Spine. Note the anterior displacement of C1, resulting in an increase in the atlantodental interspace (ADI) (*arrow*). **B. CT, Axial Atlantoaxial Joint.** In a different patient, note the low density adjacent to the atlantoaxial joint (*arrows*), indicating significant facet joint effusion. *COMMENT:* Spontaneous atlantoaxial subluxation can follow a throat infection, most commonly tonsillitis, or even tonsillectomy. The mechanism is uncertain, though facet joint distension as seen on the CT scan is thought to be the underlying pathophysiological event leading to this radiographic appearance.

The level of pain may be mild to agonizing. Known precipitants include coryza, pharyngitis, rheumatic fever, tonsillitis and tonsillectomy, tuberculous adenitis, and syphilitic pharyngeal ulcer. (6,7)

There is no consensus on the pathophysiology, but the condition is most likely caused by hematogenous extension of the infection, producing muscle spasm, joint effusion, and ligamentous laxity, especially of the atlas transverse ligament. Pathologically, there is localized osteopenia with bone softening and decalcification of the fibro-osseous junction at the insertion of the transverse ligament to the atlas lateral mass. (5) A direct communication of the veins surrounding the odontoid with suboccipital and pharyngovertebral veins has been demonstrated, which provides the anatomic basis for bloodborne dissemination of the infection. (8) Once atlas displacement has occurred, resolution to normal alignment is infrequent. The associated torticollis similarly does not resolve. Initial traction and pain control for up to 6 weeks, followed by neck bracing, has been advocated. (7) Surgical fusion in situ is usually required for painful recalcitrant cases. Cervical manipulation is contraindicated. (3)

Imaging Features. The key finding is abnormal widening of the anterior atlantodental interspace on the lateral projection (> 5 mm in children and > 3 mm in adults), often best demonstrated on flexion projections. (Fig. 18-26) Neither the odontoid process nor the lateral atlantoaxial joints show erosive changes. On the frontal projection, rotation of the atlas on the axis (*rotary subluxation of the atlas*) is commonly present as evidenced by the right to left disparity in apparent width of the lateral masses and lateral atlantoaxial spaces. (9,10)

On axial CT the widening of the anterior atlantodental interspace can be confirmed, though scanning with the neck flexed is sometimes required. Persistent rotary fixation of the atlas can be confirmed if images obtained in right and left rotation show a lack of movement. MRI is helpful for assessing any compromise of the upper cervical cord, though anterior atlas displacements of up to 10 mm can be tolerated without neurological compromise. (11,12) The transverse ligament may be shown to be disrupted and distended. MRA should be included in such cases to assess the vertebral arteries because atlas displacements can compromise vertebrobasilar flow. (11,12)

RETROPHARYNGEAL ABSCESS

Synonyms. None.

Clinical Features. The development of an abscess in the prevertebral soft tissues of the neck is an uncommon condition, which is more prevalent in children. (1,2) The most common mechanism is local extension from a ruptured suppurative retropharyngeal lymph node. (3) Other less common causes include adjacent vertebral osteomyelitis, penetrating injury such as from endoscopy, traumatic or foreign body perforation, surgery, tonsillitis with complicating quinsy, lymphadenopathy, endocarditis, dental surgery, and lung and genitourinary infections. (1,3,4) *Staphylococcus aureus* is the most common pathogen, in at least 90% of cases; Gram-negative infections make up the majority of remaining cases. (2,3) *Mycobacterium tuberculosis* and fungal infections are uncommon. (2)

The onset is usually acute with pain, dysphagia, torticollis, and fever. Leukocytosis and elevated erythrocyte sedimentation rate (ESR) are the main laboratory findings. (1,4) Complications include thrombosis of the internal jugular vein, airway obstruction, mediastinitis, pericarditis, sepsis, spinal osteomyelitis, and epidural abscess. (5)

Imaging Features. In the early phases, plain films are insensitive. Therefore, retropharyngeal abscess requires MRI for demonstration and monitoring of its clinical course, especially to exclude coincident spinal osteomyelitis or extension into the mediastinum of the chest. (1,5,6) Plain film findings include widening of the prevertebral soft tissue spaces (in excess of either 7 mm at the C2 level or 22 mm at the C6 level). (1–3) Characteristically, the displaced soft tissue–air interface with the pharynx remains smooth but convex over at least two or three spinal segments. (1) (Fig. 18-27) Contained air is occasionally seen, especially in cases complicating previous perforation. Close scrutiny of all disc spaces for evidence of associated osteomyelitis should be made. (5)

CT similarly confirms the location of the abscess as a low attenuating density, often with heterogeneous enhancement. (3,6) MRI, particularly on T2-weighted images, confirms edema and

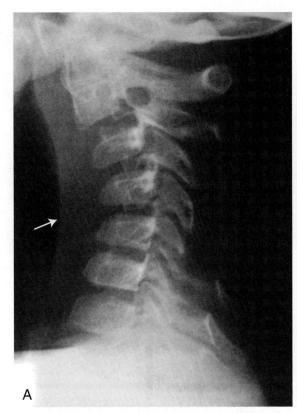

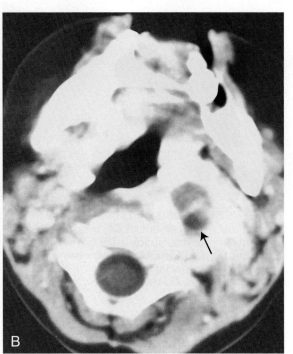

Figure 18-27 **RETROPHARYNGEAL ABSCESS. A. Lateral Cervical Spine.** Observe the increase in the retropharyngeal soft tissues at C2–C4 (*arrow*). **B. CT, Axial Neck.** Note the localized area of low density in the left retropharyngeal space, representing an abscess (*arrow*). *COMMENT:* This patient's presenting symptom was an inability to straighten her neck (torticollis). This is responsible for the poorly positioned radiograph. Retropharyngeal abscess, especially in children, can complicate cervical lymphadenitis from a throat infection or other inflammatory causes. Torticollis, in combination with fever and dysphagia, is an important clinical feature suggesting this diagnosis.

its location. (2,6) Postcontrast CT or MRI studies further define the extent of disease and reveal any evidence of complications, such as spinal infection. (1,6)

CALCIFIC TENDONITIS OF THE LONGUS COLLI

Synonyms. Retropharyngeal tendonitis, longus colli tendonitis, retropharyngeal calcium deposition disease, hydroxyapatite deposition disease of the longus colli, calcific retropharyngeal tendonitis, prevertebral tendonitis.

Clinical Features. Retropharyngeal tendonitis is an uncommon disorder of the neck characterized by deposition of hydroxyapatite crystals (HAC) into the superolateral portion of the longus colli muscle near its attachment to the anterior arch of the atlas. (1) Both acute and chronic forms have been described. The acute form presents with a characteristic clinical triad of neck pain and stiffness with dysphagia. Rarer cases in the lower cervical spine have been recorded. (2) There is occasional fever, elevated ESR, and mild leukocytosis. Peculiar to the condition is the synchronous onset of symptoms with radiologically demonstrable calcification, followed by resolution within 6 weeks of disappearance of the calcification. The age of onset is typically between 30 and 60 years, with a peak incidence of 50 years. (2,3) There is no gender predominance. Palpation of the anterolateral neck in the submandibular region reveals exquisite tenderness.

Symptomatic relief can be obtained with analgesic and anti-inflammatory medications. There are no sequelae, though additional acute episodes can occur. The chronic form shows characteristic calcification without prevertebral soft tissue swelling or symptoms; however, there is predisposition to subsequent acute episodes. (2,3)

Imaging Features. The characteristic plain film findings are soft tissue swelling and calcification anterior to the atlantoaxial region, best depicted on the lateral projection. (Fig. 18-28) The prevertebral swelling increases soft tissue interspace anterior and inferior to the atlas. The causative calcification appears as a variable density anterior and inferior to the anterior arch of the atlas. The appearance ranges from subtle and veil-like to a dense, amorphous opacity that can be singular or multiple. (4–6) Other causes for calcification in this location should be considered, including ossification in the stylohyoid ligament, accessory ossicles, and degenerative calcifications.

CT is definitive in identifying the presence and location of the calcification inferior to the atlas, which may not be visible on plain film. MRI studies most commonly show a crescenteric fluid collection anterior to the vertebral bodies, extending over two to three segments and sharply limited anteriorly by the deep cervical fascia. (4) On gadolinium administration, there is no enhancement of the margins of the effusion, which is a helpful differential finding to exclude abscess or any other fluid-containing lesion. Diffuse edema of the longus colli on T2-weighted studies has also been described, with the calcification appearing as low signal areas. (2)

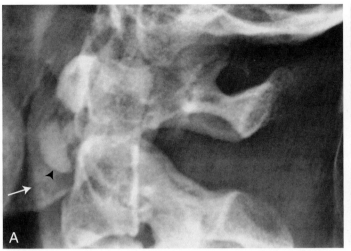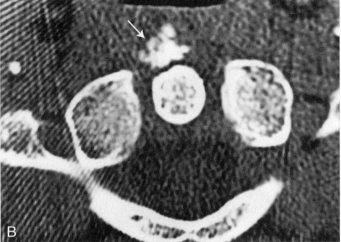

Figure 18-28   **CALCIFIC TENDONITIS OF THE LONGUS COLLI.**
A. Lateral Cervical Spine. Note the distension of the retro-pharyngeal space (*arrow*). An area of increased density is present just inferior to the anterior arch of C1 (*arrowhead*).
B. CT, Axial Atlantoaxial Joint. This study confirms the presence of calcification in the tendon of the longus colli muscle as it attaches along the inferior aspect of the C1 anterior arch (*arrow*). *COMMENT:* The combination of a large retropharyngeal space with focal calcification in this region is characteristic of calcific tendonitis of the longus colli. The condition is usually self-limiting, with symptoms subsiding once the calcification spontaneously disappears.

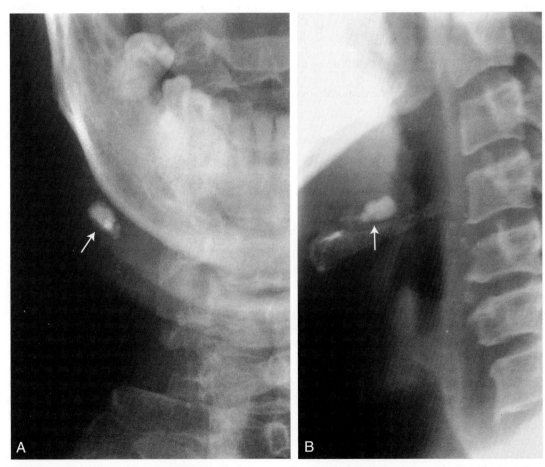

Figure 18-29   **SUBMANDIBULAR GLAND CALCULUS. A. AP Open Mouth.** Note the dense, smooth calcification in the soft tissues adjacent to the mandible (*arrow*). **B. Lateral Cervical Spine.** Inferior to the mandible, the calculus is confirmed to be in the anatomic location of the submandibular gland (*arrow*). *COMMENT:* In at least 80% of cases submandibular calculi will contain enough calcium to be visible on plain film.

SALIVARY GLAND CALCULUS (SIALOLITHIASIS)

Synonyms. None.
Clinical Features. Calculus is the most common cause for intermittent, recurrent swelling of the salivary glands. At least 80–90% of salivary gland stones occur in the submandibular gland, 10–20% in the parotid, and 1–7% in the sublingual glands. (1) In 25% of cases more than one stone will be present. Symptomatic stones usually lie within the duct. Infection followed by inflammatory stenosis within the duct leads to stasis of viscid secretions, precipitating the formation of calculi composed of calcium phosphate and carbonate. Many stones are asymptomatic and found incidentally on dental or cervical spine radiographs. (1) When symptomatic, moderate to severe pain occurs in the region of the enlarged gland, with excessive salivation. Provocation of the symptoms occurs with eating, especially citrus substances. A stone within the submandibular gland can often be bimanually palpated in the floor of the mouth.
Imaging Features. At least 80% of submandibular and 60% of parotid calculi are radiopaque on plain films, and have high attenuation values on CT. (1) (Fig. 18-29) Consistent demonstration on conventional radiographs requires complete, high-quality images, including posteroanterior (PA), oblique, and orthopantomographic views of the mandible. Intra-oral radiographs may also be required. Serendipitous discovery on cervical studies may occur, especially when submandibular stones are present below the level of the mandible. (2,3) CT is far more sensitive in identifying calculi, which are homogeneous, oval shaped, and smooth in outline. Sialograms can be technically difficult, if contrast filling of the duct is impaired by occlusion of the duct's orifice. However, the study may be beneficial and necessary for the demonstration of radiolucent stones. (1)

THYROID DISEASE

Synonyms. None.
Clinical Features. Thyroid disease includes a number of inflammatory and neoplastic conditions. Disorders of the thyroid are often suggested when tracheal deviation, calcification, or soft tissue mass findings are revealed during radiography of the cervical or thoracic spine, shoulder girdle, or chest. (1,2) Myriad symptoms may occur with thyroid disease, largely depending on whether decreased activity (hypothyroidism) or increased activity (hyperthyroidism) of the functional tissue results. (2,3) Mass effects secondary to thyroid enlargement may also produce symptoms related to compression of the trachea, esophagus, or other local structures. Musculoskeletal symptoms related to altered endocrine function include generalized non-specific myalgias and arthralgias, tiredness, malaise, and fractures (acute and insufficiency) from osteoporosis. (3) Enlargement of the thyroid (goiter) may compress the thoracic inlet with facial engorgement and respiratory distress provoked by elevation of the arms (Plummer's sign). (4,5) The most common thyroid abnormalities associated with imaging findings are multinodular goiter and carcinoma. (4–6)
Imaging Features. The key findings suggesting thyroid abnormality on plain film examination of the cervicothoracic region are calcification, soft tissue mass, and displacement of the trachea. (3) (Fig. 18-30) Ultrasound is usually the tech-

nique of choice for initial further investigation. In addition to detection of nodules and cysts, ultrasound can also provide guidance for real-time fine-needle biopsy. CT is especially useful for determining substernal extension of disease and aiding in differential diagnosis of other causes for a paratracheal mass. (6,7) Nuclear medicine with technetium-99 (^{99}Tc) pertechnetate provides functional information on gland and nodule activity and also identifies ectopic thyroid tissue and substernal extension. (8)

The diagnosis of carcinoma on imaging criteria remains problematic. Therefore, biopsy is required for confirmation. (6) Imaging features suggesting malignancy include diffuse calcification within a mass, no uptake on nuclear medicine (*cold nodule*), rapid interval growth between follow-up examinations, tracheal or laryngeal cartilage dissolution, and lymphadenopathy. (6,9,10)
Soft Tissue Mass. A soft tissue mass is usually radio-opaque on plain film. Substernal extension occurs anterior to the trachea in 75% of cases, displacing the trachea posteriorly and laterally with no definite side predominance. (2,11) Typically on the frontal projection, the mass can be seen both above and below the clavicle, placing the lesion in the anterior mediastinum (*cervicothoracic sign*). The remaining 25%, which lie posterior to the trachea, almost always lie to the right of the trachea. (2)

CT examination shows the paratracheal position and slightly higher attenuation characteristics of the thyroid gland, and can also reveal any mass effects (compression or displacement.) (6,7) Ultrasound shows a diffuse enlarged gland and is able to identify cysts and solid nodules. (9) Solid nodules on ultrasound are hypoechoic or isoechoic. (9,12)
Calcification. Calcifications may be irregular, solid, or ring-like. Irregular calcifications have no specific structure or pattern and may be pinpoint (*stippled*), granular, or more coarse. (3) These have a higher association with malignancy, with up to 60% of papillary carcinoma (most common cancer of the thyroid), 25% of follicular, and 15% of anaplastic cell types demonstrating calcification. (11) More solid and thin curved calcifications are more commonly benign and related to previous hemorrhage or lie within cyst walls. Solid types are dense and round but sometimes irregular in outline. Curvilinear arc or ring-like calcifications are typically smooth and thin.

Laryngeal cartilage calcifications should not be confused with those of the thyroid gland, carotid, or other surrounding vessels. (Fig. 18-31) Cartilage calcifications are virtually ubiquitous in the adult population and may even be seen in young children. No disease entity has been linked to the presence of these calcifications. The most commonly observed calcification is within the thyroid cartilage, especially the superior cornu, which is characterized by two parallel ascending lines of calcification diverging from the midline. These are often misconstrued as vascular calcifications. (13) (See Chapter 3.) Within the cornu, separated segments are frequently present with apparent interposed pseudo-joints. The cricoid cartilage is typically seen on lateral projections as a more amorphous conglomerate of calcification that extends anteriorly as a ring-like density. The arytenoid can calcify as a triangular dense homogenous opacity at the base of the epiglottis. (14)
Tracheal Deviation. With thyroid mass or enlargement, the adjoining tracheal wall is smoothly indented with narrowing of the lumen. The trachea at the cervicothoracic junction is usually displaced from the midline over at least 2 cm. (2) In retrosternal thyroid extensions there is more generalized tracheal deviation, extending below the clavicles. (2)

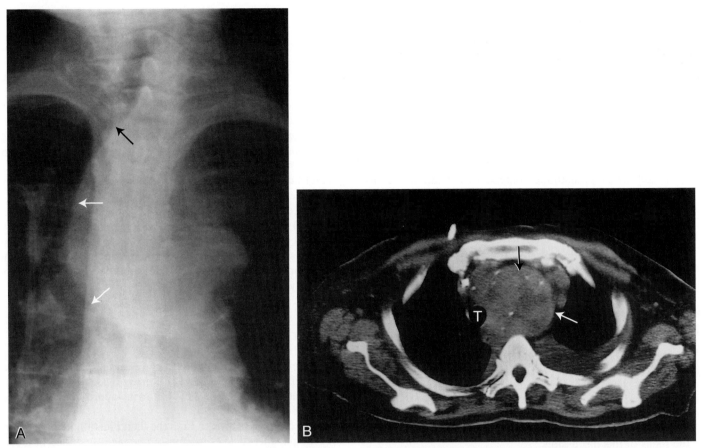

Figure 18-30 **SUBSTERNAL THYROID, GOITER. A. PA Chest.** Observe that the trachea is displaced laterally (*arrows*) owing to an adjacent soft tissue mass in the anterior mediastinum, representing a goiter. **B. CT, Axial Chest.** Note the small focal areas of calcification within this mass (*arrows*).

The displacement of the trachea (*T*) is well demonstrated. *COMMENT:* The most common cause for tracheal deviation is thyroid goiter but it can also be the result of lymphadenopathy, thymoma, teratoma, and volume loss in the upper lobe (i.e., radiation fibrosis, tuberculosis, atelectasis).

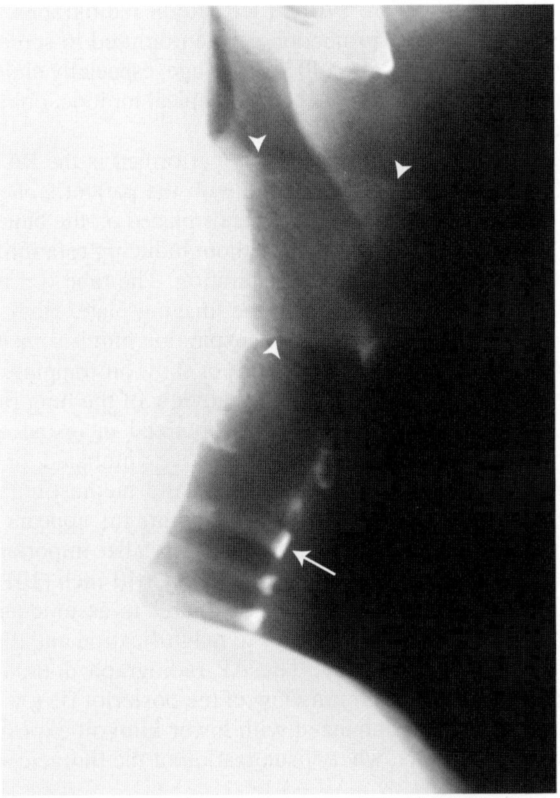

Figure 18-31 **THYROID CARTILAGE CALCIFICATION. Lateral Cervical Spine.** Note the broad mineralized plate of the thyroid cartilage (*arrowheads*). The tracheal ring cartilages can be defined through the tracheal air shadow (*arrow*). *COMMENT:* This represents normal physiologic calcification and should not be confused with a pathological finding or be deemed clinically significant.

THE THORAX: MASQUERADERS OF MUSCULOSKELETAL DISEASE

INTRODUCTION

Many disorders of the thorax manifest musculoskeletal symptoms. In addition, the anatomic contents of the thorax are, to varying degrees, demonstrated on musculoskeletal images. In this section emphasis is directed to the most common disorders of the lungs and, to a lesser extent, the heart. The discussion is divided into three sections: imaging modalities and principles of interpretation, fundamental imaging signs, and review of common diseases.

PRINCIPLES OF CHEST IMAGING

All modalities have application in the assessment of chest disorders. The most common studies employed are chest radiographs, CT, and nuclear medicine. Ultrasound (echocardiography), MRI, nuclear medicine, and coronary angiography of the heart and aorta are the mainstays of cardiac diagnosis. Chest radiography and CT are the focus of this discussion.

Chest Radiography

Basic Techniques

The basic projections are PA and left lateral radiographs. (See Chapter 1.) The lateral projection is often omitted in screening chest evaluation in patients < 40 years of age, especially children. Supplemental examinations include AP, apical lordotic, obliques, lateral decubitus, and expiration films.

PA. The most common routine study performed is the PA projection. The optimum positioning is with the patient's chest in contact with the imaging plate and hands placed on the buttocks. The shoulders are rolled forward without inducing rotation, and respiration is suspended in full inspiration. The tube is a minimum of 72 inches (183 cm) from the imaging plate. High kilovoltage (> 100 kVp) is preferred. An expiration film is sometimes obtained to accentuate a pneumothorax or show air trapping.

AP. The AP projection is a suboptimal view of the lung fields, heart, and mediastinum but is often obtained in instances of acute trauma or unconscious, uncooperative, intubated, or frail patients. The apparent size of the heart and mediastinum are enlarged in this projection; and the diaphragm appears elevated, more convex, and less distinct. It is also important to note that AP films are often performed with a 40-inch (101 cm) focal–film distance when patients are unable to assume an upright posture. This also contributes to magnification and distortion of mediastinal anatomy. The AP radiograph does, however, provide a more optimum view of the posterior ribs, whose details can be further enhanced with lower kilovolt exposures. In instances of trauma, when visualization of the thoracic spine

is important and when a lateral view is often not possible, purposeful overexposure is frequently used.

Lateral. A 72-inch (183 cm) focal–film distance is used. With the patient's arms elevated, the left side of the thorax is placed against the bucky and exposed during full inspiration. Placing the left side closest to the film minimizes magnification of the heart. This projection is used primarily to demonstrate the trachea, hila, retrosternal space, spine, and posterior lung bases. Assessment of the posterior costophrenic angles is also important because free pleural fluid will be detected first in this most dependent portion of the chest cavity.

Apical Lordotic. Obtained in the AP projection with a 72-inch (183 cm) focal–film distance and with the patient leaning back, this view projects the clavicles and first rib above the apical lung field. It is specifically used for detailed examination of the lung apex, upper mediastinum, hila, and middle and lingular lobe pathology.

Interpretation

The systematic analysis of the structures of the chest is vital to lesion detection. Although there is no step-by-step convention for interpretation of chest films, the following approach is suggested. (Table 18-4)

Patient Demographics. Find the identification label and confirm the patient's details, such as name, age, sex, date of study, and any additional information available.

Analysis of Technique. Four aspects of the frontal chest radiograph are assessed: patient position (AP vs. PA; upright

Table 18-4	Systematic Approach to Interpretation of Chest Films
Patient demographics	Cardiac borders (shape, size,
Name	definition)
Age	Hilar position, pulmonary
Date	artery size
Analysis of technique	Aortic position (size,
AP or PA	contour)
Inspiration (diaphragm	**Diaphragms**
position)	Position
Rotation	Shape
Exposure	**Skeletal components**
Overview	Ribs
Identify the obvious	Sternum
Coverup assessment	Shoulder girdles
Lung fields	Spine
Fissure identification	**Review areas**
Opacity, radiolucency	Subdiaphragm (abdomen)
Bronchovascular markings	Retrocardiac area
Hila	Chest wall (skin line, axilla,
Localization of abnormality	breast shadow)
(lobar anatomy, zone	Shoulder girdles
description)	Neck
Mediastinum	**Summary**
Anatomical divisions (ante-	Findings, diagnosis,
rior, middle, posterior)	differential diagnosis
Heart and great vessels	Additional studies
Cardiac size	(previous, supplemental)

vs. supine or semirecumbent), adequacy of inspiration, degree of rotation present, and adequacy of exposure.

AP or PA. To avoid interpreting cardiomegaly and other projectional artifacts on AP exposures, confirmation of patient position is critical. Clues that an AP projection has been performed include the scapulae projected over the lung fields, the clavicles appearing more curved and inferiorly angled, visibility of the chin over the neck outline, well-demonstrated cervical disc spaces, the presence of cardiac monitor leads, and a parallel position of the humerus to the lateral chest wall. These films should be marked by the technologist as *supine, AP,* or *portable.* Portable films and those marked *supine* are typically performed with a 40-inch (101 cm) focal–film distance, which must be taken into consideration in assessment of the lung parenchyma and cardiovascular structures.

Inspiration. An adequate inspiration is obtained when 10 posterior ribs or 7 anterior ribs can be counted above the diaphragm. Incomplete inspiration elevates the hemidiaphragms, which can simulate subpulmonic effusion and basilar congestion, while widening the mediastinum and enlarging the heart. These findings closely mimic those of congestive cardiac failure.

Rotation. In a study with no rotation the medial ends of the clavicles at the sternoclavicular joints should be equidistant from the upper thoracic spinous processes. Rotation displaces the heart and obscures the cardiac margins, simulating adjacent atelectasis, consolidation, or mediastinal shift. The mediastinum appears widened and the aortic contour distorted.

Exposure. As a general rule the thoracic disc spaces should be just barely visible through the cardiac silhouette. Clearly depicted pedicles, spinouses, and vertebral details usually indicate that the film was overexposed for evaluation of lung parenchyma. By noting the adequacy of the exposure, abnormalities of the lung fields can be better assessed and more accurate comparison among sequential or comparison studies can be made.

Overview. It is important to take some time to obtain a general overview of the film, at a distance farther away than the normal interpreting distance. The film is then generally examined for any obvious abnormality, followed by an abbreviated perusal of the lung fields, heart, mediastinum, and skeleton. A useful approach is to cover the film with the x-ray jacket and slowly move it down to facilitate left to right lung field comparisons (*coverup assessment*). Any questionable areas should be noted for more careful review, but the overview inspection of the entire film should be completed before the more detailed study of individual components is begun.

Detailed Study

Lung Fields. Two important findings to look for are changes in density and/or pattern. *Density,* of course, refers to the radiopacity of tissue. *Pattern* refers to the size or distribution of parenchymal markings in the lung fields associated with bronchi, vessels, and interstitial tissue. Either of these two factors may change focally, locally, or generally. Parenchymal abnormalities that have focal (i.e., solitary nodules) or local (i.e., segmental or lobar disease) effects are often first noted by comparing the symmetry of the lung fields. A careful left to right comparison of the chest, first as a whole and then interspace by interspace, is therefore recommended as a useful means of detecting focal or local abnormalities.

For more generally distributed pathologies, alteration of the general density of lung parenchyma must be gauged as either increased or decreased relative to the "expected" density. This can be more difficult and is usually based on the reviewer's experience in reading chest radiographs, although consideration of the relative density of other tissues on the film (i.e., mediastinum, musculoskeletal, and abdominal tissue) can also be helpful. In generalized disease, pattern changes in the distribution of the bronchovascular markings and interstitial tissues are often the principal observation.

Any abnormality should be localized to a lobe whenever possible, though descriptive terms such as *upper, middle,* and *lower* zones can be used. It should be noted that these "zones" do not correspond accurately with the lobar anatomy. The horizontal (minor) fissure of the right lung separates the upper from the middle lobe and is seen on the PA view between the anterior fourth to sixth ribs. The oblique (major) fissure is seen on the lateral view, separating the lower from the upper and middle lobes and extending from approximately the T6 vertebra to the anterior third of the diaphragm.

Mediastinum. The anatomic space and its contents separating the two lungs is the mediastinum, which is divided on the lateral projection into three divisions: anterior, middle, and posterior. Recognition of their location and knowledge of their contents provide the basis for accurate diagnosis.

The anterior mediastinum occupies the space between the anterior pericardium (heart) and sternum. The contents include the thymus, lymph nodes, and blood vessels, and it is the most common site for the thyroid gland to occupy when it enlarges. The posterior mediastinum is located posterior to the heart and anterior to the spine, containing the descending aorta, inferior vena cava, and esophagus. While technically not considered part of the anatomic posterior mediastinum, the spine and paravertebral soft tissues are, for imaging purposes, included as contents of this division. The middle mediastinum lies between the anterior and posterior mediastinum and is occupied by the heart, root of the aorta, and hila, including the mainstem bronchi and pulmonary arteries as well as lymph nodes.

Heart and Great Vessels. The heart size is estimated on the PA projection by evaluation of the cardiothoracic ratio (transverse diameter of the heart divided by the intrathoracic diameter), which normally should be < 50%. The heart margins are smooth and sharp, except at the cardiac apex where a common epicardial fat pad may blur its contour. Identification of the components of the cardiac silhouette should be made, starting at the right cardiophrenic angle and moving to the right atrium, ascending aorta, superior vena cava, aortic arch (aortic knob, aortic knuckle), descending aorta, aortopulmonary window, pulmonary trunk, left atrial appendage, left ventricle, and apex.

The hilar shadows are largely composed of the proximal portion of the pulmonary arteries, lymph nodes, and the mainstem bronchi. The level of the left hilum is normally slightly higher than the right because the left pulmonary artery passes over the left mainstem bronchus, whereas the right pulmonary artery courses below the mainstem bronchus on that side. Fibrotic retraction of lung parenchyma and atelectasis are common causes of displacement of the hila. Common causes of hilar enlargement include neoplastic or inflammatory lymphadenopathy and vascular abnormality.

Diaphragms. The right hemidiaphragm is 1–2 cm higher than the left, owing to the liver, and represents the anterior attachment and cupola of the diaphragms. The superior border is convex and slopes upward from the lateral chest wall. Slight to moderate elevation or irregularity of the contour is usually a normal variant (referred to as *eventration*). The left diaphragm is commonly elevated owing to gas in the splenic flexure. The lateral costophrenic and medial cardiophrenic angles are typically acute and sharp and should be carefully examined for "blunting" as a sign of pleural fluid.

Skeletal Components. The thoracic spine and discs, ribs, shoulder girdles, and sternum are all displayed to varying degrees and should be systematically examined.

Review Areas. Many abnormalities can be identified beyond the more obvious structures of the lungs, heart, and skeleton.

Subdiaphragm (Abdomen). Below the diaphragm, crescenteric air collections can be a clue to a perforated hollow viscus (pneumoperitoneum), such as a duodenal ulcer. Position of the magenblase (air in the fundus of the stomach) is also a useful indicator of subdiaphragmatic pathology. Dilated bowel loops from obstruction, calcified gallstones, hepatomegaly, and splenomegaly are some of the more common conditions identified on a subdiaphragmatic search.

Retrocardiac Area. Abnormalities of the heart, left lower lobe, descending aorta, esophagus (hiatus hernia), and vertebral and paravertebral soft tissues can be obscured by the density of the heart. Often an attempt to "look through" the heart density will detect an abnormality that otherwise would be missed.

Chest Wall. The breast shadows should be present bilaterally in women and if visible in men may suggest gynecomastia, asthenia, or emphysema. The skin line over the lateral chest wall should be smooth and occasionally may harbor collections of air as a sentinel sign of underlying pneumothorax. Asymmetry in axillary contour can be seen with mastectomy. Surgical clips can also provide some insight to previous disease.

Shoulder Girdles. Bone and joint abnormalities at the shoulder girdles may assist in the diagnosis of chest abnormalities, especially rheumatoid arthritis, metastatic disease, and multiple myeloma.

Lung Apices. Owing to overlap of the clavicles and upper ribs, apical disease can easily be obscured. Pleural thickening, fibrosis (tuberculous, radiotherapy), granuloma, bullae, and carcinoma (Pancoast's tumor) can all be observed in the lung apices, often requiring careful scrutiny and a supplemental apical lordotic projection.

Neck. The main radiographically visible structure in the neck is the trachea, which should be midline. Causes for its displacement include upper lobe fibrosis or collapse, tension pneumothorax, thyroid enlargement, lymphadenopathy, and mediastinal tumor. Calcifications are common and can occur within lymph nodes and thyroid goiter. Surgical clips can be markers of thyroid, parathyroid, laryngeal, or sympathetic ganglion surgery and can provide clues relevant to chest disease.

Summary. After the various components of the chest radiograph are assessed individually, the findings must be summed to either arrive at a diagnosis or to establish a differential list of the most likely diagnoses. It is also extremely important to review any previous studies that may be available. If a previous diagnosis has been established, any change in the condition should be noted. If a diagnosis is not established from the current examination alone, review of the earlier studies may assist in this process or in the building of a differential diagnosis.

It often is the nature of the conditions included in a differential list that will direct the next steps of the clinician. The workup for a vascular pathology, for instance, will differ from the laboratory work and advanced imaging studies that would be necessary in consideration of neoplastic or infectious diagnoses. The following sections will demonstrate how various imaging modalities can be applied to establish or to refine the diagnosis.

Computed Tomography

Basic Techniques

Imaging of the chest with CT remains the pre-eminent method for definitive diagnosis, guiding biopsy procedures, and monitoring the course of disease. Five basic protocols of chest imaging are described here, though with the advent of multislice technology these procedures are being expanded and refined.

Routine Intravenous Contrast CT. The most common protocol employed in chest imaging is intravenous contrast CT. At least 75 mL of non-ionic iodinated contrast is injected through an antecubital vein. Between 20 and 40 sec after the beginning of the injection, helical axial images are acquired from the lung apex to the upper abdomen. The patient must suspend inspiration while the images are acquired. Two windows are usually evaluated: one of them highlights the lung parenchyma (*lung windows*) and the other highlights the mediastinal contents (*mediastinal windows*). This study may be used to evaluate suspected lung abnormalities, such as pneumonia, collapse, mass, pleural effusion, and mediastinal pathology.

Routine Non-Contrast CT. The same helical acquisition as described above is occasionally employed without contrast when there is a history of contrast reaction, poor venous access, or determination and characterization of calcification is required. Analysis of a pulmonary nodule may include fine sections before contrast to assess for the presence of calcium as a sign of a benign process. Investigation of coronary artery calcification is performed without contrast with rapid multislice acquisitions.

High-Resolution CT. Non-contrast, non-helical thin section axial acquisitions of 1–1.5 mm are obtained at 10-mm intervals from the lung apices to the bases. These high-resolution CT (HRCT) studies are performed supine and prone at inspiration. In instances of air trapping, expiration studies are included. This technique is employed when fine structural detail is required, such as in the evaluation of interstitial lung disease. Because the portions of the lung between slices are not imaged it is an incomplete study and may not register lesions < 1 cm.

CT Angiogram. Timing image acquisition to the location of the largest concentration of contrast (*bolus*) within the vascular space allows depiction of these vessels. The most common settings for CT angiogram (CTA) are in the evaluation of the aorta for dissection and the pulmonary arteries for embolism. With multislice techniques graphic three-dimensional images can be presented, often avoiding the use of invasive angiography.

Virtual Endoscopy. Multislice technology using multiple detector rows allows rapid acquisition of thin sections, which can be used to produce startling images in any plane as well as three-dimensional images. Structures such as the tracheobronchial tree and vessels can be viewed from an endoluminal perspective. Virtual endoscopy is employed in the evaluation of stenoses, mass lesions, and status of stents.

Interpretation

Evaluation of the multiple CT images of the chest requires a systematic approach to the various anatomic components displayed and an understanding of the imaging protocol used.

Protocol Analysis. When contrast is used, timing of the examination can be assessed by the relative increase in density of contrast within the respective vessels: dense aorta–left atrium–pulmonary trunk are features of an arterial phase, whereas increased density of the inferior vena cava denotes a delayed acquisition. If the patient has low cardiac output or the scan is performed too early, most of the intravascular contrast will be visible in the superior vena cava, subclavian, and brachiocephalic veins and only little will be seen elsewhere.

Anatomic Components. Systematic assessment of the various structures is undertaken on either the lung or the mediastinal windows.

Lung Windows. The lung parenchyma is analyzed for aeration as determined by the relative radiolucency and lung size. The bronchi are individually assessed for wall thickness and size relative to the accompanying vessel, which is normally in a ratio of 1:1. The size and distribution of the vessels are analyzed. The pleural surfaces, including the fissures, can be seen as thin smooth linear opacities.

Mediastinal Windows. The mediastinal window images show the lung fields as very black and largely undiagnostic for parenchymal disease; however, calcification, necrosis, and cavitation may be detected if present. The trachea and mainstem bronchi are shown to advantage, as are the mediastinal vessels. This is the optimum window to assess for lymphadenopathy. The heart chambers, myocardium, and pericardium are all identifiable. Bone detail of the thoracic cage and spine can be examined on this window but usually requires specific bone window settings for accurate analysis.

FUNDAMENTAL SIGNS OF CHEST DISEASE

The number of diseases associated with imaging changes of the chest is immense; however, the imaging findings are often not unique—considerable overlap exists among various conditions and categories of conditions. Certain predominant imaging features have been grouped into categories or patterns that are associated with disorders affecting a particular type of tissue (e.g., alveolar or interstitial) or involving a particular mechanism (e.g., atelectasis) of pathology. Consequently, many clinicians advocate the concept of *pattern recognition,* to assist in simplifying the myriad changes observed in these many dis-

eases. In this section an abbreviated overview of these patterns is presented.

Alveolar Disease

Synonyms. Consolidation, air space disease.

Description. Pathologically, alveolar disease represents filling of the alveolar sacs with fluid, pus, cells, blood, or protein. Generally, it is a sign of more acute disease with a broad spectrum of causes. Local alveolar disease within or of a whole lobar segment is a feature of bacterial pneumonia, infarction, contusion, aspiration, and acute radiation damage. More diffuse and even bilateral alveolar opacification are features of pulmonary edema, aspiration, proteinosis, hemorrhage, and adult respiratory distress syndrome.

Identification of the characteristic signs of alveolar disease is crucial for developing an accurate list of differential diagnoses. (Table 18-5) Analysis includes confluent areas of increased radiopacity with blurred peripheral margins (*fluffy*), except when the process abuts a pleural or fissural interface, where it will be sharply demarcated. As the involved alveolar spaces take on fluid density, there will be obliteration of contained vascular markings and loss of border definition between the involved lung and other fluid-dense anatomy (e.g., heart and abdomen). This results in the classic *silhouette sign.* Air-containing branches of the bronchial tree surrounded by fluid-filled alveoli become visible as radiolucent, branching lines, resulting in the *air bronchogram sign* or the *air alveologram sign,* also characteristic of alveolar disease. (1,2)

Interstitial Disease

Synonyms. None.

Description. The lung interstitium is made up of a network of connective tissue that invests the arteries, veins, bronchi, and lymphatics centrally and peripherally envelops the lung in a fibrous sheath. It essentially acts as the skeleton of the lung, providing mechanical support, and has three continuous compartments: the axial (proximal to the hilus), parenchymal (hilus to the secondary lobules), and peripheral (subvisceral pleural space). The term *interstitial markings* on chest radiographs refers to linear (reticular) markings formed by the branching bronchovascular structures and their surrounding peribronchovascular soft tissue.

High-resolution CT is the gold standard technique for defining interstitial lung disease. (3,4) Increase in interstitial fluid, cellular infiltration, fibrosis, and granuloma formation all act to increase the volume and thickness of these structures, which produces radiographically definable changes. Though seen in some acute presentations, such as pulmonary edema and lymphangitis carcinomatosis, it is often a pattern of more chronic disease. Inter-

Table 18-5	Imaging Signs of Alveolar Disease
Opacity (patchy or confluent)	
Indistinct margins (fluffy), except at pleura	
Limited by fissures (lobar distribution)	
Loss of vascular markings	
Air bronchogram sign	
Air alveologram sign	
Silhouette sign	
Rapid onset, rapid clearing	

stitial lung disease has > 100 causes and is characterized by a number of imaging signs. (2) (Table 18-6)

Atelectasis

Synonyms. Volume loss, collapse, underinflation.

Description. Atelectasis is a sign of disease rather than being a primary disease in itself. When present, a search for a cause should be attempted, including identifying abnormalities that may be within the bronchial wall or lumen (intrinsic) or outside of the bronchus (extrinsic). Mechanisms of atelectasis include obstruction (bronchial pathology), passive (adjacent mass compression or pneumothorax), adhesive (surfactant inactivation), and cicatrization (scarring). In children the most common intrinsic cause of atelectasis is a mucus plug or foreign body. In adults < 40 years of age atelectasis commonly results from a mucus plug, foreign body, or benign tumor. In adults > 40 years atelectasis is most often associated with carcinoma. (4,5)

Three forms of atelectasis are recognized: an entire lung, an entire segment, or part of a segment (subsegmental). In the absence of pneumothorax or massive pleural effusion, total lung collapse indicates pathology close to the carina and proximal to the hilum. Common causes are carcinoma, bronchial adenoma, foreign body, misplaced endotracheal tube, and lymphadenopathy. Segmental collapse similarly is characterized by bronchial occlusion near the segmental origin; endoluminal pathology is usually neoplasm or mucus plug. (5,6) Partial collapse has more distal obstruction and may be the result of neoplasm, mucus plug, or scarring. This is most common at the lung bases and creates a linear, horizontal density (*discoid atelectasis,* Fleischner lines). Transitory subsegmental atelectasis may occur secondary to diaphragmatic splinting associated with pain. (4)

The imaging signs of atelectasis include increased opacity, bronchovascular crowding, displacement signs (mediastinal, hilar or tracheal shift, altered position and shape of adjacent fissures, diaphragmatic elevation), loss of the cardiac or diaphragmatic margins (silhouette sign), and occasionally an air bronchogram sign. (2,5,7) (Table 18-7)

Pulmonary Nodule

Synonyms. Coin lesion, lung spot, cannon-ball lesion. (4,6)

Description. The term *pulmonary nodule* applies to any lesion of the lung that is opaque and round to oval in shape. Nodular lesions can be singular (solitary pulmonary nodule) or multiple.

Table 18-6	Imaging Signs of Interstitial Disease

Hazy lung fields (ground glass opacification)
Kerley B lines
Reticular markings
Honeycomb appearance
Nodules
Generalized non-lobar distribution
Irregular cardiac outline (shaggy heart)
Prominent bronchovascular markings
Thickened bronchial walls (cuffing)
Pleural thickening, variable effusion

Table 18-7	Imaging Signs of Segmental and Lobar Atelectasis

Increased opacity
Bronchovascular crowding
Displacement signs
   Mediastinal, hilar, or tracheal shift
   Altered position or shape of adjacent fissures
   Diaphragmatic elevation
Silhouette sign
   Loss of the cardiac or diaphragmatic margins
Air bronchogram sign

Size can be a few millimeters to many centimeters. The peripheral margins of the lesion can be well defined or irregular. The differential diagnosis is broad and includes postinfection granuloma, active infection, primary or secondary tumor, vasculitis, pneumoconiosis, and granulomatous disease. (4,8)

Cavitating Lesion

Synonyms. None.

Description. A localized air-filled lesion surrounded by a visible wall constitutes a lung cavity. Thin-walled lesions are more commonly benign, whereas a thick, irregular wall is commonly a sign of malignancy. Thin-walled lesions include bullae, posttraumatic lung cyst, and pneumatocele. (6) Thick-walled lesions are more commonly abscesses, vasculitis, or tumors with internal necrosis. (6) Most cavitating tumors are of the squamous cell carcinoma type. (8)

Necrotic internal debris and fluid in a cavity will sometimes produce a characteristic air–fluid level. Fungal infections, especially *Aspergillus,* may create a radiographically visible agglomeration of hyphae, referred to as a *fungus ball* or *mycetoma,* within an area of cavitated lung. (9,10)

Adenopathy

Synonyms. None.

Description. Enlargement of lymph nodes is a cardinal sign of chest disease. Their location not only allows identification but also provides crucial clues for diagnosis. All 14 classified locations (*stations*) can be isolated by CT. The most common adenopathy sites identifiable on chest radiographs are retrosternal, paratracheal, carinal, hilar, bronchopulmonary, and retrocrural. (11) Lymph node enlargement on chest radiographs produces opaque solid masses that have smooth and sometimes lobulated margins. Retrosternal nodes widen the mediastinum on the frontal study and obliterate the normal radiolucency of the anterior *clear space on the lateral study.* (9,10) Paratracheal adenopathy produces a widening of the normally < 5 mm of soft tissue to the right of the tracheal outline. Hilar adenopathy is difficult to differentiate from the pulmonary artery but appears as a solid, sharply marginated mass. (8) Bronchopulmonary nodes are within the lung tissue distal to the hilus and when enlarged, as classically in sarcoidosis, produce an elongated, lobulated mass that is separated from the cardiac silhouette by radiolucent lung tissue. Retrocrural nodes on frontal studies produce a characteristic widening of the normally thin diaphragmatic crura seen through the cardiac silhouette. (4,6,11)

Pleural Effusion

Synonyms. None.

Description. Fluid within the pleural space may be a transudate or exudate or blood. When the parietal and visceral pleura remain closely apposed the pleural space is a potential area with a net negative pressure, which maintains lung inflation. When fluid accumulates in the space the surface tension produced by the closely apposed pleural layers acts to draw the fluid upward in a decreasing thickness. On erect chest studies this is seen as the characteristic *meniscus sign* of a sweeping, concave fluid level. (2,8) The normally acute costophrenic angles are "blunted" from the fluid; 300 cc is required to affect the lateral sulci and only 50 cc to blunt the posterior recess. For this reason early pleural effusion is best seen on the lateral study. (2) If pneumothorax co-exists, the fluid will layer, giving a horizontal air–fluid level (*hydropneumothorax*). (5,11) Causes are many and include cardiac failure, trauma, malignancy, and infection. (12)

Named Signs of the Chest

Numerous signs that assist in the diagnosis of chest disease have been described. Only the most common and important are listed in the following sections. (Table 18-8)

(*text continues on page 1766*)

Table 18-8	Common Named Imaging Signs of the Thorax		
Sign	**Definition**	**Significance**	**Plain Film**
Air bronchogram	Alveolar opacification surrounding air-filled bronchi (*arrow*)	Pus (pneumonia) Blood (hemorrhage) Fluid (transudate) Cells (tumor) Collapse (anectasis)	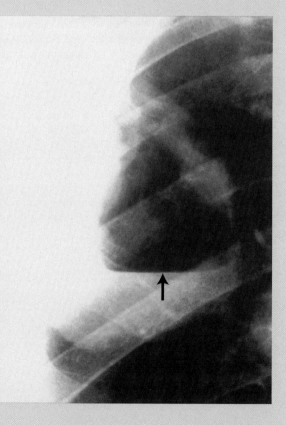
Air–fluid level	Horizontal interface of air and fluid within a mass (*arrow*)	Cavitation of the mass	

CT	Diagnosis
	Right middle lobe pneumonia

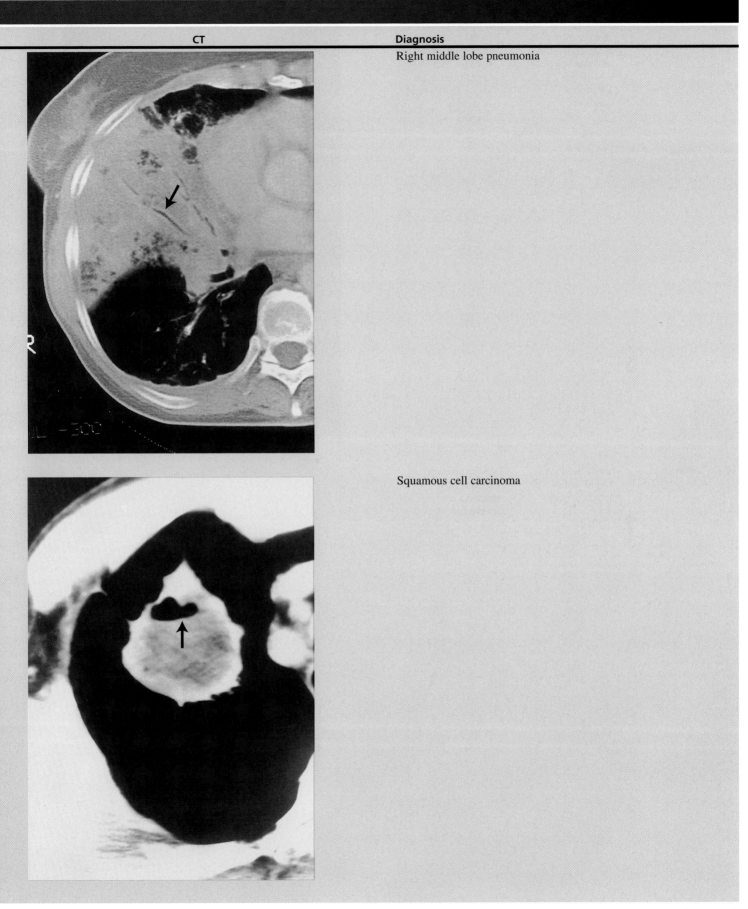

Squamous cell carcinoma

Table 18-8 | **Common Named Imaging Signs of the Thorax** (*continued*)

Sign	Definition	Significance	Plain Film
Cervicothoracic	Continuation of the margin of the mass above the clavicle suggests a posterior location (*arrows*)	Mass lies partially in the posterior mediastinum because the superior margin above the clavicle is sharply defined	
Coin lesion	Smooth-bordered, round, solid lesion (*arrow*)	Tumor (primary, secondary) Abscess Granuloma	

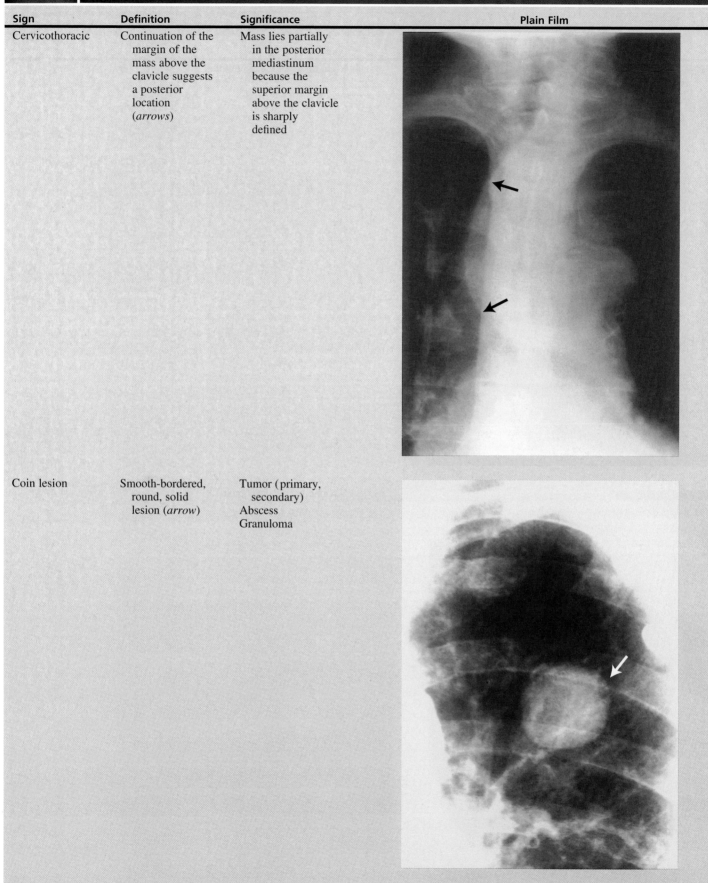

Substernal thyroid (goiter)

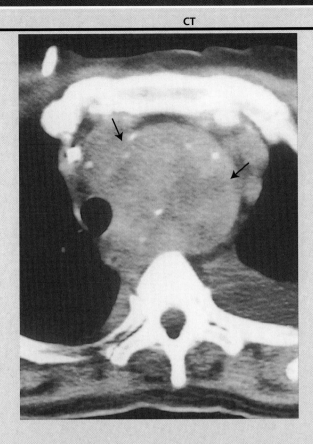

Metastatic carcinoma

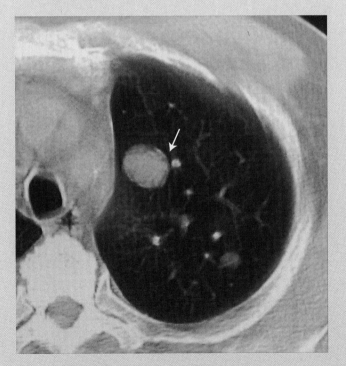

(continued)

	Table 18-8	Common Named Imaging Signs of the Thorax (*continued*)

Sign	Definition	Significance	Plain Film
Extrapleural	Opaque convexity projecting with smoothly tapering concave margins that blend into pleural contour (*arrows*)	Pleural disease or mass lesion of the rib (most common: tumor, hematoma) Intercostal space (vascular, neurogenic)	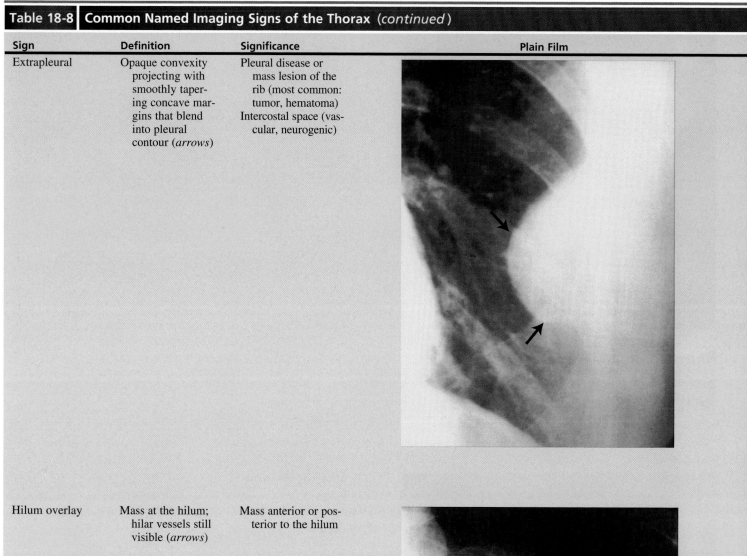
Hilum overlay	Mass at the hilum; hilar vessels still visible (*arrows*)	Mass anterior or posterior to the hilum	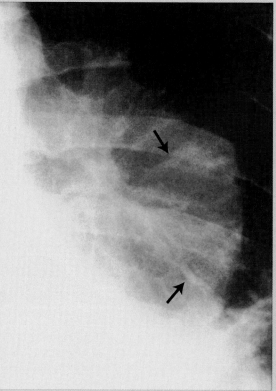

CT	Diagnosis

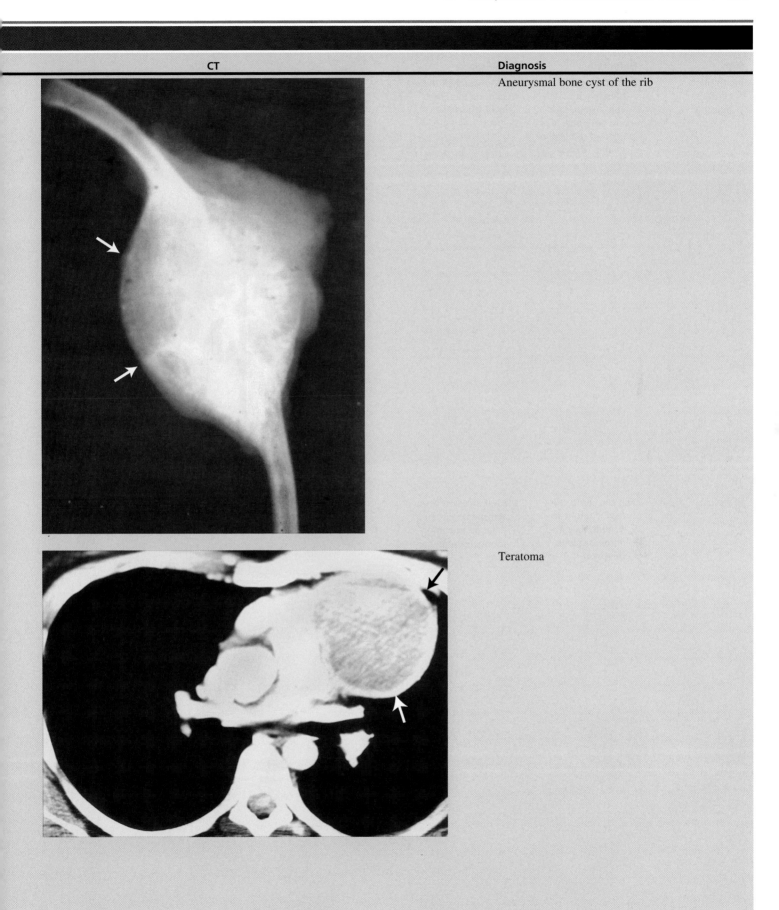

Aneurysmal bone cyst of the rib

Teratoma

Table 18-8	Common Named Imaging Signs of the Thorax (*continued*)		
Sign	**Definition**	**Significance**	**Plain Film**
Incomplete (border) margin	Part of margin blends with adjacent tissue, making only one edge of the lesion visible (*arrow*)	Lesion attached to the skin on the chest wall (fibroma)	
Meniscus	The sweeping concave contour in a blunted costophrenic sulcus (*arrows*)	Pleural effusion from transudate or exudate; no pneumothorax present	

CT

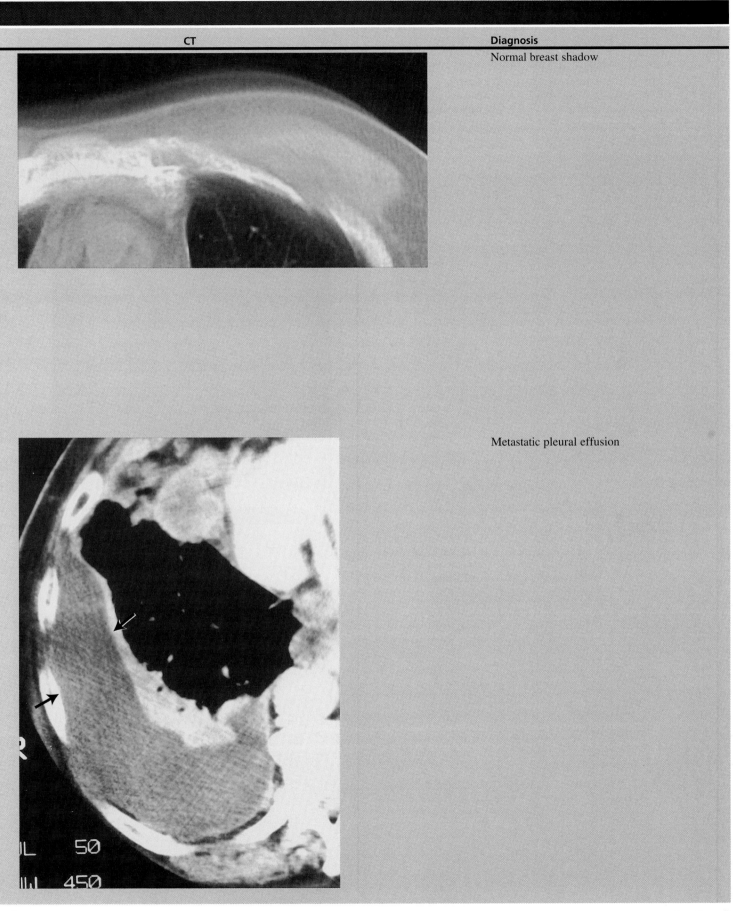

Diagnosis

Normal breast shadow

Metastatic pleural effusion

Table 18-8 | Common Named Imaging Signs of the Thorax (*continued*)

Sign	Definition	Significance	Plain Film
Paraspinal line	Displacement of the lung–vertebral interface away from the spine (*arrows*)	Paraspinal mass, including tumor, abscess, hematoma, and extramedullary hematopoiesis	
Silhouette	Loss of the normally well-defined, sharp contour of the heart, aortic outline, and diaphragm (*arrow*)	Enables anatomic localization of a water-based lesion by virtue of direct contact with adjacent structures	

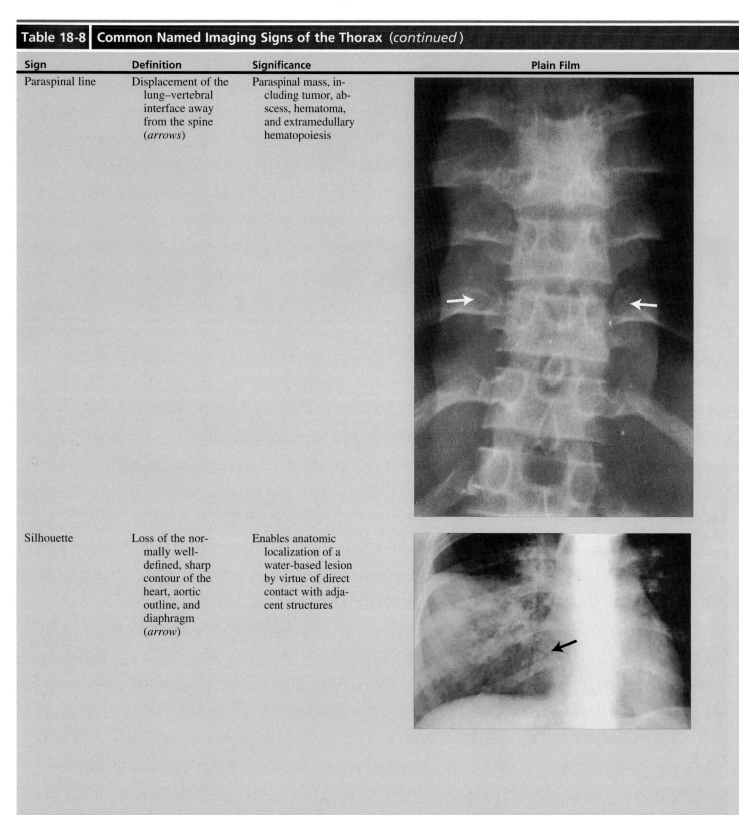

CT	Diagnosis

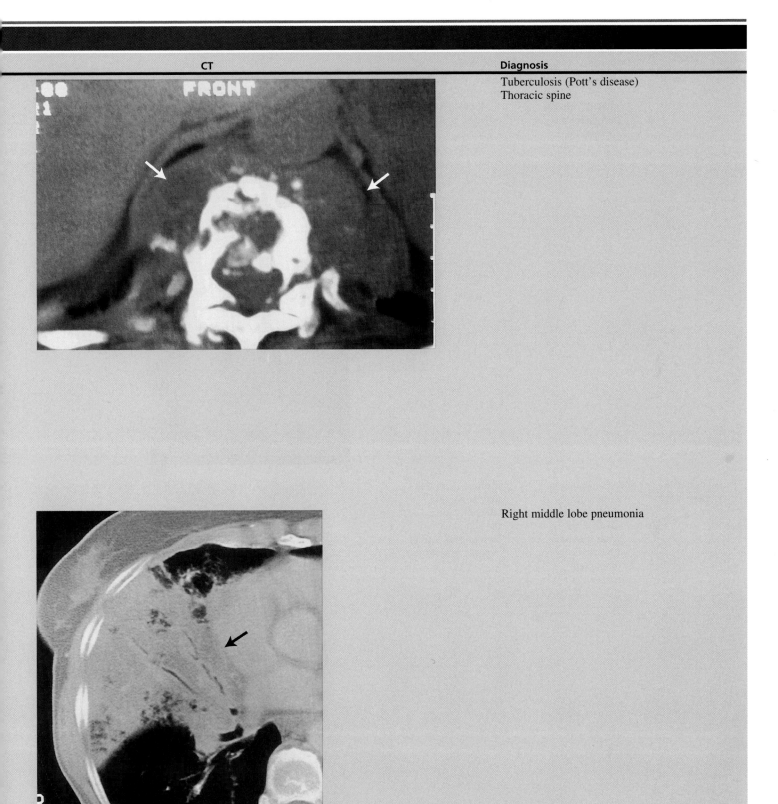

Tuberculosis (Pott's disease)
Thoracic spine

Right middle lobe pneumonia

(continued)

Table 18-8	Common Named Imaging Signs of the Thorax (continued)		
Sign	**Definition**	**Significance**	**Plain Film**
Spreading edge	A pulmonary nodule with an irregular, spiculated peripheral margin (*arrow*)	Usually implies a malignant lesion that infiltrates into the adjacent tissue	
Thoracolumbar (iceberg sign)	The paraspinal line in the lower thoracic region diverges away from the spine toward the diaphragm (*arrows*)	Paraspinal mass that may be largely situated within the abdomen (lymphoma, spinal abscess, aneurysm)	

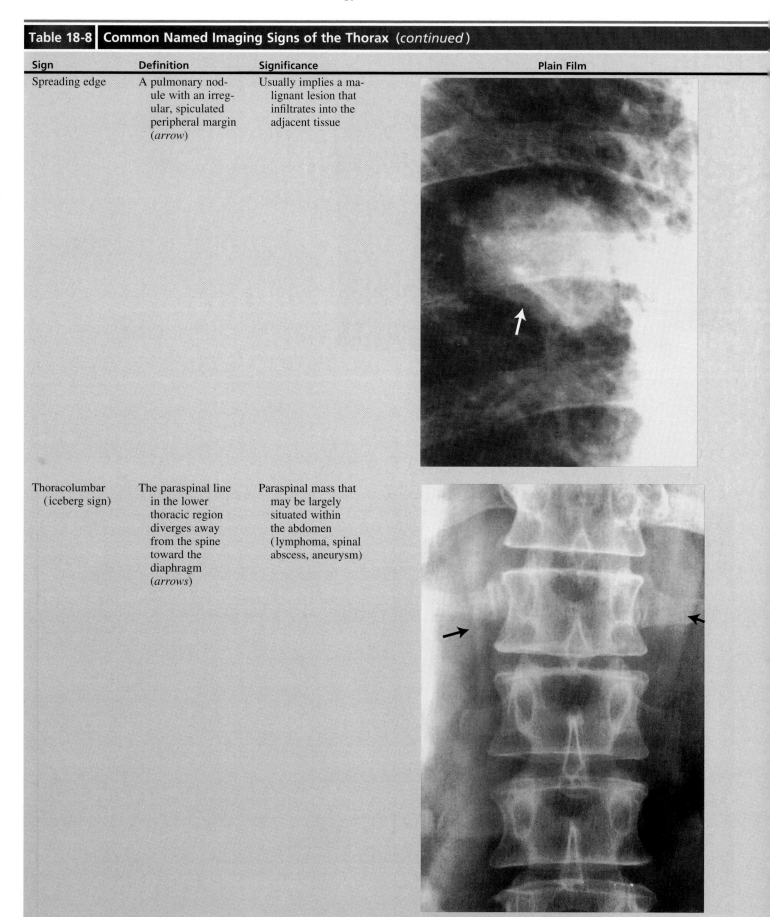

CT	Diagnosis
	Bronchogenic carcinoma

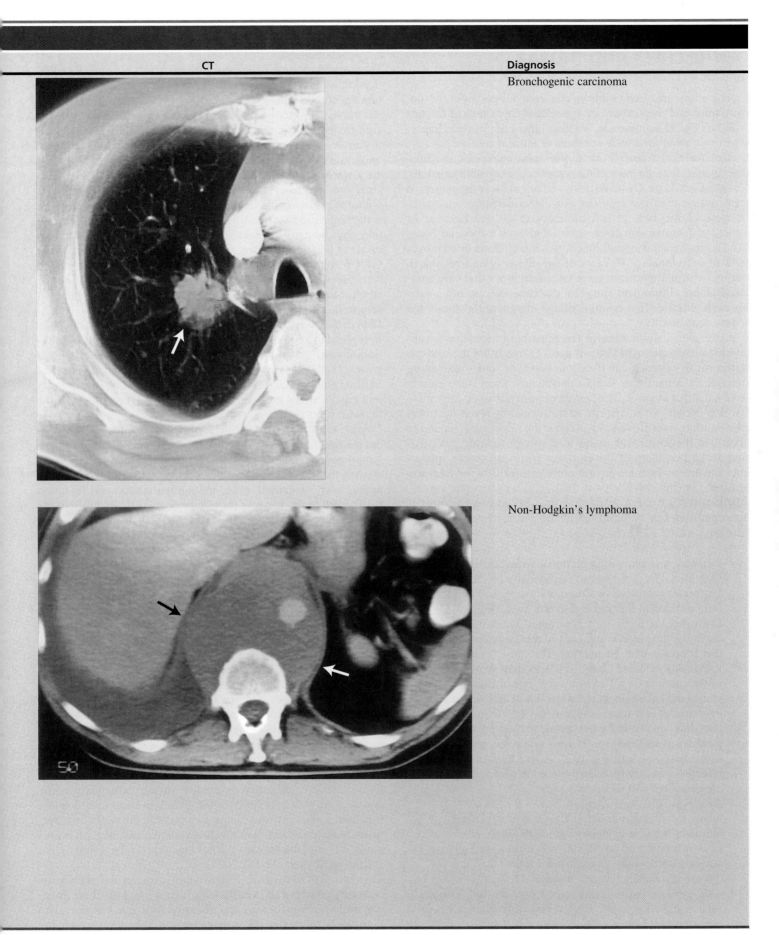

Non-Hodgkin's lymphoma

COMMON CALCIFICATIONS OF THE CHEST AND THORAX

Calcifications are often visible on conventional studies of the thoracic spine and chest. Many are age-related physiological variants with no clinical significance, whereas others can provide important information for a wide spectrum of clinical entities.

Costochondral Calcifications. The most common costochondral calcifications are those of the anterior costochondral junctions.

Costal Cartilage Ossification. *Ossification* is the preferred term, rather than *calcification,* for costal cartilage anomalies because of the lack of inflammatory cause and because of structural features that show cortex and even trabecular bone. (1) The first costochondral junction is mineralized in well over 90% of individuals > 40 years of age and is often irregular in outline with radiolucent transverse linear zones that can simulate fracture. Prominent spur-like excrescences are often visible at the inferior first costal cartilage margin at the site of the radiolucent line. (1)

Generally, calcification in the remaining cartilages is uncommon in people < 30 years of age. (2) Age is not the sole criterion for developing calcification, however, and some young individuals demonstrate florid mineralization and some elderly have a distinct absence. The pattern of mineralization appears to develop initially at the first rib. At the remaining levels the lower ribs (tenth to twelfth) usually precede the upper ribs (second to sixth). In the lower ribs males tend to demonstrate calcification at the periphery of the cartilage (*railroad tracks* appearance), whereas females have a more central (*tongue-like*) extension. (1) (Fig. 18-32)

Abnormalities of Calcified Rib Cartilages. Numerous abnormalities can be observed in the calcified costochondral cartilages. (2)

- *Trauma.* A fracture through the opacified cartilage can be identified. Dislocations can occasionally be seen. Exuberant calcification after thoracotomy and child abuse (non-accidental trauma) is also observed. (Fig. 18-33)
- *Costochondritis (Tietze's syndrome).* Acute painful hypertrophy of the costal cartilages is a relatively common entity that is benign and self-limiting. The cause is unknown. (3) Previously calcified costal cartilages may show dissolution of the calcium on CT examination, and ultrasound demonstrates the enlargement to be smooth in outline without evidence of any mass component. (4,5) Painful costochondritis involving the left second to fourth costochondral junctions is referred to as Tietze's syndrome, after the author of the first description in 1921. Active bacterial or fungal infection can also produce dissolution of calcification with an associated soft tissue mass. (3)
- *Heavy calcification.* There is anecdotal evidence that heavy calcification in individuals < 40 years of age, although found in asymptomatic individuals, can be seen in association with ankylosing spondylitis, malignancy, autoimmune disease, chronic renal failure, and thyroid disease (especially Grave's disease). (1,2)
- *Enlargement.* Diffuse enlargement without calcification is seen in rickets (*rachitic rosary*) and with calcification in acromegaly. (3,6)
- *Tumors.* Excessive calcification at a single junction can be seen in chondrosarcoma, osteochondroma, and enchondroma.

Tracheobronchial Cartilage Calcification. Prominent calcification is observed in the cartilage rings of the trachea and larger bronchi with advancing age. (Fig. 18-34) These produce a striated *dot-dot appearance* on plain film studies. (5,7) It is of no clinical significance and is not related to tracheomalacia. In newborns it can be observed with chondrodysplasia punctata (stippled epiphyses). (5,7)

Laryngeal Cartilage Complex (Thyroid Cartilage) Calcification. The most common calcification in the thyroid region is within the surrounding laryngeal cartilages. The thyroid cartilage is the largest and most easily seen of these. On the frontal projection, thyroid cartilage calcification appears as paired calcareous bands obliquely divergent, overlapping the lateral masses of the C4–C6 vertebrae (see Chapter 3). (4,8) Unskilled clinicians sometimes erroneously ascribed these insignificant findings to atheromatous plaque of the vertebral arteries, leading to unnecessary testing and anxiety for the unfortunate patient.

Thyroid Gland Calcification. Calcifications within the thyroid gland are common and usually lie within the walls of long-standing benign colloidal cysts, often as part of a multinodular goiter. (5,7) These wall calcifications are thin and curvilinear, outlining a circular lesion. (Fig. 18-35) More diffuse flocculent calcifications are seen with follicular cell carcinoma of the thyroid. (3,8)

Lymph Node Calcification. Lymph nodes are found throughout the neck and chest in predictable locations. Within the chest, lymph nodes parallel the tracheobronchial tree and are named according to their locations: paratracheal, pretracheal, retrotracheal, prevascular, subcarinal, hilar, and intrapulmonary. (9) Infection is the most common cause for calcification—usually tuberculosis and, in endemic locations, histoplasmosis. (10) Such calcifications are dense, often multiple, and typically involve the paratracheal or hilar nodes. (4,6,10) (Fig. 18-36) The combination of a calcified hilar node and a calcified peripheral granuloma in the lung parenchyma is referred to as a *Ranke complex* and is diagnostic of previous primary tuberculosis. (10) Other causes for nodal calcification include silicosis, sarcoidosis, fungal disease, and radiotherapy, especially in lymphoma, all of which can produce peripheral *eggshell* calcification. (11-13)

Aortic Calcification. Calcified atheromatous plaque is common in the aortic arch. On a frontal chest or thoracic spine study this will appear as a complete or incomplete (*thumbnail sign*) circular curvilinear calcification. (14,15) (Fig. 18-37) The thoracic aorta is fixed at its cardiac origin and at the diaphragm. With advancing age the aorta elongates and "uncoils," causing the arch to ascend into the upper thorax and create a prominent left-sided indentation on the trachea. (4,8) Calcification in the wall of the ascending aorta is a traditional sign for syphilitic aortitis. (14) Occasionally calcification is evident in the descending aorta. Aortic aneurysm, especially of the arch, will show calcification. If calcified atheromatous plaque is present in the wall of the aortic arch, the thickness of the wall beyond the calcification is normally < 5 mm; thicknesses greater than this can be a sign of dissecting aneurysm. (11,14)

Cardiac Calcification. Extensive atherosclerosis within the coronary arteries can occasionally be observed on chest imaging studies. (Fig. 18-38) Quantification (*calcium scoring*) with high-speed multislice CT is being increasingly advocated in the

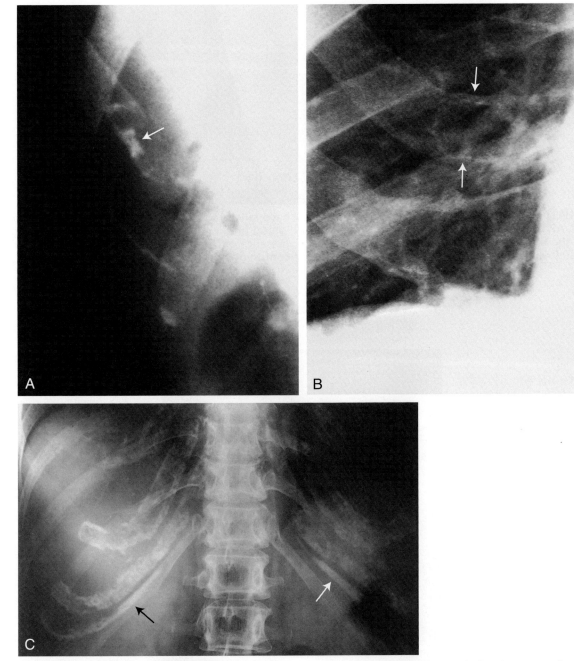

Figure 18-32 **COSTOCHONDRAL CALCIFICATION. A. Female Pattern, PA Chest.** Observe the central calcification extending from the anterior rib into the costal cartilage (*arrow*). **B. Male Pattern, PA Chest.** Note that peripheral calcification extends from the anterior rib (*arrows*). **C. Extensive Calcification, AP Abdomen.** In this male patient there is extensive bilateral costal cartilage calcification extending from the anterior lower rib margins to the sternal edge (*arrows*). *COMMENT:* The pattern of calcification exhibited can assist in the forensic identification of gender. No clinical significance for the amount of costochondral calcification shown in panel C has been documented.

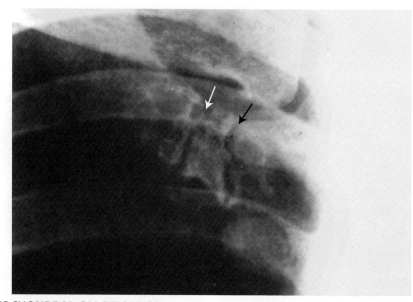

Figure 18-33 FIRST COSTOCHONDRAL CALCIFICATION, PSEUDO-CLEFT. AP Thoracic Spine. Observe the prominent calcification of the first rib costal cartilage. Note the two radiolucent pseudo-clefts (*arrows*), representing areas that have failed to calcify. *COMMENT:* This is a common physiological finding on thoracic spine and chest radiographs. The presence of these radiolucent pseudo-clefts should not be confused with fracture.

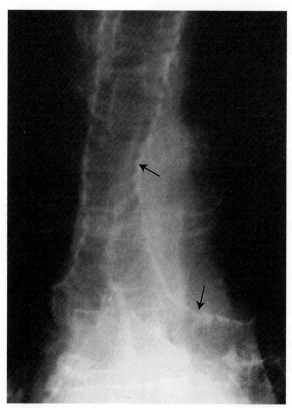

Figure 18-34 TRACHEAL CARTILAGE CALCIFICATION. AP Thoracic Spine. Observe the extensive cartilage calcification of the tracheal and mainstem bronchial rings (*arrows*). *COMMENT:* This is a common physiological finding that is usually age related and does not predispose the patient to tracheomalacia or other airway abnormalities.

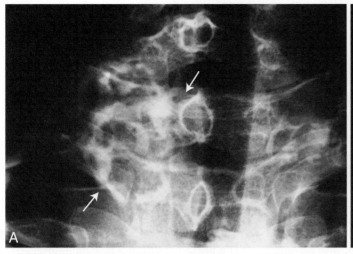

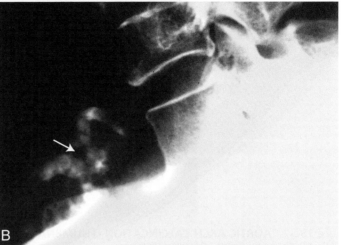

Figure 18-35   **MULTINODULAR GOITER CALCIFICATION.**
A. AP Cervicothoracic. Note the dense calcification within the soft tissues adjacent to the trachea (*arrows*). **B. Lateral Cervical Spine.** Observe the calcifications inferior to the laryngeal cartilage, adjacent to the trachea (*arrow*). *COMMENT:* Calcifications within the thyroid gland are common and rep-

resent previous hemorrhage into thyroid cysts, which are often associated with a multinodular goiter. These dense and curvilinear calcifications are usually benign. Infrequently, thyroid carcinoma can produce more diffuse, poorly defined calcification that usually has a granular appearance.

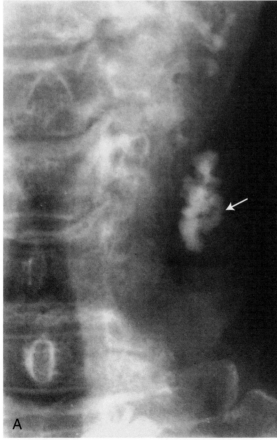

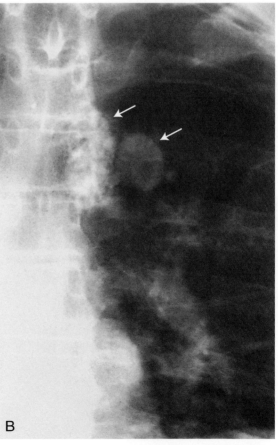

Figure 18-36   **LYMPH NODE CALCIFICATION. A. Cervical Nodes, AP Lower Cervical Spine.** Note the dense conglomerate calcification with a lobulated external contour lateral to the cervical spine and within necrotic lymph nodes (*arrow*). **B. Paratracheal Nodes, PA Chest.** Observe the dense flocculent calcification from previous granulomatous disease in

two paratracheal lymph nodes (*arrows*). This is most likely related to prior tuberculosis. *COMMENT:* These calcifications are common findings on thoracic and chest radiographs and are of no clinical significance. Peripheral ring eggshell calcification can occasionally be seen in association with sarcoidosis, silicosis, and radiotherapy for lymphoma.

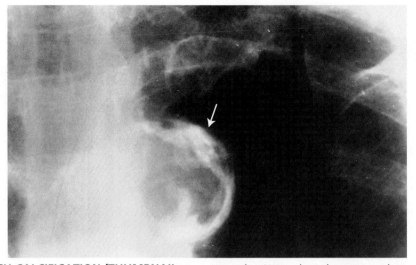

Figure 18-37 **AORTIC ARCH CALCIFICATION (THUMBNAIL SIGN). AP Thoracic Spine.** Observe the dense, curvilinear calcification in the aortic arch (*arrow*). This has occurred within a subintimal atherosclerotic atheroma. *COMMENT:* This is a common finding on both chest and thoracic spine radio-graphs. Note that the external contour of the tunica media and adventitia of the aorta lie within a few millimeters of the calcification. During aortic dissection, thickening of this wall away from the calcified plaque may sometimes be seen on a chest radiograph.

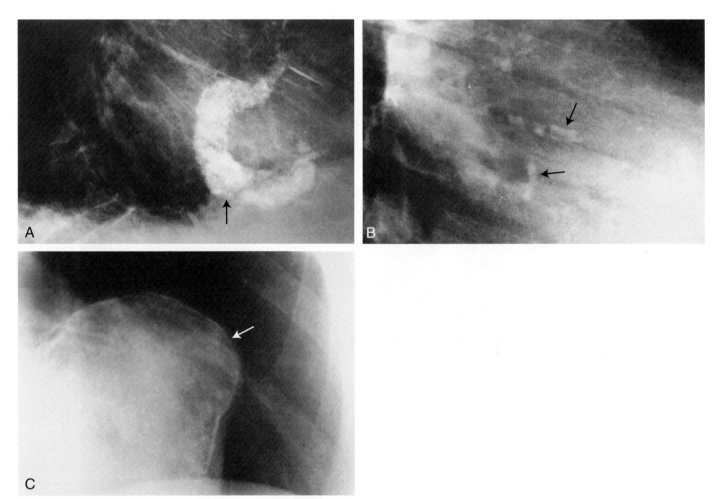

Figure 18-38 **MISCELLANEOUS CARDIAC CALCIFICATIONS. A. Mitral Valve Calcification, Lateral Chest.** Note the circular calcification (*arrow*) in the typical location for mitral valve annulus. **B. Coronary Artery Calcification, Oblique Chest.** Observe the branching calcifications (*arrows*) overlying the cardiac shadow, representing calcified atheroma.

C. Ventricular Aneurysm, PA Chest. A localized distortion of the left ventricular outline is present with peripheral calcification characteristic of aneurysm (*arrow*). *COMMENT:* These calcifications, demonstrated throughout the heart, are relatively uncommon plain film findings.

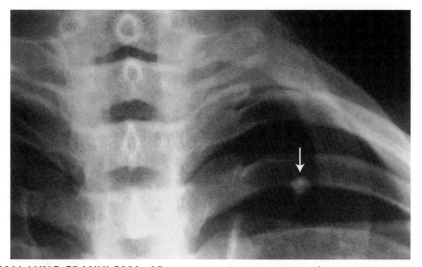

Figure 18-39 **PARENCHYMAL LUNG GRANULOMA. AP Thoracic Spine.** Observe the round, dense granuloma in the lung apex (*arrow*). There is no associated parenchymal fibro- sis. *COMMENT:* These are common asymptomatic lesions in the chest, usually the result of previous tuberculosis or histoplasmosis.

assessment of cardiac infarction risk. (16) Valvular calcification can be seen, even occasionally on plain film, within the mitral and aortic valves. (3,5,11) Pericardial calcifications can be observed in asbestos lung disease, in postinflammatory disease, and as a sequela of trauma. (4,17) Thick calcifications may restrict cardiac contractility and precipitate restrictive pericarditis. Postinfarction ventricular aneurysms often develop peripheral curvilinear calcifications.

Pleural Calcification. Pleural calcifications are commonly seen as part of previous asbestos exposure, are typically thick and irregular, and are most common at the lung bases. (17,18) Trauma and post-tuberculous empyema are other known causes of pleural calcification. (10)

Lung Parenchyma Calcification. Postinflammatory granulomas, especially from previous tuberculosis, are commonly identified in the lungs. Typical size ranges from 1 to 5 mm, although larger granulomas may be seen. Tuberculous granulomas > 5 mm are sometimes referred to as *tuberculomas.* (10,16) (Fig. 18-39) Diffusely distributed, multiple calcifications ranging from 1 to 3 mm are sometimes described as *miliary* (after the millet seed). This is usually an indication that hematogenous spread has occurred and is most often the result of tuberculosis. (10,11)

Though calcification within a pulmonary nodule is generally thought to be an imaging marker of a benign process, a pre-existing calcified lesion can be enveloped by a primary cancer (*scar carcinoma*), usually adenocarcinoma. (4,8) Calcified neoplastic lesions include the benign tumor hamartoma, which displays an irregular *popcorn pattern* of calcification in approximately 15% of cases. (11,19)

Extrapleural Chest Wall. Miscellaneous calcifications can be observed within axillary lymph nodes and the breast. Mammary calcifications should be investigated with dedicated mammography and ultrasound because of their association with malignancy. Mammary augmentation implants often show peripheral calcification in a pseudo-capsule. (4,8) Calcified larvae of the pork tapeworm (*Taenia solium;* cysticercosis) can be seen as rice-like or cigar-shaped muscle calcifications that have their long axes paralleling that of the muscle fibers. (11,19) (Fig. 18-40) Calcinosis

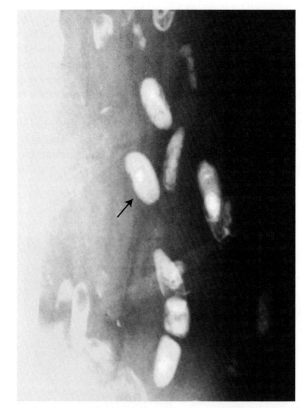

Figure 18-40 **CYSTICERCOSIS. PA Chest/Axilla.** Note the multiple oval, or cigar-shaped, calcifications present throughout the soft tissues of the upper arm (*arrow*). *COMMENT:* These represent calcified encysted larvae from parasitic infestation, which occasionally are identified by the detailed inspection of skeletal muscles. Owing to the high rate of central nervous system involvement, MRI evaluation of the brain is indicated when cysticercosis is diagnosed.

universalis or diffuse calcification of the chest wall may occur in diffuse collagen diseases (including lupus, scleroderma, and dermatomyositis) and chronic renal failure. (3,5,11,19)

VASCULAR DISEASES OF THE CHEST

The most important vascular disorders of the chest that can present with clinical features of musculoskeletal disease are pulmonary edema, pulmonary embolism, aneurysms, and dissection of the thoracic aorta. Imaging of these entities has undergone significant change and provides the essential information for accurate diagnosis.

Pulmonary Edema

Clinical Features. Accumulation of excessive transudate fluid within the lungs in either the interstitium or the alveolar sacs is referred to as pulmonary edema. (1) This can be classified as acute or chronic and often presents with a spectrum of findings from both presentations. Causes can be associated with the heart (*cardiogenic pulmonary edema*) or can be extracardiac (*non-cardiogenic pulmonary edema*), such as renal failure, head injury, and aspiration. (2,3) The underlying pathophysiology is caused by abnormal capillary hydrodynamics within the alveolus, with effects on hydrostatic pressure, colloid osmotic pressure, capillary permeability, and/or lymphatic drainage. (4,1) The most common clinical presentation is increasing shortness of breath, orthopnea, and dependent edema of the legs. (2,1)

Imaging Features. Chest radiography usually provides the clues for diagnosis; CT is used only when the diagnosis remains obscure. (1,3,5) Acute pulmonary edema is characterized predominately by centrally located alveolar signs, with hazy or fluffy increased density in a perihilar distribution, creating a *bat-wing* or *angel-wing* pattern. There is relative sparing of the more peripheral zones of the lung fields. (1,5) (Fig. 18-41) Air bronchograms become evident as the edema becomes more opaque. This type of edema most commonly follows acute myocardial infarction and, if the patient survives, can disappear within 24–48 hr. (5)

In the more common chronic form of pulmonary edema, interstitial signs predominate, with hazy lung fields, dilated lymphatics (Kerley B lines), thickened bronchial walls, upper lobe venous distension, and small pleural effusions. (4–6) (Fig. 18-42) Congestive cardiac failure is the most common cause of chronic pulmonary edema, and the diagnosis is often supported by the co-existence of cardiomegaly. (1,5,7)

Pulmonary Embolism

Clinical Features. Pulmonary embolism (PE) is an occlusive disease of the pulmonary arteries caused by mobile thrombi, usually from the lower limbs, migrating via the venous return to the pulmonary circulation. (8,9) The classic clinical triad seen in one third of patients is hemoptysis, pleural friction rub, and lower limb thromboembolism. (9) Other clinical findings include shortness of breath, pleuritic chest pain, cough, and tachycardia. (10) It is important to note that many cases are asymptomatic. (10) Greater than 50% involve the lower lobes of the lungs, and multiple sites are present in at least two thirds of cases. (8,9) More than 90% of cases are the result of deep vein thrombosis in the lower limbs. (8,9)

Known associations for the development of deep vein thrombosis include immobilization, dehydration, malignancy, and clotting disorders. (8,10) Long-distance travel has been more recently publicized as a common cause, owing to constriction of lower leg venous return from prolonged sitting on

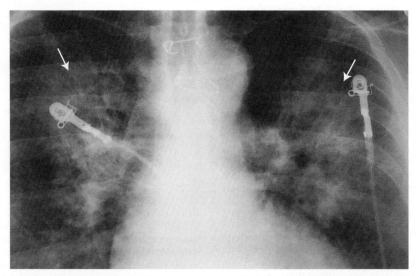

Figure 18-41 ACUTE PULMONARY EDEMA. PA Chest. Observe the bilateral and symmetric alveolar densities in the perihilar zones, creating a characteristic bat-wing appearance (*arrows*). *COMMENT:* This appearance is the consequence of peripheral vasoconstriction (which diverts blood centrally), resulting in transudation of the alveolar spaces. This pattern of acute pulmonary edema commonly follows a cardiogenic cause, such as an acute myocardial infarction. This is a transient phenomenon, which usually disappears over 24–48 hr.

airplanes, buses, or cars (*traveler's thrombosis*). (8,10) Fat emboli may also precipitate pulmonary embolus in patients who have suffered recent long bone fractures or in conjunction with orthopedic surgery, such as hip replacement. In the presence of a right to left shunt, such as an atrial septal defect, an embolus may pass into the cerebral circulation and precipitate a stroke (*paradoxical embolus*). (10)

Imaging Features. Plain chest radiography plays a limited role in diagnosis, although some signs have been described. (9,11) In embolism without infarction (90% of cases) atelectasis, pleural effusion, segmental oligemia (Westermark's sign), local widening of an artery (Fleischner's sign), and an abrupt tapering of an occluded vessel (knuckle sign) can be seen. (9,10) In cases of associated infarction, wedge-shaped consolidation that regresses from the periphery (melting sign), cavitation, pleural-based opacity with a medial convex border (Hampton's hump), and pleural effusion can be identified. (10,12)

The most definitive study for emboli to the level of at least the fifth order of arterial branching is helical CT with contrast (CT pulmonary angiogram). (12,13,14) Emboli are visualized as filling defects in contrast-filled vessels or as abrupt truncation of the expected branching pattern of a vessel. Involvement of larger vessels is particularly life-threatening. (12,14) (Fig. 18-43) A nuclear medicine ventilation–perfusion (V/Q) scan has been the mainstay of diagnosis previously, but yields a high percentage of intermediate to low probability results. This study will reveal a disparity between the degree of aeration and the blood supply of the involved portion of the lung (called a V/Q *mismatch*). (9) Ultrasound of the lower limb veins can show the venous thrombosis accurately and is routinely obtained in suspected cases of PE. (9,10,12)

Aneurysms of the Thoracic Aorta

Clinical Features. Dilatation of the aortic diameter to > 4–5 cm is the usual criterion for the diagnosis of aneurysm. (15) Known

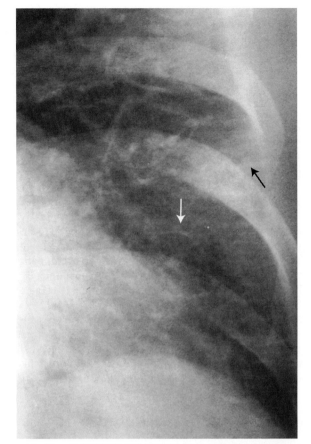

Figure 18-42 CHRONIC PULMONARY EDEMA. PA Chest. A close-up of the lung base demonstrates pulmonary congestion with a hazy appearance to the aerated lung, multiple Kerley B lines (*arrows*), and a small pleural effusion. *COMMENT:* Pulmonary congestion secondary to congestive cardiac failure displays the features seen here. Ancillary findings include upper lobe venous distension and peribronchial thickening.

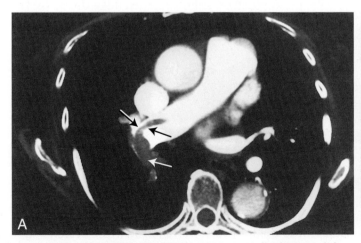
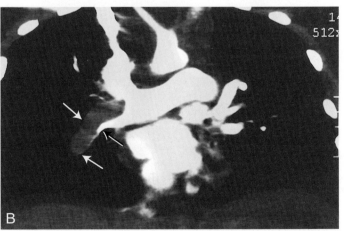

Figure 18-43 PULMONARY EMBOLISM. A. Helical CT, Axial Chest. Note the multiple filling defects in the pulmonary artery, representing large pulmonary emboli (*arrows*). **B. Coronal Reconstruction CT, Chest Angiogram.** The pulmonary emboli are clearly identified as well-defined radio- lucent areas within the opacified vessels (*arrows*). *COMMENT:* Helical CT angiography is the standard method for detection of emboli in the pulmonary vessels, ranging in size from the large arteries down through the fourth- and fifth-order branching.

causes include hypertension, coronary artery disease, trauma, and collagen diseases. Males are affected three times more commonly, with a peak age of around 65 years. (16) Many cases remain asymptomatic and are found incidentally on chest imaging. Symptomatic presentations most commonly are substernal, back (mid-thoracic), or shoulder pain. Other changes can be hoarseness (recurrent laryngeal nerve compression), stridor, dyspnea, dysphagia, and facial engorgement (superior vena caval compression). (16) Tracheal tug synchronous with the heartbeat impulse as seen on fluoroscopy (Troisier's sign) is occasionally elicited. (17,18)

Imaging Features. Age-related dilatation and tortuosity can at times be difficult to differentiate from aneurysm as the aorta "uncoils," producing accentuated curves and dilatation. Typical senile changes are usually made up of five features: the ascending aorta sweeps to the right, the aortic arch lies close to the clavicle, the tracheal indentation is more prominent, the diameter of the arch is enlarged between 3 and 4 cm, and the descending aorta is tortuous in its course and projects more laterally into the thoracic cavity. (19) (Fig. 18-44) The location of the aneurysm may suggest the origin: ascending aorta suggests syphilis and causes of cystic medial necrosis (e.g., Marfan's syndrome) and aortitis (e.g., ankylosing spondylitis), aortic arch location is associated with atherosclerosis and trauma, and the descending aorta is more commonly involved with trauma and collagen disease. The definitive imaging technique is spiral CT, which produces aortogram images. (19,20)

The imaging signs of aneurysm depend on location. (19,20)
Ascending Aorta. The convex aortic shadow is displaced to the right and superiorly and frequently exhibits a peripheral rim of thin, curvilinear calcification when the aneurysm is in the ascending aorta. On the lateral projection the aneurysm lies in a substernal location. (19,21)
Aortic Arch. The aortic arch is the most common site for aneurysm formation, making up > 90% of cases. (7,20,22) The trachea is displaced laterally; the diameter of the arch is > 4–5 cm with sharp margins, occasionally with peripheral curvilinear calcification; and the left mainstem bronchus is displaced inferiorly. (22) (Fig. 18-45) Post-traumatic pseudo-aneurysms typically occur just below the aortic arch, where shearing and torsion forces at the attachment of the ligamentum arteriosum precipitate media tearing and possible aneurysm formation. Such post-traumatic aneurysms may develop slowly over years and remain clinically silent, usually developing thin peripheral calcification. (19) (Figs. 18-45 and 18-46)
Descending Aorta. Lesions in the descending aorta are infrequent and best seen on lateral chest or thoracic spine projections. Care should be taken not to confuse age-related tortuosity and generalized dilatation, in which the descending aortic shadow is displaced to the left and is often undulating in contour. (19)

Dissection of the Thoracic Aorta

Clinical Features. Spontaneous separation between the intima and adventitia, usually with tearing of the intima, allows blood to accumulate within the media. Extravasation may remain local, migrate distally, re-enter the circulation (*double-barreled aorta*), or progress to full-thickness rupture. (16) Males are affected in a ratio of 3:1, with peak occurrence at 60 years of age. (15,16) Known associations include hypertension (90% of cases), collagen disease, vasculitis, aortic stenosis, pregnancy, trauma, and coarctation. (16) Presentation is usually acutely symptomatic, with marked severe anterior or posterior chest pain radiating to the neck, head, and thoracic spine. Occasionally, low back pain will be reported. In severe cases

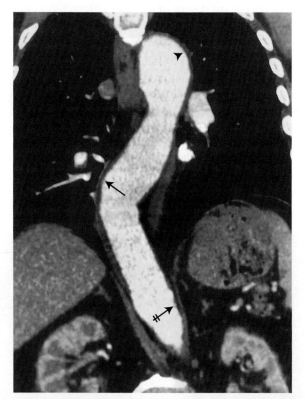

Figure 18-44 UNCOILED AORTA. CT, Coronal Chest Angiogram. A selected coronal slice reconstructed from a CT angiogram demonstrates the course of the descending thoracic aorta. There is arch dilatation (*arrowhead*), kinking to the right (*arrow*) at the midpoint of the vessel, and then a return left as the descending aorta approaches the diaphragm (*crossed arrow*). *COMMENT:* Increased tortuosity of the aorta is a common age-related change, often associated with hypertension, that can occasionally be confused with aortic aneurysm.

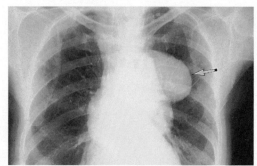

Figure 18-45 ARCH PSEUDO-ANEURYSM, DUCTUS INSERTION. PA Chest. Note the sharply defined soft tissue mass adjacent to the transverse aorta (*arrow*). The descending aorta can be seen through the mass. *COMMENT:* Without cross-sectional imaging (e.g., CT) this finding may be confused with a mediastinal mass. However, this is the typical location for post-traumatic aortic pseudo-aneurysm distal to the left subclavian artery.

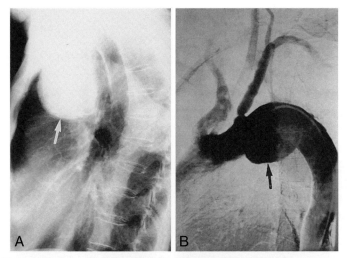

Figure 18-46   ARCH PSEUDO-ANEURYSM, DUCTUS INSERTION. A. Lateral Chest. Note the round density of the pseudo-aneurysm anterior to the trachea (*arrow*). **B. Digital-Subtraction Arch Aortogram.** The saccular pseudo-aneurysm is clearly outlined distal to the origin of the left subclavian artery (*arrow*). Also observe the focal stenosis at the origin of the left subclavian artery. *COMMENT:* Severe closed thoracic trauma, resulting in a tear of the wall of the aorta from traction of the ductus arteriosus remnant (ligamentum arteriosum), is the usual cause for this condition.

there is rapid progression to hemodynamic shock, pericardial tamponade, and death. Absent or asymmetric upper limb pulses may suggest the diagnosis. (16) Aortic dissections are classed by the DeBakey classification system: type I (~ 30%), (entire aorta); type II (< 20%), ascending aorta only; type III (50%), descending aorta only. (7,16,20)
Imaging Features. Chest radiographs may suggest the diagnosis but are often inconclusive. (19) CT angiography of the aorta is the most sensitive non-invasive method for detecting and documenting its extent. (16,19,20) (Fig. 18-47) Ultrasound is also sen-

sitive for the ascending aorta but does not allow accurate distal documentation. (16,19)

Chest radiographs may show a wide mediastinum, a wall thickness beyond calcification of > 5–10 mm, loss of arch definition, disparity between aortic segmental diameters, lung apex opacification, and pleural effusion. (19) Both CT and MRI clearly show the site of extravasation and usually the intimal flap at the site of entry. (15) Angiography has been traditionally used to make the diagnosis. (16,19)

AIRWAY DISEASE

Three major disorders of airways disease: asthma, emphysema, and bronchiectasis are reviewed here. Although the clinical manifestations do not often mimic musculoskeletal disease, they are included in this chapter because of their common incidence and because some radiographic manifestations may also be apparent on films taken for musculoskeletal diagnoses. Complications from these conditions or their treatments that may reflect on the musculoskeletal system include fatigue, osteopenic complications (such as vertebral compression and rib fractures from chronic corticosteroid use or chronic coughing), and occasionally hypertrophic osteoarthropathy. (1,2)

Asthma

Clinical Features. Asthma is an episodic disease characterized by reversible bronchoconstriction secondary to hypersensitivity to a variety of stimuli, both intrinsic and extrinsic. (3,4) Episodes of acute breathlessness with reduced airflow are typical. (5,6)
Imaging Features. Chest radiography is often employed to exclude complications such as pneumothorax, pneumomediastinum, atelectasis, pneumonia, and aspergillosis. (6–8) Acute asthma may demonstrate hyperlucent lung fields, flattened hemidiaphragms, a deep retrosternal space, and thickened bronchial walls. (9,10)

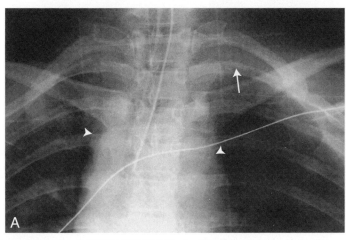

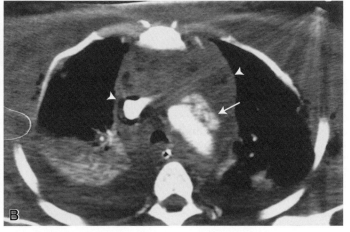

Figure 18-47   AORTIC RUPTURE. A. AP Chest. Note that the mediastinum is widened (*arrowheads*), the aortic contour is absent, and there is an apical pleural cap (*arrow*). **B. Contrast-Enhanced CT, Axial Chest.** At the level of the aortic arch note the contrast extravasation beyond the vessel wall (*arrow*).

Accumulated blood distends the mediastinum (*arrowheads*). *COMMENT:* Aortic dissection should be considered when radiographs show a widened mediastinum in a patient with post-traumatic chest pain that radiates to the back.

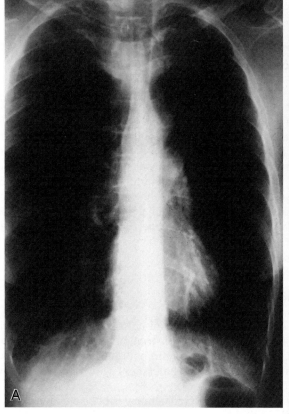

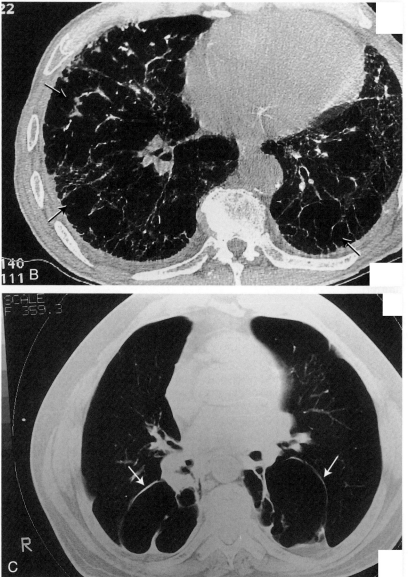

Figure 18-48 **EMPHYSEMA. A. Pulmonary Emphysema, PA Chest.** Note that the hemidiaphragms are low in the chest, though not significantly flattened. The lung fields are over-exposed relative to the mediastinum, and the heart is relatively small. **B. Pulmonary Emphysema, High-Resolution CT, Axial Chest.** Multiple emphysematous bullae are readily identified (*arrows*). **C. Bullous Emphysema, CT, Axial Chest.** Observe the large thin-walled cystic air cavities in the superior segments of both lower lobes (*arrows*). *COMMENT:*

Pulmonary emphysema is associated with smoking (centrilobular emphysema) and is most commonly confined to the upper lobes. The presence of large bullae may result in significantly reduced functional lung tissue, which can frequently be seen on plain film radiographs (vanishing lung disease). The visualization of small bullae on high-resolution CT is the optimum method for detecting pulmonary emphysema in its earliest stages.

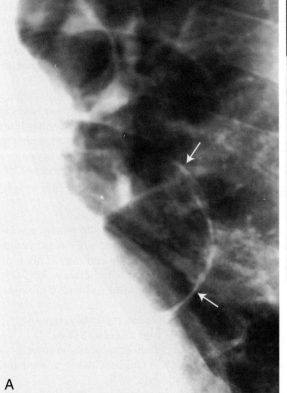

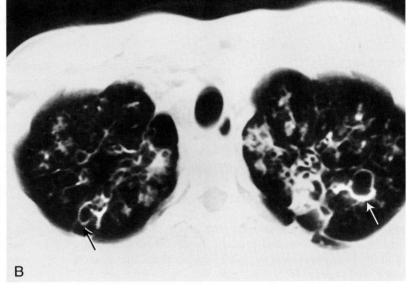

Figure 18-49 **BRONCHIECTASIS. A. PA Chest.** Note the multiple thin-walled cystic structures (*arrows*). **B. CT, Axial Chest.** The cystic bronchiectatic changes are well demonstrated. The thickened walls and bronchial dilatation (compared with the diameter of the adjacent vessels) is characteristic (*arrows*). *COMMENT:* Cystic bronchiectasis is the most severe form of the disease. The CT scan was obtained from a patient with cystic fibrosis and demonstrates characteristic complicating bronchiectasis predominantly involving the middle and upper zones. Bronchiectasis of the lower zones has the same findings.

Chronic changes may show features of bronchiectasis and scars. CT shows the same changes but is especially useful for identifying complications. (6,11,12)

Emphysema

Clinical Features. The term *emphysema* encompasses those diseases characterized by abnormal permanent expansion of air spaces distal to the terminal bronchioles with loss of the alveolar walls and supporting elastic fiber network. Four categories are recognized: centrilobular, panacinar, cicatricial, and paraseptal. (13)

- *Centrilobular emphysema* is the most common form and is closely associated with smoking, involving the middle to upper lobes of the lung and sparing the peripheral alveoli within a single acinus. (14)
- *Panacinar emphysema* is found with α_1-antitrypsin deficiency involving all lobes, but is more severe in the lower lobes where all alveoli within an acinus are affected.
- *Cicatricial emphysema* occurs secondary to fibrotic scarring from infection or other causes of structural lung distortion. (7,11)

- *Paraseptal emphysema* often has an undefined cause and occurs as a focal area of emphysema that abuts a pleural surface or fissure. (7,11)

When the emphysematous spaces greatly enlarge and become confluent, large thin-walled, air-filled cavities arise (referred to as *bullae*). When bullae are the predominant feature the condition is referred to as *bullous emphysema* (vanishing lung disease). (8,12,15) Presenting symptoms and signs typically include progressive dyspnea, increased AP dimension of the thorax (*barrel-chested* appearance), and increased resonance on percussion of the chest. At rest, patients may appear frankly hypoxic with associated peripheral edema (*blue bloater*) or relatively well perfused but dyspneic (*pink puffer*).

Imaging Features. Chest radiography is moderately sensitive but highly specific in the diagnosis of emphysema. The definitive imaging modality is high-resolution CT scan. (13,16,17) Plain film findings include hyperlucent lung fields, depressed, flat hemidiaphragms, wide intercostal spaces, and a deep retrosternal space. (14,18) (Fig. 18-48) Bullae are recognizable as thin-walled cysts that, if infected, may have an air–fluid level. (14) The heart is often small, and the vascularity is diminished, especially peripherally. The pulmonary arteries can enlarge, which, with a rapid tapering of the peripheral vessels, signals complicating pulmonary hypertension. On high-resolution CT the emphysematous spaces are > 1 cm and encircle the centrilobular artery. (8,16,17)

Bronchiectasis

Clinical Features. Irreversible dilatation of the bronchi can occur secondary to congenital defects of the bronchial walls, immotile cilia, immune deficiency, postinfection, obstruction, aspiration, and fibrosis (*traction bronchiectasis*). (19,20) It is a common finding in cystic fibrosis. (19) The main symptoms are persistent cough with purulent sputum, especially in the morning, hemoptysis, and shortness of breath. (21) More than 50% of cases involve the posterior basal segments of the lower lobes. (7,11,20)

Imaging Features. Chest radiographic findings are often absent, though thick-walled bronchi, linear or circular shadows in the lung bases, and contained mucus plugs that branch (*gloved finger sign of Simon*) may be seen. (6,7) The CT criteria for diagnosis include the bronchus being larger than the accompanying vessel (*signet ring sign*), bronchial wall thickening, and bronchi visible within 1 cm of the pleura. (8,12,22) (Fig. 18-49) Three types are described according to their appearance:

- *Cylindrical.* The most common and least severe type, characterized by thick parallel walls (*tram tracks*).
- *Varicose.* Rare variety, exhibiting a "beaded" appearance.
- *Saccular.* Most severe type, with progressive ballooning distally that creates cystic clusters (a *string of pearls*) and occasionally air–fluid levels. (9,11,22)

ALVEOLAR DISEASE

Pneumonia

Clinical Features. Pneumonia is inflammation within the lung tissue beyond the airways, involving the respiratory bronchioles, alveoli, and surrounding interstitium. (1,2) Pneumonia may occur secondary to bacteria, viruses, fungi, parasites, and chemical irritants. (3,4) These all demonstrate various patterns of inflammation, depending on the target tissue, type of immune response, and virulence of the responsible agent. The major symptoms are cough, fever, productive sputum, chest pain, myalgias, and dyspnea. (4) The principal pathogens accounting for the majority of community-acquired pneumonia are *Staphylococcal pneumoniae* (most common, 90%), *Haemophilus influenzae, Klebsiella, Mycobacterium,* and *Mycoplasma.* (3,5,6) Pneumonia occurs frequently in otherwise healthy individuals but is more common in debilitated, elderly, and immunocompromised individuals. (5) Pneumonia that recurs in the same segmental distribution or fails to resolve may be the presenting finding of underlying neoplasm or immunosuppression, such as in HIV. (5,7)

Imaging Features. Plain chest radiography is the mainstay in diagnosis and monitoring progress. The radiographic latent period from the onset of symptoms to visible radiographic changes is usually only days but always lags behind the initial clinical

presentation. CT is used when complications are suspected or there is the suspicion for underlying disease, such as malignancy. (8–10)

Two basic image patterns of pneumonia are recognizable by their own specific signs: alveolar and interstitial. These can occur in so-called pure and mixed forms. (10)

Alveolar Pneumonia Pattern. The alveolar pattern is characteristic of acute bacterial pneumonias, with rapid onset and rapid progression and resolution. The opaque changes show blurred peripheral margins (fluffy); may abut a pleural interface but generally do not cross it; contain confluent areas of opacity; and obliterate contained vascular markings with the presence of air bronchogram, air alveologram, and silhouette signs. (2,6,8,10) (Fig. 18-50)

- *Bronchopneumonia* is the term applied to patchy involvement of a lobe that is interspaced with unaffected parenchyma and surrounds larger bronchi centrally. This is a combination of alveolar and interstitial disease, beginning in the bronchi and then spilling over to involve proximal alveoli. (2,6)
- *Lobar pneumonia* occurs more peripherally, rapidly becomes confluent, and is true alveolar disease.
- *Round pneumonia* appears radiographically as a well-defined, mass-like density in children owing to immaturity of the collateral flow pathways. (6,9)
- *Abscess formation* is characterized as a mass lesion, which often develops internal cavitation. (2,8)

Interstitial Pneumonia Pattern. More typical of viruses, mycoplasma, and pneumoocystis, the interstitial pattern of pneumonia is more difficult to identify. (5) The radiographic signs may consist of hazy lung fields (ground-glass opacification, dirty lung fields), increased reticular markings, generalized non-lobar distribution, prominent bronchovascular markings, and thickened bronchial walls (cuffing). (1,5,8,10) (Fig. 18-51)

Tuberculosis

Clinical Features. Tuberculosis (TB) is a chronic bacterial infection caused by *Mycobacterium tuberculosis* and is characterized by the formation of granulomas that undergo caseous necrosis and incite a cell-mediated hypersensitivity immune reaction. (11,12) In developed countries there has been a marked decrease in the incidence of the disease, a trend that has not transferred into the remainder of the world. (13) At-risk populations include the elderly, the urban poor, minority groups, the immunodepressed (especially with HIV), and individuals with underlying pulmonary conditions such as silicosis. (13,14) The pathogenesis of the disease involves a complex sequence of events beginning with bacterial inhalation followed by lodgment in the bronchial mucosa, ingestion by macrophages, and transfer to regional lymph nodes where they may be contained or traverse into the bloodstream to disseminate systemically. (1,12) This may produce musculoskeletal involvement, including the spine (Pott's disease) and extremity joints. (15)

Presentations depend on the stage of dissemination: primary, secondary, pneumonia, and extrapulmonary. Primary tuberculosis is the initial exposure to the pathogen and is found mainly in children. They remain largely asymptomatic through the course

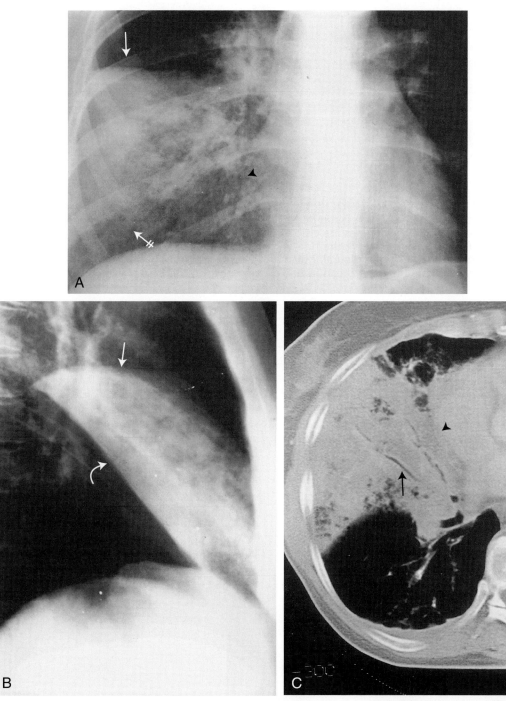

Figure 18-50   **ALVEOLAR PNEUMONIA, RIGHT MIDDLE LOBE. A. PA Chest. B. Lateral Chest.** Note the dense opacification throughout the right middle lobe, which is limited superiorly by the horizontal or minor fissure (*arrows*) and posteriorly by the oblique or major fissure (*curved arrow*). The right atrial heart border is obscured (silhouette sign) (*arrowhead*). Subtle radiolucent bronchi can also be seen within the consolidation (air bronchogram sign) (*crossed arrow*). **C. CT, Axial Chest.** The air bronchogram sign can be seen in greater detail (*arrow*). Observe the contact of the alveolar infiltrate with the right atrial heart border (*arrowhead*). *COMMENT:* These radiographic findings are characteristic of right middle lobe pneumonia.

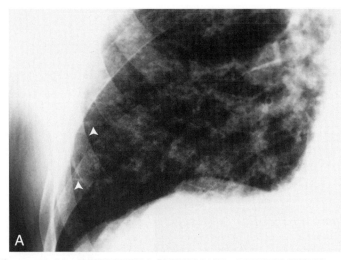 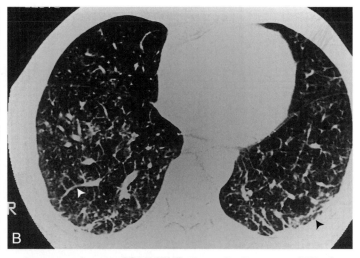

Figure 18-51 INTERSTITIAL PNEUMONIA, *PNEUMOCYSTIS CARINII*. A. PA Chest. Note the diffuse hazy increase in density within the lung base. Interstitial Kerley B lines are visible laterally (*arrowheads*). **B. CT, Axial Chest.** Observe the fine bilateral interstitial markings extending to the pleural interface (*arrowheads*), with some ground-glass opacification of the parenchyma. *COMMENT:* These findings are difficult to identify on plain film radiographs and frequently require CT correlation for diagnosis. The differential diagnosis for interstitial lung disease is extremely broad, and the final diagnosis often requires biopsy and careful clinical correlation. The diagnosis in this case was made with bronchoscopy.

of the condition, which subsequently becomes quiescent. (6,12,13) Secondary (*reactivation*) tuberculosis is the resurgence of infection from the previous primary lesions, typically initiated when immunity is reduced. Reactivation precipitates a chronic wasting disease (hence the older term *consumption*) associated with weight loss, fever, and sweats. (12,13,16) The onset of hemoptysis is often a sign of erosion into a terminal branch of a bronchial artery (Rasmussen aneurysm) and may require embolization. Tuberculous pneumonia can occur in adults not previously infected. (13)

Imaging Features. Imaging signs parallel the stages of the disease and require a combination of plain film and CT study for full characterization. (1,9,10)

The predisposition of the disease for the upper lobes is well known and often provides the first clue to diagnosis. (17) In primary TB the diagnostic features are a poorly defined upper lobe infiltrate with ipsilateral lymphadenopathy (*primary complex*).

A healed primary complex is identified with a peripheral focal calcified granuloma (*Ghon's focus*) and an ipsilateral calcified lymph node, a combination referred to as a *Ranke complex*. (17,18) (Fig. 18-52) The apical healed lesion is sometimes referred to as a *Simon's focus.* (9,18)

The hallmark of secondary or reactivation TB is the formation of cavitation, with 85% of cases involving the apical and posterior segments of the upper lobe. (17,18) (Fig. 18-53) This may be more acute with surrounding infiltrate and smooth, thin-walled cavities. In more chronic cases cavitation can remain, but lung findings exhibit predominately fibrotic changes with volume loss; pleural thickening; and sometimes calcification, linear parenchymal scars with hilar retraction, and mediastinal shift (including tracheal deviation). (6,9,17) The combination of parenchymal scarring with calcification is designated *fibrocalcific tuberculosis.* (2,18)

When TB pneumonia occurs in sites other than the upper lobe location there is a propensity for cavitation. After reactivation

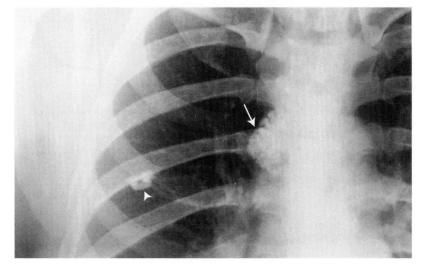

Figure 18-52 RANKE COMPLEX. PA Chest. Note the peripheral calcified granuloma (Ghon focus) (*arrowhead*) in combination with an ipsilateral calcified hilar lymph node (*arrow*). *COMMENT:* These tandem calcifications are signs of previous healed primary tuberculosis. (Courtesy of James R. Brandt, DC, DABCO, Coon Rapids, Minnesota.)

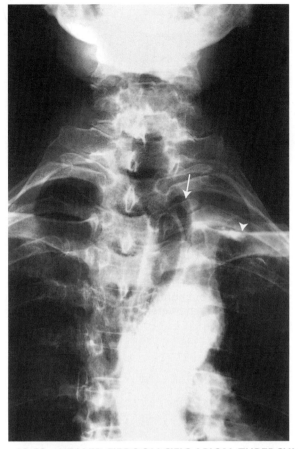

Figure 18-53 HEALED FIBROCALCIFIC APICAL TUBERCULO-SIS. AP Cervicothoracic. Note that the trachea shows marked deviation from its normal course (*arrow*). There is atelectasis of the left lung apex with associated pleural thickening and a focal calcified granuloma (Ghon focus) (*arrowhead*). *COMMENT:* When tracheal deviation is present, an investigation for its underlying cause includes loss of lung volume (e.g., scarring from tuberculosis or radiotherapy), tension pneumothorax, goiter, and lymphadenopathy. In addition, torticollis and poor positioning with the neck rotated can produce the pseudo-appearance of tracheal deviation.

a prominent tuberculous pleural effusion (*empyema*) can occur. Occasionally a granuloma of 5–30 mm is encountered (*tuberculoma*), which simulates a neoplasm; only the presence of calcification suggests its benign nature. (6,9,10)

INTERSTITIAL LUNG DISEASE

Interstitial lung disease (ILD) is a common category of lung pathology with a multitude of causes. Imaging, especially HRCT, is required for characterizing the condition and guiding the diagnostic process. Frequently the causes for the observed changes remain non-specific, requiring histopathological correlation for definitive diagnosis. Three entities are reviewed, which typify the imaging features of ILD: sarcoidosis, asbestosis, and idiopathic pulmonary fibrosis. These diagnoses also have musculoskeletal implications. (1–4)

Sarcoidosis

Clinical Features. Sarcoidosis (Boeck's sarcoid) is a chronic, multisystem granulomatous disease of unknown origin characterized by the formation of non-caseating granulomas. (5–7) It is a disease that has a predilection for females in a ratio of 3:1, with an onset between 20 and 40 years of age. (6) Symptoms are typically dry cough, malaise, fevers, chest pain, iritis, and erythema nodosum of the shin. In the acute form, fever, arthralgia, and erythema nodosum can occur, with a chest radiograph showing bilateral hilar adenopathy (Lofgren's syndrome). (6–10) In the chronic form, 50% of cases are asymptomatic, and the diagnosis is made from the chest radiograph. In 5–20% of cases, lytic bone lesions in the hands and feet occur. (1,6,7)

Imaging Features. Four stages of pulmonary sarcoidosis are described based on radiographic findings. Stage 0 is normal imaging; stage 1, bilateral hilar adenopathy; stage 2, bilateral hilar adenopathy with lung infiltrates; stage 3, pulmonary infiltrates only; and stage 4, extensive fibrosis with bullae and cavitation. Chest radiographic findings are frequently diagnostic and, in 75% of cases, sufficient for diagnosis. (1,4–6)

The intrathoracic adenopathy characteristically targets the right paratracheal and bilateral hilar lymph nodes (1-2-3 sign, pawnbroker sign, Garland's triad). (2,7,11) (Fig. 18-54) The enlarged nodes extend beyond the hila with a lobulated margin and demonstrate a clear zone of separation from the cardiac silhouette (*potato nodes*). (11) CT study will often show less extensive adenopathy of other mediastinal nodes. In long-standing sarcoidosis peripheral eggshell calcification can be seen in the involved nodes. (6,7) Parenchymal changes include fine nodules and increased reticular markings (reticulonodular ILD) as well as non-specific alveolar infiltrates; in advanced cases architectural distortion and cystic cavities (*honeycomb lung*), predominantly in the middle to upper zones, are seen. (1–3,7)

Asbestosis

Clinical Features. Inhalation of inorganic foreign particles can result in various lung reaction patterns that are grouped under the heading of *pneumoconiosis*. (12) Those that incite changes that are irreversible, even if exposure to the agent is ceased, are sometimes referred to as *malignant pneumoconioses* and include asbestos (asbestosis), silica (silicosis), and coal (anthracosis). (12) A number of different asbestiform fibers are found, but those linked to pulmonary disease are the blue-black (crocidolite) and brown (amosite) forms. Exposure occurs during the manufacture, mining, and handling of these asbestos materials, which are commonly used in insulation, brake linings, textiles, construction, and gaskets. (1,13)

The latent period for appearance of changes after exposure is usually at least 10 years but is often as long as 20–40 years. (13,14) The incidence and severity of disease is usually related to the intensity and duration of exposure. Complicating carcinoma (squamous and adenocarcinoma) is 10 times more common after asbestos exposure, and 90 times greater when combined with smoking. (4,12,15) There is also a strong association between asbestos exposure and mesothelioma, a malignant neoplasm of the pleura.

Imaging Features. Chest and spine radiographs are useful for initial diagnosis and for monitoring progress. (13,14) Calcified pleural plaques are the radiographic hallmark of asbestosis. The

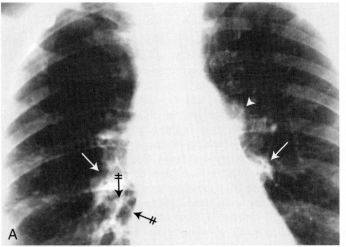

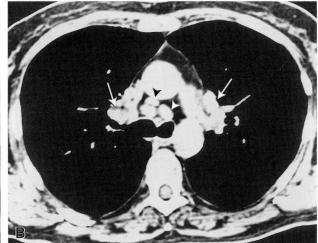

Figure 18-54 PULMONARY SARCOIDOSIS. A. PA Chest. Note the lymph node enlargement in the right paratracheal and hilar regions bilaterally (*arrows*) (1-2-3 sign, pawnbroker sign, Garland's triad). In addition, the fullness of the aorto-pulmonary window (*arrowhead*) indicates lymphadenopathy. Note the radiolucent lung separating the mediastinum from the enlarged nodes, confirming these are beyond the hilum (*crossed arrows*). **B. CT, Axial Chest.** The hilar (*arrows*) and paratracheal nodes (*arrowheads*) are easily identified. *COMMENT:* Bilateral lymphadenopathy (potato nodes) extending beyond the pulmonary hilum with sparing of the anterior mediastinum is characteristic of stage 1 pulmonary sarcoidosis.

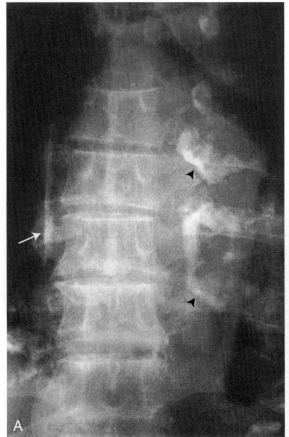

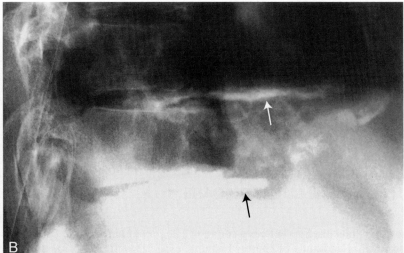

Figure 18-55 ASBESTOS-RELATED PLEURAL CALCIFICATION. A. AP Thoracic Spine. Observe the linear calcification in the paraspinal pleura (*arrow*). More extensive plaque formation is present on the contralateral side (*arrowheads*). **B. Lateral Thoracic Spine.** Note the calcified pleural plaques on the hemidiaphragms bilaterally (*arrows*). *COMMENT:* This roentgen sign is frequently the first diag- nostic finding of asbestosis that is detected and is often observed incidentally on either chest or thoracic spine radiographs. This is highly indicative of asbestos exposure. Less common causes of pleural calcifications are tubercu- lous empyema, trauma, talcosis, and postpneumothorax therapy.

pleural calcifications are often first identified on spinal radiographs rather than chest images, owing to higher technical contrast. (13,14,16) HRCT is the technique of choice for defining early changes. (13,16) Two types of changes are described: pulmonary asbestosis and asbestos-related disease. (15,17)

Pulmonary asbestosis is characterized by chronic progressive diffuse interstitial parenchymal fibrosis. The changes are most severe in the subpleural zones of the lower lobes. (15) On chest radiographs, reticular shadows radiating down from the hila create an irregular outline to the heart (*shaggy heart*). (13,14) Less common signs are small, irregular nodular opacities and irregular fibrosis with distortion but no adenopathy. (14) On HRCT, subpleural lines, subpleural dots, parenchymal bands, honeycombing, thickened septae, and occasional bullae are present in the lower lobes. (13,16)

Asbestos-related changes include pleural plaques (65%), diffuse pleural thickening (20%), and pleural calcification (50%) as well as benign pleural effusions (20%). (14–17) Pleural changes most commonly occur at the seventh to twelfth rib levels and over the diaphragmatic surfaces. (14,16,17) (Fig. 18-55)

Complications that can be seen on imaging are mesothelioma, carcinoma, and round atelectasis. (12,15) Mesothelioma is heralded by a lobulated, diffuse thickening of the pleura that encases the lung. (12,15) Carcinoma is recognized by the development of a mass lesion, whereas round atelectasis caused by the folding of the lung on itself is most commonly subpleural at the posterior lung bases and contains whorled vessels (*comet tail*). (3,11,12,15)

Idiopathic Pulmonary Fibrosis

Clinical Features. Chronic progressive interstitial fibrosis of the lung, when of unknown cause, has been ascribed various terms, including cryptogenic and, most commonly, idiopathic pulmonary fibrosis (IPF). (18,19) There is an equal gender distribution with a typical onset in the 5th–6th decades. (19) Progressive exertional dyspnea, coarse lung base crepitations, and finger clubbing are the characteristic clinical triad. (18,19) The identical clinical syndrome and imaging features can be displayed in a wide spectrum of known causes, including drugs, collagen vascular disease, and histiocytosis. (4,18,20)

Imaging Features. Imaging, although non-specific, quantifies the changes and confirms disease presence. On chest radiographs the changes are typically bibasal with hazy lower lung fields; shaggy heart contour; and increased reticular markings, which can become diffuse, creating a honeycomb appearance. (3,19) On HRCT, subpleural lines, subpleural dots, parenchymal bands, honeycombing, thickened septae, and occasional bullae are present in the lower lobes. (4,19) (Fig. 18-56) Active disease is marked by the appearance of ground-glass opacification of the lung parenchyma. (1,2,19)

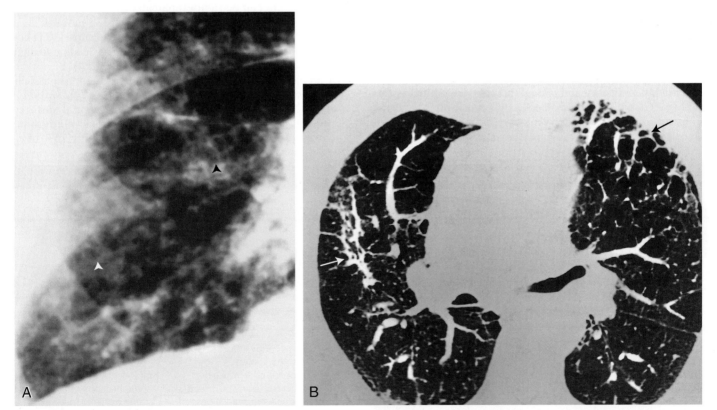

Figure 18-56 IDIOPATHIC PULMONARY FIBROSIS. A. PA Chest. Note the widespread reticular changes throughout the lung base (*arrowheads*) without pleural effusion. **B. CT, Axial Chest.** The interstitial fibrosis is characterized by thickened linear densities throughout both lungs (*arrows*).
COMMENT: Idiopathic pulmonary fibrosis is one of the most common causes for diffuse interstitial lung disease but frequently cannot be distinguished radiographically from other disorders. Similar findings are seen in sarcoidosis, histiocytosis, pneumoconiosis, and collagen diseases (such as rheumatoid arthritis and scleroderma).

TUMORS OF THE LUNG

Carcinoma of the lung is the most common cause of cancer-related death in males and females. There are numerous histologic types of lung tumors, all of which can present differently, have different prognoses, and exhibit varying imaging features. (1–3) (Table 18-9)

Imaging is essential for diagnosis, staging, guiding biopsy, and monitoring progression in response to therapy. (1) Up to 30–50% of lung tumors are asymptomatic at the time the patient presents; they are discovered incidentally on imaging. (3,4) Central tumors present with cough, wheeze, pneumonia, hemoptysis, or dysphagia. Peripheral tumors are characterized by chest pain (often pleuritic), dyspnea, and cough. Metastatic disease involving bone, liver, adrenals, or brain can be the presenting finding in > 30% of cases. (1,4)

Adenocarcinoma. Adenocarcinoma is the most common cell type in women and men as well as non-smokers, accounting for at least 50% of cases. (5,6) They occur peripherally and in almost 70% of cases occur in the upper lobes. (6) Alveolar cell carcinoma is a rare subtype of adenocarcinoma that can produce a pneumonia or pulmonary edema-like presentation. (6–8)

Squamous Cell Carcinoma. The second most common cell type (30–35%) is squamous cell carcinoma. Males predominate, and there is a strong association with smoking. (3) It frequently is diagnosed by sputum cytology when the lesion is radiologically occult. (9,10) It has the slowest growth rate and best prognosis. This cell type is the most common form to cavitate and to cause an apical mass (Pancoast's tumor). (3,9,11)

Small Cell (Oat Cell) Carcinoma. Strongly related to smoking, small cell carcinoma carries the worst prognosis. (12,13) The name is based on the histologic appearance of small, oval (oat) shaped cells. This type is most likely to present with marked mediastinal adenopathy and a small primary lesion that is frequently not found. (12,13) Small cell carcinoma is often the cause for obstruction of the superior vena cava. This is the most common cell type associated with paraneoplastic syndromes, including gynecomastia, Cushing's syndrome, acromegaly, hyperparathyroidism, and myasthenia. (12–14)

Large Cell Carcinoma. Large cell carcinoma is closely linked with smoking, exhibits rapid growth potential, and shows early metastasis. (15) The mediastinal adenopathy is often large at presentation. (15,16)

Carcinoid. Carcinoid tumors were previously designated as *bronchial adenomas.* (13) They represent neuroectodermal tumors, probably arising from the Kultschitsky cells in the bronchial mucosa. (17) They are typically small endobronchial tumors involving lobar (75%), mainstem (10%), and peripheral bronchi (15%). (17–19) At least 90% of cases are histologically benign. (18) Carcinoid syndrome is uncommon, though occasionally Cushing's syndrome may occur. (17,18)

Lymphoma

Malignant transformation within the lymphatics is categorized into Hodgkin's lymphoma (HL) and non-Hodgkin's lymphoma (NHL) based on the presence or absence of the Reed-Sternberg cell. (20)

Clinical Features. The classification of lymphoma is complex and beyond the scope of this chapter. Afflicted patients can present with musculoskeletal symptoms and night sweats (21), but most commonly enlarged lymph nodes will be reported by the patient or palpated during physical examination. (20,22)

Imaging Features. Chest radiography remains the mainstay for disease detection and progression. Controversy remains on the sensitivity of chest radiography as a screening method because lesions < 2 cm can be radiographically occult. (23) Low-dose helical CT studies detect lesions as small as 1–2 mm, which can affect early treatment before metastases have occurred. CT, however, will detect small insignificant granulomas, leading to higher rates of biopsy and unnecessary surgery. (11,23,24)

Carcinomatous lesions most commonly present as parenchymal masses with irregular margins (*spreading edge, corona radiata*). (2,19) (Fig. 18-57) Extension to the pleural surface in peripheral lesions is associated with a thin zone of attachment (*pleural tail*). (11,23,24) Cavitation occurs in only 15% of car-

Table 18-9	Primary Malignant Tumors of the Lung					
Cell Type	**Incidence (%)**	**Age (years)**	**Male:Female Ratio**	**Location**	**Clinical Findings**	**Imaging Findings**
Adenocarcinoma	50	30–50	1:2	Peripheral; upper lobe (70%)	Few symptoms; "scar" carcinoma; rapid growth rate; early lymph node spread	Mass often lobulated; < 4 cm; does not cavitate
Squamous cell	30–50	50–60	9:1	Central (60–80%); apex (5%)	Smoking related; hemoptysis; recurrent pneumonia; short of breath; Pancoast's syndrome	Spiculated mass; > 4 cm; cavitation; osteoarthropathy (5–10%); lymph node metastasis; apical mass; bone destruction
Alveolar cell carcinoma	2–5	30–50	1:1	Diffuse, bilateral	Persistent dyspnea; profuse frothy sputum	Widespread alveolar infiltrates
Small cell carcinoma	15	50–60	10:1	Central	Smoking related; early metastases (80%); paraneoplastic syndromes	Small central mass; large lymphadenopathy; superior vena cava obstruction
Large cell carcinoma	5	50–60	10:1	Central	Smoking related; early metastases; rapid growth	Mass lesion > 4 cm; large lymphadenopathy
Carcinoid tumor	5–10	30–50	1:1	Central (80%); peripheral (20%)	Rarely carcinoid syndrome; hemoptysis; atelectasis-pneumonia (90%, benign)	Round lesion; < 2 cm; 20% metastasize to nodes; 5% metastasize to bone

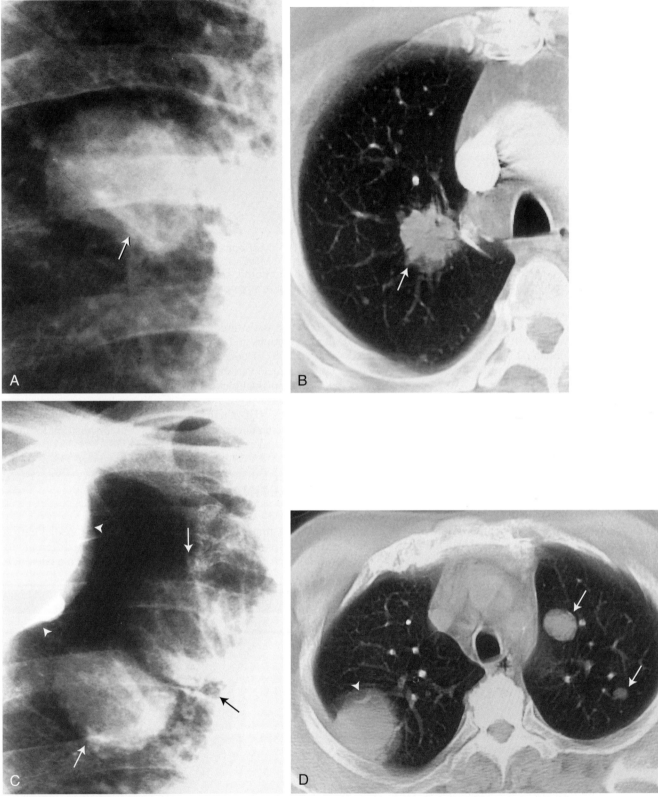

Figure 18-57   **CARCINOMA OF THE LUNG. A. Primary Bronchogenic Carcinoma, PA Chest.** Note the single solid nodule with irregular margins (spreading edge sign) (*arrow*). **B. Primary Bronchogenic Carcinoma, CT, Axial Chest.** The mass lesion is clearly depicted and demonstrates the irregular spreading edge sign (*arrow*). **C. Metastatic Carcinoma, PA Chest.** Observe the three round, well-defined nodules (*arrows*) and adjacent extrapleural mass (*arrowheads*). **D. Metastatic Carcinoma, CT, Axial Chest.** Two parenchymal nodules (*arrows*) and the extrapleural mass (*arrowhead*) are seen. *COMMENT:* A solitary coin lesion can be caused by either a primary or secondary carcinoma. Additional causes include abscess, granuloma, and vasculitis (i.e., Wegener's granulomatoses).

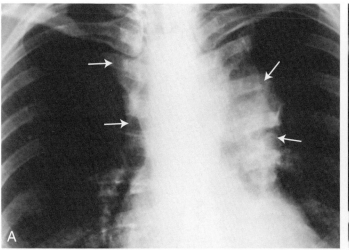

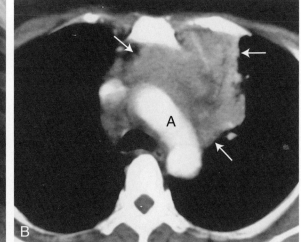

Figure 18-58 HODGKIN'S LYMPHOMA. A. PA Chest. Note that the upper mediastinum is diffusely widened (*arrows*). **B. CT, Axial Chest.** Observe the massive lymphadenopathy in the retrosternal space (*arrows*), extending to the aorta (*A*). This is the most common thoracic manifestation of Hodgkin's disease. *COMMENT:* Causes for an anterior mediastinal mass include **t**hymoma, **t**eratoma, retrosternal (**t**hyroid) goiter, and **H**odgkin's lymphoma (*the "three Ts and an H"*).

cinomas; however, 80% of these will be the squamous cell type. (10,23,24) Approximately 40% will be central masses in the perihilar zones, producing a unilateral full or enlarged hilum, which requires CT for differentiation from other mass lesions, lymph node, and pulmonary artery. (4,19)

Lymphadenopathy is best examined with CT and is critical for staging and assessing resectability. (1) CT evidence of pathologic adenopathy requires the node to be > 1 cm in the short axis. Positron emission tomography (PET) scans are the most sensitive method for detecting lymph node involvement and recurrence. (4,19)

Distal atelectasis and pneumonia are found in more than one third of cases. (1) A classic sign is the combination of a right hilar mass and collapse of the right upper lobe, creating elevation of the horizontal fissure into a serpiginous contour (Golden's reversed S sign). Elevation of the diaphragm on the side of hilar mass often denotes phrenic nerve paralysis. (4,8,19) Carcinoma in the lung apex (Pancoast's tumor) is often overlooked on chest and shoulder radiographs and is visible as a lack of lung aeration and variable degrees of bone destruction of the upper posterior ribs and upper thoracic vertebrae. (11,24) MRI is important for assessing cord and brachial plexus involvement. (4,19)

Lymphoma presentations typically are large to massive lymphadenopathy. NHL can involve all mediastinal and hilar nodes. (23) HL more characteristically exhibits a predisposition to anterior mediastinal adenopathy. (3,22) (Fig. 18-58)

MEDIASTINAL LESIONS

The mediastinum is the anatomic site where the medial lung surfaces converge in the midline; it is occupied by different structures. Three compartments are described based on a lateral chest

Table 18-10	The Mediastinum		
Division	**Boundaries**	**Contents**	**Disease**
Anterior	Retrosternal and anterior heart	Lymph nodes	Lymphoma (non-Hodgkin's)
		Thymus	Thymoma
		Blood vessels	Teratoma
		Fat	Lipomatosis
		Thyroid	Thyroid substernal extension
Middle	Anterior heart and anterior vertebrae	Trachea/hila	Carcinoma
		Lymph nodes	Lymphoma (non-Hodgkin's)
		Pulmonary arteries	Dilatation
		Heart	Aneurysm
		Aorta	Aneurysm
		Aortic arch	Aneurysm
		Esophagus	Hiatal hernia
Posterior	Anterior vertebrae and posterior ribs	Thoracic vertebrae	Tumor
		Intervertebral discs	Abscess
		Nerve roots	Tumor, meningocele
		Sympathetic chain	Tumor
		Lymphatics	Lymphoma
		Descending aorta	Aneurysm
		Lymph nodes	Lymphoma (Hodgkin's)
		Thoracic duct	Lymphoma (Hodgkin's)

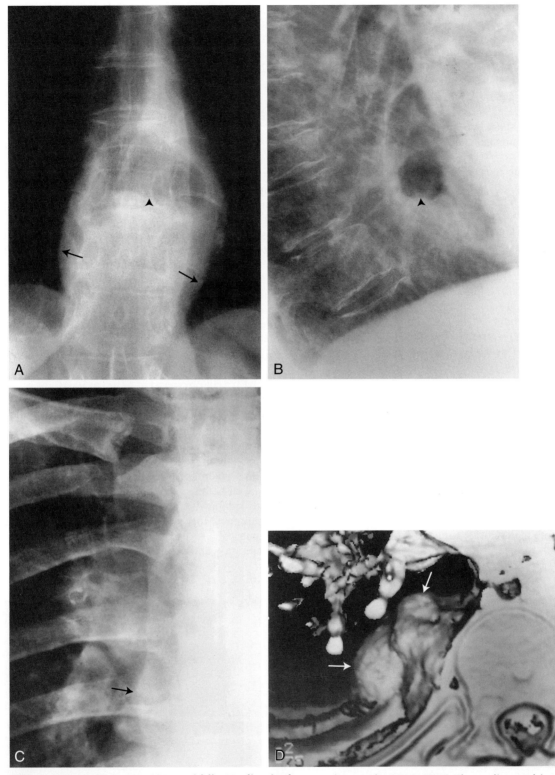

Figure 18-59 **MEDIASTINAL MASSES. Middle Mediastinal Mass, Hiatal Hernia. A. AP Thoracic Spine. B. Lateral Thoracic Spine.** Note the fusiform enlargement of the mediastinal contours (*arrows*) overlying the thoracic spine. An air–fluid level is present within the hiatal hernia (*arrowheads*). **Posterior Mediastinal Mass, Non-Hodgkin's Lymphoma. C. AP Thoracic Spine.** On the radiograph note the subtle displacement of the paraspinal line (*arrow*). **D. Three-Dimensional CT, Axial Chest.** CT reveals a lobulated paraspinal mass larger than suggested by the plain film (*arrows*). *COMMENT:* The radiographic differentiation between posterior and middle mediastinal masses is based on whether or not the lesion overlies the spine. The middle mediastinum lies anterior to the spine, whereas the posterior mediastinum includes the spine. Disorders of the vertebral column, such as neurogenical lesions, lymphoid and bone tumor masses, abscess, and hematoma, arise in the posterior mediastinum and commonly displace the paraspinal–pleural interface. (Panels A and B courtesy of Mark P. Tapper, M.Chiro.Sc., Canberra, Australia)

radiograph: anterior, middle, and posterior. (1,2) (Table 18-10) The radiographic limits of these do not correspond to those divisions made by anatomists. Chest and spine radiographs depict all of these divisions, though CT and MRI may be required to assist in diagnosis. (3,4)

Anterior Mediastinum. The most common abnormalities of the anterior division are **t**hyroid (substernal), **t**eratoma, **t**hymoma, and **H**odgkin's lymphoma (*three Ts and an H*). (5–7) On the lateral projection the radiolucent space beneath the sternum is opacified. Tracheal deviation is common, and the mediastinum appears widened. (4,6,8)

Middle Mediastinum. The most common disorders of the middle mediastinum are at the hila, where carcinoma and lymphadenopathy predominate. (9) These appear as radiopaque dense mass lesions. Hiatal hernia may appear as an inferiorly placed soft tissue mass with an air–fluid level, adjoining the diaphragmatic surface. (1,2,9)

Posterior Mediastinum. The majority of lesions that occupy the posterior mediastinum are either vertebral or neurogenical in nature. (1) Examples are vertebral tumors with soft tissue mass, infections with paravertebral abscess, and nerve tumors such as neurofibroma and ganglioneuroma. On the frontal projection careful scrutiny of the lung–pleural–vertebral interface (*paraspinal line*) may show displacement as a subtle sign of abnormality. (1,2,4,8) (Fig. 18-59)

DIAPHRAGM

The diaphragm is the musculotendinous partition separating the chest and abdominal cavities and is primarily responsible for respiration. Muscle fibers converge to the central tendon from three peripheral attachment sites: the diaphragmatic crura arising from the upper lumbar vertebrae, xiphoid process of the sternum, and lower sixth to twelfth ribs. It is innervated by the phrenic nerve. Abnormalities of the diaphragm can produce anterior and posterior chest pain, thoracolumbar pain, and referred pain to the shoulder. The normal diaphragm and its abnormalities are clearly demonstrated by plain film radiographs and CT. (1,2,3)

Normal Diaphragm

The diaphragm, though an anatomically singular structure connected across the midline by the central tendon, is often on imaging studies described as two *hemidiaphragms*. (1) The right hemidiaphragm is usually higher than the left by 1–2 cm owing to the presence of the liver. (1) Each hemidiaphragm is curved superiorly (*cupola*) and forms a sharp acute angle with the lateral ribs (*lateral costophrenic sulcus* or recess) and thoracic spine (*posterior costophrenic sulcus* or recess). The crura can often be seen to extend laterally to the upper three lumbar vertebrae. (1) On full-suspended inspiration the dome of the diaphragm typically projects below the tenth posterior and seventh anterior ribs on the PA chest radiograph. (1,4) Expiration studies allow the diaphragm to ascend and become more convex in contour. (1,4,5)

Normal Diaphragmatic Variations

Differences in position, shape, and contour of the diaphragm are commonly encountered on imaging studies. (Fig. 18-60) The relative position of each diaphragm is prone to individual variation. Patients with large body habitus or obesity have elevated diaphragms, whereas asthenic body types often have diaphragms well below the posterior tenth ribs. (6) Prominent gas within the splenic flexure of the colon may elevate the left hemidiaphragm. Most normal diaphragms are convex in shape and symmetrical. (1,4) The normal diaphragmatic excursion between inspiration and expiration is 3 cm. (1,4) Flattening of the

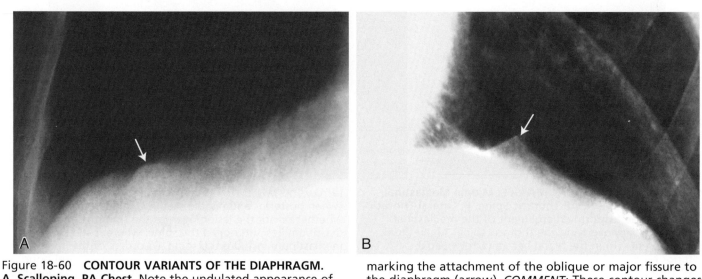

Figure 18-60 **CONTOUR VARIANTS OF THE DIAPHRAGM. A. Scalloping, PA Chest.** Note the undulated appearance of the hemidiaphragm as a result of peripheral costal diaphragmatic attachments (*arrow*). **B. Tent, PA Chest.** Observe the sharp angular shadow extending into the basal lung field, marking the attachment of the oblique or major fissure to the diaphragm (*arrow*). *COMMENT:* These contour changes should not be confused with dysfunction of the diaphragm. Occasionally the tent configuration is more prominent, with pleural effusion or atelectasis in the upper lobe.

cupola is a sign of air trapping, most commonly from emphysema. (4) A small angular density from the diaphragm (*tenting*) is often seen at the site where the oblique (major) fissure inserts and is sometimes associated with previous inflammatory pleural disease. (4) An undulating scalloped (*humping*) appearance to the entire diaphragm is commonly seen in normal patients, in thin individuals, and occasionally in patients with emphysema owing to prominence of the costal insertion sites. (4,5,7) Occasionally there is clinically insignificant interposition of the hepatic flexure of the colon between the liver and the diaphragm (Chilaiditi's syndrome). (2,8) The thickness of the normal left hemidiaphragm is < 5 mm and can be estimated by the tissue thickness between the stomach fundus and lung base. (3,5)

Functional Variations

Pain over the lower chest due to pleurisy, rib fracture, pneumonia, and other inflammatory conditions can produce splinting (spasm) of the diaphragm, which results in elevation and flattening of the diaphragm, especially more laterally. (2,3) Hiccups (singultus) can be observed under fluoroscopy as a sudden contraction of the diaphragm.

Eventration. The diaphragm is congenitally thin and allows for apparent herniation of abdominal organs into the chest. It is only at operation or occasionally on CT that accurate differentiation between eventration and rupture or absence of the diaphragm can be ascertained. (2,4)

Hernia. Three classic herniations are described: esophageal hiatus hernia, Morgagni's hernia, and Bochdalek's hernia. (9–11) Sliding esophageal hernias are the most common and are readily identified by the contained air and frequent air–fluid level. (5,10)

Rupture. Acute traumatic ruptures are more common on the left because of the protective effect of the liver. (12,13) The rupture may occur in the cupola at the musculotendinous junction or at the crura. (13) Even with CT most are initially overlooked, unless contained bowel is seen. (12) The signs for diaphragmatic discontinuity are subtle. (13) The risk of strangulation and infarction to herniated bowel loops necessitates a surgical consult for repair in most cases.

Paralysis. Interruption of the phrenic nerve anywhere throughout its course such as in the neck, thoracic inlet, or near the lung hilus results in a markedly elevated and curved hemidiaphragm. (14) Confirmation of paralysis is made with fluoroscopy or ultrasound, which shows a paradoxical ascending of the diaphragm on respiratory inspiration. (14,15)

Calcification. The most characteristic cause for diaphragmatic calcification is asbestosis. (16) Other less common causes include tuberculous empyema and talcosis; it can also be a sequela to trauma. (17) In asbestosis the calcification is usually observed only after 15–20 years following exposure. (16)

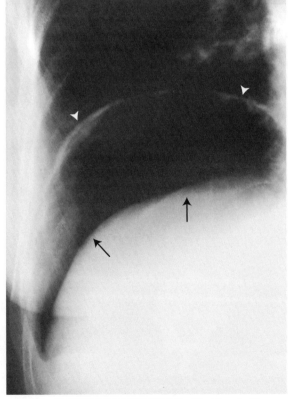

Figure 18-61 PNEUMOPERITONEUM. PA Chest. Observe the prominent crescent of air between the thin diaphragm (*arrowheads*) and the dome of the liver (*arrows*). *COMMENT:* This finding is visible only on upright studies and is most commonly the result of perforation of a sigmoid diverticulum, gastrointestinal ulcer, tumor, or recent laparotomy.

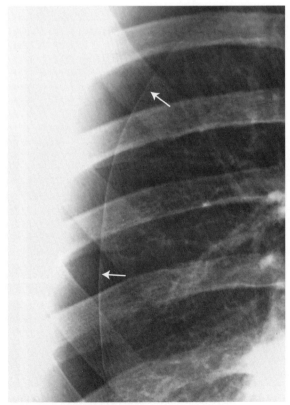

Figure 18-62 PNEUMOTHORAX, PA Chest. Note the retracted pleural interface (*arrows*). There is also an absence of vascular markings beyond the pleural line. *COMMENT:* These characteristic findings of pneumothorax can be accentuated by obtaining an expiration chest radiograph.

Subphrenic Abscess. Infection below the diaphragm may be suspected when the diaphragm is elevated and more convex in shape with an associated pleural effusion. (3,5) Occasionally gas formation may be visible in the subphrenic space. Both CT and ultrasound are confirmatory. (3,7)

Pneumoperitoneum. In the upright position, air within the abdominal cavity will rise to lie beneath the diaphragm and is best seen on the right because of the contrasting density of the liver. (Fig. 18-61) This usually signifies rupture of a hollow viscus, especially bowel perforation secondary to gastric or duodenal ulcer, diverticular disease, or cancer of the colon. (2,5)

Pneumothorax

Pneumothorax describes the entry of air into the (normally) potential space between the visceral and the parietal pleura. Several mechanisms are possible. Air may enter via abnormal communication with the bronchoalveolar space, as in rupture of a bleb or bulla of the lung. This so-called spontaneous pneumothorax is a common cause for presentation of otherwise healthy younger individuals who become acutely dyspneic while engaged in some physical

activity. Air may also enter the pleural space as a result of a penetrating chest wall injury, and rarely abdominal disease can establish communication from the bowel to the pleural space. Air usually settles at the apex in the erect position. (18) (Fig. 18-62)

Careful attention to detail and good radiographic quality are both necessary to visualize the delicate pleural line and altered peripheral density that make the diagnosis possible on PA chest radiographs. Supine radiographs or upright chest films in patients with pleural adhesions may demonstrate air over the diaphragm, which shows the posterior costophrenic recess more clearly. When bilateral, the diaphragm may be seen clearly across the midline. (18)

Retrocrural Lymphadenopathy

Behind the crura lie the thoracolumbar vertebrae, aorta, azygos and hemiazygos veins, and numerous lymph nodes. In diseases such as lymphoma the crura can be displaced laterally, producing a characteristic density that diverges from the upper lumbar vertebrae. (3) (Fig. 18-63) The same appearance can be produced

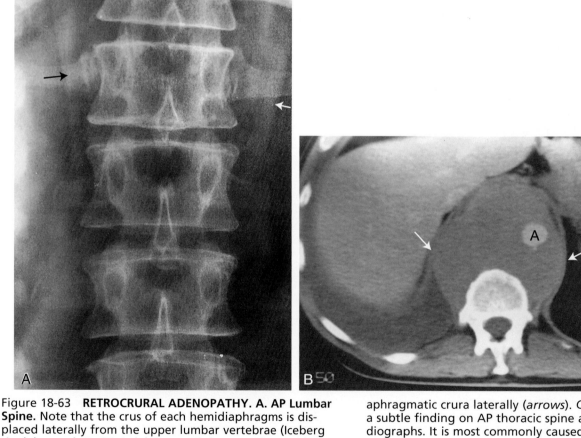

Figure 18-63 **RETROCRURAL ADENOPATHY. A. AP Lumbar Spine.** Note that the crus of each hemidiaphragms is displaced laterally from the upper lumbar vertebrae (Iceberg sign) (*arrows*). **B. CT, Axial Upper Abdomen.** Observe the large mass encasing the aorta (*A*) and displacing the di-aphragmatic crura laterally (*arrows*). *COMMENT:* This can be a subtle finding on AP thoracic spine and lumbar spine radiographs. It is most commonly caused by lymphoma, particularly of the non-Hodgkin's variety, which was the diagnosis in this patient.

by bony tumors and abscesses of the spine, neural tumors, and even varices. (2,5,7)

THE ABDOMEN: MASQUERADERS OF MUSCULOSKELETAL DISEASE

INTRODUCTION

A great variety of abdominal diseases and pathologic processes can manifest as musculoskeletal complaints. The single most common presentation is pain, which may be generalized or localized within the spine, paraspinal, pelvic, and lower limb regions. Focused imaging of these regions for the evaluation of musculoskeletal disorders includes various organs and their coverings, vessels, and adjacent tissues, which need to be interpreted. Conversely, when imaging is performed to investigate the abdominal and pelvic contents, musculoskeletal structures must also be scrutinized. This may seem obvious at first glance; but practitioner bias, based on area of interest and specialty, can lead one to overlook important findings of the visualized structures. Given the plethora of abdominal conditions that can present with musculoskeletal symptom patterns, precedence in this section is given to the more common clinical conditions. This discussion is divided into three sections: imaging modalities and principles of interpretation, fundamental imaging signs, and an overview of organ-specific conditions.

PRINCIPLES OF ABDOMINAL IMAGING

All modalities have application in the assessment of abdominal disorders. The most frequently employed studies are abdominal radiographs, CT, and ultrasound. These will be the focus of this presentation. MRI is being used more frequently, especially in the assessment of the liver, biliary tree, adrenals, and pelvic organs.

Abdominal Radiography

Basic Techniques

The basic plain film abdominal radiographic assessment includes three views—AP supine, AP erect, and PA chest. The abdominal films are performed at a 40-inch (101-cm) focal–film distance. Today, tomography is seldom used because of the availability of CT.

AP Supine. Performed in full expiration, the AP supine projection includes the lung bases and entire abdomen to the level of the pubis. This film has been referred to by various terms, such as *flat plate* and *KUB* (kidneys, ureters, and bladder). As the initial part of an intravenous urogram, it is sometimes referred to as a *scout film.*

AP Erect. The same examination (as the AP supine) is preferably performed standing but owing to patient immobility can be done in the side-lying position, preferably with the right side up

(left lateral decubitus). The major reason for the erect study is to allow air to rise within the bowel or peritoneal cavity, which permits an improved assessment of the bowel for obstruction or perforation (pneumoperitoneum).

PA Chest. The PA chest is performed erect to allow identification of any free air below the hemidiaphragm (pneumoperitoneum) and to assess for lung base pathology that may be the cause of referred pain to the abdomen.

Interpretation

Systematic assessment is important, as in all imaging, to minimize interpretive error. The following schema is suggested.

Patient Demographics. Ensure that the patient's details and any labels on the film are recognized.

Analysis of Technique. Identify the views and assess them for adequacy of exposure, rotation, the field of view, and phase of inspiration. Although the films should be clearly labeled, the presence of horizontal air–fluid interfaces in the bowel, especially in the gastric fundus (magenblase), may help discriminate between a recumbent and an upright study.

Overview. Review the studies from a distance to identify anything obvious, such as a mass, calcification, or abnormal bowel pattern. Use of the coverup method (described earlier in this chapter) is helpful.

Detailed Study. Identification of each organ outline should be attempted, such as the liver, spleen, kidneys, and bladder. These can usually be identified by the thin layer of fat outlining their external borders. Gas patterns are crucial for identifying the small bowel (by the presence of the complete thin folds of the plicae semicircularis) and the large bowel (by the incomplete and thicker haustral folds). The outline of the psoas muscles should be evaluated for definition, shape, density, and symmetry, all of which can provide clues of disease in the retroperitoneum. The diaphragms, crura, lung bases, and costophrenic sulci must be assessed.

Layers of muscle and fat along the lateral abdominal wall create a *flank stripe,* which should also be checked for symmetry, definition, and contour. Any calcification is assessed as to its origin and significance. Finally, all bone and joint structures on the study are reviewed. The presence of any artifacts that may indicate previous surgery, trauma, or the residue of any earlier contrast studies should also be noted and weighed along with other findings during subsequent diagnostic considerations.

Ultrasound

Basic Techniques

The advantage of ultrasound is the ability to specifically examine anatomy in real time, which often is required for localizing and characterizing an abnormality. In addition, there is no ionizing radiation involved. An array of sonographic probes may be used, depending on the depth of penetration required and the organ being examined. Essentially all organs are interrogated systematically in at least two planes: longitudinally and transversely and from edge to edge. Finally, vascular flow either of the vessels or the masses is assessed.

Interpretation

The basic principles of interpretation include identification of the plane of examination, the organ, the organ's size and external contours, intrinsic anatomic details, and abnormalities. Tissues are displayed and described according to their reflectivity of the sound waves (*echogenicity*). Calcified lesions (e.g., calculi) and gas are characteristically echogenic, reflecting the sonic beam strongly and showing a bright white surface with posterior shadowing (dark). Fluid-filled lesions, such as cysts, are hypoechoic because sound waves pass through relatively unimpeded, appearing as dark areas with a bright posterior margin (*posterior acoustic enhancement*). The normal gallbladder and urinary bladder are good examples of this phenomenon.

Solid lesions of lower density than normal tissue will appear darker than the surrounding tissue (*hypoechoic*) but if of the same density may be almost non-visible (*isoechoic*). Normal fat planes appear as linear bright zones, caused by the high reflectivity of the fat–tissue interface. It is the technique of choice in diseases of the biliary system (gallbladder, bile ducts), spleen, appendix, and pelvic contents.

Computed Tomography

Basic Techniques

An array of protocols are available and are tailored for distinct clinical situations. State-of-the-art CT scanning is performed with multislice helical scanning. This can allow for reconstruction into any plane (or even three dimensions)—rapidly with no loss of detail—producing startling anatomic resolution. Unless directly contraindicated, the bowel is opacified with oral contrast in virtually all cases to assist in identifying pathology. Four basic types of CT examinations are performed.

- *Non-contrast.* This is used to identify calculi and calcification that could be obscured by radiopaque contrast administration. The most common applications for non-contrast CT are for diagnosis of renal calculi, fatty or hemosiderin infiltration of the liver, and fat-containing lesions (e.g., pelvic dermoids).
- *Intravenous contrast.* Intravenous contrast is given through an antecubital vein, and the abdominal study is obtained according to which vascular phase is required. An arterial phase that will display the aorta and its branches is timed for 20–40 sec after the injection is given. The venous phase is between 70 and 120 sec. Delayed studies can be performed after this period, for example, if contrast is required in the renal pelvis. Combining these phases can be used to assess vascularity and demonstrate occult lesions.
- *CT angiogram.* By acquiring data in the arterial phase an angiographic display of all vessels can be obtained.
- *CT colonography.* Distension of the colon with carbon dioxide via the rectum is followed by helical CT acquisition. An "endoscopic" view of the colon can then be displayed constructed to create a three-dimensional effect, allowing the interpreter to navigate the lumen from rectum to cecum.

FUNDAMENTALS OF ABDOMINAL DISEASE

Organomegaly

Enlargement of an organ may be a sign of disease and can be identified on all imaging, including plain films. The signs of organomegaly are based on two features: (*a*) identifying the outlines and applying measurements and (*b*) noting secondary displacement of adjacent structures. CT and ultrasound are the most sensitive methods for detection. (1,2)

Liver (Hepatomegaly). The normal liver is bounded by the hemidiaphragm superiorly and typically projects inferiorly to the level of the lower costal margin with the hepatic flexure and transverse colon in close apposition. Normally, only a small part of the left lobe crosses the midline. Its craniocaudal span is variable, but ranges from 12 to 14 cm. (2,3)

Erect studies, especially in the elderly, can show dramatic ptosis, with the descent of the inferior margin into the pelvis, and should not be misinterpreted as a sign of hepatomegaly. This appearance may be amplified by the exaggerated thoracic kyphosis commonly seen in older patients. A tongue-like inferior extension of the right lobe (Reidel's lobe) is a common variant that also may confuse assessment. (4,5) Massive increase in size of the right lobe is characterized by elevation of the right hemidiaphragm, inferior displacement of the hepatic flexure below the right kidney, lateral and inferior position of the transverse colon, and the tip of the right lobe extending into the right iliac fossa. (1,4,6)

CT scan confirms these displacement signs and often identifies the underlying cause. Ultrasound similarly can isolate underlying liver disease and allow measurement of the liver span. (3,7)

Spleen (Splenomegaly). The normal spleen is often not visible on plain film. It measures ~ 10 cm in length but may measure up to 17 cm. Splenomegaly displaces the gastric air bubble medially and the colon medially and inferiorly. (2)

Kidney. The normal kidney is 10–12 cm in bipolar length and is tilted medially at the upper pole to parallel to the psoas shadow (18–20°), lying between L1 and L3. Normally, there is < 1 cm right to left difference in bipolar length. (7)

Calcification

Various patterns of calcification have been described, which may assist in assigning a tissue site of origin and underlying pathology. (8,9) These include tubular calcification, cystic calcification, concretions, and mass calcifications. (8,9) (Fig. 18-64)

Tubular (Conduit, Tram Track) Calcification. Mineralization of the wall of a duct or vessel produces parallel lines that appear circular in cross section. The pattern may be complete or incomplete (dot–dash). The most common example of tubular calcification is atherosclerotic calcification in the aorta and splenic artery. (3,4,8,9)

Cystic Calcification. Within the wall of a cystic organ (e.g., gallbladder), pathologic cyst, or vascular aneurysm, thin curvilinear calcification can occur. Generally the external wall is smooth and the internal wall is more irregular. (2,5,8,9)

Concretions. Endoluminal calcifications within hollow structures (calculi) produce round to ovoid conglomerates, which usually have a continuous external surface. These often are laminated

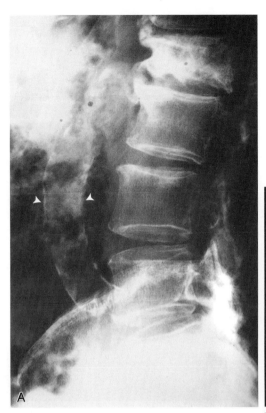

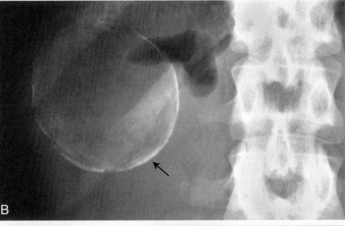

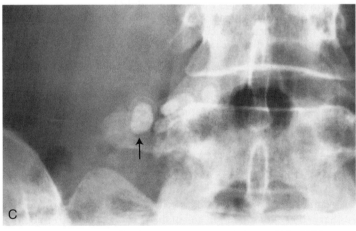

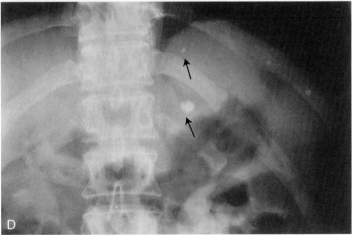

Figure 18-64 **PATTERNS OF ABDOMINAL CALCIFICATION.**
A. Tubular (Conduit, Tram Track) Calcification, Lateral
Lumbar Spine. Complete or incomplete (dot–dash) parallel
lines represent duct or vessel wall mineralization. This is
most commonly seen with aortic atherosclerosis (*arrow-heads*). In cross section these calcifications are usually circular
in shape. **B. Cystic Calcification, AP Abdomen.** Peripheral
wall calcification within cystic lesions results in characteristically thin, curvilinear arcs or circles, similar to those seen in
this hepatic hydatid cyst (*arrow*). **C. Concretion Calcification,**
AP Lumbar Spine. Intraluminal calcifications within hollow
structures (calculi) are typically round to ovoid conglomerates that usually have a continuous external surface. These
are often laminated in appearance as the result of serial
mineralized layer accumulation. Common locations for these
concretions are the gallbladder (gallstone) (*arrow*), renal
pelvis, urinary bladder, and appendix. **D. Mass Calcification,**
AP Abdomen. These types of calcifications are homogeneously
dense, as in this example of calcified splenic granulomas
(*arrows*). Other common examples are calcified fat necrosis
associated with pancreatitis and granulomas within the liver.
COMMENT: The diagnosis or differential diagnosis is formulated by identifying the pattern of calcification and placing
it in an anatomic location.

in appearance as progressive mineralized layers accumulate. Common sites include the gallbladder, urinary bladder, and appendix. Large concretions may conform to an anatomic configuration, as in the classic *staghorn calculus* that molds to the outline of the renal pelvis and calyces. (8,9)

Mass Calcification. Mass calcifications are commonly found in long-standing diseased tissue that has undergone previous necrosis. They are round and within a solid organ. (3) Granulomas within the liver and spleen, calcified necrosis associated with pancreatitis and non-functioning transplanted kidneys, and injection sites are examples. (8–10)

Gas Patterns

Accurate identification of a gas shadow is a vital clue to recognizing various disease entities. (8) While not always possible, attempts should be made to localize any gas shadow that appears abnormal.

Stomach. In the supine position, air in the body of the stomach may outline the gastric rugae as undulating parallel shadows. Erect studies produce the characteristic air–fluid level in the gastric fundus (magenblase).

Small Bowel. Normally there is little to no gas visible in the small bowel. Distension and air–fluid levels in small bowel are signs of ileus, which may be generalized or local. Localized ileus may occur in bowel sections adjacent to inflammatory abdominal disease, resulting in isolated, dilated loops of small bowel (*sentinel loops*). (6,7) The most characteristic features of a gas-filled small bowel is the demonstration of thin complete mucosal folds (plicae semicircularis), which are most prominent in the jejunum. The small bowel normally exhibits the *three–three rule*: the bowel wall should *not* be > 3 mm thick, the lumen should *not* be > 3 cm in diameter, and the folds should be < 3 mm thick and < 3 mm apart. (1,2) (Fig. 18-65) When abnormally dilated, the folds separate (*stacked coins* appearance), air–fluid levels develop as a result of secretions, and the bowel loops begin to orient in long curves and become more horizontal. (5,7) In acute obstruction, numerous dilated sequential loops lie transversely in the abdomen (*stepladder sign*). (1,4)

Large Bowel. Gas is a common physiologic finding in the colon owing to bacterial activity. The most characteristic identifying sign of normal colon filled with gas is demonstration of the haustral folds (haustrations). These typically extend incompletely across the gas-filled lumen and are thicker (> 3 mm) and more widely separated than the plicae circularis of the small bowel. (2,3,6) (Fig. 18-66) The lumen is typically 2–6 cm. In the right colon the semifluid feces produce a "speckled" appearance, contrasting with the more localized, often crescenteric gas pattern that outlines the more dehydrated bowel contents of the descending colon.

Differentiating superimposed bowel gas from osteolytic bone lesions on plain films can usually be made by identifying haustra, noting that gas crosses from bone to soft tissue or across a joint and has the crescenteric or circular shape. If a doubt persists, tilted beam studies can be performed to demonstrate relative movement of the superimposed images. (5,7)

Pathologic Gas Pattern. Collection of air within the bowel wall (pneumatosis intestinalis/coli, intramural gas) can appear linear or as small bubbles and can be a normal finding or accom-

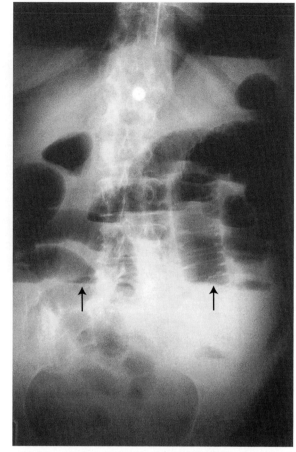

Figure 18-65   SMALL BOWEL OBSTRUCTION. Upright AP Abdomen. Observe the multiple air–fluid levels in the distended small bowel loops (*arrows*). The characteristic mucosal folds of the plicae semicircularis are visible within these distended loops. There is no gas in the rectum. A nasogastric tube is seen in the lower esophagus. *COMMENT:* Small bowel obstruction is characterized by multiple air–fluid levels in distended small bowel loops. The most common mechanical cause is postoperative adhesion; less common causes are intussusception, volvulus, and tumor.

pany necrosis. Gas within the biliary tree (pneumobilia) can be seen in the liver after sphincterotomy in the common bile duct or biliary–bowel fistula. Free gas in the peritoneal cavity (pneumoperitoneum) is best seen on the erect study beneath the right hemidiaphragm and is a sign of bowel perforation. (1,2)

Enhancement

When intravenous iodinated contrast is given with CT it has three functions: to show the blood vessels, to show organ perfusion, and to highlight lesions. It will increase the sensitivity of the study by 30–50%. (3) Any abnormality that is avascular will not enhance and will show a lower density. Conversely, a hypervascular lesion will become brighter relative to the surrounding tissue. A delayed scan shows persistent contrast enhancement in any condition in which there has been increased capillary wall permeability, including trauma, abscess, tumor, and inflammation.

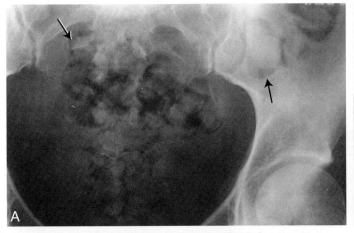
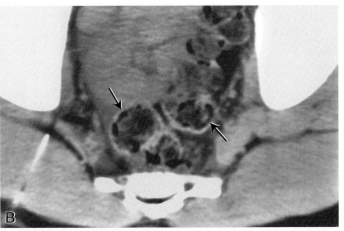

Figure 18-66   **LARGE BOWEL FECES. A. AP Abdomen.** Note the multiple segmented feces within the rectum and sigmoid colon, which are surrounded by a characteristic crescent of radiolucent air (*arrows*). **B. CT, Axial Abdomen.** Observe the segmented feces surrounded by radiolucent air crescents in the sigmoid colon (*arrows*). *COMMENT:* The differentiation of gas or fecal material from an underlying bone lesion can be made in the presence of crescentic air surrounding the fecal material, or when the density in question projects beyond the bone margin or across a joint space.

SPECIFIC ABDOMINAL DISORDERS

Liver

Musculoskeletal symptoms of liver disease are relatively uncommon, with pain over the right upper quadrant being the major complaint. Systemic complaints of malaise, anorexia, and arthralgias can be encountered. Hypertrophic osteoarthropathy with digital clubbing, arthralgia, and periosteal new bone formation in long bone diaphyses has been recorded in chronic liver disease. (1,2) Imaging is critical for detection, accurate diagnosis, and guidance for therapeutic decisions.

Liver Tumors

There are three primary malignancies of the liver.
Hepatocellular Carcinoma (Hepatoma). The most common primary malignancy of the liver is hepatocellular carcinoma, which makes up at least 90% of cases. It is most common in individuals with cirrhosis (60–90%) and hepatitis B or C. (3,4) The key laboratory test is increased serum α-fetoprotein levels. Imaging can be difficult owing to background liver disease, but ultrasound probably has the highest sensitivity for identifying the mass. CT, MRI, and nuclear medicine all contribute in difficult cases, revealing a large mass, multifocal lesions, or diffuse infiltration. (1,2)
Metastatic Disease. The most common malignant tumor of the liver is metastatic disease, which is 20 times more common than primary liver cancer. (5) Approximately 20% of all patients with known malignancy will have hepatic metastases at autopsy. (5) The most common primary sites are colon (40%), stomach (20%), pancreas (20%), breast (15%), and lung (15%). (4) More than 90% of cases present with multiple hepatic lesions. (6) Ultrasound is reported to be the most sensitive method of detection, but with new CT and MRI protocols this is probably not the case. Lesions appear round and are usually hypoechoic on ultrasound. CT shows perfused lesions on the arterial phase and decreased perfusion on the portal venous phase owing to the predominantly arterial blood supply. (Fig. 18-67)
Hemangioma. The most common benign tumor of the liver is hemangioma, accounting for 80% of cases and found in 4% of autopsies. (5) After metastatic disease, it is the second most common tumor of the liver. (2,7) It is rarely symptomatic, but when > 5 cm it may rupture, especially during pregnancy. (7) It is diagnosed almost exclusively on CT or ultrasound. (1,2) Ultrasound shows a round echogenic lesion with peripheral vascularity. CT performed dynamically with scans at 0.5, 1, 2, 5, 10, and 30 minutes show peripheral enhancement that gradually fills in centrally. (7)

Calcifications

The most frequent causes of calcifications in the liver are post-infection granulomas, hydatid cysts, and, less commonly, tumors.
Granulomas. By far the most common cause of liver calcification is granulomas. The usual causes are tuberculosis, histoplasmosis, and, less often, brucellosis. Granulomatous calcifications are typically focal, round, and solid and range in size from 1 to 10 mm. There are often co-existing splenic lesions. (2,8,9)
Hydatid Cyst. A manifestation of the parasite infection echinococcosis is the hydatid cyst. Circular irregular calcification within the wall of the cyst is characteristic. CT and ultrasound may demonstrate associated non-calcified daughter cysts; the internal membrane and "sand" of the contained cysts indicate an active lesion. (10) (Fig. 18-68)
Tumor. Calcification within tumors is relatively uncommon and best demonstrated with CT. (11) The most common liver tumors to calcify are metastatic in nature, usually mucinous adenocarcinoma of the colon and serous cystadenocarcinoma of the ovary. The pattern of calcification is finely speckled or punctate, sometimes described as psammomatous (*sand-like*) because of the histological presence of *psammoma* bodies in these lesions. (12) Primary hepatoma occasionally shows calcification, especially the fibrolamellar variety. (11)

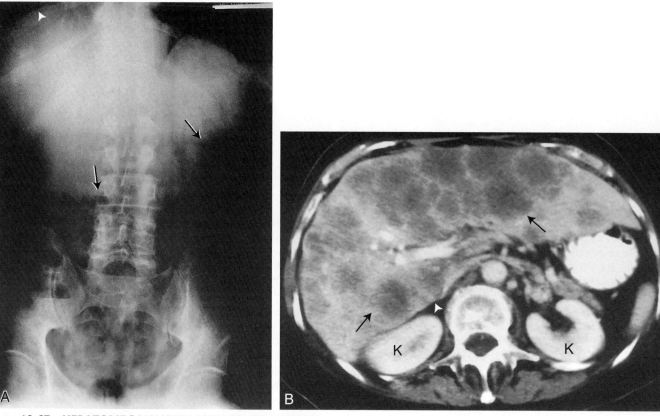

Figure 18-67 HEPATOMEGALY WITH METASTATIC DISEASE. A. AP Abdomen. Note the soft tissue density in the upper abdomen crossing the midline and inferiorly displacing the adjacent transverse colon (*arrows*). Also note the marked elevation of the right hemidiaphragm (*arrowhead*). **B. CT, Axial Abdomen.** Observe the multiple low-density lesions distributed throughout the liver, consistent with metastatic lesions (*arrows*). Note also that the liver extends across the midline and displaces the right kidney (*K*) inferiorly and posteriorly (*arrowhead*). *COMMENT:* There are many causes for hepatomegaly. In this case of clinically silent metastatic disease, the initial plain film findings of an enlarged liver prompted the referral for the abdominal CT. (Courtesy of John N. Parker, DC, Bega, New South Wales, Australia.)

Gallbladder

Cholelithiasis and Cholecystitis

Synonyms. Gallbladder calculus, gallstone, choledocholithiasis.
Clinical Features. Gallstones (cholelithiasis) are one of the most common pathologic findings at autopsy, with up to 20% of women and 8% of men over the age of 40 having at least a single stone. (13) Associated inflammation of the gallbladder wall (cholecystitis) may occur secondary to mechanical irritation, infection, or necrosis. The *Four Fs* mnemonic is sometimes used for remembering the typical patient with gallstones: female, forty, flatulent, and (with apologies) fat. The clinical triad of pain in the right upper quadrant of the abdomen, provocation of the pain on compression with inspiration (Murphy's sign), and the absence of jaundice is characteristic of gallbladder disease. (3,4,6)

Typical musculoskeletal symptoms of gallbladder disease are referred pain to the interscapular, right scapula, or shoulder regions from the splanchnic nerve or diaphragmatic irritation from inflammation to the referred cutaneous distribution of the phrenic nerve. Stones may irritate the mucosa of the gallbladder or obstruct the cystic duct, causing cholecystitis. Inflammation without stones is occasionally encountered (acalculous cholecystitis). (13) A specific type of gallbladder wall necrosis seen in diabetics

produces intraluminal and intramural gas (*emphysematous cholecystitis*). Descent of calculi into the common bile duct (choledocholithiasis) may cause obstruction, with jaundice, pain, and secondary infection (cholangitis). (4) Obstruction at the ampulla can cause pancreatitis (gallstone pancreatitis).

Three types of stones occur: cholesterol, bilirubin, and mixed. Mixed stones are the most common, constituting up to 80% of calculi, and contain variable proportions of cholesterol and bilirubin pigments. Bilirubin stones occur in < 20% of cases and are usually seen in patients with hemolytic anemia, alcoholism, or chronic biliary infection or in people of Asian descent. (4,6)
Imaging Features. Only 10–15% of gallstones will contain enough calcium to be visible on plain film radiographs. (9,13,14) Characteristically, they are round or angular with concentric laminations. Multiple stones often show flat faceted surfaces at sites of contact with adjacent stones. On occasion there will be an internal triradiate radiolucency caused by gas collections within fracture lines of long-standing, usually non-calcific, cholesterol stones (Mercedes Benz sign, crow's foot sign, peace sign). (3,4,15) (Fig. 18-69)

Biliary calculi that pass into the common bile duct (choledocholithiasis) may align in a stacked oblique arrangement in the right upper quadrant and tend to be < 5 mm in diameter. A radiodense suspension of small calcium carbonate crystals in the bile

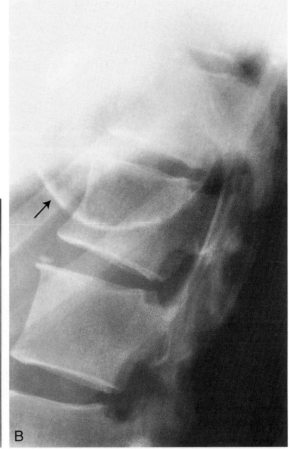

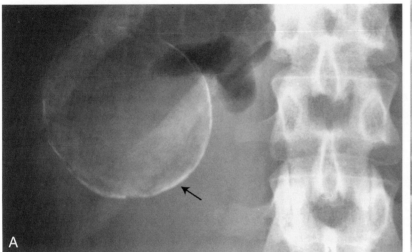

Figure 18-68 **HEPATIC HYDATID CYST. A. AP Lumbar Spine.** Note the dense calcification within the peripheral wall of the cyst (*arrow*). **B. Lateral Lumbar Spine.** The cyst wall calcification overlaps the spine, confirming that the lesion lies within the posterior aspect of the right lobe of the liver

(*arrow*). *COMMENT:* Hydatid cysts commonly calcify in both the liver and spleen, usually with thicker calcified borders than seen in this example. (Courtesy of Clive Mudgeway, DC, Whangerei, New Zealand.)

fluid (*milk of calcium bile, or limy bile*) may occasionally be seen, with a distinct flat superior border on upright plain films. (1,3,8) Rarely the gallstone may erode through the gallbladder wall and pass into the duodenum, small bowel, or colon. Once in the small bowel, a characteristic triad of findings can be seen, referred to as *gallstone ileus:* gallstone at the ileocecal junction, dilated loops of small bowel from mechanical obstruction, and gas within the biliary tree. (6,16)

Other common causes for calcification in the right side of the abdomen include renal calculus, appendicolith, costal cartilage, and hepatic granuloma. Differentiation from renal calculus is usually made on the basis of laminations, facets, and anterior location relative to the spine on the lateral projection. Appendicolith can be a difficult differentiation if the gallbladder is ptosed or the appendix lies high in association with an inverted cecum. Considerable ptosis of the gallbladder may be noted on upright radiographs, particularly in the elderly. The gallbladder may descend into the pelvis, simulating appendicolith, Meckel's diverticulum stone, gallstone ileus, or bladder stone. Costal cartilage calcifications tend to be aligned in a linear fashion, orientated superiorly and medially. Hepatic granulomas are typically homogeneous, rather than laminated. (3,6,9)

Ultrasound is the most sensitive and specific imaging modality in the assessment of gallbladder disease, with a sensitivity for

gallstone detection of at least 95%. (17) (Table 18-11) Gallstones are identified by the highly reflective surface and the acoustic shadowing behind them. Mobility of the stones can be demonstrated from upright to recumbent, unless they are impacted at the gallbladder neck in the Hartman pouch or cystic duct. (17) Cholecystitis is confirmed with pain on compression from the ultrasound probe (Murphy's sign), a gallbladder wall thickness > 3 mm, and pericholecystic fluid. (4) During the examination, the common bile duct, intrahepatic ducts, pancreas, and liver are also assessed. Imaging of the biliary tree can also be achieved by endoscopic retrograde cholangiopancreatography (ERCP), magnetic resonance cholangiopancreatography (MRCP), and CT cholangiography.

Porcelain Gallbladder

Synonyms. Gallbladder wall (mural) calcification, calcifying cholecystitis, cholecystopathic chronica calcarea.
Clinical Features. Though a relatively uncommon condition, porcelain gallbladder has clinical importance because of its association with gallbladder malignancy. It has been recorded in 0.07% of cholecystectomies (18) The macroscopic appearance of the calcification is a translucent blue hue and the wall is easily

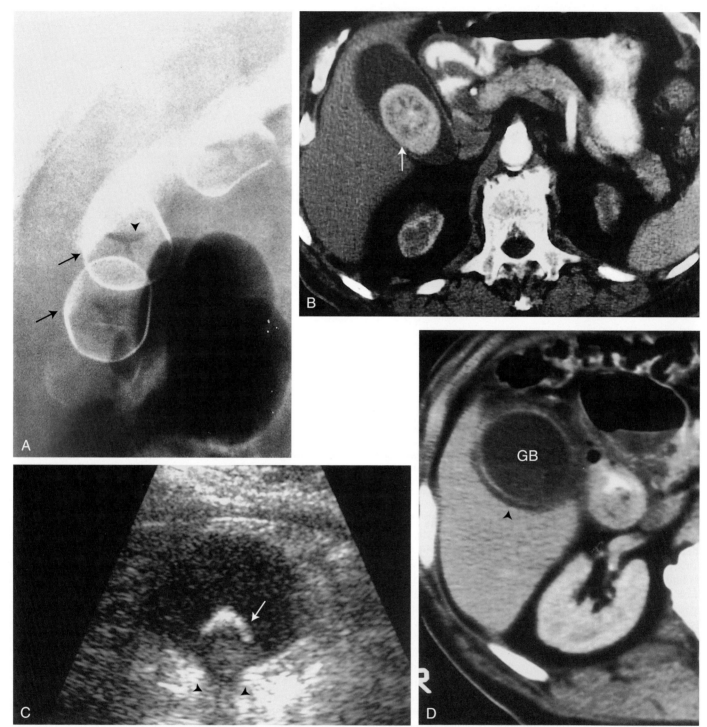

Figure 18-69 CHOLELITHIASIS AND CHOLECYSTITIS.
A. Cholelithiasis, AP Abdomen. Note the thin circular calcifications in the right upper quadrant of the abdomen, which are characteristic of multiple gallstones (*arrows*). There is a distinctive triradiate radiolucency representing gas in fissures within the stone (Mercedes Benz sign) (*arrowhead*).
B. Cholelithiasis, CT, Axial Abdomen. Observe the single large calculus within the gallbladder (*arrow*). **C. Chole-**

lithiasis, Ultrasound, Abdomen.** Note the calculus in the neck (*arrow*) and body (*arrowheads*) of the gallbladder.
D. Cholecystitis, CT, Axial Abdomen. Note the low-density crescent of pericholecystic edema surrounding the gallbladder (*GB*) wall (*arrowhead*), a sign of cholecystitis. *COMMENT:* Ultrasound is the most commonly used method for the detection of cholelithiasis, cholecystitis, and biliary obstruction.

Table 18-11	Diagnostic Imaging of Gallstones		
Modality	**Advantages**	**Limitations**	**Findings**
Plain film	Low cost; readily available	10–15% of gallstones are calcified	Laminated; faceted
Ultrasound	Rapid; high sensitivity for stones; pain provocation; complete examination	Bowel gas; obesity	Reflective stones shadowing
CT	Complete examination	Expensive; motion mis-registration; small stones; cholesterol stones	Useful for both calcified and non-calcified stones; associated pancreatitis

fractured, leading to the term *porcelain* gallbladder. Calcium is deposited in a linear manner within the muscle wall. The exact pathogenesis is unclear, though the wall is thickened and inflamed with loss of the mucosa, and the cystic duct is invariably obstructed. Despite these changes, the majority of cases are found as an incidental finding on abdominal imaging. It usually is seen in the 5th–7th decades of life and affects women in a ratio of up to 5:1. In up to 12–20% of cases, there may be an associated primary carcinoma of the gallbladder. (19,20)

Imaging Features. On plain film studies, the calcification is present as a thin, curvilinear opacity, which may outline the entire gallbladder as a pear-shaped or ovoid outline. (9) (Fig. 18-70) Less extensive calcifications occur and may be a sign of carcinomatous resorption of the deposits. (9,21) Occasionally the calcification may be bilayered owing to its presence in both the mucosa and the muscle epimysium. Small round wall calcifications can occur focally within intramural diverticula (Rokitansky-Aschoff sinuses). (21) CT is more accurate in depicting calcification. Complicating carcinoma can be seen on both ultrasound and CT as an exophytic or endoluminal mass. (1,8)

Pancreas

Diseases of the pancreas can cause musculoskeletal symptoms by a number of mechanisms. The most characteristic pain pattern is epigastric in location with radiation to the back. Back pain is typically thoracolumbar and mediated by direct inflammation or invasion of the retroperitoneum, sympathetic plexuses, and greater splanchnic nerves. Epigastric pain is mediated by peritoneal irritation. Less commonly, limb pain associated with migratory thrombophlebitis may herald the presence of carcinoma (Trousseau's sign). (6) The most important diseases are pancreatitis and carcinoma.

Pancreatitis

Synonyms. None.

Clinical Features. Inflammation of the pancreas may occur as an acute episode (acute pancreatitis) or as on-going low-grade inflammation (chronic pancreatitis), which may be punctuated by superimposed acute episodes (chronic relapsing pancreatitis). Pancreatitis may be idiopathic and familial or be secondary to alcohol, cholelithiasis, viral infection, trauma, drugs, malignancy, and metabolic disorders (such as hypercalcemia). Acute pancreatitis may produce pure edema (edematous pancreatitis), varying degrees of necrosis (necrotizing pancreatitis), or hemorrhage (hemorrhagic pancreatitis). (4) Chronic pancreatitis produces fat necrosis and saponification with calcification (chronic calcific pancreatitis) and ductal obstruction (chronic obstructive pancreatitis). (4) The diagnosis of pancreatitis rests on the correlation of history, clinical findings, laboratory results (especially elevated serum lipase), and imaging features.

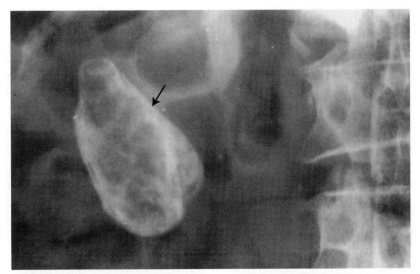

Figure 18-70 PORCELAIN GALLBLADDER. AP Abdomen.
Note the characteristic pear shape of the gallbladder, easily identified because of its densely calcified wall (*arrow*). *COMMENT:* Frequently the calcification is thinner and more subtle than this example. Plain film recognition of porcelain gallbladder is important because there is a higher incidence of associated adenocarcinoma of the gallbladder. Abdominal ultrasound or CT is performed preoperatively to identify signs of malignancy, including wall thickening, exophytic mass, liver invasion, and biliary duct obstruction.

Imaging Features. Plain film findings are often lacking in acute pancreatitis. Although not a specific sign, inflammation of the transverse colon with fluid accumulation in the phrenicocolic ligament may result in local spasm, creating an abrupt narrowing of the colon (*colon cutoff sign*). (22) Dilatation of the duodenum and proximal jejunum is a non-specific marker of localized inflammatory change (sentinel loop) that may also occur. Small pleural effusions are common. Ultrasound may be normal or may show enlargement with indistinct margins, reduced internal echoes, manifestations of fluid, or localized collections (pseudo-cysts). Arterial phase contrast-enhanced CT may show necrotic areas, characterized by local non-perfusion. Pancreatic edema and adjacent fluid collections can also be defined. (3,8)

In chronic pancreatitis the key finding on plain film, ultrasound, and CT is the presence of calcification. (6,16) (Fig. 18-71) These calcifications typically are coarse, dense, and globular, although they can sometimes be fine. They tend to occur at the L1–L2 level, although more extensive collections may form a pattern of irregular calcifications extending inferiorly and obliquely from the left upper quadrant crossing the abdominal midline. (1,23) The head is the most common site for calcification and may be the only site for these densities in 25% of cases. (23) CT and ultrasound will confirm the presence of calcifications more accurately and also show atrophy of the pancreas. Simultaneous assessment of the liver, spleen, and portal vein blood flow can be performed.

Carcinoma of the Pancreas

Synonyms. None.
Clinical Features. Carcinoma of the pancreas is the fourth leading cause of cancer-related deaths in North America. (5,24) Males are affected 2:1, with onset at 50–80 years of age, peaking at 70 years. (5) Most are pathologically scirrhous infiltrating adenocarcinomas, originating from the exocrine ductal epithelium. Two thirds involve the head, 25% the body, and 10% the tail of the pancreas. (5) Known associations include alcohol abuse, diabetes, smoking, and hereditary pancreatitis. The prognosis remains dismal, with a survival rate of < 10% at 1 year. (5,24) Symptoms include back pain, painless jaundice, thrombophlebitis, and weight loss.
Imaging Features. CT scan is the optimum method of detection, showing a spiculated mass in the pancreas with central low attenuation, biliary and pancreatic duct dilatation (*double-duct sign*), and extension posteriorly. (5) (Fig. 18-72) The key imaging feature affecting prognosis, other than distant metastasis, is the degree of encasement of the superior mesenteric artery. Greater than 50% encasement typically renders the tumor unresectable. (24)

Kidney and Adrenal Glands

Disorders of the kidney can often evoke musculoskeletal symptoms, especially back and loin pain. The most common conditions include renal calculus, carcinoma, and pyelonephritis.

Renal Calculus

Synonyms. Nephrolithiasis, urolithiasis, renal lithiasis, kidney stones.
Clinical Features. The population prevalence by age 70 may be as high as 12%, with 2–3% experiencing an attack of renal colic in a lifetime. (5) Many calculi remain idiopathic. Known causes can be classified under three broad categories: inadequate drainage, excess urinary constituents, and abnormal content. Inadequate drainage can be caused by diverticula and anomalies of the pelvicocaliceal system or ureters, such as horseshoe kidney and ureteric duplication. Excess urinary constituents occur from dehydration, hyperparathyroidism, sarcoidosis, Paget's disease, and gout. Abnormal urinary content includes cellular debris from infection, cystine, and xanthine.

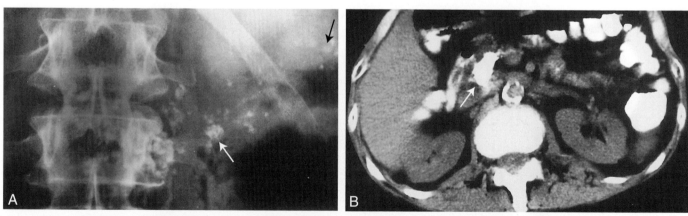

Figure 18-71 **CHRONIC PANCREATITIS. A. AP Lumbar Spine.** Note the multiple dense and irregular calcifications in the head and body of the pancreas superimposed across the L2 vertebral body (*arrows*). **B. CT, Axial Abdomen.** The calcification is confirmed within this atrophic pancreas (*arrow*).
COMMENT: Pancreatic calcification is caused by the hydrolysis of pancreatic fat that occurs as pancreatic lipases are released during pancreatitis. Common causes include impacted common bile duct calculi as well as familial tendency, coxsackie virus, hyperparathyroidism, alcohol abuse, and drug therapy (e.g., non-steroidal anti-inflammatory medications). In up to 50% of cases the cause remains unknown and, by exclusion, are diagnosed as idiopathic.

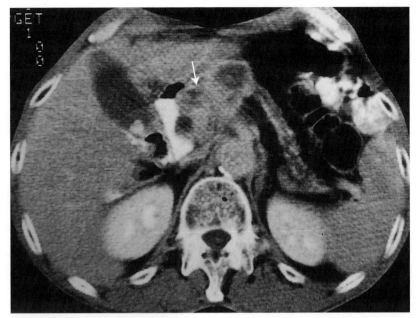

Figure 18-72   **PANCREATIC CARCINOMA. CT, Axial Abdomen.**
Observe the enlarged head of the pancreas, with compression
of the adjacent duodenum and common bile duct (*arrow*).
COMMENT: The pancreas is a difficult organ to image. CT is
the best suited modality; however, MRI may also be helpful.
The presence of gas within both the stomach and the duodenum significantly impairs evaluation by ultrasound.

Calculi are of six basic varieties: calcium oxalate, triple phosphate, uric acid, xanthine, cystine, and matrix. Each type can be
associated with specific clinical and radiologic patterns. (3,16)
(Table 18-12)

• *Calcium oxalate* stones are the most common form of
calculus and make up 75–85% of all nephrolithiases.
(16) They are more common in men, as high as
2–3:1; are typically encountered in the 3rd decade;
and are often familial. Most patients who form a
single stone continue to form additional stones every
2–3 years, an interval that may progressively shorten
with increasing age. These concretions grow as
biconcave ovals and are homogeneously dense on
imaging. (9,16)

• *Triple phosphate* (*struvite*) stones are the second most
common form and occur in 10–15% of cases. They are
composed of phosphate, combined with calcium, ammonium, and magnesium. These are usually found in women,
in a ratio as high as 5:1. They occur in combination with
urinary tract infections owing to urease-producing organisms (especially *Proteus*) and tend to form large branching
calculi that may fill the renal pelvis and calyces (*staghorn
calculi*). (3,8) These are potentially dangerous and require
surgical removal, as they can precipitate pyonephrosis and
renal failure. Infrequently, they can be extruded from the
kidney and cause psoas abscess. (25) They occur in diabetes in association with xanthogranulomatous pyelonephritis, neurogenic bladder, urinary diversion, and
indwelling catheters. (3,8)

	Incidence	Male:Female				
Type	**(%)**	**Ratio**	**Causes**	**Diagnosis**	**Imaging Findings**	**Treatment**
Calcium oxalate	75–85	3:1	Idiopathic; hyper-parathyroidism	Normal calcium; hypercalcemia	90% opaque; oval, solid	Diuretics; parathyroidectomy
Triple phosphate	10–15	1:5	Proteus infection; diabetes	Proteus; nitrite; stone analysis	100% opaque; staghorn	Surgery; antibiotics
Uric acid	5	4:1	Gout; dehydration; malignancy	Serum uric acid; stone analysis	100% lucent; hydronephrosis	Alkaline urine; uricosuric agents
Xanthine	1	1:1	Hereditary; bowel surgery	Urine oxalate; resection	90% opaque	Pyridoxine; fluids
Cystine	1	1:1	Hereditary	Stone analysis; urine cystine	90% opaque	Alkaline urine; massive fluids
Matrix	< 1	1:1	Infection; cellular debris	Stone analysis	100% lucent	Fluids; antibiotics

Table 18-12 | Clinicoradiologic Correlations of Renal Calculi

- *Uric acid* stones account for < 5% of stones. They occur characteristically in males with gout, although over half of the cases show elevated serum or urine uric acid with no known history of gout. Rarely, high cell turnover diseases such as malignancy, (especially leukemia), psoriasis, and postchemotherapy may produce uric acid calculi. They are radiolucent on x-ray imaging but detectable by ultrasound or urograms. (1,5)
- *Xanthine* stones are found in approximately 1% of cases of fat malabsorption, most commonly caused by diseases of the biliary tree, pancreas, or small bowel. High dietary intake of oxalate and ascorbic acid (vitamin C) and hereditary forms have been described. Xanthine stones are radiolucent. (1)
- *Cystine* stones are uncommon and are the result of an inherited defect in jejunal and proximal renal tubular transport. These stones contain sulfur, rendering them radiopaque. (1,9)
- *Matrix* stones are usually associated with the presence of infection or result from cellular debris that forms a solid mass of organic protein, such as mucoprotein and mucopolysaccharide. These can be radiolucent when unmineralized but often form the framework and nidus for subsequent crystal deposition, rendering them radiopaque. (1)

The classic triad for renal calculus is pain, hematuria, and visible calculus on an abdominal or lumbar spinal radiograph or CT. Pain is variable in intensity and location. It has been described as the worst pain experienced by humans, equivalent to or exceeding that of childbirth. It is a common diagnosis masqueraded by addicts to narcotics who exhibit drug-seeking behavior. (Fig. 18-73) A stone embedded within the renal parenchyma is often asymptomatic.

Once in a major or minor calyx, dull loin (flank) pain predominates. Impaction in the ureteropelvic junction (UPJ) produces *ureteric colic*—constant, agonizing pain that radiates from loin to groin, resulting in restlessness, hyperhydrosis, and emesis. (26) Progressive passage down the ureter produces pain lower in the groin into the scrotum or vulva. Once the stone enters the bladder, pain usually abates. The urethra is infrequently obstructed, and at least 60% of stones pass spontaneously. (5,16) Based on the short axis measurement of a stone, 1–2 mm, calculi usually pass without intervention, 3- to 5-mm stones have a 50% chance of unassisted passage, whereas those > 5 mm, especially if proximal in the ureter, are more than likely to require removal using a transurethral Dormia basket technique or (less likely) surgery. (26) Ureteric stents are often deployed to alleviate hydronephrosis and allow for passage over time. (1,16) In some cases, shockwave renal lithotripsy may be used to break up the stones.

Key clinical tests include serum calcium and uric acid; urine examination for hematuria, nitrites, and bacteria; stone analysis; and imaging.

Nephrocalcinosis. Nephrocalcinosis is a condition characterized by multiple small calculi deposited at the tips of the renal papillae and has multiple causes, including medullary sponge kidney (MSK), hypercalcemic disease (especially hyperparathyroidism), and renal tubular acidosis. MSK is a disease characterized by cystic dilatation of the terminal collecting ducts in which calcium oxalate calculi form. It may be unilateral, asymmetrical, or symmetrically bilateral. There is a bimodal distribution of occurrence, with peaks during adolescence and in the 3rd–4th decades. Calculi, infection, and/or hematuria are frequent presenting find-

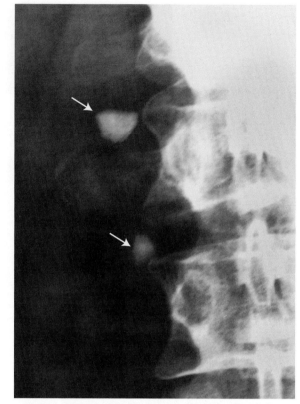

Figure 18-73 RENAL COLIC, DRUG ABUSE. AP Abdomen. Note the two renal calculi (*arrows*) in this initial film obtained on a patient presenting with renal colic. *COMMENT:* Following the initial film, the patient was given medication for pain relief. Subsequently, two small pieces of gravel secured with adhesive tape to the patient's back to simulate calculi were identified. This is a common trick for obtaining pain medications.

ings. Although familial clustering has been reported, cases are usually sporadic. On plain film imaging, the characteristic finding is multiple small opaque calculi, < 5 mm in size, orientated in a radiating fashion within the medullary pyramids (*bunch of flowers appearance*). A *calyceal diverticulum* occasionally develops small calculi that layer in the upright position. (8,16,27)

Imaging Features. Stones can be identified at any site within the kidney, renal pelvis, course of the ureter, or bladder. The radiographic appearance varies according to location. (Table 18-13) The most common sites for a calculus to obstruct the ureter are at the areas of normal constriction: at the UPJ, where the ureter passes over the iliac vessels (upper sacral level), and at the ureterovesical junction (UVJ). At least 75% of stones present in the lower ureter, especially at the UVJ. (3,16)

In the acute setting, an abdominal x-ray (KUB) is performed first because of availability, low cost, and sensitivity (the majority of stones are radiopaque). The most sensitive and specific imaging for renal calculi is a non-contrast helical CT scan, with the added advantage of visualizing other abdominal contents, which may be mimicking renal symptoms. Intravenous pyelograms (IVPs) and intravenous urograms (IVUs) have diminishing roles in stone evaluation. (3,8,16)

Plain Film. The majority of calculi are radiopaque, with a few exceptions: triple phosphate stones containing mainly magne-

Table 18-13	Plain Film Features of Urinary Calculi			
Factor	Parenchyma	Pelvicocaliceal	Ureter	Bladder
Location				
AP	T12–L3; beyond psoas edge	L1–L3; overlies psoas	L1 to pelvis; overlies transverse processes and sacral ala	Pelvic inlet; ureterovesical junction to 2 cm from ischial spine
Lateral	Overlies spine	Anterior to spine	Anterior to spine	Behind pubis
Size (mm)	1–5	1– > 20	1–5	1– > 20
Shape	Round to oval	Angular (staghorn)	Oval, irregular	Round to oval; faceted when multiple
Density	Solid	Solid or laminated	Solid	Solid or laminated
Axis	Any	Any	Superior to inferior	Any

sium ammonium phosphate (struvite), matrix stones, uric acid, and xanthine. Calculi within the renal parenchyma lie between T12 and L3 and lateral to the spine. On a lateral projection, stones commonly overlie the vertebrae and may mimic a bone island. (25) (Fig. 18-74) The stones are usually round to oval in shape when in the renal parenchyma and are often more angular or triangular when present in a calyx. A staghorn calculus is readily recognizable by its branching pattern, similar to the *antler* rack of a mature *stag;* it forms a cast-like impression of the pelvicocaliceal system. (5,13)

A calculus within the UPJ lies close to the spine, overlapping the transverse process of L2 or L3. Along the course of the ureter, calculi overlie the lower lumbar transverse processes and sacral ala. Calculi of the ureter can be mimicked by phleboliths. In the middle to distal ureter, concretions within the ascending gonadal vein are usually round and have a lucent center, whereas calculi are oval to irregular in shape and homogenously solid. (1,3) At the level of the UVJ, phleboliths within the perivesical plexus of the bladder are more difficult to distinguish from calculi, though the same criteria can be applied. Most UVJ stones lodge within 2 cm of the ischial spine. Following ultrasonographic renal lithotripsy, calculi often lodge in a stacked manner at the UVJ (*steine strasse* street, street of stones). (8,26)

CT. A non-contrast helical CT with 5-mm slice thickness display is the bare minimum technique required. (28) The size threshold sensitivity can be down to < 1 mm. Nearly all calculi are radiopaque to CT examination and depicted as a dense opacity within the kidney parenchyma, pelvis, or ureter. A stone in the ureter will be surrounded by a ring of thickened, inflamed ureteric wall, visible on CT as a *rim sign,* useful in differentiation from a phlebolith. (29) Key indirect signs include renal enlargement, perinephric inflammation (*stranding*), hydronephrosis, and hydroureter. (28) To determine if stones at the UVJ have passed into the bladder perform supine and prone views, demonstrating gravity-dependent movement.

Ultrasound. Calculi within the parenchyma show as a reflective surface (echogenic) with posterior shadowing. Most calculi down to 1 mm will be visible, but smaller calculi can be overlooked when the examination is technically impaired owing to patient size, renal scarring, improper technique, or use of the wrong probe. Hydronephrosis is well demonstrated. Calculi within the ureter are often obscured by overlying intestinal gas. Ureteric obstruction can be confirmed using Doppler technique to show no urinary flow through the UVJ (*jet sign*). Bladder calculi are readily shown as echogenic densities with posterior shadowing and may lie within the bladder diverticula. (16,27)

Carcinoma of the Kidney

Synonyms. Adenocarcinoma, hypernephroma, Grawitz tumor. **Clinical Features.** The most common form of carcinoma of the kidney is renal cell carcinoma, which makes up 90% of all renal malignancies. Males are affected 2:1, and this malignancy occurs most often between 50 and 70 years of age. (30) Known associations include smoking, phenacetin, and hemodialysis. Tumors > 5 cm at presentation will, in 75% of cases, have distant metastases. These tumors are notoriously clinically silent and present when large or with diffuse metastatic disease. (31) The known clinical triad in a male is painless hematuria, testicular varicocele, and fever. (3,8)
Imaging Features. CT and ultrasound are the definitive methods for diagnosis, usually showing a polar mass that is vascular, necrotic, and cystic. (Fig. 18-75) Calcification is visible in 15% of cases. (9,13) This may be seen on plain film but is more obvious on CT.

Miscellaneous Renal and Adrenal Disorders

Renal Cysts. Renal cysts are benign lesions found in up to 3% of autopsies and are the most common renal pathology demonstrated on imaging in patients > 50 years of age. (1,3) They occur secondary to tubular obstruction. The majority remain asymptomatic unless complicated by hemorrhage or become large enough (> 5 cm) to cause compression effects. These have no relationship to polycystic kidney disease. Ultrasound imaging is definitive in most cases, showing a thin-walled, fluid-filled lesion with posterior acoustic enhancement. No enhancement occurs in these avascular lesions with CT examination. (5,16) (Fig. 18-76)
Adrenal Hemorrhage. Adrenal hemorrhage may occur spontaneously, with birth complications, concurrent with stress, and as a complication of anticoagulant therapy. It typically heals with calcification. (Fig. 18-77)

Gastrointestinal

Inflammatory Bowel Disease

The association of inflammatory bowel disease (IBD) with musculoskeletal manifestations is well known, especially the occurrence of synovitis of the peripheral joints and ankylosing

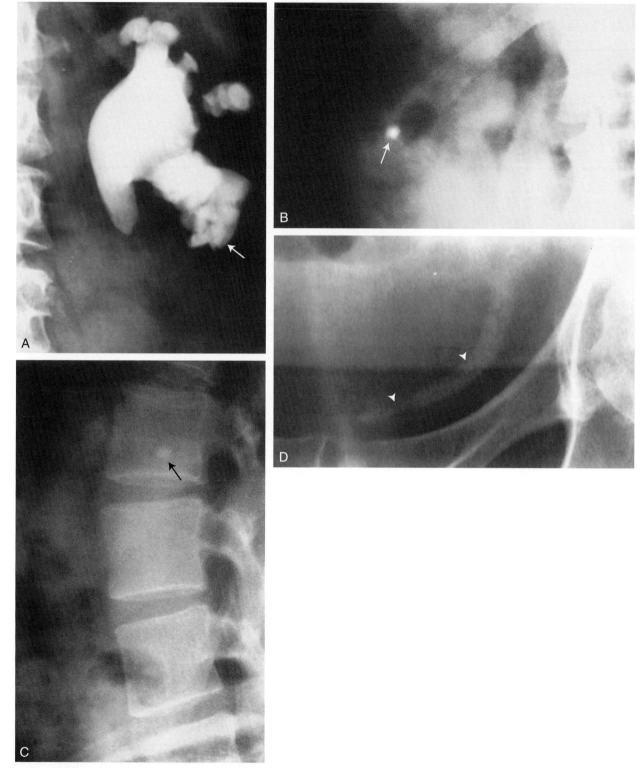

Figure 18-74 RENAL CALCULUS. A. Staghorn Calculus, AP Abdomen. Note the characteristic dense calcification forming a cast-like appearance within the renal pelvis and associated calyces (*arrow*). **B. Calculus, AP Lumbar Spine.** Observe the small dense calcification over the upper pole of the kidney (*arrow*). **C. Calculus, Lateral Lumbar Spine.** Note the small calculus over the vertebral body of L1 (*arrow*). **D. Postlithotripsy Ureteric Calculi.** Following lithotripsy, small impacted renal calculi fragments are identified in the distal ureter (*steine strasse* street, street of stones) (*arrowheads*). *COMMENT:* At least 90% of all renal calculi are visible on plain film radiographs. However, small calculi can be difficult to identify on AP projections because of overlying gas and feces. On lateral lumbar projections these may simulate bone islands. Non-contrast helical CT is the modality of choice for renal calculus demonstration.

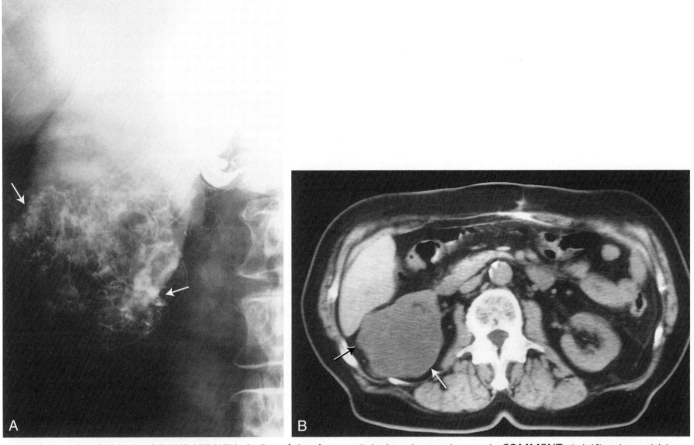

Figure 18-75   **CARCINOMA OF THE KIDNEY. A. Renal Angiogram, AP Abdomen.** Note the neovascularity distributed throughout a tumor mass originating from the lower pole of the kidney (*arrows*). **B. Axial Abdominal CT.** In a different patient observe the renal carcinoma, which is shown as a lobulated mass (*arrows*). *COMMENT:* Calcification within carcinoma of the kidney is relatively uncommon, being found in only 10–15% of cases. (Courtesy of Neils Egund, MD, Arhus, Denmark.)

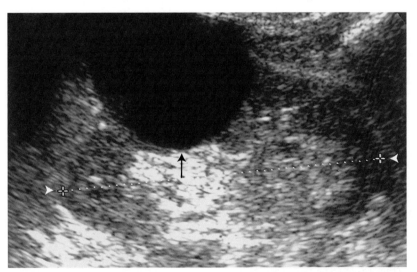

Figure 18-76   **RENAL CYST. Ultrasound, Abdomen.** Note the well-defined, thin-walled anechoic cyst extending from the renal cortex (*arrow*). The longitudinal dimension of the kidney is being measured on this study (*arrowheads*). *COMMENT:* Renal cysts are the most common abnormality of the kidney and are frequently observed incidentally on CT and ultrasound. They are usually asymptomatic, unless they are large enough or multiple and cause distension of the renal capsule. Aspiration may be necessary to reduce the symptoms. Cyst wall calcification is occasionally identified on plain film radiographs but is seen less often than calcification associated with carcinoma.

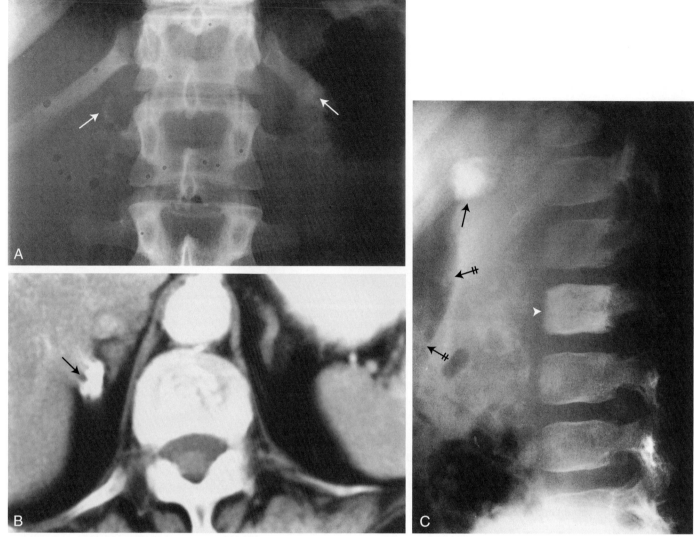

Figure 18-77 ADRENAL GLAND CALCIFICATION. A. Post-hemorrhage, AP Abdomen. Observe the subtle, finely calcified masses within the soft tissues adjacent to the T12–L1 level (*arrows*). **B. Posthemorrhage, CT, Axial Abdomen.** Note that the adrenal gland calcification appears considerably more dense on CT (*arrow*). **C. Neuroblastoma, Lateral Lumbar Spine.** Note the dense calcification in the subdiaphragmatic region (*arrow*). More diffuse calcification is present within the abdominal soft tissues anterior to the metastatic *ivory vertebra* at L2 (*arrowhead*). Note the anterior displacement of the adjacent intestinal gas shadows, confirming the retroperitoneal location of the mass (*crossed arrows*). *COMMENT:* The most common cause of adrenal gland calcification is previous hemorrhage, which characteristically has a dense structureless appearance. Calcification within the adrenal gland is associated with a number of conditions, including Addison's disease, tuberculosis, pheochromocytoma, and neuroblastoma (usually in children < 3 years old). CT examination may be employed to further evaluate adrenal gland calcifications.

spondylitis–like changes of the axial skeleton (enteropathic spondylitis). Neither these skeletal findings nor the abdominal soft tissue findings seen on plain film radiographic examination are sufficient for diagnosis. The mainstay for imaging diagnosis remains the barium contrast study. CT is also useful, both in diagnosis and identification of complications such as fistulae and intra-abdominal collections. (32,33) (Fig. 18-78) The two main presentations of IBD are ulcerative colitis and Crohn's disease. In ulcerative colitis the colon is the target site, and Crohn's disease affects the small bowel, especially the terminal ileum. Ulcerative colitis is associated with mucosal ulcerations, pseudo-polyps, and loss of the normal haustrations. Crohn's disease is characterized by strictures (*string sign*), skip lesions, cobblestone mucosal appearance, loop separation, and fistula formation. (4,8,32)

Diverticular Disease

Outpouching of colonic mucosa occurs through the sites of normal vascular perforation into the media owing to increased intraluminal pressures. The incidence of the disease increases with age, affecting 10% of the population by age 50 years and involving

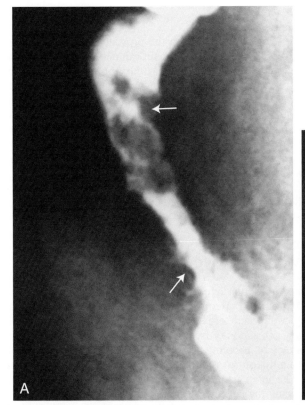

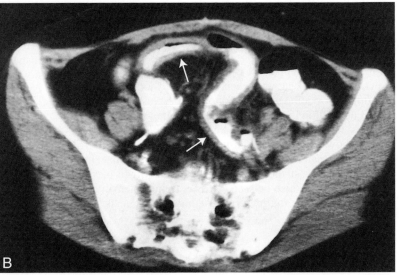

Figure 18-78 **CROHN'S DISEASE. A. Barium Series, Small Bowel.** Observe that a portion of the terminal ileum is narrowed and exhibits mucosal surface irregularity (cobblestone appearance) with linear (rose thorn) ulcers (*arrows*). **B. CT, Axial Abdomen.** Note the segment of ileum with thick walls and no mucosal detail (*arrows*). The narrowed lumen is characteristic (string sign). *COMMENT:* The most common location for Crohn's disease is the terminal ileum. Both barium-contrast radiologic examination and CT are often required for complete assessment.

> 50% after 70 years. The most common location is the sigmoid colon. Complicating infections from fecal impaction lead to inflammatory change (diverticulitis), which can precipitate perforation and pericolonic abscess. Barium enema is diagnostic, and CT and ultrasound are useful for identifying complications. (3,8,34) (Fig. 18-79)

Carcinoma of the Colon

Carcinoma of the colon is the second most frequently diagnosed malignancy, representing the third most common cause of cancer death in both men and women. Known associations include low-fiber diets, familial and hereditary polyposis syndromes,

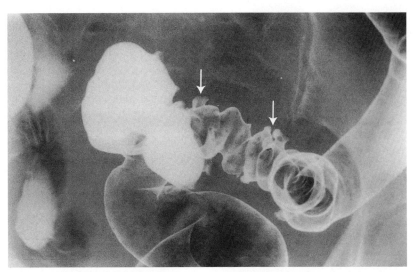

Figure 18-79 **BARIUM ENEMA, DIVERTICULAR DISEASE.** Double-contrast barium enema demonstrates multiple outpouchings (diverticula) within the sigmoid colon (*arrows*). *COMMENT:* These diverticula are round and smooth, without evidence of barium extravasation. Diverticulitis can be associated with these complicating changes.

polyps, family history, ulcerative colitis, and malignancy of the uterus and breast. The most common sites are the sigmoid, rectum, and cecum. Barium enema is the mainstay of imaging diagnosis, demonstrating a polypoid intraluminal mass or annular (*apple core*) constriction. (Fig. 18-80) CT can identify these tumors as localized wall thickening. The use of CT colonography, as it is refined, may provide a non-invasive alternative to direct colonoscopy and is rapidly replacing barium enema for early diagnosis. (4,6,16)

Appendicitis

Inflammation of the appendix is a common disorder of younger patients, with a peak age between 10 and 30 years. The appendiceal lumen is occluded by lymphoid hyperplasia, fecalith, or foreign body, allowing for stasis of the contents and development of ischemia of the appendiceal wall. Plain films are reported to show abnormalities in up to 50% of cases, with 15% showing a laminated appendicolith. (9,33) Loss of adjacent fat planes of the flank stripe and obturator and a soft tissue mass of variable size may also be seen. CT is extremely sensitive and highly specific and is the preferred method of diagnosis. (4,32) (Fig. 18-81)

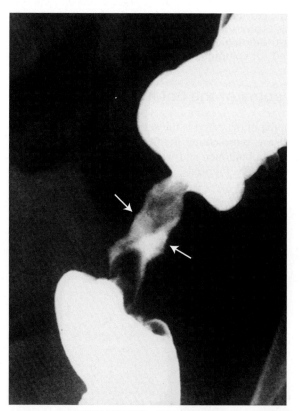

Figure 18-80 BARIUM ENEMA, CARCINOMA OF THE COLON. Note the localized concentric narrowing of the lumen in the sigmoid colon, creating an *apple-core* deformity (*arrows*). *COMMENT:* Barium enema remains a highly sensitive and specific study for identifying colon cancer and is frequently used when colonoscopy either fails or is unable to be performed.

Prostate Gland

Musculoskeletal symptoms from the prostate gland relate either to prostatitis, causing suprapubic pain mimicking that emanating from the symphysis pubis, or to primary bone pain caused by metastatic prostate carcinoma. Secondary obstruction of the bladder and renal systems may produce back and pelvic pain. Imaging of the prostate gland is best performed initially with transrectal ultrasound, which shows the size of the gland; internal architecture; presence of any calcifications; and secondary effects on the bladder, ureters, and collecting systems. Plain film examinations are useful only for detecting calculi or co-existing bony metastases. CT is used for staging purposes in the presence of carcinoma. The mass effect of prostate enlargement is often noted on contrast studies (IVP or IVU) of the urinary tract.

Benign Prostate Hypertrophy

Synonyms. Nodular hyperplasia, benign prostate hyperplasia.
Clinical Features. Benign prostate hypertrophy (BPH) is an extremely common disorder, occurring in 8% of males by age 40, 50% by age 60, and 90% by age 90. (35) Symptoms include urinary hesitancy or dribbling and delayed or incomplete micturition, often with a history of recurrent urinary tract infection. Pathologically, the inner paraurethral tissue undergoes nodular hyperplasia, sparing the peripheral glandular tissue. (8,35)
Imaging Features. The modality of choice is ultrasound, which shows enlargement of the gland. Secondary outlet obstructive changes may also be seen, including thickening and trabeculation of the bladder wall, diverticula, incomplete emptying, and hydronephrosis. (35) (Fig. 18-82) Intravenous pyelograms show a characteristic bilobed *umbrella* filling defect at the base of the bladder, a finding also seen on CT. Plain film studies show no abnormality, except in the presence of prostatic calculi, which may be displaced superiorly in a convex arch arrangement. (35)

Prostatic Calculi

Synonyms. Prostate calcification, prostatic lithiasis.
Clinical Features. Calcification within the glands and ducts of the prostate is a relatively common radiologic finding. The prevalence increases with age, especially after the 4th decade. The majority of cases are asymptomatic, though occasionally symptoms of prostatitis may occur, including dysuria and perineal or suprapubic pain. When complicated by bacterial infection, fever and pyuria may also be noted. The pathogenesis of prostatic calculi is unclear, although both bacterial prostatitis and benign prostatic hypertrophy can produce dilated glandular acini and ducts, promoting stasis of secretions, proteinaceous deposition, blood clots, and the accumulation of infected debris. Dystrophic calcification of this material may occur, referred to as *corpora amylacea.* (13)

The distribution of the calculi is variable but is most commonly symmetric within the posterior and lateral lobes. Asymmetric calculi distribution is occasionally seen. There is no association with carcinoma of the prostate gland. Calculi are not specifically treated by removal. (8,35)
Imaging Features. On plain film studies the calcifications may be subtle and sand-like or more dense clusters of amorphous globular calcifications bridging the midline, either above or behind the

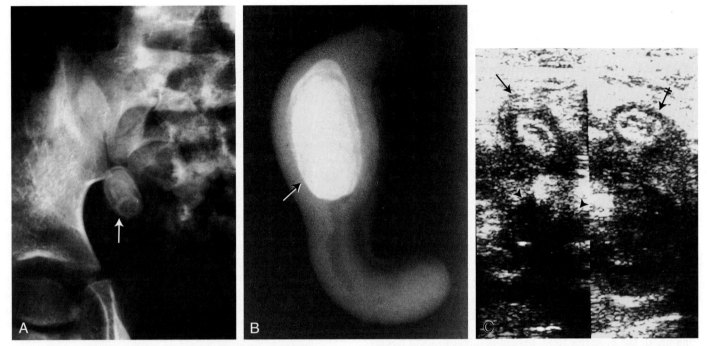

Figure 18-81   **APPENDICITIS. A. Appendicolith, AP Abdomen.** Note the laminated calculus within the appendix overlying the right iliac fossa (*arrow*). **B. Appendicolith, Surgical Specimen.** The location and fine detail of the laminated appendicolith are demonstrated (*arrow*). **C. Appendicitis with Abscess, Ultrasound, Abdomen.** Observe the target appearance of the appendix (*arrow*). The diameter of the appendix in cross section measures 17 mm; it is surrounded by a hypo-echoic (dark) fluid collection posteriorly (*arrowheads*). An important sign of inflammation is the lack of appendix wall deformity by compression of the sonographic probe through the abdominal wall (*crossed arrow*). COMMENT: Plain films may demonstrate an appendicolith in up to 15% of patients with appendicitis. CT is the preferred method of investigation because it is extremely sensitive and highly specific for findings of acute appendicitis.

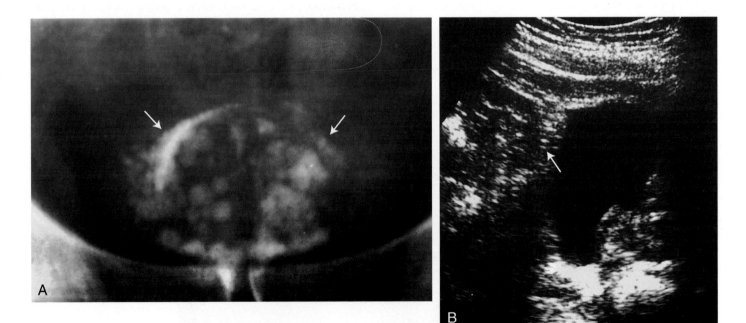

Figure 18-82   **BENIGN PROSTATIC HYPERTROPHY. A. AP Pelvis.** Observe the peripheral prostate gland calcification superimposed over the symphysis pubis and adjacent pelvic soft tissues. The calcification is present within the subcapsular space of the gland (*arrows*). **B. Ultrasound, Sagittal Abdomen.** Note that the enlarged prostate forms a prominent indentation at the base of the bladder (*arrow*). COMMENT: Prostate size and evidence of associated chronic outlet obstruction of the bladder are best assessed with ultrasound.

symphysis pubis. (Fig. 18-83) In prostatic hypertrophy the calcifications may be elevated well above the pubis and can be arranged in an arc-like fashion superiorly. (16) Overlap with the pubic bones can produce confusion with osteitis pubis, insufficiency fractures, healing fracture, and osteoblastic bone metastases.

Non-contrast enhanced CT confirms the small sand-like calcifications within the prostate gland behind the pubis. (3,16) On pelvic ultrasound calcifications are displayed as echogenic foci with posterior shadowing within the gland. Calcification within the vas deferens is virtually pathognomonic for diabetes and diverges from the midline above the pubis in a tubular pattern. On occasion the vas deferens can be traced along its course through the inguinal canal to the scrotum. (5,16) (Fig. 18-84)

Carcinoma of the Prostate

Synonyms. None.

Clinical Features. Malignancy of the prostate gland is the second most common cause of cancer-related deaths in males, and affects up to 1 in 11 over a lifetime (9%). It is rare in Asian men. It occurs only rarely < 50 years of age. The tumor arises from glandular epithelium of the peripheral subcapsular acini, most commonly in the posterior lobe. Spread is direct to local tissues such as the seminal vesicles, bladder, urethra, and rarely the rectum. (36) Lymphatic dissemination occurs to iliac and para-aortic nodes, with hematogenous spread by the Batson venous plexus to the lumbar spine, pelvis, and upper femora. The most sensitive serological marker of carcinoma is prostate-specific antigen (PSA), which provides a diagnostic and therapeutic marker far more sensitive than the previously used acid phosphatase. (36)

Four clinical presentations are described:

- Asymptomatic and discovered either on digital examination or secondary to high PSA.

- Bladder outflow obstruction symptoms (recurrent infection, biopsy for BPH).
- Surrounding tissue infiltrative effects (incontinence, constipation).
- Bone metastases (back pain, spinal cord compression, pathologic fracture, or unanticipated finding on diagnostic imaging).

Prognosis is determined by Gleason's staging (A–D), on which there remains continuing debate. (36) Essentially, microscopic malignancy-only categories (stage A) do not show spread after 10 years, though 5% do develop invasive disease. This is the most controversial stage in regard to determining what treatment, if any, is appropriate. Once a palpable nodule (stage B) is found, all cases will progress unless treated, with worsening prognosis when there is disruption of the capsule (stage C) or spread to pelvic and distal sites (stage D). At least 75% of patients present with stage C or D cancer. (36,37)

Imaging Features. Transrectal ultrasound can show a normal appearance to the prostate gland or abnormalities, such as an irregular external contour, altered internal architecture, nodule, and signs of outlet obstruction. Transrectal ultrasound has been used to more accurately identify nodules and increased vascularity and to guide biopsy of abnormal sites. MRI is the most sensitive method for demonstrating nodules and extracapsular spread. (37) CT is also commonly used for staging, when MRI is not available.

Following radical surgery impotence is common and can be treated by implant technology, which is readily recognizable on plain film and CT studies. There are no plain film features of prostate cancer other than bone or lung metastases. Nuclear bone scan is the most sensitive imaging for metastases, though MRI has been advocated as an alternative, especially in the spine, pelvis, and proximal long bones. (3,16) (See Chapter 11.)

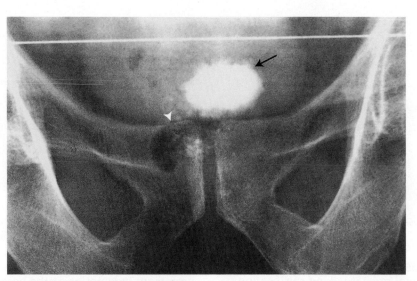

Figure 18-83 PROSTATIC AND BLADDER CALCULI. AP Pelvis. Note the large round, spiculated calcification, which represents a bladder calculus (*arrow*). The adjacent smaller sand-like calcifications are located within the prostate gland (*arrowhead*). *COMMENT:* Prostatic calcifications are commonly seen bridging the midline, either above or overlying the symphysis pubis. In prostatic hypertrophy, the calcifications may be displaced well above the pubic region. In this case, the association of prostatic enlargement with a bladder calculus suggests urinary retention with subsequent stone formation. (Courtesy of Stanley I. Innes, B.App.Sc. (Chiro), Melbourne, Australia.)

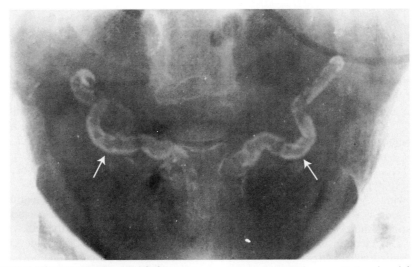

Figure 18-84 **VAS DEFERENS CALCIFICATION. AP Abdomen.** Observe the tubular (conduit) calcification bilaterally, which converges at the prostate gland (*arrows*). *COMMENT:* This finding is virtually diagnostic of diabetes mellitus.

Uterus

Uterine Fibroids

Synonyms. Leiomyoma.
Clinical Features. Fibroids are the most common tumors of women, found in 25% during active reproductive life. They are estrogen sensitive, regressing in menopause and after oophorectomy. Pregnancy often results in enlargement but regression occurs again in the puerperium. They may occur within the muscular wall (intramural), beneath the endometrium (submucosal), or in the serosa (subserosal). Histologically they are composed of smooth muscle bundles in a characteristic circular (*whorled*) pattern, which often have areas of red softening (*red degeneration*) or white hyalinization (*white degeneration*). (16) The majority involve the corpus and fundus, with < 3% at the cervix.

At least 75% of fibroids are asymptomatic, though local pressure symptoms on the bladder or rectum may produce pain or frequency. They may promote infertility, abortion, intra-uterine growth retardation, premature labor, dystocia, and postpartum hemorrhage. Abnormal vaginal bleeding is probably the most common direct clinical presentation. Malignant transformation to leiomyosarcoma occurs in < 1% of cases. (1,3)
Imaging Features. Ultrasound is the best method for detecting and assessing any effect on pregnancy. (32) Calcified fibroids are best seen on CT, though plain films of the pelvis often allow their diagnosis. (Fig. 18-85)
Plain Film. Uncalcified leiomyomas may be perceived as hazy soft tissue density masses above the bladder. Less than 10% of uterine fibroids contain enough calcium to be seen on plain film studies. (8,9,13) Three patterns of calcification are encountered: densely packed flocculent, non-confluent flocculent, and circum-

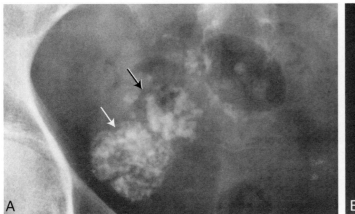

Figure 18-85 **UTERINE FIBROIDS (LEIOMYOMA). A. AP Abdomen.** Note the multiple calcified fibroids within the pelvic soft tissues (*arrows*). **B. Ultrasound Longitudinal Abdomen.** Observe the areas of increased tissue echogenicity (*arrow*) and acoustic shadowing (*arrowheads*) in this calcified intramural uterine fibroid. This distinctive appearance is the result of calcification that impairs normal soft tissue transmission of the sound waves. *COMMENT:* Less than 10% of uterine fibroids contain enough calcium to be seen on plain film radiographs. The pattern of calcification may be densely packed, flocculent, non-confluent, or circumferential. The most readily recognizable pattern of calcification is the round, densely packed form with few internal radiolucencies. Ultrasound remains the most commonly used modality for diagnosis.

ferential. Flocculent presentations are described as having a *popcorn ball* appearance on plain films. The densely packed form is the most readily recognizable, appearing round and dense with few internal radiolucencies. The less densely packed type exhibits scattered calcific foci interspersed with wide zones of radiolucency. The outer margin of the peripheral annular type calcification can be coarse or thin and may mimic a pelvic arterial aneurysm. (1,27)

Ultrasound. Transvaginal scanning greatly increases the sensitivity of the examination. (38) A fibroid may cause distortion of the uterine or endometrial surface, with variable internal density from hyperechoic to isoechoic to hypoechoic. Internal calcification results in posterior shadowing. (38)

CT. On CT most fibroids are seen as a mass that is contiguous with the uterus but demonstrating a sharp margin. (39) Variable contrast enhancement occurs. Calcification is more readily depicted on CT than on routine radiographs. (8,16)

Ovary

Musculoskeletal symptoms from ovarian disease are uncommon, though pain in the iliac fossae or lower abdomen and referred pain to the sacrum are occasionally encountered. Imaging of the pelvis, sacrum, hip, and related articulations may incidentally show ovarian-based cystic, solid, or calcified lesions. Disorders of the ovary are many and only the most important are dealt with in this section: cysts, carcinoma, and teratoma.

Ovarian Cyst

Cysts are the most common abnormality of the ovary and have a number of causes. Two broad categories of cysts exist: physiologic and pathologic. (Fig. 18-86) Ultrasound is the imaging technique of choice, preferably performed transvaginally.

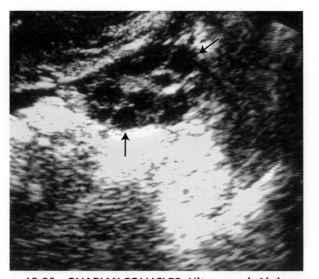

Figure 18-86 OVARIAN FOLLICLES. Ultrasound, Abdomen. Note the multiple small hypoechoic cysts within the ovary, representing normally maturing follicles (*arrows*). *COMMENT:* Cysts > 2 cm can represent developing follicles, corpus luteal cysts, or, less likely, cystadenoma and need to be followed with sequential ultrasound to document their stability or resolution.

Synonyms. None.

Physiologic Cysts. Physiologic cysts occur in response to the normal hormonal fluctuations of the menstrual cycle. Developing follicles enlarge up to midcycle (*Graafian follicle*). On release of the ovum after midcycle, a cystic structure remains (*corpus luteal cyst*), normally regressing by onset of the next cycle. (38) Cysts < 2 cm on ultrasound that have thin walls, are non-septated, and contain no solid components are not clinically relevant in most cases and resolve within 4–6 weeks. (38) If a mature follicle fails to regress, it can continue to enlarge to 4–10 cm and cause pain. However, these cysts usually resolve within two menstrual cycles (follicular cyst).

Pathologic Cysts. Suspicious imaging characteristics of ovarian cysts include thick walls, septations, solid components, progressive growth, vascularity, and co-existing free peritoneal fluid. Causes include ectopic pregnancy, endometrioma, cystadenoma/carcinoma, and abscess. (1)

Carcinoma of the Ovary

Ovarian cancer is the eighth leading cause of cancer in women and the third most common gynecologic malignancy after cervical and endometrial tumors. (40) Known associations for increased risk include family history and breast and colorectal cancer. Ovarian tumors may arise from surface epithelium, sex chords, germ cells, or metastatic origins (Krukenberg's tumors). Benign tumors constitute 80% of ovarian neoplasms and are generally found in women 20–45 years of age. (40,41) Ovarian fibroma can be associated with ascites and pleural effusions (Meigs' syndrome). The majority of ovarian tumors are derived from the surface epithelium and, depending on the dominant cell type, are classified as serous, mucinous, or endometrioid. (1,8)

Synonyms. None.

Serous Tumors. The serous type of ovarian tumor (serous cystadenoma or cystadenocarcinoma) is characterized by a large cyst containing fluid, which can be up to liters in volume. This is the most common ovarian tumor, accounting for up to 30% of both benign and malignant lesions. About 75% are benign and occur between 20 and 50 years of age. (40) They are often bilateral. Malignant lesions usually occur after 50 years of age.

Ultrasound is the best method of detection, demonstrating multiple cysts of the ovary that are > 5 cm in size, often with thick septae. (43) Large lesions can also be seen on CT. (43) (Fig. 18-87) When the septae demonstrate a nodular, thick, or solid component, the likelihood of malignancy is increased. Calcification in psammoma bodies that is visible on plain film is unusual, but may occur in 10% of cases. Calcification may be diffuse, cloud-like or smudgy densities; more focal flocculent calcification; or even fine stippled opacities. (44) On CT the calcification is usually within the solid components and only occasionally in the cyst wall. (43)

Mucinous Tumors. Mucinous tumors account for 25% of ovarian neoplasms and are often characterized by huge volumes, larger than that seen in serous types. They are principally a tumor of middle age and approximately 80% are benign. (40) Rare spread to the intraperitoneal surface results in *pseudo-myxoma peritonei* (jelly belly). Ultrasound is the preferred method for detection and characterization, though CT can also provide similar information. (42) Calcification is rare and is similar to serous types. (5)

Endometrioid Tumors. Endometrioid tumors make up 20% of ovarian tumors and are usually malignant. Up to 15% are

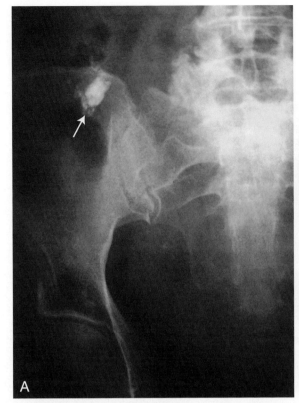

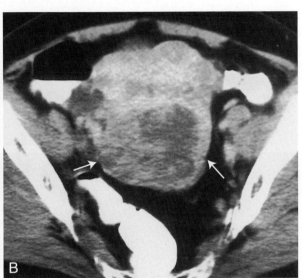

Figure 18-87   **CARCINOMA OF THE OVARY. A. AP Pelvis.** Note the irregular calcification within the ovary overlying the iliac crest (*arrow*). The absence of bowel gas centrally overlying the sacrum is caused by a soft tissue mass displacing the gas superiorly. **B. Axial Abdominal CT.** Observe the large solid mass, originating in the adnexal region, within the pelvis (*arrows*). *COMMENT:* Ultrasound is the modality of choice for the early detection of ovarian masses. CT studies are usually reserved for staging and assessing therapeutic progress.

associated with endometriosis, and up to 30% have co-existing carcinoma of the endometrium. (40) There are no specific imaging findings other than ovarian mass.

Teratoma

Synonyms. Dermoid cyst, mature teratoma, cystic teratoma.
Clinical Features. Teratomas arise from totipotential cells that migrate to abnormal sites during early embryonic development. Teratomas account for approximately 15% of ovarian tumors and are the second most common tumor of women between 20 and 40 years of age, after uterine leiomyoma (fibroids). They are the most common germ cell tumor of the ovary, and are classified into three types: mature (benign), immature (malignant), and monodermal. (40)
Mature Teratoma. The mature type is the most common form of teratoma. They are usually cystic, benign, and derived from ectodermal differentiation of totipotential cells. The major components are skin, fat, hair, and teeth, which is why they are often referred to as *dermoid tumors.* Most have structures from other germ layers, including cartilage, bone, muscle, and other body organs such as thyroid tissue. Greater than 95% contain cysts (cystic teratoma) lined with squamous epithelium and contain hair and sebaceous material. A mural-based nodule (Rokitansky nodule, dermal plug) made up of all three germ layers is frequently present and from it rare secondary malignancy can develop. (45) Malignant transformation, usually to squamous cell

carcinoma, occurs in 1–2% of cases. (46,47) Solid mature teratoma is uncommon.

Mature teratomas are characteristically found in women of reproductive age. Up to 15% are bilateral. Almost 25% are asymptomatic and found incidentally on pelvic imaging. (48) Back and pelvic pain are common symptoms, which can arise from ovarian torsion, rupture, or infection; obstruction of a ureter; or vaginal bleeding. Many cases have been described by a broad spectrum of musculoskeletal health providers in which the presenting symptoms are back and pelvic pain. (41,49) Oophorectomy is the usual treatment.

Immature Teratoma. Immature teratoma is a rare variety found in the 1st–2nd decades of life. The component tissues are primitive and can be aggressive with early metastases.

Monodermal Teratoma. A single embryonic derivative, usually thyroid (struma ovarii) or carcinoid, known as a monodermal teratoma, is rare. (3,8)

Imaging Features. Ultrasound is the imaging modality of choice for teratoma detection. It is highly sensitive and specific, does not involve ionizing radiation, and is cost effective. CT and MRI can be useful for demonstrating fat in cases in which the diagnosis remains unclear. Incidental teratoma is often observed on plain film studies of the abdomen, spine, pelvis, or hip. (8,16) (Fig. 18-88)

Plain Film. The characteristic finding on plain film is a round, soft tissue mass off the midline in the pelvis, which may be the density of water or fat and contain calcification, ossification, or teeth. Tooth formation may be elaborate and is seen in at least

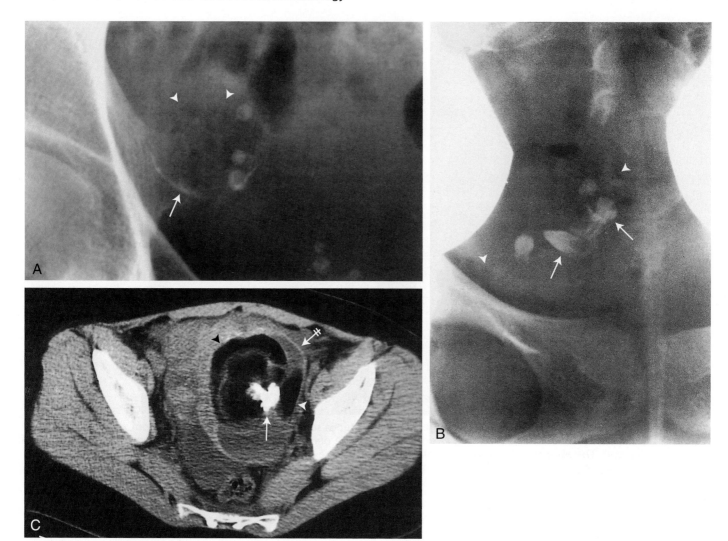

Figure 18-88   TERATOMA (DERMOID CYST). A. Fat-Containing Lesion, AP Pelvis. Observe the round radiolucency (*arrowheads*), representing fat, associated with a thin rim of curvilinear calcification (*arrow*) within a teratoma. The round radiodensities adjacent to this mass represent unrelated phleboliths. **B. Fat- and Dental-Containing Lesion, AP Pelvis.** Note the dense calcification within the pelvic soft tissues, representing malformed teeth (*arrows*). There is a surrounding area of low density caused by contained fat (*arrowheads*). **C. Fat- and Dental-Containing Lesion, Contrast-Enhanced CT, Axial Abdomen.** Note the vestigial dental elements within the Rokitansky nodule (*arrow*) surrounded by fat (*arrowheads*) and an enhancing cyst wall (*crossed arrow*). *COMMENT:* The major components of these dermoid tumors are skin, fat, hair, and teeth. Most contain materials from other germ layers, including cartilage, bone, muscle, and other body organs such as thyroid. The Rokitansky nodule is composed of tissues from all three germ layers and is frequently present when rare secondary malignancy develops. Malignant transformation can occur in 1–2% of cases.

30% of cases. (50) At least 10% will have curvilinear calcification in the cyst wall. Two thirds of all cases will be visible on plain film, and at least 40% of cases exhibit characteristics that allow a specific diagnosis of teratoma. (51) The fat present is typically radiolucent on plain film and reveals a low attenuation on CT. Use of pelvic gonadal shields may obstruct the lesion. Once identified, an ultrasound examination should be performed to confirm the diagnosis as well as to inspect the contralateral ovary for bilateral lesions. (8,50,27)

Ultrasound. Transvaginal ultrasound is the technique of choice. The sensitivity for teratoma detection with transvaginal ultrasound is at least 88%, with specificities as high as 97%. (1,48) Findings are of an adnexal mass containing cystic and solid components, echogenic foci representing fat or calcification, and occasional fluid levels. The solid Rokitansky nodule can sometimes be demonstrated on the cyst wall. Teratoma usually replaces the entire ovary. (1)

CT. The key feature seen on CT, with up to 100% specificity, is the demonstration of a cyst containing fat, calcification, and tooth formation. (52) The Rokitansky nodule can be recognized in at least 80% of cases as a solid nodule in the cyst wall, which contains fat, bone, teeth, or even hair. Fat–fluid levels occasionally are visible. Secondary malignant degeneration may be suspected in the presence of an enlarging nodule and evidence of adjacent tissue invasion. (1,16)

MRI. When the differential diagnosis of an ovarian mass is difficult, the demonstration of a high-intensity fat signal on T1-weighted MRI that disappears on fat suppression techniques is a useful finding. (53) Internal details include fat–fluid levels, hair, and mural nodules. (53)

ARTERIAL DISORDERS

Arteriosclerosis

Arteriosclerosis is the general term applied to disorders that result in "hardening of the arteries." This process is characterized by thickening and loss of elasticity of the vessel wall. There are three vascular diseases under this general heading: atherosclerosis, Mönckeberg's medial calcific sclerosis, and arteriolosclerosis.

Atherosclerosis

Synonyms. None.
Clinical Features. Atherosclerosis is the underlying process in many of the conditions that result in the highest mortality and serious morbidity of the Western world. All arteries can be affected, but it is the aorta, lower limb, coronary, and cerebral arteries that manifest the most serious consequences, such as aneurysm, claudication, limb amputation, myocardial infarction, and stroke. Atherosclerotic heart disease (coronary artery hardening) has been shown to be the leading cause of death in Canada. (1) It is unusual for only one vessel to be affected so that any patient presenting with one vascular problem frequently has widespread co-existing vascular disease and is frequently referred to as being a *vasculopathic*. (2) Known associations include hypertension, dietary factors, hereditary factors, diabetes, and smoking.

Pathologically, the lesions include the initial fatty streak, found even in young children, and atheroma. Atheromatous plaques consist of masses of cell debris, cholesterol, foam cells, and calcium capped by a fibrous cap of smooth muscle cells, macrophages, foam cells, collagen, and lymphocytes. These plaques produce clinically significant lesions by narrowing the vessel (stenosis), which may be further complicated by secondary changes, including calcification, ulceration, aneurysm, thrombosis, emboli, and hemorrhage. Other causes of vascular calcification are renal failure, hyperparathyroidism, and Wolman's disease. Vascular conditions can mimic common musculoskeletal symptoms, such as back and leg pain, neurogenic claudication, and loss of function.
Imaging Features. Initial imaging of atherosclerosis is usually performed with ultrasound. Angiograms remain the gold standard and allow deployment of therapeutic methods, including angioplasty and stent insertion. Multislice helical CT (or CTA) and MRA are also being increasingly used. Plain films may depict calcification within atheroma and in dilated walls of an aneurysm. (2,3)

Abdominal aortic calcification is the most frequently observed radiographic sign of atherosclerosis. The incidence of calcification increases with age and can be seen on conventional radiographs in 40% of individuals > 45 years of age. (4) Detection of calcified atheroma on CT scan may be present in 65% of cases, and two thirds of these patients have underlying hypertension. (5) It is a rare finding before the age of 40 and may suggest an unsuspected diagnosis of hypertension or diabetes. (6,7)

Calcification in the renal artery, often visible only on CT, is a better predictor of hypertension than aortic calcification. (7) It

has been suggested that there is a higher incidence of aortic calcification with increasing osteoporosis. (8) Advanced calcification in patients > 55 years of age is more common in patients who smoke more than one pack per day. (8) There appears to be a link between aortic atherosclerosis and increased degenerative disc disease. (9) The degree of calcification does not correlate with the degree of luminal occlusion because it does not demonstrate non-calcified atheroma, which is best assessed with ultrasound or angiography.

Gradual obstruction of the aortic bifurcation from atheroma, or sometimes acutely by a saddle embolus, produces bilateral buttock and leg pain, weakness and fatigue of the lower extremities, muscle atrophy, and impotence (in males; Leriche's syndrome). (3) (Fig. 18-89)
Plain Film Radiography. Abdominal aortic calcification on the frontal projection lies slightly to the left of midline, superimposed over the vertebrae. On the lateral view the posterior wall calcification should be 0–5 mm anterior to the L1–L4 vertebral bodies. (10) Calcified plaques appear as irregular, discontinuous (dot–dash) linear densities or, in more extensive cases, as two parallel opposing calcified walls (railroad track). Usually the earliest calcified plaques are visible anterior to the L3 or L4 segments. (Fig. 18-90) They may be displaced anteriorly by osteophytes extending from the vertebral bodies. (10,11) If the aorta is displaced > 5 mm from the spine, retro-aortic pathology, such as lymphoma or lymph node metastasis, should be suspected. (10)

With increasing age the aorta lengthens, curving more to the left and bowing anteriorly. Transverse diameter measurements of the abdominal aorta typically do not exceed 3 cm; thus values in excess should be viewed suspiciously for aneurysm. Higher up in the aorta, calcification is frequently seen within the aortic arch on thoracic radiographs as a complete or incomplete ring (thumbnail sign). (3,12,13)
Additional Imaging. Ultrasound can identify plaques as elevations in the endoluminal surface and, based on the reflectivity, distinguish between fibrous (soft) and calcified (hard) plaque. In addition, the degree of stenosis can be estimated by using Doppler techniques to measure the velocity of blood traversing the stenosis. The gold standard for diagnosis is angiography, which outlines stenoses, occlusions, and collateral circulation. Both CTA and MRA are also being used, with an accuracy approaching conventional angiography. (3,14)

- *Iliac arteries.* These are the second most common abdominal vessels to calcify. (3) The iliac arteries may be visible on the lateral view, at their bifurcation anterior to the L5 body, as a ringlike density. (Fig. 18-91) On the frontal radiograph the calcification will be linear and oriented inferior and laterally, passing into the pelvic inlet near the sacroiliac joint. Various branches of the internal iliac artery may be visible within the pelvic inlet. Calcification of the femoral artery will be superimposed over the femoral head and then pass close to the lesser trochanter. (14)
- *Splenic artery.* This is the third most frequent branch of the aorta to calcify, its incidence increasing with patient age. (15) The splenic artery is conspicuous by its location and frequently tortuous nature. The calcification usually consists of parallel, curvilinear arcs in the left upper quadrant outside of the splenic silhouette (*bag of worms*). (3) (Fig. 18-92) The finding is of no clinical significance.

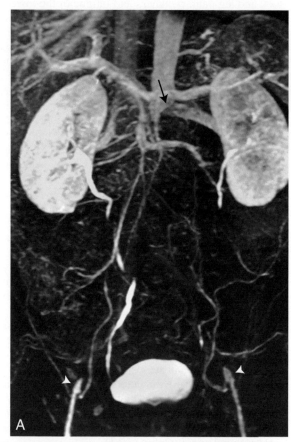

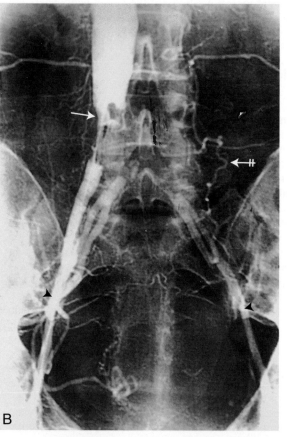

Figure 18-89 **AORTIC OCCLUSION (LERICHE'S SYNDROME).**
A. Acute Presentation, MRA, Coronal Abdomen. Note the
acute and complete occlusion of the aorta, extending from
the aortic bifurcation caudally toward the renal arteries
(*arrow*). There is some limited flow to the lower limbs by
collaterals (*arrowheads*). **B. Acute and Chronic Presentation,
Angiogram, Abdomen.** Observe the chronic atheromatous
stenosis of the lower abdominal aorta at the iliac bifurcation
(*arrow*). There are multiple compensatory collateral vessels
(*crossed arrow*) that allow flow to reach the external iliac
artery bilaterally (*arrowheads*). Acute thrombus occludes
both internal iliac arteries. *COMMENT:* Both patients presented with sudden, pulseless bilateral lower limb paralysis.
The patient shown in panel A did not survive. The patient
shown in panel B was a smoker who suffered undiagnosed
atheromatous lower limb claudication for many years; the
acute occlusion was attributed to the additional procoagulative effect of dehydration secondary to hyperemesis.
(Courtesy of Liz Thomsen, Faaborg, Denmark.)

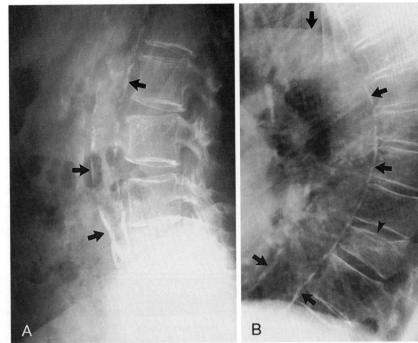

Figure 18-90   AORTIC CALCIFIC ATHEROSCLEROSIS.
A. Lateral Lumbar Spine. Note the linear calcification in the abdominal aorta (*arrows*). **B. Lateral Thoracic Spine.** Observe that similar calcification is present in the thoracic aorta (*arrows*). *COMMENT:* Incidentally, there is an old compression fracture of the T10 superior vertebral endplate (*arrowhead*). No evidence of aortic dilatation is present.

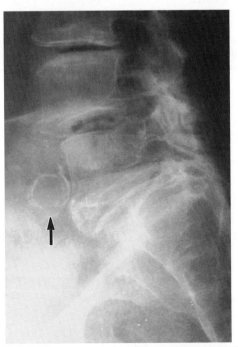

Figure 18-91   ILIAC ARTERY CALCIFIC ATHEROSCLEROSIS.
Lateral Lumbar Spine. Observe the calcified wall of the common iliac artery, which is seen en face as a complete circular density (*arrow*). *COMMENT:* This is the second most common site of atherosclerotic calcification. This lateral appearance should be correlated with the frontal projection to exclude aneurysm. (Courtesy of JoAnn Laenakker, DC, Gallatin, Tennessee.)

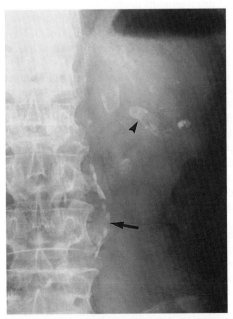

Figure 18-92   SPLENIC ARTERY CALCIFIC ATHEROSCLEROSIS.
AP Lumbar Spine. Note the tortuous calcified splenic artery (*arrowhead*) coursing medially toward the calcified aorta (*arrow*).

Aneurysms

Aneurysm Terminology

A practical understanding of the jargon associated with vascular dilatation is paramount for understanding the diagnosis, imaging features, and management options. (16)

---

aneurysm—[From the Greek for "widening."] A localized dilation of the aorta > 1.5 times the expected diameter. (17) The normal infrarenal aortic diameter between 65 and 75 years of age is ~ 2 cm, and aneurysm is equivalent to > 3 cm. (16,18) All layers of the involved vessel are intact but are thin and attenuated.

aneurysm rupture—All layers of the vessel are disrupted, often with catastrophic free flow of blood into the extravascular space. The precipitation of aneurysm rupture is unpredictable but is often related, in large part, to the cross-sectional area of the aneurysm, explained by the *La Place's Law*. The expansile stress on the vessel wall is equal to the fourth power of the radius. The practical implication of the law is that aneurysms < 5 cm often enlarge very slowly, but at around 5 cm or greater, the forces on the wall increase so that rapid expansion and the chance for rupture markedly escalates. (2,3,21,22)

atriomegaly (generalized aneurysmal disease)—Generalized dilatation of not only the aorta but of many of its branches—especially the subclavian, carotid, iliac, femoral, and popliteal vessels—exist simultaneously. (19)

dissecting aneurysm—A tear in the intima allows blood to track through the vessel wall within a *false lumen* and travel a variable distance distal, either terminating blind ended or re-entering the true lumen through a more distal intimal tear (*double-barreled aorta*). The result is a fourfold increase in risk for frank rupture. The dissecting blood (hematoma) can obstruct branch vessels or narrow or occlude the native lumen, or the dissection can extend to involve the walls of branch vessels. The external diameter of the vessel often remains unchanged. (19,20)

ectasia (dilatation)—More generalized dilatation over a longer length of the artery with less cross-sectional enlargement than an aneurysm. Tortuosity is often present as the vessel length increases.

fusiform aneurysm—A symmetric spindle-shaped dilatation involving the entire circumference of the aorta, with all parts of the wall bulging and exhibiting gradual tapering at either end to the normal diameter. (2,3)

inflammatory aneurysm—Up to 5% of abdominal aortic aneurysms have fibrosis and desmoplasia of the aneurysm wall, with a dense inflammatory, fibrotic reaction in the retroperitoneum that incorporates adjacent structures, including the ureters and duodenum. (2,3)

mycotic aneurysm—Infection of a vessel wall weakens it, producing either a true or a false aneurysm. The vessel wall may be infected by a septic embolus, by septicemia, or from direct extension from an adjacent infection. (2,3)

pseudo-aneurysm (false aneurysm)—A defect in the intima and media of the vessel wall with preservation of the adventitia allows a hematoma to form, which remains in contact with the flowing blood. Trauma, including iatrogenic, from percutaneous needle puncture, is the most common cause.

saccular aneurysm—A localized, usually eccentric outpouching of the aortic wall is present, and the adjacent wall is relatively unaffected. They are often spherical lesions, ranging from 5 to 10 cm in diameter but occasionally may be as large as 20 cm. (2,3)

suprarenal and infrarenal aneurysms—The relationship of the neck of the aneurysm to the renal arteries allows classification into either of the two types. Infrarenal types are more common and make up close to 95% of such aneurysms. This designation is crucial for determining if the abdominal aortic aneurysm is operable because suprarenal aneurysms cannot be treated owing to loss of renal perfusion during the procedure. (2,3)

Clinical Features. The first description of abdominal aortic aneurysm (AAA) was by Vesalius in the sixteenth century, and the first treatment was reported by Cooper some 300 years later. The abdominal aorta is the most common vessel for aneurysm below the diaphragm. Sites of involvement in descending order of incidence are the abdominal aorta, aortic arch, descending thoracic aorta, and, rarely, the ascending aorta. (Table 18-14) (Fig. 18-93)

Table 18-14	General Radiologic Features of Thoracic Aortic Aneurysms

Ascending aorta
  Most common cause: syphilis
    Enlarged and displaced to the right
    Peripheral rim of calcification
Transverse aorta
  Most common causes: atherosclerosis, syphilis, trauma
    Enlarged, displaced up to the left
    Trachea and esophageal shift
    Peripheral rim of calcification
Descending aorta
  Most common cause: atherosclerosis
    Left lateral displacement
    Localized bulge
    Peripheral curvilinear calcification

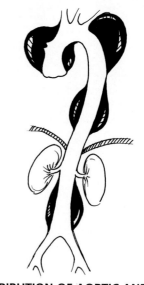

Figure 18-93 DISTRIBUTION OF AORTIC ANEURYSMS. The most common site for aortic aneurysm is distal to the origin of the renal artery and proximal to the common iliac artery bifurcation. Aneurysms at the aortic root often complicate collagen diseases and syphilis, whereas those distal to the left subclavian artery usually occur at the insertion of the ligamentum arteriosum and are typically associated with closed thoracic trauma.

AAA is probably the most common extraspinal, potentially life-threatening disorder encountered in patients presenting with back pain. (23) Numerous case reports from chiropractors and other musculoskeletal practitioners have been described. (23,24) The overall incidence of AAA is estimated at between 2% and 6% of the general population (20,25), with values reaching approximately 7.7% in individuals 65–74 years of age. (26–28) For every 5 years after the age of 65, the risk of abdominal aortic aneurysm increases 40%. (24) Males are more frequently affected by a 5:1 ratio.

Known risk factors, other than being male and > 60 years of age, are hypertension, heart disease, hyperlipidemia, peripheral vascular disease, positive family history for AAA, and cigarette smoking. (29) Smoking is the most important risk factor that can be avoided. (24) Almost 40% of AAA patients have hypertension, and 30% have heart disease. (30) There is an almost 30% incidence in male siblings of patients with AAA. (31) At least 25% of AAAs > 5 cm will rupture within 5 years, and those < 5 cm have a rupture rate of only 5%. (32) AAA on average expands by 4–5 mm per year. The largest aneurysm recorded was > 13 cm in diameter. (16,33–36)

AAA is classified according to the location of the neck (upper transition zone to a normal diameter) relative to the level of the renal arteries. This classification often determines if the dilatation can be surgically repaired. Generally, when the neck is above the renal arteries (suprarenal) the aneurysm is unresectable, whereas those with the neck below the renal arteries (infrarenal) are operable. At least 95% of cases are infrarenal.

Atherosclerosis accounts for 90–95% of AAA, with the remainder predominantly the inflammatory type. (37) One or both common iliac arteries are involved by direct extension of the AAA or as a separate aneurysm in 21–66% of cases. (38,39) Coexisting aneurysms elsewhere may include the thoracic aorta (4%), femoral arteries (3%), and popliteal arteries (2%). (3,30)

Clinical presentations are variable. Around 75% of patients with non-ruptured AAA are asymptomatic; the condition is found on physical examination or imaging examinations performed for other reasons. These same aneurysms can produce symptoms such as vague abdominal pain, back pain, lower limb ischemia and embolism, and, rarely, spinal cord ischemia or diarrhea from ischemic colitis. Severe back pain often heralds dissection, rupture, or sudden expansion. The classic clinical triad of rupture in one third of cases is sudden onset of midabdominal or flank pain, cardiovascular shock, and a pulsatile abdominal mass. (40) The most common site for rupture is through the left posterior lateral wall, which explains why back pain is so common. (41–43)

Many authors advocate routine screening for abdominal aortic aneurysm. A study involving routine ultrasound screening of men at age 65 showed a reduction in the mortality from rupture to be approximately 68% over 5 years. (17) This was attributed to early detection and increased monitoring of these patients. However, a more recent study performed on women revealed that screening and earlier identification of the aneurysm did not, in fact, reduce the incidence of rupture and mortality. (18) This is most likely attributed to the fact that the aneurysms identified on routine screening were usually asymptomatic and did not meet the criteria for surgical intervention. Unfortunately, aneurysms in women appear to progress more rapidly when expansion ensues, and a threefold increase of rupture is noted during progression. (44) Routine screening of asymptomatic women has shown to be of no clinical relevance and to be economically impractical. (18)

Frank rupture results in sudden death within minutes. Common misdiagnoses from rupture include ureteric colic, lumbar disc syndromes, pancreatitis, diverticulitis, cholecystitis, mesenteric occlusion, and peptic ulcer. On palpation, a pulsatile mass may be felt and a bruit heard in the epigastrium above the umbilicus. Confusion with a normal aortic pulsation in thin patients can be differentiated when palpation for the lateral margins of the aorta will show separation of the fingers synchronous with the pulse as a sign of aneurysm. (2,3)

Laboratory investigations are important in the management of AAA. Key studies are the ESR and creatinine levels. The ESR, if elevated, may provide a clue to the presence of an inflammatory aneurysm, which is associated with technical intraoperative difficulties, such as bowel adhesions and encasement of the inferior vena cava and ureters. (45,46) A raised creatinine level may indicate suprarenal extension or significant renal artery disease, which will need to be incorporated into the surgical plan.

The presence of a horseshoe kidney complicates the operative management because of the anomalous blood supply, which may be compromised during repair, and is best planned with either preoperative angiography or CT. (35,47) Criteria for elective surgical repair include pain symptoms, rupture, expansion of > 5 mm per year, and > 5 cm in size; however, some surgeons advocate 4 cm as the threshold size.

Elective surgery carries a 5% operative mortality, whereas emergency operations for rupture may have as high as 80% mortality within 30 days of intervention. (21,26) Careful screening of lung and kidney function should be conducted in all patients who choose elective surgery for aneurysmal repair because impairment of these two organs has been shown to be highly associated with the postoperative mortality rates. (48) It is surprising that age is of nominal concern when compared with mortality rates seen in association with lung and renal function. (48)

The operation involves cross-clamping the iliac arteries and the neck of the aorta below the renal arteries, opening the aneurysm, removing the mural thrombus, suturing the graft at both ends, and then closing the aneurysm sac over the graft to protect against aortoenteric fistulas. Today, these operations are being performed less commonly; instead, transfemoral endoluminal aortic stent placement is performed.

Imaging Findings. The commonly employed imaging modalities are plain films, CT, ultrasonography, MRI, and angiography. (Table 18-15) Incidental discovery is extremely common when plain radiographs, CT, and MRI are taken for evaluation of back pain. (34,49–51)

The imaging strategy for AAA depends on presentation. (34)

- *Clinical suspicion for AAA.* If the diagnosis is suspected purely on clinical grounds based on risk factors, palpation, or auscultation, and abdominal ultrasound is appropriate.
- *Discovery on plain film.* If the characteristic wall calcification or, rarely, vertebral body erosion is identified, further assessment with ultrasound and/or CT can be made.
- *Progress evaluation.* Patients with small aneurysms or those who are marginal surgical candidates are best monitored for progression with sequential ultrasound imaging at 6-month intervals.
- *Non-acute but symptomatic aneurysm.* The development of abdominal, back, or pelvic pain in a patient with a known AAA should have prompt assessment with CT.
- *Acute surgical emergency.* Severe pain, tachycardia, and hypotension is life-threatening and immediate laparotomy should be performed.
- *Preoperative assessment.* This is best accomplished by CTA with a helical acquisition in the arterial phase. Reformatting the acquired data allows for reconstructions in multiple planes and three-dimensional displays, which

show the relationship of the aneurysm neck to the size, mural thrombus, and the involvement of adjacent arteries (especially the iliac and renal branches). (35) Angiography is still favored by many vascular surgeons, on which similar measurements are made. Luminal diameters, location, and the state of the iliac arteries are key factors in deciding whether or not aortic graft is performed by laparotomy or by percutaneous, transfemoral endoluminal stenting.

• *Postgraft assessment.* This is usually performed with helical CTA.

Plain Film. Plain film radiography is a relatively insensitive examination for diagnosis, exclusion, or assessment of AAA. Nonetheless, the frequently asymptomatic but serious nature of this diagnosis makes it imperative to recognize any findings that

Table 18-15	Radiologic Features of Abdominal Aortic Aneurysm

Causes
   Most common: atherosclerosis (90–95%)
   Other: inflammatory, infection (mycotic), traumatic, congenital
Plain film
   Frontal projection
      L2–L4, usually on the left side
      Soft tissue mass
      Curvilinear calcification at the peripheral margin (50–85%)
      Diameter > 3 cm
      Bulging psoas margin
   Lateral projection
      L2–L4, anterior to the spine
      Soft tissue mass
      Curvilinear calcification anteriorly
      Anterior vertebral body erosions (Oppenheimer's erosions)
Ultrasound
   Echogenic mass
   Wall thickness
   Thrombosis
   Pulsation
   Adjacent abnormalities
   Monitoring progression or stability
CT
   Position relative to the renal arteries
   Points of origin and termination
   Wall integrity (rupture, dissection)
   Wall thickness
   Thrombosis, luminal size
   Leakage
   Perianeurysmal fibrosis and ureteral involvement
   Adjacent abnormalities
   Identification of horseshoe kidney
   Postsurgical repair assessment
MRI
   As for CT
   Flow abnormalities
   Accurate size measurement
   Assess visceral branch involvement
Angiography
   Detection of renal artery anomalies
   Suprarenal extension
   Additional vascular disease (iliacs, femorals)
   Patency of the mesenteric arteries
   Aortic complications (occlusion, inferior vena caval lesions)
   Identification of horseshoe kidney

may indicate the presence of aneurysm on plain film examination of the abdomen or lumbopelvic area. Calcification, the most reliable plain film finding, is seen in only 50% of patients and the calcified area may not demonstrate the full extent of an aneurysm. (16,38,52) Frontal and lateral radiographs may show calcification, but variables include film quality, body size, and aneurysm calcification position relative to the spine. Overlying gas and fecal material often obscure the calcification and only careful scrutiny may show its presence. Oblique projections are extremely useful adjunct views that can display the otherwise subtle calcification clear of the spine and the overlying bowel contents. When present on frontal films the zone for observing the wall calcification is below the renal artery (L2) and above the iliac bifurcation (L4), usually to the left of the spine (Fig. 18-94) A soft tissue density demarcated by a thin, curvilinear rim of continuous or discontinuous calcification is the most characteristic finding. Uncalcified AAA presents only as a soft tissue density, difficult to identify in most cases. The size of the aorta varies with body size and geometric magnification. (18,20,26) Measurements for determining the size of the aorta are made between the most distant calcified borders. (18,20,26)

The lateral projection, while often the most demonstrative, may be misleadingly normal. Frequently there is tight collimation anterior to the spine, which limits the field of view and may exclude the anterior margin of the lesion. In such cases the only clue may be a horizontally or obliquely oriented calcified plaque. Occasionally the lesion may extend posteriorly and overlie the spine. The close proximity of the aorta to the anterior vertebral bodies in approximately 5% of AAA cases may precipitate extrinsic anterior body erosions (Oppenheimer's erosions), which can develop in < 2 years. (24,51,53) (Fig. 18-95) Erosions are relatively uncommon because the aorta is not firmly adherent to the vertebral column and the expansion is predominantly anterior and lateral. They are more commonly found in inflammatory and contained leaking (sealed rupture) of an AAA because this will produce adherence to the spine and allow for the transmission of pulsatile impulses to create the erosions.

An additional factor is that saccular aneurysms produce more erosions than fusiform AAAs. Saccular aneurysms are most commonly associated with syphilis and are a rare occurrence in recent times. (22) These anterior vertebral body erosive defects are smooth and concave, with relative sparing of the disc–endplate region. Other causes of anterior body erosions include lymphoma, osteolytic metastasis, and subligamentous tuberculosis. (53)

Plain film signs of leakage are subtle and non-specific. On the supine plain film obliteration or lateral bulging of the psoas margin, loss of the renal outline, soft tissue extension beyond the calcified margin, ileus, and loss of the properitoneal flank stripe may be seen. (54) On the erect film blood may collect within the pelvis, creating a hazy density to the pelvic inlet, loss of the perivesical fat, and air–fluid levels in the bowel, caused by an overlying adynamic ileus. (54)

Ultrasound. Ultrasound is the diagnostic modality of choice for confirming the diagnosis, evaluating size, and monitoring progression or stability of an AAA. (16) (Fig. 18-96) It is accurate to within 3 mm of actual size of the dilatation. (16) It may show thrombus, periaortic abnormalities, dissections, cephalad and caudal extent, and complications—especially ureteric entrapment from inflammatory aneurysm with associated hydronephrosis. Usefulness of ultrasound can be limited by obesity and excessive bowel gas. Suprarenal extension cannot be directly determined, though extension above the superior mesenteric artery provides

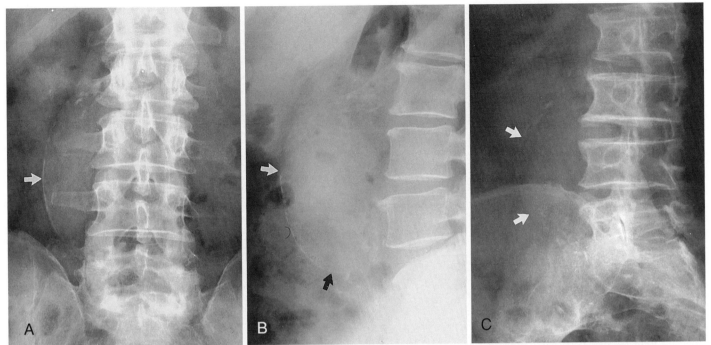

Figure 18-94 ABDOMINAL AORTIC ANEURYSM. A. AP Lumbar Spine. Note the characteristic peripheral thin rim of curvilinear calcification bordering the soft tissue density of the aneurysm (*arrow*). This location, on the left side between the L2 and L4 vertebrae, is the most common site. **B. Lateral Lumbar Spine.** Observe that the anterior margin of the calcified wall of the aortic aneurysm is visible (*arrows*). **C. Oblique Lumbar Spine.** Note that the aneurysm may become more apparent after examining the other calcified edge of the aorta (*arrows*). *COMMENT:* Only 50% of abdominal aortic aneurysms exhibit enough calcium to be visible on plain film radiographs. Tightly collimated lateral views may not include the anterior wall of the aneurysm, requiring detailed evaluation of the frontal film. The oblique film is often helpful when the lateral film is equivocal.

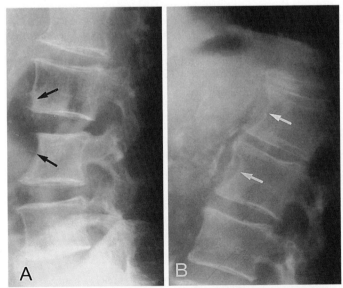

Figure 18-95 ABDOMINAL AORTIC ANEURYSM, VERTEBRAL BODY EROSIONS (OPPENHEIMER'S EROSIONS). A. L3–L4, Lateral Lumbar Spine. Note the smooth anterior erosions affecting L4 and to a lesser extent the inferior aspect of L3 (*arrows*). **B. L1–L2, Lateral Lumbar Spine.** Observe the less prominent smooth anterior erosions (*arrows*). *COMMENT:* Anterior vertebral body erosions are found in < 5% of abdominal aortic aneurysms. The differential diagnosis of these defects includes lymphoma, tuberculosis (gouge defect), and metastatic disease. (Panel A courtesy of Paul E. Siebert, MD, Denver, Colorado; panel B courtesy of Ian D. McLean, DC, DACBR, Davenport, Iowa.)

indirect evidence. (16) Rupture can be inferred by demonstrating periaortic fluid, and dissection is occasionally seen by observing an intimal flap.

CT. CT is the mainstay of imaging aneurysms. It allows the clinician to determine the extent of the AAA; to view the relationship of the aneurysm to the renal arteries; and to evaluate iliac extension, mural thrombus, rupture, distribution and amount of leakage, perianeurysmal fibrosis, and ureteral involvement. (16,35,36) (Figs. 18-96*B* and 18-97) Previous sealed rupture can be determined by the presence of a retroperitoneal hematoma below the renal artery behind the anterior renal fascia. (43) Helical acquisitions in the arterial phase allow not only for axial image display but also for reconstructions, including three-dimensional angiograms. Contrast scans delineate the true lumen of the AAA from thrombus. (16) CT is the technique of choice for examining the aorta postsurgical repair. After 7–12 weeks the fluid surrounding the graft within the aneurysm sac should be resorbed; otherwise persistent leak or graft infection may be suspected. (44,48)

MRI. Flowing blood creates a *flow void* on MRI and demonstrates the aorta as a low signal structure. Aneurysms are clearly depicted as are their complications, especially dissection, mural thrombus, and visceral branch involvement. (16,50,55) A key advantage of MRI is the simultaneous visualization of the spinal cord, which may become ischemic in the presence of thrombus or with suprarenal extension and occlusion of the artery of Adamkiewicz. (50) Three dimensional MRA assists in the assessment of renal arteries and iliac involvement.

Angiography. Placement of intravascular contrast to depict the AAA may alter the surgical approach in as many as 25% of cases. It is especially useful in the detection of renal artery anom-

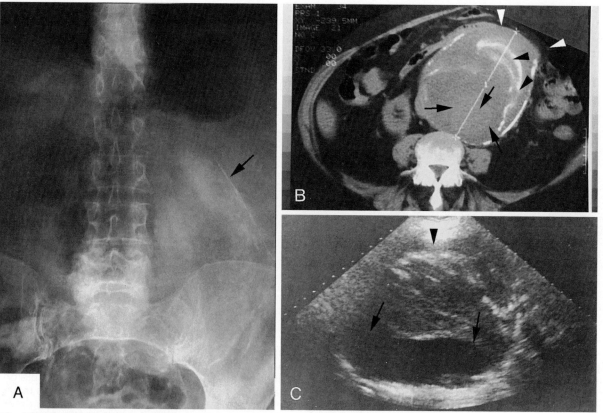

Figure 18-96 LARGE ABDOMINAL AORTIC ANEURYSM WITH EVENTUAL RUPTURE. A. AP Abdomen. Note the 14-cm aneurysm with distinctive curvilinear calcification in the peripheral wall to the left of the L2–L4 vertebral segments (*arrow*). **B. Non-Enhanced CT, Axial Abdomen.** Note that the existing lumen is extremely narrow (*arrows*). The lesion extends beyond the rim of calcification, consistent with repetitive healed dissections (*arrowheads*). **C. Ultrasound, Sagittal Abdomen.** Observe that the existing lumen (*arrows*) and anterior calcified margin (*arrowhead*) are visualized on this view. A large amount of mural thrombus can be identified between the arrows and arrowhead. *COMMENT:* This 76-year-old female presented with non-specific low back pain of non-mechanical origin, prompting plain film radiographs. Although the patient obtained a surgical recommendation, she refused and subsequently died when the aneurysm ruptured 10 months later. Elective surgery carries a 5% operative mortality, whereas emergency operations for rupture may have as high as 80% mortality within 30 days of intervention. (Courtesy of Ralph E. Brewer, DC, Denver, Colorado.)

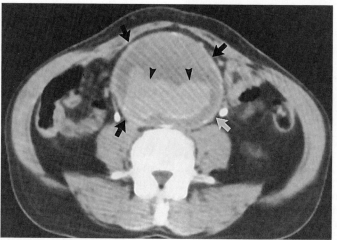

Figure 18-97 ABDOMINAL AORTIC ANEURYSM, MURAL THROMBUS. CT, Axial Abdomen. Note that after intravenous contrast injection the lumen is seen as a higher density region (*arrowheads*). The lower density tissue between the lumen and external wall represents hematoma attached to the wall (mural thrombus). *COMMENT:* Despite its large size no calcification is present within the wall (*arrows*). Mural thrombus is common in abdominal aortic aneurysm and can be the source for intermittent embolization to the lower limbs (trash foot) or can precipitate claudication. (Courtesy of Steven P. Brownstein, MD, Springfield, New Jersey.)

alies, suprarenal extension, significant lower limb disease (iliacs, femorals), patency of the mesenteric arteries, associated aneurysms elsewhere, aortic complications (occlusion, inferior vena caval lesions), and horseshoe kidney. (16) It is commonly used before endovascular stent placement to reveal if the iliac vessels are amenable to gaining access to the aorta and to derive accurate measurements for selection of the most optimum stent type and size.

Iliac Artery Aneurysm

Synonyms. None.

Clinical Features. The common iliac artery is involved in 90%, the internal iliac in 10%, and the external iliac in < 1% of lesions. (56) Aneurysms of the branches of the internal iliac artery are rare, though aneurysms of the superior gluteal artery have been recorded after ileotomy for bone graft or traumatic sacroiliac diastasis. The common iliac artery is the second most common site for aneurysm formation within the abdomen. (57) These affect males more commonly by a ratio of 4:1, with a peak incidence at 70 years of age; they are more common in vasculopathic patients. (58) Common iliac aneurysms in up to 75% of cases are continuations of AAA, with only 25% existing as isolated lesions.

The majority of iliac artery aneurysms are asymptomatic and discovered incidentally on imaging for other clinical reasons. Physical examination of the pelvis may reveal a bruit, with over half of cases exhibiting a palpable pulsation. (59) As these lesions enlarge, pressure effects on the sciatic nerve can mimic lumbar spine disc syndromes with thigh and leg pain, reflex changes, and sensory impairment. (60) Acute rupture presents with sudden, severe back and pelvic pain associated with shock. There is a high rate of mortality because of delayed diagnosis. (59) These aneurysms tend to be large when discovered, averaging 7.5–8.5 cm. (61) (Fig. 18-98)

Imaging Features. Plain film radiographs are relatively insensitive to iliac aneurysm detection, owing to the general lack of wall calcification. This is present in only 50% of cases. The aneurysm is either saccular or fusiform and outlined by thin curvilinear calcification. Overlying gas and feces frequently obscure the calcification. On the lateral film a ring-like peripheral calcification can be observed anterior to L4–L5 or lower in the pelvis. Ultrasound, CT, CTA, and angiography are important in the assessment and diagnosis of uncalcified aneurysms. (3,12)

Visceral Aneurysms

Aneurysms of the intra-abdominal visceral arteries are relatively uncommon. Over 20% of patients present with rupture, resulting in a mortality rate of 8%. (62) The remaining 80% are asymptomatic and are identified on CT and angiography and occasionally on plain film examinations when there is calcification. The visceral distribution of these aneurysms is 60% splenic, 20% hepatic, 5% superior mesenteric, 4% celiac, and the remaining 11% in other major arteries. (62,63)

Splenic Artery Aneurysm

Clinical Features. The splenic artery is the most common visceral artery aneurysm, accounting for up to 60% of such lesions. (63) It is the third most common site for aneurysm in the ab-

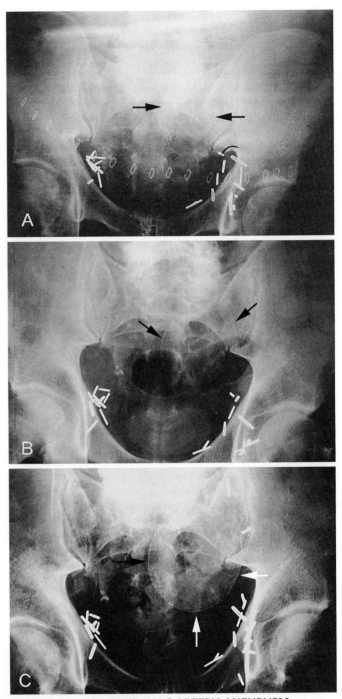

Figure 18-98 CALCIFIED ILIAC ARTERY ANEURYSM, PROGRESS OVER 10 YEARS. A. Year: 1981, Size: 4 cm; AP Pelvis. Note the subtle aneurysm wall calcification over the sacrum (*arrows*). **B. Year: 1984, Size: 6 cm; AP Pelvis.** Observe that the aneurysm has enlarged with lateral and inferior expansion (*arrows*). **C. Year: 1991, Size: 8 cm; AP Pelvis.** Note that the aneurysm continued to enlarge (*arrows*). *COMMENT:* Elective resection and grafting were successfully performed. Incidentally, the surgical clips within the pelvic soft tissues are from previous radical prostatectomy and lymph node resection for carcinoma. (Courtesy of Donald E. Freuden, DC, DABCO, Denver, Colorado.)

domen after the aorta and iliac vessels. They can be found in up to 10% of autopsies of patients > 60 years of age. (64–67) The majority of lesions are < 2 cm and involve the middle to distal artery near the splenic hilum. (68–70) These lesions are most commonly found in 5th decade, affecting females in a ratio of 4:1 but the incidence in males equalizes with progressive age. (62) The rupture rate is as high as 10%, with up to one third being fatal. Calcified aneurysms may be at a higher risk of rupture.

Known causes of splenic aneurysms include fibromuscular hyperplasia, multiple pregnancies, portal hypertension, splenomegaly, liver transplantation, pancreatitis, vasculitis, and intravenous drug use. (62,71) There is no link with commonly observed age-related arterial tortuosity. The majority of splenic aneurysms are asymptomatic, being detected incidentally on abdominal imaging, especially plain films. Symptomatic epigastric and left upper quadrant pain are the major symptoms, which may mimic peptic ulcer and are associated with probable dissection, tear, or impending rupture. (63,67,72) Not uncommonly, acute rupture occurs during pregnancy, with a mortality rate as high as 70%.

Patients requiring surgery are those with symptoms, aneurysms > 2 cm, pregnant women, and women of childbearing age. (62,70,73–75) Patients > 60 years of age with asymptomatic aneurysms < 1.5 cm can be managed conservatively, with yearly ultrasonography to monitor for progression. (67)

Imaging Features. On plain film the aneurysm wall may calcify in at least 80% of cases and be visible in the left upper quadrant as a curvilinear, almost circular *signet ring calcification.* (71) (Fig 18-99) The wall is often incomplete, at least at one site, representing the site of vessel origin. On the lateral projection this will be closely opposed to the anterior vertebral bodies or be superimposed over them. Splenic hydatid cysts may mimic an aneurysm but usually demonstrate a thicker, dense, and irregular peripheral wall of calcification. The lesion should not be confused with the more common and clinically insignificant radiologic finding of the coiled calcified splenic artery, which is not associated with aneurysm formation. Up to one third of cases have multiple aneurysms, which may give a multilobed or beaded appearance to the calcification.

CT examination should be performed in precontrast, arterial, and venous phases. The non-contrast studies confirm the location of the calcification; the arterial phase, the filling of the aneurysm; and the venous phase, arteriovenous fistula. Doppler ultrasound and angiography can also be used to confirm the aneurysm and may show arteriovenous fistula formation. (76)

Other Visceral Aneurysms

Hepatic Artery. After the splenic artery the hepatic artery is the second most common site for visceral artery aneurysm. Known causes include trauma, atherosclerosis, mycotic aneurysm, pancreatitis, intravenous drug use, Marfan's syndrome, and polyarteritis nodosa. At least 80% of these aneurysms are extrahepatic. The lesions are occasionally calcified and appear as a circular or curvilinear opacity in the right upper quadrant. (77)

Celiac Artery. Lesions in the celiac artery make up < 4% of visceral aneurysms, rarely calcify, and are usually found on angiography. The pancreaticoduodenal and gastroduodenal branches may become aneurysmal after pancreatitis and are the most lethal of all visceral artery aneurysms, with a rupture rate of 50–90%. (62)

Renal Artery. The renal artery is a relatively rare site for aneurysm formation, occurring mostly near the renal hilum. Approximately 25% of renal artery aneurysms will calcify. (78,79) The calcification is circular, ring-like (signet ring), and incomplete. The size of the lesion varies between 1 and 3 cm. On the AP film the opacity will be adjacent to the L2–L3 segments, whereas on the lateral projection it will overlie the spine. (Fig. 18-100) Lesions > 2 cm are usually treated either by placement of endovascular coils or by surgical resection.

Superior Mesenteric Artery. After splenic and hepatic aneurysms, those of the superior mesenteric artery are the third most common visceral aneurysm. (62) They are usually mycotic in origin and rarely calcify; they are visualized on CT, MRA, and angiography.

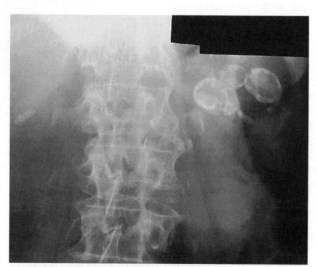

Figure 18-99 SPLENIC ARTERY ANEURYSMS. AP Abdomen. Observe the multiple circular, ring-like densities in the left upper quadrant, each representing a separate aneurysm from a coiled tortuous artery.

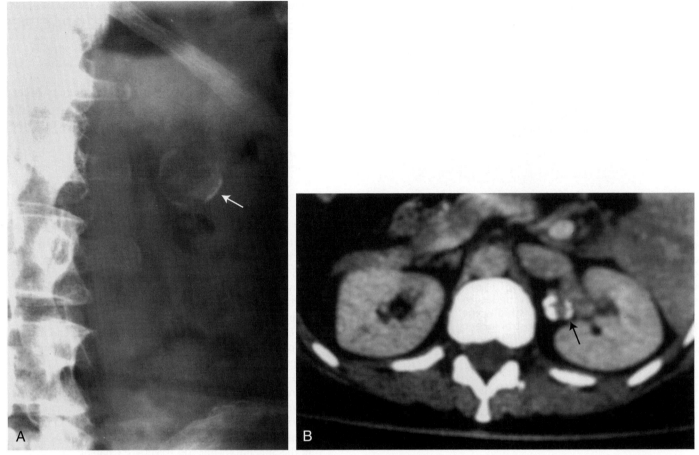

Figure 18-100   RENAL ARTERY ANEURYSM. A. AP Lumbar Spine. Note the circular calcification within the peripheral wall of an aneurysm adjacent to the T12–L1 level (*arrow*). **B. CT, Axial Abdomen.** The calcification is localized to the renal hilum, a typical location for aneurysm (*arrow*).
COMMENT: Aneurysms of the renal artery are relatively uncommon. At least 25% demonstrate mural calcification owing to their long-standing nature.

VENOUS DISORDERS

Phleboliths

Synonyms. Venous stones.
Clinical Features. Calcification of thrombi attached to the venous wall are the most common calcifications of the pelvis. (1) These are most frequently observed within the pelvic basin, particularly in proximity to the superior pubic rami, below the ischial spine. By age 40 at least one third of all individuals will have at least one pelvic phlebolith. There is an equal sex distribution. Anatomically they tend to occur in the perirectal and perivesical venous plexuses. (1,2) In males, phleboliths may be visible in the scrotal veins or the pampiniform plexus and dorsal vein of the penis and can be large. Phleboliths in females often form in the veins of the broad ligament. Histopathologic examination of phleboliths show them to consist of thickly packed layers of platelets trapped between a network of red blood cells and fibrin. (3) The calcification is composed predominantly of calcium carbonate. (4)

The significance of a phlebolith is undefined. Its pathogenesis most definitely appears related to the upright posture and sudden intermittent changes in intra-abdominal pressure acting on the poorly supported and valveless pelvic veins. (1) Phleboliths are not seen in quadruped animals. (3) There appears to be no connection between previous gastrointestinal or genitourinary disease that would predispose individuals to phlebolith formation. (5–7)
Imaging Features. Phleboliths are dense, round to oval, and well margined on imaging examinations. (Fig. 18-101) Characteristically, a central lucency is evident on plain film radiographs. (8) Usually, fewer than 6 will be visible, although occasionally up to 20 may occur. They may appear arranged in chains, especially along the upper margin of the superior pubic ramus. Infrequently, a linearly arranged group of phleboliths in the gonadal vein may overlap the sacroiliac joint region and ascend parallel but lateral to the spine. At times it is difficult to distinguish phleboliths from ureteral calculi. (8,9) A calculus is usually more angular and elongated, lacks the lucent center, and is surrounded by a thickened ureteric wall on CT. The radiolucent center and the *comet-tail sign* are perhaps the best imaging findings to aid in this differentiation. (8,9)

The radiolucent center is seen on CT, even when it is present despite on traditional radiographs; thus CT imaging is not a useful modality for this anomaly. (8) It is, however, the examination of choice to find ureteral calculi. It is rare for a phlebolith to be in the midline of the pelvic basin because of the small veins connecting both sides. In addition, phleboliths that seem to be displaced over a period of time may indicate the presence of an abnormal mass or prolapse of the uterus. (10) A phlebolith outside the pelvic basin is often associated with a soft tissue hemangioma (Maffucci's syndrome) or venous stasis.

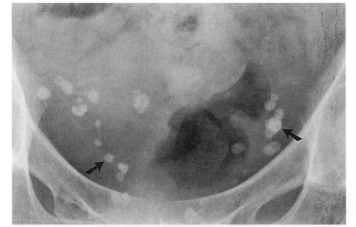

Figure 18-101   PELVIC PHLEBOLITHS. AP Pelvis. Note the multiple circular opacities (some with characteristic lucent centers) adjacent to the superior pubic rami (*arrows*). *COMMENT:* Phleboliths represent calcified organized thromboses within the perivesical plexus. The most common location for phleboliths to occur is in the lateral soft tissues of the pelvic basin, inferior to the ischial spine. They are typically round and often have a central lucency that distinguishes them from ureteral calculi. They are rarely found in the midline of the pelvis.

MISCELLANEOUS ABDOMINAL OPACITIES

Examples of miscellaneous abdominal opacities follow: (1,2)

- *Lymph node calcification.* These most commonly occur in the para-aortic location or in the mesentery. They are usually dense and mass-like in appearance, frequently with a lobulated external contour. (Fig. 18-102) (See Chapter 3.)
- *Heavy-metal injections.* These can be seen in the buttock region as well as the abdomen and appear dense and linear, representing bismuth injections into the gluteus maximus. (Fig. 18-103, *A* and *B*) (See Chapter 16.)
- *Injection granuloma.* These are most commonly seen in the buttocks as round curvilinear cystic-type calcifications. (Fig. 18-103*C*) They occur secondary to fat necrosis. (See Chapter 3.)
- *Postsurgical scar ossification.* Bone formation can occasionally be identified within surgical scars with definite cortex and internal trabeculae, especially involving the anterior abdominal wall.
- *Ingested tablets or foreign bodies.* Iron tablets and bismuth preparations can create radiopaque densities on imaging. (Fig. 18-104) These are most commonly seen in the stomach and occasionally the small bowel. Opaque objects such as coins, batteries, and sharp objects can be sequentially followed with plain film to ensure passage. (See Chapter 16.)
- *Barium retention.* After barium studies retention is often seen for months within colonic diverticula and occasionally in the appendix. (Fig. 18-105) (See Chapter 16.)
- *Bullet fragments.* These are easily identified; over time they can be physiologically degraded to produce lead poisoning. (See Chapter 16.)

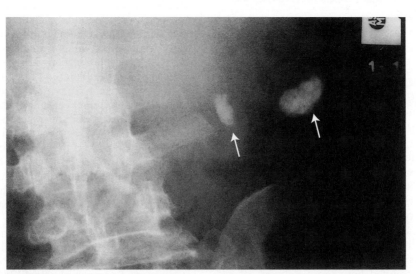

Figure 18-102   CALCIFIED MESENTERIC LYMPH NODES. AP Abdomen. Note the two dense calcifications adjacent to the transverse process and above the iliac crest (*arrows*). These are lobulated in external contour, characteristic of calcified necrotic lymph nodes. *COMMENT:* Calcified lymph nodes are a common finding throughout the abdomen. The most common locations are the mesentery and para-aortic regions. These had been previously thought to be exclusively caused by tuberculosis, though any cause of infection may be associated with this finding. They are asymptomatic and not related to malignancy.

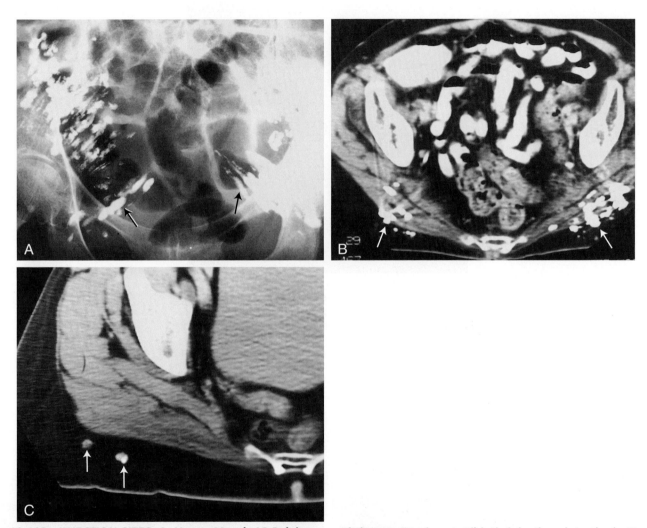

Figure 18-103 **INJECTION SITES. A. Heavy Metal, AP Pelvis.** Note the linear densities that parallel the fiber orientation of the gluteus maximus muscles bilaterally (*arrows*). **B. Heavy-Metal, CT, Axial Abdomen.** The intramuscular location of the bismuth injection sites shown in panel A is confirmed (*arrows*). **C. Calcified Fat Necrosis, CT, Axial Abdomen.** Previous antibiotic injections into the buttocks have caused focal fat necrosis with subsequent calcification in the subcutaneous tissue (injection granulomas) (*arrows*). *COMMENT:* Heavy metal is uncommonly encountered, but calcified fat necroses (injection granulomas) are frequent findings of no clinical significance.

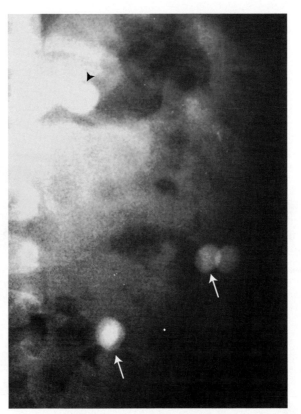

Figure 18-104 **INGESTED TABLETS. AP Abdomen.** Observe the multiple undigested tablets in the intestine (*arrows*); a single tablet remains in the stomach (*arrowhead*). *COMMENT:* Virtually any tablet, before dissolving, can be seen in the upper gastrointestinal tract. Some tablets (including iron, potassium, some vitamins, and antacid compounds) may persist through to the colon. In this child, the accidental ingestion of iron tablets was confirmed with this radiograph. (Courtesy of Anne E. Baxter, MD, Newcastle, New South Wales, Australia.)

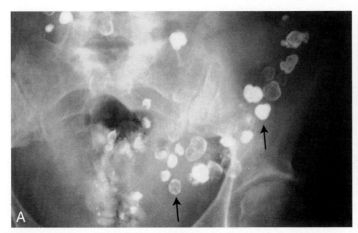

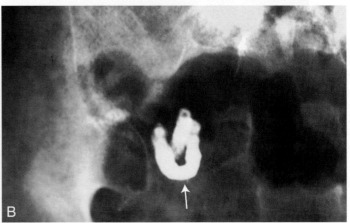

Figure 18-105 **RETAINED BARIUM. A. Diverticular Disease, AP Abdomen.** Note the multiple radio-opaque circular densities throughout the pelvis (*arrows*). They represent retained barium within diverticula from a barium study done 6 weeks earlier. **B. Appendix, AP Abdomen.** Barium is retained within the appendix (*arrow*). *COMMENT:* Retention of barium within the bowel and appendix can be present for many months and is not a precursor to diverticulitis.

MISCELLANEOUS MASQUERADERS OF MUSCULOSKELETAL DISEASE

LOWER EXTREMITY VASCULAR DISEASES

Arterial Disorders

Femoral, Popliteal, and Calf Arteries. Clinical symptoms of lower extremity arterial disorders depend on the location, the degree of the stenosis, and the ability of the individual to form collateral circulation. Frequently, such stenoses remain clinically silent because of adequate collateral circulation; however, they may present acutely as a result of thrombosis or distal embolization. Occlusion of the iliac vessels produces buttock and thigh pain; femoral lesions lead to thigh pain; and popliteal and calf obstructions cause knee, leg, and foot pain. Acute arterial obstruction is characterized in the affected extremity by the *five Ps:* **p**ulselessness, **p**allor, **p**aresthesia, **p**aralysis, and **p**ain. (1,2) Chronic stenosis is characterized by claudication and trophic skin changes, including ulceration and pain at rest.

Irregular dense calcific plaques are often visible throughout the course of the lower limb arteries. Non-calcified atheroma are common causes for lower limb claudication, which may clinically mimic neurogenic pain and claudication. (1,2) Ultrasound is used to localize and quantify the stenoses, followed by angiography, at which time balloon angioplasty or deployment of endovascular stents may be performed. (1,2) (Fig. 18-106, A and B)

Mönckeberg's Medial Sclerosis. Mönckeberg's medial sclerosis is typified by calcification within the muscle wall (tunica media) of medium to small muscular arteries. The most frequent sites affected are the femoral, tibial, radial, ulnar, digital, and genital arteries. This disorder is rare before 50 years of age. The genesis of the condition remains obscure but may be related to prolonged, sympathetic overactivity. Whatever the cause, its significance as an entity is small because no narrowing or occlusion of the lumen occurs. However, this type of peripheral vascular disease is often seen accompanying long-standing diabetes mellitus. (1,3) The most conspicuous imaging finding is the presence of circular, ring-like densities along the entire length of the vessel. This seems to give the vessel wall a coiled appearance, which is virtually diagnostic. (1,3) (Fig. 18-106, C–F)

Aneurysms

Femoral Artery Aneurysm. The femoral artery is the second most common site for aneurysm in the lower extremity, after popliteal aneurysm, and occurs mostly in the common femoral artery. (Fig. 18-107) There is a male predominance of at least 20:1. (4) The normal diameter of the femoral artery ranges from 7 to 10 mm. The average size at discovery is just > 3 cm. (4) Approximately 70% are bilateral. Co-existing aneurysms of the aortoiliac vessels are present in 85% of cases and of the popliteal artery in 45% of cases. (4)

Popliteal Artery Aneurysm. Popliteal aneurysms are the most common aneurysm found in the extremities, accounting for at least 70% of extra-axial lesions. (5) The male to female ratio is 30:1. At least 60% are bilateral, and as many as 50% of cases have simultaneous aortoiliac or femoral aneurysms. (6) Generalized atriomegaly is associated with a higher incidence of popliteal aneurysm and is seen in almost 65%. (7) Other causes include complications from previous angioplasty, graft, trauma, migrated orthopedic implants, and osteochondroma. Ischemia of the limb is common and is secondary to thrombosis in almost half the cases. A popliteal arterial diameter of > 7 mm, usually in the upper to middle course, is considered aneurysmal. The average aneurysm size is 4 cm on detection. (6) (Fig. 18-108) These aneurysms are frequently asymptomatic until they rupture or thrombose, which carries a high risk of limb loss. (6) They may be confused with a Baker's cyst in the popliteal fossa but can be differentiated on ultrasound.

Venous Disorders

Venous Insufficiency. Varicose veins, valvular incompetence, and thrombosis reduce the speed and amount of venous return and are grouped under the term *venous insufficiency.* It is a common disease, usually associated with advancing age and diabetes, and generally affects the distal lower limbs. Although the diagnosis is usually made clinically, radiologic manifestations are often specific and aid in distinguishing it from other entities.

It is most frequent between 50 and 70 years of age. A hereditary component to the disease has been identified, and females are affected at a higher rate than males. (8) Clinical findings include varicosities, skin discoloration, and trophic changes such as ulceration. It is believed that the development of tissue damage resulting from venous insufficiency is related to an inflammatory cascade, including increased endothelial permeability and infiltration of monocytes, lymphocytes, and mast cells into the surrounding connective tissues. (9) The goal of treatment is to eliminate the source of venous occlusion contributing to the patient's venous hypertension. (8,10)

Radiographic manifestations are usually present in both the soft tissue and adjacent bone of the affected region. (Table 18-16) Bone changes are generally that of thick, undulating solid or laminated periosteal new bone over the distal tibia and fibula. (Fig. 18-109) The underlying cortex and medullary cavity are usually unaffected, although the thick periosteal envelope of surrounding new bone may seemingly obliterate the usually clearly demarcated corticomedullary junction. Hypoxia appears to be the mechanism for creating periosteal irritation. (11)

Edema in the soft tissues is evidenced by a relative increase in the soft tissue density, obliteration of fascial fat planes, and displacement of the skin contour. Occasionally, a skin ulceration may be apparent as an excavation in the skin contour. Soft tissue calcification may take a number of forms, including a diffuse reticular pattern; well-defined, rounded phlebolith; or a dense branching opacity of an organized venous thrombosis. Occasionally, especially in diabetics, calcification may be apparent within the vessel wall of adjacent arteries (Mönckeberg's arteriosclerosis).

Deep Vein Thrombosis. Occlusion of a superficial vein may produce localized pain but otherwise is of little significance. Thrombosis of the deep venous system, however, has the additional and sometimes lethal association with pulmonary embolism. Risk factors include trauma, immobilization, long-distance air or vehicle travel (*travelers' disease*), clotting disorder, and malignancy. Symptoms include calf pain and swelling, which are exacerbated with foot dorsiflexion (Homans' sign).

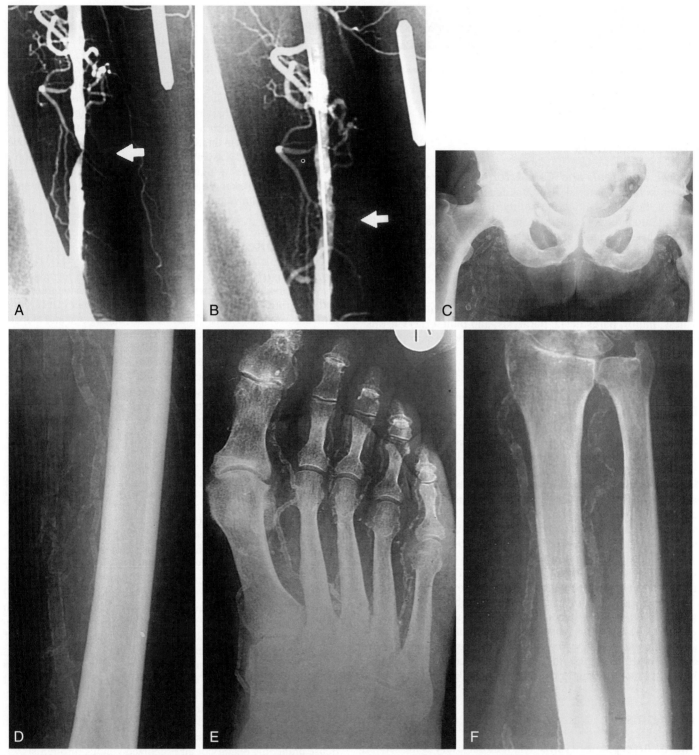

Figure 18-106 **PERIPHERAL VASCULAR DISEASE. A. Athero-sclerotic Stenosis, Angiogram, Preangioplasty Superficial Femoral Artery.** Note that a focal atherosclerotic plaque has reduced the lumen by at least 90% (*arrow*). **B. Athero-sclerotic Stenosis, Angiogram, Postangioplasty Superficial Femoral Artery.** After inflation of an endoluminal balloon, the stenotic region has been successfully dilated without evidence of complicating dissection (*arrow*). **C. Mönckeberg's Medial Sclerosis, AP Pelvis.** Note the femoral arteries and their branches. **D. Mönckeberg's Medial Sclerosis, AP Femur.** Note the superficial and profunda branches of the femoral artery. **E. Mönckeberg's Medial Sclerosis, Dorsoplantar Foot.** Note the digital arteries. **F. Mönckeberg's Medial Sclerosis, PA Forearm.** Note the radial and ulnar arteries. *COMMENT:* Endoluminal balloon angioplasty is a minimally invasive technique that can be successfully used in the treatment of atherosclerotic stenosis. Mönckeberg's medial sclerosis produced diffuse circular coiled calcification throughout the muscular wall at multiple sites. The condition represents a non-stenosing form of vascular calcification, often associated with long-standing diabetes mellitus.

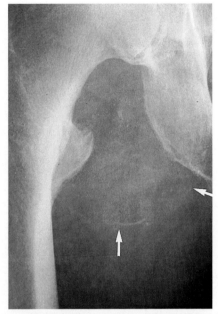

Figure 18-107 **FEMORAL ARTERY ANEURYSM. AP Hip.** Close scrutiny of the soft tissues reveals the distinctive curvilinear calcification in the wall of the aneurysm (*arrows*).

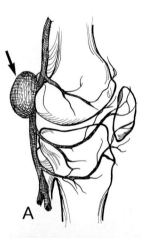

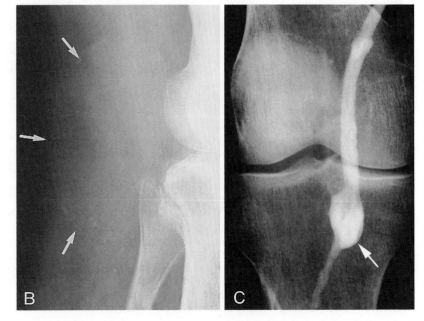

Figure 18-108 **POPLITEAL ARTERY ANEURYSM. A. Typical Popliteal Artery Aneurysm.** Most popliteal aneurysms vary in size and typically reside inferior to the adductor hiatus (*arrow*). Popliteal aneurysms in this location are the most common peripheral aneurysm. **B. Large Popliteal Artery Aneurysm, Lateral Knee.** Note the large soft tissue mass outlined by a peripheral rim of calcification (*arrows*). **C. Small Popliteal Artery Aneurysm, Angiogram, AP Lower Extremity.** Note the small saccular aneurysm (*arrow*).

Table 18-16	Radiologic Findings in Venous Insufficiency

Lower extremity
  Tibia
  Fibula
  Femur
  Metatarsals
  Phalanges
Edema
  Displaced skin contour
  Increased density
  Obliterated fascial planes
Calcification
  Dense and branching
  Diffuse and reticular
  Phleboliths
  Vascular
Periostitis
  Metaphysis and diaphysis
  Linear
  Laminated
  Undulating external surface

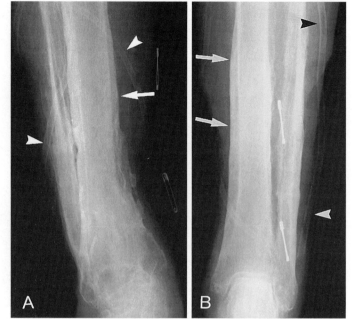

Figure 18-109 **PERIPHERAL VASCULAR INSUFFICIENCY, LOWER LEGS. A. Right Leg, AP Tibia and Fibula. B. Left Leg, AP Tibia and Fibula.** Observe the undulating, solid periosteal new bone formation at the diaphyses of the tibiae and fibulae (*arrows*). Considerable soft tissue swelling secondary to chronic venous stasis is also apparent. Note the artifact (a plastic tube) that is superimposed on the leg (*arrowheads*). *COMMENT:* Chronic venous stasis can precipitate this florid periosteal new bone formation, which may simulate hypertrophic osteoarthropathy.

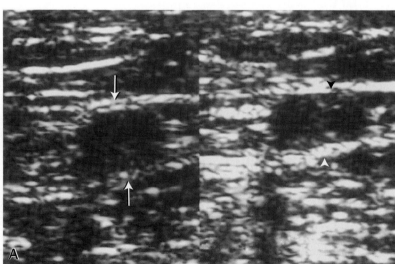

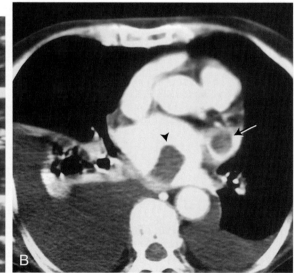

Figure 18-110 **DEEP VENOUS THROMBOSIS. A. Ultrasound, Lower Limb.** Note the thrombus within the femoral vein (*arrows*). Failure of the vein to collapse from the compression of the ultrasound head confirms the presence of endoluminal thrombus (*arrowheads*). **B. Pulmonary Embolism, Pulmonary CT Angiogram, Axial Chest.** Observe the emboli in the pulmonary artery (*arrow*) and left atrium (*arrow-head*). *COMMENT:* Lower limb ultrasound evaluation is routinely performed in patients with pulmonary embolism, as this is the most common site of thrombus formation. Ultrasound is the imaging modality of choice when venous thrombosis is suspected in a patient with painful swelling of the calf.

The diagnosis is confirmed with ultrasound, which demonstrates the thrombus and absence of venous flow. (Fig. 18-110) An inferior vena caval filter can be deployed in patients who are at high risk for pulmonary emboli in the presence of lower limb deep vein thrombosis (DVT) and who are not candidates for anticoagulation. (See Chapter 16.)

■ *References*

THE HEAD: MASQUERADERS OF MUSCULOSKELETAL DISEASE

INTRACRANIAL HEMORRHAGES

1. **Taveras JM:** *Neuroradiology,* ed 3, Baltimore, Williams & Wilkins, 1996.
2. **Osborn AG:** *Diagnostic Neuroradiology.* St. Louis, Mosby-Yearbook, 1994.
3. **Atlas SW:** *Magnetic Resonance Imaging of the Brain and Spinal Cord,* ed 2, Philadelphia, Lippincott-Raven, 1996.
4. **Grossman CB:** *Magnetic Resonance Imaging and Computed Tomography of the Head and Spine,* ed 2, Baltimore, Williams & Wilkins, 1996.
5. **Eisenberg LR:** *Clinical Imaging: An Atlas of Differential Diagnosis,* ed 4. New York, Aspen, 2002.
6. **Ramsey RG:** *Neuroradiology,* ed 3, Philadelphia, WB Saunders, 1981.
7. **Juhl HJ, Crummy BA:** *Paul and Juhl's Essentials of Radiologic Imaging,* ed 7. Philadelphia, JB Lippincott, 1998.
8. **McCort JJ:** *Caring for the major trauma victim: The role for radiology.* Radiology 163:1, 1987.
9. **Huneidi AHS, Afshar F:** *Delayed intracerebral hematomas in moderate to severe head injuries in young adults.* Ann R Coll Surg Engl 74(5):345, 1992.
10. **Adams JH:** *Pathology of non missile injury.* Neuroimag Clin North Am 1:397, 1991.
11. **Reeder MM, Bradley GW Jr:** *Reeder and Felson's Gamuts in Radiology Comprehensive Lists of Roentgen Differential Diagnosis,* ed 4. New York, Springer-Verlag, 2003.
12. **Gentry LR:** *Imaging of closed head injury.* Radiology 191:1, 1994.
13. **Kleinman PK:** *Diagnostic imaging in child abuse.* AJR 155:703, 1990.
14. **Dahnert W:** *Radiology Review Manual,* ed 5. Baltimore, Williams & Wilkins, 2003.
15. **Sadato N, Namagucui T, Rigomonti D, et al.:** *Bleeding patterns in ruptured posterior fossa aneurysms: A CT study.* J Comp Asst Tomogr 15:612, 1991.
16. **Destian S, Sze G, Krol G, et al.:** *MR imaging of hemorrhagic intracranial neoplasms.* AJNR 9:1115, 1988.
17. **Laissy JP, Normand G, Monroc M, et al.:** *Spontaneous intracerebral hematomas from vascular causes.* Neuroradiology 33:291, 1991.
18. **Cohen WA, Wayman LA:** *Computed tomography of intracranial hemorrhage.* Neuroimag Clin North Am 2:75, 1992.
19. **Besenski N, Jadro-Santel D, Grevic N:** *Patterns of lesions of the corpus callosum in inner cerebral trauma visualized by computed tomography.* Neuroradiology 34:126, 1992.

INTRACRANIAL INFECTIONS

1. **Harris TM, Edwards MK:** *Meningitis.* Neuroimag Clin North Am 1:39, 1991.
2. **Taveras JM:** *Neuroradiology,* ed 3, Baltimore, Williams & Wilkins, 1996.
3. **Ramsey RG:** *Neuroradiology,* ed 3, Philadelphia, WB Saunders, 1981.
4. **Atlas SW:** *Magnetic Resonance Imaging of the Brain and Spinal Cord,* ed 2, Philadelphia, Lippincott-Raven, 1996.
5. **Grossman CB:** *Magnetic Resonance Imaging and computed Tomography of the Head and Spine.* ed 2, Baltimore, Williams & Wilkins, 1996.
6. **Eisenberg LR:** *Clinical Imaging: An Atlas of Differential Diagnosis,* ed 4. New York, Aspen Publishers, 2002.
7. **Ashwal S, Tomasi L, Schneider S, et al.:** *Bacterial meningitis in children: Pathophysiology and treatment.* Neurology 42:739, 1992.
8. **Chang KH, Han MH, Roh Jk, et al.:** *Gd-DTPA-enhanced MR imaging of the brain: Comparison with CT.* AJNR 11:69, 1990.
9. **Demaerel PH, Wilms G, Robberecht W, et al.:** *MRI of herpes simplex encephalitis.* Neuroradiology 34:490, 1992.
10. **Osborn AG:** *Diagnostic Neuroradiology.* St. Louis, Mosby-Yearbook, 1994.
11. **Enzmann DR, Britt RH, Placone R:** *Staging of human brain abscess by computed tomography.* Radiology 146:703, 1983.

INTRACRANIAL TUMORS

1. **Ramsey RG:** *Neuroradiology,* ed 3, Philadelphia, WB Saunders, 1981.
2. **Atlas SW:** *Magnetic Resonance Imaging of the Brain and Spinal Cord,* ed 2. Philadelphia, Lippincott-Raven, 1996.
3. **Eisenberg LR:** *Clinical Imaging: An Atlas of Differential Diagnosis,* ed 4. New York, Aspen Publishers, 2002.
4. **Taveras JM:** *Neuroradiology,* ed 3, Baltimore, Williams & Wilkins, 1996.
5. **Osborn AG:** *Diagnostic Neuroradiology.* St. Louis, Mosby-Yearbook, 1994.
6. **Dahnert W:** *Radiology Review Manual,* ed 5. Baltimore, Williams & Wilkins, 2003.
7. **Grossman, CB:** *Magnetic Resonance Imaging and Computed Tomography of the Head and Spine,* ed 2. Baltimore, Williams & Wilkins, 1996.
8. **Juhl HJ, Crummy BA:** *Paul and Juhl's Essentials of Radiologic Imaging,* ed 7. Philadelphia, JB Lippincott, 1998.
9. **Reeder MM, Bradley GW Jr:** *Reeder and Felson's Gamuts in Radiology Comprehensive Lists of Roentgen Differential Diagnosis,* ed 4. New York, Springer-Verlag, 2003.
10. **Buetow MP, Burton PC, Smirniotopoulos JG:** *Typical, atypical and misleading features in meningioma.* RadioGraphics 11:1087, 1991.
11. **Maier H, Offer D, Hittmair A, et al.:** *Classic, atypical and anaplastic meningioma: Three histopathologic subtypes of clinical relevance.* J Neurosurg 77:616, 1992.
12. **Masters LT, Zimmerman RD:** *Imaging supratentorial brain tumors in adults.* Neuroimag Clin North Am 3(4):649, 1993.
13. **Vezina LG, Packer RJ:** *Infratentorial brain tumors of childhood.* Neuroimag Clin North Am 4(2):423, 1994.

VASCULAR DISORDERS

1. **Taveras JM:** *Neuroradiology,* ed 3, Baltimore, Williams & Wilkins, 1996.
2. **Eisenberg LR:** *Clinical Imaging: An Atlas of Differential Diagnosis,* ed 4. New York, Aspen Publishers, 2002.
3. **Dahnert W:** *Radiology Review Manual,* ed 5. Baltimore, Williams & Wilkins, 2003.
4. **Atlas SW:** *Magnetic Resonance Imaging of the Brain and Spinal Cord,* ed 2, Philadelphia, Lippincott-Raven, 1996.
5. **Osborn AG:** *Diagnostic Neuroradiology.* St. Louis, Mosby-Yearbook, 1994.
6. **Bagley LJ, Hurst RW:** *Angiographic evaluation of aneurysms affecting the central nervous system.* Neuroimag Clin North Am 7(4):721, 1997.
7. **Atlas SW:** *Magnetic resonance imaging of intracranial aneurysms.* Neuroimag Clin North Am 7:709, 1997.
8. **Truwit CL, Barkovitch AJ, Gean A, et al.:** *Loss of the insular ribbon: another early CT sign of acute middle cerebral artery infarction.* Radiology 176(3):801, 1990.
9. **Tomandi BF, Klotz E, Handschu R, et al.:** *Comprehensive imaging of ischemic stroke with multisection CT.* Radiographics 23:565, 2003.
10. **Bastienollo S, Pierallini A, Colinnese C, et al.:** *Hyperdense middle cerebral artery CT sign.* Neuroradiology 33:207, 1991.

11. **Brown RD Jr, Wiebers DO, Forbes G, et al.:** *The natural history of unruptured intracranial arteriovenous malformations.* J Neurosurg 68:352, 1988.

12. **Auger RG, Weibers DO:** *Management of unruptured intracranial arteriovenous malformations: a decision analysis.* Neurosurgery 30:561, 1992.

13. **Wallace RC, Bourekas EC:** *Brain arteriovenous malformations.* Neuroimag Clin North Am 8(2):383, 1998.

14. **Ramsey RG:** *Neuroradiology,* ed 3, Philadelphia, WB Saunders, 1981.

15. **Juhl HJ, Crummy BA:** *Paul and Juhl's Essentials of Radiologic Imaging,* ed 7. Philadelphia, JB Lippincott, 1998.

16. **Kesava PP, Turski PA:** *Magnetic resonance angiography of vascular malformations.* Neuroimag Clin North Am 8(2):349, 1998.

17. **Grossman CB:** *Magnetic Resonance Imaging and Computed Tomography of the Head and Spine,* ed 2, Baltimore, Williams & Wilkins, 1996.

18. **King JT:** *Epidemiology of aneurysmal subarachnoid hemorrhage.* Neurimag Clin North Am 7:659, 1997.

19. **Lasner TM, Raps EC:** *Clinical evaluation and management of aneurysmal subarachnoid hemorrhage.* Neuroimag Clin North Am 7:669, 1997.

20. **Reeder MM, Bradley GW Jr:** *Reeder and Felson's Gamuts in Radiology Comprehensive Lists of Roentgen Differential Diagnosis,* ed 4. New York, Springer-Verlag, 2003.

21. **Greiner FG, Takhtani D:** *Neuoradiology case of the day.* Radiographics 19:1098, 1999.

22. **Virapongse C, Cazenave C, Quisling R, et al.:** *The empty delta sign: Frequency and significance in 76 cases of dural sinus thrombosis.* Radiology 162:779, 1987.

THE NECK: MASQUERADERS OF MUSCULOSKELETAL DISEASE

VERTEBRAL ARTERY

1. **George B, Laurian C:** *The Vertebral Artery. Pathology and Surgery.* New York, Springer-Verlag, 1987.

2. **Hadley LA:** *Anatomico-Roentgenographic Studies of the Spine.* Springfield, IL, Charles C Thomas, 1964.

3. **Hadley LA:** *Tortuosity and deflection of the vertebral artery.* AJR 80:306, 1958.

4. **Holden A, Adler B, Song S:** *Bilateral vertebral artery tortuosity with concomitant vertebral erosion: CT and MRA findings.* Aust Radiol 40:65, 1996.

5. **Anderson RE, Shealy CN:** *Cervical pedicle erosion and rootlet compression caused by a tortuous vertebral artery.* Radiology 96:537, 1970.

6. **Cooper DF:** *Bone erosion of the cervical vertebrae secondary to tortuosity of the vertebral artery.* J Neurosurg 53:106, 1980.

7. **Glover JR, Kennedy C, Coral A:** *Tortuous vertebral artery: Onset of symptoms during pregnancy.* Clin Radiol 41:66, 1990.

8. **Thiel HW:** *Gross morphology and pathoanatomy of the vertebral arteries.* J Manipulative Physiol Ther 14(2):133, 1991.

9. **Taitz C, Arensburg B:** *Vertebral artery tortuosity with concomitant erosion of the foramen of the transverse process of the axis.* Acta Anat 141:104, 1991.

10. **Zimmerman HB, Farrell WJ:** *Cervical vertebral body erosion caused by vertebral artery tortuosity.* AJR 108:767, 1970.

11. **Freilich M, Virapongse C, Kier EL, et al.:** *Foramen transversarium enlargement due to tortuosity of the vertebral artery.* Spine 11:95, 1986.

12. **Kricun R, Levitt LP, Winn HR:** *Tortuous vertebral artery shown by MR and CT.* AJR 159:613, 1992.

13. **Danziger J, Bloch S:** *The widened cervical intervertebral foramen.* Radiology 116:671, 1975.

14. **Mokri B, Houser OW, Sandok BA, Piepgras DG:** *Spontaneous dissections of the vertebral arteries.* Neurology 38:880, 1988.

15. **Ford FR:** *Syncope, vertigo and disturbances of vision resulting from intermittent obstruction of the vertebral arteries due to a defect in the odontoid process and excessive mobility of the second cervical vertebra.* Bull Johns Hopkins Hosp 91:168, 1952.

16. **Hart RG, Miller VT:** *Cerebral infarction in young adults: A practical approach.* Stroke 14:110, 1983.

17. **Thiel H, Wallace K, Donat J, Yong-Hing K:** *Effect of various head and neck positions on vertebral artery blood flow.* Clin Biomech 9:105, 1994.

18. **Taveras JM:** *Neuroradiology,* ed 3, Baltimore, Williams & Wilkins, 1996.

19. **Ramsey RG:** *Neuroradiology,* ed 3, Philadelphia, WB Saunders, 1981.

20. **Atlas SW:** *Magnetic Resonance Imaging of the Brain and Spinal Cord,* ed 2, Philadelphia, Lippincott-Raven, 1996.

21. **Wilkinson IMS:** *The vertebral artery: Extracranial and intracranial structure.* Arch Neurol 27:392, 1972.

22. **Lewis DW, Berman PH:** *Vertebral artery dissection and alternating hemiparesis in an adolescent.* Pediatrics 78(4):610, 1986.

23. **McGregor M, Haldeman S, Kohlbeck FJ:** *Vertebrobasilar compromise associated with cervical manipulation.* Top Clin Chiro 2(3):63, 1995.

24. **Fogelholm R, Karli P:** *Iatrogenic brainstem infarction.* Eur Neurol 13:6, 1975.

25. **Caplan LR, Baquis GD, Pessin MS, et al.:** *Dissection of the intracranial vertebral artery.* Neurology 38:868, 1988.

26. **Terrett AGJ:** *Current Concepts in Vertebrobasilar Complications Following Spinal Manipulations.* Des Moines, IA, NCMIC Group, 2001

27. **Licht PB, Christensen HW, Hojgaard P, Marving J:** *Vertebral artery flow and spinal manipulation: A randomised, controlled and observer-blinded study.* J Manipulative Physiol Ther 21(3):141, 1998.

28. **Herzog W, Symons B:** *The mechanics of neck manipulation with special consideration of the vertebral artery.* J Can Chiro Assoc 46(3):134, 2002.

29. **Dvorak J, Orelli F:** *How dangerous is manipulation of the cervical spine?* Manual Med 2:1, 1985.

30. **Klougart N, Lebouef-Yde C, Rasmussen LR:** *Safety in chiropractic practice. Part II. Treatment to the upper neck and the rate of cerebrovascular incidents.* J Manipulatve Physiol Ther 19(9):563, 1996.

31. **Pratt-Thomas HR, Berger KE:** *Cerebellar and spinal injuries after chiropractic manipulation.* JAMA 133:600, 1947.

32. **Tomita K, Tsuchiya H, Nomura S:** *Dynamic entrapment of the vertebral artery by the nerve branch: A new etiology for transient cervical vertigo.* Neuro Orthop 4:36, 1987.

33. **Okawara S, Nibblelink D:** *Vertebral artery occlusion following hyperextension and rotation of the head.* Stroke 5:640, 1974.

34. **Adams KHR, Yung MW, Lye M, Whitehouse GH:** *Are cervical spine radiographs of value in elderly patients with vertebrobasilar insufficiency?* Age Aging 15:57, 1986.

35. **Hardin CA, Williamson P, Steegman A:** *Vertebral artery insufficiency caused by cervical osteoarthritic spurs.* Neurology 10:855, 1960.

36. **Husni E, Storer J:** *The syndrome of mechanical occlusion of the vertebral artery.* Angiology 18(2):106, 1967.

37. **Hutchinson EC, Yates PO:** *Cervical portion of vertebral artery: Clinico-pathologic study.* Brain 79:319, 1956.

38. **Schmitt HP:** *Anatomical structure of the cervical spine with reference to the pathology of manipulation complications.* J Manual Med 6:93, 1991.

39. **Tramo MJ, Hainline B, Petito F, et al.:** *Vertebral artery injury and cerebellar stroke while swimming: A case report.* Stroke 16(6):1039, 1985.

40. **Takakuwa T, Hiroi S, Hasegawa H, et al.:** *Os odontoideum with vertebral artery occlusion.* Spine 19:460, 1994.

41. **Hensinger RN:** *Congenital anomalies of the cervical spine.* Clin Orthop 264:16, 1991.

42. **Bernini FP, Elefante R, Smaltino F, Tedeschi G:** *Angiographic study of the vertebral artery in cases of deformity of the occipito-cervical joint.* AJR 107:526, 1969.

43. **Janeway R, Tolle JF, Leinbach LB, Miller HS:** *Vertebral artery obstruction with basilar impression.* Arch Neurol 115:211, 1966.

44. **Tokuda K, Miyasaka K, Abe H, et al.:** *Anomalous atlantoaxial portions of vertebral and posterior inferior cerebellar arteries.* Neuroradiology 27:410, 1985.

45. **Bolton PS, Stick PE, Lord RSA:** *Failure of clinical tests to predict cerebral ischemia before neck manipulation.* J Manipulative Physiol Ther 12(4):304, 1989.

46. **Greselle JF, Zenteno M, Kien P, et al.:** *Spontaneous dissection of the vertebro-basilar system: A study of 18 cases (15 patients).* J Neuroradiol 14:115, 1987.

47. **Soper JR, Parker GD, Hallinan JM:** *Vertebral artery dissection diagnosed with CT.* AJNR 16:952, 1995.

48. **Song WS, Chiang YH, Chen CY, et al.:** *A simple method for diagnosing traumatic occlusion of the vertebral artery at the craniovertebral junction.* Spine 19:837, 1994.

49. **Haynes MJ:** *Doppler studies comparing the effects of cervical rotation and lateral flexion on vertebral artery blood flow.* J Manipulative Physiol Ther 19(6):378, 1996.

50. **Combs SB, Triano JJ:** *Symptoms of neck artery compromise: Case presentations of risk estimate for treatment.* J Manipulative Physiol Ther 20(4):274, 1997.

INTERNAL CAROTID ARTERY DISSECTION

1. **Hart RG, Easton JD:** *Dissections of cervical and cerebral arteries.* Neurol Clin 1(1):155, 1983.

2. **Ozdoba C, Sturtzenegger M, Schroth G:** *Internal carotid artery dissection: MR imaging features and clinical-radiologic correlation.* Radiology 199:191, 1996.

3. **Provenzale JM:** *Dissection of the internal carotid and vertebral arteries: Imaging features.* AJR 165:1099, 1995.

4. **Davis JM, Zimmerman RA:** *Injury of the carotid and vertebral arteries.* Neuroradiology 25:55, 1983.

5. **Pitner SE:** *Carotid thrombosis due to intraoral trauma: An unusual complication of a common childhood accident.* N Engl J Med 274:764, 1966.

6. **Boldrey E, Maas L, Miller E:** *The role of atlantoid compression in the etiology of internal carotid artery thrombosis.* J Neurosurg 113:127, 1956.

7. **Parenti G, Orlandi G, Bianchi M, et al.:** *Vertebral and carotid artery dissection following chiropractic cervical manipulation.* Neurosurg Rev 22:127, 1999.

8. **Lyness SS, Wagman AD:** *Neurological deficit following cervical manipulation.* Surg Neurol 2:121, 1974.

9. **Beatty RA:** *Dissecting hematoma of the internal carotid artery following chiropractic manipulation.* J Trauma 17:248, 1977.

10. **Murthy JMK, Naidu KV:** *Aneurysm of the cervical internal carotid artery following chiropractic manipulation.* J Neurol Neurosurg Psychiatry 51:1237, 1988.

11. **Jumper JM, Horton HC:** *Central retinal occlusion after manipulation of the neck by a chiropractor.* Am J Ophthalmol 121:321, 1996.

12. **Hufnagel A, Hammers A, Schonle PW, et al.:** *Stroke following chiropractic manipulation of the cervical spine.* J Neurol 246(8):683, 1999.

13. **Peters M, Bohl J, Thomke F, et al.:** *Dissection of the internal carotid artery after chiropractic manipulation of the neck.* Neurology 45:2284, 1995.

14. **Haldeman S, Kohlbeck FJ, McGregor M:** *Unpredictability of cerebrovascular ischemia associated with cervical spine manipulation.* Spine 27:49, 2002.

15. **Terrett AGJ:** *Current Concepts in Vertebrobasilar Complications Following Spinal Manipulations.* Des Moines, IA, NCMIC Group, 2001.

16. **Russo CP, Smoker WRK:** *Nonatheromatous carotid artery disease.* Neuroimag Clin North Am 6:811, 1996.

17. **Bousson V, Levy C, Brunereau L, et al.:** *Dissections of the internal carotid artery: Three-dimensional time-of-flight MR angiography and MR imaging features.* AJR 173:139, 1999.

18. **Taveras JM:** *Neuroradiology,* ed 3. Baltimore, Williams & Wilkins, 1996.

19. **Atlas SW:** *Magnetic Resonance Imaging of the Brain and Spinal Cord,* ed 2, Philadelphia, Lippincott-Raven, 1996.

20. **Dahnert W:** *Radiology Review Manual,* ed 5. Baltimore, Williams & Wilkins, 2003.

21. **Eisenberg LR:** *Clinical Imaging: An Atlas of Differential Diagnosis,* ed 4. New York, Aspen Publishers, 2002.

SUBCLAVIAN STEAL SYNDROME

1. **Contorni L:** *The true story of the "subclavian steal syndrome" or "Harrison and Smyth's syndrome."* J Cardiovasc Surg 14:408, 1973.

2. **Fisher CM:** *A new vascular syndrome—"The subclavian steal syndrome."* N Engl J Med 265:912, 1961.

3. **Terrett AGJ:** *Current Concepts in Vertebrobasilar Complications following Spinal Manipulation.* Des Moines, IA, NCMIC Publications. 2001.

4. **Taveras JM:** *Neuroradiology,* ed 3, Baltimore, Williams & Wilkins, 1996.

5. **Ramsey RG:** *Neuroradiology,* ed 3, Philadelphia, WB Saunders, 1981.

6. **Zimmerman NB:** *Occlusive vascular disorders of the upper extremity.* Hand Clin 9:139, 1993.

7. **Fields WS, Lemark NA:** *Joint study of extracranial arterial occlusion VIII. Subclavian steal: A review of 168 cases.* JAMA 222:1139, 1972.

8. **Reeder MM, Bradley GW Jr:** *Reeder and Felson's Gamuts in Radiology Comprehensive Lists of Roentgen Differential Diagnosis,* ed 4. New York, Springer-Verlag, 2003.

9. **Atlas SW:** *Magnetic Resonance Imaging of the Brain and Spinal Cord,* ed 2, Philadelphia, Lippincott-Raven, 1996.

10. **Lacey KO:** *Subclavian steal syndrome: A review.* J Vasc Surg Nursing 15:1, 1996.

11. **Dahnert W:** *Radiology Review Manual,* ed 5. Baltimore, Williams & Wilkins, 2003.

12. **Eisenberg LR:** Clinical Imaging: An Atlas of Differential Diagnosis, ed 4. New York, Aspen Publishers, 2002.

13. **Juhl HJ, Crummy BA:** *Paul and Juhl's Essentials of Radiologic Imaging,* ed 7. Philadelphia, JB Lippincott, 1998.

STYLOHYOID LIGAMENT OSSIFICATION

1. **Dwight T:** *Stylohyoid ossification.* Ann Surg 46:721, 1907.

2. **Lipshutz B:** *The clinical importance of ossification of the stylohyoid ligament.* JAMA 79(24):1982, 1923.

3. **Eagle WW:** *Elongated styloid process.* Arch Otolaryngol 47:630, 1948.

4. **Eagle WW:** *Symptomatic elongated styloid process.* Arch Otolaryngol 49:490, 1949.

5. **Gossman JR, Tarsitano JJ:** *The styloid-stylohyoid syndrome.* J Oral Surg 35:555, 1977.

6. **Harma R, Styalgia R:** *Stylohyoid ligament ossification.* Acta Otolaryngol 224(Suppl):149, 1967.

7. **Mueller N, Hamilton S, Reid GD:** *Ossification of both stylohyoid ligaments, considerably larger on the left. Case report 248.* Skeletal Radiol 10:273, 1983.

8. **Graf CJ:** *Glossopharyngeal neuralgia and ossification of the stylohyoid ligament.* J Neurosurg 16:448, 1959.

9. **Bolton SP:** *Elongated styloid process of the temporal bone.* J Aust Chiro Assoc 17(2):69, 1987.

10. **Juhl HJ, Crummy BA:** *Paul and Juhl's Essentials of Radiologic Imaging,* ed 7. Philadelphia, JB Lippincott, 1998.

GRISEL'S SYNDROME

1. **Wetzel FT, La Rocca H:** *Grisel's syndrome. A review.* Clin Orthop 240:141, 1989.

2. **Mathern GW, Batzdorf U:** *Grisel's syndrome.* Clin Orthop 244:131, 1989.

3. **Yochum TR, Rowe LJ:** *Arthritides of the upper cervical complex.* In: R Iczak, ed, *Aspects of Manipulative Therapy,* ed 2. New York, Churchill Livingstone, 1985.
4. **Grisel P:** *Enucleation de l'atlas et torticollis naso-pharyngien.* Presse Med 38:50, 1930.
5. **Watson-Jones R:** *Spontaneous hyperemic dislocation of the atlas.* Proc R Soc Med 25:586, 1932.
6. **Werne S:** *Studies in spontaneous atlas dislocation.* Acta Orthop Scand Suppl 23:1, 1957.
7. **De Coster TA, Cole HC:** *Atlanto-axial dislocation in association with rheumatic fever.* Spine 15:591, 1990.
8. **Park WW, Rothman RH, Brown MD:** *The pharyngovertebral veins: An anatomical rationale for Grisel's syndrome.* J Bone Joint Surg 66A:568, 1984.
9. **Taveras JM:** *Neuroradiology,* ed 3. Baltimore, Williams & Wilkins, 1996.
10. **Atlas SW:** *Magnetic Resonance Imaging of the Brain and Spinal Cord,* ed 2. Philadelphia, Lippincott-Raven, 1996.
11. **Ramsey RG:** *Neuroradiology,* ed 3, Philadelphia, WB Saunders, 1981.
12. **Juhl HJ, Crummy BA:** *Paul and Juhl's Essentials of Radiologic Imaging,* ed 7. Philadelphia, JB Lippincott, 1998.

RETROPHARYNGEAL ABSCESS

1. **Craig FW, Schunk JE:** *Retropharyngeal abscess in children: clinical presentation, utility of imaging, and current management.* Pediatrics 111:1394, 2003.
2. **Parhiscar A, Har-El G:** *Deep neck abscess: A retrospective review of 210 cases.* Ann Otolaryngol Rhinol Laryngol 110:1051, 2001.
3. **Boucher C, Dorion D, Fisch C:** *Retropharyngeal abscesses: A clinical and radiologic correlation.* J Otolaryngol 28(3):134, 1999.
4. **Schmal F, Stoll W:** *Differential diagnosis and management of retropharyngeal space-occupying lesions* [German]. HNO 50:418, 2002.
5. **Jang YJ, Rhee CK:** *Retropharyngeal abscess associated with vertebral osteomyelitis and spinal epidural abscess.* Otolaryngol Head Neck Surg 119:705, 1998.
6. **Weber AL, Siciliano A:** *CT and MR imaging evaluation of neck infections with clinical correlations.* Radiol Clin North Am 38:941, 2000.

CALCIFIC TENDONITIS OF THE LONGUS COLLI

1. **Ring D, Vaccaro AR, Scuderi G, et al.:** *Acute calcific retropharyngeal tendinitis.* J Bone Joint Surg 76A:1636, 1994.
2. **Artenian DJ, Lipman JK, Scidmore GK, Brant-Zawadzki M:** *Acute neck pain due to tendonitis of the longus colli: CT and MRI findings.* Neuroradiology 31:166, 1989.
3. **Newmark H, Zee CS, Frankel P, et al.:** *Chronic calcific tendonitis of the neck.* Skeletal Radiol 7:207, 1981.
4. **Eastwood JD, Hudgins PA, Malone D:** *Retropharyngeal effusion in acute calcific prevertebral tendinitis: Diagnosis with CT and MR imaging.* AJNR 19:1789, 1998.
5. **Dahnert W:** *Radiology Review Manual,* ed 5. Baltimore, Williams & Wilkins, 2003.
6. **Juhl HJ, Crummy BA:** *Paul and Juhl's Essentials of Radiologic Imaging,* ed 7. Philadelphia, JB Lippincott, 1998.

SALIVARY GLAND CALCULUS (SIALOLITHIASIS)

1. **Silvers AR, Som PM:** *Salivary glands.* Radiol Clin North Am 36(5):941, 1998.
2. **Dahnert W:** *Radiology Review Manual,* ed 5. Baltimore, Williams & Wilkins, 2003.
3. **Reeder MM, Bradley GW Jr:** *Reeder and Felson's Gamuts in Radiology Comprehensive Lists of Roentgen Differential Diagnosis,* ed 4. New York, Springer-Verlag, 2003.

THYROID DISEASE

1. **Whittingham W, Molyneux T:** *Thyroid carcinoma detected in a chronic headache sufferer: A case report.* Chiro J Aust 24(1):23, 1994.
2. **Lazarus JH, Obuobie K:** *Thyroid disorders—An update.* Postgrad Med J 76:529, 2000.

3. **Weber AL, Randolph G, Aksoy FG:** *The thyroid and parathyroid glands. CT and MR imaging and correlation with pathology and clinical findings.* Radiol Clin North Am 38:1105, 2000.
4. **Makeieff M, Marlier F, Khudjadze M, et al.:** *Substernal goiter. Report of 212 cases.* Ann Chiro 125:18, 2000.
5. **Rodriguez JM, Hernandez Q, Pinero A, et al.:** *Substernal goiter: Clinical experience of 72 cases.* Ann Otolaryngol Rhinol Laryngol 108:501, 1999.
6. **Bockisch A, Brandt-Mainz K, Gorges R, et al.:** *Diagnosis in medullary thyroid cancer with [18F]FDG-PET and improvement using a comined PET/CT scanner.* Acta Med Aust 30:22, 2003.
7. **Jennings A:** *Evaluation of substernal goiters using computed tomography and MR imaging.* Endocrinol Metab Clin North Am 30:401, 2001.
8. **Kim SJ, Kim IJ, Kim YK:** *Tc-99m MIBI, Tc-99m tetrofosmin, and Tc-99m (V) DMSA accumulation in recurrent malignant thymoma.* Clin Nucl Med 27:30, 2002.
9. **Rakashima S, Takayama F, Wang JC, et al.:** *Radiologic assessment of metastases to the thyroid gland.* J Comput Assist Tomogr 24:539, 2000.
10. **Eisenberg LR:** *Clinical Imaging: An Atlas of Differential Diagnosis,* ed 4. New York, Aspen Publishers, 2002.
11. **Dahnert W:** *Radiology Review Manual,* ed 5. Baltimore, Williams & Wilkins, 2003.
12. **Juhl HJ, Crummy BA:** *Paul and Juhl's Essentials of Radiologic Imaging,* ed 7. Philadelphia, JB Lippincott, 1998.
13. **Jurik AG:** *Ossification and calcification of the laryngeal skeleton.* Acta Radiol Diagn 25:17, 1984.
14. **Reeder MM, Bradley GW Jr:** *Reeder and Felson's Gamuts in Radiology Comprehensive Lists of Roentgen Differential Diagnosis,* ed 4. New York, Springer-Verlag, 2003.

THE THORAX: MASQUERADERS OF MUSCULOSKELETAL DISEASE

FUNDAMENTAL SIGNS OF CHEST DISEASE

1. **Wilson AG:** *Interpreting the Chest Radiograph.* In: RG Grainger and DJ Alison, ed, *Diagnostic Radiology,* ed 3. New York, Churchill-Livingstone, 1997.
2. **Felson B:** *Chest Roentgenology.* Philadelphia, WB Saunders, 1973.
3. **Griffin CB, Primack CL:** *High resolution CT: Normal anatomy, techniques, and pitfalls.* Radiol Clin North Am 39(6):1073, 2001.
4. **Squire FL:** *Fundamentals of Radiology,* ed 5. Cambridge, MA: Harvard College, 1997.
5. **Taveras MJ, Ferrucci TJ:** *Radiology Diagnosis-Imaging-Intervention.* Baltimore, Lippincott, Williams & Wilkins, 2000.
6. **Juhl HJ, Crummy BA:** *Paul and Juhl's Essentials of Radiologic Imaging,* ed 7. Philadelphia, JB Lippincott, 1998.
7. **Proto AV:** *Pulmonary lobar collapse: Essential considerations.* In: RG Grainger and DJ Alison, ed, *Diagnostic Radiology,* ed 3. New York, Churchill-Livingstone, 1997.
8. **Eisenberg LR:** *Clinical Imaging: An Atlas of Differential Diagnosis,* ed 4. New York, Aspen Publishers, 2002.
9. **Müller NL, Fraser RS, Colman NC, Paré PD:** *Radiologic Diagnosis of Diseases of the Chest.* Philadelphia, WB Saunders, 2001.
10. **Slone RM, Gutierrez FR, Fisher AJ:** *Thoracic Imaging: A Practical Approach.* New York, McGraw-Hill, 1999.
11. **Fraser RS, Müller NL, Colman N, Paré PD:** *Fraser and Paré's Diagnosis of Diseases of the Chest,* ed 4. Philadelphia, WB Saunders, 1999.
12. **McCloud TC:** *Thoracic Radiology: The Requisites.* St. Louis, CV Mosby, 1988.

COMMON CALCIFICATIONS OF THE CHEST AND THORAX

1. **Köhler's A, Zimmer EA:** In: SP Wilk, ed, *Borderlands of the Normal and Early Pathologic in Skeletal Roentgenology,* ed 3. New York, Grune & Stratton, 1968.
2. **Ontell FK, Moore EH, Shepard JO, Shelton DK:** *The costal cartilages in health and disease.* RadioGraphics 17:571, 1997.

3. **Slone RM, Gutierrez FR, Fisher AJ:** *Thoracic Imaging: A Practical Approach.* New York, McGraw-Hill, 1999.
4. **Juhl HJ, Crummy BA:** *Paul and Juhl's Essentials of Radiologic Imaging,* ed 7. Philadelphia, JB Lippincott, 1998.
5. **Müller NL, Fraser RS, Colman NC, Paré PD:** *Radiologic Diagnosis of Diseases of the Chest.* Philadelphia, WB Saunders, 2001.
6. **Eisenberg LR:** *Clinical Imaging: An Atlas of Differential Diagnosis,* ed 4. New York, Aspen Publishers, 2002.
7. **Reeder MM, Bradley GW Jr:** *Reeder and Felson's Gamuts in Radiology Comprehensive Lists of Roentgen Differential Diagnosis,* ed 4. New York, Springer-Verlag, 2003.
8. **Taveras MJ, Ferrucci TJ:** *Radiology Diagnosis-Imaging-Intervention.* Baltimore, Lippincott, Williams & Wilkins, 2000.
9. **Ko JP, Drucker EA, Shepard JO, et al.:** *CT depiction of regional nodal stations for lung cancer staging.* AJR 174:775, 2000
10. **Hiawatsch A, Kauezor HU, Thelen M:** *Pulmonary tuberculosis— The current radiological diagnosis of an old disease.* Radiologe 40(6):507, 2000.
11. **Fraser RS, Müller NL, Colman N, Paré PD:** *Fraser and Paré's Diagnosis of Diseases of the Chest,* ed 4. Philadelphia, WB Saunders, 1999.
12. **Dahnert W:** *Radiology Review Manual,* ed 5. Baltimore, Williams & Wilkins, 2003.
13. **Squire FL:** *Fundamentals of Radiology,* ed 5. Cambridge, MA: Harvard College, 1997.
14. **Urban BA, Bluemke DA, Johnson KM, Fishman EK:** *Imaging of thoracic aortic disease.* Cardiol Clin 17(4):659, 1999.
15. **Khan IA, Nair CK:** *Clinical diagnostic, and management perspectives of aortic dissection.* Chest 122:311, 2002.
16. **Carr JJ, Crouse JR, Goff DC, et al.:** *Evaluation of subsecond gated helical CT for quantification of coronary artery calcium and comparison with electron beam.* AJR 174:915, 2000.
17. **Roach HD, Davis GJ, Attanoos R, et al.:** *Asbestos: When the dust settles: an imaging review of asbestos-related disease.* Radiographics 22:S167, 2002.
18. **Ploverosi R, Vigo M, Citton O:** *Pleural and parenchymal lung diseases from asbestos exposure. CT diagnosis.* Radiol Med [Torino]. 100:326, 2000.
19. **McCloud TC:** *Thoracic Radiology: The Requisites.* St. Louis, CV Mosby, 1988.

VASCULAR DISEASES OF THE CHEST

1. **Gluecker T, Capasso P, Schnyder P, et al.:** *Clinical and radiologic features of pulmonary edema.* Radiographics 19:1507, 1999. [Discussion 19:1532, 1999.]
2. **Perina DG:** *Noncardiogenic pulmonary edema.* Emerg Med Clin North Am 21:385, 2003.
3. **Sakal F:** *Plain x-ray diagnosis of noncardiogenic edema.* Nippon Igaku Hoshasen Gakkai Zasshi 59:367, 1999.
4. **Drake RE, Doursout MF:** *Pulmonary edema and elevated left atrial pressure: four hours and beyond.* News Physiol Sci 17:223, 2002.
5. **Matsuyama S, Ootaki M, Saito T, et al.:** *Radiographic diagnosis of cardiogenic pulmonary edema.* Nippon Igaku Hoshasen Gakkai Zasshi 59:223, 1999.
6. **Flower CDR:** *Diffuse pulmonary disease.* In: RG Grainger and DJ Alison, eds, *Diagnostic Radiology,* ed 3. New York, Churchill-Livingstone, 1997.
7. **Slone RM, Gutierrez FR, Fisher AJ:** *Thoracic Imaging: A Practical Approach.* New York, McGraw-Hill, 1999.
8. **Anderson FA Jr, Spencer FA:** *Risk factors for venous thromboembolism.* Circulation 107(23 Suppl 1):I9, 2003.
9. **Kruip MJ, Leclereq MG, van der Heul C, et al.:** *Diagnostic strategies for excluding pulmonary embolism in clinical outcome studies. A systemic review.* Ann Intern Med 138:941, 2003.
10. **Kearon C:** *Diagnosis of pulmonary embolism.* Can Med Assoc J 168:183, 2003.
11. **Hansell DM:** *Pulmonary thromboembolism.* In: RG Grainger and DJ Alison, eds, *Diagnostic Radiology,* ed 3. New York, Churchill-Livingstone, 1997.

12. **Perrier A, Nendaz MR, Sarasin FP, et al.:** *Cost-effectiveness analysis of diagnostic strategies for suspected pulmonary embolism including helical computed tomography.* Am J Respir Crit Care Med. 167:39, 2003.
13. **Garg K:** *CT of pulmonary thromboembolic disease.* Radiol Clin North Am 40(1):111, 2002.
14. **Indik JH, Alpert JS:** *Detection of pulmonary embolism by D-dimer assay, spiral computed tomography, and magnetic resonance imaging.* Prog Cardiovasc Dis 42(4):261, 2000.
15. **Ledbetter S, Stuk JL, Kaufman JA:** *Helical (spiral) CT in the evaluation of emergent thoracic aortic syndromes.* Radiol Clin North Am 37(3):575, 1999.
16. **Khan IA, Nair CK:** *Clinical diagnostic, and management perspectives of aortic dissection.* Chest 122:311, 2002.
17. **Fraser RS, Müller NL, Colman N, Paré PD:** *Fraser and Paré's Diagnosis of Diseases of the Chest,* ed 4. Philadelphia, WB Saunders, 1999.
18. **Müller NL, Fraser RS, Colman NC, Paré PD:** *Radiologic Diagnosis of Diseases of the Chest.* Philadelphia, WB Saunders, 2001.
19. **Urban BA, Bluemke DA, Johnson KM, Fishman EK:** *Imaging of thoracic aortic disease.* Cardiol Clin 17:659, 1999.
20. **Hartnell GG:** *Imaging of aortic aneurysms and dissection: CT and MRI.* J Thorac Imaging 16(1):35, 2001.
21. **McCloud TC:** *Thoracic Radiology: The Requisites.* St. Louis, CV Mosby, 1988.
22. **Creasy JD, Chiles C, Routh WD, Dyer RB:** *Overview of traumatic injury of the thoracic aorta.* Radiographics 17:27, 1997.

AIRWAY DISEASE

1. **Agusti AG, Noguera A, Sauleda J, et al.:** *Systemic effects of chronic obstructive pulmonary disease.* Eur Respir J 21(2):347, 2003.
2. **Felson B:** *Chest Roentgenology.* Philadelphia, WB Saunders, 1973.
3. **Fireman P:** *Understanding asthma pathophysiology.* Allergy Asthma Proc 24(2):79, 2003.
4. **Adams BK, Bydulka RK:** *Asthma evaluation and management.* Emerg Med Clin North Am 21(2):315, 2003.
5. **Koh YY, Kim CK:** *The development of asthma in patients with allergic rhinitis.* Curr Opin Allergy Clin Immunol 3(3):159, 2003.
6. **Muller NL, Coxson H:** *Chronic obstructive pulmonary disease, 4: Imaging the lungs in patients with chronic obstructive pulmonary disease.* Thorax 57(11):982, 2002.
7. **Fraser RS, Müller NL, Colman N, Paré PD:** *Fraser and Paré's Diagnosis of Diseases of the Chest,* ed 4. Philadelphia, WB Saunders, 1999.
8. **Müller NL, Fraser RS, Colman NC, Paré PD:** *Radiologic Diagnosis of Diseases of the Chest.* Philadelphia, WB Saunders, 2001.
9. **Cleverley JR, Muller NL:** *Advances in radiologic assessment of chronic obstructive pulmonary disease.* Clin Chest Med 21(4):653, 2000.
10. **Lynch DA:** *Imaging of asthma and allergic bronchopulmonary mycosis.* Radiol Clin North Am 36(1):129, 1998.
11. **McCloud TC:** *Thoracic Radiology: The Requisites.* St. Louis, CV Mosby, 1988.
12. **Slone RM, Gutierrez FR, Fisher AJ:** *Thoracic Imaging: A Practical Approach.* New York, McGraw-Hill, 1999.
13. **Takasugi JE:** *Radiology of chronic obstructive pulmonary disease.* Radiol Clin North Am 36(1):129, 1998.
14. **Sashidhar K, Gulati M, Gupta D, et al.:** *Emphysema in heavy smokers with normal chest radiography. Detection and quantification by HCRT.* Acta Radiol. 43(1):60, 2002.
15. **Cederlund K, Tylen U, Jorfeldt L, et al.:** *Classification of emphysema in candidates for lung volume reduction surgery: A new objective and surgically oriented model for describing CT severity and heterogeneity.* Chest 122(2):90, 2002.
16. **Newell JD:** *CT of emphysema.* Radiol Clin Noth Am 40(1):31, 2002.
17. **Bankier AA, Madani A, Gevenois PA:** *CT quantification of pulmonary emphysema: assessment of lung structure and function.* Crit Rev Comput Tomogr 43(6):399, 2002.

18. **Glerada DS:** *Radiologic assessment of emphysema for lung volume reduction surgery.* Semin Thorac Cardiovasc Surg 14(4):381, 2002.
19. **Pasteur MC, Gelliwell SM, Houghton, et al.:** *An investigation into causative factors in patients with bronchiectasis.* Am J Respir Crit Care Med 162:1277, 2000.
20. **Karakoc GB, Yilmaz M, Altintus DU, Kendirli SG:** *Bronchiectasis: Still a problem.* Pediatr Pulmonol 32(2):175, 2001.
21. **Scala R, Aronne D, Palumbo U, et al.:** *Prevalence, age distribution and aetiology of bronchiectasis: A retrospective study on 144 symptomatic patients.* Monaldi Arch Chest Dis 55(2):101, 2000.
22. **McGuinness G, Naidich DP:** *CT of airways disease and bronchiectasis.* Radiol Clin North Am 40(1):1, 2002.

ALVEOLAR DISEASE

1. **Müller NL, Fraser RS, Colman NC, Paré PD:** *Radiologic Diagnosis of Diseases of the Chest.* Philadelphia, WB Saunders, 2001.
2. **Slone RM, Gutierrez FR, Fisher AJ:** *Thoracic Imaging: A Practical Approach.* New York, McGraw-Hill, 1999.
3. **Bochud PY, Moser F, Erard P, et al.:** *Community-acquired pneumonia. A prospective outpatient study.* Medicine [Baltimore]. 80(2):75, 2001.
4. **Kamath A, Pasteur MC, Slade MG, Harrison BD:** *Recognising severe pneumonia with simple clinical and biochemical measurements.* Clin Med 3(1):54, 2003.
5. **Belleza WG, Browne B:** *Pulmonary consideration in the immunocompromised patient.* Emerg Med Clin North Am 21(2):499, 2003.
6. **Fraser RS, Müller NL, Colman N, Paré PD:** *Fraser and Paré's Diagnosis of Diseases of the Chest,* ed 4. Philadelphia, WB Saunders, 1999.
7. **Johanson WG, Dever LI:** *Nosocomial pneumonia.* Intensive Care Med 29(1):23, 2003. [Published online Dec 4, 2002.]
8. **Murray K, Gosselin M, Anderson M, et al.:** *Distribution of lung disease.* Semin Ultrasound CT MR 23(4):352, 2002.
9. **McCloud TC:** *Thoracic Radiology: The Requisites.* St. Louis, CV Mosby, 1988.
10. **Felson B:** *Chest Roentgenology.* Philadelphia, WB Saunders, 1973.
11. **Jo EK, Park JK, Dockrell HM:** *Dynamics of cytokine generation in patients with active pulmonary tuberculosis.* Curr Opin Infect Dis 6(3):205, 2003.
12. **Van Wormer LM:** *Tuberculosis: The latest.* CRNA 11(1):15, 2000.
13. **Rajagopalan S:** *Tuberculosis and aging: A global health problem.* Clin Infect Dis 33(7):1034, 2001. [Published online Aug 22, 2001.]
14. **LaRosa JA, Cutaia M:** *Urban tuberculosis: The new face of an old problem.* Curr Infect Dis Rep 5(3):246, 2003.
15. **Dass B, Peut RA, Watanakunakorn C:** *Tuberculosis of the spine (Pott's disease) presenting as 'compression fractures.'* Spinal Cord 40(11):604, 2002.
16. **Viera AJ, Bond MM, Yates SW:** *Diagnosis: night sweats.* Am Fam Physician 67(5):1019, 2003.
17. **Perkins MD:** *New diagnostic tools for tuberculosis.* Int J Tuberc Lung Dis 4(12 Suppl 2):S182, 2000.
18. **Hiawatsch A, Kauezor HU, Thelen M:** *Pulmonary tuberculosis— The current radiological diagnosis of an old disease.* Radiologe 40(6):507, 2000.

INTERSTITIAL LUNG DISEASE

1. **McCloud TC:** *Thoracic Radiology: The Requisites.* St. Louis, CV Mosby, 1988.
2. **Fraser RS, Müller NL, Colman N, Paré PD:** *Fraser and Paré's Diagnosis of Diseases of the Chest,* ed 4. Philadelphia, WB Saunders, 1999.
3. **Müller NL, Fraser RS, Colman NC, Paré PD:** *Radiologic Diagnosis of Diseases of the Chest.* Philadelphia, WB Saunders, 2001.
4. **Slone RM, Gutierrez FR, Fisher AJ:** *Thoracic Imaging: A Practical Approach.* New York, McGraw-Hill, 1999.
5. **Perez RL, Rivera-Marrero CA, Roman J:** *Pulmonary granulomatous inflammation: From sarcoidosis to tuberculosis.* Semin Respir Infect 18(1):23, 2003.
6. **Baughman RP, Lower EE, du Bois RM:** *Sarcoidosis.* Lancet 361(9363):111, 2003.

7. **Thomas KW, Hunninghake GW:** *Sarcoidosis.* JAMA 289(24):3300, 2003.
8. **Donghi M, Giura R, Antonelli P:** *Increase of serum copper concentration in Lofgren syndrome.* Sarcoidosis 12(2):147, 1995.
9. **Barnard J, Newman LS:** *Sarcoidosis: Immunology, rheumatic involvement, and therapeutics.* Curr Opin Rheumatol 13(1):84, 2001.
10. **Ponhold W:** *The Lofgren syndrome: Acute sarcoidosis* [Trans]. Rontgenblatter 30(6):325, 1977.
11. **Felson B:** *Chest Roentgenology.* Philadelphia, WB Saunders, 1973.
12. **Bonomo L, Feragalli B, Sacco R, et al.:** *Malignant pleural disease.* Eur J Radiol 34(2):98, 2000.
13. **Roach HD, Davis GJ, Attanoos R, et al.:** *Asbestos: When the dust settles an imaging review of asbestos-related disease.* Radiographics 22(Spec No):S167, 2002.
14. **Peacock C, Copley SJ, Hansell DM:** *Asbestos-related benign pleural disease.* Clin Radiol 55(6):422, 2000.
15. **Marom EM, Erasmus JJ, Pass HI, Patz EF Jr:** *The role of imaging in malignant pleural mesothelioma.* Semin Oncol 29(1):26, 2002.
16. **Ploverosi R, Vigo M, Citton O:** *Pleural and parenchymal lung diseases from asbestos exposure. CT diagnosis.* Radiol Med [Torino] 100(5):326, 2000.
17. **Chapman SJ, Cookson WO, Musk AW, Lee YC:** *Benign asbestos pleural diseases.* Curr Opin Pulm Med 9(4):266, 2003.
18. **Lindell KO, Jacobs SS:** *Idiopathic pulmonary fibrosis.* Am J Nurs 103(4):32, 2003.
19. **Green FH:** *Overview of pulmonary fibrosis.* Chest 122(6 Suppl): 334S, 2002.
20. **Nathan SD, Barnett SD, Uraban BA, et al.:** *Pulmonary embolism in idiopathic pulmonary fibrosis transplant recipients.* Chest 123(5):1758, 2003.

TUMORS OF THE LUNG

1. **Lau CL, Harpole DH Jr, Patz E:** *Staging techniques for lung cancer.* Chest Surg Clin North Am 10(4):781, 2000.
2. **Fraser RS, Müller NL, Colman N, Paré PD:** *Fraser and Paré's Diagnosis of Diseases of the Chest,* ed 4. Philadelphia, WB Saunders, 1999.
3. **Felson B:** *Chest Roentgenology.* Philadelphia, WB Saunders, 1973.
4. **Patz EF Jr:** *Imaging bronchogenic carcinoma.* Chest 117(4 Suppl 1): 90S, 2000.
5. **Strollo DC, Rosado-de-Christenson ML, Franks TJ:** *Reclassification of cystic bronchioloalveolar carcinomas to adenocarcinomas based on the revised World Health Organization Classification of Lung and Pleural Tumours.* J Thorac Imaging 18(2):59, 2003
6. **Chen R, Tatsumi A, Numoto S:** *Combined choriocarcinoma and adenocarcinoma of the lung occurring in a man: Case report and review of the literature.* Cancer 91(1):123, 2001.
7. **Cavazza A, Toffanetti R, Ferrari G, et al.:** *Combined neoplasia of the lung: description of a case of adenocarcinoma mixed with typical carcinoid.* Pathologica 93(3):216, 2001.
8. **McCloud TC:** *Thoracic Radiology: The Requisites.* St. Louis, CV Mosby, 1988.
9. **Takahashi M, Nitta N, Takazakura R, et al.:** *Many faces of squamous cell carcinoma of the lung: Its wide spectrum of radiological findings.* Curr Probl Diagn Radiol 32(2):45, 2003.
10. **Sakurada A, Sagawa M, Sato M, et al.:** *Roentgenographically occult bronchogenic squamous cell carcinoma involving mediastinal lymph nodes after removal of initial lesion by the diagnostic examination.* Lung Cancer 38(1):39, 2002.
11. **Müller NL, Fraser RS, Colman NC, Paré PD:** *Radiologic Diagnosis of Diseases of the Chest.* Philadelphia, WB Saunders, 2001.
12. **Cerilli LA, Ritter JH, Mills SE, Wick MR:** *Neuroendocrine neoplasms of the lung.* Am J Clin Pathol 116(Suppl):S65, 2001.
13. **Simon GR, Wagner H, American College of Chest Physicians:** *Small cell lung cancer.* Chest 123(1 Suppl):259S, 2003.
14. **Johnson BE:** *Management of small cell lung cancer.* Clin Chest Med 23(1):225, 2002.
15. **Takei H, Asamura H, Maeshima A, et al.:** *Large cell neuroendocrine carcinoma of the lung: A clinicopathologic study of eighty-seven cases.* J Thorac Cardiovasc Surg 124(2):285, 2002.

16. **Zacharias J, Nicholson AG, Ladas GP, Goldstraw P:** *Large cell neuroendocrine carcinoma and large cell carcinomas with neuroendocrine morphology of the lung: Prognosis after complete resection and systematic nodal dissection.* Ann Thorac Surg 75(2):348, 2003.
17. **Hage R, de la Riviere AB, Seldenrijk CA, van den Bosch JM:** *Update in pulmonary carcinoid tumors: A review article.* Ann Surg Oncol 10(6):697, 2003.
18. **Thomas CF Jr, Tazelaar HD, Jett JR:** *Typical and atypical pulmonary carcinoids: outcome in patients presenting with regional lymph node involvement.* Chest 119(4):1143, 2001.
19. **Jeung MY, Gasser B, Gangi A, et al.:** *Bronchial carcinoid tumors of the thorax: spectrum of radiologic findings.* Radiographics 22(2):351, 2002.
20. **Bociek RG, Armitage JO:** *Hodgkin's disease and non-Hodgkin's lymphoma.* Curr Opin Hematol 6(4):205, 1999.
21. **Viera AJ, Bond MM, Yates SW:** *Diagnosis: night sweats.* Am Fam Physician 67(5):1019, 2003.
22. **Yung L, Linch D:** *Hodgkin's lymphoma.* Lancet 361(9361):943, 2003.
23. **Hauke RJ, Armitage JO:** *A new approach to non-Hodgkin's lymphoma.* Intern Med 39(3):197, 2000.
24. **Slone RM, Gutierrez FR, Fisher AJ:** *Thoracic Imaging: A Practical Approach.* New York, McGraw-Hill, 1999.

MEDIASTINAL LESIONS
1. **Müller NL, Fraser RS, Colman NC, Paré PD:** *Radiologic Diagnosis of Diseases of the Chest.* Philadelphia, WB Saunders, 2001.
2. **Slone RM, Gutierrez FR, Fisher AJ:** *Thoracic Imaging: A Practical Approach.* New York, McGraw-Hill, 1999.
3. **Erasmus JJ, McAdams HP, Donnelly LF, Spritzer CE:** *MR imaging of mediastinal masses.* Magn Reson Imaging Clin North Am 8(1):59, 2000.
4. **Fraser RS, Müller NL, Colman N, Paré PD:** *Fraser and Paré's Diagnosis of Diseases of the Chest,* ed 4. Philadelphia, WB Saunders, 1999.
5. **Yung L, Linch D:** *Hodgkin's lymphoma.* Lancet 361(9361):943, 2003.
6. **Graeber GM, Tamim W:** *Current status of the diagnosis and treatment of thymoma.* Semin Thorac Cardiovasc Surg 12(4):268, 2000.
7. **Goh MH, Liu XY, Goh YS:** *Anterior mediastinal masses: An anaesthetic challenge.* Anaesthesia 54(7):670, 1999.
8. **McCloud TC:** *Thoracic Radiology: The Requisites.* St. Louis, CV Mosby, 1988.
9. **Kim Y, Lee KS, Yoo JH, et al.:** *Middle mediastinal lesions: Imaging findings and pathologic correlation.* Eur J Radiol 35(1):30, 2000.

DIAPHRAGM
1. **Suwatanapongched T, Gierada DS, Slone RM, et al.:** *Variation in diaphragm position and shape in adults with normal pulmonary function.* Chest 123(6):2019, 2003.
2. **Fraser RS, Müller NL, Colman N, Paré PD:** *Fraser and Paré's Diagnosis of Diseases of the Chest,* ed 4. Philadelphia, WB Saunders, 1999.
3. **Slone RM, Gutierrez FR, Fisher AJ:** *Thoracic Imaging: A Practical Approach.* New York, McGraw-Hill, 1999.
4. **Bellemare JF, Cordeau MP, Leblanc P, Bellemare F:** *Thoracic dimensions at maximum lung inflation in normal subjects and in patients with obstructive and restrictive lung diseases.* Chest 119(2):376, 2001.
5. **McCloud TC:** *Thoracic Radiology: The Requisites.* St. Louis, CV Mosby, 1988.
6. **Bellemare F, Jeanneret A, Couture J:** *Sex differences in thoracic dimensions and configuration.* Am J Respir Crit Care Med. [Published online May 28, 2003.]
7. **Müller NL, Fraser RS, Colman NC, Paré PD:** *Radiologic Diagnosis of Diseases of the Chest.* Philadelphia, WB Saunders, 2001.
8. **Felson B:** *Chest Roentgenology.* Philadelphia, WB Saunders, 1973.
9. **Felsher J, Brodsky J, Brody F:** *Isolated trans-hiatal colonic herniation.* J Laparoendosc Adv Surg Tech A 13(2):105, 2003.
10. **Scheidler MG, Keenan RJ, Maley RH, et al.:** *"True" parahiatal hernia: A rare entity radiologic presentation and clinical management.* Ann Thorac Surg 73(2):416, 2002.
11. **Vermillion JM, Wilson EB, Smith RW:** *Traumatic diaphragmatic hernia presenting as a tension fecopneumothorax.* Hernia 5(3):158, 2001.
12. **Shreck GL, Toalson TW:** *Delayed presentation of traumatic rupture of the diaphragm.* J Okla State Med Assoc 96(4):181, 2003.
13. **Mihos P, Potaris K, Gakidis J, et al.:** *Traumatic rupture of the diaphragm: Experience with 65 patients.* Injury 34(3):169, 2003.
14. **Stojkovic T, De Seze J, Hurtevent JF, et al.:** *Phrenic nerve palsy as a feature of chronic inflammatory demyelinating polyradiculoneuropathy.* Muscle Nerve 27(4):397, 2003.
15. **Simansky DA, Paley M, Refaely Y, Yellin A:** *Diaphragm plication following phrenic nerve injury: A comparison of paediatric and adult patients.* Thorax 57(7):613, 2002.
16. **Roach HD, Davis GJ, Attanoos R, et al.:** *Asbestos: When the dust settles an imaging review of asbestos-related disease.* Radiographics 22(Spec No):S167, 2002.
17. **Ohsaki Y, Morimoto H, Osanai S, et al.:** *Extensively calcified hemangioma of the diaphragm with increased 99mTe-hydroxymethylene diphosphonate uptake.* Intern Med 39(7):576, 2000.
18. **Weissberg D, Refaely Y:** *Pneumothorax: Experience with 1,199 patients.* Chest 117(5):1279, 2000.

THE ABDOMEN: MASQUERADERS OF MUSCULOSKELETAL DISEASE
FUNDAMENTALS OF ABDOMINAL DISEASE

1. **Myers MA:** *Dynamic Radiology of the Abdomen: Normal and Pathologic Anatomy,* ed 5. New York, Springer, 2000.
2. **Eisenberg LR:** *Gastrointestinal Radiology. A Pattern Approach.* ed 4. Philadelphia, JB Lippincott, 2002.
3. **Freeny PC, Stevenson GW:** *Margulis and Burhenne's Alimentary Tract Radiology,* ed 5. St. Louis, CV Mosby, 1994.
4. **Weill FS, Manco-Johnson ML:** *Imaging of Abdominal and Pelvic Anatomy.* New York, Churchill Livingstone, 1997.
5. **Taveras MJ, Ferrucci TJ:** *Radiology Diagnosis-Imaging-Intervention.* Baltimore, Lippincott, Williams & Wilkins, 2000.
6. **Juhl HJ, Crummy BA:** *Paul and Juhl's Essentials of Radiologic Imaging,* ed 7. Philadelphia, JB Lippincott, 1998.
7. **Squire FL:** *Fundamentals of Radiology,* ed 5. Cambridge, MA: Harvard College. 1997.
8. **Baker SR, Cho KC:** *The Abdominal Plain Film With Correlative Imaging,* ed 2. New York, Appleton & Lange. 1999.
9. **Baker SR, Elkin M:** *Plain Film Approach to Abdominal Calcifications.* Philadelphia, WB Saunders, 1983.
10. **Ring ER, Eaton SB Jr, Ferrucci JT Jr, et al.:** *Differential diagnosis of pancreatic calcification.* AJR 117:446, 1973.

SPECIFIC ABDOMINAL DISORDERS

1. **Taveras MJ, Ferrucci TJ:** *Radiology Diagnosis-Imaging-Intervention.* Baltimore, Lippincott, Williams & Wilkins, 2000.
2. **Squire FL:** *Fundamentals of Radiology,* ed 5. Cambridge, MA: Harvard College. 1997.
3. **Myers MA:** *Dynamic Radiology of the Abdomen: Normal and Pathologic Anatomy,* ed 5. New York, Springer, 2000.
4. **Eisenberg LR:** *Gastrointestinal Radiology. A Pattern Approach,* ed 4. Philadelphia, JB Lippincott, 2002.
5. **Dahnert W:** *Radiology Review Manual,* ed 5. Baltimore, Williams & Wilkins, 2003.
6. **Freeny PC, Stevenson GW:** *Margulis and Burhenne's Alimentary Tract Radiology,* ed 5. St. Louis, CV Mosby, 1994.
7. **Yu JS, Kim MJ, Kim KW:** *Intratumoral blood flow in cavernous hemangioma of the liver: Radiologic-pathologic correlation.* Radiology 208:549, 1998.
8. **Juhl HJ, Crummy BA:** *Paul and Juhl's Essentials of Radiologic Imaging,* ed 7. Philadelphia, JB Lippincott, 1998.

9. **Baker SR, Elkin M:** *Plain Film Approach to Abdominal Calcifications.* Philadelphia, WB Saunders, 1983.

10. **Singh Y, Winick AB, Tabbara SO:** *Residents teaching files: Multiloculated cystic liver lesions: Radiologic-pathologic differential diagnosis.* Radiographics 17:219, 1997.

11. **Adam A, Gibson RN, Soreide V, et al.:** *The radiology of fibrolamellar hepatoma.* Clin Radiol 37:355, 1986.

12. **Miele AJ, Edmonds HW:** *Calcified liver metastases: A specific roentgen diagnostic sign.* Radiology 80:779, 1963.

13. **Baker SR, Cho KC:** *The Abdominal Plain Film with Correlative Imaging,* ed 2. New York, Appleton & Lange. 1999.

14. **Tait N, Little JM:** *The treatment of gallstones.* Br Med J 311:99, 1995.

15. **Wright FW:** *The "Jack Stone" or "Mercedes-Benz" sign: A new theory to explain the presence of gas within fissures in gallstones.* Clin Radiol 28:469, 1977.

16. **Weill FS, Manco-Johnson ML:** *Imaging of Abdominal and Pelvic Anatomy.* New York, Churchill Livingstone, 1997.

17. **Kratzer W, Mason RA, Kachele V:** *Prevalence of gallstones in sonographic surveys world-wide.* J Clin Ultrasound 27:1, 1999.

18. **Oschner SF, Carrera GM:** *Calcification of the gall bladder ("porcelain gall bladder").* AJR 89:847, 1963.

19. **Etala E:** *Cancer de la vesicula biliar.* Prensa Med Argent 49:2283, 1962.

20. **Cornell CM, Clarke R:** Vicarious calcification involving the gall bladder. Ann Surg 149:267, 1959.

21. **Berk RM, Armbruster TG, Saltzstein S:** *Carcinoma in the porcelain gallbladder.* Radiology 106:29, 1973.

22. **Meyers MA, Evans JA:** *Effects of pancreatitis on the small bowel and colon: Spread along mesenteric planes.* AJR 119:151, 1973.

23. **Ring ER, Eaton SB Jr, Ferrucci JT Jr, et al.:** *Differential diagnosis of pancreatic calcification.* AJR 117:446, 1973.

24. **O'Malley ME, Boland GWL, Wood BJ, et al.:** *Adenocarcinoma of the head of the pancreas: determination of surgical unresectability with thin section pancreatic phase helical CT.* AJR 173:1513, 1999.

25. **Curtin JJ, Ridley NTF, Colbeck R:** *Case report: Staghorn calculus complicated by psoas abscess presenting as a flank mass in a teenager.* Br J Radiol 68:844, 1993.

26. **Morse RM, Resnick MI:** *Ureteral calculi: Natural history and treatment in an era of technology.* J Urol 145(2):263, 1991.

27. **Reeder MM, Bradley GW Jr:** *Reeder and Felson's Gamuts in Radiology Comprehensive Lists of Roentgen Differential Diagnosis,* ed 4. New York, Springer-Verlag, 2003.

28. **Katz DS, Hines J, Rausch DR, et al.:** *Unenhanced helical CT for suspected renal colic.* AJR 173:425, 1999.

29. **Traubici J, Neitlich JD, Smith RC:** *Distinguishing pelvic phleboliths from distal ureteral stones on routine unenhanced helical CT: Is there a radiolucent center?* AJR 172:13, 1999.

30. **McClennan BL, Deyoe LA:** *The imaging evaluation of renal cell carcinoma: Diagnosis and staging.* Radiol Clin North Am 32(1):55, 1994.

31. **Rowe LJ, Clarey C:** *Spinal metastases masquerading as thoracolumbar syndrome.* Chiro J Aust 29:103, 1999.

32. **Sivit CJ, Applegate KE, Stallion A, et al.:** *Imaging evaluation of suspected appendicitis in a pediatric population: Effectiveness of ultrasonography versus CT.* AJR 175:977, 2000.

33. **Lowe RA, Penny MW, Scheker LE, et al.:** *Appendicolith revealed on CT in children with suspected appendicitis: How specific is it in the diagnosis of appendicitis?* AJR 175:981, 2000.

34. **Taveras MJ, Ferrucci TJ:** *Radiology Diagnosis-Imaging-Intervention.* Baltimore, Lippincott, Williams & Wilkins, 2000.

35. **Grossfield GD, Coakley FV:** *Benign prostatic hyperplasia: clinical overview and value of diagnostic imaging.* Radiol Clin North Am 38(1):31, 2000.

36. **Gittes RF:** *Carcinoma of the prostate.* N Engl J Med 324(4):236, 1991.

37. **Yu KK, Hricak H:** *Imaging prostate cancer.* Radiol Clin North Am 38(1):59, 2000.

38. **Coleman BG:** *Transvaginal sonography of adnexal masses.* Radiol Clin North Am 30(4):677, 1992.

39. **Langer JE, Dinsmore BJ:** *Computed tomographic evaluation of benign and inflammatory disorders of the female pelvis.* Radiol Clin North Am 30(4):831, 1992.

40. **Cotran RS, Kumar V, Robbins SL:** *Robbins Pathologic Basis of Disease,* ed 5. Philadelphia, WB Saunders 1994.

41. **Atherton WW, Kettner NW:** *Benign ovarian cystic teratoma: A case report.* Top Diagn Radiol Adv Imag 26:2, 1999.

42. **Mendelson EB, Bohm-Velez M:** *Transvaginal ultrasonography of pelvic neoplasms.* Radiol Clin North Am 30(4):703, 1992.

43. **Walsh JW:** *Computed tomography of gynaecologic neoplasms.* Radiol Clin North Am 30(4):703, 1992.

44. **Castro JR, Klein EW:** *The incidence and appearance of roentgenologically visible psammomatous calcification of papillary cystadenocarcinoma of the ovaries.* AJR 88:886, 1962.

45. **Garant M, Reinhold C:** *Dermoid cyst of the ovary: Computed tomography diagnosis of an unusual case.* Can Assoc Radiol J 47:107, 1996.

46. **Peterson WF:** *Malignant degeneration of benign cystic teratomas of the ovary: A collective review of the literature.* Obstetr Gynecol Surg 12:793, 1958.

47. **Zorlu CG, Kuscu E, Caglar T, et al.:** *Malignant degeneration of mature cystic teratomas.* Aust NZ Obstet Gynecol 36(2)221, 1996.

48. **Peterson WF, Prevost EC, Edmunds FT, et al.:** *Benign cystic teratomas of the ovary: A clinico-statistical study of 1007 cases with review of the literature.* Am J Obst Gynecol 70:368, 1955.

49. **Austan F, Polise M:** *A young woman with low back pain.* J Am Acad Phys Assist 7:544, 1994.

50. **Siegel MJ, McAllister WA, Shackleford LD:** *Radiographic findings in ovarian teratomas in children.* AJR 131:613, 1978.

51. **Sloan RD:** *Cystic teratoma (dermoid) of the ovary.* Radiology 81:847, 1963.

52. **Buy JN, Ghossain MA, Moss AA, et al.:** *Cystic teratoma of the ovary: CT detection.* Radiology 171:697, 1989.

53. **Occhipinti KA, Frankel SD, Hricak H:** *The ovary. Computed tomography and magnetic resonance imaging.* Radiol Clin North Am 31:1115, 1993.

ARTERIAL DISORDERS

1. **Stone JA, Cyr C, Friesen M, et al.:** *Canadian guidelines for cardiac rehabilitation and atherosclerotic heart disease prevention: A summary.* Can J Cardiol 17(Suppl B):3B, 2001.

2. **Myers MA:** *Dynamic Radiology of the Abdomen: Normal and Pathologic Anatomy,* ed 5. New York, Springer, 2000.

3. **Taveras MJ, Ferrucci TJ:** *Radiology Diagnosis-Imaging-Intervention.* Baltimore, Lippincott, Williams & Wilkins, 2000.

4. **Boukhris R, Becker KL:** *Calcification of the aorta and osteoporosis.* JAMA 219:1307, 1972.

5. **Moynahan K, Yoshino MT:** *Aortic and renal atherosclerotic calcifications seen on computed tomography of the spine. A positive predictor of hypertension.* Invest Radiol 28:811, 1993.

6. **Lindblom A:** *Arteriosclerosis and arterial thrombosis in the lower limb. A roentgenological study.* Acta Radiol 80(Suppl):1, 1950.

7. **Monhan K, Yoshino MT:** *Aortic and renal atherosclerotic calcifications seen on computed tomography of the spine. A positive predictor of hypertension.* Invest Radiol 28(9):811, 1993.

8. **Auerbach O, Garfinkel L:** *Atherosclerosis and aneurysm of aorta in relation to smoking habits and age.* Chest 78:805, 1980.

9. **Kurunlahti M, Kerttula L, Jauhiainen J, et al.:** *Correlation of diffusion in lumbar discs with occlusion of lumbar arteries: A study in adult volunteers.* Radiology 221:779, 2001.

10. **Spirt BA, Skolnick ML, Carsky EW, et al.:** *Anterior displacement of the abdominal aorta: A radiographic and sonographic study.* Radiology 111:399, 1974.

11. **Vernon H:** *Anterior osteophytic encroachment of the abdominal aorta.* J Can Chiro Assoc 23:154, 1979.

12. **Juhl HJ, Crummy BA:** *Paul and Juhl's Essentials of Radiologic Imaging,* ed 7. Philadelphia, JB Lippincott, 1998.

13. **Reeder MM, Bradley GW Jr:** *Reeder and Felson's Gamuts in Radiology Comprehensive Lists of Roentgen Differential Diagnosis,* ed 4. New York, Springer-Verlag, 2003.

14. **Weill FS, Manco-Johnson ML:** *Imaging of Abdominal and Pelvic Anatomy.* New York, Churchill Livingstone, 1997.

15. **Sylvester PA, Stewart R, Ellis H:** *Tortuosity of the splenic artery.* Clin Anat 8:214, 1995.

16. **LaRoy LL, Cormier PJ, Matalon TAS, et al.:** *Imaging of abdominal aortic aneurysms.* AJR 152:785, 1989.

17. **Johnston KW, Rutherford RB, et al.:** *Suggested standards for reporting on arterial aneurysms.* J Vasc Surg 13:452, 1991.

18. **Liddington MI, Heather BM:** *The relationship between aortic diameter and body habitus.* Eur J Vasc Surg 6:89, 1992.

19. **Hollier LH, Stanson AW, Glovicki, P, et al.:** *Arteriomegaly: Classifications and morbid implications of diffuse aneurysmal disease.* Surgery 93:(5)700, 1983.

20. **Ramchandani P, Ball D:** *Abdominal aortic aneurysms: Diagnosis, measurement and treatment.* Postgrad Radiol 6:259, 1986.

21. **Trotter MC, Ilabaca PA:** *Ruptured abdominal aortic aneurysms: A retrospective look at a ten-year interval.* Vasc Surg 27:183, 1993.

22. **Nakagawa Y, Masuda M, Shiihara H, et al.:** *A chronic contained rupture of an abdominal aortic aneurysm complicated with severe back pain.* Ann Vasc Surg 4:189, 1990.

23. **Brown MJ:** *Prevalence of pathology seen on lumbar x-rays in patients over 50 years.* Br J Chiro 5(1–2):23, 2001.

24. **Hadida C, Rajwani M:** *Abdominal aortic aneurysms: A case report.* J Can Chiro Assoc 42(4):216, 1998.

25. **Godwin JD, Korobkin M:** *Acute disease of the aorta: Diagnosis by computed tomography and ultrasonography.* Radiol Clin North Am 21:551, 1983.

26. **Steinberg CR, Archer M, Steinberg I:** *Measurement of the abdominal aorta after intravenous aortography in health and arteriosclerotic peripheral vascular disease.* AJR 95:703, 1965.

27. **Collin J, Aranjo L:** *Oxford screening programme for abdominal aortic aneurysm in men aged 65–74 years.* Lancet 2:613, 1988.

28. **O'Kelly TJ, Heather BP:** *General practice based population screening for abdominal aortic aneurysms: A pilot study.* Br J Surg 76:479, 1989.

29. **Strachan DP:** *Predictors of death from aortic aneurysm among middle-aged men: The Whitehall study.* Br J Surg 78:401, 1993.

30. **Debakey MR, Crawford ES, Cooley DA, et al.:** *Aneurysm of abdominal aorta: Analysis of graft replacement therapy 1 to 11 years after operation.* Ann Surg 160:622, 1964.

31. **Adamson J, Powell JT, Greenhaigh RM:** *Selection for screening for familial aortic aneurysms.* Br J Surg 79:897, 1992.

32. **Nevitt MP, Ballard DJ, Hallett JW:** *Prognosis of abdominal aortic aneurysms: A population-based study.* N Engl Med J 321:1009, 1989.

33. **Schubert F:** *Giant aneurysm of the abdominal aorta.* Austral Radiol 39:58, 1995.

34. **Yochum TR, Guebert GM, Kettner NW:** *Abdominal aortic aneurysm—The total picture.* Appl Diagn Imag 1:1, 1989.

35. **Costello P, Gaa J:** *Spiral CT angiography of abdominal aortic aneurysms.* RadioGraphics 15:397, 1995.

36. **Darling CR, Messina CR, Brewster DC, Ottinger LW:** *Autopsy study of unoperated abdominal aortic aneurysms: The case for early resection.* Circulation 56(Suppl II):161, 1977.

37. **Walker DI, Bloor K, Williams G, et al.:** *Inflammatory aneurysms of the abdominal aorta.* Br J Surg 59:609, 1972.

38. **Steinberg I, Stein HL:** *Arteriosclerotic abdominal aortic aneurysms: Report of 200 consecutive cases.* JAMA 195:1025, 1966.

39. **Cabellon S, Moncrief CL, Pierre DR, et al.:** *Incidence of abdominal aortic aneurysms with atherosclerotic disease.* Am J Surg 146:575, 1983.

40. **Kiell CS, Ernst CB:** *Advances in management of abdominal aortic aneurysm.* Adv Surg 26:73, 1993.

41. **McGregor JC:** *Unoperated ruptured aortic aneurysms: A retrospective clinicopathological study over a 10 year period.* Br J Surg 63:113, 1976.

42. **Parsavand R:** *Angiographic demonstration of ruptured aortic aneurysm.* Radiology 11:577, 1974.

43. **Sterpetti AV, Blair EA, Schultz RD, et al.:** *Sealed rupture of abdominal aortic aneurysms.* J Vasc Surg 11:430, 1990.

44. **Qvardt PG, Reilly LM, Mark AS, et al.:** *Computerised tomographic assessment of graft incorporation after aortic reconstruction.* Am J Surg 150:227, 1985.

45. **Raabe R, Lawrence PF, Luers PR, et al.:** *Radiographs and clinical findings in unusual abdominal aortic aneurysms.* Cardiovasc Intervent Radiol 9:176, 1986.

46. **Vulpio C, Venuto V, Francesco F, et al.:** *Abdominal aortic aneurysm with periaortic fibrosis and ureteral obstruction—Report of two cases.* Vasc Surg 25:243, 1991.

47. **Hollis HW, Rutherford RB:** *Abdominal aortic aneurysms associated with horseshoe or ectopic kidneys: Techniques of renal preservation.* Semin Vasc Surg 1:148, 1988.

48. **Orton DF, LeVeen RF, Saigh JA, et al.:** *Aortic prosthetic graft infections: Radiologic manifestations and implications for management.* RadioGraphics 20:977, 2000.

49. **Rowe LJ:** *Abdominal aortic aneurysm* [Roentgen Briefs]. ACA Council Roentgenol 1981.

50. **Larsson EM, Heiling M, Holtas S:** *Aortic pathology revealed by MRI in patients with clinical suspicion of spinal disease.* Neuroradiology 35:499, 1993.

51. **Thorkeldsen A:** *Abdominal aortic aneurysm: A case report.* Eur J Chiro 41:95, 1993.

52. **Gomes MN, Schellinger D, Hufnagel CA:** *Abdominal aortic aneurysms: diagnostic review and new technique.* Ann Thoracic Surg 27:479, 1979.

53. **Murray RO, Jacobson HG:** *The Radiology of Skeletal Disorders,* ed 2. Edinburgh, UK, Churchill Livingstone, 1977.

54. **Loughran CF:** *A review of the plain film radiograph in acute rupture of abdominal aortic aneurysms.* Clinical Radiol 37:383, 1986.

55. **Flak B, Li DKB, Ho BYB, et al.:** *Magnetic resonance imaging of aneurysms of the abdominal aorta.* AJR 144:991, 1985.

56. **McCready RA, Pairolero PC, Gilmore JC:** *Isolated iliac artery aneurysms.* Surgery 93:688, 1983.

57. **Markowitz AM, Norman JC:** *Aneurysms of the iliac artery.* Ann Surg 154:777, 1961.

58. **Wilson NM, Collins REC:** *Ruptured common iliac artery aneurysm presenting with perianal hematoma—a case report.* Vasc Surg 24:510, 1990.

59. **Levy PJ, Sweatman CA, Davis DW, et al.:** *Ruptured solitary iliac artery aneurysms: A "silent" killer? Report of four cases and review of the literature.* Vasc Surg 27:611, 1993.

60. **Chapman EM, Shaw RS, Kubik CS:** *Sciatic pain from arteriosclerotic aneurysm of pelvic arteries.* N Engl J Med 271:1410, 1964.

61. **Lowry SF, Kraft RO:** *Isolated aneurysms of the iliac artery.* Arch Surg 113:1289, 1978.

62. **Messina LM, Shanley CJ:** *Visceral artery aneurysms.* Surg Clin North Am 77:425, 1997.

63. **Stanley JC, Thompson NW, Fry WE:** *Splanchnic artery aneurysms.* Arch Surg 101:689, 1970.

64. **Moore S, Lewis R:** *Splenic artery aneurysms.* Ann Surg 153:1033, 1961.

65. **Feldman M:** *Aneurysm of the splenic artery: An autopsy study.* Am J Dig Dis 22:48, 1955.

66. **Bedford PD, Lodge B:** *Aneurysms of the splenic artery.* Gut 1:312, 1960.

67. **Gupta AK, Ghani A, Wegener ME:** *Splenic artery aneurysms—case reports.* Vasc Surg 27:404, 1993.

68. **Shanley CJ, Shah NL, Messina LM:** *Common splanchnic artery aneurysms: Splenic, hepatic and celiac.* Ann Vasc Surg 10:315, 1996.

69. **Taylor W, Woodard DA:** *Splenic conservation and the management of splenic artery aneurysms.* Ann R Coll Surg Engl 69:179, 1987.

70. **Culver GJ, Pirson HS:** *Splenic artery aneurysm.* Radiology 68:217, 1957.

71. **Stanley JC, Fry WJ:** *Pathogenesis and clinical significance of splenic artery aneurysms.* Surgery 76:898, 1974.

72. **Spittel JA Jr, Fairbairn JF, Kincaid OW, et al.:** *Aneurysm of the splenic artery.* JAMA 175:452, 1961.

73. **Matinez E, Menendez AR, Albenedo P:** *Splenic artery aneurysms.* Int Surg 71:95, 1986.

74. **Green DR, Gorey TF, Tanner WA, et al.:** *The diagnosis and management of splenic artery aneurysms.* J R Soc Med 81:387, 1988.

75. **Berger JS, Forsee JH, Furst JN:** *Splenic artery aneurysm.* Ann Surg 137:108, 1953.

76. **Steinberg I, Finby N, Evans JA:** *Intravenous abdominal aortography in the diagnosis and differential diagnosis of aneurysms of the splenic, hepatic and renal arteries.* AJR 86:1108, 1961.

77. **Quinn JL III, Martin JP:** *Hepatic artery aneurysm, case report.* AJR 87:284, 1962.

78. **Salik JO, Abeshouse BS:** *Calcification, ossification and cartilage formation in the kidney.* AJR 88:125, 1962.

79. **Seshanarayana KN, Keats TE:** *Intrarenal arterial calcification: Roentgen appearance and significance.* Radiology 95:145, 1970.

VENOUS DISORDERS

1. **Shenult P:** *The origin of phleboliths.* Br J Surg 59:695, 1972.

2. **Steinbach HL:** *Identification of pelvic masses by phlebolith displacement.* AJR 83:1063, 1960.

3. **Dovey P:** *Pelvic phleboliths.* Clin Radiol 17:121, 1966.

4. **Culligan JM:** *Phleboliths.* J Urol 15:175, 1926.

5. **Burkitt DP:** *Hemorrhoids, varicose veins, and deep vein thrombosis: Epidemiologic features and suggested causative factors.* Can J Surg 18:483, 1975.

6. **Burkitt DP, Latto C, Janvrin SB:** *Pelvic phleboliths: Epidemiology and postulated etiology.* N Engl J Med 296:1387, 1977.

7. **Green M, Thomas ML:** *The prevalence of pelvic phleboliths in relation to age, sex, and urinary tract infections.* Clin Radiol 23:492, 1972.

8. **Traubici J, Neitlich JD, Smith RC:** *Distinguishing pelvic phleboliths from distal ureteral stones on routine unenhanced helical CT: Is there a radiolucent center?* AJR 172(1):13, 1999.

9. **Boridy IC, Nikolaidis P, Kawashima A, et al.:** *Ureterolithiasis: Value of the tail sign in differentiating phleboliths from ureteral calculi at nonenhanced helical CT.* Radiology 211(3):619, 1999.

10. **Fenlon JW, Augustin C:** *The significance of pelvic phlebolith displacement.* J Urol 106:595, 1971.

MISCELLANEOUS ABDOMINAL OPACITIES

1. **Baker SR, Cho KC:** *The Abdominal Plain Film With Correlative Imaging,* ed 2. New York, Appleton & Lange. 1999.

2. **Baker SR, Elkin M:** *Plain Film Approach to Abdominal Calcifications.* Philadelphia, WB Saunders, 1983.

MISCELLANEOUS MASQUERADERS OF MUSCULOSKELETAL DISEASE

LOWER EXTREMITY VASCULAR DISEASES

1. **Taveras MJ, Ferrucci TJ:** *Radiology Diagnosis-Imaging-Intervention.* Baltimore, Lippincott, Williams & Wilkins, 2000.

2. **Lindblom A:** *Arteriosclerosis and arterial thrombosis in the lower limb. A roentgenological study.* Acta Radiol 80(Suppl):1, 1950.

3. **Juhl HJ, Crummy BA:** *Paul and Juhl's Essentials of Radiologic Imaging,* ed 7. Philadelphia, JB Lippincott, 1998.

4. **Graham LM, Zelenock GB, Whitehouse WM Jr:** *Clinical significance of arteriosclerotic femoral arterial aneurysms.* Arch Surg 115:502, 1980.

5. **Gayliss H:** *Popliteal aneurysms: A review and analysis of 55 cases.* S Afr Med J 48:75, 1974.

6. **Whitehouse WM, Wakefield TW, Graham LM:** *Limb threatening potential of arteriosclerotic popliteal artery aneurysms.* Surgery 93:694, 1983.

7. **Chan O, Thomas ML:** *The incidence of popliteal aneurysms in patients with arteriomegaly.* Clin Radiol 41:1185, 1990.

8. **Bergan JJ, Kumins NH, Owens EL, Sparks SR:** *Surgical and endovascular treatment of lower extremity venous insufficiency.* J Vasc Interv Radiol 13(6):563, 2002.

9. **Neglen P, Raju S:** *Proximal lower extremity chronic venous outflow obstruction: Recognition and treatment.* Semin Vasc Surg 15(1):57, 2002.

10. **Schmid-Schonbein GW, Takase S, Bergan JJ:** *New advances in the understanding of the pathophysiology of chronic venous insufficiency.* Angiology 52(Suppl 1):S27, 2001.

11. **Pearse HE Jr, Morton JJ:** *The stimulation of bone growth by venous stasis.* J Bone Joint Surg 12A:97, 1930.

Mnemonics
A Learning Aid for Students of Skeletal Radiology

INTRODUCTION

All students of radiology have struggled to remember extensive lists for the differential diagnosis of various roentgen signs. The following encyclopedic list of roentgen signs with mnemonics is offered as an aid to assist the student in quick recall of some of these entities.

A *mnemonic* is defined by *Webster's Dictionary* as "something which assists or intends to assist one's memory, of or relating to memory, a technique of improving the memory, a device or code to assist memory recall."

The following list of mnemonics is divided into eight skeletal categories:

1. Congenital Anomalies (Chapter 3)
2. Skeletal Dysplasias (Chapter 8)
3. Trauma (Chapter 9)
4. Arthritic Disorders (Chapter 10)
5. Tumors and Tumor-like Processes (Chapter 11)
6. Infection (Chapter 12)
7. Vascular Disorders (Chapter 13)
8. Nutritional, Metabolic, and Endocrine Disorders (Chapter 14)

These mnemonics are presented in alphabetical order based on the roentgen signs within the appropriate category of bone disease.

A Categorical Approach to Bone Disease

mnemonic: **CATBITES**
Congenital
Arthritis
Trauma
Blood (hematological)
Infection
Tumor
Endocrine, nutritional, metabolic
Soft tissue

CONGENITAL ANOMALIES (CHAPTER 3)

Basilar Invagination

mnemonic: **COOP**
Congenital
Osteogenesis imperfecta
Osteomalacia
Paget's disease

Bilateral Madelung's Deformity

mnemonic: **RED HOT**
Radial ray dysplasias
Epiphyseal dysplasias
Dyschondrosteosis
Hereditary multiple exostosis (bayonet deformity)
Ollier's disease
Thalidomide

SKELETAL DYSPLASIAS (CHAPTER 8)

Metacarpal Sign (short fourth metacarpal)

mnemonic: **Ping Pong Is Tough To Teach**
Pseudo-hypoparathyroidism
Pseudo-pseudo-hypoparathyroidism
Idiopathic
Trauma
Turner's syndrome
Trisomy 13–18

Radial Ray Dysplasia (hypoplastic or agenetic radius)

mnemonic: **I FETCH**
Idiopathic
Fanconi's syndrome
Ellis-van Creveld syndrome
Thrombocytopenia
Cornelia de Lange's syndrome
Holt-Oram syndrome

Solitary Lytic Defect in Skull

mnemonic: **M T HOLE**
Metastasis, Myeloma
Tuberculosis, Trauma
Histiocytosis X

Osteomyelitis
Leptomeningeal cyst
Epidermoid or dermoid, Enigma (fibrous dysplasia)

Wormian Bones

mnemonic: **PORK CHOPS**
Pyknodysostosis
Osteogenesis imperfecta
Rickets in the healing phase
Kinky hair syndrome
Cleidocranial dysplasia
Hypothyroidism, Hypophosphatasia
Otopalatodigital syndrome
Primary acro-osteolysis (Hajdu-Cheney),
    Pachydermoperiostosis
Syndrome, Down's

TRAUMA (CHAPTER 9)

Rotator Cuff Muscles

mnemonic: **SITS**
Supraspinatus
Infraspinatus
Teres minor
Subscapularis

ARTHRITIC DISORDERS (CHAPTER 10)

Arthritis with Demineralization

mnemonic: **HORSE**
Hemophilia
Osteomyelitis
Rheumatoid arthritis, Reiter's syndrome
Scleroderma
Erythematosus, systemic lupus

Chondrocalcinosis

mnemonic: Three Cs
Cation disease: calcium (hyperparathyroidism), copper
    (Wilson's disease), iron (hemochromatosis)
Crystal: calcium pyrophosphate dihydrate (pseudo-gout),
    urate (gout)
Cartilage: hydroxyapatite crystal deposition disease

Chondrocalcinosis

mnemonic: **WHIP A DOG**
Wilson's disease
Hemochromatosis, Hemophilia, Hypothyroidism,
    Hyperparathyroidism (primary, 15%) Hypophosphatasia,
    Hypomagnesemia (familial)
Idiopathic (aging)

Pseudo-gout (calcium pyrophosphate dihydrate)
Amyloidosis
Diabetes mellitus
Ochronosis
Gout

Causes of Secondary Osteoarthritis

mnemonic: **NOT A PHOWIE**
Neurogenic arthropathy
Ochronosis
Trauma
Acromegaly, Avascular necrosis
Pseudogout (calcium pyrophosphate dihydrate)
Hemochromatosis, Hemophilia
Occupational
Wilson's disease
Idiopathic
Erosive osteoarthritis

Early Osteoarthritis

mnemonic: **E**arly **O**steo **A**rthritis
Epiphyseal dysplasia, multiple
Ochronosis
Acromegaly

Neurotrophic Arthropathy

mnemonic: **Six Ds**
Distension, joint (earliest finding, owing to effusion)
Density (increased subchondral bone sclerosis)
Debris (bony intra-articular fragments)
Dislocation (joint surfaces often malaligned)
Disorganization (joint components usually disrupted
    "bag of bones")
Destruction (articular bone shows loss of bone substance)

Premature Osteoarthritis

mnemonic: **COME CHAT**
Calcium pyrophosphate dihydrate arthropathy
Ochronosis
Marfan's syndrome
Epiphyseal dysplasia
Charcot joint = neurotrophic arthropathy
Hemophilic arthropathy
Acromegaly
Trauma

Protrusio Acetabuli

mnemonic: **PORT**
Paget's disease
Osteomalacia
Rheumatoid arthritis
Trauma

Spotty Carpal Bones

mnemonic: **G S RAT**
Gout
Sudeck's atrophy
Rheumatoid
Arthritis
Tuberculosis

TUMORS AND TUMOR-LIKE PROCESSES (CHAPTER 11)

Absent Greater Wing of Sphenoid

mnemonic: **M FOR MARINE**
Meningioma
Fibrous dysplasia
Optic glioma
Relapsing hematoma
Metastasis
Aneurysm
Retinoblastoma
Idiopathic
Neurofibromatosis
Eosinophilic granuloma

Blow-Out Lesion of Posterior Elements (Spine)

mnemonic: **GO APE**
Giant cell tumor
Osteoblastoma
Aneurysmal bone cyst
Plasmacytoma
Eosinophilic granuloma

Bone Tumors Favoring Vertebral Bodies

mnemonic: **CALL HOME**
Chordoma
Aneurysmal bone cyst
Leukemia
Lymphoma
Hemangioma
Osteoid osteoma, Osteoblastoma
Myeloma, Metastasis
Eosinophilic granuloma

Calcifying Metastases

mnemonic: **BOTTOM**
Breast
Osteosarcoma
Testicular
Thyroid
Ovary
Mucinous adenocarcinoma of gastrointestinal tract

Destruction of Medial End of Clavicle

mnemonic: **MILERS**
Metastases
Infection
Lymphoma
Eosinophilic granuloma
Rheumatoid arthritis
Sarcoma

Diaphyseal Lesions

mnemonic: **FEMALE**
Fibrous dysplasia
Ewing's sarcoma
Metastasis
Adamantinoma
Lymphoma, Leukemia
Eosinophilic granuloma

Diffuse Osteosclerosis

mnemonic: **FROM**
Fluorosis
Renal osteodystrophy
Osteopetrosis
Myelosclerosis, Metastases (blastic), Mastocytosis

Epiphyseal Lesions

mnemonic: **DELCO**
Degenerative subchondral cyst (geode)
Enchondroma
Lipoma
Cyst, Chondroblastoma
Osteomyelitis

Expansile Rib Lesion

mnemonic: **THELMA**
Tuberculosis
Hematopoiesis
Eosinophilic granuloma, Ewing's sarcoma, Enchondroma
Leukemia, Lymphoma
Myeloma, Metastases
Aneurysmal bone cyst

Increase in Skull Thickness

mnemonic: **HIPFAM**
Hyperostosis frontalis interna
Idiopathic
Paget's disease
Fibrous dysplasia
Anemia (sickle cell, iron deficiency, thalassemia, spherocytosis)
Metastases

Ivory Vertebra

mnemonic: **My Only Sister Left Home On Friday Past**
Myelosclerosis
Osteoblastic metastasis
Sickle-cell disease
Lymphoma
Hemangioma
Osteoporosis
Fluorosis
Paget's disease

Metastatic Lesions Involving Bone

mnemonic: **BLT** with a **K**osher **P**ickle **'N' H**ot **S**auce
Breast
Lung
Thyroid
Kidney
Prostate
Neuroblastoma
Hodgkin's disease
Sarcoma, Squamous cell

Moth-Eaten Bone Destruction

mnemonic: **H LEMMON**
Histiocytosis X
Lymphoma
Ewing's sarcoma
Metastasis
Multiple myeloma
Osteomyelitis
Neuroblastoma

Osteoblastic Metastases

mnemonic: **F**ive **B**ees **L**ick **P**ollen
Brain (medulloblastoma)
Bronchus
Breast
Bowel (especially carcinoid)
Bladder
Lymphoma
Prostate

Posterior Vertebral Body Scalloping

mnemonic: **HAMENTS**
Hurler's syndrome, Hydrocephalus
Achondroplasia, Acromegaly
Marfan's syndrome
Ehlers-Danlos syndrome
Neurofibromatosis
Tumor (meningioma, ependymoma)
Syringohydromyelia

Round Cell Tumors

mnemonic: **LEMON**
Leukemia, Lymphoma
Ewing's sarcoma, Eosinophilic granuloma
Multiple myeloma
Osteomyelitis
Neuroblastoma

Skeletal Metastases in Adult

mnemonic: **C**ommon **B**one **L**esions **C**an **K**ill **T**he **P**atient
Colon
Breast
Lung
Carcinoid
Kidney
Thyroid
Prostate

Soap Bubble Lesions

mnemonic: **FEGNOMASHIC**
Fibrous dysplasia
Enchondroma
Giant cell tumor
Non-ossifying fibroma
Osteoblastoma
Multiple myeloma, Metastasis
Aneurysmal bone cyst
Simple bone cyst
Hyperparathyroidism, Hemophilic pseudotumor
Infection
Chondroblastoma

Transverse Lucent Metaphyseal Lines

mnemonic: **LINING**
Leukemia
Illness, systemic (rickets, scurvy)
Normal variant
Infection, transplacental (congenital syphilis)
Neuroblastoma metastases
Growth lines

INFECTION (CHAPTER 12)

Button Sequestrum

mnemonic: **TORE ME**
Tuberculosis
Osteomyelitis
Radiation
Eosinophilic granuloma
Metastasis
Epidermoid

VASCULAR DISORDERS (CHAPTER 13)

Acquired Acro-Osteolysis

mnemonic: **RADISH**
Raynaud's phenomenon
Arteriosclerosis
Diabetes
Injury (burns, frostbite)
Scleroderma, Sarcoidosis
Hyperparathyroidism

Anterior Vertebral Body Scalloping

mnemonic: **LAT**
Lymphadenopathy
Aortic aneurysm
Tuberculosis

Aseptic Necrosis

mnemonic: **ASEPTIC**
Alcoholism, Atherosclerosis
Sickle cell, Storage diseases
Endogenous and Exogenous corticosteroids
Pancreatitis
Trauma
Idiopathic (Legg-Calvé-Perthes)
Caisson's disease

Avascular Necrosis

mnemonic: **PLASTIC RAGS**
Pancreatitis, Pregnancy
Lupus
Alcoholism
Steroids
Trauma
Idiopathic
Caisson's disease, Collagen disease
    (systemic lupus erythematosus)
Rheumatoid arthritis, Radiation
Amyloid
Gaucher's disease
Sickle cell disease

Osteochondritis Dissecans of Knee

mnemonic: **LAME**
Lateral
Anterior
Medial
Epicondyle

Schmorl's Node

mnemonic: **SHOOT**
Scheuermann's disease
Hyperparathyroidism
Osteoporosis
Osteomalacia
Trauma

NUTRITIONAL, METABOLIC, AND ENDOCRINE DISORDERS (CHAPTER 14)

Dense Metaphyseal Bands

mnemonic: Heavy Cretins Sift Scurrilously through
    Rickety Systems
Heavy metal poisoning (lead, bismuth, phosphorus)
Cretinism
Syphilis, congenital
Scurvy
Rickets (healed)
Systemic illness
[*also:* normal variant; methotrexate therapy]

Diffuse Periosteal Reaction in Children

mnemonic: **PERIOSTEAL**
Physiologic, Pachydermoperiostosis
E, prostaglandin
Rickets (especially, healing phase)
Idiopathic (Caffey's disease)
Osteoarthropathy (hypertrophic)
Syphilis, Scurvy
Thyroid acropachy
Excess fluorine (fluorosis)
A, hypervitaminosis; Abuse (child)
Leukemia

Frayed Metaphyses

mnemonic: **CHARMS**
Congenital infections (rubella, syphilis)
Hypophosphatasia
Achondroplasia
Rickets
Metaphyseal dysostosis
Scurvy

Generalized Sclerosis of Bone

mnemonic: **MARBLE**
Myelosclerosis, Mastocytosis, Metabolic (hypervitaminosis D,
    fluorosis, hypothyroidism, phosphorus poisoning)
Anemia (sickle cell)

Renal osteodystrophy
Blastic metastasis
Lymphoma
Enigmas (Paget's disease, osteopetrosis, melorheostosis, pyknodysostosis, tuberous sclerosis)

Heel Pad Thickening

[thickness > 25 mm (normal, < 21 mm)]

mnemonic: **MAD COP**
Myxedema
Acromegaly
Dilantin therapy
Callous
Obesity
Peripheral edema

Penciled Distal End of Clavicle

mnemonic: **SHIRT P**ocket
Scleroderma
Hyperparathyroidism
Infection
Rheumatoid arthritis
Trauma
Progeria

Vertebra Plana

mnemonic: **FETISH**
Fracture
Eosinophilic granuloma
Tumor (metastasis, myeloma)
Infection
Steroids
Hemangioma

Page numbers followed by *t* and *f* indicate tables and figures, respectively.